To Brooke   2006

From - Diana

Hami

Millie
Have fun!

Doug

To Brooke -
Happy reading!
Ryan

Principles
of Pediatric
Surgery

Editors

James A. O'Neill Jr, MD
John C. Foshee Distinguished
Professor of Surgery
Chairman, Section of Surgical Sciences
Vanderbilt Medical Center
Nashville, Tennessee

Jay L. Grosfeld, MD
Lafayette F. Page Professor
Professor and Chairman
Department of Surgery
Indiana University Medical Center
Surgeon-in-Chief
JW Riley Hospital for Children
Indianapolis, Indiana

Associate Editors

George W. Holcomb III, MD
Katherine Berry Richardson Professor of
Pediatric Surgery
University of Missouri – Kansas City
School of Medicine
Surgeon-in-Chief
Children's Mercy Hospital
Kansas City, Missouri

Jean-Martin Laberge, MD
Associate Professor of Surgery
Director, Division of Pediatric
General Surgery
McGill University Health Center
The Montreal Children's Hospital
Montreal, Quebec Canada

Don K. Nakayama, MD
Professor of Surgery
University of North Carolina
School of Medicine
Program Director of General Surgery
Residency Program
New Hanover Regional Medical Center
Wilmington, North Carolina

Robert Shamberger, MD
Interim Chief, Department of Surgery
Professor of Surgery and Senior Associate
in Surgery
Harvard Medical School
Children's Hospital
Boston, Massachusetts

Principles of Pediatric Surgery

SECOND EDITION

Eric W. Fonkalsrud, MD
Professor, Department of Surgery
UCLA School of Medicine
Emeritus Chief, Pediatric Surgery
UCLA Medical Center
Los Angeles, California

Arnold G. Coran, MD
Professor of Surgery and Head of
Section of Pediatric Surgery
University of Michigan Medical
School
Surgeon-in-Chief
CS Mott Children's Hospital
Ann Arbor, Michigan

Anthony A. Caldamone, MD
Professor of Surgery (Urology)
and Pediatrics
Director, Urology Residency
Program
Department of Urology
Brown University School of Medicine
Providence, Rhode Island

Marshall Z. Schwartz, MD
Professor of Surgery and Pediatrics
Vice Chairman, Department of Surgery
Jefferson Medical College of
Thomas Jefferson University
Philadelphia, Pennsylvania
Surgeon-in-Chief
AI duPont Hospital for Children
Wilmington, Delaware

Charles J. Stolar, MD
Rudolph N. Schullinger Professor of
Surgery and Pediatrics
Columbia University College of
Physicians and Surgeons
Director of Pediatric Surgery for
Morgan Stanley Babies and Children's
Hospital of New York
New York, New York

Ronald B. Hirschl, MD
Professor of Surgery and
Pediatric Surgery
University of Michigan Medical School
CS Mott Children's Hospital
Ann Arbor, Michigan

Daniel H. Teitelbaum, MD
Associate Professor of Surgery
University of Michigan Medical School
CS Mott Children's Hospital
Ann Arbor, Michigan

Joseph G. Borer, MD
Assistant Professor of Surgery (Urology)
and Assistant in Urology
Harvard Medical School
Children's Hospital
Boston, Massachusetts

Mark P. Cain, MD
Associate Professor of Urology
Indiana University School of Medicine
JW Riley Hospital for Children
Indianapolis, Indiana

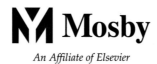

Mosby

An Affiliate of Elsevier

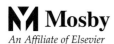
Mosby

An Affiliate of Elsevier

11830 Westline Industrial Drive
St. Louis, Missouri 63146

Notice

Surgery is an ever-changing field. Standard safety precautions must be followed but as new research and clinical experience broaden our knowledge, changes in treatment and drug therapy may become necessary or appropriate. Readers are advised to check the most current product information provided by the manufacturer of each drug to be administered to verify the recommended dose, the method and duration of administration, and the contraindications. It is the responsibility of the treating physician, relying on experience and knowledge of the patient, to determine dosages and the best treatment for each individual patient. Neither the publisher nor the editors assume any liability for any injury and/or damage to persons or property arising from this publication.

The Publisher

First Edition 1995. Second Edition 2004.

Library of Congress Cataloging-in-Publication Data

Principles of pediatric surgery.–2nd ed. / edited by James A. O'Neill Jr. ... [et al.].
   p. ; cm.
   Rev. ed. of: Essentials of pediatric surgery. c1995.
   Includes bibliographical references and index.
   ISBN 0-323-01827-0
   1. Children–Surgery. I. O'Neill, James A. II. Essentials of pediatric surgery.
   [DNLM: 1. Surgical Procedures, Operative–Child. 2. Surgical Procedures, Operative–Infant. WO 925 P957 2004]
   RD137.E86 2004   2003060189
   617.9'8–dc22

Acquisitions Editor: Joe Rusko
Developmental Editor: Janice Gaillard
Project Manager: Mary Anne Folcher
Design Coordinator: Gene Harris

CE/MVY

Printed in the United States of America.

Last digit is print number: 9 8 7 6 5 4 3 2

To our spouses and families with gratitude and love for their understanding and support without which this project could not have been accomplished.

Contributors

Joseph G. Borer, MD
Primary author of
chapters 74, 77-79

Mark P. Cain, MD
Primary author of
chapters 71, 75, 76

Anthony A. Caldamone, MD
Section editor for chapters 70-79
Primary author of chapters
70, 72, 73

Arnold G. Coran, MD
Section editor and coauthor of
chapters 1-10, 56-62, 87

Eric W. Fonkalsrud, MD
Section editor of chapters 40-55, 89
Primary author or coauthor of
chapters 40-42, 45, 50, 52, 89

Jay L. Grosfeld, MD
Section editor for chapters
19-35, 86
Primary author or coauthor of
chapters 21, 25, 28, 30, 31, 86

Ronald B. Hirschl, MD
Primary author of chapters 2, 5, 6,
10, 56, 61, 87

George W. Holcomb III, MD
Primary author of chapters 14, 16,
38, 39, 67, 69, 82, 84, 88

Jean-Martin Laberge, MD
Primary author of chapters 19, 22,
26, 27, 33, 35

Don K. Nakayama, MD
Primary author of chapters 12, 13,
36, 63, 64, 80, 81

James A. O'Neill, Jr, MD
Final editor of all chapters
Primary author or coauthor of
chapters 11, 15, 17, 18, 37, 38, 65,
66, 68, 80, 82, 83, 85

Marshall Z. Schwartz, MD
Primary author of chapters 43, 48,
49, 52, 53, 55

Robert C. Shamberger, MD
Primary author of chapters 20, 23,
24, 29, 32, 34

Charles J. Stolar, MD
Primary author of chapters 42, 44,
46, 47, 51, 54

Daniel H. Teitelbaum, MD
Primary author of chapters 1, 3, 4,
7-9, 57, 58, 60, 62

Preface

Although there are references to surgical procedures in the Bible, probably the first definitive book on surgery was written by Albucasis around 1000 AD, during the period of Arabic domination of Spain. This book was reprinted all over Europe and served as a basic reference not only for surgery but also for pediatric surgery into the 1800s. The pediatric surgical entities described were limited to treatment of fractures and common congenital malformations. Subsequent books detailing the management of a variety of pediatric surgical problems, such as those by Guersant in Paris in 1840, were really collections of lectures with strong emphasis on basic techniques of management. In the middle of the twentieth century, medical education changed to more emphasis on science and this mandated changes in textbooks. To a large degree, textbooks in a particular field of surgery reflect both practical considerations and the scientific status of the field. As biotechnology blossomed in the second half of the twentieth century, pediatric surgery was transformed by advances in the understanding of physiology, genetics, pharmacology, developmental biology, and other fields. Although pediatric surgery may be considered as both general and thoracic surgery for a particular age group, the field now clearly has its own body of knowledge, facilitating its evolution into its own specialty.

The first edition of this book was entitled, *Essentials of Pediatric Surgery* and quickly sold out. Subsequently, numerous requests for a second edition came from around the world, and this is the response. As we did for the first edition, we asked what the core elements of pediatric surgical knowledge are at this time. We agreed, however, that the essential elements now include many more basic facts. Just as other surgical textbooks have evolved over the centuries, so has this one to the extent that it is no longer appropriate to refer to it only as the Essentials; thus, the second edition of this book is now entitled *Principles of Pediatric Surgery*.

As mentioned in the accompanying Preface to the First Edition, our goal is still the same, that is, to present the core elements of pediatric surgery in a concise and clear fashion along with information from related fields that have an impact on pediatric surgical care. *Principles of Pediatric Surgery* has been designed to be useful as a source of information for pediatric surgeons, surgical residents in all specialties, and other surgeons who perform procedures on infants and children. It is also designed to serve as a concise reference in a single volume for pediatricians, neonatologists, pediatric medical specialists, and other physicians who manage the care of children.

In order to accomplish this goal, four of the five previous editors prepared the revision. (Dr. Marc Rowe, lead editor of the first edition, retired in the interim.)

Dr. Anthony Caldamone was added to coordinate the genitourinary section. Since there was so much more material to cover, however, two experienced associate editors were recruited for each of the five primary editors. In order to ensure continuity and avoid redundancy, these fifteen individuals wrote all the chapters. There was much crossover in critiquing and editing the work. All of the senior editors eventually agreed on the fundamental principles, and any significant differences of opinion were sorted out so that this edition would be authoritative. Each of the five primary editors was assigned a section of the book to edit. As a last check, to avoid redundancy, ensure accuracy, and set a single stylistic standard, the lead editor did the final editing of all chapters. *Principles of Pediatric Surgery* is a collaborative effort on the part of all involved, and primary authorship is referred to only in the Contributors' section.

Every single chapter is updated with extensive additions to the first section on physiologic and basic scientific considerations in the field of pediatric surgery, as well as to the sections on trauma, oncology, and urology. The separate chapters in the first edition, describing common pediatric surgical and endoscopic procedures, are eliminated, but all this material, including several additions, is included in the appropriate subject chapters to make it easier for the reader. Much new information on minimally invasive approaches to pediatric surgery is added to update a number of chapters. In a number of instances, discussions are provided to guide the reader in regard to whether an open or a minimally invasive approach is appropriate in a particular situation. The section on pancreatic and biliary disorders is reorganized. New additional information on transplantation is added. A new chapter on conjoined twins is included as well as basic information on otolaryngologic disorders. New suggested readings are provided, but there is no attempt to provide an extensive bibliography. Although it was our goal in this second addition to present the core information of pediatric surgery in a single volume, when we were all through we found it has become a new and different book in many respects.

Principles of Pediatric Surgery is an acknowledgment of the fact that pediatric surgeons are probably the only true general surgeons remaining in today's world. This is part of the attraction to the field and why year in and year out so many outstanding and devoted young people enter the field. This is fortunate because the vulnerable patients who depend upon pediatric surgical and medical specialists of all types deserve only the best. It is our hope that this book will help all of those physicians and surgeons who devote their lives to the care of sick and injured children.

ix

We would like to express our appreciation to our patient and efficient secretarial staff without whose help this book could not have been completed in the time allotted. We are most grateful to Donna Bock (Nashville), Sondra Davis and Terri Crist (Indianapolis), Phyllis Davis (Los Angeles), Cheryl Peterson, Amy Drongowski, and Jill Knox (Ann Arbor), Carol Simmons (Providence), Barbara Doe and Angela Lopez (Boston), Kathy Smith (Kansas City), Vassiliki Kessaris (Montreal), and Melissa Moreno-Sheehan (New York).

James A. O'Neill, Jr.

Preface to the First Edition

This book had its origin in a late-night discussion following an American Board of Surgery examination involving three of the editors of the Fourth Edition of *Pediatric Surgery*—Judson Randolph, James O'Neill, and Marc Rowe. At that time, candidate performance on the recent pediatric surgery board examination was discussed and the content of the examination analyzed. This conversation led to a question: What are the core elements of pediatric surgical knowledge? We agreed that essential elements included (1) the nine index conditions of Mark Ravitch, (2) what the American Board of Surgery identifies as "the primary components of surgery," and (3) what Pediatric Surgery Training Directors expect their residents to know at the completion of their training. In the ensuing months, the discussants continued to meet and explore the concept of the "essentials" of pediatric surgery. A questionnaire was sent to training directors and a number of other experienced pediatric surgeons asking them to list and prioritize the information that they would expect a resident to have assimilated by the end of his or her training. It became apparent after review of the responses and our previous discussions that a book that covered the essentials of pediatric surgery in a concise and clear fashion was needed. Such a book would be an important source of information for pediatric surgical residents, pediatric surgeons, and other surgeons who perform procedures on infants and children. It would also serve as a single concise reference for pediatricians, neonatologists, and other physicians who manage the pediatric patient.

Five experienced pediatric surgeons agreed to write the book. At the onset of the project, we agreed upon certain principles. First, the information had to be condensed to the point that the essentials could be adequately covered in one volume. Second, to ensure continuity and avoid redundancy, we would write all the chapters and frankly critique and edit each other's work. Although each chapter would present the concepts and approaches of the individual author, each fellow author/editor would have to agree with the fundamental principles. Surprisingly, during the development of the chapters, we found considerable agreement, and on only a few occasions were there significant differences of opinion.

Because the book is truly a collaborative effort, authorship of individual chapters is not identified. To achieve simple and clear presentations of complex concepts and information, tables, illustrations, diagrams, cartoons, and algorithms are liberally employed. Historical reviews and theoretical discussions are limited. Instead of long bibliographies, selected annotated references are placed at the end of each chapter and include classic articles as well as current studies. We believe that certain subjects that are often not included in standard pediatric surgical textbooks are important in a book dealing with the essentials. For example, a chapter was added that describes common pediatric conditions that have significant effects on the pediatric surgical patient. To increase the day-to-day practicality of the book, an entire section describing common pediatric surgical procedures—the "nuts and bolts" of pediatric surgery—was included. Neurosurgical, orthopedic, plastic, and cardiac surgical conditions that have particular significance to pediatric surgeons were also added.

As the book slowly took shape, the five of us found that certain subjects, particularly urology, required additional expertise. Dr. Curtis Sheldon became a principal contributor to the urologic section. Because the subject matter of pediatric surgery continuously and rapidly evolves, many chapters required revisions, extensive literature research, and updating. Dr. Craig Albanese greatly assisted the editors in reviewing data, researching scientific background, and identifying recent developments.

We are eternally grateful to our loyal and patient secretarial staff members who have been invaluable to us during the many months of writing, rewriting, and reviewing: Jennifer Foscoe (Pittsburgh), Colleen Kennedy (Philadelphia), Sandy Davis (Indianapolis), Jaunita Zavala (Los Angeles), and Colleen Rauch (Ann Arbor).

Every one of the exceptional young people who apply for a pediatric surgical residency writes a personal statement that includes the reasons they chose pediatric surgery as a career. The consistency of the replies is remarkable. They all wish to devote their lives to pediatric surgery because they love and want to help children, they aspire to be complete surgeons, and they see pediatric surgery as the epitome of true general surgery. This book is our attempt to aid these fine young people in their quest.

Marc I. Rowe

Contents

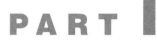

Perioperative Conditions

Neonatal and Pediatric Considerations

■ The surgery of children is predicated upon the fundamental facts that infants and children differ from adults in anatomy, physiology and particularly in their reaction to operative trauma and that the necessary adjustments of surgical procedures are not merely matters of scale.

This well-stated introduction is from the introductory paragraph of one of the first American textbooks on pediatric surgery, written by Brenner in 1938. Despite being more than 60 years old, the concepts are remarkably current in the overall approach to pediatric surgical patients. Advances in neonatal care have resulted in the survival of increasing numbers of extremely low-birth-weight infants. Their extreme prematurity predisposes these tiny, fragile infants to hyaline membrane disease (HMD), chronic lung disease (CLD), intraventricular hemorrhage (IVH), retinopathy of prematurity (ROP), necrotizing enterocolitis (NEC), intrauterine growth retardation (IUGR), apnea and bradycardia, and neurologic impairment. In addition, the entire area of neonatal survival has continued to change, even since the last publication of this book. The surgeon must provide preoperative, intraoperative, and postoperative care to extremely premature infants. Precise management and appropriate therapy often can prevent some of the aforementioned conditions and the permanent disabilities they can cause. This chapter discusses HMD and respiratory distress syndrome (RDS), bronchopulmonary dysplasia (BPD), IVH, and ROP. Two viral conditions also are discussed: respiratory syncytial virus (RSV) infections and gastrointesintal viral infections. Because these common viral illnesses may masquerade as surgical diseases, complicate existing conditions, and spread rapidly through surgical wards and intensive care units in epidemic waves, and because they preferentially attack the weakened and susceptible surgical patient, it is paramount that the surgeon become familiar with them.

PREMATURITY AND INTRAUTERINE GROWTH RETARDATION

Infants born before 37 weeks' gestation are considered premature. In general, the diagnosis of prematurity denotes a variety of associated disease processes; however, the incidence of these processes typically is stratified based on the overall birth weight. Infants who weigh 2500 g or less at birth are referred to as low-birth-weight (LBW) infants; with normal gestational age, they are referred to as having IUGR. Infants weighing less than 1500 g are referred to as very-low-birth-weight (VLBW) infants, and infants weighing less than 1000 g are referred to as extremely-low-birth-weight (ELBW) infants. Using 2001 statistics, 7.6% of live-born neonates in the United States weighed less than 2500 g. This percentage is a sizable increase from 6.7% in 1984. The rate for prematurity in blacks was more than twice that for whites. Prematurity is also higher in infants born to mothers younger than age 15 years and older than age 45 years. Infants defined as VLBW constitute 1.4% of births in the United States. Although this group comprises a small percentage of deliveries, VLBW accounts for 66% of neonatal deaths and 50% of handicapped infants. Despite a lack of reduction in LBW infants, survival has improved for them. The highest mortality is found in white boys; however, their survival has increased since the 1990s, whereas survival rates for blacks has remained unchanged. The most recent available statistics on survival based on birth weight show that for infants weighing less than 500 g, survival is 15.4%; for infants weighing 500 to 749 g, 52.4%; for infants weighing 750 to 999 g, 84.4%; and for infants weighing 1000 to 1249 g, 92.3%.

Approximately 30% of LBW infants in the United States are born after 37 weeks and have IUGR. This figure is more than double that seen in developing countries. IUGR is associated with several medical conditions that interfere with the circulation and efficiency of the placenta or with the overall growth of the developing fetus, including conditions associated with poor fetal oxygenation. The infant with IUGR is not at risk because of small size, but rather because of the consequences of malnutrition and hypoxia. Associated medical conditions include intrauterine fetal demise, perinatal asphyxia, hypoglycemia, dysmorphology, and polycythemia (with associated hyperviscosity). Infants with IUGR have an increased risk of RDS, NEC, and neonatal death. Prenatal corticosteroid use is associated with a decreased incidence of RDS and death but not NEC in these infants.

SURFACTANT AND HYALINE MEMBRANE DISEASE

The biologic and physical characteristics of surfactant, the relationship between surfactant deficiency and the pathogenesis of HMD or RDS, and the therapeutic use of exogenous surfactant to prevent and treat HMD have great significance to the pediatric surgeon. The result of effective management of HMD has led to the improved survival of these infants. As a result, the pediatric surgeon commonly cares for many small premature infants—the "micropreemie" (<1000 g body weight and <28 weeks' gestational age). These infants have multiple physiologic deficits and are vulnerable to conditions such as IVH, BPD, NEC, and patent ductus arteriosus (PDA). It is essential that the pediatric surgeon understand the more recent developments concerning HMD, surfactant therapy, and the physiologic and pathologic characteristics of the ELBW preterm infant.

Lung Development

Embryonic Stage

The lung first appears as a tiny ventral bud formed at the level of the pharynx. This bud elongates into the surrounding mesenchyme and divides into the future main stem bronchi. Branching results in the formation of conducting and lobar airways by 37 days' gestation. Segmental airways are formed by 42 days, and subsegmental bronchi are formed by 48 days. During this period, the pulmonary artery arises from branches of the sixth aortic arch. Most major lung anomalies develop during the first 50 days of embryonic development.

Fetal Stage

Fetal lung development is divided into three phases: pseudoglandular, canalicular, and saccular.

Pseudoglandular—7 to 17 Weeks

There is progressive division of the airway to form terminal bronchioles by 16 weeks. Fifteen airway generations usually result. The distal airways are lined by glycogen-rich cuboidal epithelial cells. At the same time, arteries and veins develop around the airways.

Canalicular—16 to 25 Weeks

During this stage, the lung is transformed from a previable to a potentially viable organ capable of gas exchange. The acini and the air-blood barrier form, and surfactant synthesis by the type II alveolar cells begins. Undifferentiated cells are the precursors of the type I cells, which line the lung side of the air-blood barrier, and the type II cells, which produce surfactant.

Saccular—25 Weeks to Term

Large, primitive alveoli develop, lined by squamous type I cells and cuboidal type II cells. The lung now has the potential to support gas exchange.

Birth

Alveolar development continues postnatally for 1 year. At birth, the lungs change from a fluid-filled to a gas-filled system, assuming the function of gas exchange. Fluid absorption and surfactant secretion are the two major tasks during the birth period. Fluid is absorbed directly from the alveoli under the influence of adrenergic hormones.

Surfactant Development and Function

Type II alveolar cells are responsible for surfactant secretion and metabolism. Surfactant is a lipoprotein mixture containing 80% phospholipids, 10% protein, and 10% neutral fats. Saturated phosphatidylcholine or dipalmitoylphosphatidylcholine (DPPC) are the most abundant and surface active of the phospholipids. DPPC, also called *lecithin*, can be measured in amniotic fluid, and the lecithin-to-sphingomyelin ratio can be used to determine fetal lung maturity. Phosphatidylglycerol is the second most abundant phospholipid and does not seem to be necessary for surfactant function. It also is used as a marker of lung maturity. Three lipoproteins are associated with surfactant: SP-A, SP-B, and SP-C. SP-A does not seem to be necessary for surfactant function. SP-B and SP-C are necessary and function by improving the surface activity of the surfactant phospholipids. The synthesis and secretion of surfactant are vital to the development and maturation of the immature lung; surfactant is essential for postnatal gas exchange and newborn survival. Initiation of surfactant secretion at the onset of breathing is probably the result of multiple stimuli, such as elevated catecholamine levels and lung expansion. Because surfactant synthesis and storage are present in the human late in gestation, infants born after only 25 to 26 weeks' gestation may survive.

The physicochemical boundary between respiratory gases and liquid-coated surfaces of the cells of the respiratory epithelium creates a region of high surface tension. The surface tension generated by the unequal distribution of the molecular forces at the epithelial-air interface creates forces that potentially could result in the collapse of alveoli. Surfactant decreases the surface forces at the air-liquid-cell interface and prevents collapse. Surfactant, by altering surface tension at the air-fluid-epithelial interface, exerts a profound effect on alveolar stability. The forces on the alveoli can be appreciated best by thinking of them as interconnecting spheres of different diameters—one small, one large. According to Laplace's law, the pressure pushing the surface of a sphere (alveolus) inward toward collapse is two times the surface tension divided by the radius of the sphere. If the surface tension is high or the radius is small, the pressure is increased, and there is a tendency for the sphere to collapse. Additionally, added pressure on the inner surface of the alveolus is created by the chest wall and lung tissue elasticity. These combined forces leading to collapse are balanced by the atmospheric pressure to which the inner wall of the alveolus is exposed during inspiration. Because the alveoli are not all the same size, but interconnecting large and small spheres, according to Laplace's law, the surface tension is greatest on the small spheres because of their small radius. The smaller alveoli tend to collapse, and air flows into the larger alveoli, which distend. Surfactant prevents the collapse of the small alveoli and overdistention of the large alveoli. It has the unique property of reducing surface tension in proportion to the rate and amount of surface area being compressed. As the alveolar radius decreases, in the presence of surfactant, surface tension falls precipitously, preventing collapse of the smaller alveoli. Surfactant is self-adjusting, reducing surface tension more in a collapsing, smaller radius alveolus than in a larger alveolus. The preterm infant is surfactant deficient, however. As a result, there is a collapse of small alveoli, atelectasis, and overdistention of adjacent alveoli. Patchy atelectasis and overdistention lead to the classic HMD pathology, a nonhomogeneously inflated lung.

Not only are large areas of surfactant-deficient lungs atelectatic, but also they require more opening pressure to expand. The pressure needed to open an alveolar unit is related to the radius and the surface tension. The collapsed alveolus requires more pressure to "pop" open, whereas the noncollapsed units overdistend. At high pressures, this situation can lead to barotrauma and rupture of the larger air sacs. When surfactant is added to the system, the alveoli units open at a lower pressure and fill to a greater volume at this lower pressure. The physiologic effects of surfactant explain the success in treating a surfactant-deficient condition, HMD, with exogenous surfactant. They also help to clarify the effect of prenatal administration of corticosteroids in preventing HMD. Corticosteroids induce structural maturation of the lung and may increase surfactant synthesis. In general, dexamethasone or betamethasone should be administered intramuscularly 48 hours before delivery of any fetus between 24 and 34 weeks' gestation. The incidence of HMD in preterm infants is reduced 60% to 80% by an adequate course of prenatal corticosteroids. Corticosteroid administration also reduces the incidence of other complications, including IVH, PDA, pneumothorax, and NEC.

Hyaline Membrane Disease and Respiratory Distress Syndrome

HMD is estimated to occur in 60% of infants less than 28 weeks' gestation, in 15% to 20% of infants between 32 and 36 weeks' gestation, and 5% of infants close to term. The variability is due to the remarkably wide range of timing of lung maturation. The classic clinical presentation of HMD includes grunting respirations, chest wall retractions, tachypnea, cyanosis, pallor, and increasing oxygen requirement. These signs begin within 6 hours of birth. Often symptoms begin within minutes; a delayed presentation should raise suspicion of other potential causes. In VLBW infants, the signs are masked because the infant usually is intubated at birth and mechanically ventilated. The typical radiographic features include a diffuse reticulogranular pattern and prominent air bronchograms in both lung fields caused by a combination of alveolar atelectasis and overexpansion and pulmonary edema.

This radiographic picture cannot be differentiated from neonatal pneumonia, particularly that caused by group B streptococci. For this reason, infants with this radiographic picture usually are treated with antibiotics until culture reports are returned. Most infants with HMD improve by 3 to 5 days as lung maturation progresses.

Progressive lung damage in HMD results from hypoxia, barotrauma, and a reduction in pulmonary blood flow. Pulmonary vasoconstriction, intrapulmonary shunting, and right-to-left shunts across the ductus arteriosus and foramen ovale decrease blood flow to the lungs. Secondary pulmonary damage also is caused by high oxygen levels and barotrauma from positive-pressure ventilation.

Pathologically the lungs are grossly full and "liverlike" and appear solid and airless. Interstitial edema is widespread. Hyaline membranes are the characteristic microscopic lesion. They represent a coagulum of sloughed cellular debris in a protein matrix. The membranes form at the junction of the respiratory bronchioles and respiratory ducts.

Surfactant Replacement Therapy

Stimulated by the work of Clements on surface tension, Avery wondered why infants who died with HMD never had foam in their airways. She reasoned that "the reason they lack foam is that they did not have surfactant with the capacity to reduce surface tension when surface area was reduced." In 1958, Avery showed surfactant deficiency in the lung extracts of infants with HMD. She and Buckingham identified the type II cells as the site of surfactant synthesis and the lamellar bodies as the storage units. A considerable amount of research followed, defining the composition of surfactant and its relationship to pulmonary function. Fijiwara and coworkers in 1980 performed the first successful clinical trials with surfactant replacement.

The use of exogenous surfactant has been responsible for a 30% to 40% reduction in the odds of death among VLBW newborns with RDS. In addition, in premature neonates with birth weight greater than 1250 g, mortality in a controlled, randomized, blinded study decreased from 7% to 4%. There are in general two forms of surfactant: synthetic surfactant (Exosurf; Burroughs Wellcome, Raleigh-Durham, NC), which is made of DPPC and is protein-free, and bovine surfactant extracts (Survanta; Ross Laboratories, Columbus, OH), which contain natural surfactants and associated proteins. Although it has been thought that there is a substantial difference in effect between the natural and synthetic surfactants, studies reveal no difference between Exosurf and Survanta in terms of outcome. A significantly lower risk of CLD or death at 28 days was seen in infants treated with Survanta (27%), however, compared with Exosurf (34%). A randomized, prospective, controlled study in full-term newborns with respiratory insufficiency showed an increased failure rate as defined by oxygen index greater than 40 in the control group compared with the group in whom surfactant was administered. Another controlled, randomized study showed the utility of surfactant in full-term newborns with meconium aspiration syndrome. The oxygen index minimally decreased with the initial dose, but markedly decreased with the second and third doses of surfactant from a baseline of 23.7 to 5.9. After three doses of surfactant, persistent pulmonary hypertension had resolved in all but one of the infants in the study group versus none of the infants in the control group. The incidence of air leaks and need for extracorporeal life support were markedly reduced in the surfactant group compared with the control patients. Multiple doses of surfactant also have been shown to be more efficacious in the treatment of HMD. Although acute respiratory distress is markedly improved with surfactant therapy, little impact on CLD has been noted with this therapy.

CHRONIC LUNG DISEASE AND BRONCHOPULMONARY DYSPLASIA

The introduction of mechanical ventilation in the 1960s allowed larger numbers of small, sick infants to survive HMD. In 1967, Northway and associates first described BPD, a syndrome of CLD. The affected infants were premature, had severe HMD, and had been treated with positive-pressure ventilation and high inspired oxygen concentrations. This syndrome was characterized by oxygen dependence, radiographic abnormalities, and chronic respiratory symptoms persisting for more than 28 days. The clinical and radiographic findings progressed through four stages, ending with severe CLD. In the past, BPD, or what now more commonly is referred to as CLD, was found commonly in all premature infants with HMD regardless of birth weight. The classic forms of the disease in infants with birth weight greater than 1500 g became much less frequent. With improvement in ventilatory management, the condition now is confined predominantly to surviving ELBW infants who required prolonged mechanical ventilation for HMD.

Shennan and coworkers found that continued requirement for oxygen supplementation at 36 weeks' postconceptional age is the most sensitive and specific method of predicting CLD. The criteria commonly used to establish the diagnosis of CLD is oxygen dependence for more than 28 days after mechanical ventilation and radiographic changes consistent with CLD. The incidence of CLD usually is related to gestational age and birth weight (Table 1-1). It is now unusual to find affected infants who are older than 32 weeks' gestational age.

TABLE 1-1 ■ Outcome by Birth Weight, University of Washington Medical Center, Inborn Infants, January 1989-July 1991

Birth Weight Range (g)	Infants Alive at 28 Days with BPD* (%)
600-800	87.3
801-1000	56.5
1001-1250	36.0
1251-1500	2.4
1501-2000	3.5

*BPD is defined as need for supplemental oxygen and/or assisted ventilation still present at 28 days' postnatal age.
Modified from Truog WE, Jackson JC: Clin Perinatol 1992; 19:626.

Clinical Findings

Affected infants are almost always premature, ELBW infants who have been treated by positive-pressure ventilation and high inspired oxygen concentration for more than 7 days. Additional associated factors include presence of pulmonary interstitial emphysema, male sex, low P_{CO_2} at 48 hours (suggestive of aggressive ventilator setting), PDA, and increased airway resistance in the first week of life. The characteristic radiographic appearance of CLD emerges at about 20 days of age and includes hyperinflation, homogeneity of the lung fields, and multiple fine streaks extending to the periphery. These findings and a persistent oxygen requirement or respiratory support at 36 weeks' postconceptional age are sufficient to make the diagnosis. Patients diagnosed with CLD who survive usually show gradual improvement in lung function and radiographic findings. After extubation, the infants have retractions, rales, and tachypnea for long periods. They also have slow weight gain, recurrent atelectasis, and an increased incidence of respiratory infections. Some of these infants develop right-sided heart failure (cor pulmonale).

Pathology

The pathologic findings include areas of emphysema, atelectasis, small cysts, interstitial edema, and fibrosis throughout the lung tissue. The mucosa of the airways shows widespread changes, including hyperplasia, metaplasia, and narrowing. The peribronchiolar muscles are hypertrophied.

Pathogenesis

The pathogenesis of CLD is multifactorial: Prematurity, barotrauma, and oxygen toxicity are the most important factors.

Prematurity

The incidence of CLD in mechanically ventilated infants is inversely related to gestational age. The most frequent and severe form of CLD occurs in the structurally immature lungs of infants weighing less than 1200 g. The bronchiolar and alveolar ducts display structural immaturity, abnormal pulmonary endothelial cell function, and underdeveloped vascular arborization.

Barotrauma

The near-universal association of pulmonary interstitial emphysema with the subsequent development of CLD suggests that barotrauma is an important factor in its pathogenesis. Significant factors contributing to interstitial emphysema and CLD seem to be the level of positive inspiratory pressure and the length of time the infant is exposed to intermittent positive-pressure ventilation.

Oxygen Toxicity

The clinical impression that oxygen toxicity is a major factor in CLD is supported by animal studies. The effect of oxygen on lung tissue primarily depends on oxygen concentration. Other factors include the nutritional status of the patient, lung maturation, and the presence of oxidants. High inspired oxygen alone causes atelectasis; edema and hemorrhage of the alveoli; and inflammation, thickening, and hyalinization of the alveolar membranes. The mechanism responsible for the damage is believed to involve univalent reduction of molecular oxygen with the formation of oxygen free radicals. The release of these free radicals results in widespread cellular damage. The antioxidant system is designed to combat free radical injury. Although it is well developed in term infants, this system may be incomplete in premature infants.

Infection and Inflammation

Infants requiring prolonged respiratory support in an intensive care unit have an increased susceptibility to infection. The inflammatory response triggered by either infectious agents or oxygen exposure results in activation of immune cascades and the release of inflammatory mediators, such as tumor necrosis factor, interleukins, platelet-activating factor, and nitric oxide. These agents have profound, widespread, and localized effects on lung tissue.

Other Factors

Other factors that may contribute to CLD include pulmonary edema, a possible genetic predisposition, and vitamin A deficiency. VLBW infants have low levels of vitamin A, and early studies suggested that administration of vitamin A would reduce the incidence and severity of CLD. More recent controlled studies have shown that vitamin A therapy has a slight, but relatively minimal impact on the reduction of lung disease.

Treatment

Respiratory Support

Ventilator support in susceptible premature infants should be gentle and as brief as possible. The PaO_2 should be kept at greater than 50 mm Hg but less than 80 mm Hg, and oxygen saturation by pulse oximetry should be 93% to 95%. Inspired oxygen should be kept between 0.3 and 0.5. Positive end-expiratory pressure levels of 2 to 6 cm H_2O are used to reduce the need for high oxygen concentrations. More aggressive use of oxygen therapy has come into practice in more recent years because its use has been shown to decrease the incidence of cor pulmonale and improve neurologic outcomes. Weaning should be initiated as soon as possible. Ventilator adjustments are made when peak inspiratory pressure is less than 25 cm H_2O, inspired oxygen requirements are less than 0.5, and $PaCO_2$ is 50 mm Hg. One should guide $PaCO_2$ levels to be in the range of 50 to 70 mm Hg (provided that the pH is >7.30); this allows for a decrease in excess mean airway pressures.

Fluid Management and Diuretics

Patients with CLD have interstitial and peribronchial edema and abnormal mineral and water regulation leading to hypervolemia, PDA, cor pulmonale, and pulmonary edema. Precise fluid management to avoid hypervolemia and diuretic administration improve lung mechanics. There is a rapid improvement in lung compliance, pulmonary resistance, and blood gases. Drugs such as furosemide (1 mg/kg per dose intravenously two times a day or 2 mg/kg per dose orally two times a day) also may have relaxant effects on the airway and pulmonary vasculature. Additional diuretics may include hydrochlorothiazide (2–4 mg/kg/day in two divided doses, maximum of 37.5 mg) with potassium chloride as needed. The result of prolonged use of diuretics on the long-term outcome of patients with CLD is less clear. A major side effect of prolonged diuretic use is the development of nephrolithiasis.

Bronchodilator Therapy

A highly reactive airway commonly is associated with CLD. A β-adrenergic agonist (e.g., albuterol) is administered by aerosol inhalation in a dose of 50 μg. This agent relaxes smooth muscles in the lower airways. Aminophylline (to attain serum levels of 12 to 15 mg/L) or caffeine may be administered systemically. These agents also reduce airway resistance and act as respiratory stimulants.

Other Management

Infants with CLD have an increased oxygen consumption of more than 25%, most likely because of the increased work of breathing. Malnutrition and growth retardation often develop. It is essential to maintain optimal nutrition. Total parenteral nutrition is initially necessary to avoid using the gastrointestinal tract in the sick premature infant. Early enteral feeding is important but should be balanced against the risk of NEC with infants with an immature gastrointestinal tract.

Steroid Therapy

To moderate the inflammatory response and reduce airway constriction, a short course of corticosteroids may be administered. It has been shown with meta-analysis studies that steroid therapy can lead to more rapid extubation times and a reduction in the development of CLD by 28 days of life in VLBW infants. Many frequent and potentially serious side effects have been noted in infants receiving long-term corticosteroid therapy, however. Among these adverse effects are an increase in gastrointestinal bleeding, sepsis, poor weight gain, osteoporosis, hyperglycemia, and hypertension. An additional risk is the abnormal development of the central nervous system in children receiving long-term steroid therapy. To address these concerns, many controlled randomized trials have been performed. These studies suggest that steroids should be given fairly early, before the onset of ventilator-induced lung injury. Shorter courses of steroids are preferred over longer ones, with therapies of 1 to 2 weeks being considered ideal. Use of inhalational steroids may have some benefit. Inhalational steroids are safer than intravenous steroids but do not seem as effective.

RETINOPATHY OF PREMATURITY

ROP, previously called *retrolental fibroplasia*, is the major cause of infant blindness. When recognized early and properly assigned to a disease stage, ROP can be treated effectively, and profound visual loss or blindness can be avoided. Knowledge of the pathogenesis of this condition may help reduce the incidence of the disease. It is well established that a causal relationship exists between high oxygen exposure and the development of ROP. It was shown that restrictions of oxygen levels to less than 50% in newborn infants, particularly premature infants, significantly reduced the incidence of ROP. Despite a general adoption of oxygen restriction, ROP continues to be a major problem in neonatal intensive care units. It seems that extreme prematurity itself may be an important etiologic factor in ROP.

Risk Factors

The retinal blood vessels in a premature infant undergo continued growth and development. The more premature the infant, the less developed the retinal vessels. These immature, growing vessels are susceptible to damage and the subsequent development of ROP. Extreme prematurity is a major factor in the development of ROP. The exact role played by high oxygen levels and the length of oxygen exposure is less clear. Aside from high oxygen tension, mechanical ventilation, duration of hospitalization, sepsis, shock, transfusion, IVH, and xanthine derivatives also may have a role in the development of ROP.

Pathogenesis

The retinal circulation, the circulation affected by ROP, begins as a primitive network of mesenchymal cells emanating from the area of the optic nerve. The primitive capillaries then slowly cover the retina, reaching the nasal portion by term. These growing vessels lack supporting membranes and are extremely vulnerable to insults such as hypoxia and poor perfusion. As a result of injury to these immature vessels, neovascularization occurs in the retina and surrounding vitreous. This vascular response is the early stage of ROP. If the new vessels adequately vascularize the retina and surrounding structures, the early lesions of ROP regress. If the vessels and fibrous tissue grow into the retina and vitreous, however, scar tissue forms. As this scar tissue matures and contracts, retinal detachment may develop.

Incidence

The Multicenter Trial of Cryotherapy for Retinopathy of Prematurity gathered important information on the incidence of ROP in ELBW infants. This study consisted of 4099 premature infants with a birth weight less than 1251 g from 23 centers. An internationally agreed-on grading system was used. Of the 4099 patients, 65% developed ROP: 25% had mild grade I disease, 21.7% had moderate grade II disease, and 18% had severe grade III disease. The more premature the infant, the more severe the disease. Ophthalmic morbidity is not confined to ROP. Many other abnormalities may be associated with prematurity, including strabismus, decreased visual acuity, contrast sensitivity, color sensitivity, and ocular size. Finally, myopia is a known consequence of LBW.

Therapy

The Multicenter Trial of Cryotherapy for Retinopathy of Prematurity also examined the value of cryotherapy for patients with threshold disease. Threshold disease was defined as advanced ROP identified by age 6 weeks that could be predicted to result in 50% blindness. One eye was treated, and the other acted as a control. Cryotherapy was performed in the neonatal intensive care units with the patient under local anesthesia. A cryoprobe was placed on the external eye, and the retina was frozen in different areas. The results of this study showed that a poor outcome with retinal detachment and eventual blindness occurred in 23% of the treated eyes and 46% of the nontreated control eyes. Although the exact reason for the effectiveness of this treatment is not known, it is believed that cryotherapy promotes regression of ROP by destroying the abnormal vessels and stimulating extraretinal vessel growth, causing ROP to regress.

Important Points

1. There is a marked increased risk of ROP (65.8% incidence) in ELBW infants.
2. Severe disease with profound visual loss or blindness occurs in 18% of these patients.
3. Keeping PaO_2 or transcutaneous PO_2 levels between 60 and 80 mm Hg reduces the risk of ROP in vulnerable patients.
4. All patients at risk (infants weighing <1300 g) should have ophthalmologic examinations 6 weeks after birth. If threshold disease (advanced ROP) is found and treated with cryotherapy, the risk of blindness can be reduced significantly.

INTRAVENTRICULAR-PERIVENTRICULAR HEMORRHAGE

Intraventricular-periventricular hemorrhage (IVH-PVH) is the most common acute brain injury encountered in neonates. The incidence of IVH is 50% to 75% for infants at 26 weeks' gestational age and decreases to 5% for term infants.

Pathologic Anatomy

Bleeding almost always originates in the subependymal germinal matrix and extends into the ventricular system (Table 1-2). Obliterative arachnoiditis and ventricular bleeding may produce obstructive hydrocephalus later. Extension of the hemorrhage into the cerebral parenchyma results in destruction of brain tissue.

Pathogenesis

The germinal matrix overlies the head of the caudate nucleus and is composed of neuronal and glial precursor cells (neuroblasts and glioblasts). By 26 weeks' gestation, these cells have migrated into the adjacent cerebrum, and the supportive tissue of the germinal matrix involutes, essentially disappearing by 30 weeks' gestation. From 26 to 32 weeks' gestation, the germinal matrix is a gelatinous structure nearly devoid of supportive stroma, supplied by

TABLE 1-2 ■ Grading System (Papillae)	
Grade I	Hemorrhage is localized to the germinal matrix
Grade II	Hemorrhage extends into the ventricles without enlargement
Grade III	Hemorrhage extends into the ventricles with enlargement
Grade IV	Hemorrhage extends into the brain parenchyma

a rich, primitive, vascular network. The vessels consist of a single layer of endothelial cells without smooth muscles, elastin, or collagen. Hemorrhage almost always originates from these fragile, poorly supported vessels. The germinal matrix begins to thin and involute when these neuroblast cells migrate. Involution is complete by 36 weeks' gestation, which explains why IVH is almost nonexistent beyond this gestation age.

Perinatal risk factors include hypothermia, hypotension, pneumothorax, intravenous administration of hyperosmolar fluids (sodium bicarbonate), bolus injections of albumin solution, positive-pressure ventilation, HMD, and PDA. The greatest risk factors are perinatal asphyxia and RDS. More than 50% of cases associated with perinatal asphyxia manifest IVH by the first day of life, and 90% of IVH cases manifest by the third day of life. Several factors have been associated with RDS and IVH, including the development of hypercarbia and high peak airway pressures. Infants on high-frequency oscillator therapy have been shown to have an increased incidence of IVH.

Research suggests that an increase in intravascular pressure or blood flow to the germinal matrix can cause vascular disruption and bleeding. Hemorrhagic infarction of the periependymal tissue may occur; this may lead to rupture of the infarcted area and accumulation of intraventricular blood. A sharp increase in systemic arterial and intracerebral vascular pressure can be produced by hypoxemia, hypercarbia, and sudden intravascular volume expansion. Paradoxically, episodes of hypotension may result in IVH-PVH by producing capillary leaks. Evidence suggests that use of maternal magnesium sulfate may predispose to the development of IVH.

Diagnosis

Clinical Findings

There are three presentations:

1. Catastrophic—abrupt coma, a bulging fontanelle, shock, and frequently death
2. Saltatory—signs develop over several days and include thermal instability, tremulousness, increase in muscle tone, and enlarging head size
3. Silent—50% of all hemorrhages are asymptomatic (Table 1-3)

Laboratory Findings

A low hematocrit value, hypoglycemia or hyperglycemia, hypocalcemia, hyperbilirubinemia, thrombocytopenia, and prolonged prothrombin time and partial thromboplastin time are often noted. Urinary and blood findings of inappropriate antidiuretic hormone syndrome are occasionally present. Metabolic acidosis is common with grade III and IV hemorrhages. The cerebrospinal fluid may display gross blood and an elevated protein level (>250 mg/dL).

Imaging Findings

Definitive imaging examinations, such as magnetic resonance imaging and computed tomography, require transportation of the sick premature infant. Ultrasonography is a bedside procedure and has become the imaging modality of choice. Indications for ultrasonography include infants weighing less than 1500 g or less than 35 weeks' gestation, infants requiring mechanical ventilatory support, infants who have had perinatal hypoxic episodes, and infants who are candidates for extracorporeal membrane oxygenation. Examinations are done during the first and third weeks of life and at discharge. The optimal time for a definitive ultrasound diagnosis is 1 week after the bleed. Ventricular dilation usually can be detected after 14 days.

Therapy

There is no specific therapy to reduce the morbidity and mortality of IVH-PVH. Therapeutic efforts are directed toward resuscitation and the maintenance of optimal physiologic conditions. Intravenous phenobarbital (15 to 18 mg/kg) is the primary agent to treat seizures. Serial lumbar punctures or ventricular drainage has been used for grades III and IV hemorrhage. As a result of reduced ventilator needs, use of prenatal steroids has been associated with a decreased incidence of IVH. Because barbiturates are known to have neuroprotective actions, barbiturates have been advocated in a prophylactic fashion to prevent IVH. A Cochrane review of the current literature fails to support the use of barbiturates in this fashion, however. There is some encouraging evidence that indomethacin therapy may result in a reduction of the incidence of grades III and IV IVH. Its use must be tempered with the increased incidence of renal dysfunction and possibly increased occurrence of NEC. Finally, ethamsylate, an inhibitor of prostacyclin synthesis, is a potent vasodilator and has been shown to be beneficial in reducing overall and severe IVH.

Hydrocephalus develops in 14% of infants after IVH-PVH. There is progressive ventricular dilation and elevated intracranial pressure. The most common form is noncommunicating: obstruction at the fourth ventricle or the base of the brain. Communicating hydrocephalus results from impairment of absorption of cerebrospinal fluid. In 50% of all cases, dilation is not progressive. Progression is suspected if there are episodes of apnea and bradycardia, enlarging head size, and ultrasonography changes. Symptomatic hydrocephalus should be treated with spinal needle aspiration. Serial lumbar punctures should be avoided, however, because of the increased risk of meningitis.

Further progression of fluid buildup is an indication for a shunt operation. Experience with fibrinolytic therapy given intraventricularly has suggested it may result in a decreased need for shunt operations. Several authors have administered a variety of fibrinolytic agents intraventricularly and assessed need for shunt placement.

Grade	Clinical Findings
I	Asymptomatic
II	Irritability and lethargy
III/IV	Pallor, jaundice, apnea and bradycardia, posturing, eye deviation, seizures, clonic motions

TABLE 1-3 ■ Symptoms by Grade of IVH-PVH

TABLE 1-4 ■ Morbidity and Mortality for IVH-PVH			
Grade	Hydrocephalus (%)	Mortality (%)	Impairment
I	5	0	0
II	25	<5	+
III	55	>15	+ + +
IV	80	50	+ + + +

The literature regarding its use is mixed. Ideal timing and dosing of these agents have not been established, and this therapy is not used routinely in most centers at present.

Outcome

The overall mortality for IVH-PVH is 30% (Table 1-4). There has been an overall reduction in the incidence of IVH in VLBW infants, from 40% to 50% to about 20% to 30%. In general, grades I and II hemorrhage are associated with virtually no mortality and minimal morbidity. Grades III and IV hemorrhage are associated with a high mortality and significant neurologic deficits. Finally, many other vascular lesions are associated with the premature neonate. In particular, ischemic lesions, with or without IVH, may have a significant impact on a poor neurologic outcome. These patients have a high rate of white matter lesions, such as periventricular leukomalacia. These lesions leave the area of the brain with a cystic lesion and may lead to damage to the corticospinal fibers in the internal capsule.

LONG-TERM OUTCOMES

The survivors of CLD frequently are left with chronic disabilities. Neurodevelopmental handicaps are relatively frequent (approximately 20% in infants with birth weight <1500 g) but do not seem to be more frequent than in VLBW infants requiring mechanical ventilation and intensive care who do not develop CLD. Blindness occurs in 5% of CLD patients, and hearing loss occurs in 4%. Chronic persistent pulmonary problems are common. By the time they reach adolescence or young adulthood, 76% of survivors have measurable pulmonary dysfunction, and 25% experience moderate-to-severe pulmonary dysfunction. Reviews have provided an interesting perspective on the outcomes of many prematurely born individuals. The impact of surfactant therapy and other newer neonatal modalities has been a "double-edged sword." Although the survivorship of these infants has increased, the number with long-term disabilities similarly has increased. A multicenter survey has confirmed this suspicion. The overall incidence of cerebral palsy in these infants was 12.6%. There was a statistically increased incidence of cerebral palsy in patients with IVH and CLD, and each of these conditions was noted to be an independent risk factor. For the outcomes of self-care, mobility, and social function, 11.7%, 29.5%, and 10.7% of the children scored at least 2 standard deviations below the normative means. Social function was 0.25 to 0.50 normative standard deviations lower after general surfactant availability than before general surfactant availability.

RESPIRATORY SYNCYTIAL VIRUS

RSV is the most important lower respiratory tract pathogen in infants and children. Infection by this virus is the major cause of bronchiolitis and pneumonia in infants younger than 1 year of age. Three million children younger than age 4 years are infected annually. Of children infected, 100,000 require hospitalization, and 2% to 5% develop respiratory failure. The mortality in hospitalized patients varies between 1% and 5%. Nosocomial transmission occurs via nurse-to-patient, physician-to-patient, and patient-to-patient contact. Infection does not confer protection, and reinfection rates are extremely high. RSV frequently affects the most vulnerable patients: small premature infants, immunosuppressed cancer and transplant patients, and infants with congenital heart disease or CLD.

Virus

RSV is an enveloped RNA virus that develops in the cytoplasm of infected cells. It belongs to the same Paramyxoviridae family as mumps and parainfluenza but in a seperate genus of pneumoviruses. In in vitro culture, infected cells fuse to neighboring cells and form a syncytium.

Epidemiology

The unique aspects of RSV compared with other viral diseases are its worldwide distribution, annual outbreaks, and infection in patients in the first month of life. Initial infections occur in the first 2 years of life, and most children have become infected by age 3 years. In the temperate climates of the United States, epidemics usually begin between October and December and end between April and May. The peak months are January, February, and March. RSV is responsible for 45% to 75% of all cases of bronchiolitis, 15% to 20% of cases of pneumonia, and 6% to 8% of cases of croup in infants. In urban centers and high-exposure areas, such as day care centers, infection is essentially universal by the second year of life. Reinfection occurs at a rate of 10% to 20% per epidemic throughout childhood. About 15% of infected children require physician treatment. Of infected patients who require physician treatment, 10% require hospital admission. Most admitted patients (80%) are 6 months to 1 year old. It is thought that severe illness is uncommon in the first 2 months of life because of partial protection from placenta-transferred antibodies.

Transmission

Transmission occurs via infected nasal secretions, usually in the form of large droplets. Spread is by direct contact, often via the hand or contaminated clothing. Spread is not airborne. The virus enters the patient through the nasal or conjunctival mucosa. In hospitals, spread is by patients or personnel. Physicians and nurses spread the virus through contact with infected patients and subsequent handling of other patients. Hospital staff also spread the infection by contracting the disease themselves and infecting patients. The period of viral shedding is typically 3 to 8 days, but in young infants shedding may continue for 3 to 4 weeks. In an infant ward, during an epidemic, half of the roommates and one third of the staff become infected. Intensive care units are an important site of spread, and great care must be taken to protect the most vulnerable patients in the unit. Gowns, gloves, and goggles afford maximum protection. Most important and practical, however, are avoiding contact of clothing with secretions, careful hand washing, and an awareness of the disease and its manner of spread.

Pathology and Pathogenesis

Infection travels from the site of inoculation in the eyes or nose to the oropharynx, nasopharynx, and lower respiratory tract. Children younger than age 2 years commonly develop bronchiolitis. Bronchiolitis is characterized by respiratory epithelial cell necrosis and destruction of cilia, resulting in peribronchial edema and inflammatory cell infiltration. Plugging of small airways by inflammatory and necrotic epithelial cells and edema fluid leads to areas of hyperaeration and atelectasis. If interstitial pneumonia develops, there is extensive infiltration and bronchial and alveolar cell necrosis. The cellular injury is thought to be the result of direct viral damage and secondary "immunologic" damage as a result of the release of inflammatory mediators, such as leukotrienes and products of the cyclooxygenase pathway. The release of these products may be stimulated by specific immunologic reactions, the release of a viral-specific anti-immunoglobulin E (anti-IgE), or as a result of cellular immune responses.

Clinical Features

The incubation period is usually 4 to 7 days. The illness begins with a mild cough, low-grade fever, and nasal discharge—the symptoms of a common cold. The cough becomes progressively more pronounced over 3 to 5 days. Within 5 to 6 days of the first symptoms, clinical bronchiolitis has fully developed. The work of breathing increases with retractions, nasal flaring, rapid breathing, and prolonged expiration. The chest is hyperresonant. Expiratory wheezes and rales are heard. Apnea commonly develops in infants. Radiographs of the chest show areas of hyperexpansion and atelectasis, increased bronchial markings, and scattered densities. Pleural effusions are rare. Of patients, 20% are cyanotic. Fever is inconsistent; infants are usually lethargic and afebrile. Hypoxemia is the most common reason for hospital admission ($PaO_2 \leq 50$ to 60 mm Hg on room air). A falling PaO_2 with a rising $PaCO_2$ suggests impending respiratory failure and is an indication for mechanical ventilatory support. In the rare patient who is unable to maintain adequate oxygenation with mechanical ventilation, extracorporeal membrane oxygenation has been used successfully. The mortality for severely ill infants is 1% to 5%, and death is most common in infants with underlying diseases. The usual hospital course is 5 to 7 days.

Laboratory Findings

Rapid diagnosis is made by antigen detection using immunofluorescence or an enzyme-linked immunosorbent assay (ELISA). These tests are commercially available and have diagnostic accuracy rates of 80% to 90%. Viral isolation is cumbersome and owing to the labile nature of the virus is often inaccurate.

Treatment

Mild cases are treated by supportive care. Humidified oxygen is the mainstay of therapy. The patient's oxygenation status is monitored closely for the development of respiratory failure. If wheezing is severe, a trial of bronchodilators (usually as an aerosol) is attempted. Corticosteroids and antibiotics are not helpful.

Ribavirin is a broad-spectrum antiviral agent effective against RSV, herpes simplex virus, parainfluenza, and influenza viruses. Ribavirin is given by aerosol. Its use is reserved for children with severe respiratory failure; infants with congenital heart disease, CLD, and acquired and primary immunodeficiencies; and patients who have undergone major surgical procedures, particularly organ transplantation. Ribavirin is extremely expensive, and overall efficacy based on clinical trials is controversial.

Two products are available to prevent RSV. The first is respiratory syncytial virus immune globulin (RSV-IG). This agent is prepared from human donors with a high serum titer for RSV neutralizing antibody. The second agent is palivizumab. This is a humanized mouse monoclonal antibody that is given intramuscularly. Both agents have been approved for use in children less than 24 months of age who are at risk for the development of a severe case of RSV. The indications include patients with CLD. These patients should receive medication if they have required medical treatment for CLD within 6 months of the upcoming RSV season. Patients with severe CLD benefit from treatment for the first 2 years of life. Additional indications include low gestational age (<32 weeks) without CLD. Patients with congenital heart disease or who are immunocompromised also may benefit, but clinical trials are lacking.

VIRAL GASTROENTERITIS

Viral gastroenteritis has great significance to all physicians who care for infants and children, regardless of their specialty or whether they practice in developed or developing countries. The surgeon must understand that these illnesses can be spread by the medical staff, masquerade as surgical illnesses, contribute to the pathogenesis of surgical diseases (e.g., NEC), and attack vulnerable surgical patients such as those with short-bowel syndrome or Hirschsprung's disease. In severe forms, it may lead to hypovolemia, shock, and death.

Table 1-5 lists the etiologic agents responsible for gastroenteritis in hospitalized infants in developed and developing countries. The rotaviruses are the principal etiologic agents; adenoviruses are the next most frequent pathogens in both environmental settings.

Rotaviruses

Throughout the world, 90% of infants and children younger than age 3 years develop rotavirus infections. The consequences of infection in infants in a developed country are significant, resulting in 80,000 hospitalizations and 200 deaths per year. The effect in developing countries is staggering: approximately 18 million

TABLE 1-5 ■ Viruses Responsible for Gastroenteritis					
Virus	Age Group	Incidence	Transmission	Clinical Features	Diagnosis
Rotavirus	6-24 mo	Most common and important cause of pediatric diarrhea in the world	Fecal Oral	Explosive diarrhea Vomiting Fever Dehydration common Nonbloody stools Seasonal Important cause of hospitalization	Immunoassay ELISA LA EM
Adenovirus	6-24 mo	Second most common and important cause of pediatric diarrhea in the world	Fecal Oral	Diarrhea Fever Occasional vomiting Prolonged diarrhea (9 days) Dehydration less common Year-round occurrence	EM ELISA
Norwalk- like viruses	Older children Adults	More common and important in adults	Fecal Oral Associated with food ingestion Schools Cruises Epidemic associated	Vomiting Diarrhea Cramps Headaches Low-grade fever Myalgia Short duration: 24-40 hr Not important cause of hospitalization	ELISA

LA, Latex agglutination; EM, electron microscopy.

moderate or severe cases per year and 870,000 deaths. Immunologic assays, such as ELISAs and latex agglutination assays, are commercially available as kits to detect the virus in stool specimens; ELISAs have a greater sensitivity.

In the United States, rotavirus infection appears in the fall in the Southwest, then spreads eastward, reaching the Northeast by late winter and early spring. The peak incidence is from December to April. Spread is by the fecal-oral route. Infants and young children are particularly vulnerable because of their unchallenged immune system and ease of contamination from diapers, crawling, and the tendency to put things into their mouth. Exposure is increased by close contact, as occurs in hospitals and day care centers.

Rotaviruses most commonly affect infants between age 6 months and 2 years. Younger infected infants are often asymptomatic, but a severe form in hospitals associated with NEC has been reported in epidemic outbreaks. Commonly the illness begins 1 to 3 days after exposure with explosive, watery diarrhea and often nonbilious vomiting. The diarrhea is usually not foul smelling, and the stools do not contain blood or white blood cells. Fever of 38°C is frequent. Dehydration occurs in 40% to 80% of cases but is usually less than 5%. Dehydration is isotonic and is associated with metabolic acidosis; when severe, hospitalization and intravenous fluid therapy are necessary. In mild cases, the disease is self-limited, ending in 3 to 9 days, but the child may shed the virus in the stool for 10 to 12 days after the onset of symptoms. Rotaviruses have been associated with several severe disease entities, including aseptic meningitis, NEC, Kawasaki syndrome, Reye's syndrome, and sudden infant death syndrome.

The rotavirus invades the mucosal cells of the small intestinal villi, commonly the jejunum. The mature absorptive mucosal cells are injured or destroyed and are replaced by immature mucosal cells that arise from the crypts. Functional deficits of the injured mucosal cells and immature replacement cells lead to reduced salt and water absorption. The decreased disaccharidase activity of the immature replacement cells results in carbohydrate malabsorption and osmotic diarrhea. The severity of the disease is determined by the extent of small bowel involvement. Oral hydration by glucose electrolyte fluids is usually all that is necessary to treat most dehydrated infants. A vaccine has been developed; however, because of the development of intussusception in many infants who received the vaccine, it has been taken off the market. Table 1-5 summarizes some of the characteristics of gastroenteritis secondary to rotavirus, adenovirus, and Norwalk-like viruses that cause viral gastroenteritis.

SUGGESTED READINGS

American Academy of Pediatrics Committee on Infectious Disease and Committee on Fetus and Newborn: Prevention of respiratory syncytial virus infections: Indications for the use of palivizumab and update on the use of RSV-IGIV. Pediatrics 102:1211-1216, 1998.

This article reviews the pathogenesis of RSV infections. It also discusses indications and results of prophylactic therapy for RSV.

Bernstein I, Horbar JD, Badger GJ, et al: Morbidity and mortality among very-low-birth-weight neonates with intrauterine growth restriction. Am J Obstet Gynecol 182(1, Part 1):198-206, 2000.

A careful statistical analysis was done of the neonatal risk factors associated with the finding of IUGR. An increased risk of neonatal death, NEC, and RDS was noted with IUGR.

Bhuta T, Ohlsson A: Systematic review and meta-analysis of early postnatal dexamethasone for prevention of chronic lung disease. Arch Dis Child Fetal Neonatal Ed 79:F26-33, 1998.

This article presents a meta-analysis of the risks and benefits of steroid therapy for the prevention and treatment of CLD in ventilator-dependent premature infants.

Cryotherapy for Retinopathy of Prematurity Cooperative Group: Multicenter trial of cryotherapy for retinopathy of prematurity: Snellen visual acuity and structural outcome at 5½ years after randomization. Arch Opthalmol 114:417-424, 1996.

This study reviews the outcomes of cryotherapy for infants with ROP. It also delineates many other visual impairments that these children eventually experience, including altered eye growth, reduced visual acuity, and increased risk of strabismus.

Jobe AH: Drug therapy: Pulmonary surfactant therapy. N Engl J Med 328:861, 1993.

This article reviews surfactant, its function, and therapeutic use.

Kapikian AZ: Viral gastroenteritis. JAMA 269:627, 1993.

A concise but complete review of viral gastroenteritis and its worldwide significance is presented.

MacDorman MF, Minino AM, Strobino DM, Guyer B: Annual summary of vital statistics—2001. Pediatrics 110:1037-1052, 2002.

This is the most current review of infant mortality rates, particularly as delineated by gestational age and weight.

Palmer EA, Flynn JT, Hardy RJ, et al: Incidence and early course of retinopathy of prematurity. Ophthalmology 98:1628, 1991.

Results of a multicenter trial of cryotherapy are presented, with an excellent summary of the incidence of the various stages of ROP. A population of 4099 patients was studied; 65.8% developed ROP.

Palta M, Sadek-Badawi M, Evans M, et al: Functional assessment of a multicenter very low-birth-weight cohort at age 5 years. Arch Pediatr Adolesc Med 154:23-30, 2000.

This excellent review of long-term neurologic and developmental outcomes of very-low-birth-weight infants shows that use of surfactant may increase survivorship, but also may increase neurologic developmental delay. CLD and IVH were independent risk factors for the occurrence of developmental delay.

Tortorolo G, Luciano R, Papacci P, Tonelli T: Intraventricular hemorrhage: Past, present and future, focusing on classification, pathogenesis and prevention. Child Nerv Syst 15:652-661, 1999.

This is an excellent and fairly up-to-date review of the pathogenesis and treatment of IVH in newborns.

2

Prenatal Diagnosis and Fetal Surgery

Fetal diagnosis and intervention are playing an increasingly important role in perinatal care as diagnostic tests have become more accurate and safe and as refinements in molecular analysis and in utero imaging have enhanced detection and characterization of congenital diseases and anomalies. Along with the development of the techniques of fetal and minimally invasive surgery, the ability to intervene in utero has become a clinical reality.

PRENATAL DIAGNOSIS

The frequency of major birth defects is approximately 3% among live-born infants. More than 50% of fetal defects affect the central nervous system, 20% affect the genitourinary tract, 15% affect the gastrointestinal tract, and 8% affect the cardiovascular system. A combination of tests such as maternal serum α-fetoprotein (AFP) screening alone or combined with human chorionic gonadotropin (hCG) and unconjugated serum estriol (the "triple test") and inhibin A (the "quadruple test"), amniocentesis, chorionic villus sampling (CVS), percutaneous umbilical blood sampling (PUBS), prenatal ultrasound, and in utero magnetic resonance imaging (MRI) has proved to be effective at identifying these abnormalities in utero. This identification allows for parental counseling, options for intervention or termination, and referral of affected infants to high-risk obstetric delivery centers with readily available neonatal intensive care facilities and contemporary pediatric surgical expertise. The tests also provide answers to stressful questions for parents at high risk for congenital diseases and anomalies.

Screening of maternal blood is recommended for all pregnancies to rule out elevated AFP indicative of neural tube defects and in pregnant women younger than age 35 years to assess for trisomy 18 and 21. Pregnant women who are older than age 35 years and at higher risk for chromosomal abnormalities (Table 2-1) should be offered amniocentesis or CVS instead. All women with pregnancies at risk for genetic disorders because of medical history or ethnic group should have assessment for specific markers for the disease of concern (Table 2-2).

AFP is one of the major oncotic proteins in fetal serum. Fetal defects involving lack of effective skin covering (open neural tube defects or abdominal wall defects) allow for this serum protein to be elevated in the amniotic fluid surrounding the fetus. Screening by measurement of maternal serum AFP levels should be offered to all women at 15 to 20 weeks' gestation. Maternal serum AFP levels 2 to 2.5 times the median are observed in 90% of fetuses with anencephaly and 80% to 85% of fetuses with neural tube defects with a 5% false-negative rate. Consideration must be given to the gestational age; maternal weight (heavier women have lower or more dilute AFP); any anomaly consistent with fetal edema, such as hydrops or cystic hygroma; skin defects; multiple gestations (maternal AFP may be normal at 4.5 to 5 times the median in mothers with twins); and fetal demise. If the AFP is elevated, ultrasonography should be performed to assess for fetal demise, gestational age, multiple gestations,

	TABLE 2-1 ■ Risk of Down Syndrome and Other Chromosomal Abnormalities as a Function of Maternal Age	
Age*	**Risk of Down Syndrome**	**Risk of Chromosomal Abnormality**
20	1/1667	1/526
25	1/1250	1/476
30	1/952	1/385
35	1/385	1/202
36	1/295	1/162
37	1/227	1/129
38	1/175	1/102
39	1/137	1/82
40	1/106	1/65
41	1/82	1/51
42	1/64	1/40
43	1/50	1/32
44	1/38	1/25
45	1/30	1/20
46	1/23	1/16
47	1/18	1/13
48	1/14	1/10
49	1/11	1/7

*Ages are at the expected time of delivery.
From D'Alton ME, DeCherney AH: Prenatal diagnosis. N Engl J Med 1993; 328:114.

TABLE 2-2 ■ Genetic Disorders, Ethnic Risk Factors, and Means for Diagnosis

Disorder	Ethnic or Racial Group	Screening
Tay-Sachs disease	Ashkenazi Jewish, French Canadian	Decreased serum hexosaminidase A concentration
Canavan's disease	Ashkenazi Jewish, French Canadian	DNA analysis for mutations of aspartoacyclase gene (chromosome 17)
Sickle cell anemia	Black African, Mediterranean, Arab, Indian, and Pakastani	Presence of sickling in hemolysate followed by confirmatory hemoglobin electrophoresis
α- and β-thalassemia	Mediterranean, Southern and Southeast Asian, Chinese	Mean corpuscular volume <80 μm^3, followed by confirmatory hemoglobin electrophoresis
Cystic fibrosis	Offer to whites, Ashkenazi Jews. Make available to Asians, Hispanics, African-Americans	DNA analysis of 25 *CFTR* mutations

TABLE 2-3 ■ Indications for Amniocentesis and CVS

General risk factors
Maternal age ≥35 years at the time of delivery
Elevated or reduced maternal serum AFP concentration
Maternal serum screening indicative of elevated or reduced levels of maternal serum AFP, HCG, and unconjugated estriol concentrations

Specific risk factors
Previous child with a structural defect or chromosomal abnormality
Previous stillbirth or neonatal death
First-degree relative with a neural tube defect
Structural abnormality in the mother or father
Chromosomal translocation in the mother or father
Inherited disorders: cystic fibrosis, metabolic disorders, sex-linked recessive disorders
Exposure to teratogen: ionizing radiation, anticonvulsant medicine, lithium, isotretinoin, alcohol
Infection, rubella, toxoplasmosis, cytomegalovirus

neural tube defects and other anomalies. If the elevated AFP remains unexplained after ultrasound, amniocentesis may be performed to assay the levels of AFP and acetylcholinesterase, both of which may be elevated in fetuses with spina bifida. Acetylcholinesterase allows identification of increased AFP resulting from fetal blood in the amniotic fluid because acetylcholinesterase would not be elevated in that setting. Elevated AFP levels also are observed in patients with Turner's syndrome, omphalocele, gastroschisis, sacrococcygeal teratoma, and intestinal obstruction. Maternal folic acid supplementation during the 3 months before conception and the first trimester has resulted in a remarkable 71% reduction in neural tube defects.

In contrast to neural tube defects, trisomy 18 and 21 are associated with a decrease in AFP. When combined with elevated hCG and decreased unconjugated serum estriol (the triple test), the sensitivity of detecting trisomy 21 is 65% to 70%, although detection rates are 90% for women 35 years old and older. The levels of these markers are altered, however, with maternal weight, smoking, ethnic group, and diabetes and with in vitro pregnancies. Trisomy 18 is marked by a low AFP, estriol, and hCG, in contrast to trisomy 21. The *second* trimester triple test should be offered to all mothers younger than age 35 years, with confirmatory amniocentesis performed if results are consistent with trisomy. If indicated, screening in the *first* trimester can be performed by using fetal ultrasound–determined nuchal translucency, which is increased in the fetus with chromosomal abnormalities, including Down syndrome and monosomy X (Turner's syndrome),

and in fetuses with a cardiac abnormality. Nuchal translucency measurement may be combined with pregnancy-associated placental protein A levels for Down syndrome detection with a sensitivity of greater than 70%.

Parents at risk for specific autosomal recessive disorders because of ethnic background should be offered screening for the disease. Tay-Sachs and Canavan's diseases, sickle cell anemia, and α-thalassemia and β-thalassemia screening should be offered to parents as indicated in Table 2-2. More recent recommendations suggest that screening for cystic fibrosis be offered to all whites and that screening be considered in other races. Parental blood assessment for the 25 mutations most frequently associated with cystic fibrosis in American whites (population frequency of <0.01% in the United States) is recommended. If a family history of cystic fibrosis is present, family members also may be tested and evaluation for 70 mutations performed. The presence of a specific disorder in the fetus may be shown via amniocentesis or CVS (see later) because most enzymes involved in metabolic disorders may be found in the villi or amniotic fluid cells. Genetic material from these cells can be analyzed by polymerized chain reaction, fluorescence in situ hybridization, linkage analysis, and other molecular techniques to make the diagnosis of most common inborn errors of metabolism and other disorders.

Amniocentesis

The purpose of amniocentesis is to detect the presence of metabolic disorders and chromosomal defects. Indications for amniocentesis are listed in Table 2-3. Amniocentesis is usually performed at 15 to 16 weeks' gestation and is done under ultrasound guidance to determine placental position and site of the amniotic fluid. A 20-gauge or 22-gauge spinal needle is introduced into the amniotic fluid with removal of approximately 20 mL. Results are generally available in 7 to 14 days. The technique can be performed in the setting of multiple gestations with dye injected into each amnion after sampling to prevent unrecognized repeat aspiration from the same fetus. Maternal risks are limited and include transient vaginal spotting or amniotic fluid leakage (occurring in <1% of cases). Fetal loss is estimated at 0.3% to 0.5%. Although early amniocentesis has been proposed and evaluated, performance before 13 weeks' gestation is not recommended because of the 1.3% risk of clubfoot after this procedure compared with the expected 0.1% incidence.

Chorionic Villus Sampling

CVS of the chorion frondosum allows biopsy of fetal cells for chromosomal, enzyme, or DNA analysis in the first trimester of pregnancy. Although amniocentesis and CVS are equivalent in terms of the ability to evaluate chromosomes and to assess for metabolic disorders, one must perform amniocentesis for evaluation of amniotic fluid, including AFP. CVS can be performed at 9 to 12 weeks' gestation, however, rather than 15 to 16 weeks' gestation for amniocentesis and usually takes 7 to 10 days for culture results. As such, CVS has advantages over amniocentesis in that it provides diagnoses slightly more rapidly and at an earlier stage in pregnancy.

Sampling may be accomplished by transcervical insertion of a 1.5-mm diameter plastic catheter at 9 to 12 weeks' gestation. The catheter is placed under ultrasound guidance adjacent to the placental tissue, and syringe suction is applied as trophoblastic tissue is aspirated into culture media. Alternatively a 22-gauge spinal needle may be placed via a transabdominal approach along the long axis of the placenta and the villi aspirated. The latter approach can be used at any gestational age. A transvaginal approach may be advantageous in the setting of a posterior placenta. The rate of fetal loss seems to be approximately 0.5% to 1% and does not seem to be affected by use of a transcervical versus a transabdominal approach. Although not definite, there are suggestions that performance of CVS may be associated with an increased incidence of hypoplasia or absence of the fingers or toes at a rate of 1 per 3000 compared with the general population rate. The rate appears to be higher when CVS is performed at less than 10 weeks' gestation, and as such it is recommended that CVS not be performed until later. The diagnostic accuracy of CVS is considered to be approximately equivalent to that of amniocentesis. Inaccuracies in diagnoses owing to assessment of maternal rather than fetal cells and genetic alterations in fetal cells in culture (culture artifact) may occur rarely.

Fetal Tissue Sampling and Percutaneous Umbilical Blood Sampling

The prenatal diagnosis of inherited malformations can be obtained by percutaneous sampling of fetal tissue. Biopsy of the skin and liver can be performed, allowing the diagnosis of conditions in which the genetic defect is not expressed in amniotic fluid (e.g., epidermolysis bullosum). Fetal muscle biopsy may allow diagnosis of Duchenne's muscular exstrophy. Cytogenetics under most circumstances allows a diagnosis to be made, however, making fetal tissue sampling unnecessary in most cases. A fetal loss rate of 2% to 3% is associated with fetal tissue sampling.

PUBS, also called *cordocentesis*, can be used for the prenatal diagnosis of many fetal hematologic abnormalities, including Rh or other isoimmunization problems, hemoglobinopathies such as hemophilia A or B, thrombocytopenia, chronic granulomatous disease, α_1-antitrypsin deficiency, and coagulation factor abnormalities such as von Willebrand's disease. Confirmation or clarification of chromosomal status also may be achieved. Sampling usually is performed at or beyond 18 weeks' gestation with a 20-gauge or 22-gauge spinal needle inserted under ultrasound guidance into the umbilical vein with aspiration of fetal blood. Results are usually available within 48 to 72 hours. The procedure-related rate of fetal loss after PUBS is unclear but may be 1% to 3%. Amnionitis and hemorrhage are rare. Because PUBS potentially presents a greater risk to the fetus, it should be reserved for situations needing rapid diagnosis or when safer means are unobtainable.

Preimplantation Genetic Diagnosis

Techniques are now available for evaluating oocytes and embryos 6 days after in vitro conception. The polar body from the oocyte can be biopsied and analyzed. If no known adverse gene or if a normal complement of chromosomes is present in the polar body, the oocyte can be allowed to progress to fertilization and implantation with reduced fear for expression of the recessive trait and concern for trisomy. Sex determination also can be made. This technique does not allow assessment of the paternal component, however, and relies on indirect evidence of the status of chromosomes and genes. Biopsy of a cell from a six- to eight-cell blastomere allows direct assessment of the embryonic genotype. Removal of one or two cells does not affect subsequent development.

Fetal Cell Assessment

Fetal cells may be found in maternal blood. Assessment for specific markers or genes may allow identification of the chromosomal status of the fetus. The presence of a Y chromosome in the maternal blood indicates the sex of the fetus, which would be especially important for parents with potential X-linked recessive disorders. Identification in the mother of an undesirable or even normal allele that was initially present in the father would provide information on the fetal risk for known disorders. The presence of a trisomy in the serum of the mother would indicate a fetus with trisomy. This technique may be used to identify trisomy 18 or 21. This promising technique may preclude the need for more invasive means for evaluating some fetal disorders.

Fetal Imaging

Prenatal ultrasonography is the most frequently used method of fetal imaging and is effective in determining the gestational age of the fetus, monitoring growth in high-risk pregnancies (including multiple pregnancies), and detecting many fetal anomalies. The availability of advanced real-time scanning equipment and gray-scale high resolution along with color Doppler evaluation has permitted a more precise assessment of fetal anatomy and activity. Prenatal ultrasonography has now become routine. There is a 0.5% falsely abnormal rate, however, and a 0.9% falsely normal rate found in large series. Visualization may be limited by relatively early gestational age, maternal obesity, abdominal scarring, fetal position, and oligohydramnios. Ultrasonography fails to diagnose the anomaly in 55% of fetuses with congenital diaphragmatic hernia (CDH).

Sonography also is used to evaluate amniotic fluid volume, lung development, and renal obstruction, all of which may be interrelated. The presence of normal amounts of amniotic fluid suggests that the fluid swallowed by the fetus is being excreted back into the amniotic pool by the fetal kidneys. This process begins by the fourth month of gestation and requires at least one functioning kidney. A reduced amniotic fluid volume (oligohydramnios) may reflect diminished renal function, whereas anhydramnios indicates urethral obstruction,

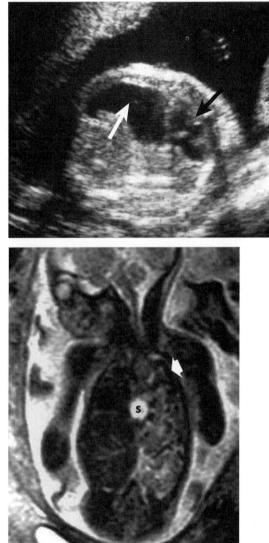

FIGURE 2-1 ■ Imaging of a fetus with congenital diaphragmatic hernia. **A,** Ultrasound. Note the stomach in the chest (white arrow) resulting in deviation of the four-chamber heart (black arrow) to the right. **B,** MRI. The stomach (S) is in the left chest as is the bowel (white arrow). (**B** from Leung JW, Coakley FV, Hricak H, et al: Prenatal MR imaging of congenital diaphragmatic hernia. AJR Am J Roentgenol 174:1607-1612, 2000.)

bilateral renal agenesis, or bilateral multicystic kidneys. In contrast, the presence of excessive amniotic fluid (>2000 mL), or polyhydramnios, may be a manifestation of impaired fetal swallowing caused by a neurologic abnormality (anencephaly), a high alimentary tract obstruction (isolated esophageal atresia, pyloric atresia, or duodenal atresia), or intrathoracic esophageal compression by a diaphragmatic hernia (Fig. 2-1A) or cystic lung lesion (cystic adenomatoid malformation).

The fetal bladder can be identified on prenatal ultrasound by 12 to 14 weeks' gestation and the fetal kidneys by 16 to 18 weeks. Serial ultrasound studies are required to document specific functional and anatomic urinary tract abnormalities. Changes in the sonogram confirm the ability of the fetal bladder to empty; separate physiologic and actual anatomic causes of hydronephrosis; and detect the presence of dilated ureters resulting from ureterovesical reflux, posterior urethral valves, or neurogenic bladder. Fetal ultrasonography also can identify other renal conditions and numerous intra-abdominal anomalies. Neurologic anomalies, such as hydrocephalus, anencephaly, microcephaly, encephalocele, and neural tube defect, have been documented on prenatal ultrasound studies.

Ultrasonography in pregnancy is the best noninvasive method for determining functional and anatomic abnormalities of the cardiovascular system. The cardiovascular structures can be visualized after 18 weeks' gestation, depending on fetal position and maternal habitus. Dynamic cardiac contractility can be evaluated, as can the presence of pericardial effusion, the four cardiac chambers, and location of the great vessels and cardiac valves. This evaluation permits the diagnosis of anomalies such as tetralogy of Fallot, hypoplastic left heart, tricuspid atresia, and double-outlet right ventricle.

Prenatal MRI may be useful for characterizing an anomaly when ultrasound has identified its presence (Fig. 2-1B). Being free from radiation, this imaging modality provides high-resolution anatomic images of potential anomalies in a safe manner for the developing fetus. The application of MRI is especially important before intended fetal intervention. Identification of the presence of the liver in the chest of a fetus with a CDH, which alters prognosis and options for treatment, is enhanced with MRI compared with ultrasonography. Likewise, MRI is especially effective at evaluating neurologic fetal anomalies.

OPTIONS AFTER PRENATAL DIAGNOSIS OF FETAL MALFORMATIONS

Following initial reports of in utero ultrasound diagnosis of congenital anomalies in the 1980s, increasingly sophisticated equipment and experience in interpretation led to the accurate prenatal diagnosis of many malformations. Prenatal diagnosis and serial ultrasound and MRI studies of fetuses with anatomic lesions make it possible to define the natural history of many anomalies, identify pathophysiologic features that affect clinical outcome, and formulate management based on prognosis.

Many complex decisions have evolved regarding management of the abnormal fetus, including safety for the mother; safety for the fetus; and family, societal, economic, ethical, and legal issues. Several hospitals have established comprehensive fetal treatment programs involving a multidisciplinary team to address considerations regarding fetal care. When a serious fetal malformation is recognized, several options are now available.

Fetal Termination

When serious malformations are diagnosed, the family may have the option to terminate the pregnancy. Several severe chromosomal, metabolic, and developmental disorders can be diagnosed in utero, including anencephaly, severe anomalies associated with chromosomal abnormalities (e.g., trisomy 13), bilateral renal agenesis, severe untreatable inherited metabolic disorders, and lethal bone dysplasias (e.g., recessive osteogenesis imperfecta).

Early Delivery

Most correctable malformations that can be diagnosed in utero can be managed by appropriate medical and surgical therapy after delivery at term when the infant is a better anesthetic and surgical risk. With most surgical disorders, it is desirable to permit the fetus to remain in utero as long as possible. Early delivery may be indicated, however, for certain fetal anomalies that require correction as soon as possible after diagnosis. The risk of premature delivery must be weighed against the risk of continued gestation. The reason for early delivery is unique to each anomaly; however, the principle remains the same: Continued gestation would have a progressive ill effect on the fetus. Preterm delivery for early decompression of the urinary tract may alleviate renal maldevelopment and maximize subsequent renal growth. Similarly, early delivery for ventricular decompression of hydrocephalus may maximize the opportunity for subsequent brain development. Congenital malformations that may benefit from induced preterm delivery for early correction ex utero include urinary tract obstruction, hydrocephalus, certain cases of gastroschisis or ruptured omphalocele, intestinal ischemia (e.g., necrosis secondary to volvulus, meconium ileus), hydrops fetalis, intrauterine growth retardation, and cardiac arrhythmias (supraventricular tachycardia).

Prenatal Treatment

Several fetal conditions may be alleviated by treatment before birth. Hydrops fetalis secondary to isoimmunization-induced hemolysis can be treated by transfusing red blood cells into the fetus. Several conditions can be improved by transplacental treatment: In the immature fetus, glucocorticoids given to the mother may increase deficient pulmonary surfactant. Cardiac arrhythmias, such as supraventricular tachycardia causing fetal congestive heart failure and hydrops, can be converted by giving antiarrhythmic drugs (e.g., digitalis) transplacentally or even directly to the fetus. Intra-amniotic thyroid hormone may be used to treat congenital hypothyroidism and goiter and to help mature the fetal lung.

In highly selected cases, fetal surgical intervention is not only possible, but also can be used successfully to treat patients with devastating congenital anomalies. Correcting an anatomic malformation in utero is more difficult than providing a missing substrate, hormone, or medication to the fetus. Anatomic malformations that interfere with fetal organ development and that alleviation of which would allow normal development to proceed should be considered for fetal intervention. Fetal wounds have been shown to heal without scar formation when surgery is performed early in the third trimester.

PRINCIPLES OF FETAL SURGERY

Maternal safety is the paramount consideration during fetal surgical procedures. Preparation of the mother begins with an indomethacin suppository and placement of an epidural catheter for analgesia. Halothane is used for intraoperative uterine relaxation and for fetal and maternal anesthesia. The uterus is exposed through a low transverse abdominal incision, and sterile intraoperative ultrasonography is used to confirm the fetal position and placental location. The hysterotomy incision is made as far away from the placenta as possible while allowing appropriate exposure of the fetus. Amniotic fluid is replaced with warmed Ringer's solution before closure of the hysterotomy.

Premature labor is the largest obstacle to a successful outcome in the postoperative course. Magnesium sulfate, indomethacin, and terbutaline are used postoperatively for tocolysis. Uterine contractions and fetal heart rate are monitored closely. After approximately 5 days, oral tocolytics are substituted for intravenous agents, then continued throughout the remainder of the pregnancy. Perioperative cephalosporin is continued for 3 to 4 days postoperatively.

There have been no maternal deaths and few maternal complications. Occasionally, patients have developed a small amniotic fluid leak from the hysterotomy site, necessitating reoperation with suture closure. After intrauterine surgery, subsequent fertility and gestation appear to be near normal. Because uterine rupture may occur after previous hysterotomy for fetal surgery, delivery by cesarean section is believed to be mandatory for subsequent pregnancies after fetal surgery.

Congenital Hydronephrosis

Unrelieved urinary tract obstruction interferes with renal development and leads to kidney damage, the severity of which depends on the type, degree, and duration of the obstruction. Infants born at term with high-grade obstruction may have advanced hydronephrosis and renal dysplasia that are incompatible with life; oligohydramnios secondary to decreased fetal urine output produces pulmonary hypoplasia, which may be fatal at birth. The hope of fetal intervention is that the life-threatening problems of respiratory and renal insufficiency will be ameliorated if the obstruction is relieved sufficiently early in gestation. For a fetus with urinary tract obstruction and oligohydramnios to be a candidate for fetal intervention, however, there must be good residual renal function at the time of diagnosis. The fetus with hydronephrosis can be managed with the following approach: If hydronephrosis is unilateral and the amniotic fluid volume is adequate, the mother should be followed by serial ultrasonography and the fetus

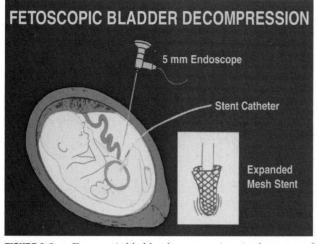

FIGURE 2-2 ■ Fetoscopic bladder decompression via placement of a vesicoamniotic expandable stent. (From www.fetus.ucsf.edu.)

treated after birth because the disease is not usually life-threatening. If bilateral hydronephrosis is present, ongoing evaluation should be performed for the presence of oligohydramnios. Development of severe oligohydramnios in the second trimester is associated with a predicted mortality greater than 90% and should be accompanied by fetal urine and ultrasound evaluation to determine the potential for normal renal and pulmonary function at birth. Urine aspirated from the fetal bladder that shows sodium less than 100 mEq/L, chloride less than 90 mEq/L, and osmolality less than 210 mOsm and a fetal kidney ultrasound that does not reveal increased echogenicity or cysts are predictive of a favorable outcome. For such a fetus, immediate delivery and ex utero decompression are recommended if the lungs are mature. For the fetus with immature lungs, in utero decompression of the bladder should be considered. For the fetus with poor predicted renal function, aggressive obstetric care or in utero decompression is not indicated.

Bladder decompression may be performed either by creation of a vesicostomy or formation of ureterostomies. The lower extremities of the fetus are exteriorized, and a transcutaneous pulse oximeter is placed on the fetal thigh. A vesicostomy is performed via a midline suprapubic incision through the fetal abdominal wall as the bladder is opened and marsupialized to the abdominal wall using interrupted nonabsorbable sutures. The rate of premature labor is substantial, and fetal survival rate is only approximately 50% to 60%. Neurologic handicaps are observed in 50% of live-born infants. Techniques for fetoscopic surgery have been developed that allow transuterine endoscopic approaches for the treatment of obstructive uropathy by endoscopic creation of a cystotomy, urethral catheter placement, ablation of obstructing posterior urethral valves, or placement of a vesicoamniotic expandable mesh stent (Fig. 2-2). A vesicoamniotic shunt also may be placed percutaneously, but the incidence of catheter dislodgment is high.

These interventions may not improve outcome. Irreversible renal dysplasia is frequently present by the time hydronephrosis is detected and intervention attempted,

and intervention may not change the prognosis for renal function. Persistent oligohydramnios is the best predictor of poor neonatal outcome. In fetal surgery candidates with predicted good renal function, 85% of surgery survivors had normal renal function. Respiratory compromise was not observed when resolution of oligohydramnios was observed after fetal intervention. Fetal surgery is indicated only in the fetus who is without other chromosomal or structural anomalies, has good renal function, has normal-appearing kidneys on ultrasound, and has a high predicted mortality because of the presence of severe oligohydramnios.

Tracheal Atresia and Stenosis

Fetuses with congenital high airway obstruction syndrome (CHAOS), typically resulting from laryngeal or tracheal atresia or high-grade stenosis, develop large echogenic lungs, flattened or inverted diaphragms, dilated airways distal to the obstruction, and fetal ascites or hydrops or both. Recognition of this entity may allow one to assess and secure the airway while the patient remains on fetoplacental support before the umbilical cord is divided. Called the *ex-utero intrapartum (EXIT) procedure*, the technique requires intensive maternal-fetal monitoring, cesarean section with maximal uterine relaxation, and maintenance of intact fetoplacental circulation (Fig. 2-3). This technique allows airway access under controlled conditions for at least 1 hour in fetuses with in utero airway interventions, such as the tracheal clip for CDH; fetuses with extrinsic lesions compressing the airway, such as bronchogenic cysts and cystic hygromas; and fetuses with intrinsic airway obstruction, such as CHAOS. Only the fetal head, shoulders, and at least one arm for monitoring are delivered while the umbilical cord remains in utero to prevent compromise of placental blood flow. For fetuses in whom airway or cardiac lesions prevent stabilization during the EXIT procedure, a technique known as *EXIT to ECMO* may be applied, in which the fetus/newborn is cannulated for extracorporeal

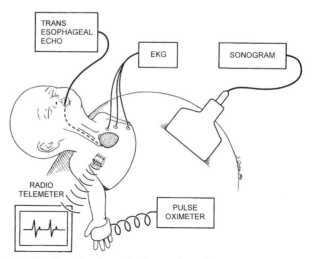

FIGURE 2-3 ■ Fetal monitoring options during an EXIT procedure. (From Mychaliska GB, Bealer JF, Graf JL, et al: Operating on placental support: The ex utero intrapartum treatment procedure. J Pediatr Surg 32:227-231, 1997.)

membrane oxygenation (ECMO) while supported by the placenta.

Congenital Diaphragmatic Hernia

CDH is a frustrating problem for the pediatric surgeon. Prenatal diagnosis of a CDH at less than 24 weeks' gestation is associated with a mortality of 58%, which includes components of fetal and postnatal demise. The mortality of liveborn infants with CDH is 37% despite maximal medical and surgical therapy.

Experimental models of CDH have shown that a surgically created diaphragmatic hernia simulates the morphologic features that correlate with fatal outcome for human neonates with diaphragmatic hernia and persistent fetal circulation. Fetal surgical repair ameliorates these pulmonary vascular changes and permits compensatory lung growth and development. Harrison and colleagues explored the effectiveness of in utero repair of CDH in humans. Surgical repair was undertaken between 20 and 30 weeks' gestation; repair after 30 weeks tended to lead to induction of preterm labor, and the fetal lung had less time to grow before birth. During the repair, the left arm of the fetus was exteriorized for monitoring, and the diaphragm was repaired with a prosthetic patch through a subcostal incision. The abdomen was enlarged to accommodate the viscera using another synthetic patch. All of the surviving fetuses showed growth of the lung in utero and had good pulmonary function after birth. A major cause of mortality at operation was the inability to reduce the liver from the fetal chest into the abdomen because of compromise of umbilical venous return in patients in whom the liver was incarcerated in the thorax. A randomized, prospective trial compared outcome in fetuses without liver herniation who were diagnosed at less than 30 weeks' gestation who underwent either open in utero CDH correction or conventional therapy. No difference in survival (fetal surgery, 75%; conventional, 86%), length of ventilatory support, or need for ECMO could be shown. These data suggest that survival in fetuses with the liver in the abdomen is fairly high and that in utero repair of a CDH is not indicated in these patients.

The combination of the presence of liver herniation, diagnosis before 25 weeks' gestation, and a lung-to-head ratio (product of the orthogonal diameters of the right lung at the level of the atria divided by the head circumference) less than 1.4 as measured on fetal MRI suggests a high mortality after birth regardless of therapy. Although repair of CDH in newborns with the liver in the thorax is not feasible, accidents of nature, such as CHAOS (see earlier) and experimental animal data suggest that lung growth can be induced via in utero obstruction of the trachea. This phenomenon has been applied to the patient with CDH to allow reversal of the lung hypoplasia without requiring the repair of the diaphragm, which uniformly leads to fetal demise in the fetus with liver herniation. Initial application of this technique involved a hysterotomy with placement of a foam plug into the trachea, which failed to induce lung growth because a seal could not be established. Subsequent patients underwent placement of clips on the trachea, which were successful at inducing lung growth. Because hysterotomy was associated with a

high rate of premature labor, however, the technique of fetoscopic tracheal occlusion via hemoclip placement was developed and has been used successfully (Fig. 2-4). The operation is performed at 27 to 28 weeks' gestation and involves a maternal laparotomy with placement of two 5-mm ports and one 10-mm port into the uterus under ultrasound guidance. A high-flow uterine irrigation system allows excellent endoscopic visualization. A suture placed in the chin and a T-bar placed into the fetal

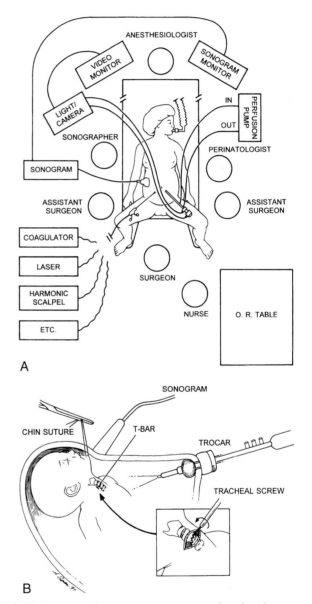

FIGURE 2-4 ■ **A,** Operating room setup for the fetoscopic tracheal occlusion procedure. **B,** Under sonographic guidance, (1) the fetus' neck is exposed and head stabilized by placing a transuterine chin suture, and (2) a T bar is placed in the fetal trachea to aid in localizing the midline fetal neck. After anterior tracheal dissection, a tracheal traction "screw" is placed in the tracheal wall allowing tracheal dissection and clip placement. (From Harrison MR, Mychaliska GB, Albanese CT, et al: Correction of congenital diaphragmatic hernia in utero: IX. Fetuses with poor prognosis [liver herniation and low lung-to-head ratio] can be saved by fetoscopic temporary tracheal occlusion. J Pediatr Surg 33:1017-1023, 1998.)

trachea allow extension of the neck and identification and retraction of the trachea. A hemoclip may be placed to occlude the trachea when dissection has provided adequate exposure. The EXIT procedure is used later to remove the clip, perform bronchoscopy and endotracheal intubation, and administer surfactant because surfactant levels appear to be reduced in experimental models of tracheal ligation. Almost all of the patients with fetoscopic clip placement showed evidence of lung growth with reasonable pulmonary gas exchange capabilities at birth. Survival was 38% in a cohort of patients with a conventional approach, 15% in the group managed with hysterotomy and tracheal occlusion, and 75% in the fetoscopic tracheal occlusion group. Preterm labor may be reduced with the fetoscopic approach, although the major complication of fetoscopy is premature rupture of membranes. More recently the fetoscopic tracheal occlusion technique has been refined and simplified to use simultaneous endotracheal and endoamniotic endoscopic visualization for placement of a gelatin-encapsulated, polymeric foam insert into the trachea. A bronchoscope is placed into the fetal trachea, which allows puncture and delivery of a wire through the anterior trachea and the uterus. The insert, which is attached to the end of the wire, is pulled into the trachea. When in place, the gelatin capsule on the insert dissolves, allowing the foam to swell and provide effective occlusion of the trachea. A prospective, controlled trial of fetal tracheal occlusion is currently under way.

Congenital Cystic Adenomatoid Malformation

Congenital cystic adenomatoid malformation (CCAM) can present as a fatal condition in a fetus or neonate or as a relatively mild lesion causing respiratory difficulty or recurrent infections in an infant or child. The former situation usually is observed with a large CCAM and is associated with the development of nonimmune hydrops in the fetus, hypoplasia of the normal lung secondary to prolonged compression in utero, and cardiac and vena caval compression. The "mirror" syndrome may develop, which is associated with placentomegaly and a maternal preeclamptic state similar to that of the sick infant and

that may jeopardize maternal health. In contrast, if the fetus is not hydropic and an isolated fetal lung lesion is present, intervention is likely to be required only after birth. Fetal MRI may allow prediction of the in utero course of a lesion by assessment of the CCAM volume ratio (CVR). The CVR is determined by measuring the three dimensions of the CCAM and applying the formula for the volume of an ellipse. This value is divided by the head circumference to correct for gestational age. A fetus with a CVR greater than 1.6 is at high risk for the development of hydrops and fetal complications, whereas these complications occur in less than 3% of fetuses with a CVR less than or equal to 1.6. Fetal intervention for CCAM should be applied in fetuses with a CVR greater than 1.6 and in fetuses who are less than 30 to 32 weeks' gestation and unlikely to have lungs mature enough for early delivery and postnatal operation.

Regression of a CCAM has been documented, although in almost all cases a remnant of the lesion can be identified on cross-sectional imaging. There seems to be a spectrum of this cystic anomaly: In the macrocystic type, cysts several centimeters in diameter can be identified on ultrasound or MRI. Cysts that are predominantly unilocular and without a substantial solid component have been treated effectively with placement of a cyst thoracoamniotic shunt, repeated serial cyst aspiration, and transuterine wire fulguration. Microcystic disease is characterized by multiple cystic lesions less than 1 cm in diameter and is managed best with pulmonary resection. In utero pulmonary lobectomy performed at 21 to 29 weeks' gestation has been successful in 13 hydropic fetuses with 8 fetuses showing hydrops resolution, impressive in utero lung growth, and neonatal survival (Fig. 2-5). This approach was unsuccessful in the other five fetuses mainly because of the development of premature labor.

Sacrococcygeal Teratoma

Fetuses with highly vascular, predominantly solid sacrococcygeal teratomas may develop a vascular steal syndrome leading to fetal demise. The blood supply to the sacrococcygeal teratoma is mainly from the middle sacral artery and the internal iliac artery. With large tumors, an arteriovenous fistula may develop with increased distal aortic

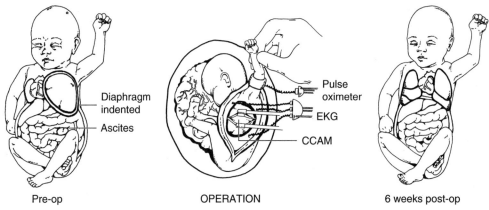

FIGURE 2-5 ■ Diagram of a left-sided cystic adenomatoid malformation in a fetus before, during, and after fetal intervention. Note the return of the mediastinum to the midline after fetal operation with reasonable inflation and growth of the left lung. (From www.fetus.ucsf.edu.)

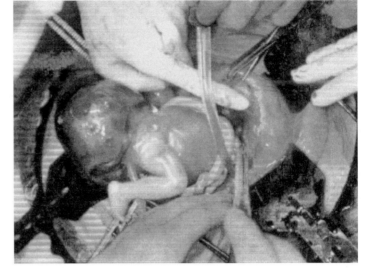

FIGURE 2-6 ■ A fetus with a large sacrococcygeal teratoma extending from the sacral region. Only the abdomen, legs, buttocks, and the tumor (arrow) have been delivered from the uterus. (From www.fetus.ucsf.edu.)

blood flow and shunting of blood away from the placenta. Development of fetal hydrops, placentomegaly, and death may ensue. The maternal "mirror" syndrome, as described previously, also may occur.

The development of hydrops indicates imminent fetal demise. Fetuses with hydrops diagnosed after 30 weeks' gestation should be delivered when pulmonary maturity is attained. Fetuses with lesions larger than 5 cm should be delivered by cesarean section to avoid dystocia, tumor rupture, or hemorrhage into the tumor. Lesions accompanied by hydrops that are diagnosed before 30 weeks' gestation usually have a poor outcome and may require surgical excision in utero. In these instances, in utero tumor debulking via open fetal operation or endoscopic laser ablation may be life-saving (Fig. 2-6). Intervention with radiofrequency ablation under ultrasound guidance to reduce tumor mass and blood flow has been successful but may result in fatal hemorrhage into the tumor. Other methods, such as interventional angiographic approaches to prevent arteriovenous shunting through the tumor, have yet to be explored.

Congenital Heart Disease

Many types of congenital cardiac disease can be diagnosed readily in utero with a high degree of accuracy. Although the fetal pathophysiology of congenital cardiac lesions is not completely understood, it seems that decreased blood flow during fetal life can result in secondary hypoplasia of vessels or cardiac chambers. Obstruction of the pulmonary or aortic valve commonly results in hypoplasia of the respective ventricle through alteration of pressure and flow relationships inside the heart. Techniques using percutaneous ultrasound–guided direct needle punctures of the heart have been used to perform balloon valvuloplasty with some success, including delivery of a neonate with a normal left ventricle after documentation of high-grade in utero aortic valve stenosis. Alternatively, open and fetoscopic fetal cardiac surgery and transumbilical fetal cardiac catheterization, guided by fetal transesophageal echocardiography, are being evaluated in animal studies.

Prenatally diagnosed complete heart block can occur without associated cardiac anomalies, is often refractory to drug therapy to increase cardiac rate and output, and often causes demise in the fetus too young for delivery. Steroids, β-agonists, and digoxin may enhance myocardial function. Percutaneous transthoracic pacing for the hydropic fetus with complete heart block or the fetus with therapy-refractory supraventricular tachycardia currently is being considered but has not been attempted clinically. The feasibility of a fetoscopic approach to transesophageal echocardiography and for pacer wire placement has been shown in sheep.

Myelomeningocele

The incidence of myelomeningocele, which previously occurred in 1 in 2000 births, has been decreasing with folic acid supplementation. This devastating anomaly is associated with lower extremity motor dysfunction; loss of bowel and bladder control; and type II Chiari malformation, in which there is downward displacement of the cerebellum with elongation of the brainstem, obliteration of the fourth ventricle, and development of hydrocephalus in 90% of patients. Fetal intervention would have application in this anomaly if the brain and spinal cord sequelae progressively developed during gestation rather than being a fixed defect. That the lesions do evolve has been suggested by documentation of lower extremity function early in gestation, which subsequently is lost in the fetus with myelomeningocele. Animal studies suggest that exposure of the spinal cord to the fetal environment results in secondary injury. In utero correction of myelomeningocele has been performed more than 220 times in four centers in the United States. Closure of the myelomeningocele in utero results in a substantial reduction in the incidence of hindbrain herniation and an associated decrease in shunt-dependent hydrocephalus from 90% to 60%. Only minor, if any, improvements in lower extremity, bowel, and bladder function are associated with in utero repair. The major complication of fetal intervention is premature labor and delivery; this and the other risks of in

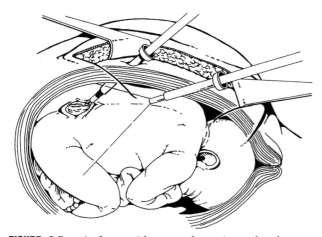

FIGURE 2-7 ■ A fetus with a myelomeningocele about to undergo in utero closure by a fetoscopic approach. (From Bruner, JP, Richards WO, Tulipan NB: Endoscopic coverage of fetal myelomeningocele in utero. Am J Obstet Gynecol 180:153-158, 1999.)

utero repair must be weighed against the benefits. A fetoscopic approach to fetal myelomeningocele may reduce this complication (Fig. 2-7). A randomized clinical trial comparing fetal surgery and routine management is under way.

Congenital Hydrocephalus

Congenital hydrocephalus secondary to stenosis of the aqueduct of Sylvius is an anatomically simple obstructive lesion with severe consequences for the developing fetal brain. Obstruction to the flow of cerebrospinal fluid produces backpressure that dilates the ventricles, compresses the developing brain, and causes neurologic dysfunction. In theory, prenatal ventricular decompression via ventriculoamniotic shunt placement may ameliorate the ongoing damage caused by obstruction and allow normal brain development to proceed. Clinical studies have shown results that are not encouraging for in utero ventricular shunting for hydrocephalus, with only 35% of fetal interventions resulting in neurologically normal individuals. A moratorium on fetal intervention for hydrocephalus is now in place.

SUMMARY

The diagnosis of fetal birth defects has achieved considerable sophistication and offers new hope for improved management of fetuses with life-threatening defects. The most invasive diagnostic and therapeutic procedures involve significant risks for the fetus and the mother, however, raising difficult ethical questions about risks compared with benefits and the rights of the fetus and the mother. Currently the success of fetal surgery has been limited. With continuing extensive investigation and cautious clinical experience, however, the utility and indications for fetal therapy should continue to expand.

SUGGESTED READINGS

The following references provide considerable background information for all aspects of fetal surgery.

Adzick NS, Crombleholme TM, Morgan MM, Quinn TM: A rapidly growing fetal teratoma. Lancet 349:538, 1997.

Adzick NS, Harrison MR: The unborn surgical patient. Curr Prob Surg 31:9, 1994.

Bruner JP, Tulipan N, Paschall RL, et al: Fetal surgery for myelomeningocele and the incidence of shunt-dependent hydrocephalus. JAMA 282:1819-1825, 1999.

Coplen DE: Prenatal intervention for hydronephrosis. J Urol 157:2270, 1997.

Harrison MR: The fetus as a patient. In O'Neill JA, Rowe MI, Grosfeld JL, et al (eds): Pediatric Surgery, 5th ed. Chicago, Mosby–Year Book, 1998, pp 33-40.

Harrison MR, Adzick NS: The fetus as a patient: Surgical considerations, Ann Surg 213:279, 1991.

Harrison MR, Mychaliska GB, Albanese CT, et al: Correction of congenital diaphragmatic hernia in utero: IX. Fetuses with poor prognosis (liver herniation and low lung-to-head ratio) can be saved by fetoscopic temporary tracheal occlusion. J Pediatr Surg 33:1017-1023, 1998.

Kitano Y, Adzick NS: New developments in fetal lung surgery. Curr Opin Pediatr 11:193, 1999.

Mychaliska GB, Bealer JF, Graf JL, et al: Operating on placental support: The ex utero intrapartum treatment procedure. J Pediatr Surg 32:227, 1997.

Simpson JL: Genetic counseling and prenatal diagnosis. In Gabbe SG, Niebyl JR, Simpson JL (eds): Obstetrics: Normal and Problem Pregnancies, 4th ed. New York, Churchill Livingstone, 2002, pp 187-219.

3

Metabolic Changes in the Critically Ill Surgical Patient

Nutritional care of the critically ill or septic postoperative patient is a great challenge. Clinically a critically ill child manifests poor enteral feeding, anorexia, and often a paralytic ileus. Alterations in use of substrate complicate this situation and may result in significant muscle wasting. Compounding these problems is insulin resistance. Insulin resistance is a characteristic problem in critically ill and particularly septic surgical patients; this results in hyperglycemia and hypertriglyceridemia. An understanding of these changes is essential for appropriate nutritional support of the pediatric surgical patient.

ESTIMATES OF THE METABOLIC RATE

Metabolic rate or energy requirements for postoperative patients can be calculated by the use of nomograms or by respirometry and indirect calorimetry. Nomograms usually provide an estimated basal energy expenditure based on age, height, and weight and allow computation of energy expended as a result of additional factors that may alter basal energy expenditure, such as postoperative stress, multiple trauma, fever, and severe infection. Table 3-1 shows nomograms currently in use.

Although several previous studies on nutritional requirements during health and disease were based on estimated energy expenditure, actual measurement is much more accurate and is becoming an important aspect of critical care management. The most commonly used method of measurement is indirect calorimetry. In this method, the amount of oxygen absorbed across the lung is assumed to be exactly equal to the amount of oxygen consumed in metabolic processes. This is the basic assumption of the Fick equation and is the reason why oxygen consumption is a valid measure of metabolism, even in patients with abnormal lung function. The energy released by oxidation of various food substrates is known from direct measurements so that the metabolic rate measured in cubic centimeters of oxygen per minute can be converted to calories per hour or per day if the substrates are known. For practical purposes, a conversion factor of 5 kcal of energy per liter of oxygen consumed is a reasonable approximation. This approximation slightly overestimates the metabolic rate but is a much more accurate approximation of the patient's

metabolic rate than a number derived from a chart or a table. A method of closed-circuit, water-sealed indirect calorimetry for infants breathing spontaneously has been developed and has shown a much wider range of energy expenditure for infants of similar weight and gestational age than that calculated by nomograms and tables. We have found that commonly used nomograms may underestimate energy expenditure by 70%.

Oxygen consumption can be measured or calculated by (1) direct volumetric change in a closed-circuit rebreathing spirometer system with carbon dioxide absorber; (2) volume and composition of exhaled gas, knowing the composition and volume of inhaled gas; and (3) oxygen content of arterial and mixed venous blood and the cardiac output, then calculating oxygen consumed by peripheral tissues by using the Fick equation. The latter method requires pulmonary artery catheterization

TABLE 3-1 ■ Basal Metabolic Rates for Normals		
Age (yr)	Males (kcal/m²/hr)	Females (kcal/m²/hr)
1	53	53
2-3	52	52
4-5	50	49
6-7	48	46
8-9	46	43
10-11	44	42
12-13	42	41
14-15	42	39
16-17	41	37
18-19	40	36
20-25	38	35
25-30	37	35
30-35	37	35
35-40	36	35
40-45	36	35
45-50	36	34
50-55	36	34
55-60	35	34
60-65	35	33
65-70	34	32
70-75	33	32
≥75	33	31

From Fleisch A: Le metabolisme basal standard et sa determination au moyen du "Metabocalculator." Helv Med Acta 18:23, 1951.

but may become more practical as miniature oximeters are added to smaller Swan-Ganz catheters. Mixed expired gas analysis is the easiest method for use in normal subjects but is not suitable for patients receiving supplemental oxygen or on mechanical ventilators because of minor variations in the inspired volume and oxygen concentration during the respiratory cycle. Direct volumetric spirometry is the best method for measuring oxygen consumption, and it lends itself to simultaneous measurement of carbon dioxide production using an infrared capnometer. With measurement of oxygen consumption and carbon dioxide production, the respiratory quotient can be determined and caloric expenditure calculated using the Weir equation.

The aforementioned methods of nutritional assessment are used to classify the nutritional status of patients at the time of injury, surgery, or critical illness. Baker and colleagues showed that a careful clinical examination is as accurate as more complex and expensive laboratory and anthropometric measurements in identifying malnutrition in stressed patients. In another excellent study, Forse and Shizgal measured body cell mass (the best standard measurement of nutritional status) and found that the depleted state could not be detected reliably based on weight-to-height ratio, triceps skin fold, midarm circumference, albumin level, total protein concentration, hand strength, or creatinine-to-height ratio. Actual measurement or estimation of metabolic rate is the best method of following the nutritional status in a critically ill patient.

ENDOCRINE ALTERATIONS AFTER SURGERY

Suits and Bottsford outlined a neuroendocrine reflex that is set in motion by significant stress; components of this reflex include an afferent arc consisting of stimuli that initiate the metabolic responses and an efferent arc that leads to volume restoration and energy-substrate production. The sequence is initiated by surgical stress, which affects the neuroendocrine reflex directly through a neural signal to the central nervous system and indirectly through the elaboration of catecholamines, the major mediators of the hypermetabolic response, and adrenocorticoids, major augmenters of this response. Components of the afferent arc involved in this system are nociceptors, chemoreceptors, and baroreceptors, all of which are capable of sending signals to the hypothalamus, where they become integrated into the physiologic response seen in the stress state.

The efferent arc is described as originating in the hypothalamus, with efferent limbs traveling through the brainstem autonomic regions and the pituitary. These brainstem autonomic areas send efferent fibers via the parasympathetic and sympathetic nervous system to the periphery, affecting neuromuscular junctions in the circulatory system and receptors at end organs, which stimulate the release of peripheral hormones. The pituitary response leads to increased adrenocorticotropic hormone, vasopressin or antidiuretic hormone, growth hormone, and prolactin release.

Neonates have well-developed neural pathways for pain; the density of nociceptive nerve endings in the skin of newborns is at least equivalent to that in adult skin. These receptors have been noted to be present throughout fetal cutaneous and mucosal surfaces by 20 weeks' gestation. The initial component of the proposed afferent arc develops early in fetal life, and the capacity for initiating a stress response is present.

In addition to the hypothalamic- and pituitary-derived endocrine factors, there are several other important substances. Mediators of this efferent pathway include endorphins, which may affect carbohydrate metabolism. Cytokines, including tumor necrosis factor-α and interleukin-6, are elevated in the neonate during stress and after surgery. Administration of tumor necrosis factor-α may mimic a postsurgical stress state. Catecholamines play a crucial role in alteration of substrate metabolism during and after surgery. Anand and colleagues reported significant increases in plasma epinephrine and norepinephrine concentrations at the end of surgery. These elevated levels are transient and may last only 6 hours after surgery. The elevation also may be blocked with halothane anesthesia. Pancreatic production of glucagon and insulin increases after surgery, and the levels have been correlated with serum glucose and epinephrine concentrations. Anand and Aynsley-Green showed that insulin levels after patent ductus arteriosus ligation in preterm infants do not rise during surgery compared with more mature neonates. Insulin does rise between 6 and 24 hours after surgery, as in older patients. In contrast to the rise in insulin, glucagon levels do not change appreciably with surgery. Cortisol levels have been shown to increase significantly in neonates undergoing even minor surgery, such as circumcision. A more detailed look at adrenocortical responses was outlined by Boix-Ochoa and coworkers, who showed that neonates did not have the normal adult circadian cycle of plasma cortisol levels, and the cortisol response to surgical stress was age dependent, with neonates mounting a quantitatively lesser response than infants. Finally, neonates less than 9 days old had a more rapid response yet released significantly lower amounts of cortisol after surgical stress.

ALTERATIONS IN METABOLIC SUBSTRATES DURING SURGERY
Energy

Using oxygen consumption measurements (Vo_2), Jones and colleagues showed that resting energy expenditure increased after surgery by 15%. This elevation lasts only 24 hours. This rise is proportionate to the operation (major versus minor) and is distinct from adults, who may show increased Vo_2 for more than 3 days. Opioids (endogenous or exogenous) may attenuate this response and may be useful to control this altered metabolic state. Previous estimates of energy needs of postoperative or septic critically ill infants may have been overestimated. Almost one third of an infant's energy needs supports growth (30 to 35 kcal/kg/day). Because a cessation of growth occurs during periods of sepsis and critical illness, a marked decrease in energy needs may ensue. In a study of critically ill, postoperative infants, the mean measured energy expenditure was only 43 kcal/kg/day. Results are extraordinarily variable, however, further emphasizing the utility of performing indirect calorimetry (if available). The use of indirect calorimetry also can yield information on the respiratory quotient (see earlier) and aid in the prevention of overfeeding.

Thermogenesis

The metabolic and thermogenic response to operative stress is age-related. Fasoli and colleagues showed that for infants during surgery there is a decreased metabolic rate and a tendency to maintain a stable body core temperature. In children, there is an increase in metabolic rate and body core temperature. In contrast to older children, the neonate is not able to respond to cold exposure by shivering. Rather the neonate uses a highly specialized tissue, brown fat, which is capable of generating heat (nonshivering thermogenesis). Albanese and coworkers showed that nonshivering thermogenesis is inhibited by anesthetic agents in animals. Termination of anesthesia results in a profound increase in this nonshivering thermogenesis.

ALTERATION IN SUBSTRATE UTILIZATION WITH SURGERY AND CRITICAL ILLNESS

In general, the amount of literature available regarding neonatal or infant metabolism during and after surgery is limited, and much has to be extrapolated from adult studies. Nevertheless, following is a summary of the changes that occur during this critical time. Table 3-2 summarizes many of the changes in substrate utilization in a neonate compared an adult in the postoperative period.

Carbohydrate Metabolism

Carbohydrate use changes dramatically at birth, from a constant supply from the placenta to the need for glucose production. In general, the neonate derives glucose from predominantly a glycogenolytic process, but also may conduct gluconeogenesis within 2 hours of birth. Hyperglycemia is a common response in the postoperative patient. This response is seen similarly in adult patients and seems to be due to a combination of increased splanchnic production of glucose and elevation of adrenaline, which activates the Cori cycle. Finally, the stabilization or decline in use of glucose in perioperative neonates also may contribute to this hyperglycemia. Anand and coworkers showed that this increase is accompanied by an increase in blood lactate and pyruvate levels, which may be used to support gluconeogenesis. Administration of a fentanyl anesthetic can block this response.

Protein Metabolism

Protein metabolism in postoperative neonates is different from that seen in adults. During initial periods of starvation, skeletal muscle is the first source of amino acids for gluconeogenesis. This source in an adult can lead to the breakdown of 500 g of lean skeletal muscle for each day of starvation. This is particularly an issue for the neonate, who has a relatively small amount of skeletal muscle. Ballard and associates suggested that a premature infant has such low amounts of skeletal muscle that he or she also will use protein from other critical sources, including the brain, liver and skin. Allowing neonates to starve for any great length of time could be extremely injurious. The response to stress and surgery is additionally distinct in that the degree of protein breakdown may exceed

TABLE 3-2 ■ Metabolic Response to Operative Stress in Adults and Neonates		
Metabolite	**Adult Response**	**Neonatal Response**
Metabolic rate and oxygen consumption	↓ Briefly, then ↑	↓ Comparable to that in adults (minimal change compared with age-matched controls)
Carbohydrate	↑ Hyperglycemia response ↑ Gluconeogenesis and ↓ glucose	↑ Glucose 2× normal immediately postoperatively (less persistent ↑ than in adults); probably secondary to glycogenolysis rather than ↑ gluconeogenesis; neonates may be unable to carry out hepatic gluconeogenesis secondary to lack of key enzyme
Protein	Negative nitrogen balance Slight ↑ protein breakdown, dependent on severity of stress; ↑ with increased severity; ↓ protein synthesis in extrahepatic tissues ↑ Amino acid utilization for gluconeogenesis, acute phase reactant synthesis, and synthesis of components of healing process ↑ Nitrogen excretion sustained 5 days	Negative nitrogen balance during the first 2-3 days Oxidation of fat stores to spare protein
Fat	Adipose tissue lipolysis → mobilization of nonesterified fatty acids and ↑ ketone body formation About 75-90% of postoperative requirements supplied by fat metabolism (10-25% by protein)	↑ Lipolysis + ketogenesis (? catecholamine stimulated) → ↑ total ketone bodies, ↑ glycerol, ↑ nonesterified fatty acids Postoperative fat utilization exceeds rate of mobilization of free fatty acids

proportionally that of the adult. In a prospective study of pediatric trauma patients, Winthrop showed that the increase in protein breakdown and nitrogen excretion greatly exceeded the measured increase in basal metabolic rate. This suggests that these patients require a significant increase in protein intake to accommodate these losses. In a study by Duffy and Pencharz, the administration of 3.9 g/kg/day versus 2.3 g/kg/day to neonates undergoing surgery was compared. These authors found the higher level of amino acids resulted in improved net protein synthesis and a reduction of endogenous protein breakdown. This high level of amino acid delivery similarly was supported by a nonoperative group of premature infants who had improved outcomes when receiving 3.5 g/kg/day of amino acids. These rates should be balanced, however, with the fact that levels may lead to a rise in blood urea nitrogen levels. Additionally, Pierro and associates showed that protein retention was almost 90% when infants were given 2 g/kg/day and 75 nonprotein calories/kg/day. If higher levels of amino acids are given, they should be monitored closely and given for relatively short periods. Administration of glucose or lipids may have equivalent protein-sparing effects. Visceral protein stores become progressively reduced over time. Because measurements of albumin may change slowly owing to its long half-life (>18 days), other measures of visceral protein status, such as prealbumin levels (half-life 2 days), better reflect metabolic derangements.

Fat Metabolism

Fat plays a major role in the delivery of energy to children. In the normal neonate, Benedict and Talbot showed that 80% of the energy requirements are fulfilled by calories derived from fat. Similarly, Kinney and colleagues showed that 75% to 90% of postoperative energy requirements are supplied by fat metabolism, and the remainder are provided by protein. Anand and coworkers showed that there was an increase in total ketone bodies and glycerol during neonatal surgery. This increase is most likely due to catecholamine-stimulated lipolysis and ketogenesis. In addition to the use of these fats for energy, they may contribute to an inhibition of glucose utilization and the commonly seen postoperative hyperglycemic state.

CONCLUSION

Neonates may be able to manifest a significant hormonal and metabolic response to surgical or traumatic stress. Although many of the physiologic changes are similar to those seen in adult patients, crucial differences in the endocrine response, the timing of these changes, and the use of substrate may have important implications for the care of infants after surgery.

SUGGESTED READINGS

Anand KJS, Brown MJ, Bloom SR, Aynsley-Green A: Studies on the hormonal regulation of fuel metabolism in the human newborn infant undergoing anesthesia and surgery. Horm Res 22:115, 1985.
This is an excellent review of neonatal surgical metabolism.

Anand KJS, Brown MJ, Causon RC, et al: Can the human neonate mount an endocrine and metabolic response to surgery? J Pediatr Surg 20:41, 1985.
This article reports a rare study in the human neonate.

Anand KJS, Hickey PR: Halothane-morphine compared with high-dose sufentanil for anesthesia and postoperative analgesia in neonatal cardiac surgery. N Engl J Med 326:1, 1992.
The effect of anesthesia on metabolism is discussed.

Boix-Ochoa J, Martinez Ibanez V, Potau N, Lloret J: Cortisol response to surgical stress in neonates. Pediatr Surg Int 2:267, 1987.
This is another rare study in human neonates.

Coran AG, Drongowski RA: Body fluid compartment changes following neonatal surgery. J Pediatr Surg 24:829, 1989.
This is the only study measuring total body water and extracellular volume in human newborns.

Coran AG, Pierro A, Schmeling DJ: Metabolism of the neonate requiring surgery. In Cowett RM (ed): Principles of Perinatal-Neonatal Metabolism, 2nd ed. New York, Springer, 1998.
This chapter is an excellent review of surgical metabolism in the neonate.

Cuthbertson DP: The disturbance of metabolism produced by bony and nonbony injury, with notes on certain abnormal conditions of bone. Biochem J 24:1244, 1930.
This classic article serves as the basis of current understanding of metabolic consequences of injury.

Wilmore DW: Catabolic illness: Strategies for enhancing recovery. N Engl J Med 325:695, 1991.
This article describes developments in hormonal manipulation (growth hormone, insulin-like growth factor, and β-adrenergic agonists) and immunomodulators (e.g., glutamine) in reversing critical catabolic illness.

Fluid and Electrolyte Management

4

In an attempt to base fluid management on a more scientific basis, a unifying concept was sought. It was concluded that maintenance fluid requirements were related directly to the metabolic activity necessary for the body to perform its vital functions. This concept is true, however, only for normal healthy subjects under stable conditions. Because there are no clinically practical devices to measure energy expenditure accurately, indirect methods were developed. In 1883, Rubner found that metabolic rate was related to body surface area. Talbot developed a system that related the volume of fluid required for maintenance to body surface area measured in square meters. Maintenance fluid needs were designated as 1500 mL/m²/24 hours. Tables were used to calculate surface area from body length and weight. As more experience with this system developed, it became apparent that there were multiple violations of the general relationship of body surface area to metabolic rate, particularly in small-for-gestational-age infants.

The caloric method was introduced next and became the standard. This method related calories catabolized to milliliters of fluid. In 1957, Holliday and Segar measured basal metabolic activity in a group of infants and children and plotted body weight against calories metabolized. Their work led to the commonly used "100, 50, 20" rule for determining fluid needs in children: 100 kcal/kg was needed for the first 10 kg of body weight. As weight increased, fluid needs and caloric needs decreased. Approximately 40 mL/100 kcal/24 hours replaces insensible losses, and 60 mL/100 kcal replaces urinary losses. Adjustments are made for exceptional situations (e.g., fever, stress). Fever increases insensible water loss from respiration and sweating. For each degree of temperature greater than 38°C, insensible water loss is increased by 5 mL/kg/24 hours. This method of calculating fluid requirements is in close agreement with several other methods based on formulas, body surface area, basal calories plus activity calories, and age. Holliday and Segar's data were based on a relatively small number of normal patients under stable physiologic conditions. Few neonates and no premature infants were studied, further reducing the accuracy and universal applicability of this system.

Other commonly used systems for calculating fluid needs of the pediatric patient include body weight, surface area, caloric factors, and multiple physiologic factors. All of these systems are based on formulas, graphs, tables, and physiologic concepts. Weight alone cannot reflect accurately the differences in body composition and physiologic characteristics of the wide spectrum of pediatric surgical patients. These systems are inadequate because their basic physiologic assumptions have inherent problems, and they are too rigid to account for the variability among pediatric surgical patients (see Chapter 3). Included in these variables are neonatal renal water needs; evaporative water losses; the growth, metabolic, and hormonal changes during and after surgery; and losses from stool, ostomies, and drains. Most of the factors cannot be measured directly but must be estimated from tables based on body weight and age. An example of the difficulties encountered in fluid care may be illustrated best by examining the postoperative fluid needs of the gastroschisis patient. It commonly had been thought that all of these infants, because of "amniotic peritonitis," required massive amounts of fluid. Rowe analyzed a group of 51 gastroschisis patients. Fluid administration in the first 24 hours postoperatively varied between 91 and 280 mL/kg (mean 147 mL/kg). Analysis showed two distinct subpopulations: a high group that received a mean volume of 180 mL/kg/24 hours and a low group. None of the previously described systems took such variability into consideration.

This chapter describes a dynamic fluid management approach that takes into account the variability and changing physiologic and pathologic factors that characterize infants and children. We focus on the newborn patient to illustrate this approach because the neonatal period is a time of profound and rapid change. The dynamic approach to fluid management avoids the pitfalls of other systems by recognizing that no single formula, rule of thumb, table, or physiologic principle can determine the fluid needs of an individual neonatal surgical patient. This approach allows constant adjustments based on the infant's responses to the fluid given. The management can be likened to a chess match, whereby each move made by either patient or physician needs to be countered by the other. The management requires initial approximations of the patient's needs, but must be assessed routinely and modified according to how the patient responds.

FETAL AND NEONATAL PHYSIOLOGY

Body Fluid Spaces

At 12 weeks' gestation, fetal total body water content is 94% of body weight, decreasing to 80% by 32 weeks and 78% by term. In the first 3 to 5 days of postnatal life, total body water decreases an additional 3% to 5%. This fluid loss results in the early observed weight loss of the newborn infant. Body water slowly decreases to adult levels of 60% at about age 1 year. Extracellular water decreases in parallel with total body water content: 60% at 20 weeks' gestation, 45% at term, and 40% at 5 days of age. It is 33% by 3 months postnatally and reaches adult levels of 20% to 25% by age 1 to 3 years. In contrast, intracellular water increases with fetal maturation, from 25% at 20 weeks' gestation to 33% by term. Postnatally, intracellular water content increases steeply to reach close to adult levels of 44% by 3 months. Many changes in these body compartments occur with neonatal surgery. The largest changes include a marked decline in extracellular water from 51.2% to 36.7%. The greatest changes were noted in gastroschisis patients, who showed a decline in both total body water (87.3% to 78.0%) and extracellular water (51.6% to 32.3%).

These compartment changes progress in an orderly fashion in utero but are interrupted when infants are born before term. At birth, premature infants still have the high total body and extracellular water of the fetus and must complete fetal and term water-unloading tasks. The premature infant's extracellular water at 28 to 32 weeks' gestation is 52% of body weight. As a result of marked natriuresis and diuresis, extracellular water falls 12% 6 to 7 days postnatally. Premature infants complete the fetal water unloading in 1 week—a task that would have taken approximately 8 weeks in utero. This postnatal reduction in extracellular fluid volume is achieved in the face of large variations in fluid intake and seems to be physiologically important in the transition from fetal to postnatal life. Preterm infants, who as a result of fluid intake in excess of renal water-unloading capacity fail to lose weight or gain weight, have an increased incidence of patent ductus arteriosus, left ventricular failure, respiratory distress syndrome, bronchopulmonary dysplasia, and necrotizing enterocolitis. A study of reports of preterm infants who develop necrotizing enterocolitis, patent ductus arteriosus, and congestive heart failure suggested that in the first few weeks of life intravenous fluid volumes greater than 170 mL/kg/24 hours may be dangerous. If one encounters neonates requiring volumes this high, monitoring must be intensified and constant vigilance maintained for signs of fluid overload.

Renal Function

Glomerular Filtration

The postnatal shift in body fluids is mediated principally through the regulation of water and sodium excretion by the kidney. The renal handling of water is related to glomerular filtration rate (GFR) and tubular function. GFR of the term newborn is 21 mL/min/1.73 m^2, which is 25% of the adult. The GFR rapidly rises to 60 mL/min/1.73 m^2 by 2 weeks, then slowly increases to adult levels by 2 years. There is a discrepancy in GFR between term and preterm infants that persists for 1 month. Despite the low GFR, all infants can handle relatively large water loads because the negative effect exerted by the low GFR is counteracted by the positive effect of the low concentrating and high diluting capacity of the newborn kidney.

Concentration and Dilution Capacity

Urine concentration and dilution are renal tubular functions. The concentrating capacity of the preterm and term kidney is well below that of the adult. In response to water deprivation, a term infant can increase urine osmolality to a maximum of 500 to 600 mOsm/kg. In contrast, the adult concentrates osmolality to 1200 mOsm/kg. The regulation of extracellular fluid osmolality is achieved principally by variations in the release of vasopressin or antidiuretic hormone (ADH), which stimulates a cyclic adenosine monophosphate–mediated increase in water permeability of the cells of the collecting tubule. Water, but not electrolytes, is reabsorbed, and the resulting urine in the lumen of the collecting tubule becomes concentrated. The stimuli for the release of ADH are an increase in extracellular fluid osmolality or decrease of the intravascular volume. The capacity to produce ADH is fully developed in term and preterm infants. It seems, however, that the collecting tubules of newborns are less sensitive to the effects of ADH than those of the adult.

Although dehydrated newborns cannot concentrate urine as efficiently as adults, water-loaded term and preterm infants have a free-water clearance well above adults. After a water load, infants can excrete a markedly dilute urine of 30 to 50 mOsm/kg, in contrast to adults, whose lowest levels are 70 to 100 mOsm/kg. Water excretion in preterm and term infants is well in excess of intake. Although term and preterm infants can increase the rate of water excretion above the rate of intake, the capacity to excrete large volumes of water may not be sufficient to meet the extrauterine demands for rapid reduction of the excess extracellular fluid volume remaining from intrauterine existence if large quantities of fluid are infused.

As just described, neonates generally respond appropriately to fluid intake and the state of hydration. The renal response is appropriate when a small volume of concentrated urine is excreted by a hypovolemic patient or a large volume of dilute urine is excreted by a hypervolemic patient. An inappropriate response is characterized by excretion of a small volume of concentrated urine despite normovolemia or hypervolemia. It is essential to determine if postoperative newborns also respond appropriately because 10% to 12% do not respond normally. Most inappropriate responders have congenital diaphragmatic hernias. Among patients with diaphragmatic hernias, 64% inappropriately retain water for the first 12 to 18 hours postoperatively.

Renal, Water, and Osmolar Excretion

Urine output and concentration are determined by the state of hydration, renal function, and osmolar load.

Osmolar load consists of endogenous and exogenous solutes, which the kidney must clear to maintain homeostasis. Endogenous solutes are metabolic byproducts and electrolytes; exogenous components are derived from intake. Renal water is the volume of water available to the kidney to excrete the osmolar load. It must be of a sufficient volume for the kidney to clear the load within its concentrating capacity. If sufficient water is not available, the osmolar substances accumulate; blood urea nitrogen (BUN), serum creatinine, and osmolality rise; and a low volume of concentrated urine is excreted. When we measure urine output, we are measuring renal water and excess urine if the intake exceeds what is needed for osmolar excretion, replacement, and metabolic function. In this case BUN, creatinine, and serum osmolality may be low, and volumes of dilute urine are passed.

We can calculate ideal urine output if the excreted osmolar load is known. Ideal urine output is the amount of water necessary for a given osmolar load to be cleared without the kidneys being required to exert their concentrating or diluting functions. The urine is excreted without tubular work at the same osmolality as serum, 280 mOsm/L. Numerous attempts have been made to estimate osmolar load in term and preterm infants. None have taken into consideration the effect of surgical trauma and diseases. In an effort to determine the ranges of ideal urine for various surgical patients, Rowe measured osmolar excretion in more than 100 newborn surgical patients during the first 3 postoperative days (Table 4-1). In the first 24 hours, the load varied between 11.6 mOsm/kg in infants with esophageal atresia and tracheoesophageal fistula and 18 mOsm/kg in premature infants with perforated necrotizing enterocolitis. Using these figures for osmolar load, one can calculate the urine output required to excrete these loads isotonically, as follows:

$$\text{Ideal urine output (mL/kg)} = \frac{\text{osmolar load} \times 1000}{280}$$

If an infant with necrotizing enterocolitis excreted an osmolar load of 18 mOsm in 24 hours, ideal urine output would be 64 mL/kg/24 hours or 2.67 mL/kg/hr. These calculations can be made only in retrospect after sufficient urine has been collected to measure the total for 24 hours. The calculations are helpful only in determining the range of ideal urine outputs for a variety of surgical patients (see Table 4-1). From the preceding discussion, it is apparent that there is no "normal" figure for urine output, and urine output alone is not a reliable guide to the state of hydration. Normal urine output is a range related to the individual and the pathologic state involved, usually 0.5 to 3.0 mL/kg/hr. Volume must be considered in relation to concentration.

Sodium Excretion

The sodium requirements range from 2 mEq/kg/24 hours in a full-term infant, to 3 mEq/kg/24 hours in a 32-week premature infant, to 4 to 5 mEq/kg/24 hours in a very-low-gestational-age or critically ill neonate. Term newborns, similar to adults, can retain sodium in the face of negative salt balance but have a diminished capacity to excrete excess sodium when in positive balance. Sodium excretion in response to a sodium load is only 10% of that of a 6-year-old child. When an excess of sodium is administered, fluid with an elevated sodium concentration is filtered through the glomerulus into the proximal and distal renal tubules. The tubular cells cannot reject the increased sodium efficiently, and reabsorption occurs despite the high intraluminal sodium. Urine with a relatively low sodium concentration is excreted. The infant rapidly reaches positive sodium balance, and hypernatremia develops.

Preterm infants have similar difficulty in handling an excess sodium load, despite the fact that, paradoxically, premature infants have a relatively higher excretion of sodium than term infants. Premature infants have a high "programmed" renal sodium output unrelated to sodium intake; when presented with a massive salt load, they cannot increase sodium excretion significantly above this relatively fixed programmed amount; and positive sodium balance and hypernatremia result.

Premature infants are "salt wasters" unless sufficient sodium is administered. The "wasting" is most marked in infants less than 33 weeks' gestation and less than 2 weeks of postnatal age. The relatively high sodium excretion and associated water diuresis in low-gestational-age infants are believed to be physiologically necessary for fetuses late in pregnancy and newborns immediately after birth to reduce total body sodium and water rapidly in preparation for postnatal development. Between 12 and 40 weeks' gestation, the total body sodium content decreases from 120 to 80 mEq/kg. In utero fetuses have an impressive sodium excretion of 8% to 15% of the sodium filtered by the glomerulus. Term infants by 3 postnatal days have a fractional sodium excretion of 1%. In contrast, preterm infants (<33 weeks' gestation) retain the high sodium excretion of the fetus, at a level of 3% to 9% of filtered sodium. The kidney of preterm infants continues the reduction of body sodium after birth to complete fetal tasks, just as if intrauterine development were proceeding. Sodium reabsorption becomes more efficient, and salt losing decreases in preterm infants between 4 and 15 postnatal

	TABLE 4-1 ■ Osmolar Load and Ideal Renal Water		
Diagnosis	**Osmolar Load (mOsm/kg/ 24 hr)**	**Ideal Renal Water (mL/kg/24 hr Urine Output)**	**Ideal Renal Water (mL/kg/hr Urine Output)**
Bowel atresia	14.70 ± 6.7	52 ± 23	2.2 ± 0.95
Esophageal atresia with tracheoesophageal fistula	11.60 ± 3.0	41 ± 10	1.7 ± 0.40
Gastroschisis	11.70 ± 8.6	42 ± 16.6	1.7 ± 0.70
NEC	17.75 ± 8.6	63 ± 30	2.6 ± 1.25

NEC, Necrotizing enterocolitis.

days. Completion depends primarily on the postconceptional age (gestational age + postnatal days) of the infant. The most premature infants achieve positive sodium balance at a lower postconceptional age but still require a longer postnatal period to adjust than less premature infants.

The recommended maintenance sodium requirement for newborn infants may be too low for preterm or critically ill infants in view of their increased sodium excretion (discussed previously). Three separate studies involving neonates of various gestational ages found that sodium maintenance requirements vary between 2 and 5 mEq/kg/24 hours. As a starting point, sodium should be administered in doses of 2 mEq/kg/24 hours to stable term infants and 3 mEq/kg/24 hours to low-gestational-age and critically ill infants. More sodium is added to cover losses in conditions such as peritonitis and intestinal obstruction. The dose is adjusted, depending on serial measurements of serum and urine sodium concentrations.

Potassium Requirements

Sodium hemostasis has been investigated extensively in neonates, but few reports of potassium balance have appeared. The usual recommended dose is 2 mEq/kg/24 hours, given sometime after the first few days of life. There has been a reluctance to administer potassium in the first 2 postnatal days or immediately after surgery, to avoid the hazards of hyperkalemia and because of fear of immature or defective renal function. In critically ill term or preterm infants, many factors may result in negative potassium balance, however, such as increased steroid and prostaglandin excretion, high urine flow rate, and the use of diuretics. To prevent hypokalemia, parenteral potassium must be administered as soon as adequate renal function has been established. We administer 1 to 2 mEq/kg/24 hours of potassium parenterally to postoperative infants when urinary output has been established, regardless of their maturation or postoperative status. We then adjust the dose, depending on serial measurements of serum and urinary potassium concentrations.

Insensible Water Loss

Insensible water loss is the invisible, continuous loss of water from the lungs (respiratory water loss) and the skin (transepithelial water loss [TEWL]). Sweating (sensible water loss) is visible and is rarely a significant route of water loss during the newborn period. Term neonates sweat only if ambient temperature exceeds 36°C and body temperature exceeds 37.5°C. Infants less than 36 weeks' gestation do not sweat in the first few days of life. By 2 weeks, even the most immature infants sweat, but the sweat glands are poorly developed, and the volume of fluid lost is low.

The major determinants of respiratory water loss are the volume of expired air, the respiratory rate, body temperature, and the humidity of the expired air. Respiratory water loss comprises about one third of total insensible water loss of term and premature infants greater than 32 weeks' gestation. In more premature infants, the proportion of insensible water loss via the respiratory system is less because of the high loss from the skin.

Respiratory water losses are 4 to 5 mL/kg/24 hours, but essentially are eliminated when infants are managed by mechanical ventilation with humidified inspired air. In infants, TEWL is the major component of insensible water loss because epithelial barrier function is proportional to the gestational age of the infant. Water molecules diffuse through the skin to reach the surface. The stratum corneum behaves as a passive diffusion barrier. The more immature the infant, the thinner and less resistant the stratum corneum, and the greater the diffusion of water molecules. The major determinants of TEWL are conceptional age and environmental conditions. For the term infant, total insensible water loss averages 12 g/kg/24 hours. TEWL accounts for 7 g/kg/24 hours and respiratory water loss for 4 to 5 g/kg/24 hours. These figures remain constant over the first 28 days of life. In very-low-gestational-age infants, TEWL may exceed renal excretion. Hammarlund measured TEWL in infants of 25 to 40 weeks' gestational age during the first 28 days of life (Table 4-2). The greatest losses were on the first postnatal day in the most immature infants (25 to 27 weeks' gestation), 129 mL/kg/24 hours. TEWL decreased steadily as postnatal age increased.

The major environmental factor affecting insensible water loss is relative humidity. There is an inverse linear relation between TEWL and ambient relative humidity. As relative humidity approaches 100%, TEWL approaches 0; conversely, as humidity falls, evaporative water loss increases. Relative humidity in incubators varies markedly between 26% and 100%, depending on the presence or absence of inhalation therapy equipment that delivers humidified gases. Of incubators, 62% have a relative humidity less than 50%. When the infant's body is covered by plastic sheets, TEWL is reduced. Water that evaporates from the skin surface is trapped in the air space between the body and the plastic. The air becomes increasingly saturated, relative humidity rises, and evaporative rate and TEWL decrease.

Exposure of infants to nonionizing radiation by infant warmers and phototherapy produces profound changes in insensible water loss. Infants nursed in an infant warmer have an increase in insensible water loss of 30% to 50%.

TABLE 4-2 ■ Transepithelial Water Loss in Newborns* Gestational Age (and Mean Birth Weight)

Postnatal age (days)	25-27 wk (0.869 ± 0.100 kg)	28-30 wk (1.340 ± 0.240 kg)	31-36 wk (2.110 ± 0.300 kg)	37-41 wk (3.600 ± 0.390 kg)
<1	129 ± 39	42 ± 13	12 ± 5	7 ± 2
1	110 ± 27	39 ± 11	11 ± 5	6 ± 1
3	71 ± 9	32 ± 9	12 ± 4	6 ± 1
5	51 ± 7	27 ± 7	12 ± 4	6 ± 1
7	43 ± 9	24 ± 7	12 ± 4	6 ± 1
14	32 ± 10	18 ± 6	9 ± 3	6 ± 1
21	28 ± 10	15 ± 6	8 ± 2	6 ± 0
28	24 ± 11	15 ± 6	7 ± 1	7 ± 1

*gm/kg/24 hr.
Modified from Hammarlund K, Sedin G, Stromberg B: Acta Pediatr Scand 72:721, 1983.

Infants exposed to phototherapy have an increased insensible water loss of 38% to 113%. All of these changes in environment need to be taken into consideration when calculating the fluid needs of a neonate.

INTRAOPERATIVE FLUID AND ELECTROLYTE ADMINISTRATION

In assessing fluid needs after surgery, it is important to calculate the volume and electrolyte concentration of all intravenous infusions administered intraoperatively by the anesthesiologist. Often in an effort to maintain "stable vital signs" and to replace evaporative water loss from exposed viscera, large quantities of normal saline, Ringer's lactate solution, blood, and plasma may have been given. As a result, adjustments may have to be made in the postoperative fluid orders to avoid fluid overload on the one hand or hypertonicity on the other. In a study of 20 newborn surgical patients, the total sodium intake during the intraoperative and immediate postoperative period was 4.7 times what usually is considered normal daily sodium intake (3 mEq/kg/24 hours). Blood chemistry measurements should be obtained immediately after surgery to identify any gross distortion of electrolyte pattern and to write the first fluid orders. Quite distinct from typical stable newborns cared for by neonatologists, reassessment of electrolytes and rewriting of fluid orders may need to be done three or four times in the first 24 hours.

Normal Saline Is Not Normal

When postoperative fluids are calculated after surgery for gastroschisis, peritonitis, and intestinal obstruction, half-normal or normal saline solutions often are administered to replace the fluid and electrolytes lost in the tissues and peritoneal cavity. After infusion of these fluids, it is not unusual for infants to develop hyperchloremia. This is because of two factors. First, saline solutions of various dilutions deliver to the infant a proportionately high chloride load. Normal saline solution has an "unphysiologic" high chloride concentration, 154 mEq/L, as opposed to the normal serum chloride concentration of 103 mEq/L. Second, despite the high level of chloride infusion, the neonatal kidney seems to reabsorb chloride avidly. To avoid hyperchloremia, some groups use half-strength Ringer's lactate solution (65 mEq/L of sodium and 54 mEq/L of chloride) to replace third-space loss. This practice is impractical for many medical centers, however. Fluid resuscitation consisting of half-normal saline with 20 mEq of potassium chloride per liter may be adequate and avoids overloading the infant with sodium and chloride. In other instances, undiluted Ringer's lactate is effective.

Opening Volume

To put the dynamic system into operation, there must be guidelines for choosing the starting volume. Ideal water requirements often have been stated to consist of the following formula:

$$\text{Ideal intake} = \text{actual intake} - \text{excess urine}$$

Additional factors need to be considered beyond an ideal intake. First, excess intake during surgery may taper the

postoperative fluid requirement. Second, increased corticosteroids, ADH, and spironolactone in the postoperative period affect the excess urine and the ability to excrete excess fluids that were administered. To accommodate for this, the examples have opening volumes or ideal water requirements for patients with three common neonatal conditions: intestinal atresia, esophageal atresia with tracheoesophageal atresia, and necrotizing enterocolitis. These volumes are expressed as mean values and include the standard deviations (SDs) in milliliters per kilogram per 24 hours. To obtain these opening volumes, fluid intake, osmolar excretion, and total urine output were measured. Ideal urine output and excess urine were calculated for each patient.

A patient with gastroschisis can serve as an example of how ideal intake figures are used to determine an opening volume. The mean volume for ideal intake for gastroschisis patients is 135 mL/kg/24 hours with an SD of 39 mL. These patients have a thick peel, the bowel is matted together by dense tissue, suggesting severe amniotic peritonitis. Urine output is low, and concentration is high. Other physical findings and laboratory findings suggest hypovolemia. One should choose a volume much higher than the mean (perhaps 1 SD + 38 mL), 135 mL + 38 mL or 173 mL/kg/hr. Orders are written for 4 to 6 hours, or 7 mL/kg/hr. If the monitoring parameters suggest continued hypovolemia (concentrated or deficient urine output or poor capillary refill) during this initial period, volume for the next 4 to 6 hours is adjusted

TABLE 4-3 ■ Range of Urine Concentration and Output in Neonatal Surgical Patients

	Range	Mean ± SD
Osmolality (mOsm/kg)	67-582	
Specific gravity	1.002-1.040	
Urine output (mL/kg/24 hr)	0.13-14.9	3.54 ± 1.97

SD, Standard deviation.

TABLE 4-4 ■ Daily Electrolyte Requirements for Pediatric Patients

Electrolyte	Daily Maintenance Requirement
For patients weighing <10 kg	
Sodium	2-5 mEq/kg
Potassium	2-4 mEq/kg
Calcium	0.5-3 mEq/kg
Phosphorus	0.5-1.5 mM/kg
Magnesium	0.25-1 mEq/kg
For patients weighing 10-30 kg	
Sodium	20-150 mEq
Potassium	20-240 mEq
Chloride	20-150 mEq
Acetate	20-120 mEq
Calcium	5-20 mEq
Phosphorus	4-24 mM
Magnesium	4-24 mEq

upward. If the infant's responses suggest hypervolemia, the volume is scaled downward.

MONITORING

Body Weight

Serial measurements of body weight are a sensitive guide to changes in total body water but may not reflect changes in blood volume accurately. Weight gain over a short period may not be caused by hypervolemia but by leakage of fluid into the tissues as a result of trauma, inadequate perfusion, inflammation, or sepsis. The fluid that escapes into the tissue is no longer in dynamic equilibrium with the intravascular and intracellular spaces. It is lost into the "third space." Capillary leak with weight gain and generalized edema is common in septic infants and is one of the components of the systemic inflammatory response syndrome and sequential multiple organ failure. Paradoxically, blood volume often is reduced. Injudicious use of diuretics in an attempt to mobilize edema often results in further reduction in blood volume without reduction of edema. Perfusion decreases, and the situation worsens. Frequently, it is necessary to increase the volume of fluid infused despite weight gain and edema to maintain an adequate circulating blood volume. Recovery from the primary condition that led to fluid leak is heralded by diuresis, weight loss, and decrease in generalized edema. This appropriate use of excess fluid administration must be balanced in some neonates whose capillary leak status is so severe as to lead to massive third spacing. In such a scenario, placing an infant on hemofiltration may be beneficial, but results in a temporary loss of urine output.

Urine Output and Concentration

Serial measurements of urine flow and concentration are the two most helpful guides to fluid management of the pediatric patient. Except in the rare occasions of inappropriate ADH-like responses, if the volume of fluid administered is low, urine output decreases, and concentration increases. Conversely, if excess fluid is given, urine output increases, and the urine becomes dilute. The problem is one of interpretation: What is an adequate urine output and appropriate urine concentration? The ranges of urine output, specific gravity, and osmolality for newborn surgical patients are listed in Table 4-3. We generally expect an output of at least 2.0 mL/kg/hr, an osmolality of 250 to 290 mOsm/kg, and a specific gravity of 1.010 to 1.013 in preterm and term newborn infants. Because of the importance of urine flow and concentration, we strongly recommend that a urinary catheter be placed in critically ill infants for hourly measurement.

Three urinary concentration properties can be measured: specific gravity, refractory index, and osmolality. Specific gravity is a measure of the weight of urinary solids per unit volume. This method is impractical in pediatric practice because of the relatively large volume of urine needed to float the specific gravity hydrometer. Refractory index is the concentration measurement most commonly used in newborn and pediatric intensive care units and is related to the concentration of total solids in solution. The refractometer measures the refractive

index, the angle at which light is bent as it passes through a solution. The refractory index is related to total solids, and total solids are related to specific gravity. The clinical refractometer is calibrated into specific gravity units—a derived measure. Only a drop of urine is required, and the measurements can be done at the bedside. Osmolality is a measure of the number of osmoles (particles or ions) of a solute per kilogram of water. It is measured by determining the freezing point depression of a fluid sample. The technique requires only 0.2 mL of urine but usually is done in a hospital's clinical laboratory. These latter determinations are not required in all patients.

To determine the relationship between refractometer, specific gravity, and osmolality, Rowe measured the urine osmolality and refractometer specific gravity of 1700 urine specimens of newborn surgical patients. The correlation coefficient was 0.824, suggesting that accuracy of refractometer specific gravity is satisfactory in most clinical situations. A specific gravity at or less than 1.002 predicts hypo-osmolality and one greater than 1.011 predicts hyperosmolality; measures between 1.004 and 1.011 are less reliable in predicting iso-osmolality.

Fractional Sodium Excretion

Measurement of fractional sodium excretion (FeNa) is a clinically useful means to determine whether a rising BUN and falling urine output is the result of renal failure or dehydration. FeNa is an index of tubular sodium reabsorption and indicates the capacity of the kidney to excrete and absorb sodium. In normal adults, if sodium intake is not excessive, almost all of the sodium is absorbed from the tubule, and the percentage that is unabsorbed, the FeNa, is usually 0.5%. Normal FeNa for term infants is less than 1%, but for premature infants it is normally 3%. When there is renal damage, the tubules cannot reabsorb sodium adequately; most of the sodium in the tubules is not reabsorbed, and FeNa increases. A level greater than 1% in term infants and greater than 3% in premature infants is abnormal.

SCENARIOS: USING BODY WEIGHT, URINE, AND SERUM MEASUREMENTS

The following scenarios help illustrate management of typical surgical neonates.

EXAMPLE NO. 1 ■ Ileal Atresia

Data. A 1-day-old term infant with ileal atresia has received 5% dextrose and 0.2N saline solution at a rate of 80 mL/kg/24 hours. Urine output is 2.0 mL/kg/hr, urine osmolality is 280 mOsm/kg, and specific gravity is 1.011.

Diagnosis. Normal hydration.

Tests. Urine output and concentration. A satisfactory volume of isotonic urine suggests a well-hydrated patient.

Action. The same fluid orders are written for another 8 hours, and volume adjustments can be guided by urine volume and concentrations.

EXAMPLE NO. 2 ■ Esophageal Atresia

Data. An 8-hour-old term infant, after operative repair of an esophageal atresia and tracheoesophageal fistula, is receiving 120 mL/kg/24 hours of 5% dextrose and 0.2N saline solution. Urine output is 3.9 mL/kg/hr, urine osmolality is 90 mOsm/kg, and specific gravity is 1.004.

Differential Diagnosis. Overhydration versus diabetes insipidus.

Tests. Body weight, hematocrit value, BUN, creatinine, and serum osmolality. To differentiate the overhydrated patient from an infant who may have diabetes insipidus as a result of intraventricular hemorrhage, the following monitoring parameters are evaluated: body weight, hematocrit value, BUN, and serum osmolality. An overhydrated patient would have an increase in body weight as a result of elevated total body water and a fall in hematocrit value, creatinine, BUN, and serum osmolality because of hemodilution as a result of elevated serum water. In contrast, there is weight loss because of a reduction in total body water in diabetes insipidus. Serum water is decreased, and the resulting hemoconcentration leads to a rise in hematocrit value, serum osmolality, and BUN.

Action. With overhydration, the volume of fluid should be cut back to a rate of 100 mL/kg/24 hours, and the urine osmolality and urine output should be monitored with an expectation that urine output will decrease and urine concentration will increase. If the patient has diabetes insipidus, the volume of free water should increase. Care must be taken, however, if the loss of serum water has resulted in significant hypertonic dehydration. In this case, dilute intravenous fluid must not be given, and hyperosmolality should be corrected gradually over 24 hours to avoid seizures and brain damage.

EXAMPLE NO. 3 ■ Short-Bowel Syndrome

Data. A 2-week-old infant with short-bowel syndrome receives 110 mL/kg/24 hours of total parenteral nutrition solution, with a glucose concentration of 20%. The urine output is 4.0 mL/kg/hr, urine osmolality is 395 mOsm/kg, and specific gravity is 1.020.

Diagnosis. Osmolar overload.

Tests. Blood and urine glucose value, body weight, hematocrit value, creatinine, BUN, and serum osmolality. To confirm the diagnosis, the urine is tested for glucose, and body weight, hematocrit, BUN, and serum osmolality are measured. Glucose in this case is the osmotically active solute that causes the diuresis and loss of free water. The diuresis results in a decrease in total body water and weight loss. As intravascular water decreases, hemoconcentration causes an increase in hematocrit value, BUN, and serum osmolality. Blood glucose is markedly elevated.

EXAMPLE NO. 3 ■ Short-Bowel Syndrome—cont'd

Action. The volume of fluid is increased and the concentration of glucose decreased. If hypertonic dehydration is present, precautions are taken to reduce the hypertonicity gradually.

EXAMPLE NO. 4 ■ Necrotizing Enterocolitis and Prematurity

Data. A 48-hour-old premature infant has perforated necrotizing enterocolitis. The gestational age is 28 weeks, and body weight is 1000 g. The infant is receiving an infusion of 10% dextrose and half-strength Ringer's lactate solution at a rate of 160 mL/kg/24 hours. Urine output is 0.2 mL/kg/hr, urine osmolality is 280 mOsm/kg, and specific gravity is 1.011.

Diagnosis. Renal failure.

Tests. Body weight, BUN, creatinine, microscopic examination of urine, urine sodium concentration, and FeNa. Oliguria in the face of isotonic urine suggests renal failure, rather than dehydration. The urine should be examined for granular casts and blood cells. With renal failure, body weight usually is increased as water is retained. BUN and serum creatinine increase. Because of tubular damage, sodium reabsorption is decreased and urine sodium excretion increased. Urine sodium levels are usually greater than 70 mEq/L, and FeNa is greater than 3% and may be 6% or 8%.

Action. If there are not gross signs of overhydration and hypernatremia, the administration of 5 to 10 mL/kg of 0.45N saline solution over 30 minutes and administration of a diuretic may be tried. If the urine output does not increase, the patient must be treated for renal failure and only replacement fluids infused. Potassium is restricted.

EXAMPLE NO. 5 ■ Congenital Diaphragmatic Hernia

Data. A 24-hour-old infant, 8 hours after repair of a congenital diaphragmatic hernia, is receiving 100 mL/kg of 5% dextrose and 0.2N saline solution. Urine output is 0.5 mL/kg/hr, urine osmolality is 420 mOsm/kg, and specific gravity is 1.030.

Differential Diagnosis. Dehydration versus inappropriate response (excess ADH).

Tests. Body weight, hematocrit value, BUN, creatinine, serum osmolality, urine sodium, and FeNa. With dehydration, if there is no capillary leak present, body weight decreases. If there is tissue damage and capillary leakage, however, body weight may increase despite intravascular dehydration. With the decrease in serum water as a result of dehydration, the resulting hemoconcentration is evidenced by a rise in hematocrit value, BUN, creatinine, and serum osmolality. Urine sodium excretion and FeNa are low.

EXAMPLE NO. 5 ■ Congenital Diaphragmatic Hernia—cont'd

If the patient is responding inappropriately, body weight increases as water is retained, and as a result of hemodilution, hematocrit value, serum osmolality, creatinine, and BUN are low. Urine sodium excretion and FeNa often increase because of the elevated blood volume. If sodium concentration is low because of hemodilution, urine sodium excretion and FeNa may be low.

Action. With dehydration, the volume of fluid administered should be increased. If an inappropriate response is present and the patient shows evidence of overhydration, the volume administered should be cut back, and urine concentration and output should be monitored continually. Usually, over 14 to 16 hours without an increased amount of fluid given, a brisk diuresis of dilute urine occurs.

SUGGESTED READINGS

Chemtob S, Kaplan BS, Sherbotie JR, Aranda JV: Pharmacology of diuretics in the newborn. Pediatr Clin North Am 36:1231-1250, 1989.

This is one of few articles dealing with the action of diuretics on the newborn.

Coran AG, Drongowski RA: Body fluid compartment changes following neonatal surgery. J Pediatr Surg 24:829-832, 1989.

This is a comprehensive study of the changes in fluid compartments after neonatal surgery.

Wilkins BH: Renal function in sick very low birthweight infants: 1. Glomerular filtration rate. Arch Dis Child 67:1140-1145, 1992.

Wilkins BH: Renal function in sick very low birthweight infants: 2. Urea and creatinine excretion. Arch Dis Child 67:1146-1153, 1992.

Wilkins BH: Renal function in sick very low birthweight infants: 3. Sodium, potassium, and water excretion. Arch Dis Child 67:1154-1161, 1992.

Wilkins BH: Renal function in sick very low birthweight infants: 4. Glucose excretion. Arch Dis Child 67:1162-1165, 1992.

The four above-listed articles constitute an excellent series dealing with several aspects of renal function in low-birth-weight infants. Wilkins discusses specific aspects using actual patient data.

Respiratory Considerations

PULMONARY MECHANICS AND GAS EXCHANGE

The approach to mechanical ventilation is best understood if the two variables of oxygenation and carbon dioxide (CO_2) elimination are considered separately.

Carbon Dioxide Elimination

Figure 5-1 and Table 5-1 demonstrate the various volumes and capacities of the lung. A capacity is formed from more than one volume. The volume of gas present in the lungs with maximal inflation is the total lung capacity (TLC). The vital capacity (VC) is the maximal amount of gas within the TLC available for ventilation. Residual volume (RV) is the air left in the lung after the VC is expired. Thus,

$$VC + RV = TLC$$

The primary purpose of ventilation is to eliminate CO_2. This is accomplished by delivering tidal volume (V_T) breaths at a designated rate. The product of V_T and rate determines the minute volume ventilation ($\dot{V}_E$). Although CO_2 elimination is proportional to $\dot{V}_E$, it is,

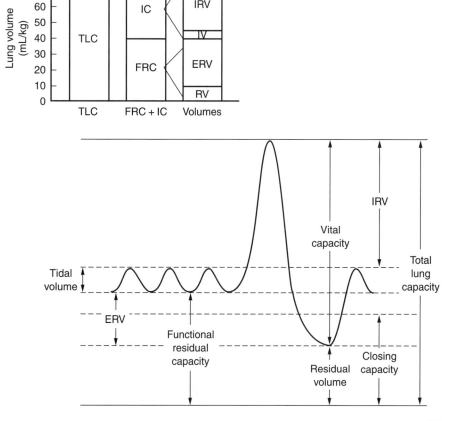

FIGURE 5-1 ■ Demonstration of the various volumes and capacities of the lung. TLC, total lung capacity; IC, inspiratory capacity; FRC, functional residual capacity; RV, residual volume; ERV, expiratory reserve volume; TV, tidal volume; IRV, inspiratory reserve volume. (Adapted in part from Hirschl RB: Mechanical ventilation in pediatric surgical disease. In Pediatric Surgery, 3rd ed. WB Saunders, 2000.)

TABLE 5-1 ■ Definitions and Normal Values for Respiratory Physiologic Parameters

Variable	Definition	Normal Value
TLC	Total lung capacity	80 mL/kg
FRC	Functional residual capacity	40 mL/kg
IC	Inspiratory capacity	40 mL/kg
ERV	Expiratory reserve volume	30 mL/kg
RV	Residual volume	10 mL/kg
Tv	Tidal volume	5 mL/kg
$\dot{V}_E$	Minute volume ventilation	100 mL/kg/min
$\dot{V}_A$	Alveolar ventilation	60 mL/kg/hr
$\dot{V}_D$	Dead space	mL = wt in lbs
$\dot{V}_D/\dot{V}_T$	% Dead space	0.33
Cst	Static compliance	2 mL/cm H_2O/kg
Ceff	Effective compliance	1 mL/cm H_2O/kg

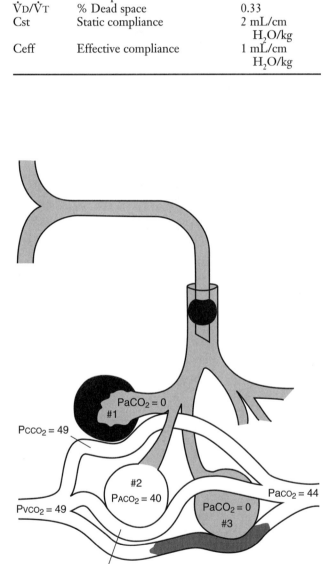

FIGURE 5-2 ■ Pulmonary dead space ($\dot{V}_D$) and ventilation/perfusion matching $\dot{V}/\dot{Q}$. $\dot{V}_D$ is a function of the conducting airways (gray), the number of nonperfused alveoli (#3), and the volume of the ventilator tubing on the patient side of the "Y." $\dot{V}/\dot{Q}$ is demonstrated as regions with high $\dot{V}/\dot{Q}$ (pulmonary embolus/thrombus: ventilation, no perfusion, #3) and low $\dot{V}/\dot{Q}$ (alveolar edema/collapse: minimal/no ventilation, reasonable perfusion, #1). (Adapted from Hirsch RB: Surgery of Infants and Children: Scientific Principles and Practice, Philadelphia, Lippincott-Raven, 1997.)

in fact, directly related to the volume of gas ventilating the alveoli. This is so because part of the $\dot{V}_E$ resides in the conducting airways or in nonperfused alveoli (Fig. 5-2). As such, this portion of the ventilation does not participate in CO_2 exchange and is termed the *dead space* ($\dot{V}_D$). In the patient with healthy lungs, this dead space consists of about one third of the tidal volume ($\dot{V}_D/\dot{V}_T = 0.33$). This fixed anatomic dead space can unwittingly be increased through the presence of extensions of the trachea such as the endotracheal (ET) tube or an extension of the ventilator tubing on the patient side of the "Y." It is critical, therefore, that endotracheal tubes be shortened as much as is reasonable and that other safeguards be applied to ensure that the anatomic $\dot{V}_D$ is minimized in the mechanically ventilated patient. In the setting of respiratory insufficiency, the proportion of dead space ($\dot{V}_D/\dot{V}_T$) may be augmented by the presence of nonperfused alveoli and a reduction in tidal volume.

The $\dot{V}_T$ is a function of the applied ventilator pressure and the volume-pressure relationship (compliance), which describes the distensibility of the lung and chest. A normal elastic lung requires less pressure to expand than a diseased or scarred lung. At the functional residual capacity (FRC), which is the static point of end expiration, the tendency for the lung to collapse (lung elastic recoil) is in balance with the tendency for the chest wall to expand. As each breath develops, however, the elastic recoil of both the lung and chest wall work in concert to oppose lung inflation. Pulmonary compliance, then, is a function of both the distensibility of the lung (lung compliance) and the distensibility of the rib cage and diaphragm (chest wall compliance). The infant's chest wall is more compliant than the lung and requires minimum force to expand it. After 6 months of age the muscles enlarge and the chest wall stiffens and compliance begins to decrease. However, a distended abdomen or tight abdominal wall closure will cause a significant decrease in compliance in spite of the strikingly compliant chest wall of the infant.

The compliance can be determined in a dynamic or static mode. Figure 5-3 demonstrates the dynamic volume/pressure relationship for a normal patient. Note that application of 25 cm H_2O of inflating pressure (ΔP) above static FRC at positive end-expiratory pressure (PEEP) = 5 cm H_2O generates a tidal volume of 40 mL/kg. The lung, at an inflating pressure of 30 cm H_2O when compared with ambient (transpulmonary pressure), is considered to be at total lung capacity (TLC). Note that the loop observed during both inspiration and expiration is curvilinear. This is due to the resistance that is present in the airways and describes the work required to overcome airflow resistance. As a result, at any given point of active flow the measured pressure in the airway is higher during inspiration and lower during expiration than at the same volume under zero flow conditions. The magnitude of flow into the airway and ultimately the alveoli during mechanical ventilation is determined by the driving pressure and the resistance to flow. In the intubated child the major determinant of resistance is the radius of the ET tube. The ET tube may be narrow simply because of the size that can be placed into the trachea, but also because of secretions. The airway radius can be reduced

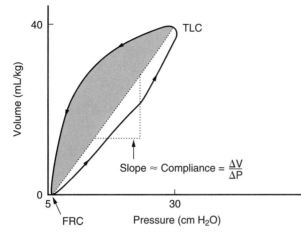

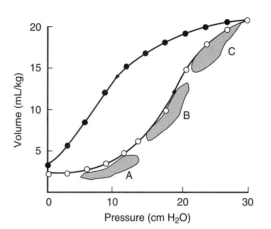

FIGURE 5-3 ■ Dynamic pressure/volume relationship and effective pulmonary compliance (Ceff) in the normal lung. The volume at 30 cm H_2O is considered total lung capacity (TLC). Ceff is calculated by $\Delta V/\Delta P$. (Adapted from Bhutani VK, Sivieri EM: Physiological principles for bedside assessment of pulmonary graphics. In Donn SM [ed]: Neonatal and Pediatric Pulmonary Graphics: Principles and Applications. Armonk, NY, Futura Publishing, 1998.)

FIGURE 5-4 ■ Static lung compliance curve in a normal lung. Effective compliance would be altered depending on whether FRC were to be at a level resulting in lung atelectasis (A) or overdistention (C). Optimal lung mechanics are observed when FRC is set on the steepest portion of the curve (B). (Adapted from West JB: Respiratory Physiology. Baltimore, Williams & Wilkins, 1985.)

by secretions or spasm. According to Poiseuille's law, for every decrease in radius, resistance increases by the fourth power. Resistance can be calculated by measuring driving pressure and dividing it by the flow of gas. When infants are weaned from mechanical ventilation, the length and radius of the ET tube adds greatly to the resistance and work of breathing. Therefore, during weaning from mechanical ventilation, when breaths per minute have been reduced to a low rate (e.g., 10 to 18 breaths per minute), the patient should be extubated rather than be required to breathe against the resistance of the ET tube.

Because of resistance, pulmonary compliance measurements, as well as alveolar pressure measurements, can only be effectively performed when there is no flow in the airways (zero flow). In Figure 5-3, this exists at FRC and TLC. The line drawn between the two points describes the "effective" compliance. The change observed is a volume of 40 mL/kg and pressure of 25 cm H_2O or 1.6 mL/kg/cm H_2O. It is termed *effective compliance* because this analysis only provides assessment of compliance between the two arbitrary points of end-inspiration and end-expiration. As can be seen from Figure 5-4, the volume/pressure relationship is not linear over the range of most inflating pressures when a static compliance curve is developed. Such static compliance assessments are most commonly performed with use of a large syringe in which aliquots of 1 to 2 mL/kg of oxygen, up to a total of 15 to 20 mL/kg, are instilled sequentially with 3- to 5-second pauses between each. At the end of each pause, zero flow pressures are measured. By graphing the data a static compliance curve may be generated that demonstrates how the calculated compliance can change depending on the arbitrary points used for assessment of the effective compliance. The compliance will change as the FRC or end-expiratory lung volume (EELV)

increases or decreases. For instance, as can be seen in Figure 5-4, at low FRC (point A) atelectasis is present and a given ΔP will not optimally inflate alveoli. Likewise, at a high FRC (point C), because of air trapping or application of high PEEP, the lung is already distended and application of the same ΔP will only result in overdistention and potential lung injury with little benefit in terms of added V_T. Optimal compliance is provided, then, when the pressure/volume range is on the linear portion of the static compliance curve (point A). Clinically, the compliance at a variety of FRC or PEEP values can be monitored to establish optimal FRC.

Typical ventilator rate requirements in patients with healthy lungs range from 10 breaths per minute in an adult to 30 breaths per minute in a newborn. The V_T is maintained at 5 to 10 mL/kg. This affords a $\dot{V}_E$ of up to 100 mL/kg/min in adolescents and 150 mL/kg/min in newborns. These settings should provide sufficient ventilation to maintain normal $Paco_2$ levels of approximately 40 mm Hg and should generate peak inspiratory pressures of between 15 and 20 cm H_2O above an applied PEEP of 5 cm H_2O. Clinical assessment by observing chest wall movement, auscultation, and evaluation of gas exchange determines the appropriate V_T.

A portion of the V_T generated by the ventilator is actually compression of gas both within the ventilator tubing and even the airways. The compliance of the ventilator tubing is 0.3 to 4.5 mL/cm H_2O. A ΔP of 15 cm H_2O in a 3-kg newborn with respiratory insufficiency and a pulmonary compliance of 0.4 mL/cm H_2O/kg would result in lung V_T of 18 mL and an impressive ventilator tubing gas compression volume of 15 mL if the tubing compliance equals 1.0 mL/cm H_2O. The relative ventilator tubing gas compression volume would not be as striking in an adult. The ventilator tubing compliance is characterized for all current ventilators and should be accounted for when considering tidal volume data. The software in many ventilators now corrects for ventilator tubing compliance when displaying V_T values.

Oxygenation

Oxygenation is determined by the fraction of inspired oxygen (FIO_2) and the degree of lung distention or alveolar recruitment, which is determined by the level of PEEP and the mean airway pressure (Paw or MAP). The MAP is equivalent to the integral of the area under the pressure-time curve during one respiratory cycle. Increases in the PEEP and MAP result in enhanced oxygenation but may adversely influence pulmonary perfusion and cardiac output, thus decreasing overall oxygen delivery (see later). The risk of barotrauma may also be increased because high levels of PEEP or MAP in conjunction with high peak inspiratory pressure (PIP) favor alveolar overdistention.

Rather than depending on the degree of alveolar ventilation as with CO_2 elimination, oxygenation predominantly is a function of the appropriate matching of pulmonary blood flow to inflated alveoli (ventilation/perfusion matching [$\dot{V}/\dot{Q}$]). Areas of ventilation but no perfusion (high $\dot{V}/\dot{Q}$), such as in the setting of pulmonary embolus, do not contribute to oxygenation (see Fig. 5-2). The common pathophysiology observed in the setting of respiratory insufficiency is that of minimal or no ventilation with persistent perfusion (low $\dot{V}/\dot{Q}$) resulting in right-to-left shunt and hypoxemia. Patients with the acute respiratory distress syndrome (ARDS) have collapse of the posterior, or dependent, regions of the lungs when supine (Fig. 5-5). As the majority of blood flow is distributed to these dependent regions, one can easily imagine the limited oxygen transfer, large shunt, $\dot{V}/\dot{Q}$ mismatch, and resulting hypoxemia that occurs in patients with ARDS. Attempts to inflate the alveoli in these regions, with interventions such as application of PEEP, can reduce $\dot{V}/\dot{Q}$ mismatch and enhance oxygenation. In normal lungs the PEEP should be maintained at 5 cm H_2O, an expiratory pressure that allows maintenance of alveolar inflation at end expiration. An FIO_2 equal to 0.50 should be administered initially. However, one should be able to wean the FIO_2 rapidly in the patient with healthy lungs and normal $\dot{V}/\dot{Q}$ matching.

The arterial oxygen (PaO_2) and arterial oxygen saturation (SaO_2) levels are measured most frequently to evaluate oxygenation. Lung oxygenation capabilities are frequently assessed as a function of the difference between the ideal alveolar and the measured systemic arterial oxygen levels

$$(A-a)DO_2 = (FIO_2 \cdot (PB - PH_2O) - PaCO_2 \cdot RQ) - PaO_2,$$

the ratio of the PaO_2 to the FIO_2 (P/F ratio), the physiologic shunt

$$\left(Qps/Qt = \frac{CiO_2 - CaO_2}{CiO_2 - C\bar{v}O_2} \right),$$

and the oxygen index

$$\left(OI = \frac{Paw \cdot FIO_2 \cdot 100}{PaO_2} \right)$$

where PB = barometric pressure, PH_2O = partial pressure of water, RQ = the respiratory quotient or the ratio of the oxygen consumption ($\dot{V}O_2$) and the CO_2 production ($\dot{V}CO_2$),

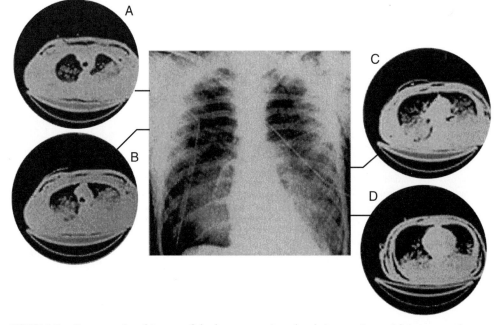

FIGURE 5-5 ■ Cross-sectional image of the lungs at various levels in a patient with acute respiratory distress syndrome. Note the diffuse infiltrates on a chest radiograph but the regional posterior, dependent atelectasis on computed tomography. The anterior, or nondependent, regions are well inflated. (Reprinted with permission from Maunder RJ, Shuman WP, McHugh JW, et al: Preservation of normal lung regions in the adult respiratory distress syndrome: Analysis by computed tomography. JAMA 255:2463-2465, 1986.)

and $C\bar{v}O_2/CaO_2/CiO_2$ = the oxygen content of venous, arterial, and expected pulmonary capillary blood, respectively.

Three variables ascertain oxygen delivery: cardiac output (Q), hemoglobin concentration (Hgb), and arterial blood oxygen saturation (SaO_2). The product of these three variables determines oxygen delivery by the relationship:

$$DO_2 = Q \times CaO_2$$

where

$$CaO_2 = [(1.36 \times Hgb \times SaO_2) + (0.003 \times PaO_2)]$$

Note that the contribution of the PaO_2 to DO_2 is minimal and is often disregarded in this equation because of the relatively large oxygen-carrying capacity of hemoglobin: under typical arterial conditions the volume of oxygen in each deciliter of blood that is bonded to hemoglobin is 20.4 mL of O_2 while only 0.3 mL of O_2 is dissolved in plasma. Normal hemoglobin contains two α and two β chains with four associated iron heme groups. Oxygen is able to reversibly form a covalent bond with the ferrous ion within the heme molecule. Arterial hemoglobin saturation is a function of the PaO_2 and the affinity of oxygen for hemoglobin, which is described graphically by the oxyhemoglobin dissociation curve (Fig. 5-6). The steep portion of the oxygen-hemoglobin dissociation curve is an important area because a small change in PaO_2 causes a relatively large change in SaO_2. At the normal physiologic PaO_2 of 100 mm Hg, SaO_2 is 100%, whereas at a normal venous PO_2 of 40 mm Hg the mixed venous oxygen saturation ($S\bar{v}O_2$) is 75%. The normal PO_2, which achieves a hemoglobin saturation of 50% (P50) is 27 mm Hg. The amount of oxygen that saturates the hemoglobin, the oxygen affinity, is affected by several factors: (1) hydrogen ion concentration or pH, (2) CO_2 pressure ($PaCO_2$),

(3) temperature, (4) 2,3-diphosphoglycerate (2,3-DPG), and (5) fetal hemoglobin concentration. As hydrogen ion concentration, arterial carbon dioxide pressure ($PaCO_2$), temperature, 2,3-DPG, or the amount of adult hemoglobin increases, oxygen affinity decreases. The oxygen-hemoglobin dissociation curve shifts to the right. When the curve shifts to the right, oxygen uptake into hemoglobin requires a higher PaO_2. In contrast, decreases in the same factors induce an increase in hemoglobin affinity for oxygen that may increase oxygen content and delivery. During normal metabolism at the tissue level, pH is low, PCO_2 has accumulated, and temperature is elevated. These conditions favor the release of oxygen from the hemoglobin molecule at the relatively low oxygen level found at the tissues. At the lung, on the other hand, conditions favor oxygen pickup rather than release: PCO_2 is lower and pH is higher.

The 2,3-DPG has a profound effect on oxygen affinity. It binds to hemoglobin, decreasing hemoglobin affinity for oxygen, making less hemoglobin available for oxygen binding. Although 2,3-DPG binds rapidly and effectively to adult hemoglobin, it interacts poorly with fetal hemoglobin. As a result, oxygen affinity of fetal hemoglobin is high and the curve shifts to the left. This provides the fetus with an effective method of extracting and releasing oxygen in the presence of low umbilical vein PO_2 levels.

The amount of oxygen delivered to the tissues is typically four to five times greater than the amount of oxygen consumed (VO_2, Fig. 5-7). The $S\bar{v}O_2$ is a direct reflection of the amount of oxygen delivered to the amount consumed (DO_2/VO_2 ratio). As DO_2 increases or VO_2 decreases,

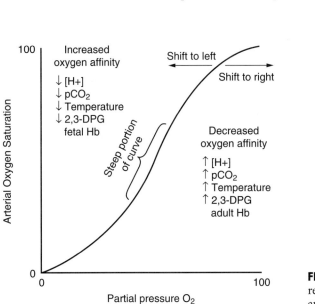

FIGURE 5-6 ■ Oxyhemoglobin dissociation curve and factors causing right and left shift of the curve. Note that fetal hemoglobin shifts the curve to the left.

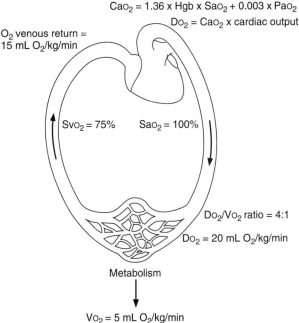

FIGURE 5-7 ■ An overview of oxygen kinetics demonstrating the relationship of oxygen consumption (VO_2), oxygen delivery (DO_2), and the mixed venous oxygen saturation ($S\bar{v}O_2$). (Reprinted with permission from Hirschl RB: Cardiopulmonary critical care and shock. In: Surgery of Infants and Children: Scientific Principles and Practice. Philadelphia, Lippincott-Raven, 1997.)

more oxygen remains in the venous blood. The result is an increase in $S\bar{v}O_2$. In contrast, if DO_2 decreases or VO_2 increases, relatively more oxygen is extracted from the blood; and, therefore, less oxygen remains in the venous blood. A decrease in $S\bar{v}O_2$ is the result. The $S\bar{v}O_2$ serves as an excellent monitor of oxygen kinetics because it specifically monitors the adequacy of DO_2 in relation to VO_2. Clinical studies suggest that the critical $S\bar{v}O_2$ before VO_2 is compromised is in the 40% to 50% range, which correlates with a critical DO_2/VO_2 ratio of approximately 2.0. Technologic advances have allowed development of a fiberoptic, continuous $S\bar{v}O_2$ monitor that accurately reflects the measured pulmonary artery $S\bar{v}O_2$. Such monitoring provides a means for assessing the adequacy of DO_2, rapid assessment of the response to interventions such as mechanical ventilation, and cost savings owing to a diminished need for sequential blood gas monitoring (Fig. 5-8). A decrease in $S\bar{v}O_2$ to less than 65% or a change in $S\bar{v}O_2$ greater than 5% to 10% should be a cause for concern. The exceptions to accuracy of $S\bar{v}O_2$ appear to be in settings in which arteriovenous shunting may be in effect in patients with cirrhosis or sepsis. Such situations in which vasoregulation is altered may lead to an observed increase in $S\bar{v}O_2$ even though the DO_2 at the tissue level remains inadequate.

In the intensive care unit, four factors can be potentially manipulated in an attempt to improve the DO_2/VO_2 ratio: cardiac output, hemoglobin concentration, SaO_2, and VO_2. Although we tend to address each factor individually, it is the combination of these four factors that summarizes the goal of interventions: sufficient oxygen delivery. One of the most efficient ways to enhance DO_2 is to increase the oxygen-carrying capacity of the blood. For instance, an increase in hemoglobin from 7.5 to 15 g/dL will be associated with a twofold increase in DO_2 at constant cardiac output. The SaO_2 can often be enhanced through application of supplemental oxygen and mechanical ventilation. Assessment of the "best PEEP" identifies the level at which DO_2 and $S\bar{v}O_2$ are optimal. Evaluation of the best PEEP should be performed in any patient requiring an FIO_2 greater than 0.60 and may be determined by continuous monitoring of the $S\bar{v}O_2$ as the

PEEP is sequentially increased from 5 to 15 cm H_2O over a short period of time. The point where the $S\bar{v}O_2$ is maximal indicates the PEEP where DO_2 is optimal. VO_2 may be elevated owing to sepsis, burns, agitation, seizures, hyperthermia, hyperthyroidism, and increased catecholamine production or infusion. Paralysis may enhance the effectiveness of mechanical ventilation while simultaneously reducing VO_2.

PULSE OXIMETRY

The pulse oximeter is one of the most important advances in noninvasive cardiopulmonary monitoring in the critically ill patient. Information with regard to oxygenation as well as heart rate and perfusion are provided in a noninvasive fashion. The measurements are continuous, so clinical changes can be rapidly detected, unlike the information obtained from intermittent arterial blood sampling.

Pulse oximeters emit light at two wavelengths, usually 660 nm (red) and 940 nm (near infrared), which is transmitted through tissue to a photodetector. The intensity of the transmitted light remains constant except for alterations in absorbency owing to the pulsatile nature of arterial inflow (Fig. 5-9). The pulsatile components are then subtracted from the nonpulsatile component. In this way only arterial blood absorbency is measured and a pulse rate determined. Because light is differentially absorbed by oxyhemoglobin (HbO_2 selectively absorbs infrared light [940 nm] and transmits red light [660 nm]) and deoxyhemoglobin (deoxyhemoglobin absorbs red light and transmits infrared light), variable absorbency at the two wavelengths allows determination of arterial hemoglobin saturation (SpO_2).

The "default" saturation for most pulse oximeters corresponds to an SpO_2 of 85%. This is often seen in low

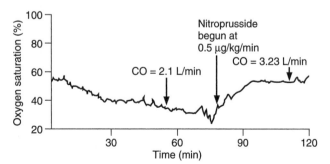

FIGURE 5-8 ■ Alterations in mixed venous blood oxygen saturation are shown as sodium nitroprusside is administered to reduce left ventricular afterload in the setting of cardiac insufficiency. (Reprinted with permission from Hirschl RB: Cardiopulmonary critical care and shock. In: Surgery of Infants and Children: Scientific Principles and Practice. Philadelphia, Lippincott-Raven, 1997.)

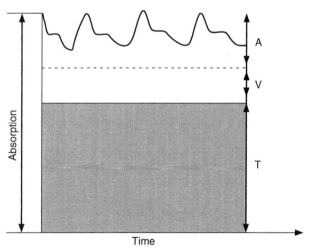

FIGURE 5-9 ■ The absorption of light for assessment of hemoglobin saturation by a pulse oximeter is illustrated. Light is absorbed by tissue (T), venous blood (V), and arterial blood (A) with the variation in light absorption resulting from alterations in arterial blood volume with each pulsation. (Reprinted with permission from Hirschl RB: Cardiopulmonary critical care and shock. In: Surgery of Infants and Children: Scientific Principles and Practice. Philadelphia, Lippincott-Raven, 1997.)

cardiac output states with poor peripheral perfusion, methemoglobinemia, and hypothermia and in states of increased vascular resistance. Therefore, the patient in whom saturation has abruptly decreased to 85% should be assessed for pulse oximeter artifact by noting whether a valid heart rate is displayed by the pulse oximeter. Movements may be interpreted as pulsations. Dampening or obliteration of the pulse wave by a circulation-supporting device such as extracorporeal membrane oxygenation (ECMO) and cardiopulmonary bypass will interfere with the accuracy of the readings. Other sources of error in pulse oximeter analysis include the presence of venous blood pulsations, the presence of nail polish, ambient room light (which affects the photodetector), and high levels of carbon monoxide (in which the oximeter overestimates the true fraction of oxyhemoglobin). Intravascular administration of methylene blue and fluorescein will induce a falsely low SpO_2 reading because of absorption of light at the investigating wavelengths.

It is fortunate that the absorbencies of fetal hemoglobin are similar to those of hemoglobin A at the two investigating wavelengths of the pulse oximeter. Therefore, the presence of hemoglobin F does not have an effect on hemoglobin saturation determination. The pulse oximeter probe is usually placed on the fingers or toes. If such probes fail to function appropriately at those sites, more central

locations such as the ears, lips, and nose may be used. Pulse oximeters can also be placed on extremities with questionable arterial perfusion to monitor for vascular compromise.

CARBON DIOXIDE MONITORING

End-tidal carbon dioxide ($etCO_2$) monitors assess the absorption of infrared light as it passes through the expired gas. Thus, $etCO_2$ monitoring is helpful to document effective ventilation of the airway after ET placement and in evaluating trends in $PaCO_2$ during ventilator manipulation. In healthy patients without respiratory insufficiency, such as those undergoing anesthesia, the maximal value assessed over a few minutes provides a relatively good approximation of the true $PaCO_2$ (Fig. 5-10). Unfortunately, $\dot{V}/\dot{Q}$ mismatch in the setting of respiratory insufficiency often results in a relative decrease in $etCO_2$ when compared with $PaCO_2$. Therefore, in those patients with respiratory insufficiency, the difference between the $etCO_2$ and $PaCO_2$ may be large, frequently changing, and useful only for trend analysis. However, the $PaCO_2 - etCO_2$ gradient and the $PaCO_2/etCO_2$ ratio are reflective of the degree of $\dot{V}/\dot{Q}$ mismatch and can be used to monitor the effects of various interventions on $\dot{V}/\dot{Q}$ matching.

MANAGEMENT OF THE MECHANICAL VENTILATOR

During spontaneous breathing, the respiratory muscles contract, the thoracic cavity expands, and a subatmospheric pressure is generated in the pleural space. This negative pressure is transmitted across the lung parenchyma, causing the lung to expand. In contrast, mechanical ventilation initiates inspiration by generating positive rather than negative pressure. The machine delivers gas into the airway, and the lungs are inflated by a pressure that is positive with respect to the atmosphere. Expiration in either case is passive and is related to the elastic recoil of the lung and thorax.

The modes of ventilation are characterized by three variables: the parameter used to initiate or "trigger" a breath, the parameter used to "limit" the size of the breath, and the parameter used to terminate inspiration or "cycle" the breath (Fig. 5-11). Gas flow in most ventilators is triggered either by time (controlled breath) or by patient effort (assisted breath). In the assist mode,

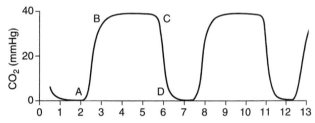

FIGURE 5-10 ■ The waveform generated by a CO_2 analyzer during tidal breathing is shown. The partial pressure of CO_2 is 0 mm Hg at the beginning of expiration (A) because of the dead space in the conducting airways. The B-C interval represents the alveolar PCO_2. The end-tidal PCO_2 is at point C. The PCO_2 then decreases during inspiration (C-D) before the cycle is repeated. (Reprinted with permission from Hirschl RB: Cardiopulmonary critical care and shock. In: Surgery of Infants and Children: Scientific Principles and Practice. Philadelphia, Lippincott-Raven, 1997.)

FIGURE 5-11 ■ Variables that characterize the mode of mechanical ventilation. (Reprinted with permission from Hirschl RB: Mechanical ventilation in pediatric surgical disease. In: Pediatric Surgery, 3rd ed. Philadelphia, WB Saunders, 2000.)

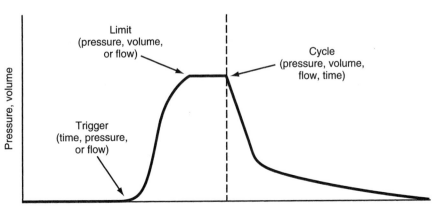

the ventilator is pressure or flow triggered. With the former, a pressure generated by the patient of approximately −1 cm H_2O will trigger the initiation of a breath. The sensitivity of the triggering device can be adjusted so that patient work is minimized. Other ventilators detect the reduction in constant ventilator tubing gas flow (bias flow) that is associated with patient initiation of a breath. Detection of this decrease in flow results in initiation of a positive-pressure breath.

Most neonatal ventilators employ time cycling, in which pressure is delivered for a preset inspiratory time (IT). With volume-cycled ventilation, inspiration is terminated when a prescribed volume is obtained. Likewise, with flow-cycled ventilation, expiration begins once the flow has decreased to a predetermined level.

The magnitude of the breath is controlled or limited by one of three variables: volume, pressure, or flow. When a breath is volume, pressure, or flow "controlled," it indicates that inspiration concludes once the limiting variable is reached. In contrast, a factor that "limits" inspiration suggests that the chosen value limits the level of the variable during inspiration, but the inspiratory phase does not conclude once this value is attained. For instance, during "pressure-limited" ventilation, gas flow continues until a given pressure limit is attained. However, the inspiratory phase does not necessarily conclude at that point. In contrast, during pressure-controlled ventilation both gas flow and the inspiratory phase terminate once the preset pressure is reached.

Pressure-controlled or pressure-limited modes are currently the most popular for all age groups, although volume-control ventilation may be of advantage in preterm newborns (Fig. 5-12). In the pressure-limited mode the respiratory rate, the inspiratory gas flow, the PEEP level, the IT:ET ratio, and the PIP are determined. The ventilator infuses gas until the desired PIP is provided, after which excess flow is diverted through a popoff value as the PIP is maintained until the prescribed IT is attained. In general, zero flow conditions are realized at end inspiration during pressure-limited ventilation. In this mode, PIP is frequently equivalent to end-inspiratory pressure (EIP) or plateau pressure. The PIP is usually set to achieve visible chest expansion. High pressures have been associated with the pathogenesis of bronchopulmonary dysplasia. Pressures exceeding 26 or 28 cm H_2O in newborns are a cause for concern. In many ventilators the gas flow rate is fixed, although newer ventilators allow manipulation of the flow rate and, therefore, the rate of positive-pressure development. Those with rapid flow rates will provide rapid ascent of pressure to the preset maximum, where it will remain for the duration of the inspiratory phase. This "square wave" pressure pattern results in decelerating flow during inspiration. Airway pressure is "front loaded," which increases Paw, alveolar volume, and oxygenation without increasing PIP. One of the biggest advantages of pressure-controlled or pressure-limited ventilation is the ability to avoid lung overdistention and barotrauma/volutrauma (see later). The disadvantage of pressure-controlled or pressure-limited ventilation is that delivered volume varies with airway resistance and pulmonary compliance and may be reduced when short inspiratory

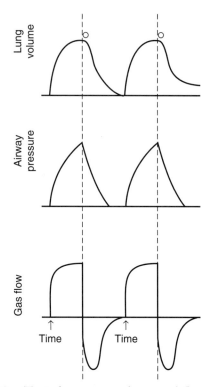

FIGURE 5-12 ■ Typical pressure, volume, and flow waveforms observed during volume-controlled ventilation (time-triggered, flow-limited, volume-cycled). *Arrows* indicate triggering variables and *open circles* show cycling variables. (From Bartlett RH: Use of the mechanical ventilator. In Wilmore DW, et al: Scientific American (R) Surgery, Web MD, New York, 1989.)

times are applied. For this reason, VT and V̇E both must be monitored carefully.

Volume-controlled or volume-limited ventilation requires delineation of the VT respiratory rate, and inspiratory gas flow (Fig. 5-13). Gas will be inspired until the preset V̇T is attained. The volume will remain constant despite changes in pulmonary mechanics, although the resulting EIP and PIP may be altered. The flow rate determines the wave pattern of a ventilator breath. A high flow rate causes a rapid rise in pressure to reach the preset volume and then a relatively long plateau at that volume and associated pressure until the end of the time cycle. At that point, flow ceases and expiration passively begins. On the other hand, a low flow rate causes a slow rise in pressure and a brief or absent plateau. If the flow rate is too low, the desired volume may never be reached during the time cycle.

Modes of Mechanical Ventilation
Intermittent Mandatory Ventilation (IMV)

IMV is time triggered, volume or pressure limited and either time, volume, or pressure cycled (see Fig. 5-13). A rate is set, as is a volume or pressure parameter. Additional inspired gas is provided by the ventilator to support spontaneous breathing when additional breaths are desired. IMV is useful in patients who do not have respiratory drive, for example those who are neurologically impaired or pharmacologically paralyzed. Work of

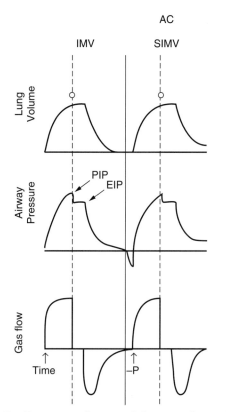

FIGURE 5-13 ■ Pressure, volume, and flow waveforms observed during intermittent mandatory ventilation (IMV), synchronized IMV (SIMV), and assist-control ventilation (AC). In this case, an end-inspiratory pause has been added. Note the difference between peak (PIP) and end-inspiratory (EIP) or plateau pressure. *Arrows* indicate triggering variables and *open circles* show cycling variables. (From Bartlett RH: Use of the mechanical ventilator. In Wilmore DW, et al: Scientific American (R) Surgery, Web MD, New York, 1989.)

breathing may be elevated in this mode in the awake and spontaneously breathing patient.

Synchronized Intermittent Mandatory Ventilation (SIMV)

In the SIMV mode, the ventilator synchronizes IMV breaths with the patient's spontaneous breaths (see Fig. 5-13). Small, patient-initiated negative deflections in airway pressure (pressure-triggered) or decreases in the constant ventilator gas flow (bias flow) passing through the exhalation valve (flow-triggered) provide a signal to the ventilator that a patient breath has been initiated. Ventilated breaths are timed with the patient's spontaneous respiration, but the number of supported breaths each minute is predetermined and remains constant. Additional constant inspired gas flow is provided for use during any other spontaneous breaths.

Assist-Control Ventilation

In the spontaneously breathing patient, brainstem reflexes dependent on cerebrospinal fluid levels of CO_2 and pH can be harnessed to determine the appropriate breathing rate. As in SIMV, the assisted breaths can be either pressure triggered or flow triggered (see Fig. 5-13).

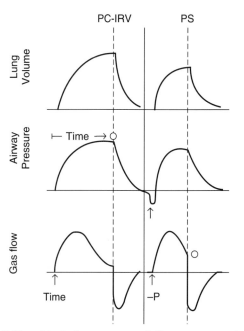

FIGURE 5-14 ■ Typical pressure and flow patterns observed during pressure-controlled inverse ratio ventilation (PC-IRV) and pressure support ventilation (PS). *Arrows* indicate triggering variables and *open circles* show cycling variables. (From Bartlett RH: Use of the mechanical ventilator. In Wilmore DW, et al: Scientific American (R) Surgery, Web MD, New York, 1989.)

The triggering mechanism sensitivity can be set in most ventilators. In contrast to SIMV, the ventilator supports all patient-initiated breaths. This mode is similar to IMV, but it allows the patient to inherently control his or her ventilation needs and minimizes patient work of breathing in adults and neonates. Occasionally a patient may hyperventilate, such as when agitated or when a neurologic injury is present. Heavy sedation may be required if agitation is present. A minimum ventilator rate below the patient's assist rate should be established in case of apnea.

Pressure Support Ventilation (PSV)

PSV is a pressure- or flow-triggered, pressure-limited, and flow-cycled mode of ventilation (Fig. 5-14). It is similar in concept to assist control in that mechanical support is provided for each spontaneous breath and the patient determines ventilator rate. During each breath inspiratory flow is applied until a predetermined pressure is attained. As the end of inspiration approaches, flow decreases to a level below a specified value (2 to 6 L/min) or a percentage of peak inspiratory flow (about 25%). At this point inspiration terminates. Although it may apply full support, PSV is frequently used to partially support the patient by assigning a pressure limit for each breath that is less than that required for full support. For example, in the spontaneously breathing patient PSV can be sequentially decreased from full support to a PSV 5 to 10 cm H_2O above PEEP. This allows weaning while providing partial support with each breath. Therefore, during PSV tidal volume may be dependent on patient effort. PSV provides excellent support and decreases the work of breathing associated with ventilation.

Pressure-triggered SIMV and pressure-support ventilation may be applied to newborns. Inspiration is terminated when the peak airway flow drops to a set percentage of between 5% and 25%. This flow cutoff for inspiration is known as the termination sensitivity, which may be adjusted: the higher the termination sensitivity value, the shorter the inspiratory time. The termination sensitivity function may also be disabled, at which point ventilation is time cycled instead of flow cycled.

Volume Assured Pressure Support Ventilation (VAPSV)

These modes attempt to combine volume- and pressure-controlled ventilation to ensure a desired tidal volume within the constraints of the pressure limit set. This mode has the advantage of maintaining inflation to a point below an injurious peak inspiratory pressure level while maintaining VT constant in the presence of changing pulmonary mechanics. Work of breathing may be markedly decreased during VAPSV.

Inverse Ratio Ventilation (IRV)

In the setting of respiratory failure one would wish to enhance alveolar distention to reduce hypoxemia and shunt. One means to accomplish this is to maintain the inspiratory plateau pressure for a longer proportion of the breath. In most circumstances the IT:ET ratio is maintained at approximately 2:1. Although some studies have failed to demonstrate enhanced gas exchange with this mode of ventilation, others have revealed an increase in Paw and oxygenation while protecting the lungs with a reduction in PIP.

Continuous Positive Airway Pressure (CPAP)

During CPAP, pressures above those of ambient are continuously applied to the airways to enhance alveolar distention and oxygenation. Both airway resistance and work of breathing may be substantially reduced. However, there is no support of ventilation. This mode requires, therefore, that the patient provide all of the work of breathing. It is to be avoided in patients with hypovolemia, untreated pneumothorax, lung hyperinflation, or elevated intracranial pressure and in infants with nasal obstruction, cleft palate, tracheoesophageal fistula, or untreated congenital diaphragmatic hernia. CPAP is frequently applied via nasal prongs, although it can be delivered in adult patients with a nasal mask.

Bilevel Control of Positive Airway Pressure (BiPAP)

Although sometimes used in the acute lung setting, this simple ventilator system is frequently used for home respiratory support, by varying airway pressure between one of two settings: the inspiratory positive airway pressure (IPAP) and the expiratory positive airway pressure (EPAP). With patient effort a change in flow is detected and the IPAP pressure level developed. With reduced flow at end expiration EPAP is reestablished. This device, therefore, provides both ventilatory support as well as airway distention during the expiratory phase. However, BiPAP ventilators should only be used to support the patient who is spontaneously breathing.

Mechanical Ventilation in the Patient with Healthy Lungs

IMV and SIMV may suffice for patients with normal lungs such as those who are post operation. If a patient is spontaneously breathing and is to be ventilated for more than a brief period, a flow- or pressure-triggered assist mode or pressure support ventilation will result in maximal support and minimal work of breathing. The normal V̇E is 100 to 150 mL/kg/min. The FIO₂ is usually initiated at 0.50 and decreased based on pulse oximetry. All efforts should be made to maintain the FIO₂ less than 0.60 to avoid alveolar nitrogen depletion, the development of atelectasis, and oxygen toxicity.

Mechanical Ventilation in the Patient with Respiratory Failure

Ventilator Induced Lung Injury (VILI)

One typically observes both a decrease in pulmonary compliance as well as FRC in the patient with acute lung injury (ALI; PaO_2/FIO_2 ratio = 200 to 300) or the acute respiratory distress syndrome (ARDS; PaO_2/FIO_2 ratio <200). These two parameters are related because the loss of FRC associated with alveolar collapse results in a decrease in the volume of lung available for ventilation and, therefore, a decrease in pulmonary compliance. As a result, higher ventilator pressures are necessary to maintain VT and V̇E. However, the adverse effects of prolonged lung exposure to high ventilating pressures (plateau pressures >35 cm H_2O) and volumes have been elucidated over the past 2 decades. The National Institutes of Health ARDS consortium showed a 9% increase in survival during low (6 mL/kg) when compared with high volume (12 mL/kg) ventilation in adult patients with ARDS. Such injury may be prevented during application of high peak inspiratory pressures by strapping the chest, thereby preventing lung overdistention, suggesting that alveolar distention or "volutrauma" is the injurious element rather than application of high pressures or "barotrauma." These data suggest that avoidance of high peak inspiratory pressures and associated excessive lung volumes should be a primary goal of any mechanical ventilatory approach to the lung.

A number of studies have demonstrated that application of PEEP or high-frequency oscillatory ventilation (HFOV) may allow avoidance of lung injury by the following mechanisms: (1) recruitment of collapsed alveoli that reduces the risk for overdistention of healthy units; (2) resolution of alveolar collapse which in and of itself is injurious; and (3) avoidance of the shear forces associated with the opening and closing of alveoli. In infants, PEEP is usually kept between 3 and 6 cm H_2O. PEEP's beneficial effects include improved oxygenation and increased FRC and prevention of atelectasis. In the older child with injured lungs a pressure of 8 to 12 cm H_2O is required to open alveoli. Alveoli will subsequently close unless the end-expiratory pressure is maintained at such pressures. This cyclic opening and closing is thought to be particularly injurious due to application of large shear forces. One way to avoid this process is through the application of PEEP to a point above the inflection pressure (Pflex) such that alveolar distention is maintained throughout

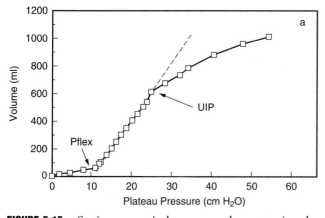

FIGURE 5-15 ■ Static pressure/volume curve demonstrating the Pflex point at approximately 12 cm H_2O plateau pressure in a patient with acute respiratory distress syndrome. PEEP should be maintained approximately 2 cm H_2O above that point. The upper inflection point (UIP) indicates the point at which lung overdistention is beginning to occur. Ventilation to points above the UIP should be avoided in most circumstances. (Reprinted with permission from Roupie E, Dambrosio M, Servillo G, et al: Titration of tidal volume and induced hypercapnia in acute respiratory distress syndrome. Am J Respir Crit Care Med 152:121-128, 1995.)

TABLE 5-2 ■ Current Favored Approaches to the Treatment of ARDS
Pressure-limited ventilation
$V_T \leq 6$ mL/kg
EIP < 35 cm H_2O
PEEP > Pflex or 8–12 cm H_2O
Permissive hypercapnia
$F_{IO_2} \leq 0.06$
$S\bar{v}_{O_2} \geq 65\%$
$Sa_{O_2} \geq 80$–85%
Transfusion to Hgb >13 g/dL
Diuresis to dry weight
Prone positioning
Extracorporeal support

the ventilatory cycle (Fig. 5-15). In addition, as mentioned previously, the distribution of infiltrates and atelectasis in the supine patient with ARDS is predominantly in the dependent regions of the lung. This is likely the result of compression caused by the increased weight of the overlying edematous lung. Application of PEEP results in recruitment of these atelectatic lung regions, simultaneously enhancing pulmonary compliance and oxygenation.

Approach to the Patient with Respiratory Failure

As a result of these new data and concepts, the approach to mechanical ventilation in the patient with respiratory failure has changed drastically over the past few years (Table 5-2). Time-cycled, pressure-controlled ventilation has become favored because of the ability to limit EIP to noninjurious levels at a maximum of 35 cm H_2O. In infants and newborns this EIP limit is set lower at 30 cm H_2O. A lung protective approach also incorporates lung distention and prevention of alveolar closure. The PEEP should preferably be maintained at least 2 cm H_2O above Pflex: a PEEP of at least 8 to 12 cm H_2O, and perhaps even greater than 15 cm H_2O, should be empirically applied in older patients. Application of increased levels of PEEP may also result in a decrease in venous return and cardiac output. As such, parameters of D_{O_2} should be carefully monitored during application of increased PEEP. One means for doing so is by attention to the $S\bar{v}_{O_2}$ whenever the PEEP is raised above 5 cm H_2O. As mentioned, one approach is to gradually increase the PEEP in increments of 2.5 cm H_2O until the desired level of oxygenation or lung protection is achieved or a decrease in $S\bar{v}_{O_2}$ to below the maximum is observed. Effective lung compliance also should be monitored to ensure that alveolar recruitment is being achieved.

If oxygenation remains inadequate with application of higher levels of PEEP, F_{IO_2} should be increased to maintain an Sa_{O_2} greater than 90%, although levels as low as 80% may be acceptable in patients with adequate D_{O_2}. As mentioned previously, one of the most effective ways to enhance D_{O_2} is by transfusion. All attempts should be made to avoid the atelectasis and oxygen toxicity associated with F_{IO_2} levels greater than 0.60. Extending F_{IO_2} to levels greater than 0.60 often has little effect on oxygenation because severe respiratory failure is frequently associated with a large transpulmonary shunt. If inadequate D_{O_2} persists, a trial increase in PEEP level should be performed or institution of extracorporeal life support (ECLS) considered.

Altering the patient from the supine to the prone position appears to enhance gas exchange, although one multicenter study suggests that even though oxygenation is improved, survival is not enhanced with this maneuver. Another means for enhancing oxygenation may be through administration of diuretics. Application of the concept of permissive hypercapnia is integral to the successful application of lung protective strategies. Pa_{CO_2} levels greater than 100 mm Hg have been allowed with this approach, although most practitioners prefer to maintain the Pa_{CO_2} less than 60 to 70 mm Hg. Bicarbonate or *tris*-hydroxymethylaminomethane (THAM) may be used to induce a metabolic alkalosis to maintain the pH greater than 7.20. Few significant physiologic effects are observed with elevated Pa_{CO_2} levels as long as the pH is maintained at reasonable levels. If adequate CO_2 elimination cannot be achieved while limiting EIP to noninjurious levels, then initiation of ECLS should be considered.

The one situation in which it may be acceptable to increase EIP to levels greater than 35 cm H_2O (30 cm H_2O in the infant and newborn) is in the patient with reduced chest wall compliance and relatively normal pulmonary compliance. Because pulmonary compliance is composed of a combination of lung compliance and chest wall compliance, a decrease in chest wall compliance, such as due to abdominal distention or chest wall edema, can markedly reduce pulmonary compliance despite reasonable lung compliance.

Weaning from Mechanical Ventilation

Once a patient is spontaneously breathing and able to protect the airway, consideration should be given to weaning from ventilator support. The FIO_2 should be decreased to less than or equal to 0.40 before extubation. Simultaneously, PEEP should be weaned down to 5 cm H_2O. The pressure support mode of ventilation is an efficient means for weaning because the preset inspiratory pressure can be gradually decreased while partial support is provided for each breath. Adequate gas exchange during a pressure support of 7 to 10 cm H_2O above PEEP in adults and newborns is predictive of successful extubation. In all circumstances, brief trials of spontaneous breathing before extubation should be performed with flowby oxygen and CPAP. Parameters during a T-piece trial that indicate readiness for extubation include the following: (1) maintenance of the pretrial respiratory and heart rate; (2) inspiratory force greater than 20 cm H_2O; (3) $\dot{V}E$ less than 1 mL/kg/min; and (4) SaO_2 greater than 95%. The weaning trial should be brief and under no circumstances longer than 1 hour because the narrow ET tube provides substantial resistance to spontaneous ventilation. In most cases the patient who tolerates spontaneous breathing through an ET tube for only a few minutes will demonstrate enhanced capabilities once the airway access device is removed. Strategies for management of the patient who has failed multiple weaning attempts are demonstrated in Table 5-3.

EXTRACORPOREAL LIFE SUPPORT

The term *extracorporeal life support* denotes the use of prolonged extracorporeal cardiopulmonary bypass, usually via extrathoracic cannulation, in patients with acute, reversible cardiac or respiratory failure who are unresponsive to conventional medical or pharmacologic management. Although *extracorporeal membrane oxygenation* (ECMO) is the traditional term associated with this technique, ECLS is the current, preferred mnemonic because the term "life support" encompasses functions other than "oxygenation," including cardiac and hemodynamic support as well as CO_2 elimination. It is important to recognize that ECLS is not a therapeutic intervention. Instead, ECLS simply provides cardiopulmonary support so that the patient is spared the deleterious effects of high airway pressure, high FIO_2, and perfusion impairment while "reversible" pathophysiologic processes are allowed to resolve either by

TABLE 5-3 ■ Management of the Patient Who Has Failed Extubation Attempts

Frequent spontaneous breathing trials
Pressure support ventilation
Caloric intake ≤10% above expenditure
Minimize carbohydrate calories
Diuresis to dry weight
Treat infection
Tracheostomy

spontaneous means or by medical or surgical therapeutic intervention.

Three prospective randomized trials have compared the effectiveness of ECLS with conventional mechanical ventilation (CMV) in full-term newborns with severe respiratory insufficiency. One of these was a randomized prospective study performed in the United Kingdom that demonstrated a significant difference in survival between full-term newborns managed with ECLS (72%) and those managed by conventional means (41%). Other studies have demonstrated a significant increase in survival among pediatric respiratory failure patients managed with ECLS (74%) when compared with carefully matched patients managed with CMV (63%).

Indications for ECLS

In the majority of newborns, pulmonary disease processes result in the pathophysiology associated with pulmonary hypertension and persistent fetal circulation (PFC).

Conventional methods such as mechanical ventilation, induced respiratory alkalosis, surfactant administration, nitric oxide administration, and high-frequency oscillatory ventilation (HFOV) may be applied to decrease the PFC and respiratory insufficiency. When these interventions fail, ECLS may allow reversal of the cycle of increasing pulmonary hypertension while minimizing the complications of high-pressure mechanical ventilation and FIO_2. In contrast to the newborn, infants and children with respiratory failure and patients of all ages with cardiac failure frequently have pathophysiologic processes that are based on parenchymal organ dysfunction.

For optimal application of ECLS, one would wish to define criteria that would allow identification of those who will ultimately succumb at the earliest moment while excluding those patients who would eventually survive by more conventional means. Two such criteria have been developed in neonates. The first is an oxygen index (OI), which is based on arterial oxygenation and mean airway pressure (MAP) and computed according to the following formula:

$$OI = (MAP \times FIO_2 \times 100)/PaO_2$$

It has been suggested that an OI greater than 40 in three of five postductal arterial blood gases each drawn 30 minutes to 1 hour apart is predictive of a mortality of 80% or more. A randomized, controlled study suggested that "early" initiation of ECLS based on an OI greater than 25, which is predictive of a 50% mortality rate, is associated with a trend toward a higher mental developmental score and a lower incidence of morbidity at 1 year of age when compared with a control group of patients in whom ECLS was initiated at an OI greater than 40. Many centers, therefore, currently consider institution of ECLS when a series of postductal arterial blood gases demonstrate an OI greater than 25 with mandatory application of ECLS when the OI is greater than 40. The other criterion used to indicate initiation of ECLS is based on the alveolar-arterial oxygen difference [(A – a)DO_2]: an (A – a)DO_2 value of greater than or equal to 610 mm Hg despite 8 hours of maximal medical management is associated with a mortality of 79% while excluding only

6% of subsequent deaths. Newborn patients with congenital diaphragmatic hernic (CDH) are frequently placed on ECLS at OI criteria equal to 25 to 30 based on a series of postductal arterial blood gases.

Criteria for high mortality risk among non-neonatal children with respiratory failure have been less well defined. Some centers employ fast entry criteria (PaO$_2$ <50 mm Hg for >2 hours) and slow entry criteria (pulmonary shunt fraction >30%) measured at an FIO$_2$ equal to 1.0 and PEEP greater than or equal to 5 cm H$_2$O to indicate need for ECLS. However, the ELSO registry would suggest that the indication for ECLS is simply classified as "failure to respond" in more than 90% of pediatric patients with respiratory failure.

Many of the "absolute" exclusion criteria have been relaxed as experience with ECLS has allowed reduction in activated clotting time (ACT) levels and refinement and standardization of various aspects of the ECLS technique:

1. Previously, an estimated gestational age of 34 weeks or less was considered a contraindication to ECLS owing to the high incidence of intracranial hemorrhage. However, ECLS has been successfully applied in the preterm newborn with an estimated gestational age of more than 32 weeks, although the incidence of intracranial hemorrhage may be as high as 40%.

2. Although intracranial hemorrhage has been considered an absolute contraindication to ECLS in the past, reasonable outcome has been demonstrated when ECLS has been instituted in the setting of grade I or II intracranial hemorrhage.

3. Mechanical ventilation for longer than 7 to 10 days in newborn and pediatric patients with respiratory insufficiency has been considered a contraindication to ECLS because of the high incidence of bronchopulmonary dysplasia and irreversible fibroproliferative lung disease. However, review of the ELSO registry data has suggested that survival in patients who have been managed with mechanical ventilation for up to 10 to 14 days may still be reasonable.

4. Cardiac arrest that requires cardiopulmonary resuscitation in the pre-ECLS period has been considered a contraindication to institution of extracorporeal support. However, survival rates of up to 60% have been observed among neonates and pediatric cardiac patients who sustain a cardiac arrest before or during cannulation. Based on these data, many centers now consider patients who sustain pre-ECLS cardiac arrest candidates for extracorporeal support.

5. To avoid application of ECLS to newborn patients with CDH and "irreversible" severe lung hypoplasia, extracorporeal support in the past was withheld from those patients who could not demonstrate a best postductal PaO$_2$ greater than 50 mm Hg. However, following the demonstration that a number of patients who met this exclusion criteria still survived, most centers will now consider any patient with CDH as a candidate for ECLS.

6. Finally, as an ethical consideration, those patients with profound neurologic impairment, multiple congenital anomalies, or other conditions not compatible with meaningful life are excluded as candidates for ECLS.

Additional relative exclusion criteria that apply specifically to pediatric patients with respiratory failure are the presence of multiorgan system failure, major burns, immunodeficiency, active bleeding, chronic lung disease, and an "incurable" disease process. Preoperative cardiac anomalies in newborns represent a relative contraindication to ECLS because they should be treated operatively, although they may be supported with ECLS until surgical intervention can be accomplished.

Methods of Extracorporeal Support

The goal of ECLS is to provide perfusion of warmed, arterialized blood into the patient. To achieve this goal, three configurations of extracorporeal blood flow are used clinically: (1) venoarterial (VA), (2) venovenous (VV), and (3) double-lumen venovenous (DLVV) bypass (Fig. 5-16). In the early experience, ECLS was almost always performed using venoarterial support because it offered the potential to replace cardiac and lung function. However, there are significant disadvantages to the use of venoarterial bypass: a major artery must be cannulated and at least temporarily sacrificed; the risk of dissemination of particulate or gaseous emboli into the systemic circulation is substantial; pulmonary perfusion may be markedly reduced; cardiac output may be compromised because of the presence of increased ECLS circuit-induced afterload resistance; and the coronary arteries are predominantly perfused by the relatively hypoxic left ventricular blood. In contrast, both VV and DLVV support provide adequate gas exchange without these disadvantages. One significant problem with VV and DLVV ECLS, however, is that a fraction of recently infused blood recirculates back into the extracorporeal circuit. As a result, oxygenation levels are relatively reduced and extracorporeal blood flow rates must be increased approximately 20% to account for this effect. The VV and DLVV extracorporeal circuit configurations also do not provide cardiac support. However, because of the numerous advantages VV and DLVV ECLS have become the preferred methods for patients of all age groups who do not require cardiac support. Even neonates, as well as older pediatric and adult patients, who require pressor support before initiation of bypass often do well with a VV or DLVV configuration once hypoxia and acidosis are resolved and high ventilator pressures reduced. The DLVV configuration of bypass has now been used in over 1200 newborn cases with a 90% survival rate; only 15% of patients required conversion from DLVV to VA ECLS. Unfortunately, double-lumen cannulas appropriate for use in patients weighing more than 4 to 5 kg are not available. However, VV ECLS with drainage from the internal jugular vein and infusion into the femoral vein is an effective means of providing support in adults and children older than 3 years of age.

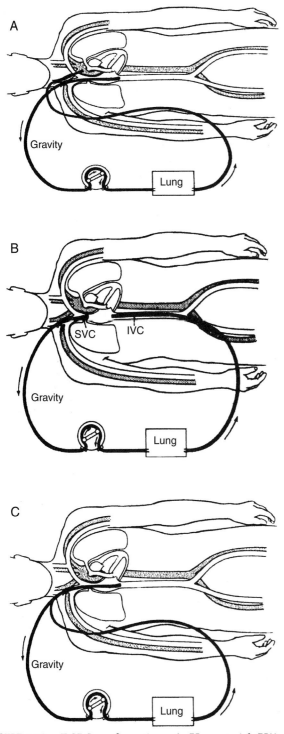

FIGURE 5-16 ■ ECLS configurations: **A,** Venoarterial (VA). **B,** Venovenous (VV). **C,** Double-lumen venovenous (DLVV). (Reprinted with permission from Hirschl RB, Bartlett RH: Extracorporeal life support in cardiopulmonary failure. In: Pediatric Surgery, 5th ed. St. Louis, CV Mosby, 1998.)

The ECLS Circuit

The ECLS circuit is composed of three basic components: a roller pump, a membrane lung, and a heat exchanger (Fig. 5-17). The remainder of the devices associated with the extracorporeal circuit serve safety and monitoring functions. Right atrial blood is drained to the pump by gravity siphon via a cannula placed through the right internal jugular vein. Roller pumps are the perfusion devices most frequently used and require continuous servoregulation and monitoring to prevent application of high levels of negative pressure to the drainage circuit and high levels of positive pressure, with a risk of circuit disruption, to the infusion limb of the circuit should occlusion occur. Application of high negative pressures to the drainage circuit results in hemolysis, damage to the endothelium of the right atrium or vena cava, and cavitation as air is drawn out of solution. To prevent generation of negative pressures a small (30 mL) distensible bladder that compresses a spring-loaded mechanical switching device that interrupts flow of power to the roller pump is frequently interposed between the venous cannula and the roller pump. The bladder remains distended as long as venous return is adequate for the current pump flow rate and the bladder pressure remains greater than −20 mm Hg. If the pump flow rate exceeds venous return or if venous drainage is impeded for any reason the bladder will collapse, resulting in discontinuation of pump flow. An alternative method for roller pump servoregulation involves the use of a pressure monitor that signals a reduction of roller pump speed or interruption of power to the pump as negative pressures are applied to the pre-pump circuit.

Once blood passes through the roller pump it is then perfused through the artificial lung. The membrane lung, which is the one most commonly used, consists of two sheets of silicone that are sealed at the edges. Oxygen gas flows through connector tubing segments at opposite ends that are in continuity with the inside of the silicone envelope. The envelope is wound up on a polycarbonate spool and blood is distributed, via a manifold, lengthwise through the interstices of the wound-up envelope. Gas exchange takes place across the silicone membrane. Membrane lungs are available from 0.4 m² to 4.5 m² in surface area: the size of the artificial lung is selected to provide total cardiopulmonary support. The size of the various ECLS components required as a function of patient weight is demonstrated in Table 5-4. Hollow fiber artificial lungs are highly efficient with regard to gas exchange, of low resistance to blood flow, and easy to prime. The disadvantage of the hollow fiber lung is the increased rate of condensation of water in the gas phase and the frequent need for replacement due to development of plasma leak.

Once through the artificial lung, blood passes through a heat exchanger as the arterialized blood is then perfused at body temperature either through (1) the internal carotid cannula into the aortic arch or (2) a femoral venous cannula or the second lumen of the internal jugular DLVV cannula into the right atrium. A bridge between the drainage and infusion tubing exists in most ECLS circuits. The purpose of the bridge is to allow temporary dissociation of the patient from the extracorporeal circuit during emergencies and during trial periods off ECLS. The volume of the neonatal circuit is 400 to 500 mL, which is one to two times the newborn blood volume. The circuit, therefore, must be primed carefully to perfuse the neonate at onset of bypass with

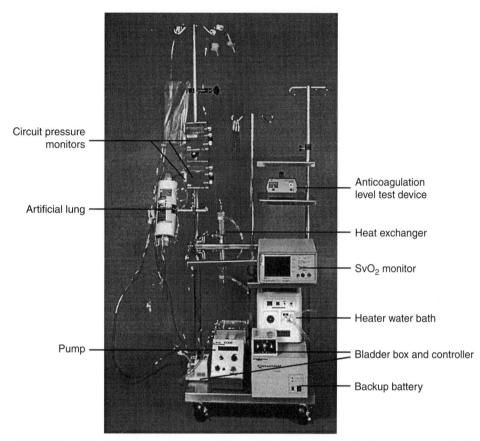

Circuit pressure monitors

Artificial lung

Pump

Anticoagulation level test device

Heat exchanger

SvO₂ monitor

Heater water bath

Bladder box and controller

Backup battery

FIGURE 5-17 ■ The ECLS circuit. (Adapted from Hirschl RB, Bartlett RH: Extracorporeal life support in cardiopulmonary failure. In: Pediatric Surgery, 5th ed. St. Louis, CV Mosby, 1998.)

blood containing appropriate pH, hematocrit, calcium, clotting factors, electrolytes, and temperature. However, ECLS may be instituted in those patients weighing more than 35 kg without addition of blood to the prime.

Patient Management on ECLS

Cannulation in general is performed in the intensive care unit. All procedures such as placement of chest tubes and appropriate intravenous, pulmonary arterial, or intra-arterial catheters are performed before cannulation and administration of heparin. Paralyzing agents are administered to prevent air embolus during placement of the venous cannula. Intravenous morphine or fentanyl and local lidocaine infiltration provide anesthesia.

The size of the venous cannula is the factor that determines the blood flow rate and, therefore, the level of extracorporeal support. As such, the largest possible venous access cannula should be placed. It should be of sufficient

TABLE 5-4 ■ Circuit Components and Prime Used for Patients of Different Size during Venovenous Support						
Weight (kg)	2–6	6–15	15–20	20–30	30–50	50+
Drainage tubing (inch)	1/4	NA	3/8	3/8	1/2	1/2
Raceway (inch)	1/4	NA	3/8–1/2	1/2	1/2	1/2
Oxygenator (m²)	0.8–1.5	NA	2.5–3.5 m²	3.5–4.5 m²	4.5 m²	4.5 m² × 2
Cannulas (Fr)	12–15 Fr	NA	Inf: 15–19	Inf: 17–21	Inf: 21	Inf: 21
	DLVV‡	NA	Dr: 15–19	Dr: 17–21	Dr: 19–23*	Dr: 21–23*
Prime	RBC: 1–2 U	NA	RBC: 3 U	RBC: 4 U	RBC: 4 U†	RBC: 5 U†
	FFP: 50–100 mL	NA	FFP: 1/2 U	FFP: 1 U	FFP: 1 U	FFP: 1 U

All cannula references are for the shortest Biomedicus cannula available in the specified size. These are only guidelines, and individual patient variables must be considered. Venovenous ECLS is not currently recommended in the 4- to 15-kg patient (< 3 years of age).
*The M# = 2.4 of the 23 Fr Biomedicus (38 cm) custom cannula is nearly the same as that of the 29 Fr Biomedicus cannula (50 cm).
†Normosol (3 L) with 12.5 g albumin and CaCl, 1 g, is usually used.
‡12 and 15 Fr double-lumen cannulas (DLVV) for VV ECLS are manufactured by Jostra and Origen. The 14 Fr DLVV cannula is manufactured by Kendall.

size to provide adequate blood flow with the assistance of a 100-cm H$_2$O gravity siphon pressure. The flow-pressure characteristics of a given cannula are determined by a number of geometric factors, including length, internal diameter, and side hole placement. The "M-number" provides a standardized means for describing the flow-pressure relationships in a variety of vascular access devices.

Transthoracic cannulation may be appropriate in the postcardiac surgery patient with cardiac and/or pulmonary dysfunction. In general, however, access for ECLS is provided by extrathoracic cannulation. The first choice of venous access is the internal jugular vein because it is a large vein that provides easy access to the right atrium through a short cannula. The femoral vein is the second choice for venous drainage access during ECLS and the first for reinfusion during VV support. In children younger than 5 years of age the femoral vein is too small to function as the primary drainage site. Therefore, the iliac vein should be considered the second choice of access in young children. A proximal venous drainage cannula (PVDC) may be placed into the proximal internal jugular vein to enhance venous drainage to the extracorporeal circuit.

The size of the reinfusion cannula is less critical than that of the venous cannula, although it must be large enough to tolerate the predicted blood flow rate at levels of total support without generating a pressure proximal to the membrane lung of more than 350 mm Hg. Infusion cannulas typically have a single end hole, whereas venous drainage cannulas have additional side holes. The first choice for placement of a cannula into the arterial circulation is the carotid artery in all age groups because it provides easy access to the aortic arch. Few complications have been associated with carotid artery cannulation and ligation in newborns, children, and adults. The second choice for arterial access is the femoral artery in those patients older than 5 years of age. In patients younger than 5 years of age, the femoral artery is of insufficient size to provide arterial access; therefore, the iliac artery is the preferred site after the carotid artery. Distal perfusion of the lower extremity arterial circulation is sometimes required when the femoral artery is cannulated, although distal perfusion is typically not required after cannulation of the iliac artery in young children.

The cannulation procedure is usually performed by direct cutdown using local anesthesia (Fig. 5-18). The patient is placed supine with the head turned to the left and a roll placed transversely under the shoulders. A 2- to 3-cm transverse cervical incision is made one finger's breadth above the clavicle over the right sternocleidomastoid muscle. Dissection between the heads of the SCM exposes the carotid sheath, which is opened as the internal jugular vein, common carotid artery, and vagus nerves are identified. Manipulation of the vein should be minimized to avoid induction of venospasm, which may preclude placement of a large venous cannula. The common carotid artery lies medial and posterior and may be safely dissected because it has no branches at this level. Heparin (100 units/kg) is administered intravenously. The tips of the arterial and venous cannulas (see Table 5-4 for sizes) will be optimally located at the opening of the right brachiocephalic artery and the inferior aspect of the

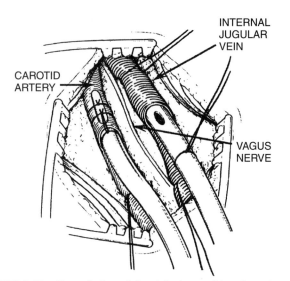

FIGURE 5-18 ■ Cannulation of the right internal jugular vein and right carotid artery for venoarterial extracorporeal support. (Reprinted with permission from Hirschl RB, Bartlett RH: Extracorporeal life support in cardiopulmonary failure. In: Pediatric Surgery, 5th ed. St. Louis, CV Mosby, 1998.)

right atrium, respectively. The cannulas are inserted a specific distance in the neonate (arterial = 2.5 cm and venous = 6 cm). The DLVV cannula must be placed such that the tip is in the mid right atrium (advanced 5 cm in the neonate) with the reinfusion ports oriented toward the tricuspid valve to minimize recirculation of reinfused blood.

Percutaneous access to the internal jugular and femoral vein is the preferred approach to cannulation in adults and children older than 3 years of age. Sequentially larger dilators are placed over a wire as the Seldinger technique allows final access of the cannula itself into these large veins. The Jostra or Origen 12 or 15 French DLVV cannula is amenable to percutaneous introduction into the internal jugular vein in neonates.

Once on extracorporeal support there typically is rapid cardiopulmonary stabilization. All paralyzing agents, vasoactive drugs, and other infusions are discontinued during use of venoarterial support, although some pressor support may be necessary when venovenous bypass is utilized. Ventilator settings are adjusted to minimal levels to allow the lung to rest and any air leaks secondary to barotrauma to seal. The S$\bar{v}$O$_2$ is conveniently monitored by a fiberoptic Oximetrix catheter placed in the venous limb of the circuit that allows determination of the adequacy of DO$_2$ in relation to VO$_2$. Pump flow is adjusted to maintain DO$_2$ such that the S$\bar{v}$O$_2$ is above the 65% to 70% range. The PaCO$_2$ is inversely proportional to the flow rate of gas ventilating the membrane lung.

Heparin is administered to prevent thrombus formation throughout the ECLS course. The level of anticoagulation is monitored hourly by the whole blood ACT. Many centers maintain the ACT between 180 and 200 seconds.

During the first few hours on bypass pulmonary function and gas exchange are often observed to deteriorate. This is frequently manifested radiologically as bilateral opacification of the lung fields and is likely secondary to the abrupt decrease in the airway pressures employed after onset of ECLS. Application of PEEP levels of 14 cm H_2O may reduce the development of the lung opacification. Aggressive diuresis is frequently instituted approximately 24 hours after initiation of ECLS because total-body water is increased in many patients. Renal function may be transiently impaired during ECLS; therefore, utilization of a hemofilter placed in the circuit to supplement renal water excretion may be necessary. Nutrition remains a high priority in the critically ill patient requiring ECLS and is carried out through parenteral nutrition or enteral feeding.

Over the ensuing days on ECLS, as the cardiopulmonary pathology resolves, the inflammatory process subsides, the pulmonary radiographic appearance improves, and the elevated pulmonary vascular pressures normalize, gas exchange increases across the native lung. The ECLS flow rate is weaned as gas exchange improves based on the $S\bar{v}o_2$ (Fig. 5-19). Simultaneous increases in lung compliance are frequently observed. Discontinuation of ECLS is associated with a final lung compliance of 0.8 mL/cm H_2O/kg or more. Most practitioners transiently discontinue ECLS to determine whether cardiopulmonary function is such that ECLS may be discontinued. This "trial off" is performed during venoarterial bypass by clamping the arterial and venous connectors between the bridge and the patient and allowing recirculation of extracorporeal blood flow through the bridge. Usually it is clear within the first 15 to 30 minutes whether ECLS may be discontinued, although prolonged trials of up to 2 hours may occasionally be required. During venovenous bypass the gas phase of the membrane lung may simply be capped indefinitely so that the patient remains on ECLS but without contribution of the artificial lung to gas exchange.

Once it has been determined that ECLS is to be discontinued, the cannulation site incisions are opened and the right carotid artery and/or internal jugular vein are ligated. Percutaneously placed cannulas may simply be removed and pressure applied without concern for the anticoagulation status of the patient. A number of centers have demonstrated the ability to reconstruct the carotid artery after a course on venoarterial ECLS. Controversy still exists regarding the practice of carotid artery reconstruction because there is no evidence to suggest that it is in fact necessary or beneficial because cerebral blood flow is normal on long-term follow-up. In fact, the ratio of right to left hemispheric cerebral blood flow and the blood velocities in the right and left internal caroid arteries are no different between newborns with reanastomosed or ligated common carotid arteries.

The mean ± SD duration of the ECLS course is 149 ± 162 hours for neonates with respiratory failure and 280 ± 204 hours for children with respiratory failure. Considerations for discontinuing ECLS at times other than when indicated by improvement of cardiopulmonary function include the presence of irreversible brain damage, other lethal organ failure, and uncontrollable bleeding. Those neonates with congenital diaphragmatic hernia or pneumonia and pediatric patients with cardiac or pulmonary failure may require substantially longer periods on ECLS before resolution of the cardiopulmonary process is observed.

Complications

In general, the complications associated with ECLS fall into one of three major categories: (1) bleeding associated with heparinization, (2) technical failure, and (3) neurologic sequelae, a majority of which are secondary to the hypoxia and hemodynamic instability that occurs before onset of ECLS.

Because of systemic heparinization, bleeding complications are the most common and devastating. Intracranial hemorrhage occurs in approximately 13% of neonates, 5% of pediatric patients, and 4% of cardiac patients. It is the most frequent cause of death in newborns managed with ECLS. The incidence of intracranial hemorrhage is clearly increased in patients who are premature, especially in those younger than 37 weeks' gestational age.

The most notable technical complications include the presence of thrombus in the circuit (26%), incorrect cannula positioning (6% to 15%), oxygenator failure (5% to 17%), pump malfunction (1% to 4%), and presence of air in the circuit (6%).

Results and Follow-Up

A total of 25,201 cases have been submitted to the ELSO registry since 1975. Of these, there have been 17,536 cases of neonatal respiratory failure and 2,361 cases of pediatric respiratory failure. The number of cases, diagnosis, and survival for neonatal respiratory support are all demonstrated in Table 5-5. Overall survival is 77%, with the best survival noted among those neonatal patients with the most frequent diagnoses of meconium aspiration syndrome (survival = 94%), respiratory distress syndrome (84%), and persistent pulmonary hypertension of the newborn (79%). Patients with CDH continue to have the poorest survival among those for whom ECLS is applied, likely because of the "irreversible" pulmonary hypoplasia that is associated with that condition. In fact, the survival in patients with CDH requiring ECLS has fallen from a high in 1987 of 71% to the current rate of 54%. The total number of neonatal respiratory ECLS cases peaked with 1,517 cases performed in 1992. There has since been a trend downward such that the total number of neonatal cases in 2000 was 867, likely owing to improved results with neonatal respiratory management, which includes the use of nitric oxide and HFOV.

The experience with patients with pediatric respiratory failure at the University of Michigan demonstrates a survival rate of 73% at that institution since 1988. In addition, patients in the younger age groups demonstrate greater survival rates, including a 100% survival in those infants younger than 1 year of age. The ELSO registry demonstrates that pediatric respiratory cases are accumulating at a rate of 150 to 200 cases per year with an overall survival rate of 55% (Table 5-6). One of the most frequent diagnoses is viral pneumonia, the most predominant being respiratory syncytial virus.

Multiple studies have evaluated the long-term follow-up of newborn and pediatric patients following a course on ECLS. Most have documented normal neurologic function in 70% to 80% of patients. Such studies have demonstrated that neurologic morbidity is no different in

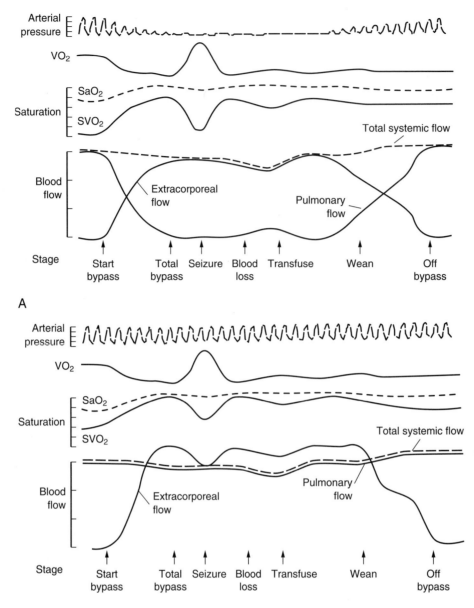

FIGURE 5-19 ▪ **A,** The dynamics of venoarterial bypass as a function of arterial blood pressure, V_{O_2}, Sa_{O_2}, $S\bar{v}_{O_2}$, and blood flow (systemic, pulmonary, and extracorporeal). The systemic arterial pressure wave is inversely proportional to the amount of extracorporeal flow, as is the amount of pulmonary blood flow. Pulmonary blood flow may increase if volume is given and the extracorporeal flow is held constant. An increase in pulmonary blood flow with transfusion may result in a decrease in Sa_{O_2} because of shunting. Total systemic flow is relatively constant unless blood loss occurs. The Sa_{O_2} is a function of the fraction of inspired oxygen blended into the ECMO lung sweep flow and remains proportional to the amount of extracorporeal flow. Changes in $S\bar{v}_{O_2}$ and V_{O_2} may be the only signs of seizure activity during ECMO support. Alterations of V_{O_2} and $S\bar{v}_{O_2}$ reflect the content, delivery, and utilization of delivered arterial oxygen from the ECMO circuit as well as the amount of hemoglobin. **B,** The dynamics of venovenous bypass as a function of arterial blood pressure; V_{O_2}, Sa_{O_2}, $S\bar{v}_{O_2}$, and blood flow (systemic, pulmonary, and extracorporeal). Because venovenous bypass removes blood from, and returns it to, the right atrium, no effect on native cardiac output is incurred. Hence, the arterial pressure wave and the pulmonary and systemic blood flow are independent of the amount of extracorporeal flow. The Sa_{O_2} is proportional to the extracorporeal flow but is at a lower level than during venoarterial bypass because of "recirculation" with admixture of oxygenated and deoxygenated right atrial blood. As with venoarterial bypass, seizure activity will increase V_{O_2} and decrease $S\bar{v}_{O_2}$. In contrast, extracorporeal flow in this instance may decrease presumably because of decreased venous return. (Modified from Chapman RA, Bartlett RH: Extracorporeal Life Support Manual for Adult Patients and Pediatric Patients. Ann Arbor, University of Michigan, 1991.)

TABLE 5-5 ■ Neonatal Cases by Diagnosis			
Primary Diagnosis	Total	No. Survived	% Survived
CDH	3939	2116	54
MAS	6086	5711	94
PPHN/PFC	2542	1999	79
RDS	1340	1126	84
Sepsis	2276	1715	75
Pneumonia	230	133	58
Air leak syndrome	88	60	68
Other	1035	679	68
Total	17,536	13,539	77

CDH, congenital diaphragmatic hernia; MAS, meconium aspiration syndrome; PFC, persistent fetal circulation; PPHN, persistent pulmonary hypertension of the newborn; RDS, respiratory distress syndrome.

TABLE 5-6 ■ Pediatric Cases by Diagnosis			
Primary Diagnosis	Total	No. Survived	% Survived
Viral pneumonia	653	404	62
Bacterial pneumonia	236	122	52
Pneumocystis pneumonia	17	7	41
Aspiration pneumonia	162	105	65
ARDS, postop/trauma	58	35	60
ARDS, not postop/trauma	241	128	53
Acute resp failure, non-ARDS	572	270	47
Other	422	218	52
Total	2361	567	55

ARDS, acute respiratory distress syndrome.

ECLS-managed when compared with CMV-managed newborns. However, children at school age demonstrate an increased risk for academic difficulties and behavioral problems when compared with their normal counterparts.

Bronchopulmonary dysplasia or supplemental oxygen requirement has been observed in 10% to 50% of patients at the time of discharge.

TRACHEAL ACCESS

See Chapter 31 (Disorders of the Upper Airway) for a discussion of intubation and tracheostomy.

SUGGESTED READINGS

Bartlett RH, Roloff DW, Custer JR, et al: Extracorporeal life support: The University of Michigan experience. JAMA 283:904-908, 2000.

Hirschl RB: Mechanical ventilation in pediatric surgical disease. In Ashcraft KW, et al (eds): Pediatric Surgery, 3rd ed. Philadelphia, WB Saunders, 2000.

Hirschl RB, Bartlett RH: Cardiopulmonary critical care and shock. In Oldham KT, et al (eds): Surgery of Infants and Children: Scientific Principles and Practice. Philadelphia, Lippincott-Raven, 1997.

Hirschl RB, Bartlett RH: Extracorporeal life support in cardiopulmonary failure. In O'Neill JA, et al (eds): Pediatric Surgery, vol 2, 5th ed. St. Louis, CV Mosby, 1998.

Zwischenberger JB, Steinhorn RH, Bartlett RH: ECMO: Extracorporeal Cardiopulmonary Support in Critical Care. Ann Arbor, MI, ELSO, 2000.

6

Cardiovascular Considerations

DEVELOPMENT OF THE CARDIOVASCULAR SYSTEM

Cardiovascular Embryology

By necessity, the cardiovascular system is the first to become functional in the embryo. The transfer and distribution of nutrients and oxygen to the rapidly developing fetus by simple diffusion from the placenta is quickly outgrown. Therefore, for the fetus to survive, the fetal heart must simultaneously develop and effectively pump blood to distribute oxygen and nutrients. Beyond the third week of gestation, angiogenic cell clusters form in the chorion, the connecting stalk, and the yolk sac, with the internal cells developing into the primitive red blood cells while the outer cells begin to form the first blood vessels. As the clusters develop into a plexus forming a primitive vasculature, the fetal straight heart tube simultaneously forms by 23 days of gestation (Fig. 6-1). As the tube grows it is forced to bend and form a loop. This looping causes the straight tube to take on the early configuration of the developed heart by 4 weeks of gestation, with the presence of primitive right and left ventricles and atria as well as a truncus arteriosus.

The septa partitioning the atria, the ventricles, and the pulmonary artery/aorta develop between 4 and 6 weeks of gestation (Fig. 6-2). Atrial separation begins when the tissue in the superior aspect of the atria joins with the growing endocardial cushion from below to form the septum primum. A communication between the two atria is maintained throughout gestation first through the ostium primum and then through the ostium secundum as the ostium primum closes. A second septum (septum secundum) forms to the right of the septum primum, which also has a hole (foramen ovale). As can be seen in Figure 6-3, the foramen ovale and ostium secundum with their overlying septa form a competent valve system that permits a right-to-left shunt but not a left-to-right shunt.

The Developing Myocardium

The development of the embryonic heart and great vessels is virtually complete by 8 weeks of gestation. Thus, any cardiac malformations have been established by that time.

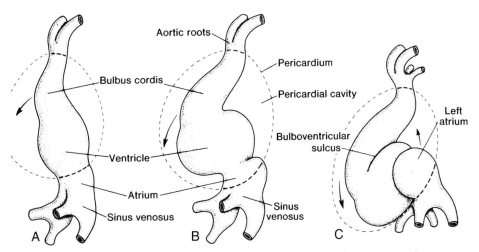

FIGURE 6-1 ■ Formation of the cardiac loop. **A,** At 22 days. **B,** At 24 days. **C,** At 26 days. *Broken lines* indicate the boundary of the pericardium. Note how the straight heart tube folds, creating the primitive atria, ventricles, and truncus arteriosus (bulbus cordis). (Reprinted with permission from Cardiovascular system: Normal development of the heart. In Langman J (ed): Medical Embryology, 3rd ed. Baltimore, Williams & Wilkins, 1975.)

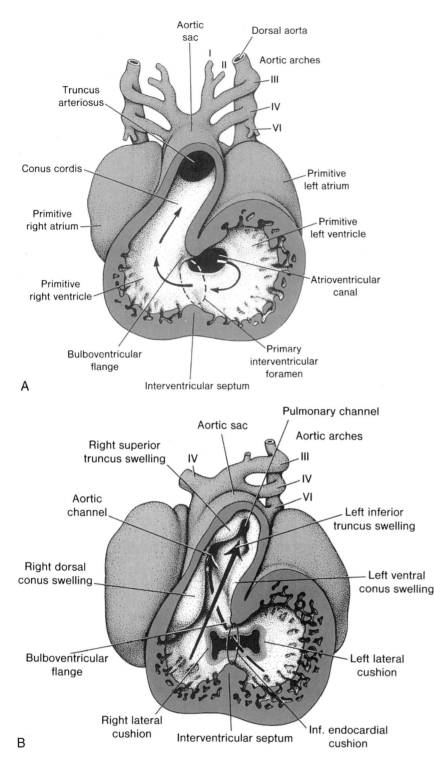

FIGURE 6-2 ■ Frontal section through the heart of a (**A**) 30-day and (**B**) 33-day embryo. The interventricular septum and the bulboventricular flange will join to form the septum between the right and left ventricles as the atrioventricular canal is divided with growth of the endocardial cushions. At the same time, swellings in the truncus arteriosus and conus cordis will fuse to form the pulmonary artery and aorta, associated with the right and left ventricles, respectively. The ring demonstrates the endocardial cushions, which are moving rapidly toward each other in the midline and will shortly fuse. (Reprinted with permission from Cardiovascular system: Normal development of the heart. In Langman J (ed): Medical Embryology, 3rd ed. Baltimore, Williams & Wilkins, 1975.)

However, myocardial maturation continues until at least 1 year after birth. To support rapid cardiac growth, the fetal and neonatal heart has a proportionally greater number of noncontractile elements (nuclei, mitochondria, and endoplasmic reticulum) than are observed in the adult heart: approximately 30% of the fetal myocardium is composed of contractile elements, whereas the adult heart is composed of about 60% contractile elements. The fetal, and to a lesser extent the infant, heart is, therefore, less compliant and less contractile than in older children. As a result, the neonatal heart responds to increased preload with little increase in cardiac output because the heart is relatively stiff and noncompliant and appears to be already working at the peak of its ventricular function curve. The neonatal heart must, therefore, rely almost exclusively on heart rate to increase cardiac output.

Fetal Circulation

Fetal growth and development occur in a relatively hypoxic environment. The placenta is the sole source of oxygen, but blood from the placenta that flows through

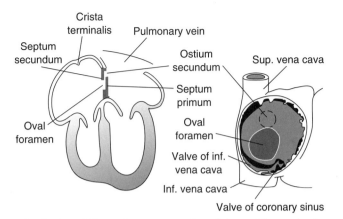

FIGURE 6-3 ■ Schematic representation of the atrial septa in the fetus and newborn. The foramen ovale and ostium secundum with adjacent septa form a flap valve that allows right-to-left, but not left-to-right, flow across the atrial septum. (Reprinted with permission from Cardiovascular system: Normal development of the heart. In Langman J (ed): Medical Embryology, 3rd ed. Baltimore, Williams & Wilkins, 1975.)

the umbilical vein into the fetus is only 65% saturated with oxygen, corresponding to a PO_2 of 35 mm Hg. This blood will mix with blood of even lower oxygen saturation that is returning from the fetal liver (57% saturated), the superior vena cava (40% saturated), and the coronary sinus (25% saturated). The fetus compensates for the hypoxia in a number of ways. First, fetal hemoglobin is 50% saturated (P50) at 18 mm Hg, whereas the P50 of adult hemoglobin is 27 mm Hg. This appears to be caused by a reduced affinity of fetal hemoglobin for 2,3-diphosphoglycerate (2,3-DPG) as compared with adult hemoglobin. This lower P50 allows for more efficient absorption of oxygen from the placenta and higher hemoglobin oxygen saturation at a lower PO_2. Second, fetal cardiac output is approximately three times greater when corrected for weight than that of adults ($\approx$450 mL/kg/min), resulting in greater blood flow to the tissues. The fetal and newborn heart, unlike the adult heart, is also resistant to hypoxia because it depends completely on carbohydrate for metabolism and contains high concentrations of stored glycogen in the myocardial tissues, allowing anaerobic glycolysis to become operative in the setting of hypoxia. In contrast, free fatty acids account for 60% of myocardial metabolism in the adult heart.

Another means for overcoming the relatively hypoxic fetal environment is the configuration of the fetal circulation, which allows partitioning of blood flow to specific areas, resulting in greater efficiency of oxygen delivery (DO_2) to the heart and brain and increased oxygen transfer from the placenta. There are three structures in the fetus that allow this phenomenon to occur: the ductus venosus, the foramen ovale, and the ductus arteriosus. The most saturated fetal blood flows from the placenta (PO_2 = 30 to 35 mm Hg) into the umbilical vein and divides into two streams: half flows through the ductus venosus into the inferior vena cava, and the rest flows into the liver (Fig. 6-4). Thus, blood within the inferior vena cava comprises desaturated blood from the lower body (one third) and relatively well-saturated ductus

venosus blood (two thirds). However, the relatively well-oxygenated blood from the ductus venosus combines with that of the left hepatic vein to form a stream within the inferior vena cava that is preferentially directed across the foramen ovale, thereby directing blood with the highest oxygen levels through the left ventricle to the heart, upper body, and brain (PO_2 = 26 to 28 mm Hg). Right hepatic vein blood, which is less well oxygenated because of mixing with blood from the portal vein, along with the poorly oxygenated inferior and superior vena caval blood flow (PO_2 = 12 to 14 mm Hg), forms a stream that is directed through the tricuspid valve and into the right ventricle. From the right ventricle this blood (PO_2 = 18 to 22 mm Hg) passes into the main pulmonary artery, where the majority shunts across the ductus arteriosus from the right to the left because (1) the pulmonary outflow is a pathway of high resistance as a result of profound pulmonary vasoconstriction and (2) the ductus arteriosus acts as a low-resistance pathway in conjunction with the placenta. Approximately 90% of the right ventricular output, therefore, passes directly across the ductus to perfuse the lower body with 65% of this relatively hypoxic blood flow perfusing the placenta. The remaining 10% of the right ventricular cardiac output passes through the pulmonary artery and through the lungs and collects in the left atrium, where it joins the left ventricular blood flow.

Because of these large shunts and the fact that the lower body is perfused predominantly by the right ventricle, the ventricles can be considered to work in parallel rather than in series as in the adult. The right ventricle ejects two thirds of the total cardiac output, most of which passes across the ductus arteriosus and perfuses the lower body and placenta with relatively hypoxic blood. The left ventricle ejects relatively highly oxygenated blood into the ascending aorta, which perfuses the myocardium, brain, head, upper limbs, and thorax. Only about 10% of its output crosses the isthmus to enter the descending aorta to meet the relatively poorly oxygenated blood that has traversed the ductus arteriosus.

Transitional and Neonatal Circulation

The circulation at birth must adjust to placental separation and the need to use the lungs for gas exchange. To do so, blood flow across the foramen ovale and the ductus arteriosus must cease as the ventricles assume an in-series configuration. This occurs as a result of an increase in systemic resistance and a simultaneous decrease in pulmonary arterial resistance. At the time of birth the low-resistance placenta is removed from the circulation, which results in an abrupt increase in systemic vascular resistance (SVR). The lungs expand, and the neonate begins to breathe the ambient air. As a result of exposure to relatively high oxygen levels along with the mechanical effects from lung expansion, the neonate's pulmonary vasculature simultaneously dilates, resulting in a marked drop in pulmonary vascular resistance. As pressures in the left atrium increase relative to the right, right-to-left flow across the foramen ovale ceases. The flap valve of the foramen ovale actually closes at 3 months of life, although the foramen is found to be probe patent in 20% of humans. In response to the alterations in systemic and

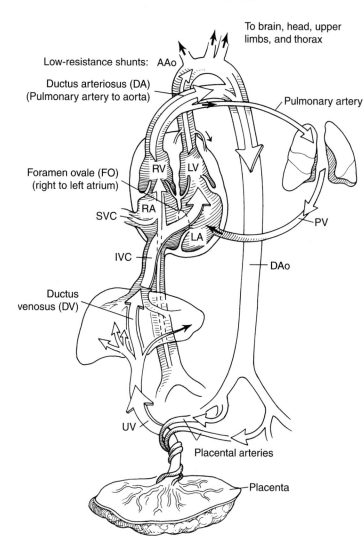

To brain, head, upper limbs, and thorax

Low-resistance shunts: AAo

Ductus arteriosus (DA)
(Pulmonary artery to aorta)

Pulmonary artery

Foramen ovale (FO)
(right to left atrium)

RV   LV

SVC   RA

LA

IVC   PV

DAo

Ductus
venosus (DV)

UV

Placental arteries

Placenta

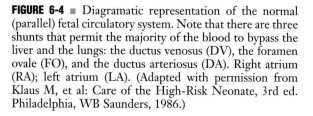

FIGURE 6-4 ■ Diagramatic representation of the normal (parallel) fetal circulatory system. Note that there are three shunts that permit the majority of the blood to bypass the liver and the lungs: the ductus venosus (DV), the foramen ovale (FO), and the ductus arteriosus (DA). Right atrium (RA); left atrium (LA). (Adapted with permission from Klaus M, et al: Care of the High-Risk Neonate, 3rd ed. Philadelphia, WB Saunders, 1986.)

pulmonary arterial resistance, blood flow across the ductus arteriosus, which in utero was right to left, now becomes left to right. At the same time, the ductus vascular smooth muscle contracts in response to increased PaO_2, specifically a PaO_2 greater than 50 mm Hg. Prostaglandins may play a role in this phenomenon because prostaglandin E_2 (PGE_2) relaxes the ductus and the concentration of PGE_2 falls precipitously after birth. The ductus arteriosus functionally closes by 10 to 15 hours and structurally closes and becomes the ligamentum arteriosum at 2 to 3 weeks after birth.

Within minutes of birth, therefore, the pulmonary and aortic circulations are thus converted from a parallel to a series arrangement, with the left ventricle now being responsible for the entire cardiac output of the neonate (350 mL/kg/min), which is much greater than that of the adult (75 mL/kg/min). Blood now flows from both the inferior and superior venae cavae into the right side of the heart and then through the pulmonary artery into the lungs. Because the pressure is now greater on the left side of the heart, there is no shunting through the foramen ovale. Shunting may transiently occur by means of the ductus arteriosus but, unlike with the in utero circulation, the shunt will be from left to right. Blood can now be

oxygenated by the lungs, and oxygenated blood is presented to the left side of the heart for distribution. The right and left ventricles, which are of approximately the same thickness at birth, begin to differentiate over the following weeks as the left ventricle thickens with exposure to the high systemic pressures and the right ventricle begins to thin.

The majority of the decline in pulmonary vascular resistance occurs in the first 2 to 3 days of life. Subsequently, PaO_2 falls at a slower rate owing to thinning of blood vessels and increase in blood vessel number, reaching adult levels by 6 to 8 weeks after birth. The manifestation of cardiac anomalies may be affected by this progressive decrease in pulmonary vascular resistance, preventing the development of obvious symptoms until the pulmonary vascular pressures have fallen to levels low enough to affect flow across a given atrial or ventricular septal defect or other anomaly.

Fetal and newborn pulmonary vessels are muscular and exquisitely sensitive to oxygen levels and, to a lesser extent, the pH of the blood. In the fetus low oxygen levels result in pulmonary vasoconstriction and reduced pulmonary blood flow. In contrast, in the newborn the relatively high oxygen environment leads to pulmonary vascular dilatation, a fall in pulmonary vascular resistance, and an increase in pulmonary blood flow. The exact mechanism that allows oxygen levels to affect pulmonary vasculature tone is unknown. It is not clear whether oxygen may have a direct effect on the musculature or act by stimulating the release of vasoactive substances such as prostacyclin (PGI_2), PGE_2, or nitric oxide (NO).

Persistent Pulmonary Hypertension of the Newborn

In the newborn period the tendency of the pulmonary vasculature to vasoconstrict in response to exogenous influences can be extremely problematic, especially in patients with meconium aspiration, congenital diaphragmatic hernia, or an abnormal distribution or smooth muscle in the pulmonary arteries. In the latter, the thickness of the muscle in the media of the pulmonary arterial system may be increased and smooth muscle may even extend into the normally nonmuscularized arterioles or capillaries. Because the transitional circulation of the newborn is very sensitive to hypoxia, acidosis, and hypercarbia, respiratory insufficiency caused by a number of disorders can result in persistent fetal circulation (PFC) with shunting through the patent foramen ovale and ductus arteriosis owing to vasoconstriction of the pulmonary vasculature and associated pulmonary hypertension (Fig. 6-5). The resulting hypoxia and hypercarbia may induce further vasoconstriction and exacerbate shunting.

Therapy is directed toward addressing any predisposing disease and correcting hypoxia, hypercarbia, and acidosis, usually with intubation and mechanical ventilation. Treatment may include pharmacologic paralysis, maintenance of systemic pressure to retard right-to-left shunting with pressor administration, exogenous surfactant administration, and hyperventilation to reduce pulmonary vasoconstriction by maintenance of PaO_2 slightly greater than 100 mm Hg and $PaCO_2$ approximately 25 mm Hg. However, the latter may be counterproductive and can no longer be recommended because high ventilator pressures are often required, which can be associated with ventilator-induced lung injury (VILI) and the development of chronic lung disease. NO is an endogenous mediator that serves to stimulate guanylate cyclase in the endothelial cell to produce cyclic guanosine monophosphate, which results in relaxation of vascular smooth muscle (Fig. 6-6). NO is rapidly scavenged by heme moieties. As such, inhaled nitric oxide (iNO) serves as a selective vasodilator of the pulmonary circulation because it is inactivated before reaching the systemic circulation. It is diluted in nitrogen and then mixed with blended oxygen and air and administered in doses of from 1 to 80 parts per million (ppm). Multiple studies have confirmed the utility of iNO in increasing oxygenation in newborns with pulmonary hypertension associated with various diagnoses. The Neonatal Inhaled Nitric Oxide Study (NINOS) demonstrated a reduction in oxygen index and a decrease in the use of extracorporeal life support (ECLS) from 55% to 39% among newborns without congenital diaphragmatic hernia with pulmonary hypertension who were treated with either 20 or 80 ppm of iNO. In contrast,

FIGURE 6-5 ■ The pathophysiology of persistent fetal circulation. Venous blood returning to the right heart preferentially flows (shunts) through the patent foramen ovale (PFO) or the patent ductus arteriosus (PDA) in the setting of severe pulmonary hypertension. This results in hypoxia, hypercarbia, and acidosis, which induce further increases in pulmonary hypertension and worsen the shunt. A vicious cycle of pulmonary hypertension and deteriorating gas exchange develops and can lead to the demise of the patient if not interrupted. (Reprinted with permission from Hirschl RB, Heiss K: Cardiopulmonary critical care and shock. In Oldham KT, et al [eds]: Surgery of Infants and Children: Scientific Principles and Practice. Philadelphia, Lippincott-Raven, 1997.)

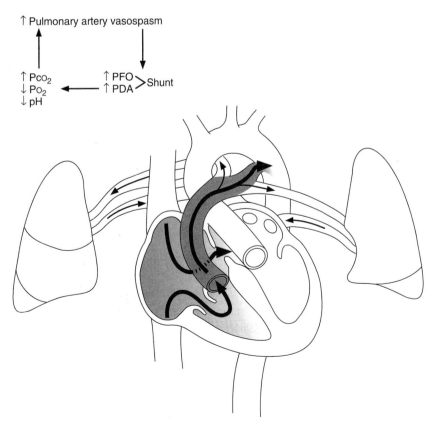

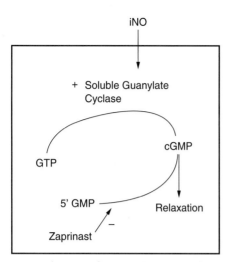

FIGURE 6-6 ■ Mechanism of action of iNO in inducing vascular smooth muscle relaxation. Zaprinast is a phosphodiesterase inhibitor that may increase the potency and duration of the effect of iNO. (Reprinted with permission from Hirschl RB: Innovative therapies in the management of newborns with congenital diaphragmatic hernia. Semin Pediatr Surg 5:255-265, 1996.)

those patients with congenital diaphragmatic hernia demonstrated no effectiveness from iNO administration in a similar study. As described in Chapter 5 (Respiratory Considerations), extracorporeal life support (ECLS, ECMO) may provide life-saving support to newborns with persistent pulmonary hypertension that is refractory to other therapies.

CARDIOVASCULAR MONITORING

Physical Examination

Although monitors are an essential part of the care of the pediatric patient, they are designed to supplement rather than to replace the clinical evaluation of perfusion and intravascular volume. Warmth and color of extremities, capillary refill, assessment of oral and ocular mucous membranes, axillary moistness, urinary output measurement in the patient without renal insufficiency, and the fullness of the anterior fontanelle in the newborn and infant may be integrated with data gained by invasive and noninvasive monitoring to assess the cardiopulmonary status.

Heart Rate

One of the basic procedures is electrocardiographic (ECG) monitoring. ECG monitoring should be used routinely in all critically ill patients to assess heart rate and to monitor for evidence of dysrhythmias, metabolic abnormalities, and myocardial ischemia. However, once routine monitoring raises suspicion for an abnormality, the 12-lead ECG is a much more specific and complete means of evaluation. Typically, ECG leads in older patients are placed on the right upper chest, the left upper chest, and the left lower chest in the anterior axillary line.

The heart rate of the newborn normally varies considerably to adapt to the body's constantly changing metabolic needs and stresses. At 1 week a term infant's heart rate can rise as high as 160 beats per minute when active and awake and 120 beats per minute during quiet, deep sleep. Brief periods of slow rates, as low as 93 beats per minute, are normal. Term infants have an average rate of 145 beats per minute by 3 months and 134 beats per minute at 6 months. The autonomic system is made up of parasympathetic and sympathetic components. The parasympathetic system is fully developed at birth, but the sympathetic system does not completely mature until 4 to 6 months of age. Consequently, vagal reflexes initiated by stimuli such as surgical trauma and airway manipulation may lead to profound bradycardia.

Blood Pressure

Noninvasive blood pressure is measured in critically ill patients using sphygmomanometry; however, invasive means of blood pressure monitoring are preferred in the critically ill patient. The approximate systolic blood pressure is first identified during cuff deflation, after which the cuff should be reinflated to a point just above this level. Subsequent slow deflation of the cuff is performed as the systolic pressure is identified at the point where the first of the Korotkoff sounds are audible. The diastolic pressure is noted at the point where those sounds disappear or are abruptly muffled. A Doppler probe may be useful to ascertain systolic blood pressure in the setting of hypotension, elevated peripheral vascular resistance, and/or poor perfusion by identifying return of pulsatile arterial flow distal to a deflating proximal extremity blood pressure cuff. Automatic blood pressure devices may be programmed to accurately and automatically measure blood pressure at various intervals. The deflating cuff identifies the presence of minute alterations in cuff pressure that are associated with the appearance and disappearance of the Korotkoff sounds and the mean blood pressure at the point of maximum amplitude of such changes.

Mean arterial blood pressure measured directly from an arterial catheter is the most accurate of the systemic pressures measured and the best measurement on which to base clinical decisions. Mean pressure is calculated by assessing the integral of the pulse wave contour during one complete cardiac cycle. The mean arterial pressure measurement is more accurate than isolated systolic and diastolic measurements because mean arterial pressure is less affected by artifacts such as catheter whip and because it does not vary if pressure is measured from a central or a peripheral artery. Distal arteries have a higher systolic and lower diastolic pressure than larger centrally positioned vessels such as the aorta. Mean pressure can also be approximated by adding one third of the pulse pressure (systolic pressure − diastolic pressure) to the diastolic pressure. Arterial access for monitoring is discussed in detail later in this chapter.

Mean blood pressure at birth is 66 mm Hg in term infants and 35 to 40 mm Hg in infants weighing less than 1250 g. Systolic pressure increases by about 1 mm Hg per day in the first 2 weeks, then 2 mm Hg per week during the next 2 weeks. Mean blood pressure reaches 93 mm Hg by 6 months of age. The lower limit of normal systolic blood pressure in children may be approximated by the formula 80 + (2 × age in years).

Central Venous Pressure and Pulmonary Wedge Pressure Monitoring

Central venous pressure (CVP) and pulmonary capillary wedge pressure (PCWP) are two clinical measurements used to assess the volume status of critically ill patients. Low values suggest that blood volume is decreased and that filling volume of the ventricular chambers (preload) is inadequate for efficient cardiac output and tissue perfusion. However, both of these measurements are indirect and in many clinical situations are imprecise reflections of preload. According to Starling's law of myocardial function, as the initial myocardial fiber length increases, the force of contraction of the fiber increases. Myocardial fiber length can best be assessed by measuring left or right ventricular end-diastolic volume (LVEDV). Both CVP and PCWP allow evaluation of LVEDV by indirectly assessing right and left ventricular end-diastolic pressure (RVEDP, LVEDP), respectively, CVP by measuring pressure in the right atrium, and PCWP by measuring left atrial pressure (LAP).

Central Venous Pressure

CVP monitoring is commonly used in newborns and young children because of the difficulty in placing a pulmonary artery catheter and measuring PCWP in these small patients. A catheter is passed into the superior vena cava to lie at the junction of the atrium and the cava or in the atrium itself. It is usually placed percutaneously, although a cutdown may be required in smaller patients. It is assumed that right atrial pressure is an accurate reflection of right ventricular pressure and that right ventricular pressure reflects right ventricular end-diastolic volume (RVEDV) or preload. However, such conclusions are dependent on right ventricular compliance being normal. In addition, because tissue perfusion is ultimately determined principally by left ventricular output, the most significant preload to assess is left ventricular preload rather than right ventricular preload. Only if there is parallel function between the right and left ventricle, there is no pulmonary disease, and there are no shunts can it be assumed that right atrial pressure is an accurate

reflection of left ventricular volume. Fortunately such is the case in many newborns and children.

Ventilation affects right atrial and ventricular volume and, as such, measurements should be made at a constant point in the ventilatory cycle, usually at end expiration. End-expiratory pressure is the most representative of the patient's vascular volume because it is relatively independent of the ventilatory status. This is especially true during mechanical ventilation because positive pressure is least at end expiration and allows, therefore, the truest assessment of CVP. The effects of positive-pressure ventilation on the CVP can be negated by briefly taking the patient off the ventilator during pressure assessment. Normally pressures vary between 5 and 15 mm Hg. Pneumothorax, abdominal distention, and pericardial tamponade are conditions that may falsely elevate the CVP.

Pulmonary Capillary Wedge Pressure

The right atrial pressure in children often accurately represents the left ventricular volume status and, therefore, left ventricular preload. However, in the setting of sepsis, the acute respiratory distress syndrome (ARDS) with application of high ventilator pressures, pulmonary hypertension, pulmonary embolus, pulmonary fibrosis, and cardiac dysfunction, the assessment of the LAP as an approximation of LVEDV may be necessary. When a pulmonary artery catheter is passed into the peripheral pulmonary artery and the balloon just proximal to the tip is inflated, the pressure reflected by the end opening in the catheter measures pulmonary venous pressure, or the PCWP, which is the same as LAP because the pulmonary veins have no valves. It is then assumed that LAP is a reflection of LVEDP and is, therefore, related to LVEDV or preload (Fig. 6-7). Determination of the LAP is important for two reasons. First, pulmonary capillary pressure, which is a determinant of the hydrostatic forces resulting in pulmonary edema, is approximated by the LAP. A pulmonary capillary pressure greater than 25 mm Hg in normal lungs and greater than 18 mm Hg in the setting of sepsis and ARDS will frequently result in the development of pulmonary edema. Second, based on the Starling principle of the heart, one would wish to optimize LVEDP

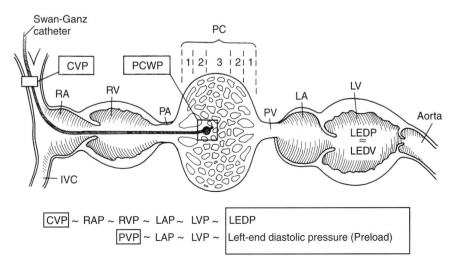

FIGURE 6-7 ■ A simplified scheme of the position of a pulmonary artery catheter and the relationship of CVP and PCWP to cardiac preload. CVP, central venous pressure; RAP, right atrial pressure; RVP, right ventricular pressure; LAP, left atrial pressure; LVP, left ventricular pressure; LEDP, left ventricular end-diastolic pressure; IVC, inferior vena cava; RA, right atrium; RV, right ventricle; PA, pulmonary artery; PCWP, pulmonary capillary wedge pressure; PC, pulmonary capillary; PV, pulmonary vein; LA, left atrium; LV, left ventricle.

as a reflection of LVEDV to enhance cardiac contractility. Unless cardiac compliance is altered, such as in congenital heart disease, sepsis, restrictive pericarditis, or cardiomyopathy or if mitral valve disease is present, the LAP will accurately reflect LVEDP and LVEDV.

By convention, PCWP is assessed at end expiration because intrathoracic pressures at this point are closest to atmospheric pressure, thus minimizing the effect of ventilation on PCWP measurements. Application of PEEP may result in overestimation of LAP. This effect is variable and less significant in the injured, noncompliant lung. In such patients, PCWP will exceed the LAP by only approximately 1 mm Hg for every 5 cm H_2O increase in applied PEEP. For this reason, and because of the potential of alveolar collapse and deterioration in gas exchange that may accompany even transient periods of ventilator disconnect in the patient with severe respiratory insufficiency, PCWP should be measured with such patients on the mechanical ventilator.

Accurate positioning of the catheter in the pulmonary artery is important for the proper assessment of wedge pressure. If the catheter is in the nondependent West's zone 1 or 2, alveolar pressure is greater than alveolar capillary pressure during at least a portion of the ventilatory cycle and, as a result, PCWP may reflect airway pressure rather than LAP. In zone 3, which is the dependent portion of the lung, alveolar capillary pressure exceeds alveolar pressure throughout the respiratory cycle. Thus, the PCWP accurately correlates with LAP. Most of the lung resides in zone 3 when the patient is supine and the majority of pulmonary artery catheters preferentially flow into zone 3 when the balloon is inflated. A chest radiograph should be performed to confirm that the tip of the catheter is located at or below the level of the left atrium.

Cardiac Output

Cardiac output is the amount of blood pumped to the peripheral tissues per unit of time, usually measured in liters per minute. It is often normalized to body weight or body surface area. When cardiac output is divided by surface area, it is referred to as the cardiac index. Measurement of cardiac output is a valuable means of assessing the functional capability of the heart. Normal PCWP and CVP suggest that the "tank is full" and preload is adequate. Cardiac output measurement is helpful in deciding whether the heart is pumping satisfactorily and, therefore, delivering oxygen efficiently. Low readings may prompt the administration of inotropic agents. Once cardiac output has been measured, SVR can be calculated by dividing the difference between the mean aortic blood pressure and the mean right atrial pressure by the cardiac output. Myocardial contractility is indirectly related to afterload, which represents the force against which the ventricle must push to eject blood, with increased afterload inducing a decrease in contractility and vice versa. A high SVR that increases afterload is most often secondary to heart failure or hypovolemia. Attempts to decrease afterload using vasodilator therapy may be beneficial when cardiac output remains reduced despite adequate volume administration.

The inotropic state of the heart reflects the ability of the heart muscles to shorten and eject blood. Ejection fraction is a common measurement of contractility.

Poor contractility can occur in the presence of acidemia, hypoxemia, sepsis, and congenital heart disease. Poor cardiac function that persists after optimization of preload, afterload, and correction of hypoxemia and acidosis necessitates the use of inotropic agents such as dopamine, dobutamine, amrinone, and epinephrine.

Clinical measurement of cardiac output is usually done using a pulmonary artery catheter and the thermodilution technique. The indicator is a cool saline solution. A bolus is injected through the right atrial port of the pulmonary artery catheter, although the indicator may be injected into any central venous port. The indicator mixes with blood in the right ventricle and is then assessed by a thermistor located at the tip of the pulmonary artery catheter. Once the initial blood temperature, the volume of injectate, the injectate temperature, and the change in blood temperature as a function of time are known, cardiac output can be determined. Before injection the right ventricle pumps warm blood into the pulmonary artery, where it meets the thermistor and is recorded. After injection the cool bolus of saline solution mixed with blood approaches the thermistor and the cooler blood temperature is measured. As the bolus passes, the blood gradually warms again. These temperature changes over time are measured by the thermistor and are recorded as a bell-shaped curve (Fig. 6-8). The area under the curve is inversely proportional to cardiac output. If the cardiac

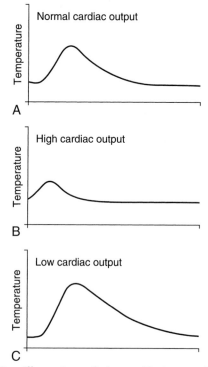

FIGURE 6-8 ▪ Illustration of thermodilution cardiac output determination during periods of normal (**A**), high (**B**), and low (**C**) cardiac output. The magnitude and duration of the change in temperature are inversely proportional to the cardiac output. (Reprinted with permission from Hirschl RB, Heiss K: Cardiopulmonary critical care and shock. In Oldham KT, et al [eds]: Surgery of Infants and Children: Scientific Principles and Practice. Philadelphia, Lippincott-Raven, 1997.)

output is high, then the decrease in blood temperature will be small and sustained only for a short period of time. In contrast, if the cardiac output is low, the decrease in blood temperature will be relatively greater and result in a longer period of temperature reduction. A microprocessor in the monitoring equipment integrates the area under the curve and calculates the cardiac output. Accuracy of the thermodilution technique relies on rapid injection rates, an accurate measurement of the injectate temperature and volume, and the absence of shunting. It is important to inject the bolus rapidly. The colder the indicator solution, the greater the signal. However, iced fluid tends to warm during passage through conduit tubing and intravascular portions of the catheter. For this reason, room temperature injectate-determined cardiac outputs are no less accurate than those assessed using iced saline injections. In general, 5-mL injectate volumes are used, except in infants and small children in whom 1-mL saline injections are preferred. In practice, cardiac output measurements are performed at least in triplicate at the same point in the ventilatory cycle, usually end expiration, with any irregular curves discarded. The remaining three individual measurements are averaged as the result with an overall accuracy of ± 10%.

Unfortunately, measurement of cardiac output by the thermodilution technique by means of a pulmonary artery catheter is usually not applicable to newborns. The smallest catheter that is equipped with a balloon to float the catheter into the pulmonary artery and ports for injection of cold saline solution and measuring of pulmonary wedge pressure is 5F. These catheters are too large for small premature infants and are difficult to place in the pulmonary artery even term infants. In addition, the presence of right-to-left or left-to-right shunts across the foramen ovale and/or ductus arteriosus interferes with the dilution of the cold saline and accurate assessment of cardiac output by the thermodilution technique. In newborns, however, CVP assessment and echocardiographic evaluation of cardiac filling often serve as reasonable assessments of volume status.

Mixed Venous Oxygen Saturation

The oxygen hemoglobin saturation in mixed venous pulmonary artery blood is referred to as the $S\bar{v}O_2$ and reflects the balance between the amount of oxygen delivered to the tissues and the amount consumed. Oxygen delivery (DO_2) is the volume of oxygen delivered to the tissues each minute and is calculated by multiplying cardiac output by the arterial oxygen content. Oxygen consumption (VO_2) is the amount of tissue oxygen consumed. As DO_2 increases or VO_2 decreases, more oxygen remains in the venous blood. The result is an increase in $S\bar{v}O_2$. In contrast, if DO_2 decreases or VO_2 increases, relatively more oxygen is extracted from the blood and, therefore, less oxygen remains in the venous blood. A decrease in $S\bar{v}O_2$ is the result. The $S\bar{v}O_2$ serves as an excellent monitor of oxygen kinetics because it specifically assesses the adequacy of oxygen delivery in relation to oxygen consumption (DO_2/VO_2 ratio). True $S\bar{v}O_2$ is best determined by assessing pulmonary artery blood because it is a composite of blood from the entire venous drainage of the body

and has been thoroughly mixed by the action of the right ventricle. This is untrue, however, if a large left-to-right shunt empties saturated blood into the right side of the heart or the pulmonary artery. Many pulmonary arterial catheters now contain fiberoptic bundles that provide continuous mixed venous oximetry data. An emitted light is reflected from circulating red blood cells and transmitted by the receiving fiberoptic bundle to an analyzer where the data on the reflected light at three wavelengths are assessed to provide accurate determination of hemoglobin oxygen saturation. Continuous $S\bar{v}O_2$ monitoring provides a means for assessing the adequacy of DO_2, early identification of cardiopulmonary instability, and rapid assessment of the response to therapy (Table 6-1). A decrease in $S\bar{v}O_2$ to less than 65% or a reduction in $S\bar{v}O_2$ of more than 5% to 10% should be investigated by assessing the factors that determine the $S\bar{v}O_2$, cardiac output, SaO_2, and hemoglobin level, with consideration for variables that might result in an increase in VO_2. The accuracy of $S\bar{v}O_2$ monitoring may be diminished under certain circumstances where arteriovenous shunting occurs, such as in the occasional patient with cirrhosis or sepsis. Importantly, this means that in situations in which vasoregulation is altered, the $S\bar{v}O_2$ may be normal though the DO_2 at the tissue level is inadequate. Further details with regard to the $S\bar{v}O_2$ can be found in Chapter 5 (Respiratory Considerations).

SHOCK

Shock is a clinical state in which the cardiopulmonary system fails to adequately deliver oxygen to and remove metabolic waste and carbon dioxide from the peripheral tissues. However, the hypoperfusion associated with shock in the pediatric population is only associated with changes in peripheral blood pressure very late in the course. Because of a child's remarkable ability to vasoconstrict, SVR can become quite high and adequate blood pressure maintained until intravascular volume or cardiac output

TABLE 6-1 ■ Causes of Increased or Decreased S$\bar{v}O_2$		
S$\bar{v}O_2$	Cause	Condition
High (>80%)	Oxygen content increased	Inspired oxygen (FIO_2) increase
	Oxygen consumption decreased	Hypothermia, paralysis, anesthesia
	Cardiac output increased	Septic shock, vasodilation
	Left-to-right shunting	Congenital heart disease, cirrhosis
Low (<65%)	Decreased oxygen content	Anemia, respiratory failure, other causes of hypoxia
	Oxygen consumption increased	Hyperthermia, sepsis
	Cardiac output decreased	Arrhythmias, tamponade, tension pneumothorax, cardiogenic shock, high positive end-expiratory pressure

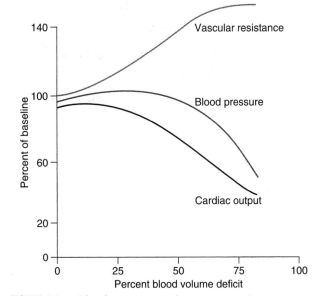

FIGURE 6-9 ■ Blood pressure, cardiac output, and systemic vascular resistance are shown in relation to progressive hypovolemia in children. Blood pressure is initially compromised after 30% to 40% volume depletion and only after all other hemodynamic reserve is exhausted. (Reprinted with permission from Hirschl RB, Heiss K: Cardiopulmonary critical care and shock. In Oldham KT, et al [eds]: Surgery of Infants and Children: Scientific Principles and Practice. Philadelphia, Lippincott-Raven, 1997.)

drops to 30% to 40% below normal levels (Fig. 6-9). At that point, blood pressure precipitously drops and vascular collapse ensues.

Low Cardiac Output States

As demonstrated in Figure 6-10, shock is usually accompanied by either a reduction in cardiac output with an increase in SVR (e.g., hypovolemic, obstructive, or cardiogenic shock) or an increase in cardiac output with a reduction in blood pressure secondary to a decrease in SVR (e.g., anaphylactic, neurogenic, endocrinologic, or septic shock; Table 6-2). A decrease in cardiac output in the setting of shock will be due to a reduction in either heart rate or stroke volume. Stroke volume, in turn, is affected by myocardial contractility, preload volume, and afterload status. Conditions with decreased cardiac output and low preload volume are usually due to hypovolemia from either hemorrhage or dehydration. Although primary cardiac disease is uncommon in pediatrics, with the exception of congenital heart disease states and occasionally cardiomyopathy, in general, it presents as increased preload accompanied by poor contractility, poor cardiac output, and decreased DO_2. Valvular heart disease, resulting from either a stenotic or regurgitant valve, may result in heart failure with a decrease in cardiac output and an increase in filling pressures. An additional cause of increased preload and decreased cardiac output is obstructive shock, which includes cardiac tamponade and tension pneumothorax. The acute filling of the pericardial space with fluid or blood or the presence of increased pressure in the hemithorax and resulting mediastinal shift result in decreased venous return

to the right side of the heart. Similar findings may be observed in patients with ARDS owing to the adverse effect of ventilator pressure on cardiac function.

Minimal monitoring in the setting of impaired perfusion would include serial blood pressure evaluations and vital signs in addition to continuous ECG monitoring. Important physical findings indicating poor perfusion or hypovolemia include poor skin turgor, cool extremities with pale color, a flat anterior fontanelle, dry mucous membranes, and capillary refill of more than 2 seconds (Fig. 6-11). More serious indicators of hypoperfusion include collapsed peripheral veins; a rapid, weak pulse; tachypneic, shallow breaths; cool extremities; and a reduction in glomerular filtration rate and renal blood flow as manifested by a reduction in urine output. A change in the level of consciousness of the patient such as restlessness, anxiety, agitation, or unresponsiveness suggests greatly impaired DO_2. Once again, it is important to recognize that hypoperfusion in children is often accompanied by a normal blood pressure until the point has been reached where complete hemodynamic collapse supervenes.

In the majority of instances in neonatal and pediatric patients hypoperfusion is secondary to low cardiac output due to hypovolemia and preload reduction. Volume resuscitation should be initiated with administration of repeated 10 mL/kg doses of crystalloid or 5% albumin (controversial) over 15- to 20-minute time periods until hypotension and hypoperfusion resolve. It is not unusual for the hypovolemic, hypoperfused patient to require 40 to 60 mL/kg of crystalloid before resuscitation is adequate. Transfusion may be required to enhance oxygen-carrying capacity when the hemoglobin value is less than 13 g/dL in neonates and less than 7 to 10 g/dL in older infants and children in whom a normal cardiac output and SaO_2 can be achieved. A hemoglobin level greater than 13 g/dL should be maintained in those patients with compromise in SaO_2 or cardiac output to optimize DO_2 (Fig. 6-12).

A CVP of more than 10 to 15 mm Hg is usually associated with sufficient volume repletion. Persistent shock despite volume administration should lead one to suspect ongoing blood loss or additional causes of hypotension such as cardiac tamponade, tension pneumothorax, adrenocortical insufficiency, sepsis, neurogenic shock, or anaphylaxis (see later). The presence of additional organ system failure and/or persistence of hypoperfusion despite adequate resuscitation may be an indication for pulmonary arterial catheter placement for purposes of assessing pulmonary arterial and LAP, $S\bar{v}O_2$, and cardiac output. Such invasive information is critical in establishing the contribution of alterations in cardiac output or vascular tone to the shock state and the need for pharmacologic intervention. In patients who are too young for pulmonary artery catheter monitoring or in whom the etiology of cardiac insufficiency remains unclear, echocardiography is a safe and noninvasive method for assessing cardiac function, ventricular filling, and the presence of congenital heart disease or pericardial effusion.

An increased heart rate is the child's most common and effective way of increasing cardiac output and DO_2. However, extremes in cardiac rate induce their own form of pathophysiology. For example, pathologic tachycardia can prevent adequate time for complete atrial filling and

SHOCK

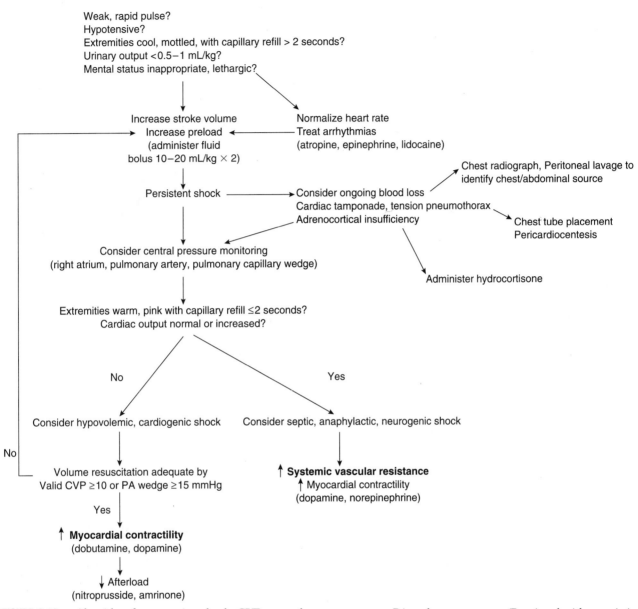

FIGURE 6-10 ■ Algorithm for managing shock. CVP, central venous pressure; PA, pulmonary artery. (Reprinted with permission from Hirschl RB: Cardiopulmonary critical care and shock. In Oldham KT, et al [eds]: Surgery of Infants and Children: Scientific Principles and Practice. Philadelphia, Lippincott-Raven, 1997.)

	Cardiac Output	Pulmonary Capillary Wedge Pressure	Systemic Vascular Resistance
TABLE 6-2 ■ Hemodynamic Profile during Various Conditions			
Septic shock*	↑	↓	↓
Cardiogenic shock	↓	↑	↑
Hypovolemia	↓	↓	↑

*Hyperdynamic phase.

can impair cardiac output. Arrhythmias contributing to the hypoperfused state should be treated. Arrhythmias can be classified into those that are too fast, too slow, or disorganized/absent and into those that are atrial or ventricular in origin (Fig. 6-13). Atrial tachyarrhythmias typically are caused by either sinus tachycardia or supraventricular tachycardia (SVT), which can be differentiated by absent or abnormal P wave and a higher rate (>220 beats per minute in infants or >180 beats per minute in children) in the setting of SVT (Fig. 6-14). Sinus tachycardia is usually associated with an underlying

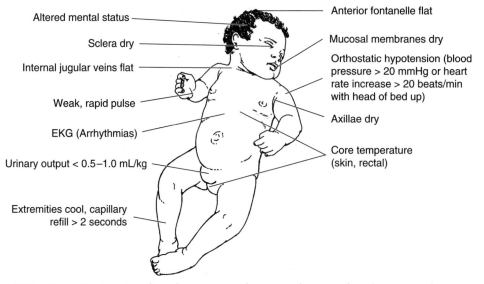

FIGURE 6-11 ■ Noninvasive clinical parameters that are indicative of inadequate perfusion or hypovolemia.

cause (fever, agitation, hypovolemia, pain, tamponade, tension pneumothorax) that must be identified and treated. Most children maintain hemodynamic stability with SVT that, therefore, can be treated with adenosine (first dose: 0.1 mg/kg, maximum 6 mg; repeat dose: 0.2 mg/kg, maximum 12 mg) on an emergent, rather than urgent, basis. Ventricular tachycardia is more hazardous and should be managed promptly with intravenous amiodarone (5 mg/kg) or lidocaine 1 mg/kg followed by a 20- to 50-µg/kg/minute lidocaine infusion (see Fig. 6-14).

Any arrhythmia associated with hemodynamic instability should be immediately attended to by synchronized cardioversion or defibrillation at a first dose of 0.5 to 1 J/kg and a second at 2 J/kg. Bradyarrhythmias are often

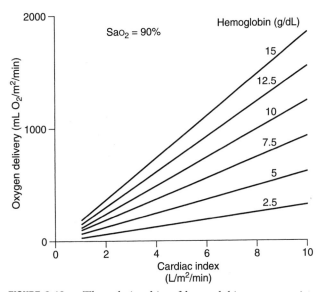

FIGURE 6-12 ■ The relationship of hemoglobin concentration and cardiac index to oxygen delivery at a constant $SaO_2 = 90\%$. Note the strong influence of hemoglobin concentration on DO_2. (Adapted with permission from Hirschl RB, Heiss K: Cardiopulmonary critical care and shock. In Oldham KT, et al [eds]: Surgery of Infants and Children: Scientific Principles and Practice. Philadelphia, Lippincott-Raven, 1997.)

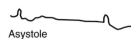

Sinus tachycardia

Supraventricular tachycardia

Ventricular tachycardia

Course ventricular fibrillation

Fine ventricular fibrillation

Asystole

FIGURE 6-13 ■ Electrocardiographic findings demonstrating the regular rhythm and P, QRS, and T sequence of sinus tachycardia at 180 beats per minute; the rapid, regular rhythm of supraventricular tachycardia at 320 beats per minute; the wide QRS complex of ventricular tachycardia; the disorganized depolarizations of coarse ventricular fibrillation and fine ventricular fibrillation; and the flat line ECG of asystole. (Adapted with permission from Chameides L: Textbook of Pediatric Advanced Life Support. Dallas, American Heart Association, 1994.)

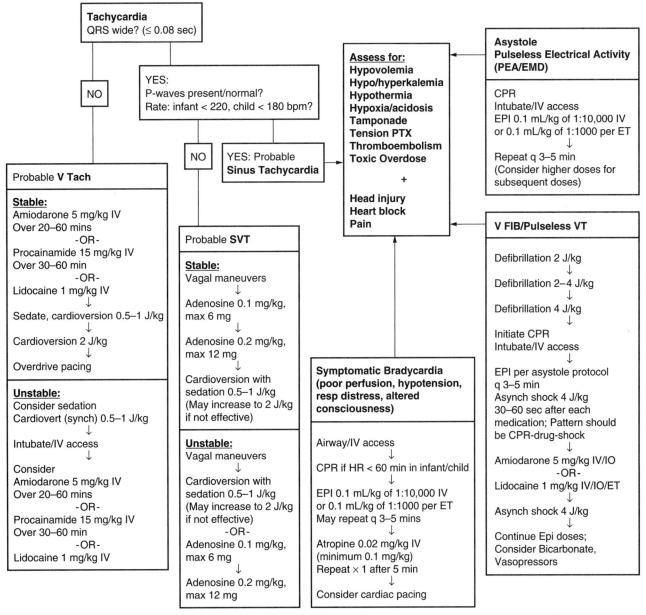

FIGURE 6-14 ■ Cardiac arrest algorithms. Protocols are demonstrated for patients in asystole; pulseless electrical activity (PEA) or electromechanical dissociation (EMD); bradycardia; ventricular fibrillation (V FIB); pulseless ventricular tachycardia (VT); stable ventricular tachycardia (V TACH) or V TACH with hemodynamic compromise; and supraventricular tachycardia (SVT). J, Joules; synch, synchronous; asynch, asynchronous; EPI, epinephrine. (Adapted with permission from Pediatric Advanced Life Support (PALS): Year 2000 Guidelines Analysis. Circulation, Supplement for August 22, 2000, vol 102, pp 291-342.)

secondary to inadequate ventilation and oxygenation (see Fig. 6-14). Less often, slow rhythms may be secondary to vagal stimulation, sinus node abnormalities, heart block, hypercalcemia, or hypermagnesemia. Vagal maneuvers such as ice water applied to the face or having the patient perform the Valsalva maneuver should be attempted first. Administration of epinephrine, 0.1 mL/kg of 1:10,000 IV or 0.1 mL/kg of 1:1000, through the endotracheal tube will usually result in an increase in heart rate and contractility. If it does not, atropine, 0.02 mg/kg with a minimum dose of 0.1 mg/kg, should be given. Atropine should be administered primarily when bradycardia is thought to

be secondary to increased vagal tone or primary atrioventricular block. If medical therapy is not effective at resolving the bradycardia, cardiac pacing may be required. Bradycardia in a child is often a reflection of a prearrest state. If not corrected, the low heart rate can progress to asystole. As such, the appearance of bradycardia in a pediatric patient should prompt immediate and aggressive resuscitative measures.

For patients in cardiogenic shock (low cardiac output and high SVR), appropriate intravascular volume resuscitation is best followed by administration of the synthetic, selective β-adrenergic agent dobutamine (Table 6-3).

Myocardial contractility, stroke volume, and cardiac output typically increase and the PCWP falls. Infusions are titrated from initial doses of 2 to 5 μg/kg/min until the desired effect is achieved or a maximum of 20 μg/kg/min is reached. Minimal alteration in heart rate or SVR is noted with dobutamine, although myocardial oxygen consumption is usually increased. Epinephrine at doses of 0.1 to 1.0 μg/kg/min may be used to provide potent α- and β-adrenergic effects in patients who are unresponsive to either dopamine or dobutamine infusions.

Patients with cardiogenic shock and elevated SVR may benefit from administration of a systemic vasodilator to reduce cardiac afterload resistance, decrease myocardial stroke work, and increase stroke volume. In addition to cardiac output, the associated reductions in right and left atrial pressure may enhance gas exchange if myocardial dysfunction is associated with pulmonary edema. A systemic vasodilator such as sodium nitroprusside (initial dose: 0.2 to 0.5 μg/kg/min; maximum 10 μg/kg/min) may be utilized in conjunction with pressors to enhance myocardial function and cardiac output (Table 6-4). Milrinone is a phosphodiesterase inhibitor that effectively enhances cardiac contractility while inducing systemic arterial vasodilation. The loading dose of milrinone is 50 μg/kg over 10 minutes followed by a continuous infusion at between 0.375 and 0.75 μg/kg/min.

TABLE 6-3 ■ Cardiovascular Inotropic Agents

Drug	Dosage	Action	Adverse Reaction	Comments
Dopamine	2-5 μg/kg/min IV	Dopamine agonist Increases renal and splanchnic arterial blood flow Peripheral venoconstriction	Tachydysrhythmias	Treat extravasation with phentolamine (Regitine) Ensure that volume status is appropriate before modcrate or high doses
	5-10 μg/kg/min IV	β-Adrenergic agonist Increases cardiac output and heart rate Peripheral vasodilation	Hypotension Tachycardia	Preterm infants or neonates may not respond to conventional low-dose renal therapy and
	10-20 μg/kg/min IV	α-Adrenergic agonist Systemic vasoconstriction Decreases renal blood flow Increases blood pressure and myocardial oxygen consumption	Hypertension Cardiac arrhythmias Renal failure	may require higher doses Tolerance may develop with prolonged use (>3 days) Toxicity accentuated in the presence of hepatic or renal dysfunction
Dobutamine	2-20 μg/kg/min IV	β₂-Adrenergic stimulant Increases myocardial contractility Peripheral vasodilation	Tachycardia that may be more pronounced in younger children Hypotension from vasodilation Hypertension Dysrhythmias	Less effect on heart rate in comparison with dopamine Often used in conjunction with dopamine
Isoproterenol (Isuprel)	0.1-1.0 μg/kg/min IV	Pure β-adrenergic agent Increases contractility and heart rate Peripheral vasodilator	Hypotension Tachycardia Tachydysrhythmias	Do not use with digoxin
Norepinephrine (Levophed)	0.05-1.0 μg/kg/min IV	Adrenergic inotrope Profound vasoconstrictor Increases myocardial contractility and peripheral vascular resistance	May cause tissue and organ ischemia	May need to be used in combination with a vasodilator
Milrinone	50 μg/kg IV over 10 min then 0.375-0.75 μg/kg/min	Phosphodiesterase inhibitor	Dysrhythmias	Long half-life (4-6 hours)
Epinephrine	0.1 mL/kg of 1:10,000 IV, IO, or 0.1 mL/kg of 1:1000 ET every 3-5 min IV infusion 0.1-1.0 μg/kg/min	α and β Stimulant Increases peripheral vascular resistance Increases myocardial contractility Increases heart rate Increases mesenteric and renal vasoconstriction Bronchodilator	Tachydysrhythmias Ventricular dysrhythmias Renal ischemia Bradycardia	Ineffective if pH is <7.1 Higher dose required in the presence of acidosis

These drugs have a varied affect on systemic vascular resistance. IV, intravenous; IO, intraosseous; ET, per endotracheal tube.

TABLE 6-4 ■ Vasodilators Used to Reduce Systemic Vascular Resistance and Cardiac Afterload				
Drug	Dosage	Action	Adverse Reaction	Comments
Nitroprusside (Nipride)	0.5-10 μg/kg/min	Antihypertensive Reduces afterload	Hypotension Metabolic acidosis Thrombocytopenia Cyanide toxicity	Increases intracranial pressure Nitroprusside is metabolized to thiocyanate Cardiac output may increase, decrease, or be unchanged depending on preload and afterload Rebound hypertension may occur when weaning
Prostaglandin E_1	0.05-0.1 μg/kg/min	Maintains patency of ductus arteriosus Potent pulmonary vasodilator with some peripheral effects	Apnea Fever Seizures Cutaneous vasodilation Inhibition of platelet aggregation Hypoglycemia Hypotension Hypercalcemia	Apnea may occur several hours after the initiation of prostaglandin E_1 infusion

Normal or High Cardiac Output, Decreased Systemic Vascular Resistance States

Systemic hypotension with normal or increased cardiac output and decreased vascular resistance is known as distributive shock and includes such conditions as sepsis, anaphylaxis, adrenocortical insufficiency, and neurogenic shock. Although myocardial function may be compromised in early sepsis after exposure to an infectious source, the pathophysiology is dominated by the release of vasorelaxing mediators that induce a decrease in systemic vascular tone. Patients with anaphylaxis to an inhaled, ingested, or intravenously administered substance or neurogenic shock due to a high spinal cord injury are noted to be warm and well perfused but with a low blood pressure in the absence of tachycardia. The hypotension may not respond to volume alone, requiring pressor administration to attain an acceptable blood pressure. Normal adrenocortical function is required to support vascular tone. Patients with adrenal insufficiency can experience vascular collapse, requiring administration of hydrocortisone to facilitate return of normal vascular tone and perfusion.

Patients with hypotension and reduced SVR are managed best initially with a continuous intravenous infusion of dopamine. Dopamine is an endogenous catecholamine that results in enhancement of renal and splanchnic blood flow at doses between 1 and 5 μg/kg/min. β-Adrenergic receptor effects become apparent between 5 and 10 μg/kg/min, and α-adrenergic receptor–induced vasoconstriction develops at doses between 10 and 20 μg/kg/min. Therefore, dopamine provides enhancement of myocardial contractility at lower doses but splanchnic and peripheral vasoconstriction at higher infusion rates. Complications of dopamine administration are relatively few. These include the induction of arrhythmias, peripheral ischemia at high infusion rates, and skin loss after extravasation. At times, dopamine infusion may be inadequate to produce the desired hemodynamic response. Such patients may benefit from the infusion of norepinephrine to further enhance vasoconstriction and increase blood pressure.

Doses in the range of 0.05 to 1.0 μg/kg/min are typical. Total-body oxygen consumption and carbon dioxide production increase between 15% and 30% with the use of dopamine, epinephrine, and norepinephrine in normal adults. In the setting of anaphylaxis, treatment includes administration of diphenhydramine, 1 to 2 mg/kg, and/or epinephrine, 0.01 mL/kg of 1:1000 by subcutaneous or intramuscular injection. In the setting of hypotension due to adrenocortical insufficiency, hydrocortisone, 1 to 2 mg/kg, should be administered.

Treatment of Metabolic Acidosis

Lactic acidosis is often observed in the setting of shock as the glycolytic pathway production of adenosine triphosphate predominates. Because of the untoward effect of metabolic acidosis on both myocardial function and the efficacy of administered inotropes, a pH less than 7.20 should be corrected by hyperventilation if the $Paco_2$ is more than 40 mm Hg and/or by administration of intravenous sodium bicarbonate, 1 to 2 mEq/kg (Table 6-5). The total bicarbonate deficit may be calculated by the following:

Total HCO_3^- deficit (mEq) = Base deficit (mEq/L) × Weight (kg) × 0.3. One half of this dose may be given over 1 to 2 hours followed by administration of the reminder over the ensuing 24 to 48 hours if indicated. Administration of sodium bicarbonate in the setting of hypoventilation may result in hypercarbia due to production of CO_2. Therefore, in patients in whom hypercarbia may be of concern, *tris*-hydroxymethylaminomethane (THAM) may serve as an effective buffer in the setting of metabolic acidosis. A 3.6% solution of THAM (tromethamine) may be administered at a dose of 3 to 5 mL/kg. The total dose over 24 hours should not exceed 40 mL/kg. Adverse effects may include hypoglycemia, as well as hyperkalemia, hypervolemia, and hypernatremia; for this reason, THAM should be utilized with caution in patients with renal insufficiency.

Optimizing $S\bar{v}o_2$

The use of a fiberoptic, continuous $S\bar{v}o_2$ monitor as part of pulmonary artery catheterization may enhance the

TABLE 6-5 ■ Agents Used to Correct Metabolic Acidosis

Drug	Dosage	Action	Adverse Reaction	Comments
Sodium bicarbonate	Initial dose 1 mEq/kg IO or IV Subsequent doses depend on pH: mEq sodium bicarbonate = weight (kg) × base deficit (mEq/L) × 0.3 Administer half of calculated deficit initially	Increases plasma bicarbonate Buffers excess hydrogen ion Increases blood pH	Hypercarbia Hypokalemia Decreased ionized calcium Decreased oxygen release from hemoglobin Hyperosmolality Hypernatremia Hypervolemia Intraventricular hemorrhage in neonates Rebound metabolic alkalosis	Sodium bicarbonate crosses the blood-brain barrier more rapidly in infants than adults In neonates, must use 4.2% solution because hyperosmolarity may cause intraventricular hemorrhage in neonates Infants/children should receive sodium bicarbonate only when adequately ventilating
Tromethamine (THAM)	Loading dose: 3-5 mL/kg IV infused over 5 min or dose = weight (kg) × 0.1 × base deficit (mEq/L) Maintenance dose: 3-16 mL/kg/hr as continuous infusion	Hydrogen ion acceptor	Venospasm Transient hypocalcemia or hypoglycemia Alkalosis Respiratory depression Thrombophlebitis	Hypoglycemia may occur when administered to preterm or term neonates Use in place of sodium bicarbonate for metabolic acidosis when serum sodium or P_{CO_2} is elevated Contraindicated in anuria, uremia, and chronic respiratory acidosis Do not administer for periods > 24 hr

ability to optimize V_{O_2} and D_{O_2} relationships. For instance, the "best PEEP" may be determined by continuous monitoring of the $S\bar{v}_{O_2}$ as the PEEP is sequentially increased from 5 to 15 cm of water over a short time period. The point where the $S\bar{v}_{O_2}$ is maximal indicates the PEEP where oxygen delivery is optional. The result of various interventions designed to increase cardiac output such as volume administration, infusion of inotropic agents, administration of afterload-reducing drugs, and correction of acid-base abnormalities may be assessed by the effect on the $S\bar{v}_{O_2}$. For example, the patient who responds to inotropic agent administration with an increase in V_{O_2} without a simultaneous increase in cardiac output may demonstrate a reduction in $S\bar{v}_{O_2}$. Likewise, the effects of transfusion or ventilator manipulation on oxygen kinetics can be assessed. Therefore, continuous monitoring of $S\bar{v}_{O_2}$ may allow assessment of the impact of various interventions on cardiac output and D_{O_2}.

Extracorporeal Life Support

Extracorporeal life support (ECLS, ECMO) may be used to provide both cardiac as well as respiratory support and is described in detail in Chapter 5 (Respiratory Considerations). ECLS involves the use of extrathoracic vascular cannulation and a modified heart-lung machine to allow prolonged extracorporeal support. ECLS should be used in the setting of acute, reversible respiratory and/or cardiac failure unresponsive to optimal ventilator and pharmacologic management. Specific criteria for initiation of ECLS in pediatric patients with cardiac insufficiency include clinical signs such as decreased peripheral perfusion, oliguria (urine output < 0.5 mL/kg/hr), core hypothermia, and hypotension despite administration of inotropic

agents or volume resuscitation. ECLS is applied in pediatric cardiac patients in the setting of cardiogenic shock (20%), cardiac arrest (20%), and acute deterioration (10%), whereas an additional 20% of patients are placed on ECLS directly in the operating room owing to inability to wean from heart-lung bypass. The ECLS device may be thought of as a D_{O_2} device that may be used to enhance and, in some situations, provide total D_{O_2} in the patient with cardiopulmonary insufficiency. Venoarterial ECLS may provide total cardiac support. ECLS is especially efficacious, therefore, in the management of the patient who is in cardiogenic shock. ECLS may also be useful in the setting of septic shock in which administration of vasoactive agents may increase vascular tone while adequate perfusion and oxygenation are provided by the ECLS device. Table 6-6 demonstrates the current results for pediatric cardiac support with ECLS in the Extracorporeal Life Support Organization (ELSO) registry.

TABLE 6-6 ■ Extracorporeal Life Support Organization (ELSO) Registry Summary Data on Cardiac Failure Cases Managed with ECLS

Primary Diagnosis	Total	No. Survived	% Survived
Congenital defect	3475	1309	38
Cardiac arrest	130	34	26
Cardiogenic shock	126	52	41
Cardiomyopathy	324	159	49
Myocarditis	141	85	58
Other	728	282	39
Total	4924	1921	42

Cardiac Arrest

The response to an unplanned cardiac arrest begins with institution of the ABCs of cardiopulmonary resuscitation (CPR). Unresponsiveness and breathlessness should be established. As soon as possible, the airway is cleared, endotracheal intubation is performed, and breathing is

instituted. If carotid or brachial artery pulses are absent, external cardiac massage is instituted by chest compression. In the newborn, the two hands thumb-encircling technique should be used with compression of the chest to approximately one third its depth. If intravenous access is not available, resuscitation medications such as epinephrine

TABLE 6-7 ■ Medications Used in the Setting of Cardiac Arrest				
Drug	**Dosage**	**Action**	**Adverse Reaction**	**Comments**
Lidocaine HCl	Bolus: 1 mg/kg IV, ET, IO Infusion: 20-50 μg/kg/min	Antidysrhythmic agent for ventricular dysrhythmias Increases electrical stimulation for threshold of ventricles without depressing the force of ventricular contraction	Myocardial depression Bradycardia Hypotension	Contraindicated in severe heart block When administered ET use 1:1 dilution
Amiodarone	5 mg/kg IV/IO Max: 15 mg/kg/day	Increases cardiac action potential duration Vasodilation	Hypotension Bradyarrhythmias Pneumonitis, hepatotoxicity with long-term oral use	
Atropine sulfate	0.02 mg/kg IV, ET, IO Minimum dose: 0.1 mg/dose Maximum single dose: 0.5 mg infant/child, 1.0 mg/dose adolescent	Anticholinergic Increases heart rate Decreases vagal tone Enhances atrioventricular conduction	Tachycardia Increases myocardial oxygen consumption, dry mouth Tachydysrhythmias	May double for second dose
Calcium chloride 10%	20 mg/kg IV/IO	Increases myocardial contractility	Gastrointestinal irritation Bradycardia Hypotension	Cannot be given IM or SC Treat extravasation with hyaluronidase Administration of calcium in hypocalcemic preterm neonates results in increased heart rates, myocardial contractility, and blood pressure In preterm infants, calcium gluconate may be preferable because of slower release (multiply $CaCl_2$ dose × 4 to obtain equivalent calcium gluconate dose)
Epinephrine	Bradycardia, arrest: 0.1 mL/kg of 1:10,000 IV, IO; 0.1 mL/kg 1:1000 ET Infusion: 0.1-1.0 μg/kg/min; titrate to effect	α and β Stimulant Cardiac stimulant and bronchodilator Increases peripheral vascular resistance Increases myocardial contractility Increases heart rate Increases mesenteric and renal vasoconstriction	Tachydysrhythmias Ventricular dysrhythmias Renal ischemia Hyperglycemia Bradycardia	Ineffective if pH is < 7.1 Higher dose required in the presence of acidosis Protect medication from light
Bicarbonate	1 mEq/kg			Base on blood gas assessment
Dextrose (Glucose)	0.5-1.0 g/kg IV, IO 2-4 mL/kg of 25% 5-10 mL/kg of 10%		Hyperglycemia Rebound hypoglycemia	Should not administer in concentration > 25%
Naloxone (Narcan)	≤ 5 years old or ≤ 20 kg: 0.1 mg/kg IV, SC, IO > 5 years old or > 20 kg: 2 mg	Narcotic agonist	Hypertension Tachycardia	Should be administered cautiously to neonates of mothers known to be physically dependent on opioids; abrupt and complete reversal may precipitate an acute withdrawal syndrome Available in neonatal dilution (0.02 mg/mL)

and lidocaine may be administered through the endotracheal tube. When doing so, medications should be diluted with up to 5 mL of normal saline and injected into the endotracheal tube to be followed by application of five positive-pressure breaths. During cardiac arrest, intravenous fluids should be administered to correct hypovolemia; positive-pressure ventilation and oxygen should be provided to correct hypoxemia; and sodium bicarbonate should be administered in an initial dose of 1 mEq/kg as directed by blood gas analysis to correct metabolic acidosis. Other medications of use in cardiac arrest include epinephrine to increase SVR, blood pressure, and myocardial contractility and automaticity, and amiodarone or lidocaine for the child with ventricular tachycardia or ventricular fibrillation (Fig. 6-14). Suggested doses and frequency of dosing during cardiac arrest are demonstrated in Table 6-7. If ventricular fibrillation is present, external defibrillation should be performed with an initial setting of 2 J/kg. If unsuccessful, this should be repeated immediately with 2 to 4 J/kg and then 4 J/kg. It is critical that the underlying etiology of the cardiac arrest is identified: the four Hs and the four Ts include hypovolemia, hypoxemia, hypothermia, hyperkalemia (and other metabolic disturbances), tension pneumothorax, tamponade, toxins, and thromboembolism that constitute some of the most common causes of cardiac arrest in children. Pulseless electrical activity (PEA) or electromechanical dissociation (EMD), indicated by the presence of organized electrical activity on ECG with ineffective myocardial contraction, is relatively commonly observed during cardiac arrest. Possible causes include tension pneumothorax, cardiac tamponade, hypovolemia, and hypocalcemia. Algorithms for the management of specific cardiac rhythm disturbances during CPR are shown in Figure 6-14.

VENOUS ACCESS

Peripheral Intravenous Access

By far the most common form of venous access, peripheral intravenous (IV) catheters, are placed percutaneously in most inpatients and those undergoing all but the most minor of operative procedures. Peripheral IV access devices are typically the "over-the-needle" type with the thin-walled catheter on the outside of the needle. Once the vein is distended by a tourniquet placed proximal to the intended access site, the needle is introduced into the vein on the upper or lower extremity or, occasionally, the scalp. As blood return is encountered, the catheter is advanced over the needle into the lumen of the vein. Because the needle extends slightly beyond the tip of the catheter one must be careful to slightly advance the needle and catheter as a unit once blood return is noted or the blunt catheter may not be within the lumen of the vein when it is advanced. This is especially important with larger catheters. IV catheters are commonly available in sizes from 24 gauge up to 14 gauge in increments of two. IV catheter dressing changes are usually performed every 72 hours, and in many institutions it is recommended that catheters be changed every 72 hours except in those patients in whom it proves to be difficult to establish access. Catheters placed under emergent conditions should be replaced within 24 hours. Thrombophlebitis may occasionally

occur and is typically treated with antibiotics and non-steroidal anti-inflammatory agents: excision of a vein with purulent thrombophlebitis is rarely required. To prevent this complication, IV catheters should be changed at the first sign of local erythema. Sloughing of skin from infusion of vasoactive drugs, especially in newborns, is a risk. Treatment of areas of extravasation of such drugs out of the vein with local infiltration of phentolamine within 12 hours may be effective at preventing skin slough. In neonates, 1 mL of a solution of 0.25 to 0.5 mg/mL is injected in five divided doses of 0.2 mL subcutaneously around the site of extravasation to a maximum total dose of 0.1 mg/kg or 2.5 mg total. In older patients, 1 to 5 mL of 0.5 to 1 mg/mL solution is injected in five divided doses subcutaneously around the site of extravasation to a maximum dose of 0.1 to 0.2 mg/kg or 5 mg total. New safety devices allow retraction of the needle once the IV catheter has been placed to protect health care workers from accidental needlesticks. IV catheters typically are effective for a period of a few days to a week.

Peripherally Inserted Central Venous Catheters (PICC)

Stable venous access on the order of a few weeks can be accomplished with a catheter that is placed through a peripheral vein on the upper extremity, although the lower extremity can be used as well in infants and advanced into central venous position. PICC lines commonly are available in sizes from 2 to 7F (3F = 1 mm). Access to the peripheral vein, most commonly the basilic or cephalic vein, is performed using an "over-the-needle" peel-away catheter that is large enough to admit the PICC line. Once intravenous access is achieved with the peel-away device, the PICC line is trimmed to a length that will allow the tip to lie in central position (Fig. 6-15). The two wings of the peel-away catheter are then pulled apart, splitting and removing the catheter with the PICC line alone remaining in the vein. In some cases in which difficulty may be encountered with obtaining peripheral venous access with the relatively large diameter peel-away catheter, a standard IV catheter can be introduced into the vein, which can then be exchanged over a guidewire for the peel-away sheath. PICC lines should be cleansed and dressed every 3 days. They are effective at providing venous access for administration of home antibiotics or parenteral nutrition because of the stability of the access combined with safety.

Central Venous Catheters

Central venous catheters or "lines" are, in general, polyurethane catheters that are placed into the large central veins (subclavian, internal jugular, femoral vein) by a percutaneous, Seldinger technique. The vessel is punctured by a thin-walled needle and a guidewire is inserted and passed into the appropriate location. Subsequently, the needle is withdrawn. The catheter is then threaded over the guidewire into the vein, and the guidewire is removed. With larger catheters a dilator may be passed over the guidewire in and out of the vein to enlarge the skin entrance and tract. Occasionally, these catheters can be placed by cutdown into central position by means of the facial, external jugular, cephalic, or saphenous vein.

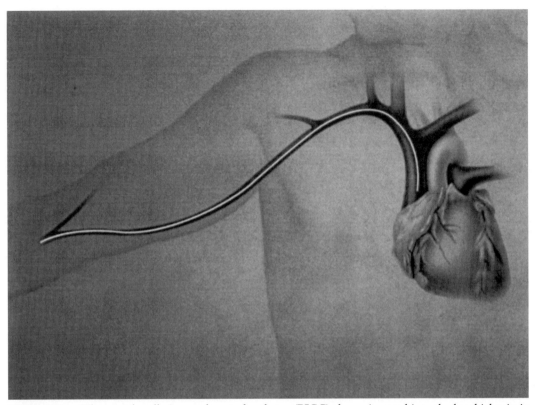

FIGURE 6-15 ■ The peripherally inserted central catheter (PICC) shown inserted into the brachial vein in the antecubital fossa and extending centrally to the superior vena cava near its junction with the right atrium.

Central catheters provide stable access and can be used to administer parenteral nutrition, vasoactive drugs, and a variety of other pharmaceuticals that should not be administered into a peripheral vein. Central venous catheters can also be used to measure right atrial pressure to assess volume status. Percutaneous central catheter placement is associated with pneumothorax in less than 1% of cases and with hemorrhage in even less. Colonization of the catheter results in 1 to 10 bloodstream infections for every 1000 catheter-days. Central catheters provide stable access for use by patients at home and are effective over a period of weeks. Care must be taken to avoid leaving the external end of the catheter open to the atmosphere: entrainment of air resulting in air embolus may occur.

Broviac Catheters and Infusaports

Broviac catheters are Silastic, cuffed, tunneled catheters that are placed into central position with the intent of providing chronic venous access for months to years. Broviac insertion has now become one of the most common procedures performed by the pediatric surgeon. The catheter can be inserted into the central venous system by cutdown of the great veins or their tributaries (facial, external jugular, cephalic, saphenous veins) or by using a percutaneous Seldinger technique (Fig. 6-16). Broviac catheters are usually available in sizes from 2.7F to 12F and have one to three lumens. The soft Silastic catheter is difficult to advance over a wire. As such, when using a

percutaneous Seldinger approach, a peel-away sheath with an internal dilator is passed over the guidewire; the guidewire and dilator are removed; the catheter is cut to the appropriate length and introduced through the peel-away sheath; and the peel-away is removed as it is split. Broviac catheters must be flushed daily with heparin. Unfortunately, they are external devices that are unpleasant for young patients and can be pulled and accidentally removed especially by young children. Even though there is ingrowth of tissue into the cuff, which reduces the incidence of catheter infections, the rate of Broviac catheter sepsis remains relatively high at 0.4 to 1.5 episodes per 1000 days of use. The Broviac catheter infection rate is even higher at 7 to 9 episodes per 1000 days of use in those patients with short gut syndrome and who require frequent access for parenteral nutrition and drug administration.

The Infusaport was developed for those requiring infrequent access for blood aspiration, chemotherapy, or administration of blood products. The "port" is a metal or plastic device with a diaphragm on the top that is placed in the subcutaneous position and anchored to the underlying fascia (Fig. 6-17). The Silastic catheter attached to the port is placed into central position in the same fashion as with a Broviac catheter. Thus there is no external device, which is an enhancement of patient lifestyle and reduces the incidence of infection to 0.07 episodes per 1000 days of catheter use. The port is accessed through the overlying skin using a Huber needle with a hole on

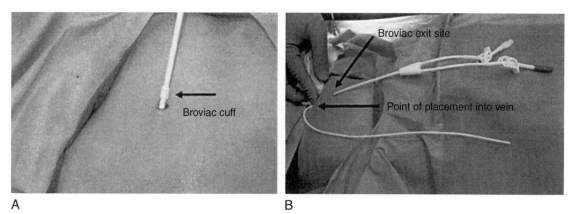

FIGURE 6-16 ■ The Broviac cuff being placed into the exit site (**A**). After insertion of the cuff into the exit site with tunneling of the catheter, the Broviac catheter is being readied for insertion into the external jugular vein by cutdown (**B**). The Broviac is laid out as it will sit once placed into the vein.

the side so that the outlet of the needle is not obstructed by the base of the port. The need for periodic needlesticks with port access may be frightening or painful for young children, which may make the Broviac catheter the preferred form of access in some patients.

Dialysis Catheters

Thin-walled, double-lumen catheters may be placed into the central venous system to provide dialysis for renal failure; for plasmapheresis for treatment of sepsis, neuropathies, or autoimmune disorders; or for stem cell harvest (Fig. 6-18). The flow required through these devices is only 3 to 5 mL/kg/min. The catheters are typically available in sizes from 10F to 14.5F and are placed percutaneously into the femoral, subclavian, or internal jugular vein. A Permacath cuffed, double-lumen catheter can be placed in similar fashion to a Broviac catheter to provide access for long-term hemodialysis.

Pulmonary Arterial Catheters

For large catheters, such as a pulmonary artery or Swan-Ganz catheter, special devices containing sheath introducers are used. Once the introducer has been placed into proper position by the Seldinger technique, it remains in place and acts as a port for the pulmonary arterial catheter. The sheath introducer has a hemostatic valve on the end through which a dilator or pulmonary artery catheter can

be passed. A side port in the introducer sheath is used for additional venous access.

A 5F pulmonary artery catheter is appropriate for patients weighing up to 25 to 30 kg and a 7F catheter is appropriate for older patients. Most catheters have five lumens: (1) a port for injection of either 0.5 or 1.5 mL of air into an inflatable balloon at the tip of the catheter; (2) a thermister probe near the tip that allows determination of core body temperature and thermodilution cardiac output; (3) a fiberoptic bundle for determination of pulmonary arterial $S\bar{v}O_2$; (4) a port distal to the inflatable balloon that allows assessment of pulmonary artery pressure when the balloon is deflated and LAP when inflated; and (5) one or two additional proximal infusion/pressure monitoring ports usually placed in the right ventricle and/or right atrium.

Pulmonary arterial catheters are most often placed by means of a subclavian or internal jugular approach. In young children (< 2 years old) the femoral venous approach may make transcardiac passage of the catheter easier. Once venous access is established through the introducer

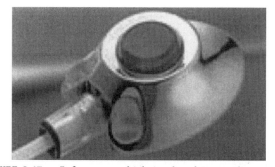

FIGURE 6-17 ■ Infusaport, which is placed in a subcutaneous pocket and accessed using an angled Huber needle.

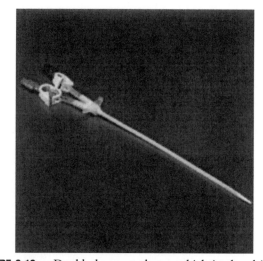

FIGURE 6-18 ■ Double-lumen catheter, which is placed into a central vein and used for hemodialysis, plasmapheresis, or stem cell harvest.

catheter, the balloon is inflated and tested, and all monitoring infusion ports are flushed and zeroed. The balloon is inflated as the catheter is gently advanced: right atrial, right ventricular, pulmonary arterial, and finally, pulmonary wedge waveforms should be observed (Fig. 6-19). A chest radiograph should be obtained to document correct placement.

Complications are few but can be life threatening. The balloon should remain inflated during passage of the catheter through the right side of the heart to reduce the incidence of arrhythmias. Treatment of arrhythmias is rarely required, and lidocaine should only be administered if sustained ventricular tachycardia is induced at the time of placement. Rupture of the pulmonary artery is a rare, but lethal, complication, which may be manifested by hemoptysis and/or cardiopulmonary collapse following balloon inflation during a wedge pressure measurement. Those patients with pulmonary arterial hypertension and coagulation deficiencies are at highest risk. This complication may be avoided by maintaining the tip of the catheter less than 2 cm lateral to the spine on radiography in adults and proportionally less in children; by inflating the balloon with the minimal volume necessary to achieve a wedge tracing; and by minimizing the frequency of wedge pressure assessment. The distal port of the catheter should be continuously monitored for permanent wedging, which can lead to pulmonary infarction. If permanent wedging is observed, the catheter should be withdrawn until appropriate pulmonary arterial and wedge tracings are observed during deflation and inflation of the balloon, respectively.

Umbilical Vein Catheterization

Umbilical vein catheterization is a simple procedure that allows rapid placement of a large-bore catheter into the central venous system. Disadvantages include a high incidence of catheter sepsis, tip malposition, danger of liver abscess, portal vein thrombosis, and perforation into the peritoneal cavity. This route is mainly indicated when central venous access is necessary in the immediate newborn period. Cannulation is usually possible up to 7 days after birth.

The large, thin-walled umbilical vein lies in the cephalad aspect of the cord stump (Fig. 6-20). The stump is cut

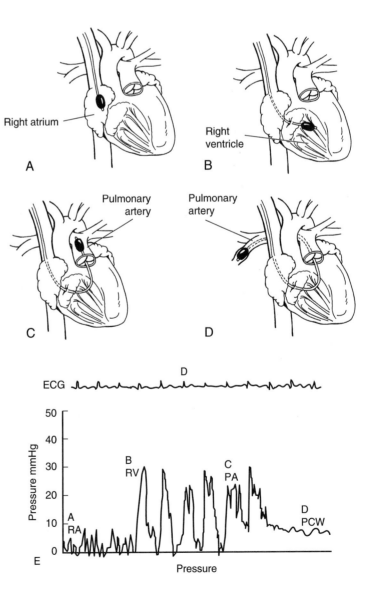

FIGURE 6-19 ■ Pulmonary artery catheter placement. Vascular pressure waveforms may be used to monitor passage of the catheter through the (**A**) right atrium (RA), (**B**) right ventricle (RV), and the (**C**) pulmonary artery (PA), and into the wedged position in the (**D**) pulmonary artery (PCW). Pulmonary capillary occlusion pressure reflects left atrial filling pressure. (From Hirschl RB, Heiss K: Cardiopulmonary critical care and shock. In Oldham KT, et al [eds]: Surgery of Infants and Children: Scientific Principles and Practice. Philadelphia, Lippincott-Raven, 1997.)

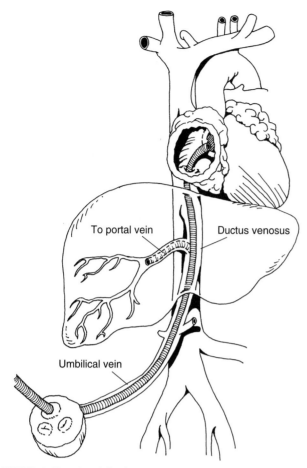

FIGURE 6-20 ■ Umbilical vein catheterization. The drawing illustrates passage from the umbilical vein into the portal circulation or through the ductus venosus into the inferior vena cava to the right atrium. The tip of the catheter should be in the inferior vena cava, just at the entrance to the right atrium as proven by radiography.

1 or 2 cm above the skin surface and stabilized with forceps or a hemostat. Blood clots are removed from the vein lumen, and a saline-filled umbilical catheter with attached syringe (5F for term newborns and 3F for premature newborns) is inserted. To avoid air embolism the catheter should never be left open to the atmosphere. During passage, if blood cannot be aspirated, the catheter is withdrawn while maintaining gentle suction to extract a possible clot. In 60% of cases the catheter passes from the umbilical vein, through the ductus venosus, into the inferior vena cava. If not, the catheter may pass into the portal vein and become lodged in a portal venous radicle. It should never be left in the portal system because of the danger of thrombosis. Once the inferior vena cava is entered, the catheter generally goes upward toward the heart, and as it is advanced, it will pass into the right atrium. The position must be checked by radiography of the chest and abdomen.

Central Venous Access Sites

Cutdown Access

Central venous access may be obtained by cutdown or by percutaneous means. A single cutdown incision made

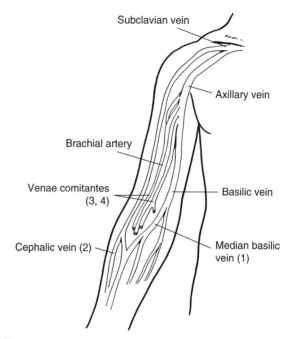

FIGURE 6-21 ■ Four-in-one cutdown. The median basilic vein (1), the cephalic vein (2), and the two deep veins (3,4) can be exposed by one incision.

from the center of the antecubital fossa to its medial border allows rapid exposure of four relatively large veins: the median basilic, the cephalic, and two venae comitantes of the brachial artery (Fig. 6-21). Central access may be easily gained through these peripheral veins. However, most commonly, access by cutdown is obtained through the external jugular vein, the common facial vein, the cephalic vein, or the saphenous vein at the saphenofemoral junction. The external jugular vein is superficial, usually visible, and of sufficient size to accommodate a relatively large catheter (Fig. 6-22). The external jugular vein joins the subclavian vein just under the middle of the clavicle and has a more direct, straight path to the superior vena cava in neonates and infants than in children and adolescents. The cephalic vein, which joins the subclavian vein after running through a triangle formed by the anterior head of the deltoid muscle, the uppermost pectoralis major muscle fibers, and the clavicle, provides another access point to the subclavian vein (Fig. 6-23) A transverse incision is made just below the clavicle in the depression made by the chest wall and the humerus. The groove between the anterior deltoid and pectoralis major muscles is opened and the vein encountered and followed to the point where it dives under the clavicle. In this area it is relatively large and easily cannulated. A catheter can be passed directly into the subclavian vein and then centrally to the superior vena cava. The facial vein may be accessed through an incision that is made parallel and approximately one fingerbreadth below the mandible at the level of the hyoid to avoid the mandibular branch of the facial nerve as it lies along the lower border of the mandible. The facial vein provides a reliable route to central venous catheterization because it enters the internal jugular directly (Fig. 6-24). The common facial vein

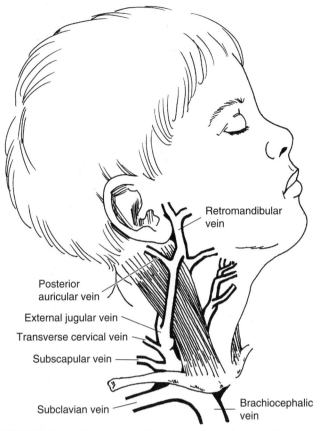

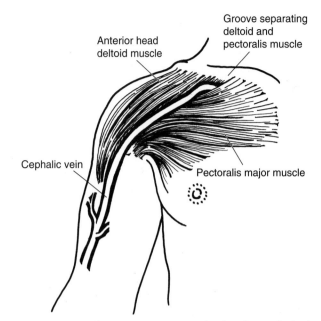

FIGURE 6-23 ■ The most important landmark to find the cephalic vein is the groove formed by the fibers of the anterior head of the deltoid muscle and upper fibers of the pectoralis major muscle. Care must be taken to note that the fibers of the deltoid run in an oblique direction and those of the pectoralis run transversely.

FIGURE 6-22 ■ The course of the external jugular vein. It passes under the clavicle and at that point joins the subclavian vein.

FIGURE 6-24 ■ Anatomy of the facial vein.

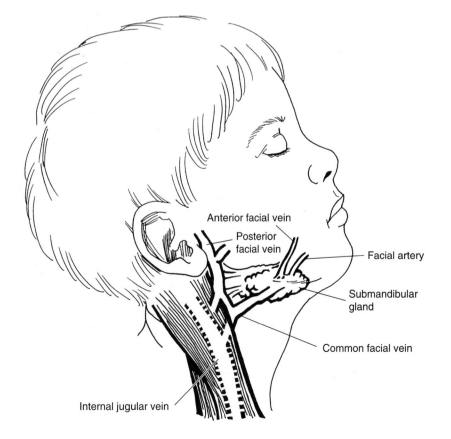

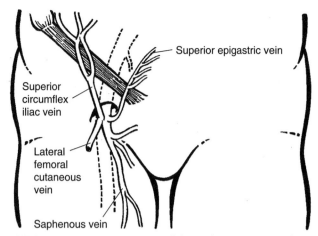

FIGURE 6-25 ■ Venous anatomy of the saphenous vein cutdown at the groin illustrating that the saphenous vein, just as it joins the femoral vein, is large and easily cannulated.

should be traced back to the internal jugular vein before cannulation to ensure proper identification.

The femoral vein may be cannulated through the saphenous vein, which is easily identified in the antero-medial subcutaneous tissues of the upper thigh/groin (Fig. 6-25). A saphenofemoral venous cutdown is a simple and rapid procedure with a high success rate and a low complication rate that can even be used in preterm infants. It allows access to the iliac veins and the inferior vena cava. To expose the saphenous vein, an incision is made just below the inguinal crease medial to the femoral arterial pulsation. The vein is encountered in the subcutaneous tissues traveling in an upward and lateral direction toward the fossa ovalis.

Under the rare circumstances where central venous cannulation through the upper or lower extremity great veins is impossible, the central system can still be cannulated through the azygos vein by placement of a catheter through one of the right posterior intercostal veins. The posterior intercostal veins lie above the intercostal artery and nerve in the subcostal groove. This neurovascular bundle is deep to the external and internal intercostal muscles and superficial to the innermost intercostal muscle and pleura. The lower eight right intercostal veins directly join the azygos vein, which enters the chest through the aortic hiatus. It runs to the right of the vertebral column and arches forward over the root of the lung to join the superior vena cava.

Percutaneous Access

Percutaneous access to the central veins is most commonly performed through the subclavian, internal jugular, or femoral veins. The choice of access site should be considered carefully in patients who might require ECLS because the internal jugular vein is commonly used for access, patients with congenital heart disease who may require bypass or repeated access for catheterization or biopsy, and those with renal failure who may require upper extremity arteriovenous fistulas for hemodialysis.

The subclavian vein is a reliable route for central venous access in even the smallest infants with the success rate of central passage in adults of between 70% and 98% being only slightly lower in infants (Fig. 6-26). Coagulopathy or thrombocytopenia is a contraindication. The incidence of pneumothorax varies between 1% and 5% but is increased with chronic lung disease or high ventilator pressure settings. The right subclavian vein is preferred for cannulation because the thoracic duct is vulnerable to injury as it joins the left subclavian vein at its junction with the internal jugular vein. Also, the dome of the

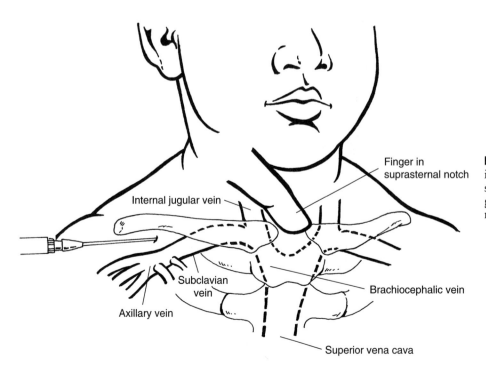

FIGURE 6-26 ■ Subclavian puncture in an older infant. The finger in the substernal notch is an important guide to the proper angle of advancement of the needle.

pleura is higher on the left and more susceptible to injury. The patient should be placed in the Trendelenburg position and a roll placed under the back. In children, a 21-gauge needle is used to access the subclavian vein. The needle is inserted just lateral to the point where the first rib and the clavicle come into approximation. The needle is advanced while aspirating with the syringe in a superior and medial direction under the clavicle as the vein is encountered. Once the needle is within the lumen of the vein, as evidenced by free return of blood during aspiration, a wire is passed through the needle, the needle is removed, and the catheter is placed over the wire into the central venous position in the superior vena cava or right atrium. Care must be taken to avoid air embolism during all portions of the procedure.

The internal jugular vein provides direct access to the right atrium. The right internal jugular vein is the preferred site because it is larger, farther away from the carotid artery, and runs directly into the innominate vein and then continues in a straight path to the superior vena cava. The left internal jugular vein is close to the thoracic duct and joins the subclavian vein at almost right angles, making central cannulation more diffcult. As mentioned previously, the dome of the pleura is higher on the left, increasing the risk of pneumothorax with left cannulation. Internal jugular cannulation should not be performed if a tracheostomy is present, ECMO is contemplated, or there is increased intracranial pressure. Because of the anatomy and mobility of the neck, it is difficult to secure the catheter following nontunneled central catheter placement for long-term use. The internal jugular vein is most frequently accessed from a point one to two fingerbreadths above

the clavicle between the heads of the sternocleidomastoid. The patient is placed in 15 degrees of Trendelenburg, and the head is turned approximately 30 degrees to the left. The two heads of the sternocleidomastoid are palpated if they are not visible (Fig. 6-27). The needle is inserted at the level of the cricoid cartilage just above the apex of the triangle and directed downward and lateral toward the ipsilateral nipple at an angle of 30 to 45 degrees. As the needle is advanced, aspiration of the syringe is performed until venous entry is signaled by a flash of dark blood. The needle is then advanced for 2 mm and cannulation accomplished, usually through the Seldinger technique. An alternative approach is posterior to the sternocleidomastoid with the needle entering the skin at the junction of the lower and middle thirds of the posterior margin of the sternocleidomastoid while the needle is oriented toward the sternal notch. Cannulation of the internal jugular vein has a high success rate and an incidence of pneumothorax of less than 0.1%. Venous and arterial bleeding can be controlled by compression, and the internal jugular vein may be used cautiously even if coagulopathy is present.

The femoral vein is located medial to the artery in the groin. The vein may be identified by aspiration with a 21-gauge needle at a 30- to 45-degree angle approximately 1 fingerbreadth medial to the palpated femoral artery and 1 to 2 fingerbreadths below the inguinal ligament (Fig. 6-28). The common femoral vein is large and superficial and has a constant relationship medial to the femoral artery, making it easy to locate for percutaneous puncture. Femoral vein catheterization in pediatric and adult patients carries a low complication rate and a high success rate.

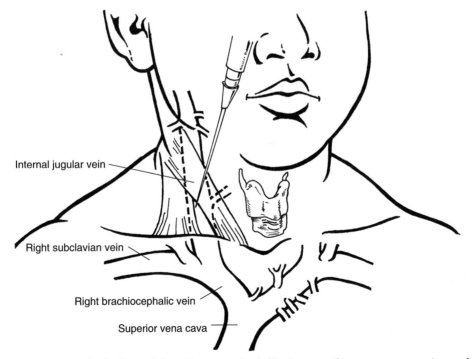

Internal jugular vein

Right subclavian vein

Right brachiocephalic vein

Superior vena cava

FIGURE 6-27 ■ The high medial or "between the bellies" approach to percutaneous internal jugular vein puncture. Note that the insertion of the needle is at the apex of the triangle formed by the two muscular heads of the sternomastoid muscle and the clavicle. The cricoid cartilage serves as a landmark.

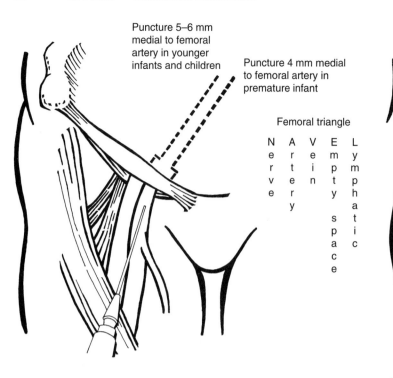

Puncture 5–6 mm
medial to femoral
artery in younger
infants and children

Puncture 4 mm medial
to femoral artery in
premature infant

Femoral triangle

N A V E L
e r e m y
r t i p m
v e n t p
e r   y h
  y   a
        s t
        p i
        a c
        c
        e

FIGURE 6-28 ■ The anatomy of the common femoral vein. The drawing illustrates the relationship between femoral artery pulsations and the femoral vein as a guide to puncture.

Intraosseous Needle Placement

In the infant and child younger than 2 years of age, in whom intravenous line placement may be especially difficult, an alternative access includes intraosseous needle placement. The long bones of infants and young children contain vascular red marrow. Fatty, yellow marrow appears by age 4 years, and by 18 years there normally is no red marrow. The proximal and distal tibia and the distal femur are the common infusion sites. The proximal tibia is preferred. Insertion is made at the midline of the flat surface of the anterior tibia, 1 to 3 cm below the tibial tuberosity (Fig. 6-29). The needle is directed distally in a 40- to 60-degree angle away from the growth plate. Other alternative sites include the distal tibia, which is often used in older children, at a point posterior to the saphenous vein and proximal to the medial malleus. Insertion into the femur is best accomplished at a point 2 to 3 cm above the external condyle cephalad at a 10- to 15-degree angle. In an infant younger than 18 months of age, an 18- to 20-gauge disposable bone marrow needle is sufficient; in those older than 18 months, a 13- to 16-gauge needle is used. The needle is angled away from the growth plate as a screwing motion is utilized to pass the needle through the cortex of the bone. A "give" is noted as the needle passes into the marrow cavity. Bone marrow may then be aspirated and drugs infused. Infusion of fluid and drugs into the bone marrow (intraosseous infusion) is an effective emergency route when venous access cannot be rapidly established. Any solutions that can be infused intravenously can be administered through the marrow. Previous studies have documented that drugs infused into the marrow appear in the right atrium within 1 minute of administration. If no marrow is aspirated, saline solution is injected and the adjacent tissue palpated for extravasation. Gravity infusion through a 20-gauge needle allows flow rates of 11 mL/min; application of a pressurizing apparatus

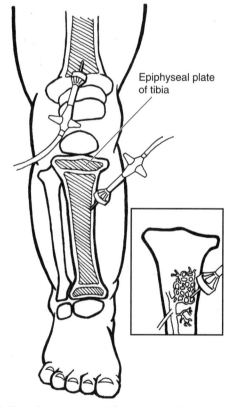

Epiphyseal plate
of tibia

FIGURE 6-29 ■ Intraosseous infusion into tibia or femur. The proximal tibia is the preferred site for infusion. The needle is directed distally at a 40- to 60-degree angle away from the growth plate. *Inset,* Multiple venous sinusoids flow into a central venous sinus and then into the systemic venous system.

increases the rate to 24 mL/min. With an 18-gauge needle, rates with gravity infusion are 24 mL/min and rates with a pressurizing device are 41 mL/min. Optimum infusion time is 2 hours, at which point venous access must be established. In addition, marrow aspiration samples may be evaluated for blood gas and electrolyte data and may be sent for typing and crossmatching for blood transfusion. Complications of intraosseous cannulation are rare and include rare fractures, development of osteomyelitis, and compartment syndrome if drugs and fluid are inadvertently infused into the muscle compartment. Insertion should be avoided in areas of local infection. To prevent infusion extravasation, needle placement should be away from a fracture and previously attempted puncture sites. Marrow infusion is contraindicated in osteogenesis imperfecta and osteopetrosis.

ARTERIAL ACCESS

Systemic Arterial Catheters

Arterial catheter placement is indicated in those patients who require frequent blood pressure monitoring and in those who require more than two or three blood gas samples per day. The most common arterial access site utilized in non-neonates is the radial artery followed by the posterior tibial and femoral artery. Peripheral arteries are best used because of the low complication rate should thrombosis occur. However, the femoral artery has frequently been cannulated using the Seldinger technique in

children with few complications. Samples from the right radial artery represent blood from the aorta proximal to the ductus arteriosus.

The sites for arterial cannulation in children are evenly split between the percutaneous and cutdown methods. Percutaneous insertion should be attempted primarily in most cases. Typical catheter sizes for arterial cannulation include 24 or 22 gauge in neonates, 22 gauge in large infants and children, and 20 gauge in older children and adolescents. Two methods of percutaneous cannulation are commonly used: (1) the direct cannulation method and (2) the transfixion technique (Fig. 6-30). With both techniques the artery is located either by palpation, Doppler probe, or transillumination. A skin puncture is made just proximal to the head of the radius and the cannula directed proximally at a 30-degree angle. With the transfixion technique the needle frequently abuts the head of the radius, which is directly under the artery. Withdrawal of the catheter and needle may demonstrate a flash of blood, at which point the apparatus is then advanced slightly until blood return stops. This signifies that the posterior wall has been punctured. The needle is removed, and the cannula is slowly withdrawn until the blood flow resumes. The catheter is then advanced into the artery. In the direct puncture method, the cannula is advanced with constant observation of the hub to detect blood return. Once blood is encountered, the plastic catheter is slowly advanced into the artery. At times a wire, such as a 0.0015-inch diameter wire that fits through a 24F catheter, may be used in a

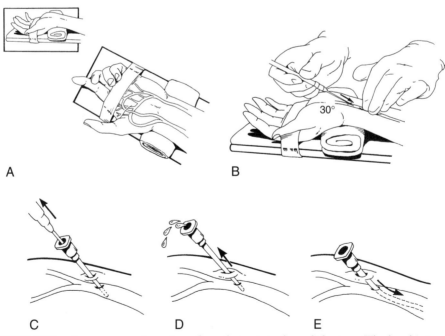

FIGURE 6-30 ■ Percutaneous insertion of a catheter into the radial artery. The hand is taped securely to an armboard with a roll placed under the wrist (**A**). The radial pulse is palpated and the needle/catheter guided at approximately a 30-degree angle through the artery (**B**). As the needle/catheter is withdrawn and passes into the artery, blood may be observed to flow into the hub. The needle/catheter is then advanced a second time and the needle removed (**C**), the catheter withdrawn until blood return is observed (**D**), and the catheter advanced down the lumen of the artery (**E**). (From Hirschl RB, Heiss K: Cardiopulmonary critical care and shock. In Oldham KT, et al [eds]: Surgery of Infants and Children: Scientific Principles and Practice. Philadelphia, Lippincott-Raven, 1997.)

Seldinger fashion to advance the catheter into the artery when difficulties are encountered with placement.

The technique of arterial cutdown of the radial or posterior tibial artery is most often utilized in neonates and infants when percutaneous puncture is unsuccessful. A transverse incision is made over the artery and the vessel exposed (Fig. 6-31). The radial artery is often located deeper than one might expect, frequently lying directly on the head of the radius. Once exposed during cutdown it is unusual to observe or palpate pulsations in the artery because of spasm. Cannulation is by puncture of the vessel by a needle and catheter device. An appropriately sized over-the-needle catheter is introduced directly down the lumen of the artery and the needle is removed. The catheter is advanced into the artery only if blood flow returns from the catheter. Otherwise, the catheter is slowly removed until blood flow return is noted, at which point the catheter is advanced. It is rare that ligation of the artery is required. Once the radial arterial catheter is in place, it is perfused continuously with saline or heparin saline flush. Care should be taken when flushing the catheter in bolus fashion because studies have demonstrated that flush may appear in the carotid artery distribution after injection of only 0.3 to 0.75 mL of flush into the radial artery of a neonate. No medications, except for heparin and papavarine, should be administered through any arterial line.

The umbilical artery provides an excellent site for arterial access in neonates with umbilical artery catheters being placed in up to 30% of neonates who are admitted to the neonatal intensive care unit. Catheterization of the umbilical artery is a rapid, easy method that allows placement of a relatively large-caliber catheter into the aorta. Placement is easiest in the first few hours of life and is only possible for about 4 days after birth. This technique allows postductal sampling for blood gas levels and pH determination, as well as direct measurement of aortic blood pressure. An incision on the inferior aspect of the umbilicus 1 to 2 cm above skin level should allow identification of one of the two thick-walled umbilical arteries

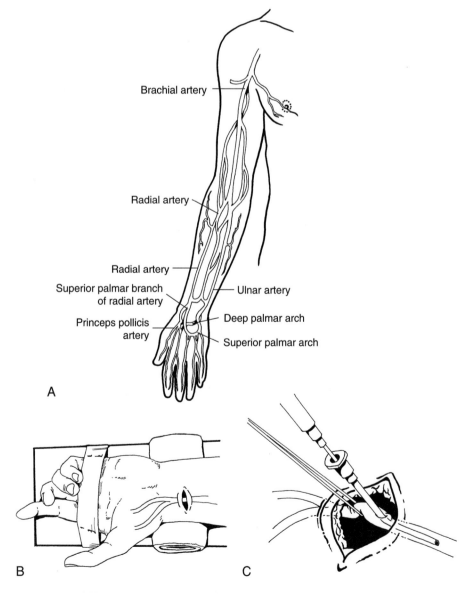

Brachial artery

Radial artery

Radial artery

Superior palmar branch of radial artery

Princeps pollicis artery

Ulnar artery

Deep palmar arch

Superior palmar arch

A

B

C

FIGURE 6-31 ■ The anatomy for radial artery catheterization, illustrating the deep palmar and superficial palmar arches and the position of the radial and ulnar arteries (**A**). Insertion of a catheter into the radial artery by the cutdown technique. A 1-cm incision is performed over the area of the radial artery just proximal to the wrist (**B**). The artery is identified on the head of the radius and retracted distally with a suture as a needle/catheter is advanced into the lumen of the artery (**C**). Ligation of the artery is usually not necessary. (From Hirschl RB, Heiss K: Cardiopulmonary critical care and shock. In Oldham KT, et al [eds]: Surgery of Infants and Children: Scientific Principles and Practice. Philadelphia, Lippincott-Raven, 1997.)

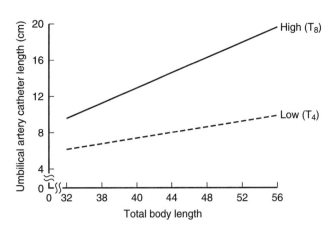

FIGURE 6-33 ■ Predicted length of umbilical venous catheter to be inserted such that the tip will be in the right atrium. The height of the umbilical stump should be included in the final catheter length determination. (From Hirschl RB, Heiss K: Cardiopulmonary critical care and shock. In Oldham KT, et al [eds]: Surgery of Infants and Children: Scientific Principles and Practice. Philadelphia, Lippincott-Raven, 1997.)

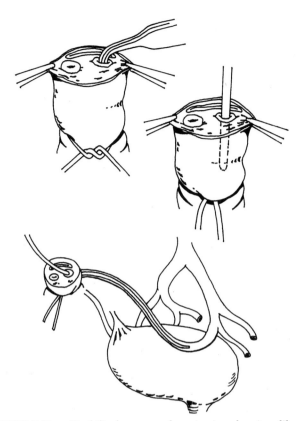

FIGURE 6-32 ■ Umbilical artery catheterization showing dilatation of the vessel and passage of the catheter. Catheters are usually placed high in the aorta at the level of the diaphragm on radiography.

that lie in the inferior aspect of the umbilical stump (Fig. 6-32). The stump is encircled with a loosely tied umbilical tape to reduce bleeding. The lumen of the artery is dilated by inserting a curved forceps and allowing it to spring open. A 3.5F (preterm or small neonate) or 5F catheter is gently advanced into the artery after flushing with heparinized saline. Resistance is often met at a point 5 to 6 cm from the umbilicus as the catheter passes from the hypogastric artery into the iliac artery. Resistance can usually be overcome by exerting light, steady pressure. Once in the internal iliac artery the catheter usually enters the common iliac artery and the aorta. Occasionally, the catheter turns downward into the external iliac artery and then distally into the lower extremity. If the artery cannot be located or cannulated in the umbilical stump, another option is to perform an infraumbilical curvilinear incision with identification of the umbilical artery in the space of Retzius that exists posterior to the linea alba and anterior to the peritoneum.

The final catheter position should be either above the mesenteric vessels in the area of the diaphragm (T9 to T11) or below the renal vessels (L4). Advancing the catheter a length equivalent to 0.65 times the distance between the umbilicus and the shoulder plus the length of the umbilical stump will place the catheter in the L4 vertebral region. The data from Figure 6-33 may be used to determine the insertion length of the umbilical artery catheter. Regardless of the method, the position must be radiographically verified.

Complications of arterial catheter placement are surprisingly low. Sepsis related to arterial catheters occurs in less than 1% and in 2% to 5% of cases with radial and umbilical artery catheters, respectively. With the use of modern catheters, aortic thrombosis appears to have decreased in the setting of umbilical artery catheter placement, and most series now report a 3% to 5% incidence. Mesenteric, renal, and lower extremity vascular occlusion resulting in tissue necrosis appears to be related more to emboli than to thrombosis. The incidence of adverse thromboembolic events appears to be greater in those patients with a low (L4 or lower) abdominal umbilical artery catheter. Overt aortoiliac thrombosis accompanied by decreased lower extremity blood flow and hypertension may be managed with umbilical artery catheter removal, heparin administration, supportive care, and antihypertensive therapy. Observation with systemic heparin administration will often result in improvement in limb perfusion. Consideration should be made toward angiography and/or thrombolytic therapy through the umbilical artery catheter before it is removed. Treatment with fibrinolytic therapy or surgical thrombectomy should be considered if limb-threatening ischemia, cardiac or renal failure, visceral compromise, or systemic acidosis is present (see Chapter 83). The potential for chronic ischemia and limb-length discrepancy after acute vascular injury should be recognized.

The incidence of radial artery thrombosis in the pediatric age group is less than 5%, and digital necrosis is seldom reported. The Allen test is still commonly recommended but impractical in infants and young children. It may be prudent to evaluate the arterial supply to the hand by a modified Allen test using Doppler ultrasonography. The Doppler probe is placed over a digital artery in the web space, which can be assessed for disappearance of Doppler signals when the radial artery is occluded. In a 1-year follow-up of pediatric patients with radial artery thrombosis from cannulation, recanalization and return of pulsations were present in most patients.

SUGGESTED READINGS

Hirschl RB, Bartlett RH: Extracorporeal life support in cardiopulmonary failure. In: Pediatric Surgery, 5th ed. St. Louis, CV Mosby, 1998, pp 89-102.

This chapter provides a complete definitive description of ECMO, indications, techniques and outcomes.

Hirschl RB, Heiss K: Cardiopulmonary critical care and shock. In Oldham KT, et al (eds): Surgery of Infants and Children: Scientific Principles and Practice. Philadelphia, Lippincott-Raven, 1997.

This chapter provides an in-depth discussion of intensive care for infants and children due to a variety of disease states.

Klaus M, et al: Care of the High-Risk Neonate, 3rd ed. Philadelphia, WB Saunders, 1986.

This classic text provides extensive background information on newborn organ systems and how they respond to serious illness.

Langman J: Medical Embryology, 3rd ed. Baltimore, Williams & Wilkins, 1975.

This is an excellent classic reference source on organ development.

Pediatric Advanced Life Support (PALS): Year 2000 Guidelines Analysis. Circulation, Supplement for August 22, 2000, vol 102, pp 291-342.

These are the current consensus guidelines for cardiopulmonary resuscitation.

7

Nutritional Support

In the 1980s and 1990s, pediatric surgeons began to focus on critical nutritional assessment and management. This focus was stimulated by developments in enteral nutrition, elemental diets, and parenteral nutrition. The introduction of parenteral nutrition by Dudrick in 1968 has been the most significant factor in making physicians aware of their patients' nutritional needs and problems. Nutritional requirements often are overlooked, however, as the physician focuses on the major disease process. In the United States, the highest incidence of malnutrition occurs in hospitalized patients, which adversely affects recovery from illness or injury. Protein breakdown and catabolic response are greater after trauma or major surgery than after simple starvation, which complicates nutritional management further. Nutritional management of infants and children must differ from that of adults because of growth considerations. Because the most challenging and distinct nutritional care is for infants, this chapter focuses mainly on the nutritional requirements and management of this patient group.

NUTRITIONAL REQUIREMENTS

Water

Water is second only to oxygen as essential for existence; lack of it results in death in a matter of days. The water content of infants is higher than that of adults (75% of body weight in infants versus 65% in adults) (Fig. 7-1). Fluids provide the principal source of water; however, some is provided by the oxidation of food and body tissues. Requirements for water are related to caloric consumption, so infants must consume much larger amounts of water per unit of body weight than adults. In general, calorie requirements (kcal/kg/day) are matched to the amount of fluid needs (mL/kg/day) (Table 7-1).

The daily consumption of fluid by healthy infants is equivalent to 10% to 15% of their body weight, in contrast to only 2% to 4% by adults. In addition, the natural food of infants and children is much higher in water content than that of adults; the fruit and vegetables consumed by infants and children contain about 90% water. Only 0.5% to 3% of fluid intake is retained by infants and children. About 50% is excreted through the kidneys, 3% to 10% is lost through the gastrointestinal tract, and 40% to 50% is insensible loss.

Energy Needs

Energy requirements vary depending on age and physiologic status of the child. Periods of active growth and extreme physical activity increase energy requirements. The average distribution of kilocalories in a well-balanced diet is as follows: protein, 15%, fat, 35%; and carbohydrate, 50%. Table 7-2 lists the kilocalorie requirements at different ages.

Protein

The requirement for protein in infants is based on the combined needs of growth and maintenance (see Table 7-2). Two percent of the infant's body weight, compared with 3% of the adult's body weight, consists of nitrogen. Most of the increase in body nitrogen occurs during the first year of life, which explains the major protein requirements that occur in infancy. The nutritional value of protein is based not only on the amount of nitrogen available, but also on the amino acid composition of the protein. A total of 20 amino acids have been identified, of which nine are essential in infants (Table 7-3). New tissue cannot be formed unless all of the essential amino acids are present in the diet simultaneously; the absence of only one essential amino acid results in a negative nitrogen and protein balance. Protein requirements in premature infants may be higher than in term infants and range from 4 to 3.5 g/kg/day. These added protein loads must be balanced against the immaturity of the renal system, and the possible development of uremia should be monitored. Three amino acids have been considered potentially essential in the neonate. Deficiencies in these amino acids may be due to an immaturity of enzyme systems. Premature infants are at particular risk. Specialized crystalline amino acid solutions should be used in premature infants on prolonged (>2 weeks) parenteral nutrition.

Carbohydrate

The greatest part of the body's caloric needs is supplied by carbohydrate. Carbohydrates are stored chiefly as glycogen in the liver and muscle but account for no more than 10% of body weight. The infant's liver and muscle mass is proportionally much smaller than that of the adult; the infant's glycogen, or carbohydrate reserve, is significantly smaller. Glycogen is converted to glucose in

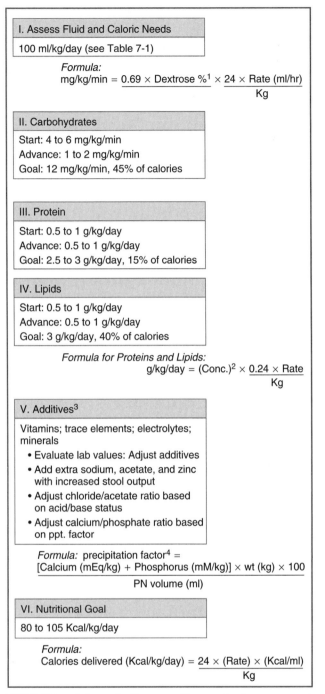

I. Assess Fluid and Caloric Needs

100 ml/kg/day (see Table 7-1)

Formula:
$$mg/kg/min = \frac{0.69 \times Dextrose\ \%^1 \times 24 \times Rate\ (ml/hr)}{Kg}$$

II. Carbohydrates

Start: 4 to 6 mg/kg/min
Advance: 1 to 2 mg/kg/min
Goal: 12 mg/kg/min, 45% of calories

III. Protein

Start: 0.5 to 1 g/kg/day
Advance: 0.5 to 1 g/kg/day
Goal: 2.5 to 3 g/kg/day, 15% of calories

IV. Lipids

Start: 0.5 to 1 g/kg/day
Advance: 0.5 to 1 g/kg/day
Goal: 3 g/kg/day, 40% of calories

Formula for Proteins and Lipids:
$$g/kg/day = \frac{(Conc.)^2 \times 0.24 \times Rate}{Kg}$$

V. Additives[3]

Vitamins; trace elements; electrolytes; minerals
- Evaluate lab values: Adjust additives
- Add extra sodium, acetate, and zinc with increased stool output
- Adjust chloride/acetate ratio based on acid/base status
- Adjust calcium/phosphate ratio based on ppt. factor

Formula: precipitation factor[4] =
$$\frac{[Calcium\ (mEq/kg) + Phosphorus\ (mM/kg)] \times wt\ (kg) \times 100}{PN\ volume\ (ml)}$$

VI. Nutritional Goal

80 to 105 Kcal/kg/day

Formula:
$$Calories\ delivered\ (Kcal/kg/day) = \frac{24 \times (Rate) \times (Kcal/ml)}{Kg}$$

FIGURE 7-1 ■ Schematic diagram of how to begin to approach writing parenteral nutrition orders for a neonate. Fluids should be adjusted based on the infant's gestational age and body weight.
[1]Dextrose concentration should be used as the percent number (i.e., 20 for 20%).
[2]The concentration in this formula should be written as the percent number (i.e., 4.25 for 4.25%).
[3]See relevant tables for each of these additives.
[4]If the amino acid concentration is greater than 1.5%, the precipitation factor should be less that 3. If the final amino acid concentration is greater than 1% but less than 1.5%, the precipitation factor should be less than 2; for an amino acid concentration less than 1%, calcium and phosphate should not be added. Adjustments to this formulation are needed if additives (e.g., cysteine) are placed in the parenteral nutrition.

TABLE 7-1 ■ **Daily Fluid Requirements**

Weight	Volume
Prematures <2 kg	150 mL/kg
Neonates and infants 2-10 kg	100 mL/kg for first 10 kg
Infants and children 10-20 kg	1000 mL + 50 mL/kg >10 kg
Children >20 kg	1500 mL + 20 mL/kg >20 kg

Note. Normal adults have a nutritional requirement of 150 nonprotein kcal for every gram of nitrogen administered. This probably increases under conditions of stress and trauma, but the exact ratio in these situations is not known. Studies have indicated that for infants this ratio is probably 230:1 after major surgery.

TABLE 7-2 ■ **Kilocalorie and Protein Requirements**

Age (Yr)	Kilocalories (kcal/kg body weight)	Protein (g/kg body weight)
0-1	90-120	2.0-3.5
1-7	75-90	2.0-2.5
7-12	60-75	2.0
12-18	30-60	1.5
>18	25-30	1.0

TABLE 7-3 ■ **Essential Amino Acids**

Threonine
Leucine
Isoleucine
Valine
Lysine
Methionine
Phenylalanine
Tryptophan
Histidine*
Tyrosine†
Cystine†

*Essential only in infancy.
†May be essential in premature infants.
Note. Glutamine, a major energy source for intestinal mucosal cells and other rapidly proliferating cells, may be an important part of the amino acid requirements. Presently, glutamine is not included in most amino acid solutions. In addition, arginine seems to have specific immunomodulation properties, which may be important in the postoperative and post-traumatic state. Protein requirements vary with the age of the patient, being highest for neonates (see Table 7-2). Total plasma protein levels in normal children range from 6 to 7.5 g/100 mL, with lower values in newborn and premature infants.

the liver and is metabolized throughout the body tissues either anaerobically to lactic acid or aerobically to carbon dioxide and water. Aerobic metabolism results in a much greater production of energy in the form of adenosine triphosphate (ATP). Delivery of carbohydrates greater than the body can use results in hyperglycemia and lipogenesis (see Chapter 3).

Fat

Fats comprise the other major source of nonprotein calories for the body. Simple lipids are the most abundant

TABLE 7-4 ▪ Intravenous Trace Minerals Preparation					
	Zinc (as sulfate)	Copper (as sulfate)	Manganese (as sulfate)	Chromium (as chloride)	Selenium (as selenious acid)
PTE-5* (1 mL)	1 mg	0.1 mg	25 μg	1 μg	15 μg
Recommended dose: 0.2 mL/kg/day of PTE-5 in neonates and children.					

*American Pharmaceutical Partners

fats in the body and food. The most common are the triglycerides. Naturally occurring fats contain straight-chained fatty acids, saturated and unsaturated, varying in length from 4 to 24 carbon atoms, with most containing 16 to 18 carbon atoms.

Humans do not synthesize linoleic acid, an 18-carbon chain with two double bonds; it must be supplied in the diet and is considered an essential fatty acid. Deficiency of this fatty acid results in dryness and thickening of the skin with a typical rash and desquamation. These deficiencies in neonates are critical because lipids are needed for central nervous system development. As long as the diet contains 1% to 2% of administered kilocalories in the form of linoleic acid, deficiency does not occur. There is some question as to the essentiality of linolenic acid; however, evidence indicates that linolenic acid is essential. A child on long-term parenteral nutrition with a fat emulsion that contained 78% linoleic acid and only 0.5% linolenic acid developed neurologic defects that seemed to improve on an emulsion that contained 54% linoleic acid and 8% linolenic acid.

Linoleic aicd is an ω-6 fatty acid, whereas linolenic acid is an ω-3 fatty acid. The metabolism of ω-6 fatty acids such as linoleic acid through the cyclooxygenase pathway results in the formation of prostaglandin E_2 and thromboxane A_2, both of which have immunosuppressive properties along with many other metabolic acid and coagulant activities. The provision of fat in the form of ω-3 fatty acids results in less production of prostaglandin E_2 and thromboxane A_2 and possibly in less immunosuppression, which could be detrimental in the postoperative, post-traumatic, or septic patient.

Minerals, Vitamins, and Other Nutrients

Rapidly growing infants need more minerals in general than do adults; this is especially true for phosphorus and calcium because of their exceptional rate of skeletal growth. The ash content of the fetus is low and at birth constitutes only 3% of body weight. It increases continuously throughout childhood, absolutely and relatively. The mineral content in adults is 40 times greater than in newborns, whereas the body weight is only 23 times greater. For each 1 g of protein retained, 0.3 g of mineral matter may be deposited. The important electropositive elements required by the body are calcium, magnesium, potassium, and sodium; the important electronegative ones are phosphorus, sulfur, and chloride. Iron, iodine, and cobalt occur in various important organic complexes throughout the body. The trace elements with known

metabolic actions are fluoride, copper, zinc, selenium, and manganese. Silicon, boron, nickel, arsenic, molybdenum, and strontium seem to be required by the body, but their specific metabolic functions are not well known (Table 7-4).

Vitamins are required in minute amounts for normal cellular metabolism. They must be supplied wholly or in part exogenously. B-complex vitamins function as coenzymes in various biochemical reactions, but the specific mode of action of the other vitamins is still relatively obscure. The fat-soluble vitamins are vitamins A, D, K, and E. The water-soluble vitamins are thiamine, riboflavin, folic acid, vitamin B_{12}, pyridoxine, nicotinic acid, biotin, pantothenic acid, and vitamin C. Because storage of fat-soluble vitamins occurs within the body, excess intake can lead to abnormalities. Likewise, a defect in fat absorption is likely to produce a deficiency of the fat-soluble vitamins.

Transport of fatty acids across the mitochondrial membrane is necessary for a normal oxidative process. Carnitine is required for this mitochondrial transport. Premature infants lack adequate amounts of carnitine. Standard parenteral nutrition solutions do not contain carnitine. Deficiency may be manifested by a hypertriglyceremia. Neonates on courses of parenteral nutrition longer than 1 to 2 weeks should receive carnitine supplementation. Infants and children may have L-carnitine added to their total parenteral nutrition (TPN) at a dose of 5 to 10 mg/kg/day to normalize plasma carnitine concentrations and improve fatty acid oxidation. Monitoring total and free plasma carnitine concentrations is recommended whenever carnitine is supplemented.

NUTRITIONAL ASSESSMENT AND MONITORING

Many infants and children who require operative intervention have malnutrition as a result of either a variety of feeding disorders or the underlying disease process for which they need surgery. Nutritional assessment is a crucial aspect of the initial evaluation of all surgical patients, and the incidence of malnutrition in surgical patients has been well documented in several reviews. In one review by Mullen, 95% of all surgical patients had one abnormal nutritional parameter, and 35% had three indicators of malnutrition. In a select group of children with congenital heart disease, Cameron showed that the prevalence of chronic malnutrition was similarly high at 65%, and the incidence increased to 80% in patients who were infants. Although a significantly malnourished patient can be identified easily, patients with mild-to-moderate malnutrition are frequently difficult to identify. A baseline assessment begins with a subjective global assessment (SGA). This assessment is easy to obtain and has a high degree of reliability with regard to the determination of degree of malnutrition. An SGA consists of a history and physical examination and should include an evaluation of weight loss (>10%), anorexia, or vomiting and physical evidence of muscle wasting. The last-mentioned finding is assessed best with documented atrophy of the deltoid or quadratus femoris muscles. Patients at particular risk for malnutrition include patients with large open wounds with the concomitant loss of protein and increased metabolic needs, with extensive burns, with blunt trauma, and with sepsis. Beyond this initial screening, a variety of indices can be used to assess further the child's nutritional status. Despite advances in nutritional assessment, a clinical evaluation of the patient's status can be as reliable as more sophisticated testing.

Growth and Development

A concern unique to the pediatric patient is growth and development. The term newborn grows at a rate of 25 to 30 g/day over the first 6 months of life, leading to a doubling of the birth weight during this time. The average infant triples his or her birth weight by 12 months. By age 3 years, the weight is four times the birth weight, and by completion of the first decade, the weight increases by 20-fold. Body length increases by 50% at the end of the first year of life and increases threefold at the end of the first decade. The preterm infant's growth pattern is distinct from term infants. Most nutrients are accumulated by the fetus in the third trimester of pregnancy. Fat accounts for only 1% to 2% of body weight in a 1-kg infant compared with 16% in a term (3.5-kg) infant. An anticipated loss of 15% of a preterm infant's birth weight is usual in the first 7 to 10 days of life compared with a 10% weight loss for a term infant. After this initial period of weight loss, a preterm infant less than 27 weeks' gestation gains weight at a slower rate of approximately 10 to 20 g/day because he or she has not yet entered the accelerated weight gain of the third trimester. This is in contrast to a 27- to 40-week gestational age infant, who could gain 35 g/day. Monitoring of growth should use a standardized growth curve. The most commonly used is that of the National Center for Health Statistics, which was updated in 2001.

Other parameters that can be useful for measuring nutritional status include bone age and dental status. Periods of stress, infection, major medical illness, and malnutrition all can result in an arrest of normal growth and development. A commonly used marker of such a period is the presence of growth arrest lines found on a skeletal survey. These lines are transversely oriented, thickened portions of trabecular bone found in the metaphysis, often in the distal femur and proximal tibia.

Visceral Protein

Enzymes, clotting factors, albumin, globulins, transport proteins, and visceral organ cell structures all are composed of visceral (nonmuscle) proteins. Visceral protein deficits adversely affect the patient's ability to mount an immune response and to heal wounds. Deficits in serum albumin levels and transferin reflect an impairment in hepatic synthesis as a result of a limited substrate supply.

Because serum albumin has a half-life of 20 days, it is not a sensitive indicator of malnutrition or protein repletion. Transferrin, a carrier protein involving iron metabolism with a 9-day half-life, is a much better indicator of protein status. It is more expensive to measure, however, is not as readily attainable, and is not useful in septic patients or patients with iron deficiency. The total lymphocyte count provides a general guide to the patient's ability to respond to infection. Lymphocytes are destroyed rapidly, and protein is required for the formation of new cells. Consequently the absolute lymphocyte count is a useful measure of the status of protein reserve.

Protein also is required for synthesizing the cells and mediators involved in the response to various skin antigens. Although skin-test reactivity is a manifestation of lymphocyte-mediated immunity, the reactivity is probably a measure of the general status of host defenses rather than lymphocyte activity itself. Many chronically and acutely malnourished patients convert from a reactive to a nonreactive state of anergy. Reactivity can be restored by nutritional repletion, making these skin tests an indirect measure of nutritional status. Christou and colleagues showed that neutrophil chemotaxis (or the lack of it) correlates with cutaneous sensitivity to recall antigens, suggesting that other immunologic tests also may be indirect measures of the patient's nutritional state.

Measure of a patient's nitrogen balance is a useful means of determining daily nitrogen requirements and the effectiveness of ongoing nutritional therapy. The goal for growth or repair is a daily positive balance of 4 to 6 g in adolescents or adults and proportionately less in infants and small children. A 24-hour urine collection is necessary, which makes the balance study difficult to obtain. Protein intake, whether enteral or parenteral, needs to be recorded accurately for calculation of nitrogen balance.

ENTERAL NUTRITION

Early nutritional support of critically ill and surgical pediatric patients is essential to avoid the added problems of severe nutritional depletion. The type of nutritional support depends on the form and extent of stress affecting the individual child. From the standpoints of the physiologic efficiency of use and the economy of administration, enteral feedings are preferable and should be the first choice in patients with adequate function of the gastrointestinal (GI) tract. Many postsurgical patients do not have a fully functional GI tract, however, to permit full enteral feedings. Combined enteral and parenteral nutrition should be used in these patients. Much literature has condemned the use of parenteral nutrition, but a meta-analysis by Braunschweig showed that enteral nutrition (EN) is associated with a similar or higher rate of complications compared with parenteral nutrition.

Enteral feedings are begun after the resolution of the postoperative ileus, which is manifested by disappearance of the bilious green color of the gastric aspirate, a decrease in volume of the gastric aspirate, and the passage of stool. The return of bowel sounds is a helpful sign in older children and adolescents but is not as sensitive or reliable in determining the disappearance of ileus in infants. Small volumes of sugar water or dilute formula are initiated in infants or small children by mouth or nasogastric tube. In older children and adolescents, clear liquids are initiated in a similar fashion, following the adage that the stressed and recovering GI tract tolerates increases in volume much more readily than increases in osmolarity. As patients are advanced through progressive stages of increased concentration of formula or liquids and solids toward normal feeding, inability to tolerate increased osmolarity, if it occurs, usually is manifested by cramps and diarrhea. Inability to tolerate increased volume usually is evidenced by vomiting or increased residuals in the nasogastric tube.

Feeding Access

If it is not possible to provide all nutrient needs by mouth despite an intact GI tract, tube feedings are recommended. When the decision has been made to begin nutritional support by feeding tube, the risk of aspiration determines whether the tube should be placed in the stomach or jejunum. Gastric feeding is always preferable because it enables normal digestive processes and hormonal responses to occur; provides for easier tube insertion; allows tolerance of larger osmotic loads with less frequent distention, cramping, or diarrhea; and results in a lower likelihood of the dumping syndrome compared with jejunal feedings. Transpyloric tube placement is indicated in patients with a high risk of aspiration, such as patients with delayed gastric emptying or gastroesophageal reflux or patients who are comatose with a depressed gag reflex. Verification of the location of the tube is mandatory before beginning enteral tube feedings. Simple insufflation of air into the tube is not sufficient, in that auscultation over the stomach can pick up sound transmitted by a tube inadvertently placed into the bronchial tree. The simplest means of confirming tube placement is by aspirating gastrointestinal contents using a small syringe. Gentle aspiration is important because small-bore soft tubes tend to collapse with negative pressure. If gastric or intestinal contents cannot be aspirated through the tube, radiographic confirmation is mandatory.

Gastric feedings can be provided using either a nasogastric tube (NGT) or a gastrostomy tube (GT). The NGT is appropriate for short-term intervention. Additionally, provision of NGT feedings before placing a GT allows the physician to assess feeding tolerance and the significance of gastroesophageal reflux. Potential drawbacks of NGT feeds include complications of gastroesophageal reflux and voluntary or involuntary removal of the tube. Long-term use of an NGT may be accompanied by nasal erosions and sinusitis. Silastic weighted tubes (i.e., Dobhoff, Biosearch Medical Products, Somerville, NJ) may be passed distal to the pylorus. Passage of a weighted feeding tube may be facilitated using a prokinetic agent, such as metoclopramide. Fluoroscopic or endoscopic intervention may be necessary if spontaneous passage does not occur. Tubes often are passed distal to the pylorus in an effort to avoid complications of gastroesophageal reflux. The utility of this modality is controversial, however. Feeding tubes may be passed into the jejunum by various routes, including nasoenterically, via an indwelling surgical GT, or surgically. Jejunal tube feeding may allow earlier initiation of postoperative feedings because the

jejunum functions within 12 to 24 hours after surgery. Long-term use of jejunal tubes is plagued with problems, however, including involuntary dislodgment of gastrostomy-to-jejunal tubes and obstruction owing to inspissation of feedings. Short-term complications of surgically placed jejunal tubes include intra-abdominal abscess and bowel infarction. Long-term complications include intestinal obstruction and peritonitis. When using tubes passed distal to the pylorus, continuous drip feedings are recommended to prevent the development of diarrhea and other symptoms of dumping.

A GT offers a more secure and manageable access site for EN when long-term alimentation (>8 weeks) is anticipated, as in patients with severe head trauma. If abdominal exploration is required in the treatment of the trauma patient, a GT may be placed at that time; otherwise a percutaneous GT may be placed even in young infants. The safety and utility of a gastrostomy in pediatric surgery patients has been well documented. The potential mortality and high morbidity also have been described if the tube gastrostomy is not performed correctly. When considering operative placement of a feeding gastrostomy, the physician always should evaluate the patient for gastroesophageal reflux, which, if present, frequently is made worse by the addition of the GT. This is particularly important in the case of brain-damaged children, for whom uncontrolled reflux is particularly dangerous. Preoperative evaluation is indicated and generally consists of a barium swallow and limited upper GT series, followed by a 24-hour pH monitoring if the barium swallow is normal. If these tests are positive for reflux, a fundoplication should be performed at the time of gastrostomy. If poor gastric motility and slow emptying also are documented, some believe a pyloroplasty should be added to the procedure.

When an abdominal exploration is required in pediatric patients, catheter jejunostomy reportedly has provided an early and relatively safe postoperative route for EN. Complications with jejunostomy tubes commonly have been reported, however, and we have preferred a combination of early parenteral nutrition followed by NGT (or nasojejunal tube) feedings later as needed.

Enteral Formulas

Standard premature infant formulas are milk-based formulas that provide 22 to 24 calories/oz. A portion of fat is provided as medium-chain triglycerides (MCT) to compensate for the limited bile salt pool. The carbohydrate is composed of glucose polymers and lactose to optimize carbohydrate absorption in the presence of limited lactase activity. These formulas also provide increased amounts of vitamins, calcium, and phosphorus compared with infant formulas. These formulas allow the increased nutrient needs to be met in a limited volume. Additionally, the increased calcium and phosphorus help prevent osteopenia. Standard infant formulas are derived from either milk or soy protein (at a concentration of 20 calories/oz). These may be used for all healthy infants. If a child is gaining weight poorly, the calorie concentration can be increased by adding relatively less fluid to either the concentrate or the powder. Alternatively, additives are available for the major energy nutrients. Composition of infant and pediatric formulas is summarized in Tables 7-5 and 7-6.

TABLE 7-5 ■ Infant Formulas

Formula*	kcal/mL	Protein (g/L)	Protein (% kcal)	Osmolarity (mOsm/kg)	Protein Source	Carbohydrate Source	Carbohydrate (% kcal)	Fat Source	Fat (% kcal)	Indications
Similac Special Care (Ross)	0.81	22	11	280	Nonfat milk, whey	Lactose, corn syrup solids	42	MCT oil, soy oil, coconut oil	47	Prematurity
Neosure (Ross)	0.73	19	10	250	Nonfat milk, whey	Lactose, corn syrup solids	42	MCT oil, soy oil	48	Prematurity, post-discharge
Enfamil (Mead Johnson)	0.67	14	9	300	Whey, nonfat milk	Lactose	43	Palm olein, soy oil, coconut oil, sun oil	48	Standard
Similac (Ross)	0.67	14	8	300	Nonfat milk, whey	Lactose	43	Soy oil	49	Standard
	0.81	22	11	380	Nonfat milk, whey	Lactose	42	Coconut oil	47	
Prosobee (Mead Johnson)	0.67	20	12	200	Soy isolate, methionine	Corn syrup solids	42	Palm olein, soy oil, coconut oil, sun oil	48	Lactose intolerance, galactosemia
Isomil (Ross)	0.67	17	10	200	Soy isolate, methionine	Corn syrup, sucrose	41	Soy oil, coconut oil	49	Lactose, malabsorption, galactosemia
Nutramigen (Mead Johnson)	0.67	19	11	320	Casein hydrolysate, cystine, tyrosine, tryptophan	Corn syrup solids, modified cornstarch	44	Palm olein, soy oil, coconut oil, sun oil	45	Protein intolerance
Pregestimil (Mead Johnson)	0.67	19	11	320	Casein hydrolysate, cystine, tyrosine, tryptophan	Corn syrup solids, modified cornstarch, dextrose	41	MCT oil, corn oil, soy oil, safflower oil	48	Protein intolerance, cystic fibrosis, neonatal, cholestasis, short-bowel syndrome
Alimentum (Ross)	0.67	19	11	370	Casein hydrolysate, cystine, tyrosine, tryptophan, methionine	Sucrose, modified tapioca, starch	41	MCT oil, safflower oil, soy oil	48	Protein intolerance, neonatal cholestasis
Neocate (Scientific Hospital Supplies)	0.69	20	12	342	Free amino acids	Corn syrup solids	47	Safflower oil, corn oil, soy oil	41	Food allergy, protein intolerance, short-bowel syndrome

MCT, medium-chain triglyceride; CHO, carbohydrate.
*Ross Laboratories, Columbus, Ohio; Mead Johnson Nutritionals, Evansville, Indiana; Scientific Hospital Supplies North America, Gaithersburg, Maryland.

TABLE 7-6 ■ Pediatric Formulas

Formula*	kcal/mL	Protein (g/L)	Protein (% kcal)	Osmolarity (mOsm/kg)	Protein Source	Carbohydrate Source	Carbohydrate (% kcal)	Fat Source	Fat (% kcal)	Indications
Pediasure (Ross)	1.0	30	12	<310	Sodium caseinate, whey protein	Hydrolyzed cornstarch, sucrose	44	Safflower oil, soy oil, MCT oil	44	Standard, oral feeds, tube feeds
Kindercal (Mead Johnson)	1.06	34	13	310	Sodium caseinate	Maltodextrin, sucrose	50	Canola oil, MCT oil, corn oil, sunflower oil	37	Standard, oral feeds, tube feeds
Boost (Mead Johnson)	1.06	43	17	610–670	Milk	Corn syrup, sucrose	53	Canola oil, corn oil, sunflower oil	30	Standard, oral feeds, tube feeds
Peptamen, Jr. (Clintec)	1.0	30	12	260 (unflavored) 365 (flavored)	Hydrolyzed whey	Maltodextrin	55	MCT oil	33	Short-bowel syndrome, cholestasis, pancreatitis
L-Emental (Hormel)	0.8	24	12	630	L-Amino acids	Maltodextrin, modified starch	63	MCT oil, soybean oil	25	Short-bowel syndrome, IBD, pancreatitis
Elecare (Ross)	1.0	30	15	551	L-Amino acids	Corn syrup solids	44	Safflower oil, coconut oil, soy oil	42	Malabsorption, food allergies
Suplena (Ross)	2.5	30	6	600	Sodium caseinate, calcium caseinate	Hydrolyzed cornstarch, sucrose	51	Safflower oil, soy oil	43	Renal failure

MCT, medium-chain triglyceride; CHO, carbohydrate.
*Ross Laboratories, Columbus, Ohio; Mead Johnson Nutritionals, Evansville, Indiana; Clintec Nutrition Division, Baxter, Deerfield, Illinois; Hormel Healthlabs, Plymouth, Minnesota.

Standard formulas are milk-based proteins and contain lactose as the carbohydrate source. There are only limited reasons to use soy formulas. These generally contain corn syrup solids as a carbohydrate source. Isomil also contains sucrose. Soy formulas are indicated to manage galactosemia and primary or secondary lactase deficiency (e.g., postenterocolitis). Soy formulas should not be used in patients with a documented allergy or intolerance to milk protein because one third of infants who have an allergen-induced reaction to cow's milk are also intolerant of soy. A protein hydrolysate or elemental formula is recommended in infants who have a milk-protein intolerance. Protein hydrolysates include Nutramigen (Mead Johnson), Alimentum (Ross), and Pregestimil (Mead Johnson). These formulas may be particularly helpful in patients with an injured GI tract (recovering from necrotizing enterocolitis) or with short-bowel syndrome. Alimentum and Pregestimil also provide significant amounts of fat as MCT, which can be useful in patients with a chylothorax. For infants, Neocate (Scientific Hospital Supplies) is the only amino acid–based formula available. Children older than age 12 months who continue to be intolerant of milk protein may respond well to Peptamen, Jr. (Clintec), which is a whey protein hydrolysate. If an amino acid–based formula is needed in children older than age 12 months, options include Neocate 1+ (Scientific Hospital Supplies), L-Emental (Hormel), and Elecare (Ross). Neocate 1+ and Elecare have long-chain triglycerides. Of the fat in L-Emental, 68% is derived from MCT. An elemental diet can be infused that can be absorbed fully in 30 to 40 cm of small intestine Likewise, the drainage from a proximal fistula can be "refed" by this route, considerably easing the task of fluid and electrolyte replacement.

Administration of an enteral feeding regimen is more certain of success when a few simple guidelines are observed. First, as previously indicated, the GI tract generally tolerates increased volume more readily than increased osmolarity; cramps, diarrhea, and subsequent poor absorption can be avoided by initiating quarter-strength or half-strength formula and advancing gradually. Second, administration of formula by continuous drip is tolerated better than by bolus feeding, and the threat of gastroesophageal reflux, vomiting, and subsequent aspiration is reduced greatly. Third, care must be taken to ensure that the enteral formula does not become contaminated, either during preparation or while hanging at the bedside. Expiration time should be observed, and a low threshold should be maintained for obtaining fresh formula. Finally, the use of pectin, Metamucil, diphenoxylate hydrochloride with atropine sulfate (Lomotil), paregoric, and loperamide hydrochloride (Imodium) in patients with short-bowel syndrome often permits enteral feeding to succeed when almost certain failure would result without the use of one or more of these agents. Cholestyramine, with its ability to bind bile acids (which can cause a colonic secretory diarrhea) is extremely helpful in patients who have lost a bulk of their ileum. The concept of gradually advancing the diet and fine-tuning is the key to ultimate success in these often complicated patients.

The rapid development of today's high technology and enteral pharmacology has resulted in increasingly more effective enteral nutrition with better absorption and fewer side effects than was possible a few years ago. EN is possible in most patients earlier than previously recognized; it can provide protein and other special nutrients equivalent to that supplied by TPN and can be furnished at a greatly reduced cost.

TOTAL PARENTERAL NUTRITION

The history of intravenous nutrition began when Wren administered alcohol intravenously in 1665. Parenteral administration of fat was studied in animals by Menzel and Perco in 1869. After attempts in Japan during the 1920s and 1930s, the first successful intravenous administration of a fat emulsion occurred in the United States in the 1950s, when Lipomul was investigated clinically. Major toxic reactions caused Lipomul to be removed from the market, however. Intravenous fat emulsions became a reality in 1962, when Wretlind introduced the soybean oil emulsion, Intralipid.

In 1904, enzymatically digested protein was administered intravenously. Today the most frequently used protein hydrolysates are prepared from casein and fibrin. To avoid metabolic acid complications, these hydrolysates have been replaced by crystalline amino acid solutions.

Although a report of TPN in an infant was published in 1944, the technique was unsuccessful in infants and children until 1968, when Dudrick described his success with the technique in beagle puppies and subsequently in an infant and adults. Pediatric surgical patients have particular nutritional needs that often exceed those of the typical term or preterm infant. Probably the most distinctive impact of TPN on surgical neonates can be exemplified by its use in patients with gastroschisis. The survival of infants with this disease increased from less than 70% before 1967 to greater than 90% in the 1970s, with TPN being a crucial factor with this improved rate of survival. With a careful selection of patients, meticulous attention to technical details, and constant monitoring of patients, the complications of the technique can be minimized and the efficacy maximized.

Dudrick's intravenous nutrition used a markedly hypertonic solution of glucose and amino acids infused through a central venous catheter. This method still is used by most institutions in the United States. In the 1980s and 1990s, however, other techniques of intravenous nutrition, especially in children, were introduced. Peripheral intravenous nutrition using less hypertonic solutions of glucose with or without fat solutions now is employed in many pediatric institutions. In essence, there are two basic approaches to intravenous nutrition in infants and children: central infusion or peripheral infusion of parenteral nutrition, with peripheral infusion having the limitation of decreased caloric delivery. Each of these techniques is effective in producing nitrogen retention and weight gain. In a difficult patient, both techniques may be required over a long period.

Indications

TPN is indicated when the GI tract must be bypassed because of severe injury or malabsorption; this includes infants with congenital anomalies such as bowel atresias, gastroschisis, volvulus, meconium ileus, and severe Hirschsprung's disease. Additionally, patients with specific GT disorders, including short-bowel syndrome, intractable diarrhea, protracted vomiting, necrotizing enterocolitis, motility disorders, inflammatory bowel disease, enteric fistulas, and bowel obstruction, may require parenteral feedings for a prolonged period. Enteral feedings also may need to be withheld temporarily in premature infants with severe respiratory distress syndrome, in children who are acutely ill secondary to aspiration pneumonia, and in children with severe mucositis secondary to chemotherapy.

Indications for Preoperative Nutrition

In adults, provision of enteral feedings preoperatively for 2 to 3 weeks may reduce postoperative wound infections, anastomotic leakage, hepatic and renal failure, and length of hospital stay. Data for parenteral nutrition support are less clear. A meta-analysis showed only a marginal benefit of preoperative parenteral nutrition in mildly or moderately malnourished patients. Benefit has been noted, however, in severely malnourished patients, who developed fewer noninfectious complications if receiving perioperative parenteral nutrition. An increased infection rate in patients receiving parenteral nutrition could not be explained completely by the use of central venous catheters, however, suggesting that use of TPN may predispose patients to increased infectious complications. Unless there are clear indications of severe malnutrition, a delay in operative management to provide preoperative TPN is not indicated. An extrapolation of these findings to neonatal patients is difficult. Because of similarities in the metabolic response to surgery, however, it seems reasonable to apply these same conclusions to pediatric patients.

Indications for Postoperative Nutrition

Use of aggressive postoperative nutritional support is more controversial. In adults, the provision of enteral nutrients may reduce the rate of sepsis and lower costs. Nutrient intolerance can be a limitation, however. These data suggest that, when used, postoperative nutrition should be started early, using a combination of TPN and EN until the GI tract fully recovers.

The effect of TPN on postoperative healing is unclear because studies are contradictory. In the postoperative period, there are higher infection rates in patients on TPN. In patients fed enterally, GI intolerance limits use in some patients. In children, TPN may improve nitrogen balance and augment insulin-like growth factor levels. Clinical outcomes (e.g., hospital stay or incidence of postoperative infections) for children receiving TPN may not change, however.

Because results in the area of postoperative nutritional support are not clear, aggressive postoperative feedings are recommended only in patients who can receive EN without complication. Postoperative parenteral nutrition should be restricted to infants who would not tolerate even a short period of starvation or older children who probably would not start EN for at least 5 to 7 days.

Composition of Solutions

Central Nutrition

TPN is a source of fluids, electrolytes, macronutrients (amino acids, dextrose, lipid emulsions), and micronutrients (multivitamins, trace minerals). Daily electrolyte requirements for neonatal and pediatric patients are discussed in Chapter 4. Sodium in TPN should be provided in sufficient amounts to promote protein synthesis and tissue development. The maximum concentration of sodium in TPN should not exceed the equivalent of normal saline (154 mEq/L). Potassium concentrations should not exceed 80 mEq/L with a maximum potassium infusion rate of 0.5 mEq/kg/hr for an infant or child and 20 mEq/hr for an adult. These are maximal infusion levels, and with these concentrations and infusion rates, a patient should be placed in the intensive care unit on a cardiac monitor. The chloride-to-acetate ratio is adjusted based on the acid-base status. Acetate is converted in vivo to bicarbonate at a 1-to-1 molar ratio. A high acetate-to-low chloride ratio helps correct the metabolic acidosis resulting from diarrhea or high fistula output. A high acetate ratio may be used effectively to help balance acid-base status in a patient on high ventilator settings who is experiencing passive hypercapnia. This is particularly the case in neonates who, because of immature renal function, may not be able to correct a respiratory acidosis. A low acetate-to-high chloride ratio minimizes the bicarbonate load in patients with metabolic alkalosis, which may be secondary to excessive nasogastric drainage. Careful monitoring of acid-base balance should be done because large changes may occur in only a couple of days. Calcium and phosphate requirements to support growth in infants and children are greater than in adults. Bone mineralization is optimized at a ratio of 2.6 mEq of calcium to 1 mM of phosphorus. Corticosteroids and loop diuretics increase calcium requirements. Chemical incompatibility limits the amount of calcium and phosphorus that can be added to TPN. Calcium and phosphorus can be added safely to TPN when the concentrations provided satisfy the following equation:

$$\text{Calcium (mEq)} + \text{phosphorus (mM)} \leq 30$$
$$\text{(per 1000 mL of TPN)}$$

The needs for optimal tissue and bone growth may not be met unless calcium and phosphorus also are provided enterally.

Amino acids are a source of nitrogen for protein synthesis. If total calories are limited, however, amino acids are metabolized as an energy source with a caloric value of 4 Kcal/g. Administration in neonates should begin at 1 g/kg/day and be advanced as tolerated to a maximum of 2.5 to 3.0 g/kg/day (higher in premature infants). Amino acid requirements in older children are based on the recommended dietary allowances (RDA), which are adjusted for specific clinical conditions. They usually range from 1 to 1.5 g/kg/day. Patients on dialysis or hemofiltration should receive higher doses of amino acids to account for filter losses. In contrast, patients with liver failure may require limitation of amino acids to avoid hepatic encephalopathy. Pediatric-specific amino acid solutions

TABLE 7-7 ■ Examples of Neonatal and Pediatric Intravenous Amino Acid Formulas			
	Trophamine 10%*	Aminosyn-PF 10%†	Aminosyn 10%†
Amino acid concentration	10%	10%	10%
Nitrogen (g/100 mL)	1.55	1.52	1.57
Essential amino acids (mg/100 mL)			
Leucine	1400	1200	940
Isoleucine	820	760	720
Valine	780	673	800
Lysine	820	677	720
Methionine	340	180	400
Phenylalanine	480	427	440
Threonine	420	512	520
Tryptophan	200	180	160
Nonessential amino acids (mg/100 mL)			
Alanine	540	698	1280
Arginine	1200	1227	980
Histidine	480	312	300
Proline	680	812	860
Serine	380	495	420
Taurine	25	70	
Tyrosine	240	40	44
Aminoacetic acid (glycine)	360	385	1280
Glutamic acid	500	620	
Aspartic acid	320	527	
Cysteine	<16		
Electrolytes (mEq/L)			
Sodium	5	3.4	
Potassium			5.4
Chloride	<3		
Acetate	97	46.3	148
Osmalarity (mOsm/L)	875	829	1000

*McGaw Laboratories.
†Abbott Laboratories.

have an amino acid profile that is essential for the developing child (Table 7-7). Their use has led to greater weight gain and improved nitrogen balance compared with the use of standard solutions.

Hydrous dextrose is a major source of calories and carbon skeletons for tissue accretion. Its caloric value is 3.4 Kcal/g. Small amounts of carbohydrates prevent breakdown of somatic protein stores and act as protein-sparing substrate. The newborn has relatively limited glycogen reserves (34 g). Relatively short periods of fasting can lead to a hypoglycemic state. Stable infants should receive approximately 40% to 45% of their total caloric intake as carbohydrate. Parenteral nutrition for the neonate should begin at approximately 6 to 8 mg/kg/min of dextrose to maintain adequate serum glucose levels. Less glucose in a young neonate leads to hypoglycemia owing to inadequate hepatic production of glucose. Older neonates and children tolerate greater loads of glucose that are administered through a central venous catheter (10 to 14 mg/kg/min). The dextrose infusion may be advanced at a daily rate of 2 mg/kg/min until the nutritional goal is reached with a maximum rate of 10 to 15 mg/kg/min. This is approximately equivalent to initiating 10% dextrose at 100 mL/kg/day and advancing the dextrose concentration 2.5% per day to a concentration of 20% dextrose. Higher concentrations of dextrose may be provided, however, if total fluids must be restricted.

Intravenous lipid emulsions are a condensed source of calories and are used to prevent or treat essential fatty acid deficiency. They should provide patients 30% to 50% of the non-nitrogen caloric needs. The maximal intravenous fat dose provided should be 3 g/kg/day. Gradually increasing the daily intake of fat from 0.5 or 1.0 g/kg/day does not seem to improve lipid clearance. Lipid clearance is improved, however, if the daily lipid volume is provided over 24 hours rather than a part of the day. The 20% lipid emulsion is better tolerated than the 10% emulsion because of its lower phospholipid-to-triglyceride ratio (0.06 and 0.12). Linoleic acid is essential for older children and adults and neonates. Deficiencies of linoleic acid may occur in 2 days in the premature infant who has limited stores. Deficiencies in older children may take considerably longer. Fatty acid deficiency may be detected by a raised serum level of 5,8,11-eicosatrienoic acid, low levels of linoleic and arachidonic acids, and an eicosatrienoic-to-arachidonic (triene/tetranene) ratio greater than 0.4. Administration of intravenous lipid emulsions at a dose of 0.5 to 1 g/kg/day prevents essential fatty acid deficiency. The 30% lipid emulsion is approved for use only in total nutrient admixtures (3-in-1 TPN solutions). Examples of intravenous lipid emulsion formulas are shown in Table 7-8.

Pediatric multivitamin formulas for intravenous administration provide a combination of water-soluble

TABLE 7-8 ■ Examples of Intravenous Lipid Emulsion Formulas

	Soybean Oil Lipid Emulsions						Soybean and Safflower Oil Lipid Emulsions	
	Intralipid*			Liposyn III†			Liposyn II†	
Total fat (%)	10	20	30	10	20	30	10	20
Linoleic acid (%)		50			54.5			65.8
Oleic acid (%)		26			22.4			17.7
Palmitic acid (%)		10			10.5			8.8
Linolenic acid (%)		9			8.3			4.2
Stearic acid (%)		3.5			4.2			3.4
Egg yolk phospholipids (%)		1.2			1.2			1.2
Glycerin (%)		2.25	1.7		2.5	1.7		2.5
kcal/mL	1.1	2	3	1.1	2	3	1.1	2
Osmolarity (mOsm/L)		260	200	284	292	200	276	258
Phospholipids-triglycerides ratio	0.12	0.06	0.04	0.12	0.06	0.04	0.12	0.06

Note. Linoleic and linolenic acids are essential fatty acids. Egg yolk phospholipids are used as emulsifiers, and glycerin is used to adjust tonicity.
*Clintec Nutrition.
†Abbott Laboratories.

and fat-soluble vitamins added daily to TPN, based on RDA and American Medical Association guidelines. Standard pediatric trace mineral formulations contain zinc, copper, manganese, chromium, and selenium. Zinc requirements are increased in patients with chronic diarrhea because of increased losses and decreased absorption. Accumulation of copper and manganese may occur with chronic severe cholestasis. Restriction of these minerals may be necessary to prevent their accumulation. Copper restriction in cholestasis may result in pancytopenia secondary to copper deficiency. To provide proper dosage, monitoring blood concentrations of trace minerals is recommended whenever a trace mineral is restricted or supplemental doses are used. Heparin may be added to TPN at a concentration of 0.5 to 1 u/mL to maintain the patency of the venous catheter and to minimize vein irritation. Additionally, heparin is a cofactor of lipoprotein lipase, an enzyme released from the vascular endothelium that enhances the clearance of lipid particles. Heparin should be avoided in patients with thrombocytopenia and active bleeding. Histamine-2 receptor blockers (e.g., ranitidine) for stress ulcer prophylaxis and human regular insulin for glycemic control also may be added to TPN.

Peripheral Nutrition

Parenteral nutrition can be delivered through a peripheral vein if central venous access is not available. This solution contains 2% amino acids and 10% glucose, which yields 0.40 kcal/mL. Electrolytes, vitamins, and trace elements are added to the infusate to provide the recommended daily requirements. The addition of heparin and lipids decreases irritation to the peripheral veins. The advantage of peripheral TPN has diminished with improved venous access and the almost exponential use of peripherally inserted central catheters (PICC) in neonates and children. One disadvantage of peripheral TPN is the large amount of fluid needed for reasonable caloric delivery. In general, for infants, 160 to 200 mL/kg of body weight per 24 hours is administered intravenously, providing

64 to 80 kcal/day. In older children, the volume is reduced according to the caloric needs. The addition of lipids improves caloric delivery.

Methods: Venous Access and Administration

On a temporary basis, delivery of concentrated TPN may be accomplished via a central venous catheter. If delivery is needed beyond a 7-day period, a more defined mode of access should be sought. For needs between 1 week and 3 months, a PICC is ideal. Because venous access is a premium in small infants, physicians should preserve veins typically used for a PICC (antecubital fossa in children and saphenous vein in neonates). For longer term access, or when a PICC cannot be obtained, a tunneled Silastic catheter may be used. Use of these tunneled catheters has the theoretical advantage of preventing bacteria from entering the bloodstream. The greatest advantage of this tunneling is the bio-ingrowth of tissue into the Dacron cuff, which prevents catheter dislodgment. Insertion of catheters, whether at the bedside or in the operating room, must be performed under strict aseptic conditions. A more detailed discussion of venous access is given in Chapter 6.

The infusate must be delivered at a slow, uniform rate to ensure proper use of the glucose and amino acids. In small infants, this is accomplished most readily by the use of a constant infusion pump. Delivery of appropriate calories and nutrients demands constant re-evaluation by the physican. Strict aseptic technique should be followed. The greatest cause of bloodstream infections comes from breaks in the infusion line. Entry into this line should be done sparingly and only after preparing the connection for at least 1 minute with povidone-iodine.

MONITORING NUTRITIONAL SUPPORT

When a specialized EN or TPN regimen has been started, metabolic assessment is performed on an ongoing basis to evaluate the effectiveness of therapy. Essential clinical

TABLE 7-9 ■ Guidelines for Blood Laboratory Monitoring of Nutritional Support in Critically Ill Pediatric Patients					
	Initial	Daily	2-3 ×/Week	Weekly	As Indicated
Glucose	X	X	X		
BUN, creatinine	X	X	X		
Na, K, Cl, CO$_2$	X	X	X		
AST, ALT, LDH, alkaline phosphatase, total and direct bilirubin, GGTP	X			X	
Magnesium, calcium, phosphorus	X		X		
Albumin, total protein	X			X	
Triglycerides	X*			X	
Hgb, Hct, CBC, platelets, PT	X				X
Cu, Zn, Se, Cr, Mn, Fe					X
TIBC, ferritin					X
Vitamin concentrations					X
Chemsticks					X
Ammonia					X
Blood cultures					X

*Measured when goal lipid infusion reached.

measurements include daily body weight, weekly body length and head circumference in infants and small children, and accurate intake and output volumes. The urine is monitored for urine glucose levels and ketones, initially with each void and once each nursing shift after the patient is stable. Table 7-9 lists the recommended blood tests and frequency of monitoring. More frequent monitoring of some parameters may be necessary in patients with specific abnormalities, as in children with kidney or liver diseases. The judicious and sparing use of blood tests is important in infants and small children, however, because of their small total blood volume and the increased risks of blood transfusion. In addition to monitoring various blood chemistries, one must pay careful attention to subjective and objective clinical parameters. Improved muscle strength, wound healing, overcoming systemic infections, improved respiratory function, and subsequent weaning from the respirator all may indicate improved nutritional status.

Weight changes during parenteral nutrition vary with the patient's overall clinical condition. If infants or children are severely depleted at the start of treatment, adequate weight gain may not be observed for several days. Patients who are not severely malnourished or septic can be expected to exhibit weight gains more comparable with those of normal infants and children. Increased metabolic demands, such as from severe trauma or sepsis, result in a flatter growth curve that may be calculated to some extent by daily determination of energy needs using indirect calorimetry, if available. Adequate weight gain should average 15 to 25 g/day in neonates and infants or 0.5% of total body weight in kilograms per day in older children and adolescents. Greater weight gain suggests excess fluid administration and fluid retention.

Urine output should be maintained at 1 mL/kg/hr or more; the urine specific gravity should be kept between 1.005 and 1.015, and glucosuria should be prevented.

If increased gradually, the large amount of intravenous glucose is well tolerated in most pediatric patients without the need for exogenous insulin. The neonate, particularly if premature, may need exogenous insulin delivery to allow for acceptable tolerance of TPN. Blood glucose levels generally remain in the high-normal range, and, if hyperglycemia and glucosuria occur, slowing the infusion rate or lowering the concentration of glucose temporarily usually solves the problem unless the patient is septic. TPN usually results in a greater excretion of solutes in the urine than observed during eternal feeding, but this increased load does not exceed the concentrating ability of a normal kidney. Water balance, even in the face of high rates of TPN administration, usually is maintained.

The transition from parenteral to oral-enteral nutrition is an important and often difficult time nutritionally for recovering patients. If this recovery phase is not managed well, patients may lose a hard-earned nutritional advantage. During prolonged TPN, patients may develop hallucinations of taste and smell and become unduly preoccupied with food at mealtime. At the same time, TPN frequently suppresses appetite, and the physician should offer reassurance that appetite will return when the TPN is tapered and stopped. Although it is important that during the transition from TPN to EN nearly full caloric requirements be supplied before parenteral support is discontinued, it is often necessary to cut back half of the daily amount of TPN to stimulate a patient's appetite and desire to eat.

COMPLICATIONS OF NUTRITIONAL SUPPORT

Although intuitively parenteral nutrition would seem to be associated with a greater degree of complications and morbidity, a meta-analysis has shown that EN complications may exceed those of TPN. Nevertheless, the following discussion centers on TPN because this may present a greater challenge to the surgeon in terms of overall management.

Technical Complications

The incidence of technical complications caused by the placement of central venous lines in infants and children has been reduced greatly by careful attention to technique and by radiographic confirmation of catheter position. The incidence of cardiac arrhythmias caused by catheter irritation has been reduced greatly by placing the tip of the catheter at the junction of the superior vena cava and right atrium rather than in the heart.

Catheter dislodgment is notoriously common and frustrating in small neonates. Although suturing is temporarily effective, use of a Dacron cuff in the subcutaneous position allows the catheter to become more securely fixed. Additionally, the frequency of catheter changes may be reduced to every 72 hours for tunneled Silastic catheters and every week for PICCs.

Although use of Silastic materials has reduced the incidence of thrombosis, this complication is still frequent. Although evidence of thromboembolism has been noted at autopsy in children dying with central venous catheters in place, clinical manifestations of this complication are rare. Pulmonary embolism occasionally has been reported in an infant or small child who has had a central venous catheter for a prolonged period. Thrombotic occlusion of the catheter may be managed with the use of tissue plasminogen activator (general dose is 1 mg/mL with sufficient amount to fill the catheter and dwell time of 2 hours). This procedure may be repeated several times unless systemic thrombolysis is induced. Children who have had a catheter in place for a prolonged period may develop an occlusion resulting from calcium precipitates or lipid deposits. Calcium may be dissolved effectively with the use of small amounts of 0.1N hydrogen chloride, and lipid deposits may be treated filling the lumen of the catheter with 70% ethanol.

The use of peripheral parenteral nutrition is associated with phlebitis and the potential of a significant skin slough. Both of these complications can be reduced by the simultaneous infusion of a fat emulsion. In addition to reducing the osmolarity and increasing the pH of the solution, infusion of fat seems to provide additional direct mechanical protection of the vein from phlebitis.

Septic Complications

Sepsis is one of the most frequent and serious complications of centrally infused parenteral nutrition in infants and children. Long-term central venous catheters are well-documented sources of bacteremia and septicemia. Microorganisms may enter the bloodstream (1) along the catheter tract, starting at the skin exit site; (2) via a contaminated intravenous solution; (3) by breaks in sterility at the catheter hub–blood drawing or cleaning intravenous tubing; or (4) from a distant septic site or the GI tract. The catheter in this case acts as a foreign body focus for bacterial growth. The most important factors in reducing the incidence of septic complications are placement of catheters under strict aseptic conditions and meticulous care of the catheter sites, particularly the

access hub. In addition, use of the catheter for parenteral nutrition alone and strict avoidance of using the catheter for drawing blood, giving blood products, or administering medications minimize the risk of contamination and mechanical failure. The absence of parenteral nutrition teams in many hospitals has left the responsibility of following care guidelines to nurses and physicians.

Catheter sepsis in a patient receiving parenteral nutrition is suggested by fever, unexplained glucosuria, or occasionally a leukocytosis. Infection is confirmed by culturing microorganisms from blood obtained through the central venous catheter or from another venous site. The Centers for Disease Control has established official guidelines for the documentation of an intravenous line infection. If the patient is not toxic, the catheter should be left in place during the initial 24 to 48 hours of evaluation because approximately 50% of febrile patients with central catheters turn out to have another source for their fever. If no other site of sepsis is found, in general a temporary catheter should be removed. For implanted Silastic catheters, intravenous antibiotics clear most infections. Broad-spectrum antibiotics should be started initially after cultures are obtained. The antibiotics can be adjusted when sensitivities are known. Gram-positive organisms may be cleared in 90% of patients; gram-negative organisms can be eliminated in 80% to 85% of patients. Fungal infections are particularly difficult to clear and have been associated with many fatalities. In general, most patients should have a catheter infected with a fungal organism removed. Duration of antibiotics should continue for approximately 10 days, and repeat cultures should show a clearance of infection.

Because febrile patients frequently are those most in need of nutritional support, it is important to have a protocol for managing central catheters in these high-risk patients. Because parenteral nutrition is never an emergency procedure, a febrile patient should undergo thorough investigation of the source of fever before initiating central TPN. TPN should never be initiated during the early stages of uncontrolled infection, particularly during recurrent septicemia. If TPN is begun while a patient is febrile, periodic blood cultures should be drawn until the patient becomes afebrile (i.e., every 1 to 3 days).

Peripheral parenteral nutrition has the advantage of eliminating most of the septic and technical complications inherent in central venous catheters. None of our infants and children managed with peripheral intravenous feeding developed invasive sepsis related to parenteral nutrition.

Metabolic Complications

Although almost every conceivable metabolic abnormality has been reported during TPN, Table 7-10 lists the more common ones. Serious consequences may ensue if these complications go undetected for any length of time. Careful monitoring with appropriate adjustment of the parenteral nutrition solution allows most patients to tolerate TPN well.

Hyperglycemia

An elevated blood glucose level may appear during initial TPN. Hyperglycemia is primarily the result of excessive

TABLE 7-10 ■ Potential Metabolic Complications Resulting from TPN	
Electrolyte imbalance	Hyper/hyponatremia
	Hyper/hypokalemia
	Hyper/hypochloremia
	Hyper/hypocalcemia
	Hyper/hypomagnesemia
	Hyper/hypophosphatemia
Complications related to carbohydrate administration	Hyper/hypoglycemia
	Hyperosmolarity and associated osmotic diuresis with dehydration, leading to nonketotic hyperglycemic coma
Complications related to protein administration	Cholestatic jaundice
	Azotemia
	Hyperchloremic metabolic acidosis (with protein hydrolysate)
Complications related to lipid administration	Hyperlipidemia
	Alteration of pulmonary function
	Displacement of albumin-bonded bilirubin by plasma-free fatty acid
	Overloading syndrome characterized by hyperlipidemia, fever, lethargy, liver damage, and coagulation disorders, reported in adults but seen rarely in children
Trace element deficiencies	Zinc
	Copper
	Chromium
Essential fatty acid deficiency	If lipids not used; manifested by skin rash

or rapid dextrose infusion. Prematurity, sepsis, stress, surgery, diabetes, and corticosteroid therapy may exacerbate hyperglycemia. Elevated blood glucose may appear with TPN initiation, but endogenous insulin secretion usually adjusts within 48 to 72 hours. Uncontrolled hyperglycemia may be treated by adding regular insulin to TPN. This may be done if hyperglycemia persists or blood glucose concentrations exceed 175 mg/dL. Treatment of hyperglycemia has received increased attention in more recent years because many iatrogenic infections have been attributed to patients having a blood glucose level exceeding 180 mg/dL. Patients stable on TPN who suddenly develop a blood glucose level greater than 200 mg/dL or who require increasing doses of insulin should be evaluated for other causes of this finding, particularly sepsis.

Hypoglycemia

Although symptoms of hypoglycemia, such as diaphoresis, confusion, or agitation, have been reported when TPN is abruptly terminated, we rarely have observed this complication in children despite many accidental interruptions of infusions. Nevertheless, 10% dextrose should always be administered when the TPN solution is interrupted for any reason, and parenteral nutrition should be tapered gradually when nutrition by vein no longer is required. Patients undergoing major surgical procedures frequently become less glucose tolerant because of endogenous hormone secretion or insulin resistance. We recommend that the parenteral nutrition infusion rate routinely be decreased by half, when the patient is taken to the operating room. The infusion usually can be brought back to the preoperative rate within 24 hours after surgery, provided that the blood glucose concentration has returned to an acceptable range after the first phase of surgical convalescence. Cycling of TPN often requires a period of increasing and decreasing the rate for 1 to 2 hours before and after the full rate of infusion is given. Premature infants may not even tolerate this slow decrease in TPN and may develop hypoglycemia. Careful monitoring of blood glucose levels in these patients is required.

Hyperkalemia

Patients receiving TPN may develop an elevated serum potassium concentration if they are not adequately anabolic and are unable to use fully the administered potassium. Other causes of hyperkalemia include decreased renal function, low cardiac output with metabolic acidosis, tissue necrosis, and systemic sepsis. Potassium should be reduced or withheld from the TPN solution until the underlying problem is resolved.

Hypokalemia

As a patient on TPN becomes anabolic and begins to synthesize new protein, there is an obligatory requirement for intracellular potassium. Intravenous potassium is administered at the level of 2 to 4 mEq/kg/day in infants and small children or at 40 mEq/kg/L in older children and adolescents. Higher doses may be required, but this becomes evident if the patient's serum potassium concentration is monitored on a regular basis. Hypokalemia, along with a decline in magnesium and phosphorus, may be seen with the refeeding syndrome (initiation of feedings in patients who have had a long-standing depletion of nutrients). Monitoring of these values is crucial in such malnourished patients.

Trace Element Deficiency

Zinc deficiency during long-term TPN has been well documented in children and is more likely to occur in patients with diarrhea. It usually is manifested by hair loss, a seborrheic type of dermatitis around the nose and mouth, and occasionally ileus. Copper deficiency results in hypochromic, normocytic anemia; neutropenia; depigmentation of the skin and hair; hypotonia; psychomotor retardation; and osteoporosis. Chromium deficiency, although rare, can produce a diabetes-like syndrome. Selenium deficiency, a potential complication of long-term TPN, is manifested by muscular pain and cardiomyopathy. These deficiencies rarely are observed in patients routinely receiving trace metal additives in the infusate.

Hyperlipidemia

Most patients receiving a fat emulsion have normal serum triglyceride and cholesterol levels. A few who receive TPN for longer than 1 month have serum triglyceride levels in the range of 300 to 350 mg/dL (normal 50 to 150 mg/dL) and serum cholesterol values of 150 to 250 mg/dL (normal 100 to 150 mg/dL). These elevations seem to be of little consequence and return to normal when the fat infusion is discontinued.

Liver Dysfunction

Although abnormalities in liver functions such as elevations in aspartate aminotransferase (AST), lactic dehydrogenase (LDH), alanine aminotransferase, and bilirubin levels have been reported within 2 to 14 days after beginning TPN, histologic examination of the liver does not reveal any consistent pathologic change. The elevations are variable and intermittent, and levels return to normal in most cases when TPN has been stopped. The abnormalities seen in patients receiving intravenous fat are essentially the same as abnormalities seen in patients on fat-free parenteral nutrition regimens. Histologically, intravenous fat pigment usually is seen in the Küpffer cells of the liver in most patients receiving intravenous fat for longer than 1 month. The significance of this pigment deposition is not yet known. Cholestatic jaundice associated with TPN is far more common in premature infants than in older children or adolescents and may be related to the immaturity of the biliary excretory system in infants. Although this cholestatic jaundice usually clears within 2 to 3 weeks after cessation of intravenous nutrition, in some severe cases, the infant develops hepatic failure and dies. The pathophysiology of this severe liver damage is not clear, and no treatment for it is available.

Fluid Overload and Overfeeding

Fluid overload in the form of pulmonary edema, peripheral edema, or congestive heart failure is rare in patients treated according to the techniques discussed earlier, provided that proper selection and monitoring are carried out. Studies using the nonradioactive isotope deuterium oxide showed that total body water during parenteral nutrition does not increase, but rather decreases, concomitant with an increase in body weight. This strongly supports the hypothesis that weight gain during parenteral nutrition is from tissue accretion rather than water retention.

Overfeeding can lead to many adverse consequences. The administration of too much dextrose may lead to an osmotic diuresis and subsequent dehydration owing to serum glucose levels exceeding renal tubular reabsorption threshold. Immunologic suppression also has been associated with overfeeding and is believed to be due to an inactivation of the complement system and a depression of neutrophil activation in the presence of hyperglycemia. Overfeeding also may affect the liver adversely because excessive glucose, which is not oxidized, is converted into fat (lipogenesis). These changes may lead to elevated serum triglyceride levels and hepatic steatosis, which may be injurious to the liver. Finally, overfeeding, with the development of lipogenesis, leads to high carbon dioxide production as reflected by an elevated respiratory quotient. Although the respiratory quotient for a pure lipogenic state is 2.75, any respiratory quotient value exceeding 1.0 represents overfeeding. A respiratory quotient this high may exacerbate ventilatory impairment in a critically ill (ventilator-dependent) child. Avoidance of overfeeding may be difficult because estimates of nutritional needs in the intensive care unit setting can be difficult, and reliance on RDA values may result in overfeeding of these children. Overfeeding these critically ill patients also may lead to fluid retention, which may compromise respiratory function further. Although previous recommendations have had physicians increase lipid delivery in these patients, it is more prudent to make an overall reduction in the amount of caloric delivery.

HOME PARENTERAL NUTRITION

In some patients with short-bowel syndrome, intestinal pseudo-obstruction, or chronic inflammatory bowel disease, there is a need for partial parenteral nutrition or TPN in the home. Home parenteral nutrition (HPN) for infants and children provides well-documented psychological, social, and economic advantages over continued hospitalization, provided that careful selection and training of patients and parents have taken place and continued backup support is available. The major indications for HPN are (1) a primary diagnosis indicating that normal growth and development will not occur without supplemental parenteral nutrition and (2) the potential need for 30 days or more of conventional parenteral nutrition. Restrictions on HPN also have been instituted by many third-party payers, and this may have a significant impact on which patients may use this service. When a Silastic central venous catheter has been placed, a detailed protocol for HPN is adapted to each patient and family, describing, stepwise, the method of infusion and catheter care. When the patient is stable with optimal parenteral nutrition volume and concentration given over 24 hours, an adaptive phase is begun. This phase consists of decreasing the duration of infusion by 2 hours each day, while holding the total daily volume constant by an appropriate increase in the infusion rate. Cycling of TPN ideally should be 10 to 12 hours. Smaller neonates may become hypoglycemic with such reductions, however. Careful monitoring of blood glucose levels should be done during the times the infusion is off.

The cost of an HPN program is one half to one third in-hospital cost of parenteral nutritional support, and further savings accrue when patients or their families learn to mix their nutrient solutions at home. A team approach consisting of the physician, nurses, and pharmacist is essential to successful HPN therapy.

SUGGESTED READINGS

August DA, Teitelbaum DH (eds): Guidelines for the use of parenteral and enteral nutrition in adult and pediatric patients. J Parenter Enteral Nutr 26:1SA-138SA, 2002.

This issue extensively reviews the current indications and supporting literature for the care of infants and children receiving parenteral and enteral nutrition.

Campos AC, Paluzzi M, Mequid MM: Clinical use of total nutritional admixtures. Nutrition 6:347, 1990.

This study shows the utility of using admixtures of lipid, protein, and dextrose in TPN solutions. These systems facilitate home usage and cycling with no increase in complication rates.

Cerra FB: Nutrient modulation of inflammatory and immune function. Am J Surg 161:230, 1991.

This article discusses the use of ω-3-based fatty acids rather than ω-6 oils (the main component of all major lipid sources today) as immunomodulators of the inflammatory response to injury and illness. The theoretical basis of downregulation of the inflammatory process by modifying the eicosanoids is discussed in detail.

Drongowski RA, Coran AG: An analysis of factors contributing to development of total parenteral nutrition–induced cholestasis. J Parenter Enteral Nutr 13:586, 1990.

This article updates knowledge of the various factors contributing to TPN-associated cholestasis.

Klein S, Kinney J, Jeejeebhoy KN, et al: Nutrition support in clinical practice: Review of published data and recommendations for future research directions. J Parenter Enteral Nutr 21:133-156, 1997.

This is a detailed meta-analysis of published literature regarding the use and efficacy of nutrition support in a variety of clinical settings.

Moore FA, Feliciano DV, Audrassy RJ: Early enteral feeding, compared with parenteral, reduces post operative septic complication. Ann Surg 216:172, 1992.

A multicenter, prospective study, enrolling 230 severely stressed patients, tested one TPN glucose-based solution against one enteral solution (EN). This large study showed significantly fewer septic complications in the EN group versus the TPN group (18% versus 35%) with a P=.01. This well-done study shows that EN has significantly fewer associated septic complications. This study implies that disruption of GI metabolism and immunology may be the cause of certain septic problems in the stressed patient.

Physioloy of Infection

8

HOST DEFENSES OF THE NEONATE

The neonate is born with a host-defense system that is functional in the perinatal period and undergoes progressive maturation postnatally. The host-defense or immune system provides a means by which neonates can recognize and eliminate foreign antigen. It is made up of two components: nonspecific and specific. Nonspecific immunity, innate immunity, includes mechanisms that operate without requiring prior exposure to antigen—that is, "experience" is not necessary. Included are the mucocutaneous barriers, natural killer cells, phagocytes, and complement system. Specific immunity is keyed to antigen presentation and exposure—that is, experience is necessary. It comprises cell-mediated (T lymphocyte) and humoral (B lymphocyte and immunoglobulin) systems. Although each system is referred to as a separate entity, they complement and supplement each other, often communicating via various cellular factors.

Newborns, in particular premature infants, are vulnerable to infection during the first 6 weeks of extrauterine life because of an inexperienced and immature immune system. Although components of the system may be seen within the first trimester, the completely developed immune system remains deficient until at least 8 years of age. This inexperience results from the neonatal immune system's development and maintenance within a sterile intrauterine environment, which in most cases precludes antigen presentation. Immunologic immaturity is manifested by qualitative and quantitative deficits in both components of the defense system, even though many of the essential elements are present at birth. The degree of immunologic immaturity varies directly with gestational age and accounts for the high incidence of infections and infection-related mortality in the premature and very-low-birth-weight infant.

NONSPECIFIC IMMUNITY

Polymorphonuclear Neutrophil System

The most primitive host-defense mechanism involves the ingestion and killing of microorganisms by phagocytic cells. To understand the defects in this and other neonatal host defense systems, a review of the steps leading to microbial killings is necessary.

The polymorphonuclear neutrophil (PMN) is the first line of defense against microorganisms that penetrate the mucocutaneous barrier. These cells migrate from the bone marrow and bloodstream to the site of the invading organism—a process termed *chemotaxis* (Fig. 8-1A). This process occurs through a specific set of sequences guided by cell adhesion molecules. PMN recruitment begins by a rolling of the cell onto the endothelium overlying the area of infection. This is followed by a slowing of the rolling, which is mediated by a selectin-mediated process. If sufficient numbers of other adhesion molecules are present, the PMN enters a static phase and adheres to the surface of the endothelium. These adhesion molecules include intracellular adhesion molecules (ICAM-1 and ICAM-2) on the endothelium and lymphocyte function–associated antigen-1 (LFA-1, also called *CD11a/CD18*) and macrophage antigen-1 (MAC-1, also called *CD11b/CD18*) on the PMN. These surface interactions lead to a loss of tight adhesions between endothelial cells and the subsequent transendothelial migration of the PMN (Fig. 8-1B). When within the extravascular tissue, the cell moves along a chemotactic gradient until the microorganisms are encountered.

Most microorganisms must be opsonized or coated before PMN recognition and engulfment (phagocytosis) occur. Opsonins are a group of plasma proteins consisting chiefly of immunoglobulins and complement (C3) fragments that promote phagocytosis by binding to specific receptor sites on the PMN. These sites activate cytoskeleton contractile elements, which initiate an investigation and engulfment. When the offending organism is phagocytosed, the PMN can exert its primary function of microbial killing by binding the phagosome to various granules. It deploys its microbicidal activity by one of two mechanisms: oxygen-dependent and oxygen-independent killing. Oxygen-independent killing uses cellular lysozome, lactoferrin, and acid. Oxygen-dependent killing relies on the chemical reactions of nicotinamide-adenine dinucleotide phosphate (reduced form) (NADPH) to convert molecular oxygen to superoxide radicals, hydrogen peroxide, and reactive hydroxyl radicals. These molecules

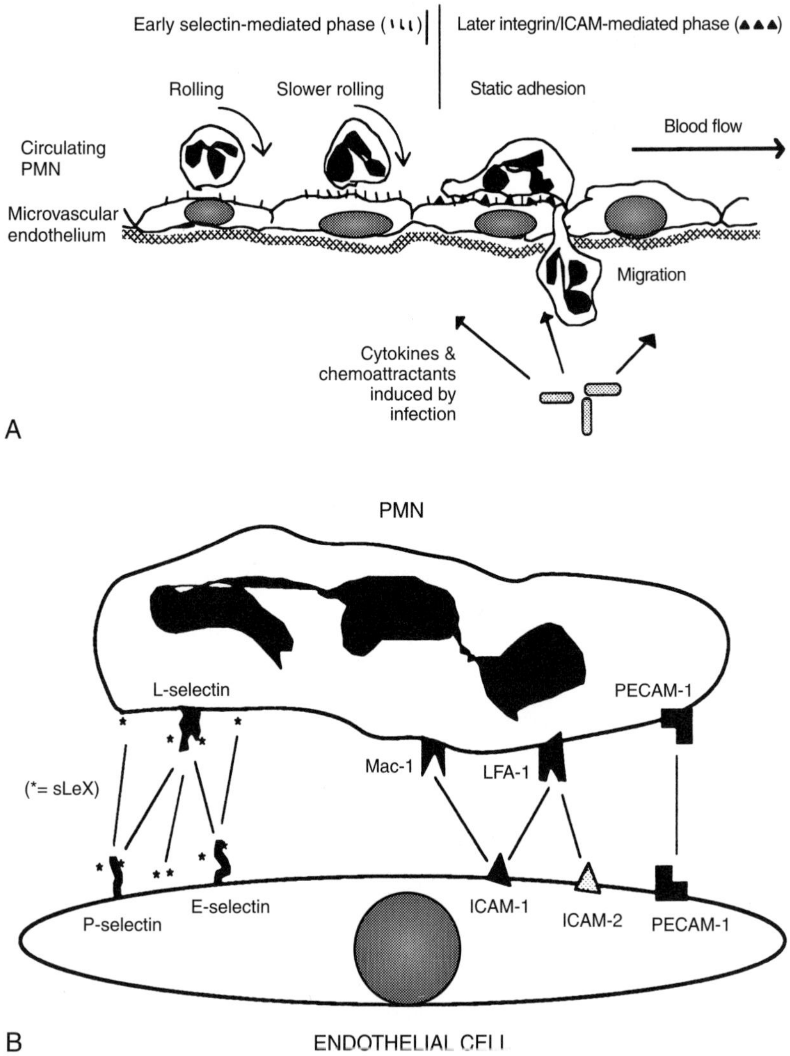

FIGURE 8-1 ■ These two panels show events that occur in the process of neutrophil (PMN) recruitment to a site of activation and the binding of the PMN to endothelial cells. **A,** A circulating PMN begins the process of binding to the endothelium, which is overlying an area of inflammation. The process is a series of steps, including rolling, slowing, and binding. **B,** The specific cell surface binding that allows the PMN to bind to the endothelium. Note the surface ligands on the PMN and endothelium (see text). When bound, the PMN may pass through the endothelial layer and enter the area of infection (see Fig. 8-3). (From Tosi MF, Cates KL: Immunologic and phagocytic responses to infection. In Feigin RD, Cherry JD [eds]: Textbook of Pediatric Infectious Diseases, vol 1, 4th ed. Philadelphia, WB Saunders, 1998, pp 24 and 25.)

require the presence of NADPH oxidase. A deficiency or mutation of this enzyme leads to the development of chronic granulomatous disease (see later). These reactions are capable of killing many gram-negative and gram-positive bacteria, fungi and viruses.

The neonatal PMN system, in contrast to the adult PMN system, has quantitative and qualitative deficiencies. The greatest deficiencies are present in premature infants. Quantitatively the neonate's total peripheral granulocyte count is comparable with that of a normal adult, but the neutrophil storage pool, which consists of band and metamyelocyte forms, is markedly reduced. This loss of total body neutrophil mass is most apparent in infants born before 32 weeks' gestation. Neonates, when faced with a bacterial challenge, often develop neutropenia and a left shift, signifying rapid depletion of an already reduced neutrophil storage pool. Similarly, qualitative defects in PMN function are not obvious in either term or preterm infants unless challenged by a high number of bacteria in vitro. Neonatal neutrophils have decreased bactericidal capacity for *Escherichia coli* and *Staphylococcus aureus* at neutrophil-to-bacteria ratios of 1:100 but not at ratios of 1:1.

In vitro studies have shown that there are a variety of primary functional defects in PMNs. In particular, PMNs from premature infants have a deficit in MAC-1 and to some degree LFA-1. This deficit impairs the ability of these cells to adhere to endothelium and gain access to the site of infection. Additional defects have been noted in the ability to slip effectively between endothelial cells because of an inability to change shape properly.

Mononuclear Phagocyte System

The mononuclear phagocyte system is composed of bone marrow precursors for circulating monocytes and mature tissue macrophages. After bone marrow stimulation, the monocyte circulates in the blood for approximately 72 hours, relocates at a predetermined tissue (e.g., the Küpffer cells or hepatic macrophages), then differentiates into a mature macrophage. The mononuclear phagocyte's microbicidal function is similar to that of the PMN. The macrophage is unique, however, because it (1) possesses a tissue débridement function; (2) serves a crucial role in wound healing; (3) is a major source of cytokines, particularly after stimulation with endotoxin; and (4) serves as a link between the specific and nonspecific immune systems via antigen processing and presentation to T and B cells.

The migration of monocytes to areas of infection is delayed and decreased in newborns. This situation is believed to be the result of impaired chemotactic activity and poor adhesion to endothelial cells, which may explain the poor healing of cutaneous abscesses in neonates. Phagocytic and microbicidal activity is equal to that of adults, however.

Complement System

The importance of the complement system lies in its role as facilitator of PMN bacterial killing by producing opsonic proteins and potent neutrophil chemoattractants. Additionally, complement proteins themselves can form a membrane attack complex capable of bactericidal activity in the absence of immunoglobulins.

The complement system consists of more than 30 specific plasma proteins that regulate the inflammatory response and cause bacteriolysis. It can be activated by either an antibody-dependent mechanism or an antibody-independent mechanism (Fig. 8-2). In either case, complement proteins are generated that may affect PMN function. C3b is a potent opsonin and may activate the alternate pathway into producing more opsonin; additionally, C5a is the most potent chemotactic factor for PMNs and other phagocytic cells. C5b, when complexed with C6, C7, C8, and C9, leads to functional lytic activity. Classic activation, which is antibody dependent, requires either IgM or IgG; IgG derived from the infant or infant's mother may serve as a source of complement activation.

Complement protein levels and activity correlate directly with gestational age and birth weight. Because there is little placental passage of complement proteins, neonates must rely on postnatal production. Most complement components are decreased slightly in term infants, but there is a greater deficiency in preterm infants. Similarly, complement activity is approximately 50% of that of an adult in term infants and 10% to 30% of adult levels in preterm infants. These defects amplify the deficiencies in the PMN and monocyte systems, rendering the term, and especially the preterm, infant's phagocytic cells incapable of efficiently arriving at the site of the infection and killing the offending organisms. Although the neonate has deficiencies in complement activity, these rarely lead to major immune deficiencies.

Mucocutaneous Barriers

Under normal circumstances, the skin and mucous membranes of neonates permit postnatal colonization but resist bacterial invasion. All newborns become contaminated with vaginal flora during labor and delivery (except during cesarean section delivery). After the first bath (which removes maternal microorganisms), bacterial colonization begins after contact with nursing personnel and family members. Within 3 days, the nares, throat, and skin of the well infant are colonized with gram-positive microorganisms. Within 1 week, anaerobic bacteria and members of the Enterobacteriaceae family colonize the gastrointestinal (GI) tract. The GI tract flora in formula-fed infants becomes predominantly *E. coli*, whereas that of breast-fed infants is a mixture of *E. coli* and lactobacilli.

The bacterial flora of a sick neonate maintained in an intensive care unit (ICU) is entirely different. These infants are subjected to broad-spectrum antibiotics, which alter their "normal" flora and allow colonization by a wide variety of multiple drug-resistant organisms that are housed in ICUs (e.g., coagulase-negative staphylococci and *Pseudomonas*). Infection occurs when the normal mucocutaneous barriers are either altered or bypassed, as occurs with the placement of transcutaneous catheters and endotracheal tubes. Coagulase-negative staphylococci are one of the most common pathogens that infect critically ill newborns with an altered mucocutaneous barrier. Bacteria have an ability to cross mucocutaneous surfaces first by adhering to the epithelium and second by crossing the barrier. Many mechanisms have evolved that allow bacteria to adhere to the epithelium. These include the generation of s-pili and p-pili from *E. coli*, which bind to the epithelium. The body has developed many countermeasures to prevent this adherence, including the formation of mucoproteins, which retard this adherence. In the case of *E. coli*, mannose is expressed by epithelial cells and prevents typical *E. coli* from binding. In the case of enterotoxigenic *E. coli*, the bacteria for colonization factors 1 and 2, which are resistant to mannose and can adhere, eventually invade the epithelium. Coagulase-negative staphylococci elaborate a slime factor, or exopolysaccharide matrix, which allows *Staphylococcus epidermidis* to adhere to foreign bodies and to inhibit phagocytosis and antimicrobial activity.

Preterm infants are especially vulnerable to infection by coagulase-negative staphylococci and other colonizing

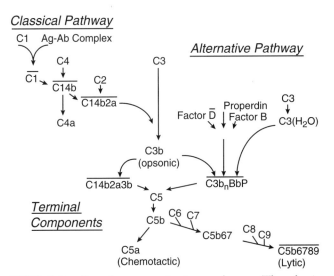

FIGURE 8-2 ■ Complement activation pathways. The classic pathway complexes C1 with an antigen-antibody (Ag-Ab) complex to activate the cascade. In the alternative pathway, there is no dependence on specific antibody, but rather an initiation by microbial surface macromolecules. Note the common path of C3 required in both pathways. (From Lewis DB, Wilson CB: Developmental immunology and role of host defenses in neonatal susceptibility to infection. In Remington JS, Klein JO [eds]: Infectious Diseases of the Fetus and Newborn Infant, 4th ed. Philadelphia, WB Saunders, 1995, p 64.)

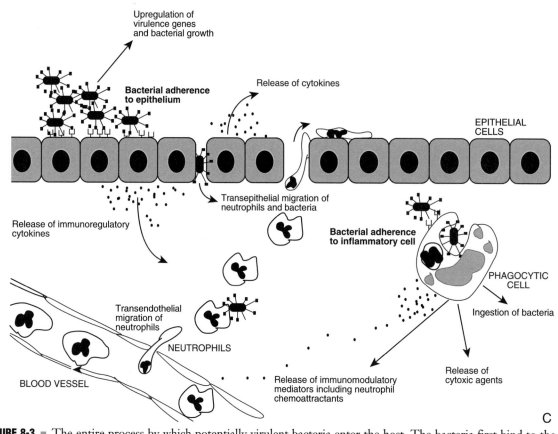

FIGURE 8-3 ■ The entire process by which potentially virulent bacteria enter the host. The bacteria first bind to the intestinal epithelium and secondarily invade across this layer. When the organism binds to the epithelium, many cytokines are released, which break down the epithelial barrier **(A)**. The bacteria invade, and another series of cytokines are released, which begins the recruitment of immunoregulatory cells to migrate to this area of the bowel **(B)**. Bacteria adhere to the PMN via opsonization, and the organism is phagocytosed and killed **(C)**. (Adapted from Abraham SN, Sharon N, Ofek I: Adhesion of bacteria to mucosal surfaces. In Ogra PL, Mestecky J, Lamm ME, et al [eds]: Mucosal Immunology, 2nd ed. San Diego, Academic Press, 1999, p 38.)

organisms for several reasons. First, their skin is thin and fragile and may peel away with a minimum amount of handling, rendering them prone to easy penetration by colonizing organisms. Second, their gut barrier (Fig. 8-3) serves as a defense system that prevents enteric bacteria from invading the body. This barrier is physiologically and immunologically immature. Physiologic components of the gut barrier include gastric acid, pepsin, nonzymogen pancreatic proteins, pancreatic proteases/lipases, peristalsis, the mucus layer, and a colonization-resistance system that primarily consists of intrinsic anaerobic bacteria. The epithelium itself prevents bacteria from entering by maintaining a tight junction between epithelial cells and maintaining the integrity of the cell wall, so as to prevent transcellular passage of organisms. The immune component of the gut barrier (and all mucosal surfaces) is composed principally of secretory IgA (sIgA, i.e., IgA found in external secretions, such as tears, saliva, breast milk, the gut), with a small contribution by immunoglobulin M (IgM) and immunoglobulin G (IgG). sIgA functions principally as an "antiseptic paint" by selectively coating and aggregating bacteria, preventing their attachment to, and invasion of, the gut epithelium. Finally, the intestine contains a fully organized immune system

(gut-associated lymphoid tissue [GALT]), which prevents pathogens from gaining entry into the host. In addition to protecting the neonate, the GALT also continually samples foreign antigen, such as bacteria from the intestinal lumen via specialized epithelial cells called M-cells, which overlie Peyer's patches. These cells allow for antigen processing and the continued development of a competent gut immune system. Many of the components of the gut barrier are deficient in neonates. Gastric acid and pepsin secretion are low and do not reach adult levels until approximately 4 weeks of age. Relative pancreatic insufficiency exists throughout the first year of life, providing a lower than normal secretion of pancreatic enzymes. Coordinated peristaltic activity develops late in gestation and may not be fully developed until the eighth month of gestation. In the absence of breast-feeding, there are only trace amounts of IgA and gut-associated IgG and IgM during the first week of life. For these reasons, the gut barrier of newborns, particularly preterm newborns, is less efficient at preventing bacterial passage across the gut mucosa. Additionally, the epithelial barrier itself, predominately maintained by epithelial tight junction, is far less competent in newborns compared with mature adults.

SPECIFIC IMMUNITY

B Lymphocytes and Antibodies

B lymphocytes are characterized by the presence of cell-surface immunoglobulin. They are produced in the fetal liver and bone marrow and are activated by direct antigen recognition or T-helper cell stimulation. Activation results in differentiation into antibody-producing plasma cells. The plasma cells reside in the lymph nodes; the spleen; the mucosal linings of the bone marrow; and GI, genitourinary, and respiratory tracts. The manufactured antibodies they produce comprise a broad family of glycoproteins called *immunoglobulins*. There are five major classes (isotypes) of immunoglobulins: IgG, IgA, IgM, IgD, and IgE. Additionally, there are four subclasses of IgG (IgG1, IgG2, IgG3, IgG4) and two subclasses of IgA (IgA1, IgA2). Immunoglobulins have two identical heavy chains and two identical light chains. These form two amino termini, or Fab regions, for antigen recognition. The carboxy terminus, or Fc receptor, can bind to B cells, or it can be used for complement activation.

Antibodies contribute to the neonatal host-defense system by their ability to opsonize bacterial pathogens and neutralize viruses. When bound to bacteria, they can activate the classic complement cascade. Immunoglobulins also are important for neutralization of viruses and toxins and for antibody-dependent cytolysis. Infants are born with a relative immunoglobulin deficiency with the exception of IgG, which is maternally derived via transplacental passage. Fetal production of IgA and IgM is limited because of the lack of in utero antigenic stimulation and occurs only in the setting of intrauterine infection (Table 8-1). Maternally derived IgG steadily is broken down by the neonate. It reaches a nadir at 3 to 4 months, by which time neonatally derived IgG begins to reach appreciable levels. IgA (serum and secretory) and IgM production begin predominantly at birth. IgA reaches adult levels by 6 to 8 years, and IgM reaches adult levels by approximately 2 to 4 years.

The serum level of transported maternal IgG varies directly with gestational age, and although term infants may have normal levels at birth, premature infants are born with, or may develop, a profound hypogammaglobulinemia. In addition, two of the four IgG subclasses (IgG2 and IgG4) are particularly deficient in all neonates

TABLE 8-1 ■ Serum Concentration of Immunoglobulins in Term and Preterm Infants						
	IgG	IgA	sIgA	IgM	IgE	IgD
Term	Normal	↓	Absent	↓	↓	↓
Preterm	↓	↓↓	Absent	↓↓	↓↓	↓↓

as a result of impaired placental transport. This fact is important because antibodies to capsular polysaccharide antigens of many pyogenic bacteria often are contained in the deficient IgG2 and IgM fractions. This deficiency contributes to the neonate's susceptibility to overwhelming infections with organisms such as *E. coli*, group B streptococci (GBS), *Klebsiella pneumoniae*, *Streptococcus pneumoniae*, and *Haemophilus influenzae*. Because the neonate's antibody profile depends on the profile of antibodies in the maternal circulation, the absence of type-specific maternal antibodies is believed to be a risk factor for sepsis from pathogens such as GBS, varicella-zoster virus, and herpes simplex virus. During overwhelming sepsis, neonates display antigen-specific incompetence, particularly to pneumococci and *H. influenzae*. This phenomenon seems to be secondary to defective B-lymphocyte and plasma cell differentiation and T lymphocyte–mediated facilitation of antibody synthesis.

The absence of IgA, IgM, and IgG2 and lack of antigen-specific antibody render the term neonate susceptible to infection. Preterm neonates are particularly vulnerable because of a profound deficiency of all immunoglobulin isotypes and subclasses.

T Lymphocytes

T cells are essential for the development of cell-mediated immunity. In contrast to PMNs, macrophages, or even B cells, T cells do not recognize free antigen. Instead, they respond to antigen when it is present on the surface of antigen presenting cells, such as macrophages, monocytes, Langerhans' cells, or dendritic cells (Fig. 8-4). When presented with antigen, T cells indirectly may augment or suppress the immune response by serving as helper or suppressor cells. This refers to the type of cytokine-mediated response that is derived from

FIGURE 8-4 ■ Principal fashion in which T lymphocytes bind and are presented foreign antigen by antigen presenting cells (APC). There are two classes of major histocompatibility complexes (MHC), which present the antigen, class I for CD8⁺ T cells and class II for CD4⁺ T cells. (Adapted from Lewis DB, Wilson CB: Developmental immunology and role of host defenses in neonatal susceptibility to infection. In Remington JS, Klein JO [eds]: Infectious Diseases of the Fetus and Newborn Infant, 4th ed. Philadelphia, WB Saunders, 1995, p 22.)

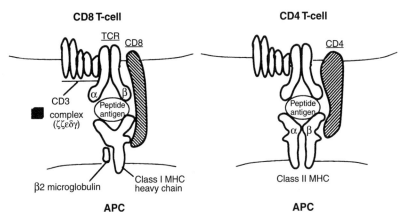

such presentation. T cells can exert direct bactericidal activity, however, only in the presence of cells that are infected with intracellular parasites or viruses.

At birth, the absolute number of T cells is normal or even increased, and their functional activity is near normal. Neonatal T cells may not be capable, however, of producing all the cytokines that now are recognized as crucial in the immune response. Newborns display diminished T-cell production of a class of cytokines called *colony-stimulating factors* (CSF) (see Neonatal Septicemia). This deficiency is potentially detrimental to neonates because these cytokines are the major regulators of increased peripheral blood cell (e.g., neutrophils and platelets) production during the septic state. Diminished neonatal T-cell production of other cytokines, such as migration-inhibition factor, interferon-γ, and lymphotoxin, also has been reported. CD8+ T cell–mediated cytotoxicity, delayed hypersensitivity, and T-cell help for B-cell differentiation also are diminished in the newborn.

Breast Milk and Host Defense

Breast-feeding may decrease the risk of neonatal infection. Breast-feeding provides protection from lower respiratory tract illness, otitis media, bacteremia, meningitis, and necrotizing enterocolitis. Human milk provides an array of humoral and cellular anti-infectious factors and essential nutrients. Milk includes antibodies, such as sIgA and small amounts of IgM and IgG, and cellular immune factors, such as macrophages, lymphocytes, and polymorphonuclear leukocytes. Additionally, it provides components of the complement system. Lactoferrin and other proteins, such as lysozyme, interferon, migration-inhibiting factor, epidermoid growth factor, α-fetoprotein, and oligosaccharides, interact with and bind offending organisms. Strong evidence exists for the protective role of sIgA, the main immune component of the enteromammary-bronchomammary axis. The origin of IgA-secreting plasma cells in the mammary gland is believed to be in the GALT (primarily Peyer's patches) and to a lesser degree in the bronchus-associated lymphoid tissues. The axis begins when antigens, such as bacteria, are transported from the mother's gut lumen to the intestinal Peyer's patches. Macrophages recognize and process the antigen within the Peyer's patches. T cells in the submucosa are activated by macrophage-antigen complex, undergo proliferation, and release cytokines that activate B cells. The resting B cells, which normally express IgM on their cell surface, now are activated to undergo an isotype switch from IgM to IgA. IgA-committed B cells leave Peyer's patches, enter the regional lymph nodes, and travel through the lymphatic circulation and into the bloodstream. These cells then "home" to various exocrine glands (mammary, salivary, lacrimal) and mucosa-associated tissues (respiratory, GI, and genitourinary tracts). Terminal differentiation into IgA-secreting plasma cells takes place. Peyer's patches lymphocytes also are capable of undergoing direct antigen-driven stimulation to proliferate, migrate, differentiate, and repopulate the intestinal lamina propria with cells that secrete specific IgA antibodies.

Bacteria are sampled in the mother's gut and presented to B cells that then home to the breast. These cells secrete specific IgA into the milk. The inexperienced infant drinks the milk and now has specific sIgA to bacteria that an "experienced" mother has been exposed to. The American Academy of Pediatrics recommends that breast-feeding continue for the first 12 months of an infant's life, although the predominant immunologic benefits are derived within the first 2 weeks of nursing.

NEONATAL SEPTICEMIA
Incidence and Etiology

Systemic bacterial infections in the first month of life are a major cause of morbidity and mortality. The incidence of sepsis is related directly to gestational age. There is a 1:250 incidence of sepsis in preterm infants, whereas term infants have a 1:15,000 incidence. Despite the availability of potent and specific antimicrobial therapy, mortality rates are 15% to 50% when sepsis occurs during the first week of life and 10% to 20% if it occurs after the first week. Mortality is approximately the same for each of the major bacterial causes of neonatal sepsis and varies inversely with birth weight and gestational age.

Neonatal sepsis generally is classified as early (during the first week of life) or late (after the first week). Early infections occur after fetal or perinatal exposure to microorganisms colonizing the maternal genital tract (intrapartum infection, often with delayed rupture of membranes). Many of these are opportunistic. The organisms can be cultured readily not only from the cervix or vaginal canal of normal pregnant women, but also from the external environment and the skin and GI tract of normal individuals. The predominant pathogens of early-onset neonatal sepsis in the United States are GBS and *E. coli*, although there are regional differences. Other organisms associated with early neonatal sepsis include *Listeria monocytogenes* and other streptococci. Meningitis is a frequent sequela of early-onset bacteremia in newborns and most commonly is caused by GBS, gram-negative bacilli, and *L. monocytogenes*. Chronic congenital infections (TORCH [toxoplasmosis, rubella, cytomegalovirus, and herpes simplex] infections) also occur early but are transmitted hematogenously from the mother to the developing fetus (intrauterine infection).

Late-onset infections are primarily nosocomial. Coagulase-negative staphylococci (*Staphylococcus epidermidis*) is the predominant organism. Other pathogens, including *S. aureus*, *Enterococcus*, gram-negative bacilli (*Pseudomonas*, *Klebsiella*, *Serratia*), and fungi (*Candida*, *Malassezia*), are currently common nosocomial pathogens in neonatal ICUs. Their role as nosocomial pathogens is related to the increasing survival of a population of very-low-birth-weight infants with prolonged hospitalizations.

Clinical Manifestations

Weight gain and oliguria are often the first indicators of sepsis. These signs have been ascribed to a capillary leak phenomenon that results in an increase in total body water, leading to anasarca and hyponatremia. Other nonspecific signs of neonatal septicemia are nonspecific and include lethargy, irritability, poor feeding, or the suggestion by nursing staff that the newborn is not doing as well as previously. Hypothermia is as common as hyperthermia, particularly in premature infants, who frequently experience irregular fluctuations of body temperature. Tachypnea, cyanosis, apnea, tachycardia, bradycardia, and hypotension also may be noted. Focal neurologic signs, tremors, seizures, or a full fontanelle may develop in septic neonates with or without meningitis. The onset of jaundice in the first 24 hours of life, in the absence of a primary hemolytic disorder, suggests septicemia, most often caused by gram-negative bacilli, particularly *E. coli*. More recently, a loss of normal heart rate variability has been shown to be an accurate predictor of neonatal stress and suggestive of neonatal sepsis.

Laboratory Evaluation

Isolation of bacteria from blood, cerebrospinal fluid (CSF), or urine is the most specific way to diagnose bacterial sepsis. Nearly one third of neonates with proven sepsis have concomitant meningitis. Conversely, a small but significant number of infants with meningitis have negative blood cultures. Lumbar puncture often is required in the work-up of neonates. To avoid an excessive number of these tests, it generally is recommended that a lumbar puncture be performed for all symptomatic infants and for asymptomatic neonates who have laboratory values indicative of sepsis (see next paragraph). Similarly, greater than 20% of neonates with fatal sepsis fail to have positive blood cultures even though they are later proved to be culture positive at autopsy. In general, a positive blood culture is found in only 50% to 80% of all neonates presenting with sepsis. Other laboratory abnormalities may be needed to make the diagnosis of sepsis without a positive blood culture. Immunologic assays that detect bacterial antigens in body fluids are helpful in providing a rapid specific diagnosis before culture results return in infants with infections caused by GBS, *S. pneumoniae*, *Neisseria meningitidis*, or *H. influenzae*. These techniques include countercurrent immunoelectrophoresis, latex agglutination, and enzyme-linked immunosorbent assays, with the last-mentioned being the most sensitive. Finally, urine cultures should be obtained in patients who present with late onset of neonatal sepsis because cultures obtained earlier than 72 hours have a low yield. Typically, these cultures should be obtained via a straight catheterization or by a suprapubic tap.

Hypoglycemia may accompany septicemia. It is encountered more frequently during infections caused by gram-negative bacilli than by gram-positive organisms. Although leukopenia (<2500 white blood cells/mm^3) or leukocytosis (>25,000 white blood cells/mm^3) supports the diagnosis of neonatal infection, the differential white blood cell count is of greater utility. Commonly a leftward shift with an increased number of bands and metamyelocytes accompanies a normal peripheral white blood cell count during infection. Additionally, a depressed white blood cell count is seen more frequently than an elevation. A ratio of immature-to-total neutrophils is helpful. Ratios greater than 0.2 suggest sepsis, and a ratio greater than 0.4 is highly suggestive. A depressed platelet count may be noted during gram-negative septicemia, although a normal platelet count does not exclude the diagnosis. Finally, several investigators have found that an elevation in C-reaction protein is a useful measure of neonatal sepsis (levels >1.0 mg/dL).

Pathogenesis of Septic Shock

Septic shock in newborns and adults is a distributive form of shock resulting in a generalized blood flow maldistribution. It traditionally has been recognized as a consequence of gram-negative bacteremia, but it also may be caused by gram-positive organisms, fungi, and probably viruses and parasites. It begins with a nidus of infection that triggers systemic and metabolic responses through activation of cellular and plasma mediators. The infecting nidus may consist of endotoxin (capsular polysaccharide), proteases, lipid moieties from gram-negative bacteria of peptidoglycans, exotoxins, and hemolysins from gram-positive bacteria.

Endotoxin, a lipopolysaccharide component of the outer membrane of gram-negative bacilli, is implicated as a prime initiator of adult and newborn septic shock. Endotoxin induces the activation of several humoral pathways, such as the alternate complement pathway, the coagulation and kinin system via factor XII activation, the arachidonic cascade, and endogenous opioid peptide release. Deregulation of the production of cytokines by macrophages and T cells is believed to be responsible for the endotoxin-induced activation of cellular inflammatory systems via the activation of neutrophils, endothelial cells, and monocytes. Activated neutrophils are responsible for vascular and tissue injuries and the production of platelet-activating factor. Endothelial cell activation exposes substrate that can activate the coagulation cascade and can initiate local production of nitric oxide. Endotoxin-activated monocytes produce additional cytokines, such as tumor necrosis factor (TNF), interleukin (IL)-1, IL-6, IL-8, and interferon-γ; and macrophage-derived nitric oxide. TNF is believed to play a pivotal role in the pathophysiologic changes in shock caused by gram-negative (endotoxin-induced) and gram-positive organisms. Its effects are protean. It causes release of granulocyte-monocyte colony-stimulating factor (GM-CSF), IL-1, IL-6, and interferon-γ and induces vascular endothelial damage.

Activation of these humoral and cellular pathways results in the systemic and metabolic responses to sepsis. Distributive changes in systemic and microcirculatory blood flow occur, contributing to impaired oxygen use. The release of vasoactive substances may contribute to the loss of normal vascular autoregulation with subsequent hypotension. Capillary leak is common, with resultant tissue edema and limited oxygen diffusion from the capillaries to the mitochondria. Activation of the coagulation cascade may precipitate disseminated intravascular coagulation, which is associated with a high mortality in septic neonates. The hypermetabolic response results in significant energy expenditure mediated by the interaction of cytokines and the neuroendocrine axis (this should be distinguished from the well-described hyperdynamic state of cardiac function in adult septic shock to which there is no clearly documented neonatal counterpart). If early intervention is not initiated, multiple system organ failure and death may ensue (see Treatment of Neonatal Sepsis).

Treatment of Neonatal Sepsis

Neonates with suspected sepsis must be treated immediately and empirically until culture results become available. The choice of antibacterial agents is based on knowledge of the prevalent organisms responsible for neonatal sepsis and their patterns of antimicrobial susceptibility. When septicemia is suspected in the first 5 days of life (early-onset disease) and a causative agent is unknown, the combination of ampicillin and an aminoglycoside commonly is used, although an increasing number of physicians now are using ampicillin in combination with a third-generation cephalosporin (e.g., cefotaxime). Additionally, because of the better penetration of the CSF, cefotaxime has an advantage over aminoglycosides in infants suspected of having meningitis. When late-onset septicemia is suspected, the chosen antibiotics must provide coverage for organisms that may be acquired from the environment, such as *S. aureus*, *S. epidermidis*, selected gram-negative bacilli, and fungi. Accordingly the initial combination of drugs is generally vancomycin and an aminoglycoside. Adjustment is made depending on subsequent culture results.

Physiologic factors unique to neonates may preclude the use of certain drugs, while requiring altered dosage schedules for others. These factors consist of an expanded extracellular fluid volume, paucity of body fat, immaturity of hepatic enzyme systems, and decreased glomerular filtration—all of which may affect profoundly the absorption, conjugation, inactivation, and excretion of antibiotics in the newborn period. In general, the less mature the infant is gestationally, the lower the renal clearance and hepatic metabolism of antibiotics. For these reasons, therapeutic monitoring of plasma drug concentrations (particularly during aminoglycoside and vancomycin therapy) and renal and hepatic function is necessary to ensure therapeutic efficacy, while minimizing toxicity.

When sepsis is ruled out based on a combination of test results, negative cultures, and a normal clinical appearance, antibiotics may be terminated in 48 hours. Antibiotic treatment of proven neonatal septicemia generally is continued for 10 days. A longer period of treatment may be required depending on the clinical response of the patient. Patients with GBS or *Listeria* meningitis respond best to 14 days of treatment, and gram-negative meningitis requires 3 weeks of treatment after the CSF has been sterilized. Special consideration should be given to neonates who continue to seem septic despite broad-spectrum antibiotic coverage and negative cultures. These infants may be harboring fungi, particularly *Candida*, and consideration should be given to instituting empirical treatment with antifungals until culture results are available. Table 8-2 lists the commonly used antimicrobials for neonatal sepsis.

Supportive management of septic neonates begins with the institution of appropriate quantities of intravenous fluids, electrolytes, and glucose. Most septic infants develop intestinal ileus and require gastric decompression

TABLE 8-2 ■ Commonly Used Antibiotics for the Treatment of Neonatal Sepsis

Antibiotic	Dosage	Route	Schedule	Toxicity	Comments
Penicillin G	100,000-150,000 U/kg/day (N,P)*	IM, IV	q8h-q12h (N,P)	Allergic reactions Rare nephrotoxicity	Use highest dose in meningitis
	100,000-300,000 U/kg/day†	IM, IV	q6h-q8h	Rare neuromuscular blockade High doses may cause seizures	
Ampicillin	100-150 mg/kg/day (N,P)	IM, IV	q8h-q12h (N,P)	Rubella-like rash Elevated transaminase levels Nausea, vomiting, diarrhea Rare interstitial nephritis	Penicillin of choice combined with an aminoglycoside in the prophylaxis and treatment of infections with group B streptococci, group D streptococci (enterococci) and *L. monocytogenes*
	150-300 mg/kg/day	IM, IV	q6h-q8h		
Aminoglycosides	Adjust according to peak serum concentration		Adjust according to trough serum concentration	All potentially nephrotoxic and ototoxic Loop diuretics potentiate ototoxicity	Monitor peak and trough serum concentrations Excessive peak concentrations are associated with ototoxicity; excessive trough concentrations are associated with nephrotoxicity
Gentamicin	5 mg/kg/day (N,P)	IM, IV	q18h (N,P)	Nephrotoxicity Ototoxicity Neuromuscular blockade	Poor CSF penetration Peak <10.0 μg/mL (5-10 μg/mL) Trough <2.0 μg/mL
	7.5 mg/kg/day	IM, IV	q8h-q12h		

TABLE 8-2 ■ Commonly Used Antibiotics for the Treatment of Neonatal Sepsis—cont'd					
Antibiotic	**Dosage**	**Route**	**Schedule**	**Toxicity**	**Comments**
Tobramycin	4-5 mg/kg/day (N,P)	IM, IV	q12h (N,P)	See gentamicin	Peak <10.0 μg/mL Trough <2.0 μg/mL
	5-7.5 mg/kg/day	IM, IV	q6h-q8h		
Cephalosporins				Phlebitis with IV infusions	All produce a positive direct Coombs' reaction (unknown clinical significance) Not effective against group D streptococci (enterococci)
Cefazolin	40 mg/kg/day (N,P)	IM, IV	q12h (N,P)	Nephrotoxicity Neutropenia	Poor CSF penetration
	60 mg/kg/day	IM, IV	q8h-q12h	Allergic rash Thrombocytopenia	
Cefotaxime	100-150 mg/kg/day (N,P)	IV	q12h (N,P)	Nephrotoxicity Neutropenia Mildly elevated transaminase levels Eosinophilia	Penetrates CSF well Use highest dose in meningitis
		IV	q6h-q8h		
Cefuroxime	30 mg/kg/day (N,P)	IM, IV	q12h	Transient anemia, leukopenia, and thrombocytopenia	Penetrates CSF well
	60 mg/kg/day	IM, IV			
Ceftazidime	100 mg/kg/day (N,P)	IV	q12h	Nephrotoxicity Transient bone marrow suppression Mild elevation of transaminase levels	Greatest activity against *Pseudomonas* of all the cephalosporins
	150 mg/kg/day	IV	q8h		
Ceftriaxone	50 mg/kg/day (N,P)	IM, IV	q24h	Mild diarrhea Eosinophilia Increased prothrombin time	Do not use as sole drug in infections caused by staphylococci or pseudomonal organisms
	50-75 mg/kg/day	IM, IV			
Vancomycin	20-40 mg/kg/day (N,P)	IV	q12h (N,P)	Nephrotoxicity-synergism with aminoglycosides Ototoxicity Neutropenia Rapid infusion (<30 min) results in transient rash of upper body ("red man syndrome") and hypotension	Adjust dosage and schedule based on peak and trough serum concentrations Peak 25-40 mg/mL Trough <10.0 mg/mL Effective against *S. epidermidis* and methicillin-resistant *S. aureus*
	30-60 mg/kg/day	IV	q6h-q8h		
Clindamycin	10-20 mg/kg/day (N,P)	IV	q12h (N,P)	Nausea, vomiting, diarrhea	Pseudomembranous colitis in adults and adolescents but rarely in children
	20-40 mg/kg/day	IV	q6h-q8h		
Metronidazole	15 mg/kg/day (N,P)	IV	q12h	Vomiting, diarrhea Phlebitis	Effectively penetrates CSF Minimal experience in neonates
	15-30 mg/kg/day	IV	q8h		
Amphotericin	Initial dose 0.25 mg/kg. Increase in 0.25-0.5 mg/kg increments to maximum daily or QD dosage of 1 mg/kg	IV	q24h-q48h	Febrile reactions Flushing Nephrotoxicity Hypokalemia Hypomagnesemia Anemia	Administer slowly over 4-6 hr Protect from light Monitor renal function
Fluconazole	6-12 mg/kg/day depending on intensity of infection, intervals depending on age	IV	Varies	Nausea Rash Dizziness	Treatment of susceptible fungi, most active against *C. albicans*

*(N,P), dose for neonates (<1 week old) and premature infants. Not intended for infants <2 kg.
†Dose for term infants (>1 week of life).

to prevent aspiration. Meticulous attention to temperature control, oxygen requirements, and urine output and concentration is paramount. Pharmacologic therapy with inotropic, chronotropic, or pressor agents may be necessary for cardiovascular support.

With improved neonatal care, the rate of case fatality in neonatal sepsis has decreased by 32% since the 1980s. Several adjuvant therapies have been advocated in attempts to improve these results further. Use of intravenous immune globulin (IVIG) has proven efficacy among children with infections from congenital or acquired immunodeficiency states. Although it seemed to follow that IVIG would be useful in neonatal sepsis, clinical studies have shown conflicting data. Two meta-analyses have shown a slight but small reduction in serious infections in neonates treated with IVIG. There was no decrease in mortality or serious morbidity, however. The overall conclusion is that although use of IVIG is safe and has slight efficacy, it does not produce sufficient benefit to warrant routine administration.

The most recent advancement in adjuvant therapy has been in the augmentation of cellular immunity. Because PMNs are functionally inefficient in neonates and the total body mass is markedly lower than in older infants, strategies to increase PMN functionality and numbers would seem a likely successful strategy. Use of colony-stimulating factors has been examined in several clinical trials. Two basic strategies have been used. First is the use of colony-stimulating factors in patients who are already septic. Randomized clinical trials have shown that granulocyte colony-stimulating factor (G-CSF) intervention in septic, neutropenic neonates has no toxicity and can increase neutrophil counts significantly. It has not been shown definitively, however, that G-CSF therapy has an impact on survival.

The second approach for colony-stimulating factor therapy is as a prophylaxis for patients at high risk for sepsis. Use of GM-CSF has been employed in at least three controlled trials of neonates who were thought to be at risk for neonatal sepsis. GM-CSF was used because it was believed to have greater efficacy in promoting phagocyte proliferation and function than G-CSF. Two of the three studies showed a significant benefit, with GM-CSF being able to be prophylactic against the development of septic complications. Although not incorporated into routine practice, these studies offer some cogent argument to begin the use of GM-CSF in high-risk patients. It seems that small-for-gestational-age infants derive the greatest benefit.

ACQUIRED IMMUNODEFICIENCY SYNDROME

In contrast to the early predominance among homosexual men, one of the most significant increases in human immunodeficiency virus (HIV) infection and acquired immunodeficiency syndrome (AIDS) is occurring in adolescents. Half of the estimated 5.3 million new HIV infections in the world occur in adolescents and young adults (15 to 24 years old). Within the United States, 25% of new cases are in 13- to 21-year-olds. Of the approximately 432,000 people reported to be living with

HIV in the United States, 5575 are children younger than 13 years old. The age of childhood HIV has changed significantly. Between 1984 and 1992, HIV in children was rising almost exponentially. From 1992 to the present, there has been a nearly 50% decline, however, despite a relatively stable number of children born to HIV-positive mothers. This is due to the use of postexposure prophylaxis with antiretroviral agents, screening, treatment of gravid mothers, and advancement in educational programs, all leading to a marked reduction in the number of newborns with HIV. Another tremendous decline in HIV-positive children has occurred since the loss of the numerous HIV-infected children who developed AIDS from the use of blood products before the universal screening of these products, beginning in 1985. Despite these trends, an understanding of the pathophysiology and care of HIV-positive children is essential.

Handling of Infants with Human Immunodeficiency Virus

When the infected infant has had his or her first bath and maternal blood has been cleaned off, the infant can be handled normally except for precautions in handling the infant's blood and body fluids. Infection is not transmitted by casual contact. Respiratory or separate room isolation is inappropriate for either the mother or the infant. Breast-feeding is not recommended because breast milk contains the virus. Universal precautions for blood-containing products and tissue should be observed; however, urine and saliva (<1 infectious particle/mL) contain extremely low levels of virus and are in such a range that routine use of gloves for handling them is not advised.

Transmission in Neonates

The most common form of HIV transmission is vertically from infected mothers. Rates of transmission in untreated mothers range from 12% to 30%. This transmission may occur intrauterine, intrapartum (during the passage through the birth canal and from exposure of maternal blood), or postpartum (via nursing). HIV may be passed to the fetus by 10 weeks' gestation; in utero transmission accounts for 30% to 40% of all vertically transmitted cases. Many of these cases may be avoided with the administration of antiretroviral therapy during pregnancy. Intrapartum passage is the most common form of transmission and accounts for 60% to 70% of cases; many cases can be avoided with elective cesarean sections. Nursing accounts for approximately 10% to 15% of cases and is clearly the most preventable. A meta-analysis of 15 prospective studies showed that elective cesarean section decreased vertical transmission by 50%. Transmission was reduced by 87% when elective cesarean section was combined with prenatal, intrapartum, and neonatal zidovudine therapy. Transfusions of blood products now account for only 3% to 6% of all transmissions of HIV in children.

Pathogenesis

HIV uniquely binds to the CD4$^+$ cell surface molecule. This marker is on primary helper T lymphocytes and in other organs, including portions of the brain, including microglia, astrocytes, and oligodendroglia, and placental tissue. The infection in the brain accounts for the well-known neurologic deterioration observed in children. When bonded, the virus infects the cells. In the case of lymphocytes, these cells migrate to lymphoid tissue. This accounts for the lymphadenopathy characteristic of the acute viral syndrome. After 2 to 4 months, the level of culturable virus decreases, and the patient enters a latency period that may last 8 to 12 years. Although little is observed clinically, there is a high rate of viral turnover, with more than 1 billion $CD4^+$ cells being depleted each day. The body attempts to balance this with $CD8^+$ T lymphocytes acting against structural and regulatory viral proteins. Additionally, neutralizing antibodies are generated during the infection and seem to suppress viral replication during the latency phase.

Clinical Course

Children may show one of three clinical patterns. Approximately 15% to 25% of newborns develop a rapid disease in which the median survival is 6 to 9 months. This typically is seen with early intrauterine infections. Most children (60% to 80%) have a slow progression with a median survival of more than 6 years. These patients typically develop HIV via the intrapartum period and by testing are typically HIV negative in the first week of life. Fewer than 5% of children have minimal or no progression of the syndrome and have a prolonged survival. The typical patient presenting with the initial viremia has lymphadenopathy, parotitis, hepatomegaly, and splenomegaly. Moderate symptoms occur in patients who have the disease for more than 2 months and have recurrent or chronic diarrhea, fevers, and recurrent infections (hepatitis, herpes simplex stomatitis, pneumonitis, candidal esophagitis) and some visceral involvement, including cardiomegaly and nephropathy. In severe, advanced disease, patients develop serious bacterial infections (sepsis, meningitis, pneumonia) and malnutrition, chronic diarrhea with or without cryptococcosis, and encephalopathy. Typical associated organisms include *S. pneumoniae* and *Salmonella*. Other pathogens such as *Staphylococcus*, *Enterococcus*, *Pseudomonas aeruginosa*, *H. influenzae*, and other gram-negative or gram-positive organisms also may be seen. Also included are atypical mycobacterial infections, oral candidiasis, and *Pneumocystis carinii* pneumonia.

The incidence of central nervous system involvement in perinatally infected children is 40% to 90%, with a median onset at 19 months of age. The development of central nervous system involvement is more common in children. It may be associated with a loss of developmental milestones, mental deterioration, and progression marked spasticity and gait disturbance. Commonly, encephalopathy is an indication for feeding tube placement (gastrostomy tube), particularly when associated with malnutrition. Diarrhea and weight loss are common reasons for nutritional intervention.

Diagnosis

Detection of HIV relies on either the presence of antibody to HIV or the presence of virus. In a child older than 18 months of age, the presence of IgG antibody to

HIV by two separate tests confirms the diagnosis of HIV infection. The delay until this age is to exclude the possibility that the antibody was derived from a maternal source. HIV detection by polymerase chain reaction techniques is useful for detection in younger children. Approximately 40% of infected neonates test positive using viral assays in the first 2 days of life, and 90% test positive by 2 weeks of age. Serial testing should be done because infants who do test positive benefit from early initiation of antiretroviral treatment.

Treatment

Use of antiretroviral agents has been proved to have a significant impact in patients with HIV. The goal of the treatment is to inhibit retroviral replication. The advantage is to reduce the destruction of the patient's immune system, while preventing replication, which may lead to the development of resistance to the antiretroviral agents. The use of these agents is difficult because multiple drugs are required, each with their own potential range of side effects and toxicities. For a successful result, patient adherence to the treatment regimen is crucial. Two basic arms of therapy are the reverse transcriptase inhibitors and protease inhibitors. Patients are given two different reverse transcriptase inhibitors, a nucleoside reverse transcriptase inhibitor and a non-nucleoside reverse transcriptase inhibitor. The two transcriptase inhibitors and the protease inhibitors act at different points of the viral replication cycle; the agents act on actively replicating and nonreplicating viruses.

OTHER IMMUNOLOGIC DISORDERS

Although an extensive discussion of pediatric immune deficiency syndromes is beyond the scope of this chapter, this section discusses three additional immune disorders in which surgically relevant processes are seen that may involve the pediatric surgeon.

Chronic Granulomatous Disease

The pediatric surgeon frequently is asked to care for chronic granulomatous disease. Patients with this disorder have a defect in the nicotinamide-adenine dinucleotide phosphate (reduced form) (NADPH) oxidase complex. Although neutrophils can migrate to a site of infection and phagocytose organisms, they lack the ability to kill these cells because they have an absence of the oxidative burst necessary to destroy the organism. Diagnosis of an infection conventionally was performed with a nitroblue tetrazolium test. Currently, many chemiluminescence tests can show oxidative burst of PMNs and help make the diagnosis. Patients with chronic granulomatous disease are at risk for staphylococcal, gram-negative, enteric bacteria, pseudomonal, yeast, and nocardial infections. Patients frequently develop large infiltrates of the lungs and liver. Despite the patient receiving adequate antibiotic agents, the surgeon often has to perform a wide débridement and excision of infected tissue, or the process fails to clear.

DiGeorge Syndrome

DiGeorge syndrome comprises an association of an abnormal facies, a pure T-cell deficiency owing to a lack of thymic tissue, hypocalcemia (owing to a loss of parathyroid tissue), and congenital heart disease. Most cardiovascular abnormalities are from an interrupted aortic arch or a truncus arteriosus. Patients with this disorder have a defect in the embryonic tissues of the branchial arches and abnormalities of the neural crest tissue.

Complement Deficiencies

Complement deficiencies are seen in approximately 0.03% of the general population, although many of these may be transient in nature. The most profound deficiency is a loss of C3, which, although rare, is the main factor for activating the complement cascade. Because of the key role of complement in opsonization, most patients with a complement deficiency are at risk for the development of infections secondary to encapsulated organisms. Most patients develop a meningococcal infection.

SUGGESTED READINGS

Bernstein HM, Calhoun DA, Christensen RD: Use of myeloid colony-stimulating factors in neonates with septicemia. Curr Opin Pediatr 14:91-94, 2002.

This is an excellent review of the current clinical experience with myeloid colony-stimulating factors, including recombinant G-CSF and rhGM-CSF.

Centers for Disease Control and Prevention: Guidelines for the use of antiretroviral agents in pediatric HIV infection. MMWR Morb Mortal Wkly Rep 47 (RR-4):1, 1998.

A very good review of potential antiretroviral agents that can be used in patients with HIV as well as babies born to mothers with HIV.

Centers for Disease Control and Prevention: Report of the NIH panel to define principles of therapy of HIV infection and guidelines for the use of antiretroviral agents in HIV-infected adults and adolescents. MMWR Morb Mortal Wkly Rep 47 (RR-5):1, 1998.

Review of the use of antiretroviral agents for adolescents with HIV or exposure to HIV.

Faye A, Burgard M, Crosnier H, et al: Human immunodeficiency virus type 2 infection in children. J Pediatr 130:994, 1997.

A very good review of the pathogenesis and natural history of infants and children with HIV.

Gessler P, Luders R, Konig S, et al: Nenoatal neutropenia in low birthweight premature infants. Am J Perinatol 12:34038, 1995.

This study on a large number of low-birth-weight infants shows the low level of neutrophils in neonates.

International Perinatal HIV Group: The mode of delivery and the risk of vertical transmission of human immunodeficiency virus type 1—a meta-analysis of 15 prospective cohort studies. N Engl J Med 340:977, 1999.

This is an excellent study on the prevention of vertical transmission of HIV.

Modi N, Carr R: Promising stratagems for reducing the burden of neonatal sepsis. Arch Dis Child Fetal Neonatal Edit 83:F150-F153, 2000.

This article provides an excellent discussion of some of the newer adjuvant therapies to treat and prevent neonatal sepsis.

Quie PA: Antimicrobial defenses in the neonate. Semin Perinatol 14:2, 1990.

This is an overview of the specific and nonspecific antimicrobial defense systems of neonates. Specific neonatal infections and immunodeficiency are discussed.

Trotta PP: Cytokines: An overview. Am J Reprod Immunol 25:137, 1991.

This is an overview of the various types of cytokines with attention to physicochemical and biologic properties.

Hematologic Considerations

Hematologic considerations encompass an enormous scope during the care of the pediatric surgical patient. Included in this is the care of the anemic infant, diagnosing and caring for coagulation abnormalities, anticoagulation, and transfusion.

ANEMIA

In general, the newborn is found to be in the polycythemic range (hemoglobin: 16.0 g/dL and hemocrit > 60%, respectively) at birth. These values level off, and a physiologic anemia is commonly noted at age 3 to 5 months (hemoglobin: 9.0 to 10.0 g/dL; hematocrit: 30% to 33%). The etiology of this "physiologic anemia" is more than likely multifactorial. Included is the fact that iron is stored but is not well utilized in the first few months of life. Other anemias have a multitude of potential mechanisms. Findings of anemias in surgical patients is quite common. Understanding the etiology and treatment may be more complex. The first step in understanding why an infant or child is anemic is based on a good differential diagnosis. In general, anemias are best understood by breaking them down into various categories of etiology. Table 9-1 lists potential causes of childhood anemias. Determination also depends on some basic laboratory studies. This includes determination of a complete blood cell count, mean corpuscular volume (MCV), red cell distribution width (RDW, an indicator of various red blood cell structures), ferritin, and serum iron level. Occasionally, vitamin B_{12}, folate, and total iron-binding capacity studies may be needed.

TABLE 9-1 ■ Etiology of Childhood Anemia Based on Adjusted Reticulocyte Count (ARC)	
Increased Red Cell Production (ARC < 2)	**Increased Red Cell Production (ARC > 2)**
Deficiency of Hematopoiesis	**Hemolytic Anemias: Normocytic**
Microcytic anemias,	Isoimmune
Defective heme synthesis	ABO or minor
Iron deficiency	Antigen incompatibility
Anemia of chronic disease	Autoimmune
Lead poisoning	Idiopathic
Copper deficiency	Postinfectious
Defective globin synthesis	β-Thalassemia
α-Thalassemia	Nonimmune
β-Thalassemia	Microangiopathic (DIC, HUS, TTP)
Macrocytic anemia	Vitamin B_{12} deficiency
Defective DNA synthesis	
Folate deficiency	**Intracorpuscular Defects**
Vitamin B_{12} deficiency	Intrinsic membrane
Metabolic drugs (e.g., methotrexate)	Hereditary spherocytosis, elliptocytosis, stomatocytosis
	Hemoglobinopathies
Bone Marrow Failure	Sickle cell
Normocytic	Enzymopathies
TEC	G6PD
Chronic renal disease	
Parvovirus B-19	
Macrocytic	
Congenital red cell aplasia (Diamond Blackfan syndrome)	
Fanconi's anemia	
Chronic liver disease	

TEC, transient erythroblastopenia of childhood, a pure red blood cell aplasia; DIC, disseminated intravascular coagulation; HUS, hemolytic-uremic syndrome; TTP, thrombotic thrombocytopenic purpura: G6PD, glucose-6-phosphate dehydrogenase deficiency.

Additionally, an adjusted reticulocyte count (ARC) should be determined to ascertain if an adequate erythropoietic response is attained:

$$ARC = \frac{\text{Hematocrit (measured)}}{\text{Hematocrit (expected)}} \times \text{Reticulocyte count}$$

Should the child have a persistent anemia, a further work-up with review of the peripheral smear, quantitative hemoglobin electrophoresis, and hematology consultation should be obtained.

Iron-Deficiency Anemia

Iron-deficiency anemia may typically be seen in the first 6 to 24 months of life. Iron deficiency may complicate physiologic anemia. The cause of this anemia is inadequate intake of nutritional iron. Most infants require dietary iron supplements for the first year of life. Infants absorb iron in the duodenum (90%) and proximal jejunum (10%). Particularly at risk are those infants who receive whole cow's milk, those with exclusive breast-feeding for more than 1 year (without vitamins), and those infants receiving iron-free or reduced-iron formulas. There is actually very little evidence that iron-restricted formulas have much basis for general use, so they should generally be avoided. Iron deficiency may also be caused by chronic blood loss commonly seen in surgical patients in neonatal intensive care units in whom multiple laboratory studies are performed. Iron deficiencies are also quite common in premature neonates who are on prolonged courses of parenteral nutrition. Treatment consists of 3 to 6 mg/kg/day of oral iron, which may need to continue for up to 3 months.

Aplastic Anemia

Aplastic anemia is a blood dyscrasia characterized by decreased bone marrow production of platelets, white blood cells, and erythrocytes. In half the cases, aplastic anemia is the result of a toxic effect from a chemical (antibiotics or other drugs) on the bone marrow. Aplastic anemia in patients receiving chloramphenicol is not dose related. It is most frequently related to an idiosyncratic reaction that may be associated with a genetic predisposition to marrow injury. In the majority of cases of aplastic anemia the cause remains unknown. Surgical procedures in these patients increase the risk of developing opportunistic infection and require careful management of blood component therapy. Aplastic anemia may be cured by a bone marrow transplant.

Hemolytic Anemias

Hemolytic anemia is a condition in which red blood corpuscle survival is reduced to one eighth of normal, a level beyond the ability of the bone marrow to compensate. It may be the result of genetically related abnormal red blood cell morphology, hereditary metabolic derangements in red blood cell metabolism, or idiopathic formation of autoantibodies against red blood corpuscles. The most common forms of hemolytic anemia are hereditary spherocytosis, sickle cell disease, thalassemia major, glycolytic red blood cell enzyme deficiencies (e.g., pyruvate kinase, hexose kinase) hemoglobin C disease, and autoimmune hemolytic anemias.

Hereditary spherocytosis is an autosomal dominant disorder characterized by an abnormal elliptical red blood cell shape that results in erythrocyte entrapment in the spleen and destruction by hemolysis. The diagnosis is suspected by the appearance of anemia, splenomegaly, jaundice (resulting from hemolysis), and a positive family history. The diagnosis is confirmed by an abnormal osmotic fragility test. Lessening of jaundice is the result of diminished red blood cell production (aplastic crisis), causing severe anemia that requires transfusion. This condition is frequently complicated by spleen-related biliary tract disease (see Chapter 69). In most cases the treatment of choice is elective splenectomy at 5 years of age unless a hemolytic crisis at an earlier age requires frequent transfusions. Gallstones are detected by ultrasound examination and managed by cholecystectomy, usually at the time of splenectomy.

Sickle Cell Anemia

The gene for sickle cell disease is present in 8% to 10% of American blacks and in a higher percentage in Africans. It is also found to a lesser extent in Greeks, Italians, and Saudi Arabians. Sickle hemoglobin is less soluble in a deoxygenated state and can form crystal polymers that distort the red blood cell membrane. Homozygous disease (occurring in 1 in 625 individuals) is manifested by a painful abdominal crisis or by bone and joint pain caused by a vaso-occlusive episode or progressive hemolytic anemia and splenomegaly. The patient has a normocytic anemia and sickle cells in the peripheral blood smear. Patients will have a quantitative hemoglobin electrophoresis with 0% hemoglobin A, 85% to 95% hemoglobin S, 2% to 3% hemoglobin A2, and 5% to 15% hemoglobin F. The diagnosis is confirmed by a positive Sickledex prep demonstrating sickle cells at a low oxygen tension. Prenatal diagnosis of sickle cell disease can now be diagnosed by amniocentesis and DNA analysis.

A number of complications may accompany sickle cell disease. An appreciation for these problems is essential to discerning surgical from nonsurgical processes. Acute hemolytic crisis or aplastic crisis may require urgent splenectomy. An aplastic crisis is caused by a viral suppression of red blood cell precursors in the bone marrow and is often associated with parvovirus B19. This will be manifested by a severe anemia and reticulocytopenia. Transfusion is essential until the bone marrow recovers. In acute splenic sequestration, the spleen suddenly becomes engorged with red blood cells, leading to the loss of significant blood volume. Splenic sequestration typically occurs between 6 months to 2 years of age. Hyperhemolytic crisis occurs in patients with sickle cell disease who also have a glucose-6-phosphate dehydrogenase deficiency and are exposed to an oxidative stress.

An even more devastating complication is a vaso-occlusive crisis secondary to microvascular infarcts. These infarcts may occur in any organ and may be induced by infection, cold exposure, dehydration, venous stasis, or acidosis. Such a process occurs in areas of slow venous flow. Pain may occur in long bones, vertebrae, the sternum, central nervous system, lungs, penis, myocardium, and intestine. Acute chest syndrome, which is one of the most lethal conditions associated with sickle cell anemia, is caused by a vaso-occlusive crisis of the lungs. Dactylitis consists of painful swellings of the dorsum of the hands and feet from small infarcts in the small bones of the extremities. Patients with a vaso-occlusive crisis may present with abdominal pain, which typically resolves with oxygen, hydration, and transfusions. On rare occasions, the intestine may infarct; therefore, the pediatric surgeon must observe patients carefully during such a crisis. In addition to the liberal use of intravenous fluids (1.5 times maintenance), opioid analgesics and the occasional use of nonsteroidal anti-inflammatory agents may be employed. The acute chest syndrome will require exchange transfusion, oxygen, and occasional use of antibiotics. Often it is difficult to distinguish acute appendicitis from a vaso-occlusive abdominal crisis in these patients. Computed tomography is often helpful in this situation.

As a consequence of microinfarction and congestion, the spleen will eventually infarct by 4 to 6 years of age. Thus, patients are at risk from overwhelming sepsis secondary to encapsulated organisms. Additional complications include osteomyelitis (typically secondary to *Salmonella*), leg ulcers, hyposthenuria, priapism, and biliary tract disease. The presence of stones in the gallbladder and bile ducts may result in cholecystitis and gallstone pancreatitis. Elective laparoscopic cholecystectomy is the procedure of choice for gallstones.

Other Anemias

Other deficiencies of hematopoiesis include the thalassemias, nutrient deficiencies, and anemias of chronic diseases. The thalassemias are not uncommon disorders and are categorized into α and β subgroups. These thalassemias result from a reduced synthesis of the α- or β-globin chain of hemoglobin, respectively. The α-thalassemias are caused by deletions of portions of the α genes, whereas the β-thalessemias are caused by an error in transcription or translation of the mRNA. Thalassemias can fall into either one-gene deletion, which is silent; two-gene deletions, which are thalassemia minors; and hemoglobin H or three-gene deletions. Children with thalassemia major (also referred to as Mediterranean anemia or Cooley's anemia) present with microcytic, hypochromic, hemolytic anemia in early infancy requiring early and repeated transfusion. These children develop hepatosplenomegaly and iron overload, resulting in damage to the heart, liver, pancreas, and endocrine organs. Hemolysis results in biliary tract disease as well. Recent experience with hypertransfusion therapy in early infancy has shown suppression of extramedullary hematopoiesis, thus reducing the risk of early complications. These conditions are further discussed in depth in Chapter 67 (Gallbladder Disease) and Chapter 69 (The Spleen).

Additional Surgical Considerations

In the past, 10.0 g/dL was considered the minimum safe hemoglobin level for a general anesthetic in neonates and infants. In recent years, however, advances in anesthesia, intraoperative monitoring, and attempts to avoid unnecessary blood transfusion have reduced the level considered adequate for a margin of safety to 8.0 to 8.5 g/dL in most pediatric centers. Oral iron therapy can be administered for elective preoperative cases and will raise the hemoglobin level approximately 1.5 g/dL/week. Acute blood loss resulting in anemia, shock, and the need for urgent transfusion therapy is covered in detail in the section on trauma.

Prevention or the reduction of transfusions with the use of recombinant human erythropoietin has been shown to be beneficial in several clinical settings, including the treatment of children with hematologic or solid malignancies. The benefit of erythropoietin in the settings of trauma or critical care is being studied.

Packed red blood cells should be given for a low hemoglobin level. Although in previous years a 10-mL/kg level of transfusion was given for infants and small children, many groups have become more liberal with the volume, using 15 mL/kg or more, provided that the volume does not exceed 1 unit of packed red blood cells. This facilitates boosting red blood cells while limiting the exposure to the child to a single donor. Fresh-frozen plasma consists of plasma separated from the red blood cells. Each milliliter of fresh-frozen plasma contains 1 IU of coagulation factors and inhibitors. In general, fresh-frozen plasma can be given in a dose of 10 to 20 mL/kg over a 1-hour period.

Children whose families are Jehovah's Witnesses present a potential dilemma. Without exception, minors must be transfused during a life-threatening episode without regard to parents' preferences. If the surgeon has time, a court-granted permission may help in terms of relations with the patient's family. Nevertheless, a number of strategies may be used to boost the level of red blood cell volume. Such benefits include a reduction in transfusion-related immune deficiencies, economic advantage, and prevention of viral transmission. Strategies should include preoperative autologous blood procurement, intraoperative red cell salvage hemodilution, and use of meticulous hemostasis. A unique approach to improving hemostasis has been the use of recombinant factor VIIa (NovoSeven) in the setting of uncontrolled bleeding. This product has been used in hemophilic patients with inhibitors and in nonhemophilic patients with uncontrolled bleeding during surgical procedures or with major trauma.

HEMOSTASIS AND THROMBOSIS

Hemostasis depends on normal function and integrity of the blood vessels and coagulation system and on platelet-vessel interaction. Abnormalities in hemostasis may lead to hemorrhage or thrombosis in association with either decreased or increased hemostasis. The majority of bleeding disorders in the newborn period are the result of coagulation protein deficiencies or thrombocytopenia.

Platelets

Platelets are produced in the bone marrow by precursor megakaryocytes. The normal platelet count in term neonates is $250,000/mm^3$ (which is similar to that for adults and older children). Platelet counts of $100,000/mm^3$ are observed in 10% to 20% of premature infants. Thrombocytopenia in the newborn has diverse causes (Table 9-2). It is often observed in premature infants who have multiple medical complications. Low platelet counts in this group of patients are frequently accompanied by an increased incidence of hemorrhagic events, high morbidity and mortality, and an increased risk of intraventricular hemorrhage. Thrombocytopenia may also be observed in infants with infections, whether bacterial or viral or intrauterine or postnatal. In addition, it can be associated with disorders such as respiratory

TABLE 9-2 ■ Laboratory Findings in the Newborn Period			
	Hemophilia	Vitamin K Deficiency	DIC
PTT	P	P	P
PT	N	P	P
Fibrinogen	N	N	L
FSPs	Negative	Negative	Positive
Platelet count	N	N	L

PTT, Partial thromboplastin time: PT, prothrombin time; P, prolonged; N, normal; L, low; FSPs, fibrin-split products; DIC, disseminated intravascular coagulation.

TABLE 9-3 ■ Blood-Clotting Factors	
I	Fibrinogen
II	Prothrombin
III	Thromboplastin
IV	Calcium
V	Proaccelerin (labile factor)
VI	Activated factor V (term not used)
VII	Proconvertin (stable factor)
VIII	Antihemophilic factor
IX	Plasma thromboplastin component—Christmas factor
X	Stuart-Prower factor
XI	Plasma thromboplastin antecedent
XII	Hageman factor, contact factor
XIII	Fibrin-stabilizing factor

distress syndrome, necrotizing enterocolitis, hyperviscosity, and maternal idiopathic thrombocytopenic purpura. Thrombocytopenia may result from certain maternal medications such as sulfa drugs, phenytoin (Dilantin), cimetidine, digoxin, chlorothiazides, and acetaminophen. Finally, congenital disorders such as Wiskott-Aldrich syndrome, Fanconi's anemia, and platelet trapping in a hemangioma may be associated with thrombocytopenia.

Platelet dysfunction may develop even with a normal platelet count in infants of mothers who took aspirin, meperidine (Demerol), or promethazine (Phenergan). Aspirin inhibits release of adenosine diphosphate and interferes with platelet aggregation. This effect can last as long as 5 to 10 days after aspirin ingestion.

In addition to occurring with certain drugs, acquired platelet abnormalities can occur after the ingestion of some food, spices, and vitamins. Platelet dysfunction is also observed in patients with chronic renal failure, after cardiopulmonary bypass, and in association with myeloproliferative and lymphoproliferative disease. Desmopressin transiently corrects the bleeding time in patients with renal failure.

Coagulation Factors

The coagulation system consists of procoagulants, anticoagulants (inhibitors), and the fibrinolytic system. In most situations, hemostasis is in balance so that appropriate clot formation and dissolution occur in response to injury. Decreased procoagulant activity and increased fibrinolysis result in excessive bleeding, whereas decreased inhibitor activity or defective fibrinolysis will lead to thrombosis. Procoagulants are a series of proteases and accessory factors that interact to form thrombin, which in turn converts fibrinogen to a fibrin clot. Procoagulants include (1) contact factors (factor XI—plasma thromboplastin antecedent, factor XII—Hageman factor, prekallikrein [Fletcher] factor, and high-molecular-weight kininogen); (2) vitamin K–dependent factors (factor II—prothrombin, factor VII—proconvertin, factor IX—plasma thromboplastin component or Christmas factor, and factor X (Stuart-Prower factor), protein C, and protein S; (3) consumable factors that are depleted during the clotting process (factor I—fibrinogen, factor II—prothrombin, factor V—proaccelerin activator globulin, factor VIII—antihemophilic factor, and factor XIII—fibrin-stabilizing factor); and (4) a variety of other factors, including factor III (tissue thromboplastin factor) and factor IV (calcium) (Table 9-3).

Procoagulation Process

There are two different pathways for initiating the coagulation process: the intrinsic and extrinsic pathways (Fig. 9-1). The intrinsic pathway is stimulated when factor XII reacts with subendothelial collagen. Following this step, sequential interaction with other factors (factors XI, IX, VIII, and platelet factor 3) results in activation of factor X. The extrinsic pathway is stimulated when injured tissue releases tissue thromboplastin (factor III), which reacts with factor VII to activate factor X. The intrinsic and extrinsic pathways both activate factor X through different reactions, but beyond this step the clotting pathways are identical. Activated factor X, factor V, and platelet factor 3 function together to convert factor II (prothrombin) to thrombin. Thrombin then converts factor I (fibrinogen) to fibrin in the form of a loose clot. Factor XIII (fibrin-stabilizing factor) changes the loose friable clot into tight fibrin polymers. The definitive clot is composed of platelet aggregates and tight fibrin polymers. The concept shown in Figure 9-1 represents an over-simplification of the actual coagulation process, which may rely on both intrinsic and extrinsic components simultaneously.

Anticoagulation Processes

The coagulation process is controlled by a series of protease inhibitors (anticoagulants) that limit clot formation or extension (Fig. 9-2). Antithrombin III interacts with endogenous heparin on the endothelium as well as with exogenous heparin to neutralize the actions of factor Xa, as well as activated factors XII, XI, and IX. Protein C is activated by thrombin in the presence of thrombomodulin (an endothelial cell receptor). Activated protein C in the presence of protein S inhibits the activity of factors V and VIII and slows fibrin formation. Protein S acts as a cofactor for protein C. Both protein C and protein S are vitamin K–dependent plasma proteins.

Alteration of Coagulation Factors with Age

The levels of fibrinogen and factor VIII in newborns are similar to those in older children and adults, whereas the levels of factors V and XIII are only mildly decreased. Levels of other coagulation factors may vary with gestational age. Levels of vitamin K–dependent factors II, VII,

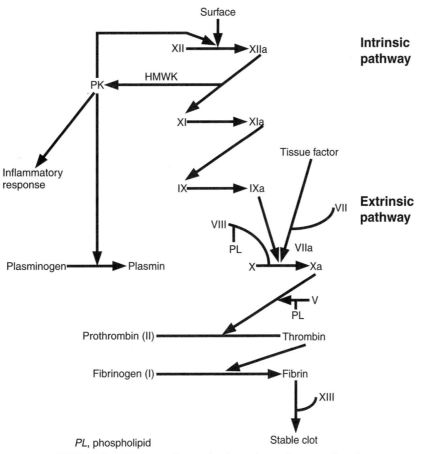

PL, phospholipid

FIGURE 9-1 ▪ Diagram shows clotting scheme (procoagulants).

and X in the term newborn are only 50% of adult levels, whereas factor IX levels are 30% of adult levels. These low levels in term infants are probably related to immature hepatic function and decreased factor synthesis and are even lower in premature infants. Because neonates are vitamin K–deficient, this may also play a role in the decreased levels to vitamin K–dependent coagulation factors. All the coagulation proteins reach normal levels between 3 and 6 months of age.

The levels of natural inhibitors—protein C, protein S, and antithrombin III—are all decreased at birth. This is balanced by the decreased levels of vitamin K–dependent coagulation factors observed at birth. Protein C levels are 30% of adult levels at birth and 40% at 6 months of age; they continue to increase, reaching normal levels in early childhood. The newborn's protein S levels are 50% of normal adult levels; adult concentrations are reached at 2 months of age. Protein S exists in the circulation as free protein S, and a portion is bound to a C4b-binding protein. Only free protein S has anticoagulant activity and is active before protein C and antithrombin III. Antithrombin III levels in neonates are also 50% of adult levels and become normal at age 6 months.

Disorders of Coagulation
Evaluation of the Bleeding Patient

In neonates, bleeding is most commonly caused by inherited coagulation disorders, vitamin K deficiency,

occasionally isolated platelet disorders, and disseminated intravascular coagulation (DIC). In most instances only patients with DIC are seriously ill, whereas those with coagulation factor disorders and vitamin K deficiency present as otherwise normal-appearing infants. These disorders may be manifested by large ecchymoses or by localized bleeding from a large cephalohematoma, the gastrointestinal tract, or the umbilical cord; they may also result in excessive bleeding after circumcision in the neonatal unit. A family history of bleeding, a history of maternal medications or illnesses during pregnancy, and documentation that vitamin K was actually administered is important to obtain. Vitamin K deficiency may also be seen in patients with severe diarrhea, cystic fibrosis, biliary atresia, and hepatitis. A clotting disorder should be suspected in older infants and children if bleeding occurs after a surgical procedure, a dental extraction, or a laceration that has been recently sutured, or if there are petechiae or an ecchymosis greater than 5 cm.

The platelet count, prothrombin time (PT), and partial thromboplastin time (PTT) are the frontline tests used to evaluate bleeding. The platelet count will document instances of thrombocytopenia. An evaluation of the size of the platelet on the peripheral smear may be useful, because large platelets are often indicative of rapid production and destruction, whereas thrombocytopenia in the presence of normal-sized platelets reflects reduced bone marrow production. In neonates the bleeding time is difficult to evaluate and is not usually tested.

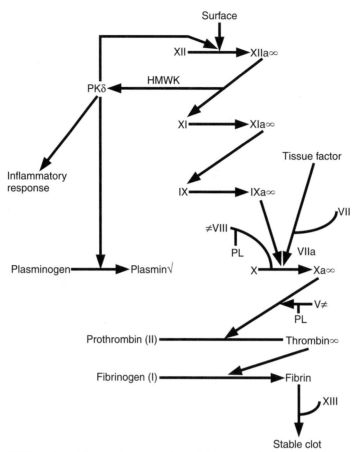

FIGURE 9-2 ■ Scheme of anticoagulants-inhibitors. Inhibitors: ∞, AT-III; ≠, protein C; δ, C1 esterase; √, A2 antiplasmin.

The bleeding time is a good way to assess the interaction of platelets with vascular endothelium but not in infants and children with thrombocytopenia. In older infants and children with normal platelet counts, the bleeding time may be useful in identifying platelet dysfunction and von Willebrand's disease (vWD).

Both the PT and PTT may be slightly prolonged in normal healthy newborns because of relative deficiencies of certain of the coagulant factors at birth, and they may be further prolonged in premature infants. Any questionable abnormality of PT and PTT in neonates must therefore be compared with what is interpreted as a "normal newborn level" in the institution in question (see Table 9-2). The PT measures the extrinsic activation of factor X by factor VII in addition to factors II, V, and fibrinogen and, when abnormally elevated, usually indicates the presence of an acquired defect. The PTT measures the intrinsic pathway concerning activation of factor X by factors XII, XI, IX and VIII, as well as the final coagulation reactions involving factors II and V and fibrinogen.

DIC must be suspected in ill-appearing patients with thrombocytopenia and abnormally prolonged PT and PTT. A fibrinogen level and a test for the presence of fibrin-split products (FSPs) and D-dimers should be obtained to separate liver disease from DIC as the cause of clotting dysfunction. The fibrinogen level is decreased in liver disease, and increased D-dimer levels and degradation of fibrinogen and fibrin to split products is seen in DIC;

occasionally, however, D-dimer levels may be elevated in cases of liver disease, especially when DIC coexists with liver failure. As a general rule, factor VII is usually decreased in patients with severe liver disease, and FSPs are almost never present in patients with primary clotting factor deficiencies or vitamin K deficiency. In patients with suspected isolated clotting factor deficiencies, measurements of specific clotting factor levels should be obtained (see Table 9-2).

Evaluation of the Hyperthrombotic Patient

Deficiencies in anticoagulant proteases may lead to thrombotic syndromes including splenic infarct, deep vein thrombosis of the lower extremity, mesenteric venous thrombosis, and pulmonary emboli (Table 9-4). The basic work-up of a patient in whom such a disorder is suggested consists of a high index of suspicion. Such clotting tendencies may result from either a deficiency of thrombosis inhibitors (antithrombin III, protein C, protein S), dysfibrinogenemias, or dysfibrinolysis. These disorders now comprise the majority of thrombotic events in childhood when no other mechanical causes are found. Many of these are inherited in an autosomal dominant fashion; however, a negative family history does not preclude one of these disorders. The initial work-up of these disorders is complex but it should initially start with a thrombin time (TT) and euglobulin clot lysis time. If the TT is prolonged, dysfibrinogenemia is likely and

TABLE 9-4 ■ Hereditary Thrombotic Disorders				
Disorder	Genetics	Estimated Frequency	Screening Tests	Usual Plasma Level, % of Normal
Resistance to activated protein C	AD	1:800 to 1:5000	DNA screening or functional assay of aPTT	NA
Prothrombin gene polymorphism	AD	1:50	Genetic testing for polymorphism 20210A	NA
AT-III deficiency	AD (heterozygote)	1:5000	AT-III heparin cofactor assay (S-2238) AT-III antigen	35–60
HCF-II deficiency	AD (heterozygote)	Rare	HCF-II assay with dermatan sulfate	40–50
Protein C deficiency	AD (heterozygote)	1:10,000	Protein C activity using thrombomodulin and S-2366 chromogenic substrate	40–60
Protein C deficiency	AD (homozygote)	Rare	As above plus protein C antigen assay	0–5
Protein S deficiency	AD (heterozygote)	1:20,000	Antigen activity assays	40–60
Dysplasminogenemia	AR, AD	Rare	ELT: chromogenic assay for plasminogen	40–50
Dysfibrinogenemia	AD	Rare	Thrombin time, reptilase time	Abnormal
Decreased tPA release	AD	Rare	tPA assay after stress	

AD, Autosomal dominant; AR, autosomal recessive; AT-III, antithrombin III; ELT, euglobulin lysis time; HCF-II, heparin cofactor II; tPA, tissue plasminogen activator.

should be confirmed by specific fibrinogen testing. A prolonged euglobulin clot lysis time is suggestive of a dysfibrinolysis. Specific assays for plasminogen, tissue plasminogen activator (t-PA), and t-PA inhibitor will be needed. If both TT and euglobulin clot lysis times are normal, the patient should be checked with specific tests for antithrombin III, protein C, and protein S and also be assessed for factor V Leiden mutation.

Resistance to Activated Protein C. The most common inherited procoagulant disorder is resistance to activated protein C. This disorder was first recognized in 1993 and comprises up to 45% of patients with venous thromboembolic events. Activated factor V is normally degraded by protein C. Patients with a mutated factor V (factor V Leiden) are resistant to protein C. The mutation is found in up to 7% of the Swedish population and is passed on in an autosomal dominant fashion. The disorder may also occur in an acquired fashion during a stressful event such as trauma or surgery.

Prothrombin Gene Polymorphism. The prothrombin gene polymorphism 20210A is the second most common congenital defect that is associated with an increased risk of thromboembolism. This mutation causes an increase in plasma concentrations of prothrombin, the precursor of thrombin. The disorder is most common in Mediterranean populations (4% to 5%) and is rare in nonwhite groups.

Protein C deficiency may be familial and is inherited by an autosomal dominant heterozygous condition with incomplete penetrance and variable expressivity or an autosomal homozygous recessive form seen in infants with skin lesions suggestive of purpura fulminans as a result of microvascular thrombosis. These cases must be treated early with sodium warfarin (Coumadin). An acquired

protein C deficiency may also occur in liver disease, malignancy, infections, and postoperative states.

Another thrombotic disorder is antithrombin III deficiency. This is one of the more common deficiencies, being found in 0.01% to 0.05% of the general population. Protein S deficiency may similarly prevent normal clot inactivation. Each of these deficiencies may comprise 4% to 5% of unexplained thrombosis in a young patient.

Thrombotic tendencies may also occur from disorders of the fibrinolytic system. The function of the fibrinolytic system is to lyse clots (fibrin) by the action of the terminal enzyme plasmin. Fibrinolytic activity is mediated by plasminogen after its activation to plasmin. Plasmin degrades factors V and VIII as well as fibrinogen. These well-regulated reactions limit the extent of fibrin formation and maintain vessel patency. Patients with a dysfibrinolysis have an inherited deficiency in plasminogen, defective release of t-PA, or abnormally high levels of t-PA inhibitors. All of these result in a deficiency in the ability to lyse fibrin.

Dysfibrinogenemias now comprise more than 100 separate qualitative abnormalities, most of which are inherited in an autosomal dominant fashion. The most common dysfibrinogenemia is caused by an abnormal fibrin monomer polymerization combined with resistance to fibrinolysis. This appears to be associated with a decreased ability of plasminogen binding.

Treatment of most of these disorders should consist of heparin anticoagulation (low doses for prophylaxis or moderate doses for an actual thrombotic event). This should be followed by long-term therapy with warfarin. If anticoagulation is contraindicated in patients with an antithrombin III deficiency, then antithrombin concentrate should be used. Fresh-frozen plasma may be used in such cases with protein C or S deficiencies. Females should be counseled against the use of oral contraceptives.

SPECIFIC DISORDERS OF HEMOSTASIS

Hemorrhagic Disease of the Newborn

Since the routine administration of prophylactic vitamin K to almost all newborn infants at birth, hemorrhagic disease of the newborn (HDNB) is rarely encountered. HDNB is defined as any bleeding problem related to vitamin K deficiency and decreased activity of factors II, VII, IX, and X. Vitamin K–dependent clotting proteins are synthesized in the liver but are biologically inert until activated by vitamin K. Vitamin K is obtained from the diet and intestinal bacterial synthesis. Both may be limited in the first few days of life. As maternally derived stores of vitamin K rapidly disappear, bleeding may occur after the first day of life (second to seventh day). The platelet count is normal, but the PT and PTT are abnormally elevated. Because breast milk is a poor source of vitamin K, breast-fed infants who do not receive vitamin K are at greatest risk. Administration of 1.0 mg of aqueous vitamin K intravenously will usually return the PT and PTT toward normal and resolve bleeding in 4 to 6 hours.

If clinical bleeding and coagulation tests do not improve, liver disease or a specific coagulation factor deficiency must be suspected. Early hemorrhagic disease that occurs in the first 24 hours of life may be observed in infants of mothers with seizure disorders taking phenytoin or phenobarbital. Late hemorrhagic disease occurring in older infants between 1 and 3 months of age is manifested by central nervous system bleeding or extensive ecchymoses and is attributed to poor intestinal absorption of vitamin K. This poor absorption may be related to cystic fibrosis, biliary atresia, celiac disease, prolonged use of total parenteral nutrition, and chronic diarrhea with malabsorption. Prolonged diarrhea for longer than 1 week in breast-fed infants may also be a predisposing factor.

Clotting Factor Deficiencies

Hemophilia A and B

Clinical manifestations of these two hemophilia conditions are similar enough that they are covered together (Table 9-5). Classic hemophilia A or factor VIII deficiency is the most common hereditary coagulation disorder and occurs in 1 in 5000 males. Factor VIII circulates in the plasma as a complex of two separate peptides: factor VIII coagulant protein and vWF. The function of factor VIII is to facilitate the generation of fibrin. The vWF has two functions: (1) to act as a carrier to transport factor VIII and (2) to act as a bridge and facilitate platelet adhesion to injured endothelium. Classic hemophilia is a sex-linked disorder with the gene carried on the X chromosome. It affects only male children and is characterized by decreased levels of factor VIII coagulant activity and normal amounts of the carrier protein (vWF).

Factor IX deficiency or hemophilia B (also known as Christmas factor) is clinically indistinguishable from hemophilia A and accounts for 15% of all cases of hemophilia (1 in 25,000 males). This is also a sex-linked disorder that occurs only in males, and a positive family history is noted in 65% of cases.

Other than the type of factor replacement, the clinical course of the two processes are similar. Bleeding caused by hemophilia in neonates is usually limited to a cephalohematoma or bleeding from the gastrointestinal tract or the umbilical cord or after a circumcision and is rarely severe. In older children bleeding varies according to the severity of the disease (e.g., mild, moderate, or severe) from mild soft tissue bleeding and frequent joint hemorrhages to severe life-threatening central nervous system hemorrhage. Mild cases have more than 10% factor VIII or IX activity and have few spontaneous hemorrhages but are at risk after trauma or surgery. Moderate cases have 2% to 10% factor activity. Severe cases have less than 2% factor VIII or IX activity with frequent, and often severe, spontaneous hemorrhages two to four times per month. This variation suggests that there may be a wide range of factor VIII gene mutations. Gene mutations may also

TABLE 9-5 ■ Hereditary Hemorrhagic Disorders Caused by Coagulation Factor Deficiencies

Disorder	Population Frequency	Genetics	Bleeding Tendency	
			Heterozygote	Homozygote
Factor XI	Variable	AR	None to mild	Mild to moderate
Factor IX	$10–20/10^6$	X-linked recessive	Mild in carrier	Mild to severe in hemizygote
Factor VIII	$60–100/10^6$	X-linked recessive	Mild in carrier	Mild to severe in hemizygote
Factor X	$0.5/10^6$	AR	None	Moderate
Factor V	$0.5/10^6$	AR	None	Moderate
Factor II	$0.5/10^6$	AR	None	Moderate
Factor VII	$0.5/10^6$	AR	None	Moderate
Dysfibrinogenemia	$1.0/10^6$	AD	Variable	Variable (some with thrombotic tendency)
Factor XIII	$0.5/10^6$	AR	None	Severe
α_2-Antiplasmin	Rare	AR	None to mild	Severe
von Willebrand	Variable	AD/AR	Mild to moderate	Severe

AR, Autosomal recessive; AD, autosomal dominant.

explain the occurrence of cases of sporadic hemophilia without a family history. Some of the carrier females have significantly reduced coagulation factors and may behave like mild cases.

The diagnosis is suspected in boys with bruising or bleeding and an abnormal PTT but normal PT and platelet count. The definitive diagnosis is made by obtaining specific factor levels.

Treatment has undergone tremendous advances in the past 10 years. Patients treated with older factors VIII or IX had a very high risk of developing hepatitis B, C, or D as well as infection with human immunodeficiency virus. Of hemophiliacs receiving plasma-derived factor between 1979 and 1984, 90% developed acquired immunodeficiency syndrome. An additional problem that is associated with usage of the factor is the development of factor VIII inhibitors (circulating antibodies usually in the immunoglobulin class that neutralize factor VIII coagulant activity). The development of recombinant technology has resulted in the preparation of factor VIII from recombinant DNA and obviates reliance on pooled plasma as a source, excludes viral transmission, and reduces, but does not eliminate, the risk of inhibitor antibodies. Such inhibitors may occur in 15% of hemophilia A and 1% of hemophilia B patients.

Treatment utilizes desmopressin acetate for very minor hemorrhages. Desmopressin will triple or even quadruple the initial factor VIII level for hemophilia A but has no effect on factor IX levels. Caution should be exercised with its use in that desmopressin has an antidiuretic effect, and fluids and electrolytes should be monitored. Aminocaproic acid (Amicar) may be used for oral bleeding, such as for dental procedures. For more serious bleeding or major surgery, recombinant factor VIII concentrate will be needed. Recombinant purified factor VIII and IX concentrates are the agents of choice. For active bleeding or preparation for a major surgical procedure, the factor level is brought up to 100%. Minor surgery or minor trauma will require factor levels between 30% to 50%. After an initial loading over the first 24 hours, lower levels may be set. Plasma factor levels should be determined 10 minutes after the administration of the factor. The following formulas can be used in calculating required dosages for infusion:

Factor VIII units required =
% factor VIII activity desired × weight (kg) × 0.5

- Each unit of recombinant factor VIII infused per kilogram of body weight will yield a 2% increase in plasma factor VIII level. The half-life of factor VIII is approximately 12 hours, and therefore infusion is required every 12 hours.

Factor IX units required =
% factor IX activity desired × weight (kg) × 1.2

- Each unit of recombinant factor IX infused per kilogram of body weight will yield a 0.8% increase in plasma factor IX level. Because factor IX has a longer half-life, infusions are required every 24 hours.

Current practice includes intrauterine detection of a male infant in a pregnant carrier female at risk at 13 to 16 weeks of gestation by amniocentesis and prenatal diagnosis of hemophilia A by chorionic villus sampling or fibroblast DNA sampling at amniocentesis.

Although hereditary deficiencies of practically all clotting factors have been described, these are extremely rare and beyond the scope of this discussion.

Von Willebrand disease (vWD) is an autosomal dominant disorder related to a deficiency in von Willebrand factor (vWF), which also results in decreased factor VIII levels. The vWF gene is located on the short arm of chromosome 12 and is a large multimeric plasma glycoprotein. Fifteen percent of vWF is produced in megakaryocytes and contained in platelet alpha granules, whereas 85% is secreted into the plasma from its major site of production in the endothelial cell. vWD is the most common inherited bleeding disorder in humans, being present in approximately 1% of the general population. More than 20 distinct clinical and laboratory subtypes have been identified. Type I is the most common quantitative deficiency (80% of cases) and presumed to be the result of heterozygous inheritance of one normal and one deficient allele. This results in a mild bleeding diathesis caused by decreased amounts of structurally normal vWF. Type II is probably a mutation with decreased amounts of abnormally structured vWF, and type III is a relatively rare autosomal recessive homozygous form of type I with barely detectable levels of vWF. This is a more severe form of the disease than the others, behaving more like a moderate form of hemophilia. The vWF has two major functions: (1) it serves as a carrier for factor VIII and circulates as a tightly associated complex and stabilizes its activity and (2) it also plays a crucial role in mediating platelet adhesion to injured subendothelium, acting as a bridge between platelet glycoprotein Ib and glycoprotein IIb/IIIa and subendothelial elements such as collagen, to which it binds, and heparin.

The diagnosis of vWD is achieved by demonstrating a normal platelet count and PT, prolonged bleeding time and PTT, and direct measurements of vWF and factor VIII, which are both significantly decreased to 15% to 40% of normal levels. It is difficult to evaluate the bleeding time in newborns, and therefore testing for vWD should be deferred until infants are at least 1 month of age. Additionally, a functional assessment may be made by the ristocetin cofactor assay, which uses the antibiotic ristocetin to induce vWF to bind to platelets.

Highly purified factor VIII concentrates that have been specially processed to remove any potential viral transmission (e.g., Humate P) contain vWF and will correct the factor VIII deficiency and treat the bleeding tendency. Desmopressin, 0.3 μgm/kg, intravenously causes release of factor VIII and vWF from endothelial stores and may be useful in the treatment of bleeding in type I vWD. Desmopressin is ideal for minor or moderate surgical procedures. It is not useful in type III vWD and is contraindicated in type IIb vWD and pseudo-vWD. Pseudo-vWD refers to a platelet type of vWD caused by an increased binding of the vWF to the platelet membrane, thus decreasing the plasma concentration of vWF.

As noted earlier, desmopressin also has no efficacy in children with hemophilia B.

Disseminated Intravascular Coagulation

Disseminated intravascular coagulation is associated with a variety of conditions in neonates, including sepsis, shock, acidosis, hypoxia, hypothermia, and maternal abruptio placentae and placenta previa. The underlying factors include a physiologic or structural change in endothelial cell function, resulting in activation of both coagulation and fibrinolysis. Platelets and factors II, V, VII, and fibrinogen are consumed when fibrin is formed. The stimulation of fibrinolysis generates the release of FSPs, which inhibit the normal conversion of fibrinogen to fibrin. DIC occurs in sick infants (more commonly in premature infants) and is characterized by diffuse bleeding in the form of petechiae, oozing from puncture sites, and gastrointestinal hemorrhage. DIC is not an uncommon presentation in neonates suffering from necrotizing enterocolitis with perforation or necrotic bowel. In rare cases there is diffuse thrombosis and skin necrosis. The laboratory findings include a decreased platelet count and prolonged PT and PTT. Factors V and VIII and fibrinogen are decreased and FSPs and D-dimers are increased. The treatment requires vigorous treatment of the underlying cause of DIC, correction of acidosis, hypoxia, and so on, and administration of antibiotics in septic patients. Fresh-frozen plasma and platelet transfusion may be required. If serious bleeding continues, an exchange transfusion may be necessary. In cases with thrombosis, intravenous heparin is administered followed by fresh-frozen plasma and platelets.

SUGGESTED READINGS

Bilgin K, Yaramis A, Haspolat K, et al: A randomized trial of granulocyte-macrophage colony-stimulating factor in neonates with sepsis and neutropenia. Pediatrics 85:446-455, 2001.

This paper describes the successful use of GCSF to stimulate neutrophil function in patients who are septic and/or immunosuppressed.

Glader BE, Amylon MD: Hemostatic disorders in the newborn. In Taeusch HW, Ballard RA, Avery ME (eds): Diseases of the Newborn, 6th ed. Philadelphia, WB Saunders, 1991.

This textbook chapter clearly describes the recognition and management of hemostatic disorders in newborns.

Hathaway WE: New insights on vitamin K. Hematol Oncol Clin North Am 1:367, 1987.

This excellent review concerning vitamin K in infancy describes the problems associated with this vitamin deficiency in regard to hemorrhagic diseases of the newborn and other coagulation-dependent factors.

Manco-Johnson MJ, Abshire TC, Jacobson LJ, et al: Severe neonatal protein C deficiency: Prevalence and thrombotic risk. J Pediatr 119:793, 1991.

This article clarifies the clinical presentation, risks, and management of infants with protein C deficiency.

Manno CS: Difficult pediatric diagnosis: Bruising and bleeding. Pediatr Clin North Am 38:637, 1991.

This clinically relevant review of normal hemostasis and hematologic disorders in infants and children is worthwhile reading.

Martlew VJ: Peri-operative management of patients with coagulation disorders. Br J Anesth 85:446-455, 2000.

An excellent review of how to manage patients with coagulation disorders who require operation.

Smith WZ: Major surgery without blood transfusion. Curr Anesthesiol Crit Care 11:42-50, 2000.

This paper describes how to avoid intraoperative transfusion by a variety of methods and alternatives even with major surgery.

Taylor RW, Manganaro L, O'Brien J, et al: Impact of allogenic packed red blood cell transfusion on nosocomial infection rates in the critically ill patient. Crit Care Med 30:2249-2254, 2002.

The immunosuppressive risk of blood transfusion is discussed in depth in this authoritative article.

Zoubek A, Krongerger M: Early epoetin alfa treatment in children with solid tumors. Med Pediatr Oncol 39:459-462, 2002.

These authors describe anticipatory treatment of anemia in immunosuppressed children with malignancy.

Special Considerations in Pediatric Anesthesia

PREANESTHETIC PREPARATION

Lack of understanding, inability to rationalize, separation anxiety, transference of stress from the parents, fear of strangers, and pain make preanesthetic planning unique in young children. Thus, preoperative education of parents and children along with selective administration of preanesthetic sedation can improve the operative experience.

Preanesthetic Sedation

Sedatives allay anxiety, facilitate induction of anesthesia, and reduce the amount of anesthetic agents required. However, some premedicants expose the patient to potential adverse drug complications and can delay recovery from anesthesia. Most anesthesiologists believe that children younger than 1 year of age do not need preoperative sedation. In general, healthy children 1 to 5 years of age require sedative premedication when separating from their parents. Although preoperative sedatives may be of benefit in healthy children older than 3 years of age, many will not require such medications if they are optimally managed psychologically. Interestingly, behavior of unsedated children who are optimally managed psychologically compares favorably with those of premedicated children. As such, the anesthesiology and surgical teams should direct their effort to ensuring optimum psychologic preparation of the patient and to providing a suitable preoperative environment that will reduce fear and anxiety. Preoperative visits by the anesthesiologist; parental education; and tours, videos, and books are helpful in familiarizing children and their parents with the hospital, operating room, and various procedures. Large playrooms with ample toys may allay anxiety. The perioperative process should involve minimum parental separation. Anesthesiologists also can reduce preoperative anxiety by carefully tailoring the mode of induction of anesthesia.

Despite these efforts at reducing fear and providing a comfortable environment, some children will remain anxious. In such cases, oral midazolam, 0.5 mg/kg, in a cherry syrup to hide the bitter taste of the oral drug, may be administered to induce sedation and anxiolysis. A fentanyl lollipop (5-15 µg/kg) may be used, although nausea and vomiting may be a problem. As an alternative, midazolam (0.2-0.3 mg/kg) may be administered nasally. Injections should be avoided because of the pain and fear associated with needles, although ketamine is frequently used intramuscularly in patients who have behavior problems, who are agitated, or who have congenital heart disease. Children with mental retardation tend to be difficult to manage during induction of anesthesia and may benefit from a sedative premedication. Sedatives should not be given to patients who have airway or ventilation problems or those with central nervous system disorders. In patients with congenital heart disease, sedation can influence pulmonary systemic vascular resistance and cardiac output. In most patients with congenital heart disease, premedication with narcotics will improve oxygen saturation. However, patients with congenital heart disease who receive sedation should be carefully monitored after premedication. Table 10-1 lists some of the commonly used preanesthetic sedative agents and their characteristics.

Anticholinergic Drugs

Anticholinergic agents abolish vagal reflexes caused by anesthetic agents and other stimuli and block excess secretions. Infants and children require anticholinergic drugs before surgery because the parasympathetic system dominates the autonomic nervous system, especially until the sympathetic system matures at approximately 6 months of age. Neonatal cardiac output is principally determined by heart rate, and stimuli that induce a vagal response will cause bradycardia and a decrease in cardiac output. In addition, anticholinergic agents should be administered before succinylcholine because this muscle relaxant is associated with bradycardia in infants and children.

Most anesthesiologists choose atropine as the drug of choice because of its effectiveness in blocking cholinergic effects on the pediatric heart. The typical dose is 0.02 mg/kg, with minimum dose of 0.1 mg to avoid potential paradoxical bradycardia. It is usually given intravenously during induction of anesthesia to avoid the discomfort of an intramuscular injection and to allow the drug to be most effective when anesthetic and muscle-relaxing agents are being administered and vagal stimulation is prominent. Glycopyrrolate (Robinul) is also popular because it causes less tachycardia and has fewer central nervous system effects than atropine. Among the procedures occurring during induction and surgery that cause intense vagal stimulation are laryngoscopy, intubation, and manipulation of abdominal viscera and eye muscles.

TABLE 10-1 ■ Medications Used for Preinduction Sedation before General Anesthesia and for Conscious Sedation for Diagnostic Studies and Minor Procedures

Drug	Type	Dose and Route	Adverse Effects	Comment
Morphine	Narcotic Analgesic	0.05 mg/kg IV	Respiratory depression Postoperative vomiting Hypotension	Used commonly for congenital heart disease Clearance prolonged in neonates
Fentanyl	Narcotic Analgesic	1 µg/kg IV 5-15 µg/kg PO	Chest wall rigidity Bradycardia Nausea/vomiting	Fast onset, short half-life Few hemodynamic changes Incorporated into a lollipop for PO use (Oralet)
Pentobarbital	Sedative	2-6 mg/kg PO 2-6 mg/kg rectally	Slowly metabolized in infancy	Does not provide analgesia Not to be used in age < 1 year
Midazolam (Versed)	Neuroleptic	0.05-1.0 mg/kg IV 0.2-0.3 mg/kg IN 0.5 mg/kg PO	Decrease blood pressure	Fast onset, short-acting Anxiolytic Amnestic Allows smooth induction Bitter taste
Ketamine	Anesthetic	6 mg/kg PO 4-6 mg/kg IM 0.5-2 µg/kg IV	Emergence reactions with hallucinations, delirium following anesthetic doses	Rapid onset (<5 minutes) Analgesic and amnestic Effective in patients with cyanotic heart disease Induction of dissociative anesthesia at doses of 6-10 mg/kg IM
Chloral hydrate	Hypnotic Neuroleptic	50-75 mg/kg PO	Bitter taste Nausea and vomiting	Minimal respiratory depression

PO, orally; IM, intramuscular; IV, intravenous; IN, intranasal.

Table 10-2 lists the common anticholinergics and their characteristics.

GENERAL ANESTHESIA

Induction of Anesthesia

Making the child comfortable and reducing fear during induction of anesthesia is paramount. Presence of a parent tends to reduce patient stress and anxiety. Monitoring should be kept to a minimum to avoid instilling anxiety in the child. Electrocardiographic leads and pulse oximetry can usually be placed without disturbing the patient. Induction of anesthesia can be accomplished primarily by administration of intravenous agents or inhalational anesthetic agents given by mask.

Mask Induction

The most common induction technique is accomplished by exposing the patient to an inhalational anesthetic with a mask. No needles are necessary, and the intravenous

TABLE 10-2 ■ Anticholinergic Agents Used for Premedication

Drug	Dose and Route	Adverse Effects	Major Action	Comment
Atropine	0.02 mg/kg IV/IM (minimum 0.1 mg/kg)	Congenital heart disease may reduce cardiac output due to tachycardia Reduces mucociliary action Affects temperature regulation, sweating Relaxes esophageal sphincter and may increase gastroesophageal reflux Produces erythematous rash as a result of histamine release	Vagolytic, highly effective	Rapid onset, short period of effectiveness (<1 hour) Because of drying secretions and effects on mucociliary action not used with cystic fibrosis Affects temperature regulation; not used with fever
Glycopyrrolate (Robinul)	0.01 mg/kg IV		Minimal central nervous system effect Effective at drying secretions	Does not cross blood-brain barrier Produces less tachycardia than atropine Decreases gastric acid

IV, intravenous; IM, intramuscular; PO, orally.

line can be placed after the child is asleep. Because children are frightened by a mask over their face, rapport must be established. A clear plastic mask lessens anxiety. A number of preparations are available to coat the mask and hide the smell of the anesthetic agents. These preparations include fruit and bubble gum flavors. Anesthesia can be induced in children while they are sitting on the anesthesiologist's lap or lying on the litter before being moved to the operating table. Many anesthesiologists prefer to blow anesthetic agent across the patient's nose and mouth using the hose rather than the mask. The usual anesthetic agent for induction is sevoflurane with oxygen because airway irritation is lessened and uptake of the drug and emergence from anesthesia are both faster with sevoflurane when compared with inhalational agents (Table 10-3). As anesthesia is induced patients may pass through an excitement stage in which they will become transiently combative. Once induction has been accomplished, usually signified by the child no longer having a reaction to voice command and having absence of eyelid reflex, an intravenous (IV) line is inserted and necessary drugs are administered. The airway is then controlled, as outlined in Chapter 31.

Intravenous Induction

Intravenous induction has the decided advantage that it is rapid, does not require use of a mask, lessens the risk of an excitement phase, and decreases the risk of laryngospasm. IV induction is especially applicable to older patients and those of all ages with IV access already established. If an IV line is not in place, mask induction is preferred to avoid the pain of the needlestick and the difficulty of obtaining venous access in an awake, moving patient. The pain of a needlestick may be reduced by applying a mixture of lidocaine 2.5% and prilocaine 2.5% (EMLA cream) to the dorsum of the hand at least 60 minutes before placement of the IV line. ELA-MAX, which consists of 4% liposomal lidocaine, needs to be placed only 15 to 30 minutes before the procedure. Whenever intravenous induction is used, children must be preoxygenated to avoid hypoxia. Propofol is the most commonly used intravenous drug for induction. It is rapid acting, taking as little as 60 seconds for induction (see Table 10-3). The agent has a short effect, lasting only 8 minutes, and the cardiovascular effects are minimal. Ketamine has also been used for intravenous induction in high-risk cardiovascular patients. Thiopental may be used in those with increased intracranial pressure.

Cardiac Anesthesia

Patients with congenital heart disease of hemodynamic instability present unique problems because of the vasoactive and negative inotropic effects of many narcotics and volatile agents. Anesthetic inductions in children with congenital heart disease are dependent on specific cardiac defects and the presence or absence of an IV line. Typically, induction will be performed with sevoflurane, IV or IM ketamine, and barbiturates; or high-dose fentanyl (15-25 µg/kg). Administration of pressor agents before induction should be considered.

Problems during Induction of Anesthesia

Induction can be one of the most dangerous periods during the course of the patient's stay in the operating room. Among the most significant problems are loss of airway, laryngospasm, and regurgitation from a full stomach.

Loss of Airway

During induction, as children relax, the tongue muscles become lax and the tongue may fall into the retrolingual area, causing airway obstruction. This can usually be alleviated by pulling the child's mandible forward (so-called chin lift). Airway obstruction can usually be avoided by allowing infants to lie in a neutral position; the "sniffing position" is best for children. Control can also be achieved by inserting an oral or nasal airway.

The Difficult Airway

Difficult airway access can be predicted in children with the Pierre Robin syndrome and other congenital abnormalities. Other children with difficult airway access can be identified by history or Mallampatti score. With proper forethought and care, a smooth induction and good outcome is to be expected. Awake intubations, while preferred in such patients, are not tolerated by infants and children outside the newborn period. The best approach, therefore, is to perform intubation while the patient is spontaneously breathing under sevoflurane anesthesia. If muscle relaxants are used during manipulation to achieve airway access, the short-acting agent succinylcholine is best. The approach to the difficult airway is discussed further in Chapter 31.

Laryngospasm

Laryngospasm is usually initiated by laryngoscopy or insertion of an endotracheal tube or bronchoscope or by the presence of secretions on the vocal cords during light anesthesia. The patient becomes difficult to ventilate, and paradoxical movements of the chest may be observed in the spontaneously breathing patient. A mask can be placed tightly over the face and positive-pressure ventilation with 100% oxygen administered with application of positive end-expiratory pressure even up to 20 cm H_2O. Succinylcholine easily breaks laryngospasm.

Regurgitation

When agitated, as many as 50% of infants and children may regurgitate during anesthesia. The infant stomach is large, and infants have relatively high intra-abdominal pressure. Many anesthetics and muscle relaxants cause relaxation of the gastroesophageal sphincter. Fear, anxiety, and trauma delay gastric emptying for many hours. A slight head-up position reduces the incidence of regurgitation. The anesthesiologist should avoid pressure on the abdomen and be alert to gastric distention caused by the face mask. A tube should be passed into the stomach only if gastric distention is noted because stimulation by a nasogastric tube may cause vomiting. Suction should always be available.

TABLE 10-3 ■ Inhalational and Intravenous Agents Used to Induce and Maintain Anesthesia

Drug	Advantages	Disadvantages	Use
Nitrous oxide	Pleasant odor Rapid uptake and distribution Hypnotic and analgesic Minimal respiratory depression	Decreases blood pressure Decreases heart rate Nitrous oxide in blood decreases O_2 affinity for hemoglobin Nausea and vomiting Nitrous oxide diffuses into air-containing space faster than original gases leave, resulting in problems in pneumothorax, bowel obstruction, diaphragmatic hernia, internal ear operations	Widely used to supplement other inhaled or IV agents
Isoflurane	Rapid induction Rapid and smooth emergence Does not affect cardiac output No sensitivity to epinephrine No seizures Bronchodilation Arrhythmias are rare Little effect on intracranial pressure Inexpensive No hepatotoxicity	Unpleasant odor Cough and laryngospasm on induction Depresses ventilation and requires controlled ventilation Hypotension due to vasodilation Potentiates D-tubocurarine and pancuronium Can cause bradycardia in infants unless premedicated	Almost never used for induction because of odor Good for maintenance because inexpensive and less effect on heart rate and cardiac output; easy to control depth of anesthesia
Sevoflurane	Sweet smell Rapid induction and emergence Mild effect on blood pressure, heart rate, or cardiac output No sensitivity to epinephrine Arrhythmias are rare Little effect on intracranial pressure No hepatotoxicity Minimal airway reactivity	Decreases ventilation; requires ventilatory support Expensive	Good for induction
Propofol	Rapid onset and short half-life	Painful on injection Does not provide complete anesthesia; must be supplemented by another agent Long-term infusion may be associated with metabolic acidosis	IV induction of anesthesia 2.5-3.0 mg/kg Maintenance 50-200 µg/kg/min
Thiopental	Rapid onset and short duration Few hemodynamic effects	Bronchoconstriction	IV induction of anesthesia 6-7 mg/kg
Ketamine	Sympathomimetic agent Bronchodilation	Emergence reactions Increased secretions	IV induction in congenital heart disease, reactive airway disease
Fentanyl	Narcotic		IV induction of anesthesia 15-25 µg/kg
Sufentanil	Narcotic		IV induction of anesthesia 10-20 µg/kg

Full Stomach

In patients with a full stomach the operation should be delayed or a local or regional block substituted for the general anesthetic if possible. It is impossible to completely empty the stomach with a nasogastric tube. In patients who are considered to have contents in the stomach or who have other problems that might result in

a full stomach, such as bowel obstruction, delayed gastric emptying, ileus, or increased intra-abdominal pressure, rapid-sequence induction is indicated. This type of induction begins with breathing 100% oxygen for several minutes. A tonsil suction should be ready. In those patients with pyloric stenosis, the stomach should be emptied by a wide-bore catheter. During induction of anesthesia, cricoid pressure should be applied (the Sellick maneuver). Cricoid pressure obliterates the esophageal lumen and prevents vomitus from reaching the airway. The patient then undergoes rapid-sequence induction using a sedating agent and a paralyzing agent, with endotracheal intubation performed once muscle relaxation has been achieved. Ventilation is initiated and cricoid pressure discontinued once access to the airway has been ensured. Rapid-sequence induction is discussed in depth in Chapter 31.

Special Situations

The patient with a critical airway caused by tracheal stenosis or the presence of a foreign body should undergo induction of anesthesia with a volatile agent while maintaining spontaneous respirations until the airway is secured and the foreign body removed. Patients with anterior mediastinal masses present unique problems: cardiogenic shock with cardiac arrest may occur during induction despite adequate airway control. This phenomenon appears to be related to cardiac obstruction by the mass or the effects of the mass on venous blood return to the heart, which may be induced by chest wall relaxation, especially with use of muscle-relaxing agents. Those patients with compromise of more than 50% of the tracheal lumen are especially at risk. One should attempt to avoid general anesthesia but should have the availability of extracorporeal life support (ECLS/ECMO) or cardiac bypass if general anesthesia is required.

MAINTENANCE OF GENERAL ANESTHESIA

Inhalation and Intravenous Anesthetics

Once anesthesia is induced and the patient intubated, the anesthesiologist must maintain anesthesia and analgesia for the patient and satisfactory working conditions for the surgeon. Anesthetic and adjuvant drugs must be chosen to ensure analgesia, unconsciousness, and muscle relaxation. Alveolar ventilation, tissue oxygenation, and cardiopulmonary and nervous system stability must be maintained. Pediatric anesthesiologists commonly use muscle relaxants and inhalation anesthetics supplemented by intravenous narcotics, otherwise known as balanced anesthesia, rather than using a single volatile agent to produce deep surgical anesthesia. Balanced anesthesia allows use of narcotics, muscle relaxants, and volatile agents to maximize the safety of each of these agents while providing the most stable form of anesthesia. Table 10-3 lists the characteristics of commonly used inhalational and intravenous anesthetic agents.

Muscle Relaxants

Muscle-relaxing medications consist of those that are depolarizing agents, such as succinylcholine, and nondepolarizing agents, such as pancuronium and rocuronium. Depolarizing agents act at the neuromuscular junction to depolarize the muscle; they also do not allow the muscle to repolarize. Thus, disorganized fasciculations are observed as all the muscles are activated. In contrast, nondepolarizing agents compete with acetylcholine at the neuromuscular junction to prevent muscle activation. The short-acting depolarizing agent succinylcholine and the intermediate nondepolarizing agents atracurium and vecuronium are commonly used during pediatric anesthesia. The duration of the effect of atracurium and vecuronium is 20 to 30 minutes. Long-acting agents include pancuronium and rocuronium. The characteristics of muscle relaxants are listed in Table 10-4.

The paralysis caused by nondepolarizing relaxants should be reversed at the end of each operation unless postoperative mechanical ventilation is planned. To reduce the likelihood of prolonged muscular paralysis, the degree of neuromuscular blockade should be monitored with a nerve stimulator during the course of the operation, and the patient should be given only enough of the selected agent to achieve the desired degree of block, typically no or one twitch out of a train-of-four response during nerve stimulation. To reverse paralysis, a fast-acting parasympathetic blocking agent such as atropine with a dose of 0.02 mg/kg is administered just before the rapid-onset acetylcholinesterase inhibitor edrophonium (Tensilon) at 0.5 to 1.0 mg/kg. Alternatively, the slower-onset glycopyrrolate (Robinul) at a dose of 0.01 mg/kg can be given before the antiacetylcholinesterase drug neostigmine (Prostigmin) at a dose of 25 to 80 µg/kg. The parasympathetic blocking agent is administered just before the acetylcholinesterase inhibitor to prevent undesired parasympathetic effects while allowing an increase in acetylcholine activity at the neuromuscular junction. The effectiveness of reversal is judged by muscle strength, adequacy of ventilation, and response to nerve stimulation. Minimum criteria for withdrawing assisted ventilation should be good muscle tone, flexing of the arms and legs, and adequate respiratory efforts. Absence of tetanic fade on nerve stimulation is one indication of adequacy of reversal. Many premature infants require mechanical ventilation after the use of muscle relaxants.

REGIONAL ANESTHESIA

In recent years there has been a resurgence of interest in regional anesthetic techniques in children. The factors fueling this renewal of interest are (1) the effective postoperative pain relief without sedation that is associated with regional anesthesia, (2) the fact that regional anesthetics may provide analgesia yet avoid the risk of the postoperative respiratory dysfuction associated with general anesthetics and muscle relaxants, and (3) the ability of regional techniques to reduce the requirement for other anesthetic agents. The disadvantages of using a regional anesthetic in children are (1) the special training and skills required and (2) when used independently the patient remembers the operative procedure and is aware of noises and activities in the operating room. Table 10-5 lists the dosages and some of the characteristics of commonly used local anesthetics. Neonates are more susceptible to toxicity from local anesthetics because with these agents the half-life is increased in the first 6 months of life. Thereafter, children eliminate local anesthetic drugs at the same rate as adults. Body weight is the safest and simplest basis to determine the maximum recommended dose.

TABLE 10-4 ■ Muscle Relaxing Agents

Agent	Type	Dose	Metabolism, Recovery Time	Side Effects	Comment
Succinylcholine	Depolarizing, short acting	Intubation: < 1 yr of age: 2 mg/kg IV >1 yr of age: 1 mg/kg IV	Plasma pseudo-cholinesterase (90%), 3-10 minutes	Muscle injury Higher doses required in infants Bradycardia Increases intraocular pressure Masseter spasm Trigger for malignant hyperthermia Increases serum myoglobulin phosphokinase and potassium	Only depolarizing agent commonly used Not reversed by neostigmine Should not use with liver disease If abnormal pseudocholinesterase, prolonged effect Not used on trauma and burn patients because of risk of hyperkalemia Cardiac arrest with Duchenne muscular dystrophy due to muscle contraction
Atracurium	Nondepolarizing, intermediate acting	0.5 mg/kg IV	Ester hydrolysis and Hofmann degradation, 20-30 minutes	Longer recovery in neonates with low body temperature	Neonates <48 hr require less drug for paralysis No circulatory effects
Vecuronium	Nondepolarizing, intermediate acting	0.1 mg/kg IV	Renal and hepatic, 9-20 minutes		Short acting No circulatory effects ten times more potent than pancuronium Safe for infants susceptible to malignant hyperthermia Potentiated by inhalational anesthetics
Pancuronium	Nondepolarizing, long acting	0.1 mg/kg IV	Renal and hepatic, 55 minutes	Tachycardia (vagolysis) Hypertension in premature newborns	
Recuronium	Nondepolarizing, long acting	0.6-1.2 mg/kg	Hepatic, 60-70 minutes	Mild increase in heart rate Mild decrease in blood pressure	Rapid onset (≈60 seconds)

IV, intravenous.

In most cases, local or regional techniques of anesthesia are combined with sedation and anesthetic agents to reduce patient anxiety and memory of the procedure. Monitored anesthesia care may be used in the operating room to provide light sedation in conjunction with local anesthetic administration at the operative site. The usual indications for performing procedures using solely local or regional anesthetics are (1) children with a family history of malignant hyperthermia (MH); (2) infants and children with neuromuscular disease with reduced respiratory reserve and weakened pharyngeal reflexes; (3) premature infants undergoing inguinal hernia repair who have a history of, or who are at risk for, apnea; (4) children or adolescents with chronic respiratory disease such as asthma or cystic fibrosis; and (5) cooperative children who must undergo emergency peripheral procedures after recent intake of food. Children who are uncooperative or who may be difficult to intubate because of anatomic abnormalities are poor candidates for a local or regional anesthetic approach.

Spinal Anesthesia

Spinal anesthesia is used occasionally for anesthesia in newborns in whom short pediatric surgical procedures less than 1.5 hours in duration are being performed in the inguinal region or lower extremities. The advantage of regional spinal over general anesthesia is the reduction in the risk of postoperative apnea associated with administration of general anesthetics in preterm newborns and infants younger than 51 weeks post conception and in full-term newborns and infants younger than 44 weeks post conception. The technique of spinal anesthesia in infants and children is similar to that of adults. The infant or child is placed in the sitting or lateral decubitus position. A 25- or 22-gauge spinal needle is introduced between the spinous processes in the midline until free flow of cerebrospinal fluid is noted (Fig. 10-1). In newborns the dural sac into which the anesthetic is to be placed ends at S3 (S1 in adults) whereas the spinal cord ends at L3 (L1 in adults). Thus, dural puncture for placement of the anesthetic should be no more cephalad

TABLE 10-5 ■ Local Anesthetics Used for Analgesia

Drug	Type	Maximum Dose	Neonatal Maximum Dose	Epidural Infusion < Age 3 Mo	Epidural Infusion > Age 3 Mo	Comment
Lidocaine	Amino Amide	4 mg/kg 5-7 mg/kg with epinephrine	5 mg/kg with epinephrine			Prolonged elimination in newborns Toxic dose: central nervous system and cardiovascular Hypersensitivity Can be used topically Combined with prolocaine to form EMLA
Bupivacaine (Marcaine)	Amino Amide	2.5 mg/kg	2 mg/kg	0.1-0.2 mL/kg/hr of bupivacaine 0.1% with fentanyl 0.5-2 µg/mL	0.3-0.4 mL/kg/hr of bupivacaine 0.1% with fentanyl 2 µg/mL	Used for caudal, epidural, and local anesthesia in infants and children Infants at greater risk for toxicity Toxicity = cardiac asystole Long duration of action Greater sensory than motor block Excellent for postoperative pain

than L3 and typically is performed in the L5-S1, L4-5, or L3-4 vertebral interspaces, where injury to the spinal cord is unlikely. Lidocaine, tetracaine, or bupivacaine may be instilled into the subarachnoid space with motor and sensory anesthesia induced below the T10 level. Lidocaine provides a short- to intermediate-acting spinal anesthetic (about 1 hour), whereas tetracaine and bupivacaine provide intermediate- to long-duration blocks (2 to 3 hours). Addition of epinephrine or phenylephrine to the local anesthetic may increase the duration of the block. Complications include back pain (5%), transient radicular

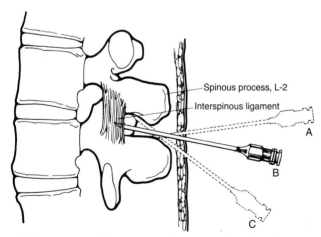

FIGURE 10-1 ■ Midline approach to the subarachnoid space. The spinal needle is inserted with a slight cephalad angulation and should advance in the midline without contacting bone (B). If bone is contacted, it may be either the caudad (A) or the cephalad spinous process (C). (Reprinted with permission from Bernards CM: Epidural and spinal anesthesia. In Clinical Anesthesia, 3rd ed. Philadelphia, Lippincott-Raven, 1997; and Mulroy MF: Regional Anesthesia: An Illustrated Procedural Guide. Boston, Little Brown, 1989.)

irritation (1.5%), and, most importantly, post–dural puncture headache in approximately 4% of children, which may require epidural injection of blood as a patch. Post-spinal anesthetic headache may be suggested in the infant or child who is irritable and cries while sitting up or standing but is more comfortable while lying down.

Caudal Blocks

Single-shot caudal epidural blocks are one of the most popular techniques for achieving perioperative analgesia in the T10 to S5 dermatome region. The block is relatively simple with a high rate of success. The sacral hiatus is first identified by the presence of the sacral cornua on either side of the hiatus (Fig. 10-2). These cornua represent the nonfusion of the S5 vertebal arch. The sacral hiatus extends from the sacrococcygeal junction up to the fused vertebral arch of S4 and is separated from the subcutaneous tissues by the sacrococcygeal membrane. The patient is placed in the lateral decubitus position. Once the sacral hiatus is identified, the index and middle finger of the palpating hand are placed on the sacral cornu and the caudal needle is inserted at an angle of approximately 45 degrees to the sacrum in between the two fingers. While advancing the needle, a decrease in resistance to needle insertion should be appreciated as the needle pierces the sacrococcygeal membrane and enters the caudal canal. The needle is then redirected so that the angle of insertion relative to the skin surface is decreased. The needle is then advanced 5 to 10 mm into the epidural space depending on the size of the child. Further advance is not attempted because dural puncture and unintentional intravascular cannulation become more likely. Once the needle is in appropriate position, a test dose of local anesthetic with 1:200,000 epinephrine is administered and the heart rate monitored to rule out intravascular injection. Bupivacaine 0.25% administered at a dose of 0.75 mL/kg is the most commonly used local

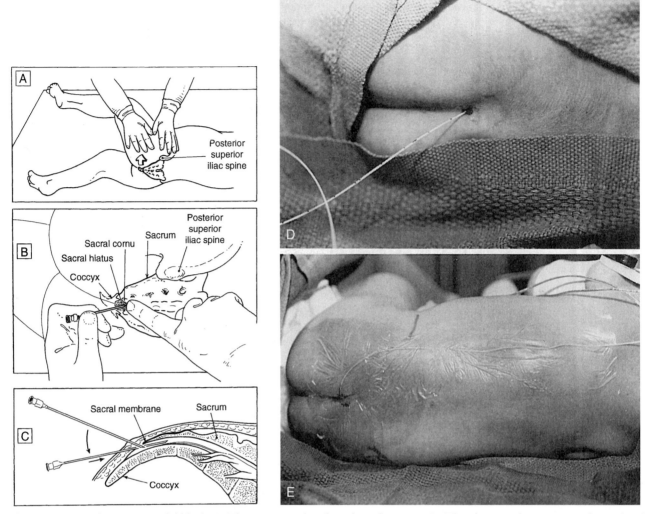

FIGURE 10-2 ■ Performing a caudal block. **A,** The patient is placed in a lateral position. **B,** The posterior iliac spines are located and the sacral cornu palpated; an intravenous needle and intravenous catheter is advanced at an angle of approximately 45 degrees until a distinct "pop" is felt as the needle pierces the sacrococcygeal ligament. **C,** The angle of the needle with the skin is reduced until parallel to the sacrum, and the needle or intravenous catheter is advanced into the caudal canal. **D,** If a continuous technique is used, the caudal catheter is advanced to the midlevel of the surgical incision (it usually readily passes in children younger than 5 years of age) and the introducing needle or catheter is withdrawn. **E,** The catheter is secured with benzoin and an occlusive dressing. (Reprinted with permission from Polaner DM, et al: Pediatric regional anesthesia. In A Practice of Anesthesia for Infants and Children, 3rd ed. Philadelphia, WB Saunders, 2001.)

anesthetic because of its relatively long half-life (mean effect of a caudal block of 5 hours). Ropivacaine is a relatively new long-acting local anesthetic with reduced cardiac and central nervous system toxicity and a higher therapeutic index when compared with bupivacaine, which may be useful for performance of caudal blocks. Clonidine may augment local anesthetics without increasing the adverse effects of respiratory depression, motor block, urinary retention, or nausea. Addition of clonidine, 1 to 1.5 µg/kg, up to a maximum of 30 µg to bupivacaine in a caudal block may enhance the duration of the associated analgesia one and one-half- to twofold. A catheter may be passed through the needle to be left in the caudal or lumbar region for control of postoperative pain. In infants and young children, the catheter may be passed up to as high as the thoracic level in the epidural space, although success with this approach may be variable.

Epidural Anesthesia

Epidural anesthesia has become an integral part of the anesthetic and postoperative pain management strategy in patients undergoing major thoracic, abdominal, and pelvic procedures. Although epidurals may be placed in older children while they are awake, a continuous epidural catheter is most often placed after induction of general anesthesia and before the procedure to provide effective analgesia for the duration of the operation. The patient is placed in the lateral decubitus position, and an 18- or 19-gauge Tuohy needle, which has a side-facing hole, is introduced between the spinous processes in similar fashion to performance of a spinal anesthetic (Fig. 10-3). However, unlike spinal anesthesia the needle does not penetrate the dura. Instead, the needle with stylet is embedded in the ligamentum flavum in the intervertebral space, at which point the stylet is removed and a saline-filled

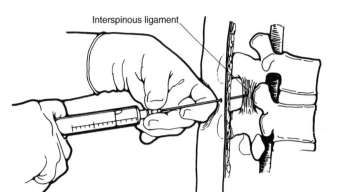

FIGURE 10-3 ■ Placement of a subdural catheter. The Tuohy needle with a side hole at the tip is placed into the ligamentum flavum (interspinous ligament), at which point the stylet is removed. The needle is advanced slowly as the plunger is gently compressed to observe loss of resistance as the needle passes into the epidural space. (Adapted with permission from Bernards CM: Epidural and spinal anesthesia. In Clinical Anesthesia, 3rd ed. Philadelphia, Lippincott-Raven, 1997; and Mulroy MF: Regional Anesthesia: An Illustrated Procedural Guide. Boston, Little Brown, 1989.)

syringe is attached. The needle is then advanced slowly as the plunger on the syringe is intermittently compressed to check for the loss of resistance that is the hallmark of entry into the epidural space. Once the space is encountered, a 20- or 21-gauge catheter is introduced through the needle into the epidural space and advanced. Infusion of long-acting local anesthetics such as bupivacaine 0.25% at rates of 0.2 to 0.4 mL/kg/hr in neonates and infants and 0.4 to 0.6 mL/kg/hr in infants and children older than 6 months of age are effective and well tolerated. Another local anesthetic, ropivacaine, is likely to become useful as an agent for epidural anesthesia. It has an anesthetic effect quite similar to that of bupivacaine, although its central nervous system and cardiovascular toxicity profile provide an increased safety margin. Clonidine, an α_2-adrenergic agonist, may be added to the epidural infusion, which nearly doubles the effect of the local anesthetic.

Addition of opioids, such as fentanyl or hydromorphone (Dilaudid), provides synergistic analgesia while minimizing adverse effects. Complications are rare and include accidental intravascular injection of local anesthetic, incidental dural puncture with possible intrathecal injection of anesthetic, and epidural abscess. Bupivacaine and other local anesthetics usually provide good sensory analgesia with minimal motor block. However, lower extremity weakness and inability to walk occur in a substantial number of children. Urinary retention is a problem with epidural local anesthetic administration, and bladder catheterization is often required. Relative contraindications to epidural catheter placement include anticoagulation and sepsis.

The risk of neurologic deficits after lumbar epidural catheter placement is low, even in the heavily sedated or anesthetized child. However, with a thoracic approach, injury to the spinal cord is possible if the needle is advanced too far. Contact of the needle with the spinal cord will elicit symptoms in the awake patient, thus avoiding injury. However, most children will not tolerate placement of epidural catheters while they are awake, and catheter placement is considered to be more safely performed in the anesthetized child who is not moving. There is controversy, therefore, whether thoracic epidural catheter placement should be performed under anesthesia in children. With an experienced pediatric anesthesiologist the risk of neurologic injury is small, and the advantages of postoperative pain management with a high lumbar or low thoracic epidural far outweigh the risks. As such, in most children's hospitals high lumbar and thoracic epidural catheters are placed fairly routinely under anesthesia.

Nerve Blocks

Blocks used in children include penile blocks in which the dorsal nerve of the penis is anesthetized by injecting a combination of rapidly acting lidocaine and the slower-onset, but longer-acting bupivacaine just below the center of the pubic symphysis (Fig. 10-4). A field block around the base of the penis may supplement the dorsal penile block. An ilioinguinal/iliohypogastric nerve block is

FIGURE 10-4 ■ Dorsal penile nerve block using a subpubic approach. Note the relationship of the dorsal penile nerve. This block can be supplemented by circumferential local injection about the base of the penis. (Reprinted with permission from Sethna NF, Berde CH: Pediatric regional anesthesia. In Pediatric Anesthesia, 4th ed. New York, Churchill Livingstone, 2002; and Dalens B, Vanneuville G, Dechelotte P: Penile block via the subpublic space in 100 children. Anesth Analg 69:41, 1989.)

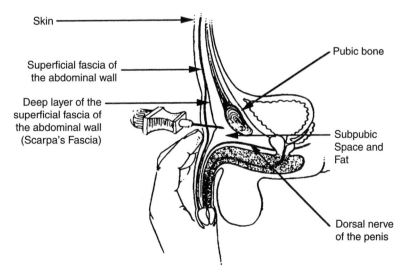

Skin

Superficial fascia of the abdominal wall

Deep layer of the superficial fascia of the abdominal wall (Scarpa's Fascia)

Pubic bone

Subpubic Space and Fat

Dorsal nerve of the penis

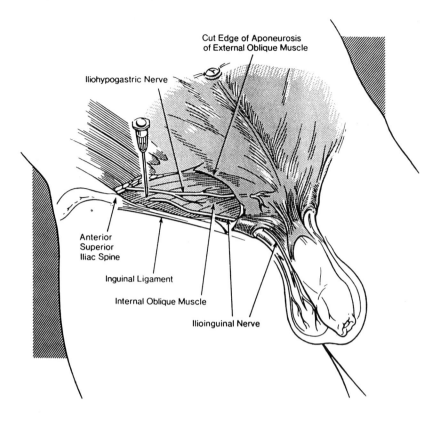

Cut Edge of Aponeurosis
of External Oblique Muscle

Iliohypogastric Nerve

Anterior
Superior
Iliac Spine

Inguinal Ligament

Internal Oblique Muscle

Ilioinguinal Nerve

FIGURE 10-5 ■ Diagram showing the course of the ilioinguinal and iliohypogastric nerve, the landmarks, and the site at which the needle should be inserted relative to the anterior superior iliac spine. These nerves can also be directly visualized and blocked during performance of an inguinal procedure such as a hernia repair. (Reprinted with permission from Sethna NF, Berde CH: Pediatric regional anesthesia. In Pediatric Anesthesia, 4th ed. New York, Churchill Livingstone, 2002; and Brown T, Schulte-Steinberg O: Neural blockade for pediatric surgery. In Neural Blockade: Clinical Anesthesia and Management of Pain, 2nd ed. Philadelphia, JB Lippincott, 1988.)

performed by infiltrating local agents below the external oblique muscle one fingerbreadth superior and medial to the anterior superior iliac crest (Fig. 10-5). Alternatively, the nerves may be directly anesthetized beneath the external oblique fascia, where they are directly observed during a hernia repair or other inguinal procedure. Peripheral nerve, upper-extremity, lower-extremity, and intercostal nerve blocks may also be performed.

METABOLIC COMPLICATIONS OF ANESTHESIA

Pseudocholinesterase Deficiency

Succinylcholine is primarily metabolized by an enzyme in the liver and plasma called pseudocholinesterase. Neuromuscular blockade induced by succinylcholine can be prolonged by a decreased concentration of pseudocholinesterase—the presence of an atypical form of the enzyme. Liver disease, pregnancy, and a number of drugs can lower pseudocholinesterase levels, but usually only with manifestations of mild increases in the duration of neuromuscular blockade.

Neuromuscular blockade can be markedly prolonged if the patient has an abnormal genetic variant of pseudocholinesterase. The activity of the normal pseudocholinesterase is inhibited to a far greater extent by dibucaine than is the variant pseudocholinesterase. Dibucaine can be used, therefore, to test for the variant pseudocholinesterase: dibucaine inhibits the normal enzyme by 80% and the abnormal enzyme by only 20%. Subsequently, many other genetic variants of pseudocholinesterase have been identified, although the dibucaine-resistant variants

are the most important forms. Pseudocholinesterase activity can also be assessed as the number of substrate molecules (μmol) hydrolyzed per unit of time.

Malignant Hyperthermia

MH is characterized by an increased metabolic rate and rhabdomyolysis after exposure to trigger agents, frequently halothane and succinylcholine. The reported incidence of MH is 1 attack per 14,000 anesthetic administrations in children and 1 in 40,000 in adults. MH is a familial disease of multigenetic inheritance, variable expressivity, and incomplete penetrance. First-degree relatives have a high risk; second-degree relatives have a lower but significant risk. MH is more common in patients in the setting of myopathies such as central cord disease, Evans's syndrome, myotonia congenita, and Duchenne muscular dystrophy.

In normal skeletal muscle, depolarization leads to calcium release and muscle contraction followed by calcium uptake and muscle relaxation. MH is a metabolic abnormality resulting in high muscle cell calcium concentration related to the fact that calcium removal appears to be inhibited or overwhelmed. The clinical manifestations and laboratory findings that result from an attack of MH are caused, therefore, by sustained muscle contraction and increased glycolysis by aerobic and anaerobic processes. The early signs of MH are masseter spasm, tachycardia, arrhythmias, tachypnea, and hypertension. As MH progresses, there is generalized muscle rigidity, rapidly rising temperature (39.5°C [103.1°F]), profuse sweating, and skin mottling. Laboratory findings uniformly include a high $PaCO_2$ (>46 mm Hg), elevated blood lactate level (>2 mL/L), and a high potassium level (>5 mEq/L). An elevated level of serum creatinine phosphokinase (>2000 U/L), myoglobinemia and myoglobinuria, pH less than 7.29, and a base deficit of –6 may also be observed. The initial episode usually begins soon after induction of anesthesia. Disseminated intravascular coagulation may develop as a complication. Severe attacks may lead to permanent neurologic sequelae. After an attack of MH, fluid shifts and myocardial damage may lead to acute pulmonary edema. Because of the myoglobinuria, unless there is a vigorous diuresis, acute renal failure may develop. Succinylcholine is a clear triggering agent. Halothane has also been specifically implicated as a trigger, but all inhalational anesthetics can act as potent stimuli.

Before the introduction of dantrolene, the mortality of MH was approximately 65%. Now with early recognition and prompt treatment, death can be prevented. Once an episode of MH is suspected, all triggering agents should be discontinued. Intravenous administration of dantrolene is the most important step in treatment, because it releases calcium from the sarcoplasmic reticulum. Dantrolene must be diluted in sterile water; the dose is 2.5 mg/kg. Repeated doses should be given until the metabolic acidosis subsides. The patient should be cooled, drapes removed, the heating apparatus turned off, and cold solutions infused through the intravenous lines. Body cavities should be filled with cold saline solution and ice packs applied to the groins and axillae. Extracorporeal bypass cooling may be used but is not usually necessary. Central venous or pulmonary artery catheters, arterial lines, and Foley catheters should be inserted. Arrhythmias should be treated when they occur. Metabolic acidosis should be addressed by administration of sodium bicarbonate, and respiratory acidosis should be treated with hyperventilation. Regular insulin, 10 U, in 50% dextrose and water may be used to lower potassium levels when they are elevated. If necessary, intravenous calcium may be given. Hypovolemia should be treated with intravenous fluids, and renal failure should be prevented by fluid infusions and diuretics. Mannitol is part of the dantrolene formulation: there is 150 mg of mannitol per milligram of dantrolene in the vial. Furosemide at a dose of 1 mg/kg can also be administered.

In suspect patients and those with a family history of MH, consideration should be given to performing a thigh muscle biopsy and in-vitro contraction test with caffeine and halothane stimulation on the specimen before anesthesia. This is the only definitive method of making a diagnosis of susceptibility to MH. Patients should ideally have the necessary operation performed with a minimum of stress, while being sedated under a local or regional anesthetic. The use of oral dantrolene prophylactically is controversial but may be useful. Nontriggering techniques of general anesthesia must be chosen. Phenothiazine, ketamine, and atropine are avoided because of their temperature-interfering effects. Although there are no completely safe agents, balanced anesthetic techniques using nonpolarizing muscle relaxants should be chosen and drugs such as diazepam, morphine, barbiturates, and nitrous oxide considered. Intravenous dantrolene is given before induction.

POSTOPERATIVE PAIN MANAGEMENT

The limited cognitive ability and language skills of infants and children may lead to underestimation and, therefore, undertreatment of postoperative pain. As such, it is imperative that pediatric surgeons and others caring for children after operations are skilled at assessing levels of pain in children. Self-reporting of pain should be used whenever possible. A number of pain scales and tools have been developed that are effective at identifying levels of pain in children. The Oucher scale has six photographs of a child's face with expressions associated with varying levels of pain intensity, which allows caretakers to quantify the severity of pain in a child. The Wong-Baker scale is composed of six drawings of faces with associated word descriptors (Fig. 10-6) and can be used in patients as young as 3 years old. Patients can point to the drawing or descriptor to indicate their level of pain. Visual analogue scales are also effective in older children. Observation of patient behavior and activity can be very telling: the FLACC pain assessment tool incorporates variables of the *Facial* expression, the position of the *Legs*, *Activity*, presence of *Crying*, and the ability to *Console* the patient in the development of a score that predicts pain levels in infants and children as young as 2 months of age (Table 10-6). Parents are often an excellent source of information regarding their child's pain status. Postoperative pain control may be achieved by any of a number of combinations of approaches and techniques, many of which have been discussed previously. Local infiltration with bupivacaine should be performed at the conclusion of most operative cases and may provide pain relief for up to 5 to 8 hours. Likewise, peripheral nerve, ilioinguinal, dorsal penile, and intercostal nerve blocks may be effective for similar durations, although addition of clonidine, which prolongs and intensifies analgesia, may increase this duration for 12 to 16 hours.

Pain relief after minor procedures may be achieved with acetaminophen (Tylenol), 15 mg/kg, and ibuprofen, 6 to 10 mg/kg, every 4 to 6 hours. The incidence of postoperative hemorrhage is not increased by the administration of ibuprofen. Codeine, 0.5 to 1.0 mg/kg, or oxycodone, 0.05 to 0.15 mg/kg, may be combined with acetaminophen (Tylenol #3, Tylox, respectively), or hydrocodone, 5 mg, may be combined with acetaminophen, 500 mg (Vicodin, Lortab), to supplement pain control as necessary, although nausea, vomiting, and constipation are frequently associated with these medications. Toradol, 0.5 mg/kg, up to 30 mg/kg maximum, may be administered intravenously for up to 5 days and is especially popular for use during and after minimally invasive procedures. Table 10-7 demonstrates the characteristics of such medications.

Intravenous opioids are used for severe pain and when children cannot take oral preparations. Opioids may be prescribed intravenously in children on an intermittent basis. Morphine is used most frequently for this purpose and is given in a single dose of 0.05 to 0.1 mg/kg, up to 5 to 8 mg/kg maximum. The half-life of morphine is

A

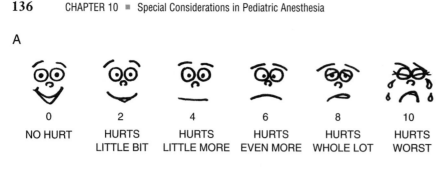

0	2	4	6	8	10
NO HURT	HURTS LITTLE BIT	HURTS LITTLE MORE	HURTS EVEN MORE	HURTS WHOLE LOT	HURTS WORST

B

Worst possible pain

10
9
8
7
6
5
4
3
2
1
0

No pain

FIGURE 10-6 ■ **A,** Wong-Baker FACES pain rating scale with a number from 0 to 10. Patients older than 3 years of age can point to the drawing or descriptor to indicate their level of pain. **B,** A number scale in a vertical position can be used by older children to rate pain. (Reprinted with permission from Wong DH, et al: Whaley and Wong's Nursing Care of Infants and Children, 6th ed. St. Louis, CV Mosby, 1999; and Merkel S, Malviya S: Pediatric pain, tools, and assessment. J Perianesth Nurs 15:408-414, 2000.)

10 to 20 hours in preterm newborns, 7.6 hours in term neonates, and 2.9 hours in older infants and children: clearance of morphine appears to normalize to adult levels by 1 month of age. In addition, there is a higher incidence of morphine-induced respiratory depression among neonates. Thus, the dosing interval of morphine should be increased in the neonate to approximately 6 hours and monitoring, which should be performed in all patients receiving intravenous narcotics, should be enhanced. Meperidine is approximately 10 times as potent as morphine. Unfortunately, the metabolite normeperidine may accumulate, leading to central nervous system symptoms, including seizures. Fentanyl is frequently administered as an infusion for analgesia in the postoperative period. The half-life is prolonged in preterm newborns to 17 hours from 7 hours in children.

In patients who are expected to experience substantial postoperative pain, continuous administration of intravenous opioids is most effective. In patients older than 7 years of age, this may be performed as patient-controlled analgesia (PCA). With this technique, a baseline rate of intravenous opioid administration is chosen. Most intravenous PCA devices consist of a microprocessor-controlled pump triggered by depressing a button. When the pump

TABLE 10-6 ■ FLACC Pain Assessment Tool

Categories	Scoring		
	0	**1**	**2**
Face	No particular expression or smile	Occasional grimace or frown, withdrawn, disinterested	Frequent to constant frown, clenched jaw, quivering chin
Legs	Normal position or relaxed	Uneasy, restless, tense	Kicking or legs drawn up
Activity	Lying quietly, normal position, moves easily	Squirming, shifting back and forth, tense	Arched, rigid, or jerking
Cry	No cry (awake or asleep)	Moans or whimpers, occasional complaint	Crying steadily, screams or sobs, frequent complaints
Consolability	Content, relaxed	Reassured by occasional touching, hugging, or talking; distractable	Difficult to console or comfort

Each of the 5 categories, (F) face, (L) legs, (A) activity, (C) cry, (C) consolability, is scored from 0 to 2, which results in a total score between 0 and 10.
Adapted with permission from Merkel S, et al: The FLACC: A behavioral scale for scoring postoperative pain in young children. Pediatr Nurs 23:293-297, 1997; and Merkel S, Malviya S: Pediatric pain, tools, and assessment. J Perianesth Nurs 15:408-414, 2000.

TABLE 10-7 ■ Agents Commonly Used for Postoperative Pain Control				
Drug	**Type**	**Dose and Route (Older Than Age 6 Mo and < 50 Kg)**	**Dose and Route (> 50 Kg)**	**Comment**
Morphine	Narcotic Analgesic	0.05-0.1 mg/kg IV q2-4h IV infusion: 5-10 µg/kg/hr for abdominal surgery, 10-30 µg/kg/hr for more extensive surgery (age < 6 mo: 0.01 mg/kg/hr IV infusion)	5-8 mg IV q2-4h 1.5 mg/hr IV infusion	Used commonly for congenital heart disease Clearance prolonged in neonates and liver and renal disease May cause hypotension Respiratory depression especially < age 6 mo
Fentanyl	Narcotic Analgesic	0.5-1.0 µg/kg IV q1-2h 0.5-2.0 µg/kg/hr IV infusion	25-50 µg IV q1-2h 25-100 µg/hr IV infusion	Fast onset, short half-life Bradycardia may occur Associated with chest wall rigidity Prolonged elimination in preterm neonates
Codeine	Narcotic Analgesic	0.5-1.0 mg/kg q3-4h PO	30-60 mg q3-4h PO	Nausea/vomiting in many patients Often combined with acetaminophen in 1:10 ratio (Tylenol #3)
Oxycodone	Narcotic Analgesic	0.1-0.2 mg/kg q3-4h PO	5-10 mg q3-4h PO	Often combined with acetaminophen (Tylox, Percocet)
Hydrocodone	Narcotic Analgesic	0.2 mg/kg q3-4h PO	5-10 mg q3-4h PO	Often combined with acetaminophen (Vicodin, Lortab)
Methadone	Narcotic Analgesic	0.1mg q6-12h IV 0.1-0.2 mg/kg q6-12h PO	5-8 mg q4-8h IV 5-10 mg q4-8h PO	Can accumulate and cause delayed sedation Useful because of prolonged duration of action
Meperidine (Demerol)	Narcotic Analgesic	0.8-1.0 mg/kg q2-3h IV 2-3 mg/kg q3-4h PO	50-75 mg q2-3h IV 100-150 mg q3-4h PO	To be avoided in young children because metabolite may cause seizures
Hydromorphone (Dilaudid)	Narcotic Analgesic	15 µg/kg q3-4h IV 2-6 µg/kg/hr IV infusion	1.5 mg q3-4h IV 0.3 mg/hr IV infusion 6 mg PO q3-4h	
Acetaminophen	Analgesic	10-15 mg/kg q4h PO 20 mg/kg q6-8h PR	650-1000 mg q4h PO maximum 2.6 g/day	Most widely used mild analgesic Excessive dosing may produce hepatic failure
Ibuprofen	NSAID	6-10 mg/kg q6h PO	400-600 mg q6h PO	
Ketorolac	NSAID	0.5 mg/kg (max 15 mg) q6h IV	0.5 mg/kg (max 30 mg) q6h IV	Not to exceed 5 days Used with caution in setting of renal impairment, risk of bleeding, gastrointestinal ulcers

PO, orally; IV, intravenous; PR, rectally.

is triggered, a preset amount of opioid is delivered into the patient's intravenous line. A timer in the pump prevents administration of an additional bolus until a specified period (lockout interval) has elapsed. Thus, individual patients can safely titrate pain medication to their own needs because the patient must have adequate levels of consciousness to press the trigger to receive additional narcotic. The baseline rate of opioid administration, the dose per bolus, the total dose over a given period of time, and the "lockout" period are prescribed (Table 10-8). Pain control by this technique is more uniform and effective when compared with intermittent nurse dosing. In patients younger than the age of 7, nurse-controlled analgesia may be used in which the nurse is responsible for pressing the button and administering a narcotic bolus above the baseline rate after assessing the patient. In select cases and with proper education, "parent-controlled analgesia" may also be effective in this age group.

A caudal block provides analgesia for a limited period (mean = 5 hours). However, placement of a small catheter into the lumbar or thoracic epidural space allows continuous or intermittent administration of local anesthetics

TABLE 10-8 ■ Typical Starting Parameters for a Patient-Controlled Analgesia (PCA) Approach in Children			
Drug	**Bolus Dose (µg/kg)**	**Continuous Rate (µg/kg/h)**	**4-Hour Limit (µg/kg)**
Morphine	20	4-20	300
Hydromorphone	5	1-3	20-40
Fentanyl	0.25	0.15	4

Lockout interval = 8-10 minutes.
Adapted with permission from Greco CD, Houck CS, Berde CB: Pediatric pain management. In Gregory GA (ed): Pediatric Anesthesia. New York, Churchill Livingstone, 2002.

TABLE 10-9 ■ American Society of Anesthesiologists Physical Status Classification

Class I	A normal healthy patient
Class II	A patient with mild systemic disease
Class III	A patient with severe systemic disease
Class IV	A patient with severe systemic disease that is a constant threat to life
Class V	A moribund patient who is not expected to survive without the operation
Class VI	A patient who is an organ donor

Adapted with permission from Malviya S, Voepel-Lewis T, Tait AR, Merkel S: Sedation/analgesia for diagnostic and therapeutic procedures in children. J Perianesth Nurs 15:415-422, 2000.

or narcotics with associated regional analgesia without systemic narcotic administration. The epidural approach is effective after large thoracic or abdominal incisions. Epidural medications are most often administered on a continuous basis (see Table 10-5). In some cases a PCA approach may be used with the patient controlling limited intermittent boluses. Simultaneous administration of systemic opioids and sedatives is given only rarely and under controlled circumstances because of the potential respiratory depression that can be induced if the patient is receiving epidural opioids. If an epidural is only infusing local anesthesia, then systemic opioids may be administered. Close monitoring, including pulse oximetry and respiratory rate, is required for all patients on epidurals and those receiving intravenous sedatives and opioids. As described previously, the disadvantages of an epidural include the need for bladder catheterization and the limitation in postoperative ambulation. Infection and spinal headache caused by subarachnoid puncture are rare, as are neurologic sequelae from placement while the patient is anesthetized. Failure of an epidural to provide adequate analgesia is observed in approximately 25% of patients.

CONSCIOUS SEDATION

It is necessary to provide sedation for diagnostic and therapeutic procedures that induce anxiety and pain in children. Studies have demonstrated that infants and children who have experienced pain with previous procedures such as bone marrow biopsies and circumcisions have increased anxiety with subsequent procedures. However, the use of conscious sedation may be the greatest source of adverse events during performance of minor procedures. Therefore, the clinician should approach conscious sedation with a high level of respect and preparation for potential adverse outcomes.

First and foremost, the patient must be treated as if he or she is about to undergo general anesthesia because a failed conscious sedation procedure often results in the equivalent. American Society of Anesthesiologists (ASA) physical status classification should be assigned (Table 10-9), especially those with ASA class III or IV have a higher incidence of failed conscious sedation procedures. A Mallempatti score, as described in Chapter 31, should be assessed by examining the oropharynx in case airway

access becomes necessary. The patient should have fasted per the guidelines for general anesthesia (see later). Finally, intravenous access should be established before initiation of conscious sedation, and blood pressure, pulse oximetry, respiratory rate, and heart rate should be documented every 5 minutes during the procedure, as should the level of sedation (Table 10-10). Resuscitation and airway access and management equipment must be available, and a person other than the surgeon who is trained in basic cardiac life support or pediatric advanced life support should be present throughout the sedation period until the child has met discharge criteria, which includes presence of baseline vital signs, oxygenation, and level of consciousness; ability to maintain a patent airway and to handle secretions; and ability to move and ambulate as age appropriate. This individual's only responsibility should be to monitor the patient's physiologic status and to support the child as necessary.

The selection of appropriate sedative drugs is critical to the success of the sedation and procedure (see Table 10-1). The goals of the procedure are to provide anxiolysis, analgesia, amnesia, and cooperation. A benzodiazepine such as intravenous midazolam, 0.5 to 0.1 mg/kg, provides anxiolysis and amnesia and is a popular drug for sedation for minor procedures. It is often combined with intravenous fentanyl, 1 μg/kg, which is a powerful analgesic and sedative. Both agents have rapid onset within 1 to 3 minutes and are relatively short-acting, making them ideal for brief procedures. Fentanyl may cause chest wall rigidity, which would require airway access and control. Both agents should be titrated carefully because synergistic respiratory depression can occur. Chloral hydrate is the most commonly used sedative for noninvasive diagnostic studies because this agent produces somnolence but no analgesia.

Reversal agents for benzodiazepines and opioids should be available in the event of excessive sedation or other adverse effects. Flumazenil antagonizes the central nervous system effects of benzodiazepines after intravenous administration of a 0.01-mg/kg dose to a maximum of 0.2 mg per dose. This dose may be repeated if there is no effect in 30 to 60 seconds, to a maximum of 1 mg cumulative. Naloxone (Narcan) is an opioid antagonist with

TABLE 10-10 ■ The University of Michigan Sedation Scale

0	Awake and alert
1	Minimally sedated: Tired/sleepy, appropriate response to verbal conversation and/or sound
2	Moderately sedated: Somnolent/sleeping, easily aroused with light tactile stimulation or a simple verbal command
3	Deeply sedated: Deep sleep, arousable only with significant physical stimulation
4	Unarousable

Adapted with permission from Malviya S, et al : Validity and reliability of the University of Michigan Sedation Scale (UMSS) in children undergoing computerized tomography. Anesthesiology 93:A1259, 2000; and Malviya S, Voepel-Lewis T, Tait AR, Merkel S: Sedation/analgesia for diagnostic and therapeutic procedures in children. J Perianesth Nurs 15:415-422, 2000.

similar rapid onset that is administered in an initial dose of 1 to 10 mg/kg. Although these agents are effective, the danger of resedation is high because of the longer half-life of most narcotics and benzodiazepines when compared with flumenazil and naloxone. As such, patients receiving a reversal agent during conscious sedation require observation and monitoring for an extended period.

OUTPATIENT SURGERY

Although outpatient or ambulatory surgery was first reported in 1909, it was not until the past few decades that there was a massive shift from inpatient to outpatient surgery. This shift was fueled by the need for medical cost containment and has been insisted on by third-party payers and government agencies. At most children's hospitals over 60% of all operations are performed on an outpatient basis. This trend has significantly reduced the total cost of many pediatric operative procedures and increased the availability of beds for patients with more complex illnesses. There are several advantages of an outpatient procedure for the pediatric patient and the family. First, anxiety associated with parent-child separation is reduced because the child and the parent can remain together during the admission, preparation, and on-call periods. In many cases the parent can be present during induction of anesthesia. The family can then be reunited as the child wakes up and recovers from the operation. Second, exposure to hospital pathogens is reduced, thus minimizing the risk of nosocomial infections: the incidence of enteric and respiratory tract infections postoperatively is reduced in patients undergoing ambulatory surgery, in contrast to those admitted to the hospital.

Many pediatric operations lend themselves to the ambulatory approach. Operations such as inguinal hernia repair and myringotomy are relatively atraumatic and have a short and uncomplicated convalescent period. Even those requiring complex postoperative care may be performed on an ambulatory preoperative basis with admission to the hospital after the procedure.

Selection of Patients for Preoperative and Postoperative Outpatient Surgery

The infant or child should be in good health. Systemic diseases, if present, should be thoroughly documented and under good control. Anesthesiologists usually will accept ASA class I and usually class II patients (see Table 10-9). Class III patients, after proper consultation and discussion with attending physicians and surgeons, are sometimes operated on an ambulatory basis. Operations are favored that have minimal blood loss, are of short duration, and do not extensively involve the airway or body cavities.

There is controversy concerning the method of managing the "ex-premature" infant. Infants who were premature are at greater risk for postoperative apnea. Postoperative apnea is also more common in full-term infants with a history of apnea and in those infants younger than 44 to 46 weeks, conceptional age (Fig. 10-7). Apnea usually occurs within 12 hours of anesthesia but may occasionally occur as late as 40 hours postoperatively. Based on the available data, reasonable recommendations

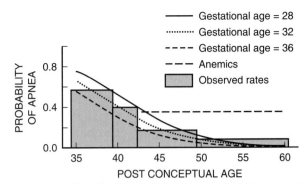

FIGURE 10-7 ■ Predicted probability of apnea for all patients, by gestational age and weeks of postconceptual age. The risk for apnea diminishes for infants born at a later gestational age. The *shaded boxes* represent the overall rates of apnea for infants within that gestational age range. Patients with anemia are shown as a separate group (*horizontal hatched line*) because the probability of apnea was the same regardless of postconceptual age or gestational age for infants with anemia. (Reprinted with permission from Coté CJ, Zaslavsky A, Downes JJ, et al: Postoperative apnea in former preterm infants after inguinal herniorrhaphy. Anesthesiology 82:809-822, 1995.)

for ambulatory surgery include overnight admission for monitoring after elective outpatient procedures in ex-premature infants (<37 weeks gestational age) who are 50 weeks or less post conception. All infants with respiratory insufficiency or history of apnea are admitted for observation.

Preoperative Preparation of the Patient and Parent

Proper preparation includes preoperative education and familiarization with the outpatient facilities, personnel, and procedures. Laboratory studies should be performed based on need because of specific diseases involving the cardiac, pulmonary, renal, hematologic, or immune systems and the medications being administered.

NPO Orders

Parents of patients who are to undergo outpatient surgery must be carefully instructed when to discontinue feedings and oral medications before the operation. Abstinence from the ingestion of all solid or semisolid foods including milk, formula, pudding, and juices containing particulate matter is necessary for 6 hours before the anticipated time of operation. Patients are allowed to take clear fluids including water, flat carbonated beverages, weak tea, Jello, Kool Aid, and transparent juices devoid of particulate matter up to 2 hours before the anticipated time of operation. Breast milk may be consumed up to 4 hours before induction of anesthesia. All essential oral medications required for cardiac, respiratory, renal, or neurologic conditions may be taken with one sip of water as close as possible to the ordinary time before the operation.

Criteria for Discharge

The patient's condition must be assessed by an anesthesiologist and should include the criteria in Table 10-11. In addition, the parent or patient should be provided

TABLE 10-11 ■ Criteria for Discharge after Outpatient Procedures

Stable and appropriate-for-age vital signs
Age-appropriate ambulation
Absence of vomiting and ability to tolerate oral fluids
Absence of bleeding
Absence of respiratory distress
Absence of pain that cannot be controlled by oral medication
Age-appropriate alertness

with written instructions and telephone numbers for contact if problems should arise.

SUGGESTED READINGS

Barash PG (ed): Clinical Anesthesia. Philadelphia, Lippincott-Raven, 1996.

Berde CH, Sethna NF: Analgesics for the treatment of pain in children. N Engl J Med 347:1094-1103, 2002.

A concise summary of current pain management in children.

Brown DL: Spinal, epidural, and caudal anesthesia. In Miller RD (ed): Anesthesia, 5th ed., New York, Churchill Livingstone, 2000, pp 1491-1519.

Coté CJ, et al (eds): A Practice of Anesthesia for Infants and Children, 3rd ed. Philadelphia, WB Saunders, 2001.

Considered one of the major texts of pediatric anesthesia; this book provides a nice overview.

Gregory GA (ed): Pediatric Anesthesia. New York, Churchill Livingstone, 2002.

One of the foremost pediatric anesthesia textbooks, which covers almost all aspects of the field.

Journal of Perianesthesia Nursing 15:383-447, 2000.

A nice reference for many aspects of conscious sedation and pain management in pediatric patients.

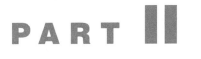

Trauma

11

The Injured Child

EPIDEMIOLOGY

Although there are many similarities between children and adults in terms of the surgical approach to traumatic injuries, there also are many differences. Since at least the 1980s, trauma has been the leading cause of death in childhood, constituting more than half of childhood mortality. In the 1- to 14-year-old age group, greater than 50% of mortality is related to accidental and deliberate trauma, 10% is related to malignancies, and 5% is related to congenital abnormalities; the remaining deaths are due to miscellaneous causes, such as infectious disease and metabolic disorders. About 20 million pediatric injuries are estimated to occur each year, involving 30% of all children, although many of these injuries are minor. Despite the fact that between 1979 and 1996 mortality from unintentional injuries decreased 45% as a result of various preventive measures, approximately 13,000 children die from trauma each year, 1 million are temporarily disabled, and 75,000 are permanently disabled. The estimated cost of all these childhood injuries is greater than $15 billion yearly. Not included in these figures are the large number of birth injuries that occur each year. Although efforts at prevention of injury in childhood have been responsible for significant reductions in mortality, much remains to be done. Although there have been remarkable improvements in the design of car seats and other restraint devices for children in automobiles, universal seat belt laws are still not enforced as much as they should be. Highway speed limits have increased steadily from 55 miles per hour to 70 miles per hour, and helmet laws for riders of motorcycles and bicycles have been repealed in many states. The improvements in childhood trauma, morbidity, and mortality have been related to several factors, including improvements in the organization of care and trauma education, a better understanding of trauma physiology as a basis for care, selective management of blunt trauma, better management of burn injury, and preventive measures.

PHYSIOLOGY AND OTHER CONSIDERATIONS IN INJURED CHILDREN

From the standpoint of the effects and responses to injury, children are similar to adults in many respects but different in others. Children younger than age 1 year, especially infants, display different metabolic characteristics, and responses may be different from those in adults qualitatively and quantitatively.

The pathophysiologic problems related to serious injury that result in mortality during the first hour or so after injury are cardiovascular, respiratory, and central nervous system in nature. Each of these problems results in significant metabolic consequences that may be progressive over hours to days after injury; this is referred to as the *systemic inflammatory response syndrome* (SIRS). If not interrupted, SIRS may result in infection and multiple system organ failure. A previously well, normal child has significant physiologic reserves, but a more rapid approach to resuscitation is needed to satisfy a relatively increased metabolic rate, particularly in very young children. Treatment is based on an understanding of the neuroendocrine and cellular responses to injury, the pathophysiologic effects of decreased cardiac output and oxygen delivery and circulatory failure, and the metabolic consequences of reperfusion after resuscitation.

Injury stimulates the central nervous system to produce a variety of endocrine substances in proportion to the extent of injury, including excessive amounts of cortisol, antidiuretic hormone, catecholamines, insulin, glucagon, renin, aldosterone, and endorphins. As produced, these substances interact and act independently. They are protective when produced in appropriate amounts, but deficient or excessive production may result in either an inadequate or a harmful physiologic response. The longer the injury goes untreated, the more prolonged and complicated the situation becomes. This response can be blunted by early effective resuscitation for a favorable outcome.

The cellular responses to shock and injury are better known now, and this information supports the prioritization in resuscitation of airway, breathing, and circulation designed to ameliorate the effects of hypoxemia caused by inadequate oxygen delivery because of impairment of respiratory function and cardiac output. Emphasis is placed on early intubation and maintenance of breathing whenever there is even a question of respiratory impairment or severe head injury, particularly because of the increased metabolic requirements of young children. With regard to maintaining and improving cardiac output, the emphasis has been placed on early and appropriate fluid resuscitation with Ringer's lactate and red blood cells as needed. Use of albumen solutions is deferred until after the first 24 hours following injury because it may be harmful before that. In addition, correction of acidosis and maintenance of normal body temperature are crucial to resuscitation because the response to resuscitation is less in the presence of severe acidosis or hypothermia. Additionally, because catecholamine production is one of the primary neuroendocrine responses to shock, it has been found that the use of epinephrine, norepinephrine, and dopamine, which have alpha and beta effects on the heart and the kidney, may be useful adjuncts in selected patients. The overall goal is to reverse the shift in cellular metabolism from aerobic to anaerobic mechanism and to eliminate the production of lactic acid because these processes may result in cellular damage that is manifested by capillary leak, organ failure, and irreversible acidosis. In severely injured patients, reperfusion may result in secondary cellular injury despite adequate resuscitation. Reperfusion injury and inadequate circulatory support may result in cellular death and the production of cytokines. Cytokines are protein products produced by multiple cellular sources. They are proinflammatory and anti-inflammatory, and the response seems to be identical in children and adults, although different quantitatively. Unregulated production of cytokines not only results in peripheral cellular and organ failure, but also in the production of acute-phase proteins, which stimulate hypermetabolism and SIRS. Numerous other inflammatory mediators are produced that also stimulate coagulation and the immune system. The prime clinical manifestations of all of these responses, if prolonged, are hypermetabolism and massive edema. Just as in adults, the best currently available therapeutic approach in this situation is the provision of adequate nutrition emphasizing protein over glucose initially and use of the gastrointestinal tract when possible.

Although the information just related stresses the relative similarities in injured children and adults, it is useful to consider the essential differences as well. The child is a different host at different times compared with the adult. An immature personality and personality characteristics that influence the psychological response to trauma vary according to age and the level of maturity of the child and the tendency to be injured. In most instances, the child is young or accident prone and usually a boy. The surgeon who cares for injured children deals with patients who often are unable to express pain and discomfort or to localize complaints. Severe pain and anxiety may produce paradoxical reactions, in which case initial evaluation and treatment are difficult. In this regard, environmental factors in the emergency department and in the hospital are particularly important if a good long-term psychological outcome is to be obtained. Depression, regression to earlier stages of development, hostile reactions, and delirium may represent untoward psychological reactions to injury. Some children become extremely difficult to manage and manifest behavioral changes whereby they tend to injure themselves, pull out necessary tubes, or disrupt dressings and intravenous lines, necessitating the use of restraints. Because children are developing individuals, all approaches to treatment, including surgical procedures, must take into account subsequent growth and development. Examples of the latter include special approaches to the management of fractures in childhood and preservation of the injured spleen.

In terms of quantitative and qualitative differences in the management of injuries in young children, one of the most important is the difference in blood volume relative to the size of the patient. A relatively small amount of blood loss may be significant and require immediate replacement in infants, whereas it might be well tolerated by adolescents.

The increased surface area-to-body weight ratio of children compared with adults results in increased evaporative water loss and heat loss, and the younger the child, the greater the loss. Additionally, children have thin skin and a relative absence of insulating fat, factors that promote hypothermia. The age of maturation of the integumentary system is about 16 years. In infants, severe hypothermia may impair the response to fluid resuscitation. Rapid administration of blood and intravenous fluids may produce hypothermia, so it is advisable to warm all solutions before infusion. Young children are highly labile relative to temperature regulation and may have rapid shifts in core temperature with a tendency to equilibrate with the environment. Temperature regulation matures at around age 10. Mention has already been made of the deleterious effects of metabolic acidosis as a factor in resuscitation. Infants in particular are prone to develop acidosis in response to shock because of their relatively increased metabolic rate.

Small children tend to have a labile peripheral circulation, which is affected by shock and hypothermia in a variable way so that clinical estimation of the adequacy of cardiac output on this basis may be difficult. In general, myocardial function is good in normal children, but peripheral vascular compensation tends to be poor. This is less of a consideration in children older than age 2 years. Another special response in the pediatric age group is the redistribution of blood flow to priority areas from the splanchnic bed when there is volume deficiency so that children are more prone than adults to develop ileus and gastric dilation. Another factor that promotes gastric dilation is tachypnea, which also is accentuated in injured children. Excessive gastric dilation may promote vomiting and aspiration, diaphragmatic elevation and respiratory distress, and inferior vena caval compression with diminution of preload and cardiac output.

The pulmonary system of children is generally well developed within a few months after birth. The high metabolic demands of infants require the pulmonary system to function at a high level, however, so there is only marginal reserve. By age 4 years, a greater margin of functional residual capacity exists. In infants and children, limitation of excursion of the chest wall, airway compromise, pneumonia, atelectasis, and risk of aspiration are greater.

The renal response to injury in children younger than age 6 years is relatively immature. In children younger than age 2 years, these limitations in renal function make them particularly susceptible to dehydration and fluid overload. Very young children produce large volumes of dilute urine as a manifestation of glomerular and tubular immaturity. Renal tubular function with regard to free water clearance is less efficient so that fluid retention occurs as large volumes of resuscitation fluids are administered. For this reason, diuresis may be prolonged so that the need to use diuretic agents in small children is greater than in larger subjects. Metabolic and nutritional requirements of infants are high, almost three times those of adults, and are reduced gradually as organ systems mature. After about 8 years of age, metabolic requirements of children are similar to those of adults. Current information related to metabolism and nutrition indicates that levels of protein intake of approximately 1.5 to 3.0 g/kg/24 hours seem to be appropriate, administered with just enough nonprotein calories to satisfy metabolic requirements. The addition of glutamine to intravenous and enteral regimens seems to diminish protein loss, while supporting the immune system. It also has been shown that the administration of recombinant human growth hormone, insulin, and insulin-like growth factor improves protein anabolism and increases glucose clearance, which may be impaired because of insulin resistance. Metabolic and nutritional requirements of infants are high, almost three times those of adults, and are reduced gradually as organ systems mature. After about 8 to 10 years of age, metabolic requirements of children are similar to those of adults.

Head injuries are not only common in childhood, but also constitute the major cause of mortality. The central nervous system is not completely developed in children, and severe injuries may result in arrest of neurologic development. The head constitutes a larger proportion of the body in children than in adults, making it a larger target for blunt trauma. Also, the incidence of multiple organ involvement with head injury is higher in children than in adults, although that may be changing with the appropriate use of restraint devices. The incidence of subdural hematoma in children is higher than in adults, but most of these are insignificant, so the need for emergency craniotomy in children is less. The most common presentation of serious head injury in children is generalized cerebral swelling. Adequate control of hyperglycemia in the head-injured child is crucial to prevent a poor outcome.

It also seems that the mechanisms of injury are different in children compared with adults. Adults have a high incidence of penetrating trauma, whereas more than 80% of children have blunt injuries. Isolated head injuries have approximately 20% mortality and a 30% incidence of long-term disability, and the mortality is 70% when a serious head injury is associated with other serious organ system injuries, emphasizing the importance of rapid resuscitation and care for small children. Motor vehicle injuries, bicycle accidents, falls, and burns are the main agents that cause serious trauma in childhood, and most children are injured in or near their homes. This is certainly the case with child abuse, which poses obvious problems in terms of diagnosis and long-term management. The gradual development of pediatric trauma centers and combined adult/pediatric centers has improved prehospital and hospital care and long-term rehabilitation.

A unique form of pediatric trauma is birth injury. The most common injuries in newborns include pneumothorax, fractures, peripheral nerve injuries, intracranial hemorrhage, and solid organ injuries. Premature infants tend to have visceral injuries, central nervous system hemorrhage, and pneumothorax. Term infants tend to have pneumothorax, long bone fractures, peripheral nerve injuries, and solid organ injuries. The most common nerves injured at birth are the facial nerve, the brachial plexus, and the phrenic nerve. The most common fractures involve the clavicle, humerus, and femur, including shaft fractures and epiphyseal separations. The most common solid organ injuries include intracapsular hematomas of the liver and spleen, adrenal hemorrhage, and occasional renal injuries. Iatrogenic trauma includes catheter perforations of the pharynx and tracheobronchial tree, vascular complications of central venous and peripheral arterial access, and skin sloughs from infiltrations.

Because 80% of pediatric injuries are blunt, many more patients are followed expectantly than would be the case with penetrating injuries as seen in adults. Additionally, certain organ systems are more vulnerable in children than in adults. The most prominent is the head, which is involved in three fourths of blunt injuries. The urinary bladder is unprotected in infants because it is not located completely within the pelvis. In addition, the liver, spleen, and kidneys have less abdominal and lower thoracic wall protection in children. The approach to airway management and resuscitation is also considerably different in children, particularly in terms of the critical nature of the small airway and relatively small blood volume.

In all age groups, mortality related to trauma has a characteristic pattern. Approximately half of all trauma deaths occur at the scene; 30% occur within a few hours of injury; and the remaining 20% occur days to weeks later, usually because of infection. Consequently, approximately half of the trauma deaths are potentially preventable with expeditious and definitive treatment.

INITIAL ASSESSMENT AND RESUSCITATION

The best available model for emergency management is the Advanced Trauma Life Support (ATLS) course. ATLS stresses the team approach to trauma management. Similar emphasis is provided by the Advanced Pediatric Life Support course.

The development of effective Emergency Medical Services and training of technicians has significantly improved prehospital care and transportation from the scene of the accident to the hospital. With the development of better systems of trauma care in many countries, children are being transported routinely to hospital emergency facilities equipped with all of the sizes of equipment required for support of the airway and circulation for patients of varying sizes and ages and different-sized splints to immobilize fractures. Specialized emergency medical technician training in pediatric care is directed at the techniques of airway management, vascular access, and fluid resuscitation of infants and children.

In the hospital emergency department, the responding team is trained to work together. One individual is designated to be in charge of the overall resuscitation effort; one is responsible for the head and neck, airway management, and technical manipulations above the chest; another is responsible for the midportion of the body and vascular access in that area; and a fourth is responsible for management of the lower part of the body, vascular access there, placement of a urinary catheter, and immobilization of fractures. Another member of the team is responsible for determining the child's history, the existence of any preexisting condition such as congenital heart disease or neurologic disease that might influence emergency evaluation and management, and the immunization status of the patient. The primary goal of initial management is to treat airway impairment and life-threatening shock first before attempting to make a diagnosis.

Emergency management of injured children is best divided into immediate life support and postinjury stabilization. The initial priorities include immobilization of the neck, establishment of an adequate airway, control of breathing, and maintenance of the circulation. Initial resuscitation has been divided into two segments: the primary and secondary surveys. The goals of the primary survey are to establish a reliable airway and adequate ventilation, to maintain the circulation, and to assess neurologic status. When the patient becomes stable in terms of the airway and hemodynamics, the secondary survey is performed, including performance of diagnostic studies and establishment of surgical priorities (Table 11-1).

Primary Survey and Management of the Airway

All children who are seriously injured, particularly children with head injuries, should be presumed to have cervicospinal injury until proved otherwise. Although cervicospinal injuries are far less common in children than in adults, it is safest to place a cervical collar on the child at the same time one establishes an adequate airway. Sandbags may be placed on either side of the head; tape securing the forehead to a backboard may be used in place of a cervical collar if one is not available. With regard to the airway, certain anatomic differences in infants and children warrant special consideration. The younger the child, the more anterior and superior the position of the larynx in the neck, and the airway is relatively small and easily obstructed. Infants have a relatively large head and a short neck compared with older children and adults. Also, these small subjects have a relatively large tongue and small mandible, which makes infants obligate nose breathers. In addition to having a relatively small larynx, the epiglottis may be soft and collapse over the airway. Foreign material in the airway is prone to cause bronchospasm because of the relatively greater amount of smooth muscle in the immature tracheobronchial tree compared with that of older children and adults. If there is any degree of upper airway compromise, particularly if compounded by bronchospasm, lung volumes tend to diminish, and high pleural pressures tend to close distal airways even more. Airway resistance becomes extremely high, and the attendant increased work of breathing may exceed a small child's reserve. Consequently, there should be a low threshold for placement of an endotracheal tube and ventilatory support.

Airway obstruction related to injury may be compounded by the presence of chronically enlarged tonsils or facial fractures. Also, obstruction may be caused by vomitus of gastric material, blood, or teeth. Other factors that may interfere with respiratory function include central nervous system injury, severe thoracic trauma, gastric dilation, and abdominal distention. Physical findings that suggest airway obstruction include increased work of breathing, nasal flaring, marked retractions, wheezing, stridor, and cyanosis. Resultant hypoxemia may cause delirium, extreme agitation, or, if advanced, mental depression.

Initially the patient's pharynx should be suctioned free of secretions and any foreign material that may be present. A simple chin lift maneuver may establish a good airway, providing mask ventilation with oxygen at a rate of 5 L/min or greater, while avoiding hyperextension of the neck. In most instances, an oral airway may be helpful to hold the tongue forward. If there is any question about persistent airway obstruction or ability to breathe, orotracheal intubation should be performed. An orotracheal tube almost always can be placed except in rare instances in which there are extensive facial or laryngeal fractures, under which circumstances needle or incision cricothyroidotomy may be required. In very small subjects, cricothyroidotomy may cause long-term damage to the larynx, so tracheostomy is a better approach if orotracheal intubation cannot be performed. It is best to use an uncuffed endotracheal tube the size of the patient's fifth fingernail or one that would be expected to pass through the child's nares. Nasotracheal intubation is also useful, especially if an airway is to be needed for several days, but this route should not be used in patients with facial fractures or patients suspected of having cervicospinal injuries because of the hyperextension necessary for nasotracheal tube placement. Tracheobronchial toilet also is expedited by placement of an endotracheal tube.

When possible, mask ventilation with 100% oxygen should be performed before placement of an endotracheal tube. In agitated patients, appropriate doses of atropine and succinylcholine may be helpful, but cricoid

---

TABLE 11-1 ■ Initial Management of the Injured Child

Primary survey
  Establishment of a reliable airway
  Ventilation
  Establishment of large-bore intravenous lines
  Support of the circulation
  Rapid assessment of neurologic status
Secondary survey (performed if patient is stable)
  Diagnostic studies
  Establishment of surgical priorities
    Mass lesion in the brain
    Chest and abdominal injuries
    Peripheral vascular injuries
    Fractures

TABLE 11-2 ■ Normal Vital Signs by Age Group*			
Age (yr)	Heart Rate (beats/min)	Blood Pressure (mm Hg)	Respirations (resp/min)
0-1	120	80/40	40
1-5	100	100/60	30
5-10	80	120/80	20

*Urinary output should average 1 mL/kg/hr in all age groups.

pressure should be applied as the endotracheal tube is being placed if muscle relaxant is administered. It is helpful to pass the tube into the right main stem bronchus until breath sounds can be heard on only one side of the thorax, then to withdraw the tube gradually until good breath sounds can be heard bilaterally to take into account the relatively short length of the trachea in children. Tube position should be confirmed by radiograph as soon as feasible. All endotracheal tubes should be fixed carefully to the skin above the mouth so that movement of the tongue and mandible does not cause dislodgment.

Table 11-2 outlines the normal range of vital signs for various pediatric age groups. If ventilation is being supported via an endotracheal tube, the rate and depth of ventilation must be appropriate for the child's age, size, and degree of airway resistance. If there are complicating thoracic injuries, these must be appropriately addressed if ventilatory support is to be effective.

Because hyperventilation is a common initial response in children who are injured and in pain, gastric dilation may present a problem. A nasogastric tube should be passed into the stomach as soon as a secure airway is established. In patients with facial fractures, the gastric tube should be placed via the mouth to avoid passage into the cranium if the cribriform plate is fractured. This helps avoid vomiting and potential aspiration and further alleviates gastric dilation, which may impair diaphragmatic movement or obstruct caval venous return to the heart. Nasogastric tube placement is also an important feature of prehospital care before transportation of seriously injured children to a trauma center.

Shock and Circulatory Support

As soon as a secure airway and ventilatory support have been established, the patient's circulation should be assessed (Fig. 11-1). The presence of shock is usually clinically apparent. Infants and children tend to have mottling of the skin, cool and pale extremities, poor capillary refill, rapid and thready pulse, poor heart sounds, and diminished neurologic response even in the absence of head injury. Neck veins are usually collapsed, but when they are distended, intrathoracic injury, particularly tension pneumothorax, must be suspected. In small children, breath sounds are widely transmitted so that clinical diagnosis of a tension pneumothorax may be obscure. Thoracentesis or tube thoracostomy on the suspected side or even bilaterally is usually a safe course to follow. It is essential, however, to differentiate a pneumothorax from a main stem intubation, causing collapse of the opposite lung, absent breath sounds, and

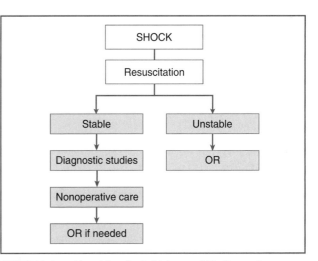

FIGURE 11-1 ■ Algorithm for initial care. OR, Operating room.

hyperresonance by percussion. If pericardial tamponade is suspected, pericardiocentesis is indicated (see Chapter 12).

The most common cause of shock in children is blood loss. Shock corresponds to loss of at least one fourth of blood volume. External bleeding usually can be controlled by pressure. Extensive lacerations of the scalp should be palpated initially, however, to determine if there is an underlying depressed skull fracture. Also, deep lacerations of the extremities may require either direct or digital compression of limb arteries until more specific measures can be taken. It is generally best to avoid tourniquets. The steps involved in initial management of shock include large-bore intravenous access, withdrawal of sufficient blood for initial laboratory studies and type and crossmatch, rapid determination of the site of volume loss when possible, and administration of sufficient fluids for resuscitation.

Intravenous access may be difficult in children because the vessels are small and extremely prone to vasoconstriction peripherally. A No. 20 or larger indwelling plastic cannula should be placed in a peripheral vein for rapid infusion of large volumes of fluids. A saphenous vein cutdown anterior to the medial malleolus at the ankle is a rapid and reliable approach for placement of a large-bore catheter. Experienced individuals may find percutaneous placement of femoral vein catheters useful as well, but it is best to avoid subclavian access in emergency situations. If venous access cannot be achieved immediately, intraosseous infusions allow rapid administration of resuscitation fluid. Routine laboratory studies include white blood cell and platelet counts, serum electrolytes and blood urea nitrogen, blood glucose, serum amylase, and type and crossmatch. When a secure intravenous line has been placed and resuscitation fluids given, additional infusion lines can be placed. If intraabdominal injury is suspected, an intravenous line should be secured above the level of the diaphragm. After that has been accomplished, central venous and arterial pressure monitoring catheters may be placed if needed.

Because blood loss is the most common cause of shock in children, this should be treated first. It should not be assumed that shock is from closed head or cardiac injury because these problems are rarely responsible for shock in children. Because shock is consistent with a volume loss of at least one fourth of blood volume, an equivalent amount or 20 mL/kg of body weight of Ringer's lactate should be administered initially along with 2 mEq/kg of sodium bicarbonate. If rapid infusion of Ringer's lactate solution restores blood pressure to normal levels that are maintained, no blood is likely to be required. If the initial infusion of 20 mL/kg of Ringer's lactate fails to restore blood pressure to a normal range or does so only temporarily, type-specific crossmatched red blood cells are required. If a child is exsanguinating and time does not permit appropriate crossmatching, type O blood should be given if type-specific blood is not available. During the time of rapid resuscitation, other members of the team should ensure that external hemorrhage has been controlled and that fractures are immobilized to prevent further loss of blood. If there is continuing evidence of hemorrhage, one must assume that there is hidden blood loss in the chest or abdomen. Acidosis should be neutralized on an ongoing basis and maintenance of body temperature should be ensured. In the case of pelvic fractures, appropriate immobilization should be ensured. If a child does not respond to these efforts, immediate laparotomy should be performed if bleeding is suspected to be intra-abdominal. If a child has had cardiac arrest, closed chest massage, control of external bleeding, and rapid fluid resuscitation usually restore the circulation. Rarely, emergency department thoracotomy, occlusion of the distal aorta, and open cardiac massage may be necessary. The last measure is probably fruitless in individuals who have had cardiac arrest in the field. Other than emergency department thoracotomy, however, all other operative procedures should be performed in the operating room rather than in the emergency department.

When airway control and adequate resuscitation have been accomplished, the final task in the primary survey is to assess the status of the central nervous system and to initiate appropriate diagnostic and therapeutic measures. Considerations relative to the central nervous system and other organ systems are detailed in the appropriate chapters in this book. Patients suspected to have severe central nervous system injury as evidenced by a Glasgow Coma Scale score of 7 or less should have immediate endotracheal intubation and ventilation. Immediately after the primary survey and, if possible, during resuscitation, a chest radiograph, a lateral film of the cervical spine, and a plain film of the pelvis should be performed. Additionally, it is helpful to assess the patient's condition initially by the Injury Severity Score and the Abbreviated Injury Scale or the Pediatric Trauma Score, all of which seem to give reliable data in children (Table 11-3).

Secondary Survey and Continuing Care

When airway control and stabilization of the circulation have been accomplished, diagnostic studies can be done, and the surgeon can determine whether immediate surgery is needed. Approximately 90% of children who have blunt trauma do not require operative intervention but need only close observation and support. It is generally best to administer broad-spectrum antibiotics when the

TABLE 11-3 ■ Injury Evaluation Scoring Systems

I. Injury Severity Score (ISS)
A. Abbreviated Injury Scale (AIS) (used to calculate the ISS)*

AIS Code	Description
1	Minor
2	Moderate
3	Serious
4	Severe
5	Critical
6	Maximum
9	Unknown

B. ISS

The sum of the squares of the highest AIS in each of the ISS body regions:
1. Head and neck
2. Face
3. Chest
4. Abdomen and pelvic contents
5. Extremities and pelvic ring
6. External

Pediatric Trauma Score†

	Category		
Component	+2	+1	−1
Size	>20 kg	10-20 kg	<10 kg
Airway	Normal	Maintainable	Unmaintainable
Systolic BP	>90 mm Hg	90-50 mm Hg	<50 mm Hg
CNS	Awake	Obtunded/ LOC	Coma/decerebrate
Open wound	None	Minor	Major/penetrating
Skeletal	None	Closed fracture	Open/multiple fractures

Note: Both the ISS and Pediatric Trauma Score scoring systems correlate with survival outcome in children.
*Each organ or body structure injured has a specific code modified by the adjacent number corresponding to the severity of injury to that structure.
†Sum of grades for each of six categories. This is a physiologically based scoring system.
BP, Blood pressure; CNS, central nervous system; LOC, loss of consciousness.

patient is first seen, but their continuation depends on further definition of the extent and type of injury. Several days of observation and evaluation are required because many forms of blunt injury are not evident at the outset. These include delayed necrosis of the wall of the jejunum or duodenum, traumatic pancreatitis, establishment of infection in an extensive pulmonary contusion, and delayed manifestations of urinary extravasation associated with renal fractures.

Patients with head injuries, facial fractures, and suspected cervicospinal fractures are evaluated best by computed tomography (CT) scan. CT scans with intravenous and intragastric contrast agents also are useful for evaluation of chest and abdominal injuries. If an injury to the thoracic aorta is suspected, helical CT with contrast or angiography is indicated. In the emergency department, focused abdominal sonography for trauma (FAST) may be useful to screen the abdomen for the presence of blood or fluid. Although diagnostic peritoneal lavage was used extensively in the past, it is rarely used now with improvements in CT. If a bladder injury is suspected, particularly in the presence of extensive pelvic fractures, a cystourethrogram should be performed using retrograde filling if necessary.

Fluid administration must be adjusted to maintain normal blood pressure, pulse, and urine output in the range of 1 mL/kg/hr. Maintenance of adequate urine output is one good indication of adequate replacement of intravascular and extravascular fluid losses. Also, resolution of acidosis further indicates adequate volume replacement. One of the problems identified with rapid, massive fluid administration for the treatment of shock is the problem of overresuscitation and production of the abdominal compartment syndrome as a feature of massive edema production. Many measures have been advised to monitor for compartment syndrome, including monitoring of bladder pressure and serial monitoring of intra-abdominal pressure along with following peak inspiratory pressures on ventilation. The emphasis on rapid, aggressive fluid resuscitation must be balanced by the avoidance of excessive resuscitation. When fluid resuscitation equals 25% of total body weight, resuscitation regimens should be reassessed to reduce the incidence of excessive resuscitation, while maintaining normal organ function. The injured patient is observed best in an intensive care unit initially with constant monitoring. Skeletal injuries should be treated by external fixation, and head and thoracic injuries should be observed carefully and treated supportively. Patients who have undergone significant periods of shock still may be unstable and require inotropic support and more specific

monitoring, including central venous pressure and pulmonary capillary wedge pressure monitoring. Central venous pressures should be maintained in the range of 5 to 10 cm of saline solution, and pulmonary capillary wedge pressures as measured by a Swan-Ganz catheter should be maintained in the range of 10 mm Hg. Patients who are thought to have adequate volume replacement but who are still hypotensive may require vasoactive drugs. Dopamine at a dosage of 2 to 10 or higher µg/kg/min may be useful, but continuous hemodynamic monitoring is required under such circumstances. The priorities in emergency management are detailed in Table 11-4 and are considered in subsequent chapters.

SUGGESTED READINGS

Advanced Trauma Life Support Program. Chicago, American College of Surgeons, 1998.

The ATLS program is an all-encompassing educational course dealing with all aspects of trauma, including initial evaluation, resuscitation, advanced diagnosis, and treatment. All individuals who treat injured children should be thoroughly familiar with this course.

Kincaid EH, Chang MC, Letton RW, et al: Admission base deficit in pediatric trauma: A study using the National Trauma Data Bank. J Trauma 51:332-335, 2001.

Acidosis is a primary indicator of mortality and an appropriate focus for aggressive treatment.

O'Neill JA: Advances in the management of pediatric trauma. Am J Surg 180:365-369, 2000.

The various factors related to improved pediatric trauma care, such as the development of specialized pediatric trauma centers and better understanding and translation of basic science advances to trauma treatment programs for children, are reviewed in this article.

Saggi BH, Sugerman HJ, Ivatury RR, Bloomfield GL: Abdominal compartment syndrome. J Trauma 45:597-609, 1998.

This excellent review thoroughly describes the various factors involved in the production of massive edema and abdominal hypertension. These observations have been extended to burns and sepsis, indicating that there are limits to resuscitation.

Turi RA, Petros AJ, Eaton S, et al: Energy metabolism of infants and children with systemic inflammatory response syndrome and sepsis. Ann Surg 233:581-587, 2001.

The authors analyze metabolic rate and support in patients with SIRS and sepsis compared with normals. The differences were minimal in infants compared with the situation in adults who are characteristically hypermetabolic, probably because infants and small children represent a two-compartment system, one for growth that can switch to one related to adaptation to injury. Children with severe injury do become hypermetabolic, however.

TABLE 11-4 ■ Priorities in Emergency Management

Immediate
  Cardiorespiratory compromise by chest, neck, and facial
    injuries
  Severe external hemorrhage
High priority
  Retroperitoneal and intraperitoneal injury
  Head and spinal injury
  Severe burns
  Extensive soft tissue injury
  Long bone fractures
Next priority
  Genitourinary injury
  Peripheral vascular, nerve, and muscle injury
  Limited soft tissue injury

12

Thoracic Injuries

Thoracic injuries in children are second only to head injuries as causes of mortality, accounting for approximately one fourth of pediatric trauma deaths. The overall mortality of chest injuries among hospitalized children is 15% to 22%. The mortality of an isolated chest injury is about 4%. The presence of an associated extrathoracic injury increases the mortality to 29%. The highest mortality (>50%) is with associated head and neck injuries, with the cause of death related to the head injury (Table 12-1).

As with all pediatric trauma, blunt injuries predominate over penetrating mechanisms (83% versus 15%). The mortality rates associated with blunt (15%) and penetrating (14%) trauma are approximately equal. The thoracic injury is the cause of death, however, in only 14% of deaths from blunt mechanisms, whereas in 97% of penetrating injuries the cause of death is the chest injury itself. Nearly three fourths of blunt injuries in children involve motor vehicle crashes (occupant, 41%; pedestrian, 33%). Street violence involving guns (60% of all penetrating chest injuries) and knives (33%) is more common in adolescents.

Anatomic and physiologic characteristics of the pediatric respiratory system work against a child with an injury to the airway or chest. The upper airway, larynx, and tracheobronchial tree are much smaller in children than in adults and are more susceptible to obstruction by saliva, mucus, blood, and foreign bodies or by collapse of the soft tissues of the mouth and tongue. The larynx is positioned higher in the neck than in adults and is tilted in a cephalad angle. Direct laryngoscopy is a difficult task, and esophageal intubation is a distressingly frequent complication. The trachea is relatively short, measuring only 5 cm in length in infants. Right main stem bronchial intubation is also a common complication of management. Distal airways, already narrow in small children, are subject to obstruction by relatively small amounts of edema or bronchospasm.

Infants and small children have a compliant chest wall, a product of thin, cartilaginous ribs and weak chest muscles. The chest wall tends to collapse rather than expand when the patient increases respiratory effort to compensate for the effects of a chest injury (seen clinically as sternal retractions). The thin chest wall offers little protection to the underlying lung and heart from blunt injury mechanisms, allowing significant lung and cardiac injuries (usually contusions) without radiographic evidence of rib fractures.

The mediastinum in children is freely mobile, an anatomic feature that magnifies the effects of a tension pneumothorax. The heart is pushed to the contralateral chest wall, collapsing the contralateral lung and impairing venous return by angulating the cavae.

INITIAL EVALUATION AND TREATMENT

Thoracic injuries directly interfere with the airway and breathing, two of the basic priorities of trauma care. The early recognition and prompt management of significant chest injuries is a major challenge in pediatric trauma care.

Assessment of the adequacy of the airway and breathing is the initial step in management. While maintaining a neutral head position to minimize motion of the cervical spine, the mouth and pharynx are examined and cleared of any foreign material. Oxygen is given by mask. If there is evidence of airway obstruction, a chin-lift or jaw-thrust maneuver may open an airway obstructed by soft tissues. If obstruction persists or if ventilatory efforts are inadequate, immediate orotracheal intubation is required. An early priority is the passage of a nasogastric or orogastric tube to alleviate gastric distention and diminish the chance of vomiting and aspiration.

A clinical assessment of the adequacy of respiratory function includes level of consciousness, tachycardia or

TABLE 12-1 ■ Mortality and Intrathoracic Organ Injured	
Organ Injured	%
Vascular injuries	50
Esophagus	43
Heart	40
Bronchi	20
Open wounds	19
Lungs	18
Diaphragm	16
Fractures	11

National Pediatric Trauma Registry data, 1985-1991.

bradycardia, skin color, and cyanosis. Bradycardia and cyanosis are late findings, reflecting severe arterial desaturation. Anxiety and restlessness, signs of hypoxia, require a work-up for respiratory distress. Sedatives should not be given. Oxygen should be provided by mask. Physical findings should be confirmed by pulse oximetry, arterial blood gas determinations, and chest radiograph.

Abrasions and contusions over the chest suggest a potential chest injury. Gentle compression of the chest locates areas of tenderness, crepitus, and instability. Physical findings that reflect significant thoracic injury include paradoxic movement of the chest wall, a sucking wound, tracheal or mediastinal shift, diminished or absent breath sounds, distant heart sounds, or subcutaneous air. If tension pneumothorax is suspected, immediate needle aspiration or placement of a chest tube without a confirmatory chest film is required. Hypotension with physical evidence of chest trauma is an indication for the immediate placement of a chest tube on the suspected side. Other details of resuscitation are given in Chapter 11.

When airway, breathing, and circulatory priorities have been addressed, diagnostic studies can be initiated. Because 95% of patients with penetrating chest injuries and nearly all patients with blunt chest trauma may be treated without thoracotomy, it is usually possible to complete specific diagnostic studies. A plain x-ray of the chest is a routine part of the secondary trauma survey. Other studies used selectively to augment and refine diagnostic information are computed tomography (CT) with intravenous contrast, bronchoscopy, esophagoscopy, electrocardiogram (ECG), echocardiography, angiography, creatine phosphokinase isoenzyme levels, pericardiocentesis, and video-assisted thoracoscopy. The applications of each of these studies are discussed subsequently.

BASIC TECHNIQUES FOR EMERGENCY MANAGEMENT

Cricothyroidotomy and Tracheotomy

Endotracheal intubation is discussed in Chapter 11. When an endotracheal tube cannot be passed (an exceedingly rare occurrence), cricothyroidotomy or tracheotomy is indicated. Cricothyroidotomy is difficult in infants because the thyroid cartilage overlaps the cricoid cartilage and obscures the cricothyroid membrane. If a surgical airway is needed, a "slash" tracheotomy quickly gives wide exposure to the upper airway. A generous transverse incision is made over the child's neck, halfway between the thyroid cartilage and the sternal notch. A vertical incision is made through the second and third, or third and fourth, tracheal rings without resecting any part of the tracheal wall. A standard endotracheal tube should be used initially for ventilation until an appropriate tracheostomy tube is available. If cricothyroidotomy is performed, it should be converted to a tracheotomy as soon as possible to avoid permanent damage to the larynx, particularly in children younger than age 6 years. Surgical airways performed under emergency conditions have a high incidence of complications.

Thoracentesis

Continued respiratory distress despite supplemental oxygen or assisted ventilation suggests the presence of a pneumothorax, hemothorax, or hemopneumothorax. In trauma management, thoracentesis is a temporizing measure allowing decompression of the thorax until a chest tube can be placed. The most direct approach is in the midclavicular line in the second intercostal space, using a plastic intravenous cannula. The cannula is left in place until a chest tube is placed in the thorax and its function is confirmed.

Tube Thoracostomy

Under certain circumstances, including tension pneumothorax, hemothorax, open chest wound, and flail chest, placement of a chest tube is required on an emergency basis before obtaining a chest film. The tube is placed into the side of the chest suspected to have pneumothorax or on the side ipsilateral to the location of positive physical findings of injury, such as abrasions, lacerations, or crepitus. A tube equal in diameter to the span of the intercostal space is inserted in the fifth intercostal space, directly lateral to the nipple, in the midaxillary line. The tube is placed obliquely to the apex, then sutured in place, dressed, and placed on suction (Fig. 12-1).

Complications of chest tube placement include empyema, undrained hemothorax or pneumothorax, improper position, recurrent pneumothorax or hemothorax after chest tube removal, and direct lung injuries. Complication rates range from 6% to 38%, depending in part on whether a surgeon, emergency physician, or prehosptial provider places the chest tube. Administration of antibiotics while the chest tube is in place decreases the incidence of infection.

Pericardiocentesis

Aspiration of the pericardial sac is indicated when pericardial tamponade is suspected because of hypotension, distended neck veins, and distant heart sounds. Careful judgment must be exercised in determining whether the procedure is best done in the emergency department or the operating room. Figure 12-2 shows the technique for pericardiocentesis. A plastic-sheathed needle is passed gently upward and slightly to the left of the xiphoid process. As soon as blood is seen, the needle is removed from the catheter and the blood aspirated. An alternate technique is to use a stainless steel needle connected to an ECG lead to minimize the risk of unintentional myocardial puncture.

SPECIFIC THORACIC INJURIES ACCORDING TO PRIORITY

Although specific injuries are discussed, they always should be considered in relation to other organ system and body region injuries that may be present (Table 12-2). Nonetheless the high mortality of patients with thoracic injuries, whether solitary or combined with other injuries, warrants an immediate and aggressive approach to management.

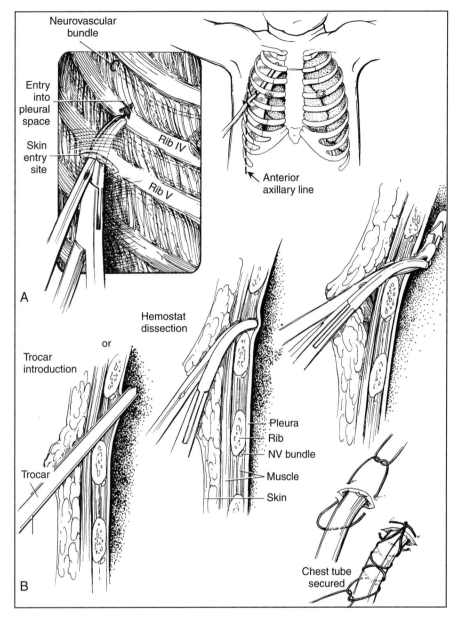

FIGURE 12-1 ■ **A,** A small hemostat is inserted through a small incision in the anterior axillary line and is tunneled upward, entering the chest above the next rib. The chest tube is inserted and secured with a suture ligature. **B,** A trocar can be used as an alternative method of insertion.

Life-Threatening Injuries

Direct Injuries of the Upper Airway

Direct injuries of the upper airway are uncommon injuries that result from direct trauma to the neck, such as "clothesline" injuries. Associated esophageal and cervical spine injuries are encountered commonly. The two most common injuries are fracture of the larynx and transection of the trachea just below the cricoid. Physical examination reveals bruises and abrasions over the anterior aspect of the neck, subcutaneous emphysema, stridor, and dyspnea. Immediate control of the airway is necessary, by either endotracheal intubation or tracheotomy, followed by primary repair of the airway and associated injuries.

Tension Pneumothorax

Pneumothorax is the most common manifestation of thoracic injury associated with an air leak. Progressive accumulation of air in the pleural space may collapse the ipsilateral lung and push the mediastinum into the contralateral hemithorax and angulate the cavae to the point where venous return becomes compromised (Fig. 12-3). Cardiovascular collapse may follow. Tension pneumothorax should be suspected in any hypotensive patient with external evidence of chest injury.

The classic physical findings of tension pneumothorax include ipsilateral absent or diminished breath sounds and hyperresonance to percussion, shift of the trachea to the contralateral side, and distended neck veins. Because infants and small children have short necks, the evaluation of tracheal position and neck vein distention is difficult. Infants with open fontanelles may have bulging of the anterior fontanelle as a sign of elevated central venous pressure. Signs of imminent cardiovascular collapse may be present, such as tachycardia; cool, clammy extremities; depressed sensorium; and hypotension. Thoracentesis is

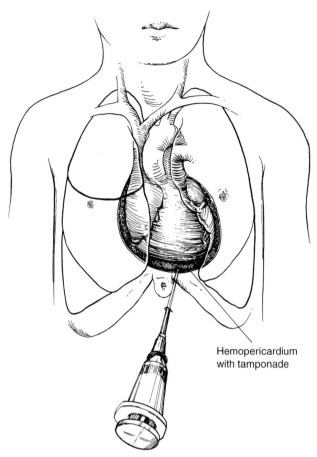

Hemopericardium
with tamponade

FIGURE 12-2 ■ The safest and simplest method of performing pericardiocentesis for diagnosis and temporizing treatment of pericardial tamponade. If significant amounts of blood are obtained, thoracotomy is in order.

always justified under these circumstances, with needle placement into the side of the chest with signs of injury, including bruising, abrasions, crepitus, or gross instability, to permit lung expansion and normal positioning of the mediastinum.

TABLE 12-2 ■ Treatment Priorities in Thoracic Trauma

Life-threatening injuries
   Airway injuries
   Tension pneumothorax
   Massive hemothorax
   Cardiac injury and tamponade
   Flail chest
   Open pneumothorax
Potentially life-threatening injuries
   Extensive pulmonary parenchymal injuries
   Tracheobronchial injuries
   Myocardial contusion
   Diaphragmatic rupture
   Esophageal rupture
   Impending aortic rupture
Less serious injuries
   Simple pneumothorax
   Traumatic asphyxia

If there is any question about the appropriate side for thoracentesis, bilateral aspiration is appropriate. Placement of an adequate-sized chest tube should follow.

Massive Hemothorax

Massive hemothorax and hemopneumothorax have pathophysiologic effects similar to those of tension pneumothorax. Massive hemothorax is caused by an injury to a major vascular structure or an intercostal artery. Although patients with tension pneumothorax have distended neck veins, patients with hemothorax lack venous distention because of hypovolemia. In the latter condition, the chest is dull to percussion, whereas in the former the chest is hyperresonant.

Initial treatment is by tube thoracostomy. The rate of bleeding determines whether urgent thoracotomy is needed. Vigorous volume replacement must be initiated before evacuating blood from the chest and decompressing what central venous pressure is present. In most cases, tube thoracostomy drainage and restoration of normal circulating blood volume is all that is required. If bleeding exceeds 20 mL per kg of body weight or threatens to reach that level over a short time, thoracotomy is indicated.

Cardiovascular Injuries and Tamponade

Blunt trauma to the chest seldom produces significant cardiac or aortic injuries in young children, probably because the mobility of the structures of the mediastinum

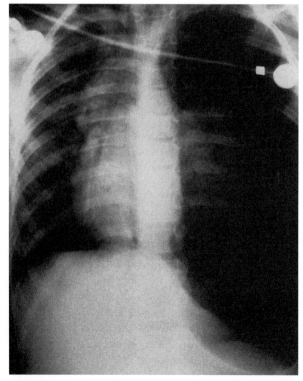

FIGURE 12-3 ■ Chest film obtained in the emergency department on an 8-year-old child who sustained severe blunt thoracic injury shows marked mediastinal shift associated with hypotension and hypoxemia typical of severe tension pneumothorax. Vital signs returned to normal after placement of a chest tube.

in younger age groups are somehow protective. With adolescent patients, cardiac and major vascular injuries associated with violent mechanisms (e.g., high-speed motor vehicle crashes, gunshots, and stab wounds) are more common.

Cardiac tamponade results from the accumulation of blood, fluid, or air within the pericardium. The most frequent cause of cardiac tamponade is penetrating injury to the heart from a gunshot or stab wound. Infrequently, barotraumas from positive-pressure ventilation may cause air to accumulate under pressure in the pericardium. Cardiac output often can be maintained until the volume of extracardiac fluid or air compresses the cardiac chambers to the point where filling is inadequate to maintain cardiac output. The patient exhibits shock with increased central venous pressure. The classic signs of cardiac tamponade are diminished heart sounds, decreased arterial blood pressure and pulse pressure, and jugular venous distinction. On chest x-ray, the cardiac silhouette may be enlarged or assume a rounded shape. Echocardiography can confirm the presence of fluid within the pericardium, but this study should be obtained only if the patient's condition allows.

Decompression of the pericardium is necessary to correct cardiac tamponade. Pericardiocentesis may relieve the condition to the point where transfer to the operating room can take place. It should be considered as a temporary maneuver, however, until the underlying injury can be repaired. Placement of a chest tube into the pericardium through a small incision just to the left of the xiphoid may be sufficient in cases of tamponade caused by pneumopericardium. Hemopericardium from the accumulation of blood leaking from a cardiac injury requires open repair, however. If time and the patient's condition permit, it is safest to perform pericardiocentesis in the operating room so that immediate thoracotomy or sternotomy can be performed with equipment and personnel available for total cardiopulmonary or left heart bypass.

Cardiac contusion is seen mainly in adolescents. It should be suspected in patients who have had significant blunt injuries of the anterior chest, if cardiac output remains low despite what is considered to be adequate restoration of blood volume, or if ectopy or arrhythmias develop on ECG monitoring. Echocardiography rules out cardiac tamponade. Although there is no absolute test for cardiac contusion, kinesis or dyskinesis on echocardiography or elevated creatine phosphokinase MB or troponin I levels confirm the diagnosis. Supportive care for myocardial contusion is the same as that for myocardial infarction, with continuous monitoring of ECG and treatment of arrhythmias and use of inotropes as needed.

Aortic rupture most often occurs below the takeoff of the left subclavian artery or at the ligamentum arteriosum. A false aneurysm develops, with blood traversing the gap in the aorta, which may be completely transected. Blood leaks from the area, leading to characteristic findings on chest x-ray, including widening of the mediastinal silhouette, flattening of the left heart contour, and an apical "cap" overlying the apex of the left lung. Fracture of the first or second rib, sternum, or

scapula reflects a violent transfer of energy to the chest, a circumstance that may put the aorta at risk for rupture. Aortic rupture often is present without any of these associated fractures, however. Although contrast-enhanced CT may show an aortic tear, aortography is the most definitive study for confirmation of the diagnosis. Immediate repair is indicated. Consideration should be given to preserve spinal cord and distal aortic blood flow either with a vascular shunt or with a left ventricular bypass.

Echocardiography also can detect patients who have traumatic ventricular septal defects or ruptured chordae from sudden compressive injuries of the heart. Clinical signs of traumatic asphyxia may be present, such as subconjunctival hemorrhages and upper body petechiae and plethora. Early repair of traumatic intracardiac defects should be performed with cardiopulmonary bypass.

Flail Chest

When significant blunt trauma results in two or more ribs being fractured in more than one location, a segment of the chest wall becomes unstable and disconnected from the solid portion of the thoracic cage, and normal respiratory excursion is impaired. The flail segment responds to the changes in intrathoracic pressure rather than to the influence of the respiratory muscles. On inspiration, the flail segment retracts inward rather than expanding outward. On expiration, it pushes outward rather than retracting. Fractures that extend over lateral and posterior aspects of the thorax also may impair diaphragmatic motion, further compromising ventilation. As the flail segment pushes in during inspiration, the mediastinum shifts toward the contralateral lung, compressing it. Because of the force required to produce multiple rib fractures, the underlying lung invariably is injured as well. Pulmonary contusion fills the alveoli with blood and edema, interfering with gas exchange and decreasing pulmonary compliance. Because the chest wall is pliable in young children, flail chest primarily is a problem in children older than age 12 years.

A flail chest in a patient with respiratory distress is usually obvious on inspection, with the involved area moving paradoxically and having overlying abrasions and ecchymoses. Pneumothorax and hemothorax often accompany flail chest. These patients require supplemental oxygen and correction of hypovolemia. Excessive fluid administration must be avoided to minimize the accumulation of pulmonary edema in the underlying pulmonary contusion. An associated pneumothorax or hemothorax should be treated appropriately. Intercostal nerve blocks with 0.25% or 0.5% bupivacaine and morphine administration are helpful to control severe pain.

Inadequate gas exchange, documented on arterial blood gas levels, associated with a significant flail requires endotracheal intubation and ventilatory support with sufficient positive end-expiratory pressure to splint the flail segment outward. Controlled ventilation is continued until chest wall stability is re-established and pulmonary contusion clears.

Open Pneumothorax

Impalement, usually the result of motor vehicle crashes, produces a gaping hole in the chest cavity through which air freely enters and exits (hence the equivalent term, *sucking chest wound*) as the patient struggles to breathe. The ipsilateral lung collapses, and the mediastinum shifts into the contralateral thorax during inspiration, further compromising ventilation. Open pneumothorax is exceedingly rare in children.

Immediate treatment is to cover the defect with petroleum gauze and a dressing taped on three sides and to place a chest tube. The wound should be débrided and closed primarily if possible. Intravenous antibiotics are indicated because the surrounding soft tissues are generally contused and are prone to infection.

Potentially Life-Threatening Injuries

Some injuries, although potentially lethal, permit sufficient time for stabilization of the patient's ventilatory and circulatory status and performance of sufficient diagnostic studies to make a precise diagnosis. If these injuries go unrecognized, however, they can prove to be fatal.

Lung Injuries

Laceration of the lung may result from penetrating trauma or when rib fractures puncture the visceral pleura. Pneumothorax or sometimes hemopneumothorax results and usually is managed easily with a chest tube. Physical findings include hemoptysis and crepitus from a fractured rib or subcutaneous air. A chest film confirms the diagnosis. Only rarely is thoracotomy needed to control a large or persistent air leak or bleeding.

Pulmonary contusions are areas of hemorrhage, edema, and atelectasis within the lung parenchyma from direct injury. With large or multiple contusions, hypoxemia may result from ventilation-perfusion mismatching. Overhydration must be avoided to minimize accumulation of fluid within the damaged area of lung. The initial therapeutic approach is supportive with supplemental oxygen, fluid restriction, and antibiotics. Assisted ventilation may be required, depending on the degree of physiologic impairment. In mild and limited cases, recovery is prompt, usually within 1 week. More extensive contusions may require 3 weeks to resolve.

After severe lung injuries, post-traumatic pseudocysts may develop within the lung. In childhood, nearly all slowly resolve over time. Some may become infected and form lung abscesses. Intravenous antibiotics and percutaneous CT-guided placement of drainage catheters are effective initial measures should a lung abscess develop. Occasionally, open operative intervention is required.

Tracheobronchial Injuries

Either penetrating or blunt injuries may disrupt the intrathoracic trachea or bronchi. In blunt trauma, tracheobronchial injury results from a sudden deceleration that avulses the main stem bronchus at the level of the carina. Also, forceful compression of the chest against a closed glottis may tear the membranous portion of the trachea, usually within 2 to 3 cm of the carina. Most injuries from blunt trauma are within 1 or 2 inches of the carina.

A major tracheobronchial injury causes hemoptysis and subcutaneous emphysema. Pneumothorax is often under tension and bilateral. A chest tube releases pleural

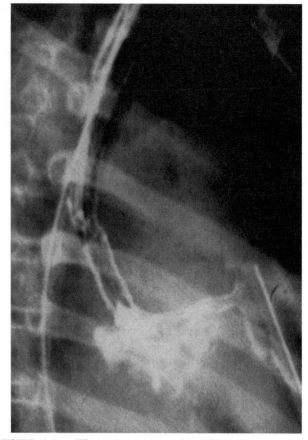

FIGURE 12-4 ■ This patient presented with blunt thoracic trauma and had a persistent massive air leak despite tube thoracostomy drainage. This metrizamide bronchogram shows an injury of the left main stem bronchus, which required emergency repair.

air that continuously drains on suction (Fig. 12-4). The lungs fail to re-expand completely after chest tube placement. Flexible bronchoscopy usually shows the injury because most are near the level of the carina. More distal injuries may require bronchography.

Tears of the intrathoracic trachea and major bronchi require direct repair. Tears located more distally often respond to high-frequency low-pressure ventilation. Bronchoscopic instillation of fibrin glue may seal distal bronchial leaks. If these measures fail, segmental resection or lobectomy may be required. If the patient's condition permits, associated pulmonary contusion should be allowed to resolve before attempting resection.

Myocardial Contusion

See earlier under Cardiovascular Injuries and Tamponade.

Diaphragmatic Rupture

Penetrating injuries may lacerate the diaphragm directly. Sudden increases in intra-abdominal pressure caused by extreme blunt forces usually rupture the diaphragm through the central tendon. Of injuries, 80% involve the left diaphragm; the remainder are right-sided or bilateral. Associated injuries, often involving the spleen or kidney, are almost always present. In about half of cases, the diagnosis is not made until days to weeks later, with gradually progressive respiratory impairment. Diagnosis usually is suggested on plain films with basilar opacification and obliteration of a clear diaphragmatic border. A nasogastric tube may identify an intrathoracic position of the stomach. CT with oral and intravenous contrast agents may help in identifying other intra-abdominal organs herniated into the chest.

If the diagnosis is made shortly after injury, the repair is done best through a laparotomy because of the high incidence of associated intra-abdominal injuries. When in the abdomen, the integrity of both diaphragms should be checked. Thoracotomy is an appropriate approach in situations in which the diagnosis has been delayed because the herniated viscera may have developed troublesome adhesions within the chest.

Esophageal Rupture

Almost all esophageal injuries are related to penetrating mechanisms and related to endoscopic or dilation procedures. Shearing injuries of the esophagus may accompany laryngeal and tracheal injuries, but intrathoracic esophageal rupture from blunt trauma does not seem to occur. Boerhaave's syndrome, rupture of the esophagus with forceful vomiting, is a problem only in adolescents, and even then it is rare.

Esophageal injury may be suspected whenever penetrating injuries appear to extend into the region of the esophagus or when endoscopic or dilation procedures have been difficult. If not recognized immediately, leakage of saliva and gastric juice into the mediastinum produces mediastinitis with fever, chest pain, and subcutaneous emphysema without pneumothorax. If esophageal injury is suspected, a water-soluble contrast esophagram must be performed. If extravasation of contrast material is found, immediate repair with wide mediastinal drainage and broad-spectrum antibiotics are in order.

Impending Aortic Rupture

Injury to the heart and great vessels has been discussed earlier. Most patients with free aortic rupture die at the scene. Patients with a contained false aneurysm on contrast CT, magnetic resonance angiography, or aortography should have urgent repair using an aortic shunt or left ventricular bypass.

Less Serious Injuries

Simple Pneumothorax

Pneumothorax with minimal lung collapse may cause a minimum of discomfort and few respiratory symptoms. The safest approach to all patients with pneumothorax is tube thoracostomy. If a patient with a pneumothorax has an injury in another body region that requires surgical repair, a chest tube always must be placed before endotracheal intubation and induction of anesthesia.

Traumatic Asphyxia

Sudden compressive injury of the chest constricts the superior vena cava and heart, causing widespread petechial hemorrhage over the upper part of the body, the conjunctivae, and brain. It is primarily a problem in children. Although the condition itself is not considered to be dangerous, the presence of traumatic asphyxia

reflects significant crushing forces. Associated intrathoracic and intra-abdominal injuries may be present along with pulmonary impairment and transient central nervous system dysfunction.

INDICATIONS FOR OPERATIVE INTERVENTION IN THORACIC TRAUMA

In nearly all cases of chest injury, tube thoracostomy drainage and ventilatory support are sufficient treatment. Of all cases of penetrating injuries of the chest, fewer than 2% of cases with pneumothorax and 10% of cases with hemothorax require thoracotomy. Table 12-3 lists the generally accepted indications for thoracotomy either on an emergency or a delayed basis.

As a general rule, emergency department thoracotomy for cardiac tamponade should be considered for children with penetrating injuries with vital signs or mentation in the field or on arrival to the emergency department. Survival from emergency department thoracotomy under such circumstances is 50%, whereas survival of patients without vital signs in the field nears zero. Survival is highest among patients with a single stab wound or low-velocity gunshot wound (e.g., an air rifle). Survival nears zero in patients with cardiac tamponade from multiple stab wounds, high-velocity gunshot wounds, or blunt trauma.

The volume and rate of blood loss in cases of massive hemothorax determine the need for thoracotomy. The risk of death increases linearly with the volume and rate of chest hemorrhage. A standard based on data derived from adults suggests that thoracotomy is indicated when total chest tube output exceeds 1500 mL in 24 hours, a volume roughly 25% to 30% of the total blood volume, or about 20 to 25 mL/kg body weight in children. With life-threatening rates of blood loss, immediate thoracotomy should be performed.

Video-assisted thoracic surgery (VATS) has a diagnostic and therapeutic role in the treatment of patients with chest trauma. The procedure seems to have particular value in situations in which recovery does not progress as

---

TABLE 12-3 ▪ Indications for Operation in Thoracic Trauma

Thoracotomy immediately or shortly after injury
  Massive continuing pneumothorax
  Cardiac tamponade
  Open pneumothorax
  Esophageal injury
  Massive air leak from tracheobronchial injury
  Aortic or other vascular injury
  Acute rupture of the diaphragm
Delayed thoracotomy
  Chronic rupture of the diaphragm
  Clotted hemothorax
  Persistent chylothorax
  Traumatic intracardiac defects
  Evacuation of large foreign bodies
  Chronic atelectasis from traumatic bronchial stenosis

expected and as a diagnostic adjunct in problem cases. One example is a persistent air leak after tube thoracostomy for pneumothorax. Thoracoscopy identifies the source and allows stapled repair of the pleural tear or segmental resection of the injured lung. Another example is failure of full lung expansion because of clotted hemothorax, risking later development of an empyema or a restrictive fibrous peel. VATS allows complete evacuation of blood clots, empyema material, and fibrin.

SUGGESTED READINGS

Black TL, Snyder CL, Miller JP, et al: Significance of chest trauma in children. South Med J 89:494-496, 1996.

This review of 1356 pediatric trauma patients over a 2.5-year period identified 82 patients with chest injuries. The data suggest that chest injuries seen in children, usually rib fractures and contusions, are not associated with a high mortality unless an associated extrathoracic injury is present.

Cooper A, Barlow B, DiScala C, et al: Mortality and truncal injury: The pediatric perspective. J Pediatr Surg 29:33-38, 1994.

This article summarizes data from the National Pediatric Trauma Registry from 1985 through 1991. Of all 25,301 reported cases, 1553 (6%) involved intrathoracic injuries.

In nearly all penetrating injuries, the cause of death was the chest injury itself.

Inci I, Ozcelik C, Nizam O, et al: Penetrating chest injuries in children: A review of 94 cases. J Pediatr Surg 31:673-676, 1996.

Tube thoracostomy alone was sufficient in the management of 79.8% of cases. Thoracotomy was performed in only 4.3% of patients.

Karmy-Jones R, Jurkovich GJ, Nathens AB, et al: Timing of urgent thoracotomy after trauma: A multicenter study. Arch Surg 136:513-518, 2001.

In this study of 157 adult patients, the risk of death increased linearly with the volume of blood loss from chest injury. The authors recommend thoracotomy for losses that exceed 1500 mL within 24 hours.

Lowdermilk GA, Naunheim KS: Thoracoscopic evaluation and treatment of thoracic trauma. Surg Clin North Am 80:1535-1542, 2000.

The indications, techniques, and possible applications of VATS in chest injuries are reviewed.

von Oppell UO, Bautz P, De Groot M: Penetrating thoracic injuries: What we have learnt. Thorac Cardiovasc Surg 48:55-61, 2000.

This is a summary of the management of 1000 patients annually with penetrating chest injuries.

Abdominal and Genitourinary Trauma

13

Most abdominal injuries in childhood are due to blunt injury mechanisms, of which nearly 60% are automobile-related (Table 13-1). Falls, bicycle injuries, and child abuse also are significant causes of injury in pediatric age groups. Abdominal injuries are present in 10% to 20% of automobile-related injuries and 5% to 15% of falls. Blunt trauma mostly affects solid organs—spleen, liver, and kidney (Table 13-2).

Many factors make children particularly vulnerable to abdominal injury. The abdominal wall and lower rib cage are relatively thin in children and provide little protection to the underlying organs. The liver and kidneys lie relatively lower in the abdomen in children, making them particularly vulnerable to direct trauma. Retroperitoneal structures, such as the kidneys and pancreas, lie only a short distance away from the anterior abdominal wall in thin children. The liver occupies a relatively large percentage of the abdominal cavity, further exposing it to injury.

Three specific blunt injury mechanisms deserve mention: handlebar injuries, lap belt injuries, and child abuse. A fall onto a set of handlebars causes a focused blow to the liver, pancreas, duodenum, or jejunum. Lap belt injuries produce a nearly pathognomonic triad of anterior abdominal abrasion, intestinal perforation, and lumbar spine fracture. Intentional injuries to infants most often involve the head and face and extremities. Evidence of torso injuries, such as rib fractures and contusions, should be sought as well. Although any intra-abdominal organ can be injured from abuse, duodenal hematoma is one that is particularly associated with deliberate injury in infancy.

Penetrating injuries primarily affect adolescent victims of violence, with gunshots predominating and a significant number of stab wounds. The spectrum of organs injured from penetrating mechanisms differs. Intestinal injuries are present in more than two thirds of penetrating abdominal injuries, with an increasing proportion of vascular injuries.

The mortality of blunt abdominal injury among hospitalized patients (9%) is higher than penetrating injuries (6%) because blunt mechanisms more often affect multiple body areas, particularly the head and chest, where injuries carry a higher risk of death. Intra-abdominal vascular injuries carry the highest mortality (47%), followed by injuries to the liver (13%), gastrointestinal tract (11%), spleen (11%), pelvis (7%), kidneys (7%), pancreas (7%), and lower urinary tract including the bladder (3%).

Examination of the abdomen is part of the secondary survey of the trauma patient. The priority is to identify an abdominal cause of significant hemorrhage or intestinal perforation. The management of injuries to individual organs is discussed later. Specific injuries

---

TABLE 13-1 ■ Mechanisms of Abdominal Injuries in Children

Mechanism	%
Blunt (86% of all injuries)	
Motor vehicle—occupant	32
Motor vehicle—pedestrian	27
Fall	13
Bicycle	12
Other	16
Penetrating (13% of all injuries)	
Gunshot wound	56
Stab wound	24
Other	20
Other (1% of all injuries)	

National Pediatric Trauma Registry data, 1985-1991. Data from Cooper A, Barlow B, DiScala C, et al: Mortality and truncal injury: The pediatric perspective. J Pediatr Surg 29:33-38, 1994.

TABLE 13-2 ■ Frequency of Abdominal Organ Injured by Injury Mechanism

Blunt		Penetrating	
Organ	%	Organ	%
Spleen	30	Gastrointestinal tract	70
Liver	28	Liver	27
Kidneys	28	Blood vessels	19
Gastrointestinal tract	14	Kidneys	10
Bladder/urethra/ureters	4	Spleen	9
Pancreas	3	Bladder/urethra/ureters	8
Blood vessels	3	Pancreas	6

National Pediatric Trauma Registry data, 1985-1991. Data from Cooper A, Barlow B, DiScala C, et al: Mortality and truncal injury: The pediatric perspective. J Pediatr Surg 29:33-38, 1994.

deserve mention. Injury to the hepatic veins, in particular the right hepatic vein, causes massive hemorrhage that may be uncontrollable. Unrecognized bleeding from the liver or spleen is a classic pitfall in trauma management and cause of preventable trauma deaths. Similarly the mortality of intestinal perforation rises sharply when treatment is delayed beyond 24 hours after injury.

INITIAL EVALUATION AND TREATMENT

The general principles of resuscitation and stabilization are outlined in Chapter 11. All patients who have sustained injury to the torso must be assumed to have intra-abdominal injury with hemorrhage. Initial priorities are the placement of large-bore intravenous cannulas and the administration of appropriate amounts of crystalloid solutions. At least one catheter should be placed above the diaphragm. A nasogastric or orogastric tube is mandatory to decrease the risk of aspiration, potentially to improve respiratory function, and to allow a more reliable abdominal examination.

Injuries of higher priority (e.g., airway injuries or tension pneumothorax) should be treated first, with the abdomen being attended to shortly thereafter. If a patient with an intra-abdominal injury continues to be hypotensive despite resuscitative efforts, immediate laparotomy is needed. If patients respond favorably to fluid resuscitation, further evaluation and diagnostic studies can be performed. Stable patients, particularly patients with solid organ injury, are often candidates for selective nonoperative management. All patients should be resuscitated and approached with urgency, as if they are being prepared for surgery. Patients undergoing diagnostic studies should be monitored continuously because clinical deterioration may occur rapidly and unexpectedly.

HISTORY AND PHYSICAL FINDINGS

After the primary survey and resuscitation, the secondary survey entails a head-to-toe search for significant injuries that may be potentially life-threatening. For the abdomen, these include any injury that causes significant blood loss or perforates the gastrointestinal or genitourinary tracts. The examination of the abdomen is guided by the history of mechanism of injury. Specific mechanisms, such as penetrating wounds, falls onto handlebars, and lap belt injuries, draw attention to specific organs. More general blunt mechanisms (e.g., child abuse and motor vehicle crashes) require an open mind to the possibility that any intra-abdominal organ can be injured. Repeated examinations are necessary because manifestations of some injuries become evident over time and become detectable only after hours or days have passed.

Examining an injured child often presents many challenges. The unconscious head-injured child is unable to cooperate with the examination or complain of pain. Crying or prolonged bag-valve-mask ventilation may cause gastric distention with abdominal distention and tenderness that may mimic a significant intra-abdominal injury. Young children, scared by the event, ambulance ride, and emergency department, may be impossible

to evaluate. Restlessness and anxiety are cardinal signs of hypoxia and not necessarily a psychological situational response. A gentle, calm approach is important to allow an adequate abdominal examination.

Inspection of the abdomen reveals abrasions and ecchymoses that may suggest underlying intra-abdominal injury. Distention of the abdomen that persists despite gastric decompression raises concerns of intra-abdominal bleeding or gastrointestinal perforation. Auscultation of the abdomen may reveal absent bowel sounds, a consequence of ileus from either peritonitis or hypotension. With resuscitation and recovery, bowel sounds should return over time. Failure of return of peristalsis suggests significant hemoperitoneum or intestinal perforation. On palpation, a reassuring finding is a soft, nondistended, and nontender abdomen. Serial examinations are still necessary because distention, tenderness, and involuntary abdominal spasm could develop as a result of localized or generalized peritonitis. Although the abdomen may be difficult to evaluate in a patient with a head injury, it still may be possible to elicit peritoneal signs even in an obtunded child. Serial measurements of abdominal girth in small children give an indication of progressive distention from hemorrhage.

Hematomas of the perineum and blood at the urethral meatus signal the presence of urinary tract injury. Compression of the pelvic ring in the anterior-posterior and lateral dimensions reveals unstable pelvic fractures. Rectal examination assesses rectal tone, the presence of blood in the rectum, and fragments of pelvis violating the rectum. Turning the patient to the side is mandatory so that the back can be visualized completely and examined.

LABORATORY STUDIES

In general, laboratory studies are supplementary to the clinical history, physical examination, and specific imaging studies. Many laboratory studies are routine, including a complete blood count, urinalysis, levels of serum electrolytes, urea nitrogen, creatinine, glucose, amylase, liver enzymes, and samples for type and crossmatch. Results require correlation with the overall clinical picture because most abnormal values may have many possible causes. Serial determination of the hematocrit has value in the estimation of blood loss, transfusion requirements, and adequacy of tranfusion therapy. A high white blood cell count reflects intra-abdominal bleeding, splenic injury, and peritonitis from a perforated viscus. Peritonitis in infants and small children may be associated with a depressed white blood cell count (<3000 cells/mL). Elevations of liver enzyme levels strongly indicate liver injury. Many patients with bleeding from other sources may exhibit elevated liver enzyme values, however. Elevations of serum amylase, a useful screen for pancreatic injury, also may be present with facial injuries that involve the salivary glands and brain injury with cerebral hemorrhage, in which case serum lipase may be useful.

The threshold of microscopic hematuria that requires further radiographic evaluation of the urinary system in children is a matter of some controversy. Nearly all normotensive children without significant injuries who have microscopic hematuria recover without surgery, and urgent imaging studies are not indicated. Bleeding after what otherwise would have been considered minor trauma suggests a structural abnormality of the kidney, however, such as hydronephrosis or a tumor. Follow-up ultrasound is necessary. The threshold for significant renal injury appears to be 50 red blood cells per high-powered field; only 2% of children with fewer than 50 red blood cells per high-powered field have significant renal injuries.

IMAGING STUDIES

Plain films of the chest, a basic part of the evaluation of the trauma patient, provide valuable information in patients with suspected abdominal injury. The patient in shock from blunt torso injury requires only a chest film to exclude intrathoracic sources of blood loss; a normal chest film indicates an intra-abdominal source. Lower rib fractures increase the risk of liver or spleen injury. Evidence of diaphragmatic rupture also increases the likelihood of associated abdominal solid organ injury. Because the abdomen extends into the lower portion of the thoracic cage, as high as the level of the nipples (fourth intercostal space), evaluation of penetrating injuries must consider the possibility of injuries to structures in the chest and the abdomen (Fig. 13-1).

Abdominal plain films that include the pelvis also are a part of the secondary trauma survey. Findings are often notoriously "soft," however, and require clinical correlation

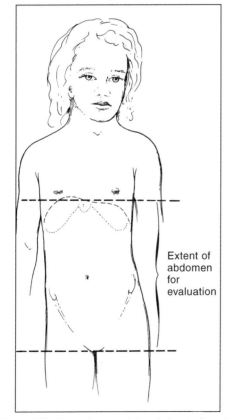

Extent of abdomen for evaluation

FIGURE 13-1 ■ The boundaries of the abdominal cavity, which must be evaluated by physical examination and imaging studies that must include the full extent of the diaphragm and pelvis.

or corroboration with additional imaging studies. Splenic rupture may push gastric or colonic air medially. Massive hemoperitoneum may create a generalized ground-glass appearance to a largely gasless abdomen. Intestinal gas escaping from a perforated viscus may accumulate in scattered collections of gas that do not conform to an expected intestinal shape. Free air from perforations often is missed because abdominal plain films in trauma patients are nearly always taken when the patient is supine and before significant volumes of gas escape from the gastrointestinal tract.

Pelvic fractures seen on abdominal plain films are important findings even though they are not associated with an increased incidence of abdominal solid organ injury. Unstable fractures that involve the main pelvic ring often are associated with severe hemorrhage that requires immediate transfusion and measures to stabilize the pelvis. A patient with a pelvic fracture associated with hematuria requires an evaluation of the lower urinary tract. Patients with either pelvic fracture or hematuria alone in the absence of other physical findings (e.g., blood at the urethral meatus) do not require routine cystography.

Intravenous pyelography (IVP) in trauma patients has largely been replaced by other imaging modalities that provide better anatomic definition, notably contrast-enhanced computed tomography (CT). The "one-shot" IVP has been advocated to assess the ipsilateral kidney quickly for significant injury and to evaluate the adequacy of function of the contralateral kidney should the injured kidney require nephrectomy. The one-shot IVP performed in trauma patients has a significant rate of false-negative results (8%), however, and an unacceptable rate of false-positive results (26%). Seldom does the functional status of the contralateral kidney determine the surgical management of the injured kidney. For these reasons, use of the one-shot IVP is unusual.

CT provides clear and accurate imaging of intraperitoneal and retroperitoneal structures and has tremendous utility in trauma evaluation. Intravenous contrast enhancement provides additional information regarding organ blood flow and continuing hemorrhage where contrast extravasation can be detected. It has particular value in abdominal solid organ injury (spleen, liver, and kidney), where it is most accurate.

More difficult is the detection of intestinal and pancreatic injuries. The volume of free air may be too small or collections may be missed on CT. Similarly, absence of leakage of enterally administered contrast material does not exclude an intestinal perforation. Often the only sign of intestinal or mesenteric injury is the presence of intra-abdominal fluid without solid organ injury. Other signs of intestinal injury include bowel wall thickening or enhancement with intravenous contrast material, mesenteric fat streaking, or bowel dilation. Overall the sensitivity of bowel injury by CT is 64% to 86% and specificity is 94% to 97%.

Pancreatic injuries are difficult to diagnose with CT unless 3-mm cuts are taken, the only sign often being an area of radiolucency within the pancreas on a single CT cut or separation of the interval between the gland and the splenic vein. Complicating CT interpretation is the small incidence of intra-abdominal fluid collections without any abdominal or retroperitoneal injury.

The role of CT in the evaluation of bladder injury is controversial. The standard approach is conventional cystography after assessment of the urethra. Some advocate delayed CT images of the pelvis 5 minutes after intravenous contrast injection with occlusion of a urinary catheter; others have noted that insufficient bladder distention using the technique may miss a perforation of the bladder dome. CT cystography fills the bladder retrograde through the urinary catheter, after which CT scan through the pelvis is performed. CT cystography provides diagnostic images equal to images provided by conventional cystography, with the primary advantage being that the test can take place at the same setting as other CT evaluations.

CT has become the modality of choice for diagnostic imaging in patients with blunt abdominal injury. Its wide acceptance is due to many factors: accurate results with few false-positive and false-negative interpretations, newer generation imaging systems that provide fine resolution images within minutes, wide availability in trauma centers and community hospitals, and ready availability of radiographic personnel to conduct the studies and interpret the results. More recently, however, it has been pointed out that radiation from pediatric CT may increase lifetime cancer mortality risk 0.18% for an abdominal scan and 0.07% for a head scan. Of the 600,000 abdominal and head CT examinations performed annually in the United States, a rough estimate is that 500 individuals ultimately might die from cancer attributable to the CT radiation. Further improvements will lie in more selective criteria of patients who need CT and active reduction of radiation exposure.

There has been some debate whether CT or diagnostic peritoneal lavage is the most appropriate study to evaluate significant abdominal injury in the immediacy of the trauma setting. The accuracy of CT and its generally ready availability has overcome two major advantages of diagnostic peritoneal lavage: its ability to detect intra-abdominal bleeding and its ready applicability. This is discussed further later.

There has been increasing use of abdominal ultrasonography as a screening tool in the immediate assessment of blunt trauma, called *focused abdominal sonography for trauma* (FAST). The immediate goal of FAST is to detect hemoperitoneum by using real-time ultrasound to search the pelvis, the right paracolic gutter, and the left upper quadrant for free fluid. More than one fifth (22%) of splenic fractures and two fifths (42%) of bowel injuries are not associated, however, with free intraperitoneal fluid (determined by CT). In part because ultrasound diagnosis of abdominal injury depends on showing free fluid, the technique has a relatively low sensitivity (62% to 78%) in detecting splenic injury in children. Although the presence of hemoperitoneum identifies an intra-abdominal source of blood loss, ultrasonography has limitations in the diagnosis of specific organ injuries.

CT and ultrasonography have been used in the follow-up assessments of patients with abdominal solid organ injury to document healing, although they have doubtful clinical utility for this purpose. In asymptomatic patients, these follow-up examinations, although reassuring to the clinician, do not provide clinically useful information. Either test is useful in situations in which pain, fever, or persistent ileus signal possible complications of nonoperative therapy, such as development of a hepatic biloma or a splenic abscess.

Magnetic resonance imaging (MRI) has been used occasionally to evaluate abdominal trauma, but it is more difficult and expensive to perform, more difficult to interpret, and more time-consuming than CT. MRI can be advantageous in the evaluation of specific injuries, however. MRI is the imaging study of choice in spinal cord evaluation, so it would be an important study in patients in whom spinal cord injury is suspected. Magnetic resonance cholangiopancreatography (MRCP) can provide diagnostic quality images of the pancreatic duct with sufficient detail to detect pancreatic ductal disruptions, early pseudocyst development, late strictures, and the exclusion of significant ductal injury.

Angiography seldom is needed but is an important technique in the control of bleeding complications associated with pelvic injuries. Selective embolization of actively bleeding pelvic vessels in these cases may be life-saving.

PERITONEAL LAVAGE

The goal of peritoneal lavage in the management of trauma is to determine whether there is blood, intestinal contents, or pancreatic juice in the free peritoneal cavity. If blood is present, the decision to perform a laparotomy still must be based on additional clinical factors, such as additional anatomic information from CT, hemodynamic stability, and ongoing transfusion requirements. CT provides accurate information in patients with solid organ injury, and in such cases peritoneal lavage would not provide any useful additional information. A hypotensive patient with blunt injury without other sources of blood loss and clear lung fields on chest film also would not benefit from peritoneal lavage because an abdominal source of blood loss needs to be excluded by laparotomy.

In current pediatric trauma practice, the primary application of peritoneal lavage is in the evaluation of the unstable patient who requires urgent operative therapy for deteriorating neurologic status or in whom the source of blood loss or clinical findings are in doubt. An example of the latter instance is the multiply-injured hypotensive patient, in whom finding the body region responsible for blood loss is an urgent issue. Another is the patient with intra-abdominal fluid on CT without solid organ injury, in whom the source of fluid could be either intestinal contents or mesenteric bleeding. Peritoneal lavage is not a reliable technique in two situations: retroperitoneal injuries and pelvic fractures, in which blood is almost always present in the peritoneal cavity.

The open technique, in which a catheter is placed into the peritoneal cavity under direct visualization, is the safest approach. In patients who have had previous abdominal surgery, a situation that may prohibit peritoneal lavage, the open technique is the only acceptable approach. In infants, a plastic-sheathed needle may be passed obliquely into either lower quadrant. In older children free from previous abdominal surgery, the Seldinger technique (placement of a guidewire through a stainless steel needle, over which a catheter is placed) gives a direct means for peritoneal lavage.

Obtaining blood or bile-stained fluid on entry in the abdomen is a positive result. If no fluid is obtained, Ringer's lactate or normal saline solution is infused through the catheter in a volume sufficient to circulate throughout the abdominal cavity, generally 100 mL in infants, 300 to 500 mL in toddlers, and 500 to 1000 mL in older children and adolescents. The effluent is obtained for blood count (>50,000 red blood cells or 500 white blood cells per mL is considered positive); amylase levels; and microscopic analysis for bile, bacteria, or intestinal contents.

DIAGNOSTIC LAPAROSCOPY

The more recent developments of laparoscopy and minimally invasive surgical techniques have led to their application in the evaluation and treatment of abdominal injuries. At this stage in the development of minimally invasive surgery, these techniques have limited applicability. Unstable patients with massive blood loss require rapid removal of clot and blood and repair or removal of injured organs, procedures that are performed best with an open laparotomy. In patients who do not require operation, elective nonoperative management of abdominal injuries has high success rates that do not depend on direct visualization of injured organs.

The greatest potential of diagnostic laparoscopy is in the patient with equivocal clinical findings or response to resuscitation, who does not clearly require an immediate laparotomy, but conversely is not completely free from symptoms. Diagnostic laparoscopy searches for a significant injury and provides video imaging for minimally invasive repair of any injuries found. Injuries not amenable to laparoscopic repair require conversion to a formal open laparotomy.

Another potential area where diagnostic laparoscopy may have applicability is in stable patients with penetrating injury. Experiences with laparoscopic evaluation of penetrating thoracoabdominal injuries indicate limitations with the technique, however. When compared with findings at open laparotomy, diagnostic laparoscopy had a sensitivity of 88% for liver and spleen injuries; 83%, diaphragm; 57%, pancreas and kidney; and 25%, hollow viscus.

PREPARATION FOR OPERATION

Because the clinical situation can change abruptly, all patients with abdominal trauma should be approached as if they will undergo surgery, whether the initial management is operative or nonoperative. Adequate intravenous access is mandatory. Fluid resuscitation sufficient to restore promptly and maintain adequate circulatory volume is an absolute priority. In patients in whom the need for laparotomy is certain, additional fluids to cover intraoperative evaporative and "third-space" losses should be anticipated and administered. Obtaining adequate amounts of typed and crossmatched blood is an urgent priority in case transfusion or operation is required. For patients who need blood before a complete type and crossmatch can be completed, O-negative or type-specific blood must be immediately available.

Patients with penetrating injury, patients who have extensive injuries from blunt trauma, and patients who arrive in shock should receive broad-spectrum antibiotic coverage with combination therapy (ampicillin, gentamicin, and clindamycin) or a third-generation cephalosporin. Antibiotics can be discontinued promptly if significant injury is ruled out later. Patients with significant intra-abdominal injury or soft tissue injuries are protected from infective complications if antibiotic coverage begins during the initial phase of trauma resuscitation and management.

Children who have been immunized for tetanus within 10 years do not require a booster immunization. In practice, patients receive boosters if they have extensive, soiled soft tissue wounds thought to be prone to tetanus. Patients not previously immunized or in whom immunity is thought to have lapsed should receive appropriate active and passive immunization.

All phases of trauma evaluation and care require measures to prevent heat loss and hypothermia. Infants are particularly vulnerable.

GENERAL INDICATIONS FOR OPERATION

The basic indications for operation for abdominal trauma are ongoing blood loss that has produced shock or will produce shock if not controlled and peritonitis from a perforated viscus (Table 13-3). The clinical challenges involve the recognition of patients who require immediate operation and patients who will recover without surgery, so-called selective management.

Patients with abdominal trauma who arrive hypotensive and remain so despite resuscitative efforts likely will require abdominal exploration, especially if the chest fields are clear on x-ray and abdominal distention is present. It is important not to wait for the development of

---

TABLE 13-3 ■ Indications for Laparotomy: Abdominal Injury

Blunt injuries
   Continued hemodynamic instability despite resuscitation
   Signs of continuing hemorrhage
   Need for blood replacement in excess of half of blood volume
   Pneumoperitoneum
   Physical signs of peritoneal irritation
   Signs of significant injury to the intestine, pancreas, bladder, ureter, renal vasculature, or rectum
Penetrating injuries
   Most gunshot wounds
   Selective operation for stab wounds with
      Hypotension
      Unexplained blood loss
      Evisceration
      Physical signs of peritoneal irritation
      Signs of significant amounts of blood or intestinal contents on peritoneal lavage or CT

hypotension before deciding to operate because hypotension is a late sign of blood loss in infants and children and is a signal of impending hemodynamic collapse. Tachycardia, an early sign of blood loss and a compensatory mechanism, is a better monitor of adequacy of resuscitation. Persistence of tachycardia despite resuscitative efforts reflects a situation that likely will require surgical correction. Prompt stabilization of vital signs with initial crystalloid resuscitation is an excellent indication that operation will not be required.

More problematic is a patient who requires transfusion because of failure of initial crystalloid infusions (20 mL/kg of Ringer's lactate as a bolus, repeated twice) to stabilize the overall clinical status, correct hypotension, or reverse tachycardia. Initial trials of nonoperative management of solid organ trauma in children set a transfusion threshold of 40 mL/kg, or about half of the estimated blood volume, with operation being recommended when the transfusion volume exceeded that amount. Because of risks inherent in transfusion therapy, including blood-borne infections and transfusion reactions, more recent emphasis has been on limiting the need for tranfusion therapy.

There are two general situations that potentially involve transfusion. First is the patient who is hemodynamically stable but becomes gradually anemic. Nearly all clinicians accept low hemoglobin concentrations without transfusion, as low as 7 g/dL, as long as the patient remains symptom-free and maintains stable vital signs. Oral iron and erythropoietin therapy can be used to return the patient's hemoglobin levels to normal over the long-term. The second is the patient who does not respond to crystalloid resuscitation and in whom blood transfusions become an early necessity within hours of surgery to maintain hemodynamic stability. These patients predictably need operative repair of the bleeding organ, and continued delay waiting for an arbitrary 40 mL/kg transfusion threshold is not warranted and risks unnecessarily increasing the total transfusion requirement.

Perforation or rupture of the stomach or bowel is an absolute indication for operation. Peritoneal irritation from intestinal contents or stool in the abdomen causes involuntary spasm and tenderness on physical examination. Repeated examinations are important because initial findings may be confounded by pain and psychological stress. Specific findings that reflect peritonitis from traumatic gastric or intestinal perforation are increasing abdominal pain, distention, leukocytosis and acidosis, and the failure of clinical improvement over time.

Free air, either on abdominal plain film or CT, difficult to detect on initial films, is an indication for operation if found. Contrast material administered by mouth or by rectum increases the sensitivity of CT in detecting intestinal perforations. Gastrointestinal contents, digestive enzymes, or bile on peritoneal lavage reflects free intestinal leakage, as does the presence of bacteria or bits of vegetable matter on microscopic examination of lavage fluid. Other indications for surgery are organ dependent and are discussed in the appropriate sections that follow.

PENETRATING INJURIES

Many studies support the selective management of abdominal stab wounds, an approach whereby laparotomy is performed only for specific clinical indications: hypotension, unexplained blood loss, evisceration, or signs of peritoneal irritation on physical examination. In one series, 50% were treated successfully without operation, whereas 8% were observed initially but later underwent delayed surgery. The nontherapeutic laparotomy rate was 8%, and the false-negative physical examination rate was 6%. Subsequent investigations noted that either peritoneal lavage or CT (with "triple contrast"—intravenous, oral, and rectal) could bring nontherapeutic laparotomy rates to nearly zero, while improving on the false-negative physical examination rates. Because retroperitoneal injuries may not produce anterior abdominal findings on physical examination, triple contrast CT is mandatory in stab wounds to the back and flank. The detection of changes in clinical status demands scrupulous serial examinations and in-hospital monitoring.

Selective management has been advocated for abdominal gunshot wounds. The traditional approach was to perform immediate laparotomy on all patients who had sustained a gunshot that penetrated the abdominal cavity. In a study of adult trauma patients with gunshot injuries, surgery was performed only for essentially the same clinical indications listed previously for stab wounds: hypotension or peritonitis on a reliable clinical examination. With this approach, 38% were treated successfully without operation, whereas 4% underwent delayed surgery. The nontherapeutic laparotomy rate was 14%, compared with 47% had all patients been explored with routine laparotomy.

BLUNT INJURIES

Selective management is the approach of choice in the management of blunt abdominal injury in clinically stable patients free from signs of ongoing blood loss or peritonitis. Success rates approach 98% for injuries that involve the kidney; 95%, spleen; 90%, liver; and 72%, pancreas. Because nonoperative approaches are so often successful in blunt abdominal trauma, special care must be taken to evaluate any new clinical finding and all changes in overall clinical status.

Laparotomy should be considered in cases of blunt trauma if the patient's condition continues to be unstable despite adequate fluid resuscitation or blood transfusion or both. Operation is mandatory with any indication that a perforated viscus is present: peritoneal irritation on physical examination; pneumoperitoneum; extravasation of contrast on CT; and bile, bacteria, vegetable matter, or increased white blood cell count on peritoneal lavage. Operative repair is indicated for intraperitoneal rupture of the bladder, renovascular avulsion or thrombosis, complex pancreaticoduodenal injury, pancreatic transection, and rectal perforations. Specific issues in selective management for each organ are discussed later in the appropriate sections.

TRAUMA LAPAROTOMY

The surgical team must be prepared to begin the operation immediately should the patient suddenly deteriorate at any phase during work-up, preparation for surgery, and anesthetic induction. A patient with marginal hemodynamic reserve may decompensate with the administration of anesthetic drugs, the institution of positive-pressure ventilation, or as the result of ongoing blood loss. Intra-arterial monitoring may be useful in hypotensive patients. Multiple large-bore intravenous cannulas are secured before the abdomen is opened. Blood for transfusion must be available in the operating room. In hypotensive patients, blood transfusions should be started and forced through warmed intravenous tubing with the help of pressure devices.

The operative field extends from the clavicles to midthigh, allowing thoracotomy if necessary and exposure of the femoral vessels for additional intravenous access. Unexplained hypotension can be addressed by the placement of a chest tube into each hemithorax and pericardiocentesis (or creation of a subxiphoid pericardial window) to diagnose and treat simultaneously an unsuspected pneumothorax, hemothorax, or cardiac tamponade. When in the abdomen, if uncontrollable bleeding is encountered, the aorta can be occluded through an anterior thoracotomy.

The abdomen should be entered through a midline incision because this permits rapid access to the abdominal cavity and wide exposure of its contents. A midline incision permits extension into a sternotomy if necessary (e.g., for a transhepatic inferior vena cava shunt to facilitate the control of massive hepatic bleeding). After complete removal of intraperitoneal blood and clots, all quadrants of the abdomen are packed with counted laparotomy pads to tamponade any active bleeding. Completion of abdominal packing is a good opportunity to allow the anesthetic team to catch up with fluid and blood infusions and to begin to normalize vital signs and for the surgical team to regroup and begin to plan which procedures will be necessary and in what order.

Evacuation of intraperitoneal blood and the orderly removal of packs from each quadrant allow direct observation of injured solid organs. The gastrointestinal tract must be run from esophagus to rectum, taking care to inspect anterior and posterior aspects of the stomach and intestine. For the stomach, this means opening the gastrocolic ligament and entering the lesser sac; for the duodenum, a Kocher maneuver is necessary. The surgeon hands each loop of small bowel to the assistant surgeon, turning it from one side to the other so that both surgeons thoroughly inspect each loop. The ascending and descending colon are inspected carefully for hematomas and squeezed to detect a perforation.

The retroperitoneum is inspected for hematomas, discolorations that indicate the leakage of intestinal juice, or abnormal fluid collections that reflect the escape of urine or pancreatic juice. Small hematomas located in the lateral aspect of the retroperitoneum that remain stable in size can be left undisturbed. Large or expanding hematomas need to be explored. Central retroperitoneal hematomas require exploration, searching for major vascular injury or injury to the transverse duodenum or pancreas. Exploration of the abdomen and retroperitoneum must be performed in an orderly, deliberate fashion so that nothing is missed.

Placement of drains depends in part on the organ injured and the degree to which bleeding has been controlled. Most splenic injuries, even injuries that have been repaired, do not require drainage. Most instances of pancreatic and duodenal injuries are drained because of the high incidence of leakage and creation of a fistula. Oozing that results from complex injuries and disseminated intravascular coagulation should be drained to evacuate further bleeding and to monitor ongoing blood loss.

Nonabsorbable monofilament synthetic suture is a logical choice to close the abdomen for at least two compelling reasons. First, shock and hypoxia delay wound healing. Second, contaminated wounds compromised by inadequate blood flow and hypoxia are at risk for wound infection and dehiscence. Primary closure is appropriate for most cases in which the patient is stable and no complicating factors are present. In contaminated wounds, the subcutaneous tissue and skin are best left open and treated with dressing changes or closed on a delayed primary basis in 3 to 4 days.

The development of massive amounts of edema and "third spacing" in the intestine, mesentery, and retroperitoneum may prevent easy primary fascial closure of the abdomen. In these cases, ill-advised closure of the fascia may create abnormally high pressures within the abdomen sufficient to prevent perfusion of the intestine, kidneys, and lower extremities. The clinical diagnosis of development of the abdominal compartment syndrome demands careful inspection of the perfusion of the intestine during the abdominal closure, the development of abnormally high ventilatory pressures after closure, and the degree of difficulty in bringing the fascial incision together. Should abdominal compartment syndrome develop, attempts at primary fascial closure should be discontinued. Placement of a prosthetic manufactured for this purpose or sterile intravenous bag material sutured to the margins of the fascial defect may be a useful temporizing measure in these instances.

MANAGEMENT OF INJURY TO SPECIFIC ORGANS

Spleen

The guiding principle in management of splenic injury is preservation of the organ whenever possible. Since King and Schumaker's 1952 report of the association of splenectomy with lethal bacterial sepsis, the importance of the spleen in resistance to bacterial infection (especially encapsulated organisms such as pneumococcus, meningococcus, and *Haemophilus influenzae*) is firmly established. The risk of postsplenectomy sepsis in trauma patients is 0.5% to 2%. The risk is highest in patients younger than age 4 years and greatest in the first 2 years after splenectomy. The risk never falls to zero on long-term follow-up. If postsplenectomy sepsis occurs, the

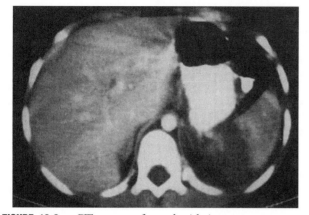

FIGURE 13-2 ■ CT scan performed with intravenous contrast material and gastrointestinal contrast enhancement shows isolated splenic rupture that resulted from blunt trauma. This patient responded to nonoperative management as do most patients with splenic injuries.

mortality is 50%. It has been estimated that adequate immunologic function of the spleen requires 30% to 50% of the original splenic mass, a consideration used to guide strategies for operative repair of an injured spleen.

Diagnosis

The spleen is the most common organ injured with blunt abdominal trauma. Any blow to the anterior abdomen, particularly to the left flank, left costal margin, or left upper quadrant, should raise the suspicion of a splenic injury. Physical examination reveals tenderness laterally in the left upper quadrant but without signs of peritoneal irritation. CT with intravenous contrast material provides anatomic detail of the extent of injury and the amount of blood in the peritoneum (Fig. 13-2).

Indications for Operation

The success rate with patients with splenic injuries who do not require laparotomy approaches 95%. As discussed earlier, the primary indication for surgery is persistent

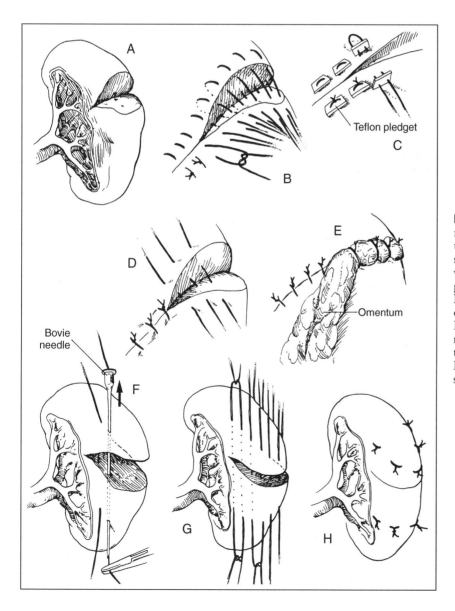

FIGURE 13-3 ■ Various options for splenic repair and preservation depending on the type and severity of the injury. **A,** Typical splenic laceration. **B,** Placement of deep vertical mattress sutures. **C,** Use of pledgets if sutures tend to pull through. **D** and **E,** Placement of simple sutures with omental flap **(E)** into a deep defect. **F,** Placement of sutures through a spinal needle so that the needle tract can be cauterized in extensive lacerations. **G** and **H,** Placement of multiple horizontal mattress sutures for long, deep lacerations.

hemodynamic instability despite resuscitation. Splenic injury grading schemes based on CT findings have been devised. In children, in contrast to adults, the grade of splenic injury by CT criteria does not predict which patients will fail selective nonoperative therapy and require operation.

Operative Considerations

Evaluation of the spleen requires the complete mobilization of the spleen, tail of the pancreas, and stomach. Division of the lateral and superior attachments of the spleen, posterior attachments of the pancreas, and attachments to the splenic flexure allows delivery of the spleen into the incision.

Splenectomy is reserved for patients with irreparable damage to the organ and patients with significant associated injuries or massive hemorrhage who would not tolerate a prolonged operation. Care must be taken to avoid injury to the tail of the pancreas when mobilizing the spleen or during splenectomy or splenorrhaphy. Ligation of the vasa brevia (short gastric vessels) must be secure, leaving a long segment of vessel on the greater curve of the stomach so that the ligature does not become dislodged during surgical manipulations or as a consequence of postoperative gastric distention.

Figure 13-3 illustrates some techniques of splenorrhaphy. As noted, the goal is preservation of at least 30% to 50% of the splenic mass to preserve its immune function. Basic principles are to ligate individual bleeding vessels within and outside of the splenic substance and careful approximation of the fractured splenic parenchyma. Absorbable cellulose and fibrin sealant and judicious use of electrocautery slow bleeding from exposed splenic substance. Simple through-and-through absorbable sutures usually can hold simple fractures or lacerations together. Teflon pledgets or a pedicle of omentum placed between the suture and the spleen keeps the thin capsule from tearing. Devascularized segments are best simply resected, especially if most of the splenic substance remains. When the spleen has multiple fractures, but most of the segments are viable, placement of an absorbable mesh bag gathers the fragments and holds them in apposition with the help of a ladder sling fashioned from absorbable suture. All patients who have undergone splenectomy or splenorrhaphy must be followed closely after operation for the possibility of continued bleeding.

Splenic autotransplantation has been advocated, but there is no clear-cut evidence that it is protective. The autotransplanted spleen elaborates immune substances,

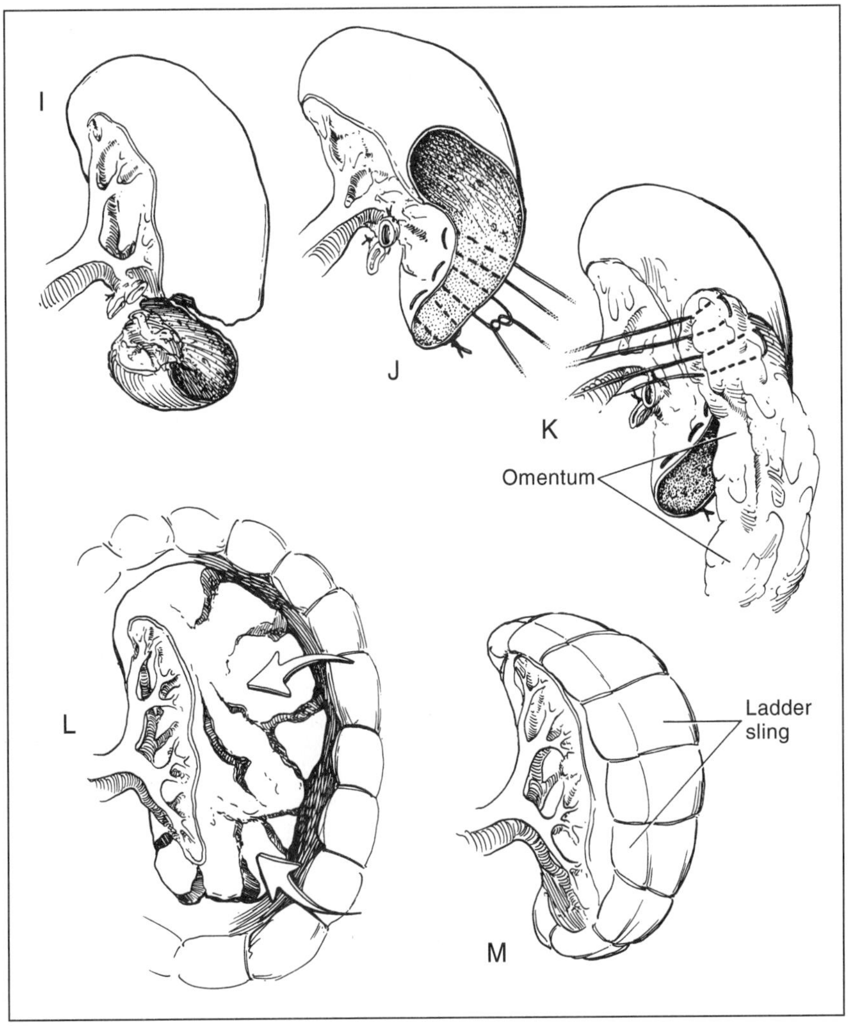

FIGURE 13-3—cont'd ■ **I-K,** Amputation of devascularized lower pole from complete fracture with placement of horizontal mattress sutures across the defect **(J)** and insertion of an omental flap to tamponade bleeding **(K). L** and **M,** Use of a sling around a severely fractured spleen.

but being outside the systemic arterial system, it loses its filter function.

Because of the risk of postsplenectomy sepsis, a patient who has lost a spleen or undergone removal of more than 50% of the organ should be given active immunization against pneumococcus, meningococcus, and *H. influenzae.* Most clinicians have the child take oral penicillin throughout the childhood years. The patient, parents, and medical personnel must know the child is without a spleen (e.g., a medical alert bracelet or necklace), and aggressive intravenous antibiotic therapy is indicated at any sign of a serious infection.

Nonoperative Considerations

Hemodynamically stable children with splenic injury frequently show an acute drop in hematocrit from a mean of 37% at presentation to 31% within the first 24 hours after injury. Values then return to values not significantly different from baseline in 1 to 2 weeks. Transfusion rates reported from large children's hospitals have decreased to 0 to 10% of patients, with blood being given almost exclusively to severely injured patients with multiple injuries.

Traditionally, patients with splenic injury were admitted to the intensive care unit and placed on strict bed rest for days to weeks. More recent practice has proved that this conservative approach is not necessary. Stable patients can be admitted to the hospital ward. Discharge follows at 48 hours if the patient is having no abdominal tenderness, is eating a regular diet, and is having stable hematocrit levels. The child is allowed to return to school with non-contact activity for 1 month. Routine ultrasonography or CT of the spleen during follow-up has little clinical utility.

Splenic pseudocyst is a late complication of splenic injury resulting from intrasplenic or subcapsular hematoma. The patient complains of left upper quadrant pain. On examination, the spleen may be enlarged. Imaging studies show a large nonperfused filling defect in the spleen. The splenic remnant is treated best by either limited segmental resection or removal of the pseudocyst wall and closure by standard suture techniques. Fever and leukocytosis signal the presence of a splenic abscess. CT-guided drainage of the abscess cavity, along with intravenous antibiotics, results in resolution of these cases.

Liver

Among intra-abdominal injuries from blunt force trauma, liver injuries have the highest risk of mortality. Serious injuries to the liver involve the inferior vena cava, hepatic veins, or intrahepatic vessels. All bleed profusely when torn. Operative exposure and control may be difficult, particularly in the face of massive bleeding from the vessel itself. When major vessels are not injured, the parenchyma generally stops bleeding, however, and allows selective nonoperative management in 90% of cases. The presence of the biliary tract complicates management: Extravasated bile may collect in a biloma, or bleeding may decompress into the biliary tree and result in hemobilia.

Diagnosis

The liver is the second most common organ injured with blunt abdominal trauma. As with the spleen, any blow to the anterior abdomen, particularly to the right upper

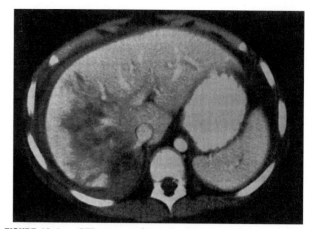

FIGURE 13-4 ■ CT scan performed after severe blunt injury of the abdomen shows a bursting injury of the liver. The patient was stable and no operative intervention was required, although most patients with injuries this severe seen immediately after injury probably would be operated on.

quadrant, costal margin, or flank, directs concern to the possibility of hepatic injury. A patient with a major liver injury with massive hemorrhage is in shock and has abdominal distention. Efforts under this circumstance must be directed toward obtaining adequate intravenous access and making plans for immediate laparotomy. Further diagnostic studies, such as CT, are not indicated. Stable patients have right upper quadrant tenderness. CT provides excellent detail of the extent of the injury and an estimate of the amount of blood in the peritoneum (Fig. 13-4). At times, angiographic embolization may be helpful either alone or as an adjunct to operation.

Indications for Operation

As noted previously, hemodynamic stability guides the necessity for operation. CT grading criteria quantify the degree of liver injury and amount of intraperitoneal bleeding. Even with the highest degree of hepatic injury (laceration extending into the region of the hepatic veins and vena cava), selective nonoperative treatment is successful in more than two thirds of cases. Patients who arrive hypotensive, have abdominal distention because of intra-abdominal blood, or require immediate blood transfusions likely will require operative control of bleeding.

Operative Considerations

A hypotensive patient needing operation because of liver injury is likely to have a complex fracture involving a large volume of the liver or one that extends into the trunks of the hepatic veins near or involving the vena cava. The trauma team must prepare for the control of all major vessels entering and leaving the liver, including the intrathoracic inferior vena cava.

On entry, sterile gauze packs placed behind, below, and on top of the liver provide initial control of bleeding. Removal of packs, one by one, allows a systematic survey of the extent of injury. Simple sutures, described earlier in the discussion of splenic injuries, suffice for simple superficial lacerations. Exploration of the deepest part of large fractures may be necessary to identify bleeding large vessels that require direct application of clips or suture. Deep wounds, such as stab wounds or gunshot wounds, may require extension to allow the full extent of the wound to be seen.

The Pringle maneuver (occlusion of the porta with the thumb and forefinger or a vascular clamp) may be required to control bleeding that persists despite packing or to identify lacerated vessels deep within a laceration. If bleeding is restricted to one lobe, hepatic resection may be necessary to control bleeding after control of the appropriate hepatic and portal branch. In general, however, in most cases, hepatic resection for trauma is more débridement of pulverized liver and suture control of individual vessels than a formal lobectomy.

Juxtahepatic and vena caval injuries are signaled by massive hemorrhage behind the dome of the liver or failure of the Pringle maneuver to control bleeding. Mortality exceeds 60% for all of these injuries. Isolated left hepatic vein injuries have the best survival, whereas injuries involving the right hepatic vein and vena cava have a mortality greater than 80%. Placement of a large catheter from the right atrium into the subhepatic cava to bypass venous return from the area of injury, attractive in theory, has not been successful in practice. In these extreme cases, total vascular isolation of the liver may be the best option to control juxtahepatic hemorrhage (Fig. 13-5). Clamps or tourniquets on the vena cava above and below the liver and across the porta hepatis may permit control of bleeding and repair of major vessels. Hepatic artery ligation has been proposed as a method to control extensive bleeding, but in nearly all cases other methods also are required. There have been reports of immediate transplantation in a few instances of irreparable hepatic injuries.

Injuries that require massive transfusion lead to consumptive coagulopathy, hypothermia, acidosis, and uncontrollable bleeding. Faced with physiologic and hematologic complications of transfusion therapy, the best course may be to pack the abdomen and to close the abdomen temporarily until conditions stabilize. Definitive surgical control of bleeding may be possible at a second-look operation 24 to 48 hours later.

Nonoperative Considerations

The nonoperative management of hemodynamically stable children with liver injury is the same as that outlined earlier for children with splenic injury. Patients who respond quickly to resuscitation and have mild symptoms can be observed briefly on the hospital ward for 48 hours, then discharged. In the absence of symptoms, follow-up ultrasound or CT in asymptomatic patients is not considered clinically useful.

Many children with liver injuries, even though successfully managed without operation, have symptoms that are slow to resolve and require a longer stay in the hospital. Fever and ileus are common and suggest the presence of bile leaking into the peritoneal cavity. Right pleural effusion may develop and require thoracentesis. Although most cases resolve over several days, the overall discomfort of the child and the possibility that a late complication is developing usually combine to keep the child in the hospital longer.

Late complications of liver injury require further radiographic studies. Persistent upper abdominal discomfort and a slow drift in hematocrit may signal the expansion of an intrahepatic hematoma. Follow-up CT helps document changes in the appearance of an intrahepatic fluid collection. Right upper quadrant discomfort, elevated

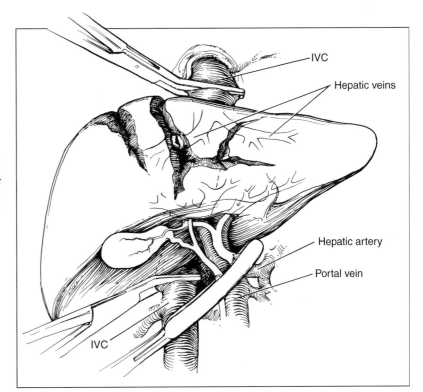

FIGURE 13-5 ■ In cases of complete hepatic rupture associated with hepatic vein or inferior vena caval laceration, total vascular isolation of the liver as shown here is extremely helpful and may be maintained for 1 hour while repair is performed.

bilirubin, and gastrointestinal hemorrhage suggest the development of hemobilia. Arteriography shows the arterial-biliary fistula and allows selective embolization to control bleeding. Leakage of bile may cause persistent fever, ileus, or jaundice. CT scan with intravenous contrast may distinguish between a laceration, hematoma, or intrahepatic biloma. Radionuclide scans may show extravasation of bile. Of patients with liver injury, 15% have delayed complications requiring surgery. Operative treatment is indicated for signs of continued bleeding, expanding hematoma, bile leak, continued hemobilia despite embolization, or development of a hepatic or perihepatic abscess.

Intestinal Injuries

Small Bowel

The major challenge in the management of an intestinal injury lies in its diagnosis. Prompt identification avoids complications and deaths. Some mechanisms of injury put the intestine at risk and suggest the likely presence of an intestinal injury: gunshot and stab wounds, falls onto handlebars, lap belts placed across the child's midsection, and being run over by an automobile. In contrast to the perforation caused immediately by a bullet or knife, one caused by blunt trauma may take 2 or 3 days to evolve. Blunt trauma shears the bowel against the vertebral column, damaging the bowel wall. A perforation may be immediate or develop gradually as an area of partial damage slowly gives way. Omentum or adjacent bowel loops may adhere to the area, limiting the leakage of air or intestinal juice and obscuring the development of peritoneal signs.

Patients with peritoneal signs require abdominal exploration. In the absence of clinical signs or in situations in which signs are equivocal, diagnosis depends on radiographic studies and peritoneal lavage (discussed earlier). Although peritoneal lavage gives the most definitive diagnosis of bowel injury, the procedure seldom is applied in pediatric trauma. Images from CT, now far more widely used, must be inspected carefully for small amounts of free air. Leakage of enteral contrast material is rarely present in children with bowel injury. Indirect findings on CT that suggest bowel injury, such as bowel wall thickening or mesenteric fat streaking, must be correlated with the overall clinical picture. If questions remain and the possibility of intestinal injury cannot be ruled out, diagnostic peritoneal lavage or laparoscopy is indicated.

All patients with free perforation of the small intestine require operation and closure of the hole. Larger areas of damage may require segmental resection and primary anastomosis. In situations in which extensive small bowel or mesenteric injury places the child at risk for short-bowel syndrome, the guiding principle is to remove only devitalized and necrotic areas and to preserve as much bowel length as possible. One such situation is when a length of bowel is stripped from its mesentery. Second-look procedures are necessary 12 to 48 hours later to assess the viability of remaining segments of bowel.

A stricture may develop in an area of a partial-thickness injury without free perforation. Obstruction occurs 7 to 21 days after the injury. Contrast radiographic studies show the area of stricture or partial small bowel obstruction. A contained perforation often gives the same clinical picture.

Duodenum

Duodenal hematomas resolve in nearly all cases, whereas duodenal perforations require repair. CT with oral contrast differentiates between the two conditions: A duodenal hematoma causes upper intestinal obstruction, whereas retroperitoneal air and extraluminal contrast identify a perforation. Intraperitoneal or retroperitoneal fluid, mesenteric enhancement, and a thickened intestinal wall, findings that indicate a small bowel perforation, do not establish perforation in the duodenum. Nearly 40% of patients with duodenal injuries have associated injuries of the pancreas.

Children with duodenal hematomas are treated expectantly, with nasogastric suction and parenteral nutrition. Resolution of the hematoma and resumption of oral feeding generally requires about 2 weeks. Obstruction that persists beyond 2 weeks should be considered for evacuation or surgical bypass of the obstruction as indicated. If a duodenal hematoma is encountered during surgery for repair of other injuries, the duodenal serosa should be incised and the clot evacuated.

Gastric juice and pancreatic enzymes put duodenal repairs at risk for dehiscence and fistula formation, so considerable judgment is necessary. In most cases, an isolated duodenal perforation can undergo simple primary closure. More complicated injuries require protection of the duodenal closure by diverting the digestive tract away from the area of injury. This may include Roux-en-Y anastomosis or a distal gastrectomy with gastrojejunostomy. Some surgeons place a duodenostomy in any patient with a duodenal repair. A jejunostomy created distal to the repair maintains enteral nutrition.

When damage to the pancreas accompanies a major duodenal injury, diverticulization of the duodenum completely isolates the area. Diverticulization includes antrectomy, Billroth II gastrojejunostomy, closure of the pylorus, repair of the duodenum, and catheter drainage of the duodenal remnant. Drainage of the biliary tract, through either a T-tube in the common duct or a cholecystostomy, controls biliary flow until the repair appears completely healed. Other experts advocate temporary closure of the pylorus without antrectomy and Billroth II gastrojejunostomy.

Wide drainage of the region of the duodenum and pancreas is recommended in all cases because of the high risk of a duodenal fistula. If a fistula occurs, drainage, restriction from oral feeding, and parenteral nutrition are needed.

Stomach

The stomach may rupture if blunt injury occurs when it is distended, such as after a large meal. Patients have abdominal distention to an impressive degree, along with generalized peritonitis. Massive amounts of free air are visible on plain film. Closure of the rent in the stomach requires débridement of the edges and appropriate two-layer closure. Feedings may resume after several days of nasogastric drainage.

Colon and Rectum

Colonic injuries are most often the result of penetrating injury. They are exceedingly rare after blunt trauma. Primary closure is safe and successful when the laceration is limited and not associated with significant peritoneal contamination. Extensive injuries, such as associated with gunshot wounds and associated with extensive abdominal contamination, are treated best by closure and protective colostomy.

Rectal injuries in children are usually impalement from child abuse or fall onto a sharp object. These injuries are treated best by proximal colostomy, irrigation of the distal rectal segment, and drainage of the presacral space.

Mesenteric Vessels

Either penetrating or blunt trauma may disrupt the mesenteric vessels. Early recognition is important. Hematoma formation or devascularization may lead to delayed necrosis of a segment of intestine. Direct repair of the disrupted vessel is necessary with major visceral vascular disruptions.

Pancreas and Biliary Tree

Pancreas

Fixed in the retroperitoneum with its midportion draped over the vertebral column, the pancreas is susceptible to blunt injury to the midsection. Pancreatic injuries frequently result from falls onto handlebars, blunt trauma from motor vehicle crashes, and child abuse. Most patients have abdominal pain and signs of peritoneal irritation. Elevations of serum amylase, present in three fourths of cases, range from normal to dramatically high. Absolute levels do not correlate with the extent of injury, however. If a patient presents 2 or more days after injury, the serum amylase level may be normal. CT findings, which include hemorrhage, retroperitoneal edema, and lucency in the area of a transection, show a pancreatic injury in a little more than half of the cases. CT may be normal, however, in 13% of cases of pancreatic injury. MRCP is an appropriate study to rule out major ductal injuries.

Most patients have contusions or transections in the midbody of the gland, where it crosses the vertebral column. Parenchymal disruptions associated with contusions generally heal without surgical repair, but resolution of the injury may take several weeks. Major disruptions of the main pancreatic duct or transection in the gland leads to formation of a pseudocyst. Injuries to the head of the pancreas often are associated with duodenal injuries.

Stable patients with an isolated pancreatic contusion should undergo selective nonoperative management with nasogastric drainage and parenteral nutrition. With resolution of pain, tenderness, and hyperamylasemia, nasogastric drainage can be discontinued. With return of gastrointestinal function, feedings may begin, first with a clear liquid diet, then with a low-fat diet. Clinical monitoring of symptoms, physical signs, and serum amylase levels continue.

If pain persists or recurs after first appearing to resolve, and signs of peritoneal irritation return, an ultrasound should be obtained to search for a pseudocyst. Pseudocysts usually develop 2 to 4 weeks after injury. Small pseudocysts (<4 cm in diameter) can be observed, with the expectation that they will resolve. Large or enlarging pseudocysts should undergo percutaneous catheter drainage. MRCP should be performed in these cases to assess the status of the duct. A large cyst resistant to catheter drainage should be addressed with laparotomy. A thick-walled pseudocyst identifiable on CT may undergo internal drainage. If it is adherent to the stomach, cystogastrostomy can be performed, whereas others can be drained into a Roux loop of jejunum. Thin-walled cysts need external drainage. Development of pain and fever suggests the development of a pancreatic abscess. CT shows extensive retroperitoneal edema with areas of liquefaction and devitalized tissue. Laparotomy is required to drain pancreatic abscess because devitalized pancreas and retroperitoneal tissue will have to be débrided. Multiple drains in the region are required.

If a pancreatic transection is known to be present, early distal pancreatectomy with preservation of the spleen is the preferred approach. Pancreatic resection avoids pancreatic fistula and pseudocyst formation. The procedure involves control of multiple tributaries from the gland to the splenic vein, a reasonably straightforward procedure when performed soon after the injury. When operation has been delayed for several days, however, inflammation in the area makes resection considerably more difficult. MRCP or endoscopic retrograde cholangiopancreatography may be useful in cases in which a transection is suspected. The results after distal pancreatectomy are excellent with little or no mortality and minimal complications except in cases in which other injuries are associated.

The various methods of operative management of major duodenal injuries (discussed earlier) are appropriate for injuries of the head of the pancreas. These methods all are preferred to pancreaticoduodenectomy because of the high attendant morbidity of the procedure. This measure may be necessary, however, in a few cases in which there is extensive damage to the duodenum and the gland, and resection is largely débridement of devitalized tissue.

Pancreatic ascites is a rare postinjury complication. Paracentesis shows fluid with high amylase content. MRCP or endoscopic retrograde cholangiopancreatography may be necessary to visualize the ductal disruption and guide operative strategy.

Extrahepatic Biliary Tree and Gallbladder

Injuries to the extrahepatic bile ducts are distinctly unusual even with penetrating injuries. Injury to the gallbladder is treated best with cholecystectomy, whereas primary repair is best for bile duct injuries. If a satisfactory primary repair is not possible, a Roux-en-Y hepaticojejunostomy should be performed. Most isolated extrahepatic bile duct injuries are not recognized for 24 to 48 hours after injury.

Bony Pelvis

Pelvic injuries are the result of intense force, usually during pedestrian or motor vehicle crashes. Extensive pelvic injuries carry a high mortality. A pelvic fracture signals a high risk for significant blood loss and associated major injuries in the abdomen and elsewhere in the body. Stupor associated with hemorrhagic shock may mask pain. A fracture of the pubic rami produces pain in the groin. Abrasions, large bruises, and large lacerations may be present. The bony pelvis may be asymmetric and unstable to anterior-posterior and lateral compression. Because lower genitourinary tract injuries so often accompany pelvic fractures, hematomas of the perineum, blood at the urethral meatus, and the location of the prostate in male victims should be sought. A shard of bone may lacerate the rectum so that rectal bleeding is an important finding.

Plain film of the abdomen, taken during the secondary survey of the trauma patient, should include the pelvis to search for a fracture. Presence of fracture requires an abdominal CT scan to evaluate for visceral injury and to help define the extent of injury to the bony pelvis. Signs of lower urinary tract injury require a urethrogram and cystogram.

Unstable pelvic fractures require immobilization with external fixation devices. External fixation is also the first step in the control of hemorrhage from a pelvic fracture. If bleeding continues, angiography is indicated with selective embolization of bleeding vessels. Should a pelvic hematoma be encountered during laparotomy for another cause, it is best left undisturbed, and external fixation and selective angiography should be attempted first.

Genitourinary Trauma

Kidney

The kidney is the second most common intra-abdominal organ injured from blunt trauma in childhood. It is far less commonly involved in penetrating trauma. Although isolated renal injury occurs, 40% to 50% of cases have associated injuries to other body regions, including the head, extremities, thorax, and other intra-abdominal organs. Renal injuries are not usually life-threatening, but immediate surgery is indicated in a few instances. The kidney with preexisting disease, particularly hydronephrosis and tumors, is particularly prone to injury. Many congenital and neoplastic problems are first discovered because of hematuria following relatively mild injuries.

Most injuries to the kidney are the result of direct blows to the parenchyma resulting in contusion, intracapsular hematoma, or fracture. Sudden deceleration may avulse the vascular pedicle or ureteropelvic junction. Even minor degrees of trauma may cause serious renal injury. Child abuse always must be considered. Renal injury causes mild abdominal and flank guarding and tenderness over the involved kidney. Gross and microscopic hematuria is generally present. There are anecdotal experiences that hematuria may be absent in disruptions of the renal pedicle, but more recent surveys indicate some degree of microscopic hematuria is present in essentially all cases of significant renal injuries.

Radiographic evaluation is usually possible. When patients must be brought to the operating room as an emergency because of hemorrhage from other structures, obtaining a one-shot IVP has been advocated to show the presence of a functioning kidney contralateral to the injury.

Although it is important to show that two kidneys are present, however, rarely does the functional status of the contralateral kidney determine the surgical management of the injured kidney. Use of the one-shot IVP is decreasing. When there is sufficient time, a CT scan with intravenous and enteral contrast should be performed.

Various classifications of renal injury have been proposed, but a simple classification of renal injuries is as follows:

1. Minor injuries, including simple contusions and confined lacerations with an intact capsule. Vital signs are stable.
2. Major injuries, including lacerations with extension through the renal capsule, with or without extravasation. Vital signs are stable.
3. Critical or emergency injuries associated with major vascular disruptions, shattered kidneys, or injuries associated with uncontrollable hemorrhage and unstable clinical signs. Immediate operation is necessary to salvage the organ or to control life-threatening hemorrhage. Most have associated intra-abdominal injuries.

Stable patients with minor or major injuries are placed on bed rest with close clinical follow-up. Daily examination of the urine monitors the degree of hematuria. When hematuria has cleared, the patient may be taken off bed rest and discharged to home on limited activity. Minor injuries do not require follow-up imaging.

Observation may be employed in stable patients with intermediate injuries in which there is extravasation of urine but no evidence of an expanding flank mass. Many patients with major injuries do not have major complications, and healing often occurs without operation. With the expansion of extravasation, continued bleeding, or evidence of infection, delayed operation is indicated. The advantage to a delayed approach is that hemorrhaging surfaces will have sealed and the need for nephrectomy is minimized.

Immediate surgery is usually necessary for a shattered kidney, renal pedicle injury, continued hemorrhage, or a penetrating injury (Figs. 13-6 and 13-7). At laparotomy, the renal pedicle is controlled before opening Gerota's fascia. Without such control, bleeding may make definition of the extent of injury impossible, necessitating a nephrectomy. If bleeding is encountered, the renal vessels are occluded, and the kidney is cooled by surrounding it with crushed ice. Necrotic tissue is débrided, bleeding vessels are ligated, and lacerations of the collecting system are closed with absorbable sutures. Parenchymal lacerations are closed with the same techniques used for other solid organs described earlier. When only a portion of the kidney has been injured, partial resection is possible because of the segmental nature of the renal blood supply. The renal pelvis and ureter must be inspected for injury. If there is any question, a nephrostomy tube should be placed and brought out the flank. Wide drainage also should be performed using Penrose drains to prevent the accumulation of urine and subsequent infection.

Renal pedicle injuries are exposed best after gaining wide exposure of the aorta and inferior vena cava on

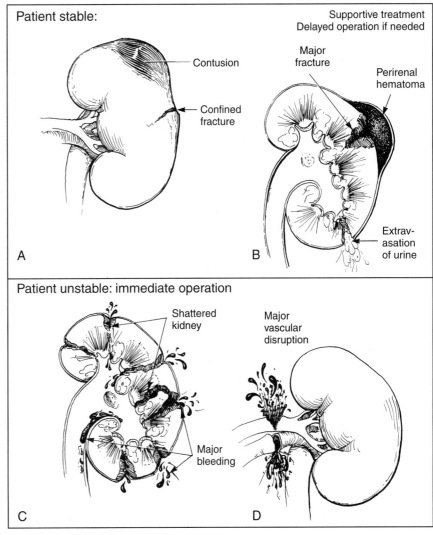

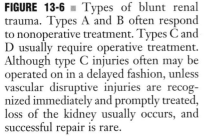

FIGURE 13-6 ▪ Types of blunt renal trauma. Types A and B often respond to nonoperative treatment. Types C and D usually require operative treatment. Although type C injuries often may be operated on in a delayed fashion, unless vascular disruptive injuries are recognized immediately and promptly treated, loss of the kidney usually occurs, and successful repair is rare.

both sides. Standard techniques for vascular repair should be used depending on the nature of the injury, but often aortorenal bypass with saphenous vein or Dove-Tex graft may be necessary. When possible, injuries to the major renal veins should be repaired. Occasionally, ligation is necessary, particularly of branch vessels.

It is rarely possible to repair major disruptions of the renal artery and save the kidney because repair must be done within hours of injury or renal necrosis develops. Additionally, many vascular disruptions go unrecognized.

Complications occur more commonly in patients who have been treated expectantly because of accumulation of blood and urine around the kidney. Late complications occur in major injuries, including development of urinoma, infection, loss of function, and hypertension. A follow-up imaging study should be done in 6 weeks to monitor the resolution of major injuries and pedicle reconstructions. All patients regardless of treatment should be followed for the possibility of delayed onset of hypertension related to the presence of necrotic or ischemic renal tissue or vascular stenosis within the kidney.

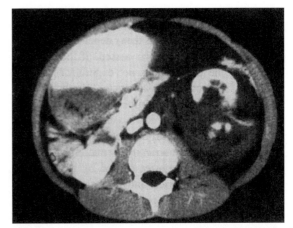

FIGURE 13-7 ▪ CT scan performed on a 6-year-old child who was hit by a car shows a massive left renal injury with a surrounding hematoma and extravasation of contrast material. Operative repair was performed to control continued bleeding and was successful in preserving two thirds of the kidney.

Urinary Bladder

Most bladder injuries are caused by extensive pelvic fractures. Penetrating injuries are rare. Bursting injuries occur if patients are injured with a full bladder. Physical signs are limited, but lower abdominal tenderness is usually elicited.

Indications for cystography include pelvic fractures to any degree, significant hematuria, blood at the urethral meatus, and ileus associated with azotemia. Cystography best establishes the diagnosis because some intraperitoneal ruptures may be missed unless the bladder is fully distended with contrast material. Additional views allow inspection of the posterior aspect of the bladder. A postvoiding study shows the presence of extravasated contrast material in the pelvis from an extraperitoneal tear. CT has been used to delineate bladder injuries. When a CT scan is performed to evaluate abdominal injuries, it is helpful to have a catheter in the bladder and to clamp it during the study. Delayed images of the pelvis 5 minutes after contrast injection may show intraperitoneal and extraperitoneal bladder injuries.

Small extraperitoneal ruptures may be treated nonoperatively with Foley catheter drainage. Close follow-up ascertains that fluid collections do not enlarge or become superinfected. Healing usually takes 2 to 3 weeks, and antibiotic coverage is needed. If the patient fails to improve, surgical repair is necessary. Intraperitoneal ruptures require repair using two-layer or three-layer closure with absorbable suture material and drainage of the prevesical space. A suprapubic tube vesicostomy may be placed, with the tube being brought out through a stab incision separate from the repair. Shards of bone from a fracture must be removed. All penetrating injuries are treated surgically.

After bladder repair, catheter drainage should continue for 7 to 10 days. Contrast study confirms the integrity of the repair. Postoperative complications include stones, fistula formation, and stenoses of the ureters or the urethra.

Urethral Injuries

Blunt injury from either a straddle injury or a pelvic fracture is the most common cause of urethral injury in childhood. Most are at the level of the membranous urethra in the male. The classic sign is blood at the meatus or presence of a perineal hematoma. A hematoma confined to Buck's fascia involves the penis. If the fascia is ruptured, the hematoma may spread along the planes of Colles' fascia, spreading over the scrotum, perineum, and lower abdomen and along the inguinal creases. The patient has difficulty voiding.

If a urethral injury is suspected, the patient first should undergo a retrograde urethrogram. If the urethra is intact to the bladder neck, a Foley catheter is passed. If the urethra is injured or if there is resistance to passing the catheter, it is best not to pass a urethral catheter. Instead a suprapubic catheter becomes necessary. Extravasation of contrast material establishes the presence of a urethral injury. Even in the absence of leakage, a partial-thickness injury may be present that leads to late stricture formation.

Most urethral injuries associated with pelvic fractures involve the posterior urethra. Associated bladder injuries are common. Definition of these injuries, similar to injuries of the anterior urethra, first involves a retrograde urethrogram, followed by cystography.

The treatment of anterior urethral injuries depends on extent and location. Partial and limited injuries may be splinted with a Silastic catheter for 2 weeks. There are two approaches to more extensive injuries. Primary repair is appropriate when the injury is associated with a large hematoma. In most cases, however, anterior urethral injuries should be treated with suprapubic vesicostomy and delayed surgical repair over a stent 3 to 6 months later.

The same general approach is used in cases of posterior urethral injuries. There has been more enthusiasm for primary repair with suprapubic diversion. The two ends of the urethra are aligned over a Silastic catheter, with delayed revision if stricture occurs. Primary repair converts a closed pelvic fracture, if present, into an open one, however, which carries a higher risk of infection. Urethral injuries in females are usually treated by direct repair, stenting, and suprapubic vesicostomy.

Genital Injury

Most blunt genital injuries in males involve the penis. Rupture of the corpus cavernosum causes hemorrhage into the surrounding tissues. A catheter passed into the urinary bladder stents the urethra. Operative exploration is indicated to evacuate the hematoma, repair the ruptured corpus, and repair the urethra, if necessary. Partial amputations should undergo reattachment.

Injury to the scrotum depends on the extent of injury. Mild contusions may be observed, but in most cases exploration is the safest course. Sonography has been suggested to ascertain the need for exploration, but surgery allows evacuation of the hematoma, control of bleeding, and repair of a ruptured testis. Scrotal closure may require débridement and cleansing first.

Injuries to the female external genitalia are almost all the result of straddle injuries. Sexual assault is important to recognize and document appropriately. Because of pain and psychological stress, a complete examination requires general anesthesia. Careful inspection of the urethra, vagina, and rectum can proceed, and appropriate fluid samples for legal inspection and bacteriology can be obtained. Urethroscopy, cystoscopy, vaginoscopy, and proctoscopy may be required. Débridement of injured tissue and repair of extensive lacerations avoid the potential for rectovaginal and vesicovaginal fistula formation. A Foley catheter should be left in place as indicated.

SUGGESTED READINGS

Albanese CT, Mesa MP, Gardner MJ, et al: Is computed tomography a useful adjunct to the clinical examination for the diagnosis of pediatric gastrointestinal perforation from blunt abdominal trauma in children? J Trauma 40:417-421, 1996.

Of 30 patients undergoing laparotomy for intestinal injuries, 11 underwent immediate operation for shock, peritonitis, or free air on plain film, and 19 underwent a laparotomy an average of 3.4 hours later because of the delayed appearance of peritonitis. Only 3 of the 19 patients had free air on CT; the remainder had dilated, thick-walled bowel loops or mesenteric infiltration. In this study,

CT was adjunctive to the clinical examination in the decision to operate for intestinal injury.

Brenner D, Elliston C, Hall E, et al: Estimated risks of radiation-induced fatal cancer from pediatric CT. AJR Am J Roentgenol 176:289-296, 2001.

Certain to be an important and controversial article, the authors estimate that increased estimated lifetime cancer mortality risks attributable to the radiation exposure from a CT scan in a 1-year-old are 0.18% for an abdominal CT examination and 0.07% for a head CT examination.

Cooper A, Barlow B, DiScala C, et al: Mortality and truncal injury: The pediatric perspective. J Pediatr Surg 29:33-38, 1994.

This article summarizes data from the National Pediatric Trauma Registry from 1985 through 1991. Of 25,301 reported cases, 2047 (8%) involved abdominal injuries. Although the mortality rate of blunt abdominal injuries is 9%, the abdominal injury itself is the cause of death in only 22% of cases. The mortality of penetrating abdominal injuries is 6%, and the abdominal injury is the cause of death in two thirds.

Jobst MA, Canty TG Sr, Lynch FP: Management of pancreatic injury in pediatric blunt abdominal trauma. J Pediatr Surg 34:818-824, 1999.

In this study, serum amylase levels were elevated in 71% of cases and did not correlate with severity of pancreatic injury. Abdominal CT was normal in 13%. Nonoperative management was successful in 46% of cases, with 27% developing pseudocysts. Of cases, 13% underwent primary distal pancreatectomy with preservation of the spleen for distal main ductal injuries.

Mehall JR, Ennis JS, Salzman DA, et al: Prospective results of a standardized algorithm based on hemodynamic status for managing pediatric solid organ injury. J Am Coll Surg 193:347-353, 2001.

Hemodynamic status, not CT grade of injury, guided the treatment algorithm of children with blunt injuries of the spleen and liver. Of hemodynamically stable patients with isolated injuries, 98% were discharged successfully without transfusion or intensive care unit observation within 48 hours of admission.

Morey AF, Bruce JE, McAninch JW: Efficacy of radiographic imaging in pediatric blunt renal trauma. J Urol 156:2014-2018, 1996.

In this study, only 2% of patients (11 of 548 patients from collected series) with less than 50 red blood cells per high-powered field had significant renal injuries, whereas 27% of patients with gross hematuria had significant renal injuries. The authors present an algorithm for the radiographic evaluation of blunt renal trauma, although some of their end points (IVP, one-shot IVP) are not used widely in present practice.

Russell RS, Gomelsky A, McMahon DR, et al: Management of grade IV renal injury in children. J Urol 166:1049-1050, 2001.

Renal injury associated with urinary extravasation can be treated with selective nonoperative management successfully in most (9 of 15 [60%]) cases. Of the remaining six patients who required intervention, only two required operation, one early and one late in the course. The others were treated successfully with percutaneous drainage or placement of a ureteral stent when necessary.

Shilansky J, Pearl RH, Kreller M, et al: Diagnosis and management of duodenal injuries in children. J Pediatr Surg 32:880-886, 1997.

CT with oral contrast accurately distinguishes duodenal hematoma from perforation. Children with duodenal hematomas require an average of 16 days to resolve upper intestinal obstruction.

Velhamos GC, Demetriades D, Toutouzas KG, et al: Selective management in 1,856 patients with abdominal gunshot wounds: Should routine laparotomy still be the standard of care? Ann Surg 234:395-403, 2001.

This report from the Los Angeles County–University of Southern California Medical Center establishes the safety and efficacy of selective management of gunshot wounds in hemodynamically stable patients free from peritonitis and in whom a reliable physical examination could be performed. The rate of successful nonoperative management (38%) is lower and the rate of nontherapeutic laparotomy (14%) is higher than rates quoted for abdominal stab wounds.

14

Musculoskeletal Injuries

Fractures in childhood, similar to head injuries, are most commonly isolated injuries, but frequently they are part of the spectrum of multiple trauma. With multiple trauma, fractures contribute significantly to the hypermetabolic response to injury. Although the definitive management of long bone fractures in extensively injured children is not an immediate priority in emergency management, all fractures should be splinted or immobilized so that long-term management is not compromised. Children at various ages have clear-cut anatomic and physiologic differences from adults. These essential differences account for some of the unusual fracture patterns seen in childhood. They also account for a different rate of healing and remodeling potential compared with that seen in adults. Depending on the preexisting state of the child, bone age may or may not keep pace with the child's actual age.

The National Pediatric Trauma Registry helps to identify trends and understand the epidemiology of pediatric musculoskeletal injuries. Data from more than 28,000 injuries evaluated at 61 children's hospitals reveal the most common injury mechanisms as follows: falls (26%), motor vehicle accidents with child as passenger (19%), motor vehicle accidents with child as pedestrian (16%), bicycle injuries (9%), stabbing (5%), and gunshot wounds (5%).

There is a distinctive fracture pattern associated with child abuse, which is described in more detail in Chapter 18. As with other forms of injury, fractures occur at least twice as often in boys as in girls.

ESSENTIAL DIFFERENCES BETWEEN CHILDREN AND ADULTS

Anatomy

Figure 14-1 details the general anatomic features of immature bone. The primary difference between children and adults relates to the status of the growth centers during the various stages of childhood. Each long bone is divided into epiphysis, physis, metaphysis, and diaphysis. The epiphysis has two layers of cartilage with an intervening secondary center of ossification with the function of restructuring the end of the bone as the joint develops. The next layer down is the physis, which is the growth plate that provides longitudinal growth and conversion of cartilage to bone in the immediate underlying metaphysis. Proceeding downward is the diaphysis, which is surrounded by periosteum, which provides circumferential bone growth. When growth is completed, the epiphysis and physis drop out and are represented solely by articular cartilage, under which are the metaphysis and diaphysis. Adult bone has limited potential for remodeling, whereas young bone has considerable potential for reshaping itself.

The relatively soft nature of pediatric bone and its tendency to be more porous than adult bone make it relatively resistant to fracture but less resistant to collapse or compression. This is why particular fractures, such as the greenstick and elevation or torus fractures, are seen in children but not in adults. Children also sustain all of the same fractures adults do. Periosteum in children is thicker and more elastic than in adults, so children more often have fractures with periosteal elevation and a lesser degree of displacement. Another difference is related to the presence of the growth center. The physis is the weakest point in the bone, and it is particularly susceptible to torsion injuries. Depending on the degree of maturity, the pattern of a fracture through the growth center varies because its resistance to force increases over time.

Physiologic Differences

Because the musculoskeletal system is a metabolically active, rapidly changing part of the body, fractured bones in children heal and remodel more rapidly than bones in adults. The rapidity of fracture healing in children is age dependent such that newborns may have stable union of a femoral fracture in 7 to 10 days, whereas it may take about 6 weeks in adolescents. The sturdy periosteum tends to maintain alignment and to form new bone rapidly. In general, the vascularity of periosteum is extensive so that nonunion is uncommon. Although pediatric bone has a great potential to remodel, this is limited primarily to fractures in and around the physis in young children. It is still important to correct bony deformities from fractures and to immobilize them to avoid healing with angulation or rotation.

Fractures that are near to or directly involve the growth plate may create a secondary disturbance in one of two ways. First, growth may be prematurely arrested when the growth plate itself is injured. This arrest in growth may

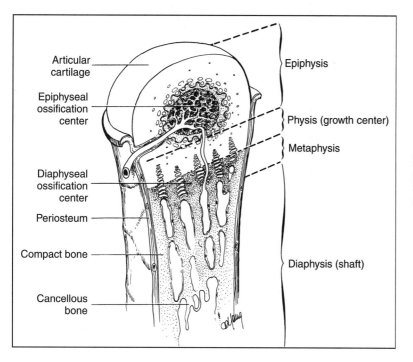

Articular cartilage

Epiphyseal ossification center

Diaphyseal ossification center

Periosteum

Compact bone

Cancellous bone

Epiphysis

Physis (growth center)

Metaphysis

Diaphysis (shaft)

FIGURE 14-1 ■ Immature bone has the capability of continuing growth, but it is more susceptible to injury of various areas because growth alteration or arrest may occur.

create a progressive limb-length discrepancy or an angular deformity of the joint. Second, growth may be accelerated when the growth plate is stimulated by the healing process. This may create an overgrowth of 1 to 2 cm after femoral shaft fractures, which occurs during the first year after injury. Because of these issues, children with significant remaining growth potential must have close long-term follow-up to ensure appropriate identification and treatment of potential problems.

History and Physical Findings

Whether children have sustained minor or major trauma, it is important to obtain a background history regarding illnesses or congenital disorders that affect bone formation and to determine whether the history is consistent with the nature of the fracture seen. If the history does not match the biomechanical forces expected to be responsible for a particular fracture or if the fracture appears to have predated the stated history, abuse must be considered, particularly if the child is younger than age 2 years. If a particular fracture is found to be associated with minor forces, metabolic bone disease and pathologic fractures must be considered. If the history indicates a crush injury or if there is any question of vascular interruption or excessive swelling, a compartment syndrome must be excluded.

The priorities of trauma management must be emphasized during the evaluation and management of any child with a high-energy mechanism of injury. The elements of the primary survey are airway protection with cervical stabilization and evaluation of breathing, circulation, disability, and exposure with environmental control to prevent hypothermia. More detailed evaluation of the spine and extremities should occur during the secondary survey.

Important physical findings in evaluation for fracture include observations regarding deformity, degree of swelling, contusions, signs of ischemia, shortening or abnormal movement, and associated soft tissue injury, which may indicate an open fracture. All bones of the skeleton should be palpated for any sign of tenderness, crepitus, or deformity. This palpation is particularly important because young children may be unable to provide a reliable history. The character of peripheral pulses should be determined with accuracy before and after immobilization of a fracture using a Doppler if necessary. Special care should be taken in the evaluation of potential open fractures. Appropriate cultures should be performed, and if there is any question, thorough exploration, débridement, and reduction should be performed in the operating room with the patient under general anesthesia.

If peripheral pulses are diminished initially, particularly in the presence of marked swelling, or if pulses diminish in amplitude on serial Doppler examination, a compartment syndrome should be suspected, particularly if the lower leg or forearm is involved. In addition to disturbances in peripheral pulses, patients may complain of pain in the extremity, paresthesia, or paralysis. Under these circumstances, compartment pressures should be measured with one of the available monitoring systems, such as the Wick or slit catheter, which is a helpful guide to determine whether fasciotomy will be needed. If there is any question, it is best to do a fasciotomy.

The mainstay of diagnosis is radiography. The observer must be knowledgeable about the normal radiographic appearance of bone at varying stages of life, realizing that cartilage is not radiopaque and that centers of ossification vary in their appearance at different ages. If there is any doubt, comparative films of the opposite extremity may be helpful but should not often be necessary for the practitioner experienced in the normal radiographic appearance of pediatric bone. It is generally necessary to take anteroposterior and lateral films and sometimes oblique views to image a fracture accurately. When obtaining films, the x-ray tube should be moved but not the injured extremity to avoid increasing the amount of damage already present. At times, other more specific studies must be obtained. Computed tomography may be required to evaluate the spine and pelvis, and arteriography may be necessary to image the potentially damaged arterial tree. Aspiration of a joint may be necessary to verify the presence of an intra-articular fracture not seen on film but associated with blood and fat particles in the joint. Magnetic resonance imaging may be needed to diagnose cartilaginous and ligamentous tears within major joints, particularly the knee.

FORMS OF MUSCULOSKELETAL INJURY IN CHILDREN AND THEIR TREATMENT

Figure 14-2 shows the different types of fractures that may be encountered in children.

General Principles of Management

As mentioned, management of fractures in the emergency department should begin by placement of an appropriate traction or splinting device until other more emergent problems are managed. Failure to immobilize a major fracture in a child who is flailing about because of pain may extend the amount of damage present, promote bleeding, and even convert a closed fracture to an open one. A variety of devices are available, but the general principle is to splint the extremity as found, immobilizing the joint above and below the fracture without excessive pressure. Neck collars and backboards help to splint spinal fractures and pelvic fractures. Traction splints reaching to the hip joints are best used for femur fractures, whereas most other fractures can be managed in simple splints or slings.

Depending on the type of fracture encountered and how much manipulation is required, a general anesthetic may or may not be required. Satisfactory position must be achieved without vascular embarrassment before healing progresses to a point that fixes the fracture in an undesirable position. A fracture in an infant may begin to heal in a few days, whereas it may take a few weeks in an adolescent. Postreduction radiographs and periodic checks must be performed to ensure maintenance of appropriate position until the healing fracture is strong enough to overcome the muscular forces specific to the particular bone. Generally, it takes 4 to 6 weeks for an upper extremity fracture to heal in a child of any age, but for a lower extremity, healing may take 1 month in a toddler and twice as long in an adolescent. Metaphyseal, undisplaced, or impacted fractures heal more rapidly than displaced fractures or fractures of the shaft of the bone, which are more frequently complete fractures. If there is an extensive soft tissue injury associated with the fracture or if the fracture is open, healing may take appreciably longer. More care must be taken with reduction of fractures of the growth plate than the shaft because of the potential for interrupting the circulation to the growth center.

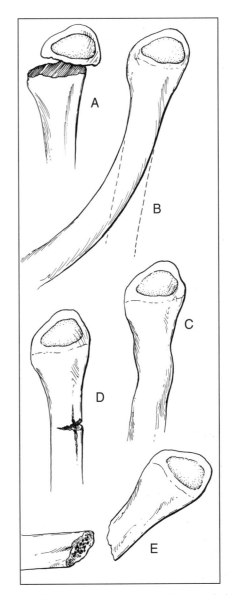

FIGURE 14-2 ■ Because bone is softer and more pliable in the pediatric age group, particularly in very young children, different types of fractures may be encountered, and treatment varies according to the type of fracture. **A**, Epiphyseal/physeal fracture. **B**, Bend or bow. **C**, Torus or buckle fracture. **D**, Greenstick fracture. **E**, Complete fracture.

As children get older, they more frequently sustain severe traumatic forces, while the character of more mature bone makes it more susceptible to fractures with a pattern of comminution, oblique displacement, and instability. Often cast immobilization is insufficient, and either internal or external fixation is required.

Generally, for vascular injuries associated with unstable fractures, circulation should be reestablished first, then the fracture stabilized, unless the anticipated manipulation for fracture reduction would be likely to disrupt a repair, under which circumstances fracture reduction is accomplished first. A potential compartment syndrome always must be considered under these circumstances.

Open fractures always should be treated in the operating room after culture and administration of broad-spectrum

TABLE 14-1 ■ Types of Musculoskeletal Injuries in Childhood

Epiphyseal and physeal (growth plate) fractures
Diaphyseal (shaft) fractures
Dislocations
Joint injuries, cartilaginous and ligamentous tears

antibiotics. After débridement and thorough irrigation and fixation of the associated open fracture, the wound is best left open and, if possible, closed in a delayed fashion 48 to 72 hours after the initial débridement procedure.

As soon as is feasible, physical therapy is initiated. Rehabilitative efforts are continued until the patient is returned to full function.

SPECIFIC INJURIES

Four general patterns of injury are seen: epiphyseal and physeal fractures, shaft fractures, dislocations with or without associated fractures, and a variety of sports injuries including injuries to articular cartilages (Table 14-1).

Epiphyseal and Physeal Fractures

Most epiphyseal and physeal fractures are caused by falls, many on an outstretched hand, which produces angulating and twisting forces. Salter and Harris classified these injuries into five distinctive patterns. Figure 14-3 depicts the Salter-Harris classification. Each of these patterns has different implications in terms of treatment and outcome. In general, type I and II fractures can be treated by closed reduction, whereas type III and IV fractures usually require open reduction and internal fixation. Type V Salter fractures are similar to type I except that they are noted to be associated with growth arrest. Type V epiphyseal fractures are uncommon, and they seem to involve the knee and ankle most frequently.

The epiphyses of various bones not only have different patterns of injury, but also they differ further depending on the age of the patient. Epiphyseal separation of either end of the clavicle may be difficult to diagnose radiographically and may be more evident on physical examination or computed tomography scan. These injuries frequently require open reduction and fixation.

Fractures of the proximal humeral epiphysis usually can be treated by immobilization in a Velpeau sling for 3 weeks. More complicated fractures with displacement may require a shoulder spica. Epiphyseal fractures of the distal humerus frequently have long-term growth disturbances, joint subluxation, and interposition of soft tissue structures between the fracture fragments. Many of these fractures require open reduction and internal fixation.

Fractures of the proximal and distal ulna usually can be treated by simple immobilization. With any degree of displacement, open reduction is usually necessary.

Fractures of the proximal radial epiphysis usually can be reduced in a closed fashion, although it may require a general anesthetic. Fractures of the distal radial epiphysis are the most common epiphyseal injury in childhood. This fracture almost always can be treated by closed reduction and immobilization for 4 to 6 weeks.

Fractures of the proximal femoral epiphysis are unusual, but when they occur, urgent reduction and fixation is necessary to reduce the risk of avascular necrosis. Fractures of the distal femoral epiphysis are important because of the degree of growth that occurs at this site. All of these fractures must be reduced carefully, usually with the patient under general anesthesia. Occasionally, open reduction is required.

Proximal tibial epiphyseal injuries are unusual depending on which portion of the proximal end of the tibia is injured and the specific type of fracture. Treatment may vary, but at times maintenance of reduction may require some form of internal fixation with pins. Just as with patients with femur fractures, patients with injuries to this portion of the tibia must be followed because of the potential problems with extremity growth. The same consideration applies with regard to fractures of the distal tibial epiphyseal plate. In most cases, closed reduction and immobilization are sufficient, but long-term follow-up is important to diagnose either total or partial growth arrest, the latter being associated with late appearance of angulation. Fractures of the epiphysis of the distal fibula and of the physes of the bones of the foot are generally treatable by closed reduction and immobilization.

Shaft Fractures

Clavicular fractures are among the most common diaphyseal fractures encountered. The diagnosis is usually evident on clinical examination, although radiographs are

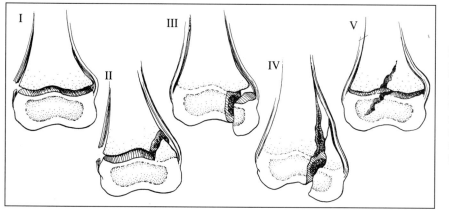

FIGURE 14-3 ■ The five forms of epiphyseal fractures generally encountered. This classification is particularly useful in determining the type of treatment that should be used and in predicting the long-term outcome, because each is associated with different degrees of devascularization of the growth plate (Salter-Harris classification; see text).

confirmatory. Most fractures can be treated by immobilization with a simple sling or figure-8 bandage. Open reduction and fixation is rarely necessary.

Humeral fractures are particularly important because of the occasional association of neurovascular injuries. The radial nerve is the one most frequently injured, depending on the type of fracture and the age of the patient. The principles of treatment include traction to correct overriding, malalignment, or angulation and either a sling or a hanging cast. Supracondylar humeral fractures at the elbow not only are common, but also they bear special consideration because of the potential for compromise of the brachial artery and the nerves about the elbow. In many instances, supracondylar fractures can be treated with closed reduction and pinning, but whenever there are signs of continuing vascular compromise or if a stable reduction cannot be obtained with traction, open exploration and vascular repair may be necessary with fracture fixation.

Fractures of the radius and ulna are extremely common in childhood, and they may take many forms as shown in Figures 14-2 and 14-3. These fractures and their treatment vary greatly, but the principles of therapy include correction of alignment, avoidance of rotational deformities, and maintenance of the interosseous space so that the ability to pronate and supinate is preserved. Most forearm fractures in children require 6 to 8 weeks of immobilization depending on their severity. Follow-up radiographs should be taken at early intervals after cast placement to detect loss of reduction.

With severe injury either from a fall or as a direct blow in a motor vehicle accident, fractures of the femoral neck and shaft of the femur are common. Although epiphyseal injuries of the femur frequently are associated with growth deficiencies, the same is not usually true of neck or shaft fractures of the femur. Initially, traction followed by placement of a hip spica is usually sufficient for the treatment of most children with neck or shaft fractures. The overall approach is influenced, however, by age, associated injuries, and the pattern of the fracture. Infants younger than 2 years are treated best with Bryant's traction for 2 to 3 weeks followed by casting. Older children should be placed in skeletal traction with the pins away from the growth center. Traction should be continued until position is satisfactory enough to permit a spica cast to be placed. Long-term follow-up is necessary to detect deficiencies or excesses in longitudinal growth. Fractures about the knee that are undisplaced may be treated by closed reduction and immobilization, but more frequently, displacement is present, and open reduction is necessary.

The same general approaches are referable to fractures of the tibia and fibula. Most patients require an anesthetic for manipulation and correction of torsion, angulation, and position. A long leg cast should be applied and left in place for 6 to 12 weeks depending on the age of the child. These fractures require long-term follow-up to detect growth abnormalities. Open reduction seldom is needed.

Fractures of the various bones of the foot are uncommon. When they do occur, they are usually nondisplaced, which permits simple immobilization with a cast with the foot in anatomic position.

Dislocations

Dislocations are less common in children than in adults because children have a greater degree of joint motion and redundancy of the joint capsule. This extra degree of joint mobility decreases over time so that joint dislocations generally occur in older children except in children with specific disorders of connective tissue, such as Ehlers-Danlos syndrome. In older children and adolescents, dislocations occur more commonly, and they may or may not be associated with adjacent fractures. The most common dislocation encountered in a young person is of the elbow joint. When associated with a radial head or ulnar fracture, reduction may be difficult, and open reduction may be required. Neurovascular injuries sometimes occur but far less commonly than in the lower extremity. Severe forms of direct trauma may result in dislocations of the hip, knee, or ankle (in that order). Dislocations of the hip should be reduced at the earliest possible time to avoid avascular necrosis of the femoral head. As with adults, the prime consideration with posterior dislocation of the knee joint is occlusion of the popliteal artery or a stretch injury of the peroneal nerve. Ligamentous repair should be performed on a delayed basis after initial reduction. Dislocation of the patella is common, and, although closed reduction and immobilization for 4 weeks often constitute successful treatment, at times operative management is necessary.

COMPLICATIONS OF FRACTURE TREATMENT

A variety of considerations related to treatment have been mentioned in the foregoing section. The main categories of complications follow (Table 14-2).

Early Ischemia

Early ischemia related to arterial damage is particularly a concern with supracondylar fractures about the elbow and knee. The brachial and popliteal arteries are the ones most often damaged. In addition, delayed ischemia may result because of progressive compartmental swelling, which first causes venous congestion, then arterial insufficiency. Compartment syndromes may be seen with fractures of the forearm or tibia, crush injuries, excessive traction, a cast that is too tight, or delay in fracture treatment. If a compartment syndrome associated with ischemia goes untreated for longer than 6 hours, permanent loss of muscle and nerve function, Volkmann's ischemic contracture, and causalgia syndrome may result. Fasciotomy of all compartments is necessary.

TABLE 14-2 ■ Complications of Fractures and Their Treatment

Early ischemia from arterial damage
Compartment syndrome
Limb growth disturbance
Injury to related vascular and visceral structures
Avascular necrosis of epiphyses
Musculotendinous fibrosis and limitation of motion
Joint instability

Growth Disturbances

Growth disturbances associated with long bone fractures are common and may be missed if follow-up is insufficient. Serial scanographs are necessary to predict the degree of inequality that might be expected at the time of maturity, and expeditious or appropriately timed epiphysiodesis or limb lengthening should be performed as indicated. The same consideration is true with regard to abnormal angulation after fracture treatment.

Bone Fragment Injury

Fragments of bone associated with fractures at times may injure adjacent structures, such as the neurovascular bundle in the leg or pelvic organs with pelvic fractures.

Avascular Necrosis

With all epiphyseal and intracapsular fractures of the femoral neck, close observation for several months should be carried out to determine whether avascular necrosis has occurred so that appropriate intervention can be initiated.

Limitation of Motion and Function

Early rehabilitation and physical therapy, appropriate timing of weight bearing, and long-term rehabilitative follow-up help to prevent limitations in motion and function, which otherwise may be associated with musculotendinous fibrosis accompanied by fractures and immobilization therapy.

SUGGESTED READINGS

Copley LA, et al: Vascular injuries and their sequelae in pediatric supracondylar humeral fractures: Toward a goal of prevention. J Pediatr Orthop 16:99, 1996.

This article describes the management of 128 consecutive children with grade III supracondylar humeral fractures, of which 17 presented with absent or diminished radial pulses.

Davidson RS, Hahn M: Musculoskeletal trauma. In O'Neill JA, et al (eds): Pediatric Surgery, 5th ed. St. Louis, Mosby, 1998, p 309.

This chapter summarizes the anatomy and physiology of childhood bone and the pathophysiology of fractures in this age group, diagnosis, and approaches to treatment.

Frankel VH, Nordin M: Basic Biomechanics of the Skeletal System. Philadelphia, Lea & Febiger, 1980.

This book is the best source of basic information on the biomechanics of the skeleton, providing the basis for understanding the results of direct and indirect trauma to bone. An understanding of the biomechanics of the skeleton also provides the basis for understanding the approaches to treatment of skeletal fractures. Special considerations for children are presented.

National Pediatric Trauma Registry: Available at www.nptr.org.

The mission of the website for the National Pediatric Trauma Registry is to collect, analyze, and disseminate information on children hospitalized for traumatic injuries in the United States.

Rang M: Children's Fractures. Philadelphia, JB Lippincott, 1983.

The classic classification of pediatric fractures is presented. This classification is used universally, so the reference is an important one.

15

Vascular Injuries

The basic approaches to and principles of management of vascular injuries are similar in children and adults now. In the past, it was considered that vascular repair in infants and children was not feasible, even after interruption of major vessels, so expectant therapy was used in the hope that collateral circulation would permit survival of an extremity. Although infants and children do have a greater capacity to form satisfactory collaterals than adults, and even though amputation rates after major vascular interruption are only approximately half of that expected in adults, the extent of limb loss with expectant therapy has been unacceptable. Also, although limbs have survived after interruption of femoral arteries, long-term growth has been impeded significantly in at least 70% of cases. These facts have led to a more aggressive approach to repair and reconstruction of injured arteries, even in infants.

SPECIAL PROBLEMS OF THE CHILD: AGE AND PHYSIOLOGY

Infants and children with vascular injuries differ from adults not only in terms of the small size of the vascular tree, but also in terms of physiology. The smaller the child, the more prone he or she is to extreme vascular spasm, which may last for 3 or 4 hours. Infants and small children have relatively small vascular volumes and a tendency to develop low flow states associated with peripheral vasoconstriction after what might be thought to be only modest hemorrhage. In polycythemic newborns, arterial spasm associated with an arterial stick easily may result in thrombosis. Diabetic mothers are particularly prone to have infants with polycythemia and hyperviscosity, which also may predispose to arterial thrombosis. Because of increased metabolic rate in small subjects compared with adults, anticoagulation with heparin may be difficult to regulate. A chronic arterial occlusion in an adult may be manifested primarily by claudication, whereas disturbance of linear growth may be the prime manifestation in children. Conversely, in the case of traumatic arteriovenous fistulas, impressive overgrowth of a limb and congestive heart failure may occur. With excessive flow, overgrowth may be evident in 1 to 2 years, whereas with deficient arterial flow, limb shortening may not be evident for 4 or 5 years. Chronically deficient flow in the lower extremity is manifested more often by growth disturbance than in the upper extremity, where claudication is more common based on follow-up of patients who underwent subclavian-pulmonary artery anastomoses as infants.

EPIDEMIOLOGY

Although blunt trauma causes 80% of all injuries in childhood, more than 90% of vascular injuries in childhood are penetrating in nature. Of all penetrating vascular injuries, about half are iatrogenic, but in children younger than age 2 years, almost 90% are iatrogenic, being related to invasive diagnostic and monitoring procedures. It is understandable that small subjects with tiny blood vessels have a high risk and incidence of injury from invasive vascular procedures. Also, many of these subjects have had these procedures performed because of cyanotic congenital heart disease, under which circumstances they may be polycythemic, have increased blood viscosity, and have low peripheral blood flow. The same is true of sick neonates, particularly low-birth-weight infants.

Cardiac catheterization is the most common procedure resulting in arterial occlusion in infants. The femoral artery is the one most frequently involved. With routine heparinization during catheterization procedures, the incidence of thrombosis has fallen, but it is still approximately 10%.

Catheterization of small peripheral arteries for monitoring purposes is routine in most pediatric intensive care units where critically ill infants and children are cared for. These arterial catheters are used for serial monitoring of blood pressure and blood sampling for precise metabolic and acid-base management of patients undergoing resuscitation or extensive operative procedures. Although risky, catheterization is safer than performance of multiple arterial punctures. Because many patients have periods of low cardiac output and low peripheral flow, thrombosis and skin sloughs are common. Catheterization of the superficial temporal artery has had such a high incidence of complications that its use has been abandoned. Provided that the patient has a patent ulnar artery, the radial artery seems to be the site of choice when an indwelling arterial catheter is needed because it has the lowest incidence of complications. The dorsalis pedis and the posterior tibial arteries are available for use; however, they usually thrombose, and the long-term implication of using these foot arteries is not known. Although the femoral artery is available, this is an undesirable site for arterial monitoring because femoral thrombosis requires operative thrombectomy. The risk of this complication is especially high if the femoral artery and vein on the same side are catheterized. Umbilical artery catheters are used routinely in low-birth-weight infants for monitoring respiratory care and for administering intravenous fluids, blood products, and various drugs; the incidence of major complications related to their use is approximately 5%. Some degree of thrombosis occurs in probably 50% of patients, but the serious complications generally occur in sick newborns who require catheters to be in place for long periods. The problems encountered with the use of umbilical artery catheters include aortic thrombosis, peripheral embolism to leg and visceral vessels, hypertension from embolism to the renal arteries, and, rarely, mycotic aneurysm. The safest location for placement of an umbilical artery catheter is approximately at the level of the fourth lumbar vertebra, and low-dose heparin should be given as an infusion through the catheter.

Although the incidence of iatrogenic penetrating injuries is highest in children younger than 2 years, iatrogenic and traumatic causes are approximately equal between the ages of 2 and 6 years. In children older than age 6 years, only one third of the injuries are iatrogenic, and the remainder are from traumatic causes of various sorts. Penetrating injuries generally are caused by knives, glass shards or other sharp objects, and gunshot wounds. About 15% of patients have arterial injuries as the result of blunt trauma. Most injuries are associated with femoral or proximal tibial fractures that are displaced, some are caused by severe direct blows to the vasculature, and some are associated with compartment syndromes caused by crush injuries. Occasionally, vascular disruption is the result of extensive soft tissue avulsion injuries.

Most serious vascular injuries are arterial. Rarely, penetrating vascular injuries involve not only an artery, but also an adjacent vein, and arteriovenous fistulas result.

Venous injuries are common but not ordinarily as clinically significant as arterial or arteriovenous injuries. Indwelling venous catheters cause venous thromboses and occasional septic or suppurative thrombophlebitis associated with sepsis. Central venous catheters are used extensively in the management of seriously ill infants and children and frequently are left in place for long periods for parenteral nutrition. Right atrial perforation is a rare complication with the use of soft Silastic catheters but, if not recognized promptly, can lead to pericardial tamponade or tension hydrothorax. Thrombosis of the jugular or innominate vein may result in unilateral swelling and edema, but superior vena caval thrombosis produces cyanosis and edema of the entire upper part of the body. In newborns, noncommunicating hydrocephalus may result from superior vena caval thrombosis and in premature newborns is occasionally lethal because of intraventricular bleeding.

PATHOLOGY

There are several manifestations of arterial injury, with different implications regarding treatment. With cardiac catheterization, the most common problem is occlusion by

thrombosis, which may result in complete occlusion of the artery or partial occlusion with narrowing. Another manifestation of arterial injury that may occur with either iatrogenic or accidental penetrating injury is formation of a false aneurysm. This may occur whenever there is a modest-sized lateral injury to an artery. At other times, the vessel may be completely transected. Finally, intimal flap disruptions may be created, particularly with blunt trauma and displaced fractures of the long bones (Fig. 15-1). Although some evidence indicates that some minimal degree intimal flap–type injuries may correct themselves spontaneously, more frequently these lesions lead to progressive occlusion over a period of hours.

Depending on the nature of the injury and the size of the penetrating instrument, arteriovenous fistulas may be large or small, single or multiple. In most instances, there

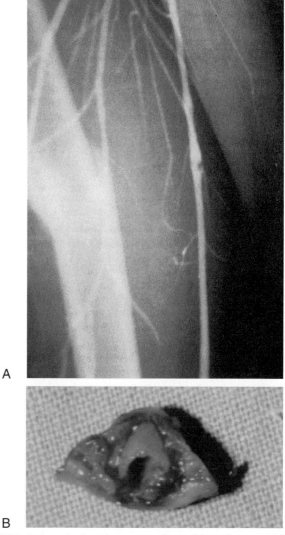

FIGURE 15-1 ■ **A,** Arteriogram performed in a 9-year-old boy who was hit by a car. The femur fracture was associated with diminished pulses. A typical intimal flap injury is shown. As with most injuries of this type, progressive thrombosis will occur, so operative repair is indicated. **B,** The pathology of the segment of artery excised and how the accumulation of blood outside the intima will result in occlusion.

is a single communication between the artery and vein with a small bridge of friable tissue between. In short order, marked dilation of both vessels occurs as flow increases.

Peripheral venous occlusions, usually thromboses, lead to immediate edema proximal to the site of thrombosis, but this is alleviated over time by recanalization and recruitment of collateral venous circulation. Injury to visceral veins of any size leads to exsanguination unless immediate control can be obtained. Penetrating injuries involving arteries and veins caused by traumatic events in the extremities usually present as extensive hemorrhage first, then thrombosis in the region of the venous laceration.

DIAGNOSIS

The initiating cause of a vascular injury, the surrounding circumstances, and the precise timing are usually available in the patient's history. Additionally, if there are predisposing factors to arterial occlusion, such as polycythemia or a low flow state, this also is usually immediately evident. Physical findings may not be diagnostic, however, of vascular injury or occlusion. Signs of vascular injury include diminished or absent distal pulses, persistent bleeding, a large hematoma, or a history of major hemorrhage associated with shock. Occasionally a thrill may be felt or a bruit heard. Generally, there is distal pallor, cyanosis, and coolness compared with the normal extremity. Muscle pain, weakness, and paralysis are late signs of arterial occlusion (Table 15-1). In the case of long bone fractures, if signs of arterial insufficiency are present after fracture reduction, arterial disruption must be suspected. Spasm often is considered to be the cause of peripheral ischemia after fracture reduction or cardiac catheterization and similar invasive procedures, but if signs of arterial compromise persist longer than 4 hours after the injury, it is safest to conclude that this is from thrombosis rather than spasm. Because arterial repair is most successful within the first 6 to 8 hours, this 4-hour time limit for consideration of spasm as the cause of ischemia is reasonable. The arteries most frequently involved in trauma include the subclavian artery beneath the clavicle, the brachial artery adjacent to the elbow or shaft of the humerus, and the region of the lower femoral and proximal popliteal artery along the distal femur. The popliteal artery may sustain a stretch injury and occlusion with posterior dislocation of the knee or occlusion from being trapped between bony fragments in a supracondylar fracture. Knowledge of the frequency of these injuries is helpful in terms of directing diagnostic efforts.

TABLE 15-1 ■ Signs and Symptoms of Arterial Injury

Penetrating wound over major vessels
Persistent bleeding
Major hemorrhage with shock
Audible bruit or thrill
Diminished or absent pulse
Distal pallor, cyanosis, coolness
Muscle pain, weakness, paralysis

Often it is unnecessary to do special diagnostic studies when there are clear-cut signs of arterial occlusion with peripheral ischemia and a history of major hemorrhage from an obvious penetrating injury. Under these circumstances, prompt operation is all that is required. In most instances, a more deliberate approach is needed, however. Palpation of peripheral pulses in small subjects is difficult, and appreciation of comparative pulse amplitude between extremities on palpation alone is inaccurate. Consequently, color Doppler flow studies have become routine for the clinical evaluation of ischemic extremities. A diminished pulse amplitude in an involved extremity is highly suggestive of ischemia, particularly if the pattern goes from triphasic to biphasic, indicating that only collateral circulation is being heard. Determination of the arterial pressure index (ankle/brachial) is helpful. If the index is less than 0.9, there is likely to be absent or markedly diminished flow in the vessel in question. Doppler flow studies can be refined further with the use of duplex scans, and they have the advantage of being noninvasive. These studies may be particularly useful for the demonstration of false aneurysms (Fig. 15-2A).

In small infants, arteriography is not always desirable because of the small size of vessels and the risk of injury to other vessels. A reasonable alternative is a radionuclide flow study with diethylenetriaminepentaacetic acid (DTPA) injected intravenously. This is particularly helpful for the evaluation of suspected aortoiliac and renal thromboses. Doppler and DTPA flow studies also are extremely helpful for postoperative monitoring of arterial repairs.

In many situations, arteriography is the preferred diagnostic approach. This is true in terms of evaluation of injuries of all visceral vessels, particularly the aorta, possible arteriovenous fistulas, and suspected arterial occlusions associated with blunt trauma with fractures or crush injuries (Fig. 15-3).

The goal of special diagnostic studies in the case of arterial injuries is to define accurately the status of the involved vessels and to expedite necessary repair in the shortest possible time. At times, it is preferable to explore an artery for strongly suspected pathology rather than to waste time working out the logistics of performing special studies.

In the case of major venous injuries, most situations demand immediate exploration and repair. On a selected basis, at times venography or cavography (or both) and duplex Doppler studies are indicated.

MANAGEMENT

With the exception of injuries to major visceral vessels associated with exsanguinating hemorrhage, bleeding can be controlled in most vascular injuries. Preferably, patients are prepared for repair by adequate replacement of blood volume, stabilization of major organ function, correction of electrolyte and acid-base abnormalities, and administration of antibiotics. Poor cardiac output predisposes to failure of repair of small arteries and veins. It is important to have adequate intravenous access for blood replacement because extensive bleeding may be encountered while gaining exposure for adequate proximal and distal vascular control. Heparin is not useful preoperatively

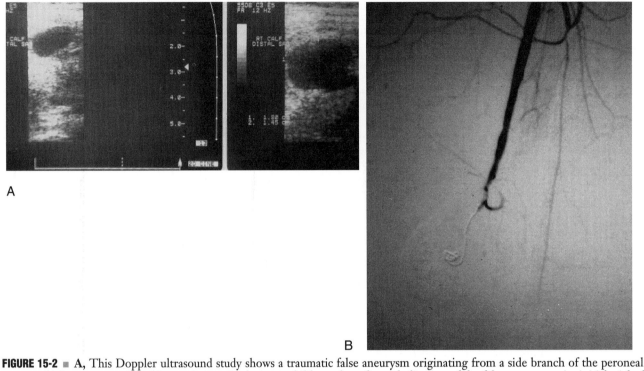

A

B

FIGURE 15-2 ■ **A,** This Doppler ultrasound study shows a traumatic false aneurysm originating from a side branch of the peroneal artery, which was patent. **B,** This arteriogram in the same child was done for embolization of the false aneurysm. An initial trial of compression was not tolerated by the patient.

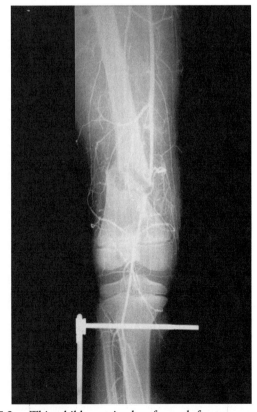

FIGURE 15-3 ■ This child sustained a femoral fracture, and distal pulses were absent after reduction. This arteriogram shows vascular interruption with reconstitution of flow beyond, via collaterals. Prompt repair was performed, and every effort was made to preserve collateral vessels.

but should be used routinely systemically and locally intraoperatively. Special consideration may need to be given in terms of anticoagulation to patients with extensive associated injuries, particularly injuries to the central nervous system.

Lesions that May Respond to Nonoperative Management

Although systemic heparinization was used frequently in the past for infants and children with signs of arterial occlusion from invasive procedures and some blunt injuries, long-term results with this treatment have proved unsatisfactory. At times, systemic heparinization is useful after the repair of small arteries, but the indications are limited.

Acute arterial thromboses, occlusion from embolism, and postoperative thromboses frequently respond to thrombolytic therapy. The agent of choice is tissue plasminogen activator (TPA) because urokinase is no longer available. If there are no contraindications, such as recent intraventricular bleeding in a premature newborn, TPA may be tried. TPA, 0.25 to 1.5 mg/hr or 0.1 to 0.5 mg/kg/hr, may be infused via an indwelling catheter just above the level of the thrombosis as defined by injection of contrast material through the catheter. Heparin should not be used during TPA therapy. Generally, some lysis of the clot can be shown within 18 hours, but if it is not seen by 48 hours, local infusion of TPA is unlikely to help. In instances in which intra-arterial infusion is not feasible, systemic intravenous therapy may be used at doses of 1.0 to 2.0 mg/hr for 48 hours. For therapy in newborns, 0.125 to 1.25 mg/hr is a reasonable dosage range.

In the case of major hemorrhage from vessels that may be sacrificed, as in the case of arterial bleeding associated with pelvic fractures, angiography followed by catheter embolization may occlude the damaged vessels effectively and control the hemorrhage. Direct injection or catheter embolization and injection of thrombin or coils also may be useful for the treatment of some false aneurysms (see Fig. 15-2B). An equally effective method of managing pseudoaneurysms on the extremity is to compress the lesion firmly so that it can be collapsed and undergo thrombotic occlusion. These forms of nonoperative therapy of pseudoaneurysms of the extremity have made operative intervention infrequently necessary. These methods should be attempted before surgical management of pseudoaneurysms of the extremities.

Under special circumstances in patients who are ill and when close observation can be accomplished, it may be reasonable to observe some arterial lesions with the expectation that spontaneous resolution may occur. These lesions include limited intimal flap disruptions, areas of arterial narrowing but with good distal flow, and some small pseudoaneurysms. Expectant therapy is risky, however, unless close monitoring can be performed with immediate intervention if required. Only minimal arterial injuries without obvious clinical manifestations should be managed in this fashion.

Operative Management

All vascular injuries except those mentioned in the preceding section should be considered for operative repair, unless there is a compelling medical contraindication. A general anesthetic should be used routinely in children. Gentle anesthetic induction should be used to prevent children from straining excessively and possibly dislodging a clot that has controlled bleeding. For isolated vascular injuries and thromboses involving small vessels, intraoperative heparinization is used at a dosage of 1 mg or 100 U/kg every 1 to 2 hours; thereafter, approximately one half the heparin dose should be repeated. Protamine inactivation is ordinarily not necessary, and the heparin effect can be allowed to diminish on its own. There is no essential difference in the technical approach to vascular repair in infants and children except that microvascular instruments and suture and magnifying loops are needed. In tiny vessels, interrupted sutures of 6-0 or 7-0 polypropylene should be used rather than running sutures to avoid narrowing the vessel and to allow for subsequent growth. Surgical exposure must be sufficient to permit wide visualization of the vasculature and prompt proximal and distal control. In the case of fractures, the order of vascular repair and fracture fixation is based on the duration of the vascular interruption and whether manipulation of the fracture after repair would disrupt it. Studies have shown that repair can be done safely either before or after fixation. If both vein and artery are injured, venous reconstruction is performed first to alleviate the effects of venous hypertension, provide better runoff, and enhance the success of arterial reconstruction. Fasciotomy is usually necessary in these instances. Thorough débridement and lavage of extensive soft tissue injuries associated with vascular trauma are important to avoid infection.

Whenever possible, patients should be positioned in the frog-leg position to permit harvesting of saphenous vein should an interposition graft or onlay patch be needed. Synthetic grafts occasionally are required but are less desirable in children. Intraoperatively the Fogarty balloon catheter is helpful for the removal of proximal and distal clot associated with the injury. Intraoperative and completion arteriography may be helpful in patients who are thought to have poor distal runoff or when more than one arterial injury is present in an extremity.

When spasm complicates arterial repair in small children, thrombosis may occur either intraoperatively or immediately postoperatively. Measures that may be used include gentle dilation of the artery by injection of heparinized saline solution or use of a Fogarty balloon catheter. Topical application of 2.5% papaverine or 1% lidocaine or intra-arterial injection of lidocaine or nitroglycerin may be useful.

More recently, endovascular techniques have been used to manage arterial injuries, particularly of the thoracic and abdominal aorta. Although there eventually may be a place for these techniques in children, unless considerations of growth can be allowed for, indications will be limited.

In patients in whom arterial reconstruction is delayed for more than 6 hours; in patients with crush injuries, multiple fractures, and extensive soft tissue injuries; and in patients with associated venous injury, it is generally best to perform fasciotomy to avoid a compartment syndrome. Usually, most venous injuries can be repaired by lateral venotomy or end-to-end anastomosis. Arteriovenous communications usually are treated by division of the fistula and reconstruction of artery and vein by lateral suture or vein patch angioplasty.

COMPLICATIONS AND RESULTS

Depending on the vessel involved, if disrupted or occluded arteries are not repaired, the amputation rate is 10% to 70%. Even if a limb survives arterial occlusion because of establishment of collateral flow, however, some disturbance in growth is likely in 80% of patients, so there is a great deal to gain from attempting repair. Based on a variety of reported series, restoration of pulse can be expected in more than 90% of patients. Although 15% of the latter lose the pulse on follow-up, limb survival occurs in more than half of this group. Mortality is related primarily to complications of associated injuries, particularly head injuries. Patients who develop compartment syndromes or who have had excessively delayed vascular repair are in danger of developing Volkmann's ischemic contracture, causalgia, and other neurovascular disorders. Available data would indicate strongly that an aggressive approach to vascular reconstruction of injured arteries in infants and children is warranted.

SUGGESTED READINGS

Frykberg ER: Advances in diagnosis and treatment of extremity vascular trauma. Surg Clin North Am 75:207, 1995.
This article reviews current diagnostic approaches taking into account that angiography is not always desirable in small children and what alternatives exist.

Frykberg ER, Crump JM, Dennis JW, et al: Nonoperative observation of clinically occult arterial injuries: A prospective evaluation. Surgery 109:85, 1991.

Frykberg and colleagues describe a controversial but occasionally useful approach to occult arterial injuries that have the potential to heal without operation. The article is important because it separates lesions that must be explored from lesions that potentially are treated nonoperatively.

Tepas JJ, Mollett D: Vascular injuries. In O'Neill JA, Rowe MI, Grosfeld JG, et al (eds): Pediatric Surgery. St. Louis, Mosby, 1998, p 337.

This chapter reviews diagnosis and management of vascular injuries commonly encountered in children.

Zenz W, Muntean W, Beitzke A, et al: Tissue plasminogen activator (alteplase) treatment for femoral artery thrombosis after cardiac catheterization in infants and children. Br Heart J 70:382–385, 1993.

This article provides a good description of thrombolytic techniques in addition to the methods described in this chapter.

Central Nervous System Injuries

16

The most common cause of death and disability after severe trauma in childhood is related to closed head injury. Much is yet to be learned regarding the effects of severe head trauma on brain development, but available studies suggest that neuropsychiatric recovery after significant head injury takes longer than 1 year following resolution of the immediate effects of the injury. Numerous studies indicate that the basic pathophysiology of head injury in children is different in many respects from that in adults. The ability to recover also differs in that children may compensate better for brain destruction.

HEAD INJURIES

When children are injured in motor vehicle accidents either as pedestrians or as passengers, head injuries are the most common form of presentation. At least half of deaths caused by head injury occur before the patient reaches the hospital. Of all trauma deaths, 25% are caused by head injury. The cost to society is enormous because of the long recovery and disability involved. The causes of head injury in order of frequency include motor vehicle–related causes, falls, accidental blows to the head, and child abuse. Severe head injuries usually are associated with motor vehicle accidents and child abuse, and mild-to-moderate head injuries generally are seen with falls and accidental blows to the head.

Head injuries may be divided into two forms: (1) primary injury, including all primary traumatic events occurring in the first few minutes after injury for which there is no treatment, and (2) secondary injury, which is potentially treatable and relates to secondary events that may compound the initial injury and progress over hours to days. The causes of secondary injury are hypoxemia, hypercarbia, shock, and increased intracranial pressure (ICP). The principal factors that promote secondary injury are hypoxemia and diminished blood flow to the brain, which are at least potentially preventable. All current therapy is directed at thoroughly evaluating the primary injury and supporting the patient to avoid secondary injury.

Pathophysiology

To evaluate various forms of head injury, it is helpful to know the mechanism of injury—that is, whether it is the result of a direct blow with injury to the skin and bone,

TABLE 16-1 ▪ Forms of Head Injury
Diffuse
Concussion
Diffuse axonal injury
Focal
Linear skull fracture
Depressed skull fracture
Subdural hematoma
Epidural hematoma
Intracerebral hematoma
Cortical contusion

acceleration and deceleration as with severe shaking in child abuse, or shearing forces. In general, the brain must have a continual supply of oxygen and glucose to function. After trauma, the brain compensates by a process of autoregulation to preserve its blood flow by cerebral vasoconstriction. In young children, the response is partly one of acute vasodilation, however, so the initial rapid increase in ICP is related to congestion of the brain as a result of increased intracranial blood volume. This response is in contrast to cerebral edema and vasoconstriction seen in adults and older children. This latter observation forms the basis for the differences in approach to the treatment of severe head injuries in infants and children compared with adults. The injuries themselves may be classified into focal and diffuse injuries. The most common serious injuries are diffuse (Table 16-1).

Forms of Head Injury

Diffuse Injuries

Diffuse brain injuries are caused by acceleration or deceleration, pedestrian injuries, and the shaken baby syndrome form of child abuse. These mechanisms cause sudden brain movement and a shearing force, resulting in damage to the white matter.

Concussion

Concussion may range from mild to severe. Mild concussion may involve only short periods of unconsciousness or loss of memory without loss of consciousness. A common minimal clinical sign of concussion is a period of amnesia.

The disturbances are generally short-lived and followed by little more than a headache. Moderate concussions usually are associated with short periods of unconsciousness associated with temporary and reversible neurologic findings. Patients may remain confused or agitated for hours to days. In severe concussion, the temporary period of unconsciousness may last 6 hours, and the temporary neurologic disturbances take several days to resolve.

Diffuse Axonal Injury

As with concussions, diffuse axonal injuries may be mild, moderate, or severe (Fig. 16-1). In these forms of injury, in addition to the white matter, there is generally evidence of myelin disruption and complete axonal tearing. The more severe the injury, the deeper the level of white matter damage.

With mild diffuse axonal injuries, the period of unconsciousness is 6 to 24 hours. Mild axonal injury is associated with cognitive deficits, which may last 1 year.

Moderate diffuse axonal injury is presumed to be present when the period of unconsciousness lasts more than 24 hours, but in which brainstem function is preserved. These injuries are associated with 15% to 20% mortality, and significant morbidity usually is seen.

Patients are considered to have severe diffuse axonal injury when unconsciousness is immediate and coma lasts longer than 24 hours without any evidence of a focal lesion. All of these patients have signs of brainstem dysfunction. Mortality is in the range of 60%, and permanent neurologic disability occurs in all patients.

Focal Injuries

Focal injuries generally occur from direct blows to the skull, but mild localized hematomas also may be seen in association with diffuse injuries. As a measure of frequency, with severe pediatric head trauma, operative intervention is required only approximately 20% of the time.

Linear Skull Fracture

Linear fractures are generally the result of falls in children younger than 1 year old. There may be no loss of consciousness. Usually the child is alert, but in a few instances, after several hours, there is a delayed onset of drowsiness and vomiting. Whenever symptoms suggestive of mild increases in ICP are present, a computed tomography (CT) scan should be obtained. Most of these patients have mild concussions, and it is rare to find a mass lesion, such as a hematoma. Supportive care is all that is required; no specific therapy is needed. In rare instances, a growing fracture is noted, indicating the presence of a leptomeningeal cyst specific to the pediatric age group. Surgery is required with appropriate cranial reconstruction.

Depressed Skull Fracture

Simple depressed skull fractures do not always require emergency surgery (Fig. 16-2). The occasional depressed skull fractures associated with focal neurologic deficits, seizures, or a changing level of consciousness should be evaluated by serial CT scans to rule out mass lesions. In most instances, the depression is less than 5 mm, and no surgery is required. The use of CT or magnetic resonance imaging (MRI) has made it possible to be selective about the repair of closed depressed skull fractures, limiting surgery to patients with depression of 1 cm or greater. Compound depressed skull fractures require emergency surgery as guided by CT to evaluate the status of the underlying brain and the possible presence of other intracranial mass lesions. Antibiotics are appropriate for these patients.

Subdural Hematoma

Subdural hematoma requiring surgery is unusual in children. The small unilateral subdural hematomas often seen in association with diffuse head injuries usually do not require evacuation. Isolated subdural hematomas associated with neurologic deficits or progressive loss of consciousness should be evaluated. Occasionally, chronic subdural hematomas are encountered, particularly in children who have been abused, and these usually require surgical intervention. Approximately 60% of children with significant subdural hematomas have associated skull fracture, whereas the others do not because of the pliable nature of the cranium in young children.

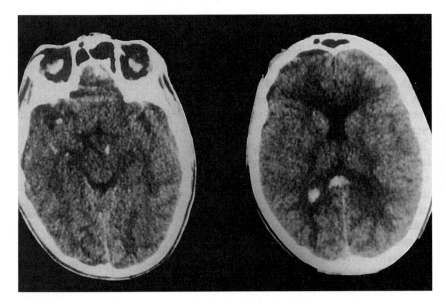

FIGURE 16-1 ▪ CT scan demonstrates characteristic findings of diffuse axonal or shearing injury in a child who sustained blunt head injury. He was unconscious with elevated intracranial pressure when this imaging study was performed.

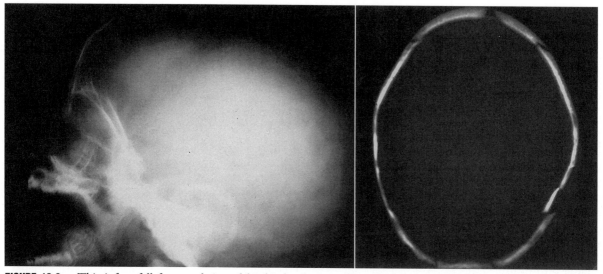

FIGURE 16-2 ■ This infant fell from a chair and hit his head on a table. On the skull film (left), a fracture is not well visualized, but on the bone windows on the CT scan, a right parietal fracture is seen. This mildly depressed fracture did not require elevation.

Epidural Hematoma

Epidural hematoma is the most treatable focal lesion one is likely to encounter (Fig. 16-3). Only 50% of children with epidural hematomas have skull fractures, although if one is seen, the hematoma is likely to be below the fracture site. In children younger than 5 years of age, in whom skull fractures are uncommon, epidural hematomas may occur in the high temporoparietal region rather than in the anterior temporal fossa over the midportion of the middle meningeal artery. Patients with epidural hematomas usually have rapid deterioration of neurologic function, but a CT scan should be obtained first if possible to exclude other associated injuries.

Intracerebral Hematoma

Intracerebral hematomas are uncommon in childhood, usually the result of a severe blow to the head or penetrating injury. Surgery is indicated for sizable hematomas associated with marked increases in ICP or brain herniation.

Cortical Contusion

Cortical contusions are lesions seen more often in older children than in infants and toddlers. These contusions are evident on CT or MRI; however, most are not extensive. They may occur either below an area of focal injury or on the opposite side of the brain as a contrecoup lesion associated with acceleration/deceleration injuries.

Assessment of Neurologic Status

The most reproducible method of evaluation of the severity of primary head injury is the Glasgow Coma Scale (GCS) (Table 16-2). The GCS must be modified in infants and in patients who are intubated because of the inability to evaluate verbal response. As part of the primary survey in the emergency department, the factors in assessment of neurologic status in order of importance include the level of consciousness, pupillary function,

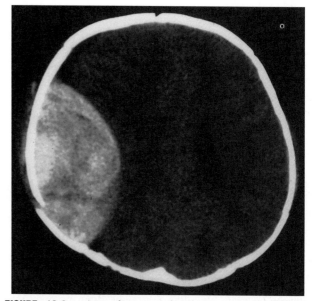

FIGURE 16-3 ■ According to the history provided, this 7-month-old infant did not wake up for her nightly feeding and began vomiting in the morning. The mother's boyfriend reported the infant fell from a chair the previous day. On the CT scan, there is a large epidural hematoma associated with a right parietal skull fracture. There is a mass effect on the right parietal brain and marked shift of the midline from right to left. The right lateral ventricle is compressed as a result of the mass effect, and the left lateral ventricle is slightly prominent. The infant was taken emergently to the operating room for evacuation of the epidural hematoma and recovered uneventfully.

TABLE 16-2 ■ Glasgow Coma Scale Score	
Eye opening	
Spontaneous	4
To speech	3
To pain	2
None	1
Best motor response	
Follows commands	6
Localizes	5
Flexion withdrawal	4
Abnormal flexion	3
Extension	2
None	1
Verbal response	
Oriented	5
Disoriented	4
Inappropriate words	3
Sounds only	2
None	1

motor responses on each side of the body, pattern of breathing, and peripheral sensation.

Consciousness must be evaluated on a continuing basis. Two levels of consciousness can be determined on examination—awareness and arousal. Appropriate verbal responses and protective motor responses to painful stimuli indicate cortical function. Signs of arousal, such as eye opening in response to stimuli, indicate brainstem function. In coma, both these elements of consciousness are lost. Lateralized paresis or paralysis of the extremities generally indicates focal injury. This injury is assessed best by testing the reflexes in both arms and legs. If a patient is determined to have progressive deterioration of neurologic function with lateralized weakness of an extremity, a mass lesion is likely; neurologic deterioration in the absence of lateralizing signs or pupillary inequality indicates a severe generalized injury or secondary brain injury related to hypoxia and ischemia of the brain.

The specifics of the GCS evaluation require that the patient not be sedated and that shock has been corrected. Otherwise, a low GCS score may not represent brain injury but rather the poor physiologic status of the patient. The GCS is not completely applicable to infants, so modifications are necessary to replace the best verbal response evaluation. Modifications include evaluation of responses to noise, light, and pain elicited by sternal rubbing. The GCS is useful in children older than age 1 year if speech is replaced by crying. In addition to neurologic examination, the nares and the external auditory canals should be examined for signs of leakage of blood or cerebrospinal fluid, which might suggest a basilar skull fracture.

Pupillary function is evaluated by size, equality, and response to light. Pupillary asymmetry should be assumed to be related to intracranial injury. Usually the larger pupil is related to third nerve compression and is on the side of the mass lesion. Absence of papillary response to light generally indicates a severe injury.

Intracranial monitoring to determine the level of ICP is another helpful measure in evaluating the continuing status of a patient with severe head injury. Cerebral perfusion studies also may be indicated under extreme circumstances. These latter two methods of physiologic monitoring may be extremely helpful guides to treatment because cerebral perfusion pressure is related to ICP, systemic blood pressure, and cerebral blood flow.

CT is the most helpful and most definitive way to assess the severity of intracranial injury. Although MRI can provide additional information, it takes longer to perform. CT provides all of the essential information necessary to make a decision regarding the presence or absence of significant intracranial injury and whether emergency operative intervention is required. MRI is more valuable for patient follow-up, although serial CT is usually sufficient and less expensive to perform.

Management

To minimize the effects of cerebral edema, patients with severe injury should not be overhydrated but should receive adequate resuscitation to provide a sufficient cerebral perfusion pressure and oxygen delivery. Otherwise, devastating secondary brain injury may result. Although vigorous support of the circulation is a key element in the supportive care of children with severe head injury, more recent therapies have evolved in the direction of trying to maintain euvolemia with a normal electrolyte balance. Fluid restriction should not be used as a primary therapy. Hypotonic solutions are not used, and hyperglycemia is avoided. Hypertonic solutions are under investigation because there is some evidence that they may be protective. Anemia is corrected with blood transfusion. When osmotic agents such as mannitol are used, the appropriate intravascular volume is maintained with isotonic fluids or plasma expanders. If operative intervention is needed because of a focal lesion, such as a compound depressed skull fracture or a significant intracranial hematoma, immediate endotracheal intubation and ventilation are needed, followed by the appropriate neurosurgical procedure. Also, endotracheal intubation and ventilation should be the first step in the management of children with a GCS score of 7 or less because a score of this magnitude indicates a severe neurologic injury. Intubation is accomplished while protecting the airway to prevent aspiration of gastric contents and while stabilizing the neck in the event of a cervical fracture. If facial injuries or a basilar skull fracture is present, a gastric tube should be passed orally.

As soon as the patient is stabilized, arterial blood should be drawn for the measurement of pH, PO_2, and PCO_2. The PO_2 should be maintained at greater than 80 mm Hg, and oxygen saturation should be maintained by oximetry at greater than 95%. In addition to these supportive measures, there are rational and sequential treatments for effectively lowering ICP in head-injured patients. The intensity of the level of treatment is calibrated to the level of injury in a particular patient; if a particular therapy is not yielding satisfactory results, escalation of therapy and intracranial monitoring is undertaken. The aim of all therapies is to raise the intracranial milieu to "normal" levels; this is often achieved by first bringing systemic physiologic parameters toward normal. Proper oxygenation and optimization of hemodynamics permit proper cerebral perfusion pressures; escalated therapies include the pharmacologic support of blood pressure and reduction of peripheral arterial resistance. Reduction of central and peripheral venous pressures further allows for perfusion of the brain. Elevation of the head of the bed and maintenance of the head in a truly neutral position allows for proper venous drainage. The use of narcotic sedation and muscular paralysis prevents excess straining and coughing, common responses to endotracheal tubes and mechanical ventilation.

Hyperventilation should be reserved for episodes of refractory intracranial hypertension. Hyperventilation should not be used prophylactically as in the past, however, because it can exacerbate cerebral ischemia. When used, the degree of hypocarbia should be limited to a P_{CO_2} of 30 to 35 mm Hg. In general, hyperventilation is reserved for patients with ICP monitors who have failed to respond to sedation, paralysis, cerebrospinal fluid drainage (when possible), and osmotic diuresis. Osmotic diuresis with mannitol should be reserved for patients with an ICP greater than 20 mm Hg. The initial dose can be a maximum of 1 g/kg bolus, which has a maximum effectiveness in approximately 20 to 60 minutes. Because mannitol can have deleterious effects on blood pressure and renal function if serum osmolarity exceeds 320 mOsm/L, the minimal dose required to improve ICP must be used; more frequent and smaller doses may be optimal (e.g., 0.25 g/kg every 2 to 3 hours). The response to osmotic diuresis can be gauged by ICP monitors.

Intracranial monitoring is reserved for patients presenting with severe head trauma (GCS score of ≤8 after cardiopulmonary resuscitation), particularly if other injuries require therapies deleterious to ICP (e.g., large volumes of fluid for hypotension, high levels of positive end-expiratory pressure for pulmonary injury). There is controversy regarding the optimal method of measuring intracranial/intraventricular pressures and regarding the outcome difference achieved by aggressive pressure measurements. Nonetheless, monitors do provide a basis for deciding the intensity and the duration of measures used to treat intracranial hypertension. Some children with severe cerebral injury show signs of inappropriate antidiuretic hormone secretion. In these situations, frequent measurements of serum electrolyte levels and osmolality are necessary. Hourly fluid balance and daily weights are key to the management of this hormonal abnormality.

The administration of corticosteroids to head-injured patients is generally not recommended. No beneficial effect of steroids has been shown convincingly. Previously, spinal cord injuries were treated with high-dose methylprednisolone, but even these protocols have been questioned in terms of efficacy (see section on spinal cord injuries). Phenytoin and phenobarbital are indicated only when seizures are noted. High-dose barbiturate therapy is reserved for patients whose head injuries have failed prior management. The use of pentobarbital to levels of burst suppression on electroencephalography reduces ICP, but this pharmacologic "coma" also reduces sympathetic tone and causes myocardial depression, often requires dopamine support, and forces reliance on ICP monitoring performance because a neurologic examination is not possible. Whether the reduction of the metabolic demand for oxygen and the reduction of cerebral blood flow are sufficient to justify this aggressive therapy cannot yet be answered. Outcome data are difficult to interpret, particularly in the severely damaged patients who comprise this treatment group. Whether comatose by the accident or comatose by pharmacologic induction, within 24 hours of admission, it is generally possible to begin intragastric feedings to support the ongoing nutritional needs of the patient.

Outcome

Mortality is related to the effects of elevated ICP in isolated head injury or to the extent of associated injuries in multiple trauma. Children with a GCS score of 3 with flaccid coma have a mortality of around 60%. In the absence of multiple trauma and shock, mortality is 10% to 20% in patients with a GCS score of 4, manifested by decerebrate coma. Children with a GCS score of 5 or more with isolated head injury usually do not die. Recovery depends, however, on the duration of coma. If coma lasts less than 3 weeks, return to reasonable independent functional activities, including school, is likely. When coma extends beyond 3 weeks, long-term neurologic and neuropsychologic deficits are usual. The better the initial care, the better the long-term function. Intensive rehabilitative efforts should be made at the outset of treatment to maximize long-term function.

SPINAL CORD INJURIES

Spinal injuries are far less common in children than in adults. In children younger than 6 years of age, however, approximately 2% with severe head injuries have cervicospinal injuries. The latter are generally high cervical injuries; lower cervicospinal injury is uncommon in young children. Falls and pedestrian injuries are the most common causes of cervicospinal injuries. In adolescents, cervical injuries occur with the same frequency as in adults, and the principles of management are the same.

Diagnosis

Although an adequate lateral cervicospinal radiograph and CT are the mainstays of evaluation, equally important is the absence of tenderness on palpation of the cervical spine (Figs. 16-4 and 16-5). Radiographs are negative in 25% or more of children with spinal cord injury, so cervicospinal tenderness and abnormalities of neurologic examination are key to diagnosis. All children with serious injuries should have cervicospinal immobilization accomplished immediately on admission to the emergency department (Fig. 16-6). It is important to differentiate so-called pseudosubluxation, related to the mobility of the upper cervical spine in children, from true dislocation. Precise diagnosis of upper cervical vertebrae injuries may require CT, particularly for the evaluation of the C1 ring. In young children, virtually all cervicospinal fractures occur between C1 and C3. Lower cervical spine fractures are encountered in children older than age 8 years.

Thoracolumbar spine injuries result from extreme flexion, axial rotation, or direct injury. Conventional radiographs are usually sufficient to show vertebral body

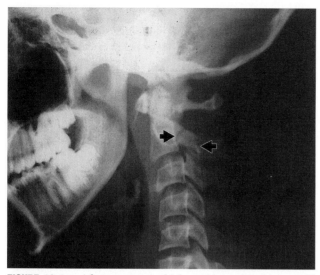

FIGURE 16-4 ■ After a motor vehicle accident, this 16-year-old patient was neurologically intact but complaining of neck pain. On the lateral cervical radiograph, there is a fracture of the posterior elements of C2 (arrows). This hangman's fracture has mild anterior displacement of C2 on C3. In addition, there is mild soft tissue swelling anterior to C2.

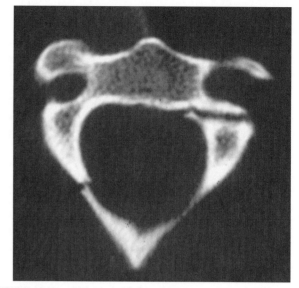

FIGURE 16-5 ■ CT scan of the patient in Figure 16-4 with a hangman's fracture reveals a nondisplaced fracture of the right lamina and the left lateral mass of C2.

collapse, malalignment of vertebral bodies indicative of dislocation, and transverse process fractures. Thoracospinal injuries frequently are associated with pneumothorax and vascular injuries, and lumbar spine fractures commonly are associated with visceral injuries, particularly when seat belt injuries are suspected. Lumbar spine fractures also frequently are associated with retroperitoneal injuries and urinary retention. CT is the best imaging modality to show bony compromise of the spinal canal by bone fragments or dislocation. Careful serial neurologic examinations are also an important part of overall evaluation of all types of spinal injuries.

Management

Initially, all patients with serious head injury and particularly patients who are unconscious should have the cervical spine immobilized. If an adequate physical examination can be performed with cooperation of the child, absence of spinal tenderness is helpful in ruling out significant injury. In the case of patients who are unconscious or if tenderness is present in the conscious patient, the immobilization collar should be left in place until appropriate flexion/extension radiographs or CT can be performed to rule out instability.

The initial goal of treatment of spinal injury is to provide stability. Then efforts must be made under

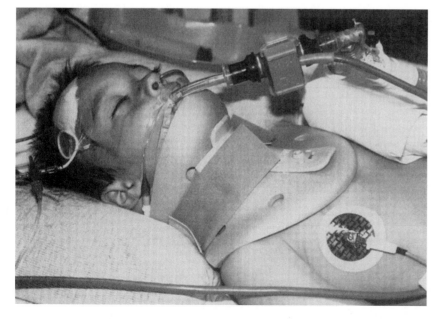

FIGURE 16-6 ■ Photograph shows the appropriate placement of a cervical collar on a patient with a suspected spine injury. This type of immobilization should be performed in all patients until cervicospinal injury is ruled out, particularly in patients who are unconscious.

appropriate control to restore proper alignment and to ensure the integrity of the spinal cord. External pin fixation either with a Halo or with tongs is appropriate initially using weights of 2 to 10 lb, depending on the age and size of the child. C1 and C2 fractures are treated by simple immobilization. Traction helps to correct alignment, but surgery may be needed if bone or disk material is seen within the spinal canal. Supportive management also includes nasogastric decompression, catheter drainage of the bladder, and avoidance of postural hypotension. Assisted ventilation may be required for patients with injuries above C5. A Halo jacket is useful for management of cervicospinal and thoracospinal injuries. At times, surgery and internal fixation are required for occasional patients who develop progressive spinal deformities. Rehabilitation efforts should be initiated at the earliest possible time to relieve spasticity, avoid decubiti and contractures, and expedite possible recovery.

The use of methylprednisolone for treatment of acutely spinal cord–injured patients is controversial. A reanalysis of previous data from the National Acute Spinal Cord Injury Study II and III failed to show compelling data to justify the use of high-dose steroids in the treatment of acute spinal cord injury. The use of methylprednisolone is not considered standard care and is not a recommended treatment. In the strictest sense, use of methylprednisolone therapy remains experimental. Similarly the optimal timing of surgical intervention in spinal cord injuries is controversial, and a debate continues regarding the efficacy of early surgical intervention.

Outcome

The outcome for patients who have only limited and non-progressive deficits initially is excellent. The outcome for children with spinal cord injury who present with complete neurologic deficit initially is extremely poor, however, with less than 5% chance of recovery.

SUGGESTED READINGS

Caron MJ, Kelly DF, Shalmon E, et al: Intensive management of traumatic brain injury. In Wilkins RH, Rengachary SS (eds): Neurosurgery, vol 2. New York, McGraw-Hill, 1996.

This chapter reviews current concepts about management of the patient with a severe neurologic injury.

Brain Trauma Foundation: Am Assn Neurological Surgeons: Indications for intracranial pressure monitoring. J Neurotrauma 17:479, 2000.

This article from the Brain Trauma Foundation discusses recommendations for intracranial monitoring in head-injured patients.

Luerssen TG: Neurological injuries in infants and children: An overview of current management strategies. Clin Neurosurg 46:170, 2000.

A concise overview of treatment options for pediatric patients with neurologic injuries is presented.

Am Assn Neurological Surgeons Guidelines: Management of pediatric cervical spine and spinal cord injuries. Neurosurgery 50:(Suppl)S85, 2002.

This article describes diagnostic and treatment options for the child with a suspected cervical spine injury.

Am Assn Neurological Surgeons Guidelines: Pharmacological therapy after acute cervical spinal cord injury. Neurosurgery 50:(Suppl)S63, 2002.

This review article describes indications and rationale for pharmacologic therapy in patients with an acute spinal cord injury.

17

Burns

Intentional and accidental injuries are responsible for 62% of deaths in children 1 to 19 years old. Motor vehicle–related accidents are responsible for 29% of childhood mortality. Burn injuries are the third leading cause of mortality in children younger than age 5 years. More than 300,000 children sustain burns each year, and approximately 75,000 are hospitalized with 1800 deaths. These figures represent a remarkable improvement over prior years because of prevention strategies and improvements in care in burn centers. Most burn injuries sustained by children occur in the home as a result of an accident, so most such injuries are potentially preventable, and this is reflected in the improved mortality statistics.

Scalds from boiling hot liquids cause most minor and major burns in children 1 to 5 years old, and boys are burned twice as often as girls. Although most injuries are due to a toddler's pulling a pot of boiling liquid off the stove or a bathtub mishap, many children younger than age 4 sustain such burns as a manifestation of child abuse.

In children older than age 5 years, flame, chemical, and electrical burns constitute the prime causes in that order. In this age group, the incidence of injury is equal in both sexes. Flame burns are the primary cause of major full-thickness injuries and are associated with the highest morbidity and morality.

PATHOPHYSIOLOGIC CONSIDERATIONS OF BURNS IN CHILDREN

Chapter 11 provides a detailed comparision of the physiologic differences between children and adults and their differential responses to injury. Most of these differences gradually diminish as growth progresses, equalizing around age 12 to 14 years. With special reference to burn injury, certain physiologic differences are of key importance. Because small children have almost three times the surface area-to-body weight ratio of adults, the degree of evaporative water and heat loss in children is greater so that fluid requirements are increased. The same consideration relating to water turnover is pertinent to all other elements of metabolic turnover so that all aspects of replacement are quantitatively greater. After burn injury, plasma cytokines (interleukin-1β and interleukin-6) are increased in proportion to burn size and time after burn, and these substances influence the metabolic and immunologic responses in the first few weeks after thermal injury. Children older than age 1 year seem to have similar responses. In severely burned children, hypermetabolism and catabolism are increased compared with baseline for at least 9 months after injury, which is longer than that measured in adults.

In addition to the disparity in surface area to body weight ratio in children compared with adults, the younger the clild, the thinner the skin and the underlying insulating fat layer. For this reason, children have greater heat loss and water loss compared with adults, resulting in a burned child in a ompromised circulatory state rapidly becoming dangerously hypothermic. The guidelines used to judge the adequacy of fluid resuscitation require additional criteria beyond those for adults. Young children are particularly prone to vasoconstriction and mottling, particularly when cold, which seriously may invalidate judgments regarding the adequacy of cardiac output based on the quality of the peripheral circulation. Broad estimations of the adequacy of cardiac output are required.

Although pulmonary function generally is good in normal children, the degree of reserve is small because of the relatively increased metabolic rate of the child. With inhalation injury, children deteriorate faster than adults, particularly in terms of upper airway edema and alveolar-capillary block. Children with severe inhalation injury may carry residual effects for many more months after recovery than generally noted in adults.

The younger the child, the less efficient free water clearance is as fluid resuscitation progresses. For this reason, children are more prone to accumulate edema than adults, and it tends to be retained longer, a factor that relates to conversion from partial-thickness to full-thickness burn and quality and timing of wound healing.

INITIAL EVALUATION

The American Burn Association has published practice guidelines for burn care, including recommendations for initial assessment. These guidelines appropriately emphasize the fact that burn patients should be evaluated similar to any other trauma patient, initially using the concept of the primary and secondary survey before a definitive care phase. The ABCs (airway, breathing, circulation) of evaluation and emergency treatment are followed with special emphasis on burn-specific components of the secondary survey. If a child has been injured in an enclosed space, if there are facial burns with singed nasal hairs or blisters inside the mouth, or if there are signs of upper airway obstruction or wheezes heard over the chest, inhalation injury must be suspected and managed appropriately.

Burns frequently are associated with other injuries, particularly from blunt trauma after motor vehicle accidents. Evaluation of the burn should be coordinated with evaluation of all other potential injuries. Although hemorrhage and intracavitary injuries may take priority over the burn, additional consideration should be given to the increased requirements for fluid replacement. A rapid history should be obtained first to determine the details of the mechanism and timing of the injury to help evaluate burn severity because scald injuries are usually partial thickness and flame burns are full thickness in nature. The historical circumstances also are important because burn injury sustained in an enclosed space may indicate

possible inhalation injury. It is important to determine any co-existing congenital or acquired diseases, the child's current immunization status including tetanus, medication history, and whether there are drug allergies. Because the surface areaa and depth of the burn are proportional to the amount of fluid replacement required, careful estimates should be made. Estimation of wound depth may be difficult if a patient is seen more than 4 hours after burn injury because the appearance may be altered by edema or changes in circulation; however, the history still may be helpful in this respect. For estimation of surface area injured in children, the rule of nines may be useful in children older than age 10 years, but some modification of the Lund and Browder chart is needed in young children because of the relatively greater surface area of the head and lesser surface area of the legs compared with older subjects (Fig. 17-1). Clinical assessment of the extent of surface area injured is easier to perform after cleansing of the wound with saline solution and appropriate débridement. Soap is not required in this process and potentially may be toxic because of absorption through the injured surface.

In addition to determining the extent and depth of the wound, the presence of circumferential burns; the involvement of the face, hands, genitalia or feet; the presence of electrical or chemical injury; and the possibility of child abuse should be emphasized in the history and physical examination. With regard to tetanus immunization, patients who have been immunized within the previous 10 years need not receive tetanus toxoid unless the burn is associated with a tetanus-prone soft tissue injury. Unimmunized patients should receive tetanus immune globulin followed by active immunization.

CARE OF MINOR BURNS

Most burns in childhood are minor in terms of extent and depth because most are scald injuries. Minor burns may be classified as partial-thickness injuries, involving no more than 10% of body surface area (BSA), or full-thickness injuries, involving no more than 2% of BSA. The latter patients can be treated with oral fluid therapy to supplement basal requirements. Intravenous fluids should be started immediately on infants who have burns involving more than 10% of total BSA (or >15% in older children). Burns involving more than 15% of total BSA would be considered major burns.

The goals of treatment of minor partial-thickness burns are to minimize the problems of pain, superficial infection, bothersome wound drainage, and prolonged convalescence. As a first aid measure, parents may be instructed to apply cold towels soaked in ice water to limited partial-thickness burns because this has been shown to reduce edema and to minimize pain, but this measure should not be used for larger injuries because dangerous hypothermia may result. Ice should never be applied directly to any burn. With regard to definitive management, just as with large burn injuries, more than one method of care is available. Depending the age of the child and the part of the body burned, one may use closed dressing care, open therapy with topical antibacterial agents, or a combination of these two methods.

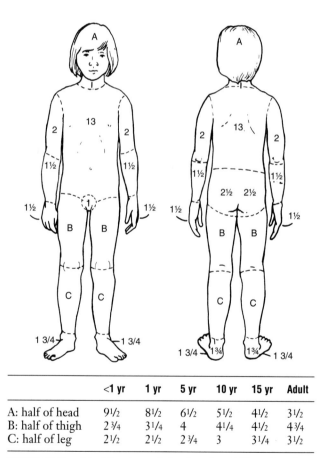

	<1 yr	1 yr	5 yr	10 yr	15 yr	Adult
A: half of head	9½	8½	6½	5½	4½	3½
B: half of thigh	2¾	3¼	4	4¼	4½	4¾
C: half of leg	2½	2½	2¾	3	3¼	3½

FIGURE 17-1 ■ Modification of the Lund and Browder chart permits estimation of percentage of body surface burned in children of various ages. It takes into account the relatively larger surface area of the head and smaller surface area of the thighs in infants and young children. (From Barkin RM: Emergency Pediatrics, 4th ed. St Louis, 1994, Mosby-Year Book, 1994.)

With small burns, blisters should be left intact because they may protect against infection, accelerate healing, and provide greater comfort than if unroofed. Débridement of blisters is probably the preferred approach for more extensive injuries. Although minor burns usually become colonized by surface bacteria, invasive infection or conversion to full-thickness injury is unlikely in this era of topical antibacterial treatment. Superficial infections may cause increased pain and delayed wound healing, however.

Two different forms of closed dressings may be used, but the dressing should be designed to provide a function similar to that of normal skin in terms of transmission of gases and water vapor from the wound surface. The traditional dressing is a layer of nonadherent petrolatum gauze followed by bulky gauze dressings changed every other day or so. The second approach, used more commonly today, is to apply a topical antibacterial cream such as silver sulfadiazine over the wound, then to cover it with a relatively light dressing changed every 12 to 24 hours. Alternately a minor burn wound may be treated open with application of topical antibacterial cream. These wounds are washed every 12 to 24 hours and the cream is renewed. Office follow-up every 5 to 7 days is generally satisfactory, and healing is usually complete within 10 to 14 days. Burns of the face and trunk are treated best open, whereas extremity burns are treated more effectively with light dressings.

Patients with full-thickness burns of limited extent may be treated to the point of eschar separation on an outpatient basis, then admitted for skin grafting, or within 48 hours they may be treated on an outpatient basis by wound excision and immediate grafting. An individualized approach to pain control is necessary and may be accomplished by appropriate adjustment of wound care and administration of oral analgesics.

HOSPITALIZATION GUIDELINES

Although guidelines have been provided for the outpatient treatment of minor burns, these guidelines are predicated on the principle that adequate outpatient follow-up can be accomplished. In any instance in which that is not possible, even children with minor burns should be hospitalized. The limit regarding hospitalization should probably be 5% BSA burn for infants younger than 1 year of age or 15% of BSA otherwise. Any patient who requires intravenous fluids should be hospitalized. Patients with burn injuries to large portions of the face, perineum, hands, or feet probably should be hospitalized initially. Children with obvious signs or even a suggestion of airway injury must be hospitalized. If there are serious social factors involved or if there is any possibility of deliberate abuse, the child should be hospitalized as well or if there is any doubt whether outpatient care can be effective. A short hospitalization of 1 or 2 days ordinarily clarifies this issue. Patients with chemical or electrical burns of any degree should be considered for hospitalization because the depth and extent of injury may be greater than is apparent. Children with burns in excess of 30% of BSA, particularly if combined with inhalation injuries, are managed best in a burn center with specialized facilities and experienced personnel because better outcomes are achieved in these centers.

CARE OF MAJOR BURNS

Major burns may be defined as any that require hospitalization. Traditionally, major burns have been defined as burns involving greater than 20% of BSA in infants and 30% of BSA in older children, burns associated with inhalation injury, or burns associated with other forms of life-threatening trauma (Fig. 17-2).

Airway Management

As part of the primary survey, immediate evaluation of the patient's airway and breathing comes first. Airway patency must be assessed and ensured initially, and the primary initial concern is progressive edema, which may result in airway compromise. If there is any question about impending upper airway obstruction, the most common form of inhalation injury in children, endotracheal intubation should be performed. Even if airway obstruction is not apparent at the outset, with ongoing fluid resuscitation, patients with burns of the head and neck region particularly may accumulate excessive edema, which may make intubation far more difficult than if it had been performed initially. When only mild manifestations of inhalation injury are present, blood gas levels can be monitored, and endotracheal intubation can be performed if signs of deterioration appear, but normal blood gas and peripheral oxygenation measurements shortly after burn injury do not rule out the possibility of an inhalation injury.

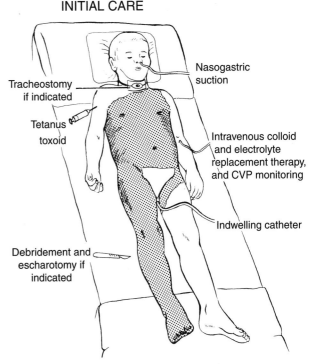

FIGURE 17-2 ▪ Immediate considerations in the resuscitative care of the severely burned child.

Intubation is indicated if upper airway patency is in jeopardy, if gas exchange or work of breathing indicates that mechanical ventilatory support is needed, or if mental status is compromised sufficiently to threaten the airway. If endotracheal intubation is expected to be required for several days, the nasotracheal route should be used if possible because it is easier to immobilize the tube under those circumstances. A nasotracheal or endotracheal tube is best kept in place with the use of fabric tape tied securely around the tube, then fixed around the patient's head because adhesive is ineffective and potentially damaging in children with facial burns. The use of an endotracheal tube and assisted ventilation is based best on clinical experience and careful clinical assessment. The diagnostic standard of inhalation injury at present is probably bronchoscopy, but this is not always practical, and a history of burn in a closed space, physical findings of singed nasal hair, carbonaceous sputum, or elevated carboxyhemoglobin levels may be all that is necessary. X-ray criteria of atelectasis or widespread infiltrates are usually not evident until 12 hours or more after the inhalation episode. Although many intricate diagnostic studies have been described, the most practical approach to diagnosis is still correlation of history and clinical findings.

The goals of management of inhalation injury during the first 24 hours after burn are to ensure airway patency and adequate oxygenation and ventilation. The use of prophylactic steroids, antibiotics, and nebulized agents is probably not warranted. Other than limiting controlled pressure ventilation to inflation pressures less than 40 cm H_2O, even to the point of accepting respiratory acidosis to a pH of 7.2, almost any method of mechanical ventilation is acceptable. In severe cases, there are data to support the use of volumetric diffusive respiration, a pressure-controlled ventilator with a superimposed subtidal oscillation, a technique that minimizes inflation pressures to avoid barotrauma. If endotracheal intubation is expected to be needed longer than 7 to 10 days, it may be prudent to perform tracheostomy, particularly in patients with profuse, thick secretions. Nasotracheal or endotracheal intubation should be the primary method of airway management, however, because of the greater incidence of tracheal and pulmonary infectious complications associated with tracheostomy. Because inhalation injury predisposes to infectious pneumonia, aseptic care techniques must be used in the management of any tube in the airway. Daily monitoring by x-ray and serial blood gas determinations should be performed because the manifestations of pulmonary damage related to inhalation injury may take several days to be manifest. Flexible bronchoscopy may be useful not only for diagnosis, but also for pulmonary toilet and treatment of atelectasis.

Any child with a significant burn and children with associated injuries usually have a tachypneic response to injury and pain, which may result in gastric dilation and vomiting with aspiration. In all of these children, a nasogastric tube should be passed early to avoid gastric distention and aspiration of gastric contents and to alleviate the potential effects of ileus associated with shock. Acute gastric dilation ceases to be a problem by 48 hours after burn unless sepsis intervenes.

Inhalation injury is a major source of mortality and morbidity. Although survival has improved remarkably in more recent years because of improvements in care, many children who have survived inhalation injuries have evidence of significant pulmonary impairment for 9 months after recovery.

Fluid Resuscitation

As part of the initial management of the burn-injured patient, adequate intravenous access must be established, preferably in nonburned extremities. If central venous access is contemplated, it probably should be deferred until after the initial phases of fluid resuscitation because of the potential complications with central venous catheter placement in the emergency setting.

More than 30 years ago, it was recognized that after burn injury and resuscitation there would be accumulation of edema not only in the burned tissues, but also throughout the body. Studies have pointed out that the cause of the capillary permeability responsible for generalized edema is the release of numerous cytokines and mediators, which cause cellular dysfunction, capillary leak, and other manifestations of injury. Interleukin-1 and interleukin-6 are prominently involved, and the magnitude of release is proportional to burn size. The primary goal of fluid resuscitation is to preserve and restore tissue perfusion without producing excessive edema beyond that which is obligatory. The new concept of burn shock is that it is hypovolemic and cellular in nature and that it is characterized by a decrease in plasma volume, extracellular fluid, and cardiac output and decreased urine output. It is known that the greatest loss of fluid from the capillary bed is in the first 4 hours after injury and that the maximum accumulation of edema is in the first 12 to 24 hours in extensive burn injuries. Numerous studies performed over the years have shown that effective replacement of plasma volume in patients with extensive burns requires sodium and crystalloid solutions. Additionally, numerous studies have shown that colloid has little effect and may be deleterious for the first 24 hours after burn. After that time, colloid has a greater capacity to be retained in the capillary bed. There is no clearly superior method of approach to fluid resuscitation in burn-injured patients, but everyone accepts the principle that one must replace the extracellular salt and water that is lost in the burn tissue and in the cells of the body. The most popular approach at present involves the use of Ringer's lactate for 48 hours after burn, decreasing the salt and water load after that time. Because it is known that the extent of edema is related to the amount and type of fluid administered, a variety of formulas have been devised, some based on carefully controlled scientific studies and others based on empirical information about how groups of patients respond to various approaches. Some formulas still use colloid initially, but most withhold it for at least 24 hours. Another point of agreement has to do with the rate of fluid administration based on studies that indicate when the maximum fluid shifts occur after injury. On this basis, one half of the resuscitation volume is administered in the first 8 hours postinjury and the other half in the succeeding 16 hours, while monitoring urine output and estimating the adequacy of cardiac output.

Adequate urine output is considered to be in the range of 0.5 to 1.5 mL/kg/hr. After the first 24 hours postburn, resuscitation volumes usually end up being one half to three fourths of the first day's requirements.

Several formulas have been devised as guidelines for fluid replacement in burn-injured patients. The most popular are the Parkland formula and the modified Brooke formula, as outlined in Table 17-1; however, there are many other approaches. Clinical research is ongoing with regard to the use of hypertonic saline solutions, which theoretically have the advantage of replacing sodium deficits, while limiting the amount of fluid administered. This has yet to be proved, and the use of hypertonic solutions in children is less well accepted. The original hypertonic saline solution used has 250 mEq Na/L, but others have used 180 mEq Na/L. Because children are particularly prone to hypertonicity, most clinicians have preferred to use Ringer's lactate solutions.

In terms of pediatric resuscitation, the most frequently used approaches have been a modification of the Brooke formula using 3 mL/kg/% burn or the approaches used at the Cincinnati and Galveston Shriners' Burns Institute (Table 17-2). The tendency toward use of large-volume

of fluid resuscitation in more recent years has been associated with the appearance of "abdominal compartment syndrome." This syndrome indicates that enough but not excessive volumes of fluid are called for based on careful monitoring. All approaches use the monitoring guidelines mentioned earlier. It also is known that significant inhalation injury increases fluid requirements 30% to 50%.

After the first 48 hours following burn when diuresis is usually under way, colloid is administered according to need with 5% albumin at 0.5 mL/kg/% burn. Maintenance fluids are required plus an additional amount for evaporative water loss (Table 17-3). Fluid replacement during this interval may be provided intravenously and enterally. Potassium supplementation usually is required at this point. The American Burn Association has published evidence-based practice guidelines that represent the current consensus regarding fluid replacement after burn injury in childhood.

To a large degree, the extent of fluid losses related to burn injury is proportional in an linear fashion to the amount of surface area burn, but it increases in a nonlinear fashion to the factors of depth and inhalation injury. Also, a child younger than age 2 years requires more fluids than older children. Although Ringer's lactate is used initially, during the second 24 hours, capillary losses may be less so that the fluid requirements often may be met with 0.5 N saline in 5% glucose at one half to three fourths of the first day's requirements.

As mentioned earlier, the primary physiologic guidelines for judging the adequacy of fluid resuscitation during the first 24 to 48 hours are an estimation of the adequacy of cardiac output and adequate hourly urine output. Continuing lactic acidosis and the possibility of mental confusion must be monitored as well, however, because these findings indicate inadequate cardiac output. Severe acidosis and hypothermia often must be corrected before burn shock can be addressed adequately by fluid replacement.

The glucose response to injury is unpredictable in infants and small children, so it is important to monitor serum glucose values serially. Because most children are hyperglycemic initially, Ringer's lactate solution should be used, but for the occasional patient who is initially hypoglycemic, additional 5% glucose may be required. Rarely, protracted hyperglycemia may require supplemental insulin administration.

TABLE 17-1 ■ Estimation of Fluid Requirements: First 48 Hours Postburn

First 24 hours
  Ringer's lactate solution: 3 mL/kg/% burn (25–35% burn); 4 mL/kg/% burn (>35% burn)
Second 24 hours
  5% dextrose in 0.45 N saline solution: one half to three quarters of first 24-hr requirements
  5% albumin solution as indicated
Guidelines for fluid replacement
  Hourly urine output
  Vital signs, central venous pressure
  Clear sensorium
  Adequacy of peripheral circulation
  Absence of lactic acidosis, hypothermia
  Hematocrit value, serum electrolyte levels, pH, glucose value

TABLE 17-2 ■ Other Approaches to Fluid Resuscitation: First 48 Hours Postburn*

| Warden (Cincinnati) | 4 mL/kg/% burn | First 8 hr
Ringer's lactate solution + 50 mEq NaHCO$_3$ + 1500 mL m² BSA
Second 8 hr
Ringer's lactate solution
Third 8 hr
Ringer's lactate solution + 12.5 g albumin |
| Herndon (Galveston) | 5000 mL/m² BSA burn + 2000 mL/m² BSA burn | Ringer's lactate solution + 12.5 g albumin |

*The same criteria for monitoring are used as in Table 17-1.

TABLE 17-3 ■ Estimation of Fluid Requirements Beyond 48 Hours Postburn, Evaporative Water Loss Phase

Daily maintenance: dextrose 5% 0.2 N saline solution according to individual needs
Evaporative water loss: dextrose 5% 0.2 N saline solution 1–2 mL/kg/% burn/24 hr
Potassium—as needed
Blood—as needed
Guidelines for fluid needs in this phase
  Daily body weight
  Daily urine volume and specific gravity
  Values for serum sodium, potassium, urea, hematocrit, osmolality

After 48 hours postburn, evaporative water loss is the prime loss involved, and because this is 85% free water, it may be replaced effectively with 5% glucose in 0.2 N saline with added potassium. Guidelines for adequate replacement during this interval include serial measurements of body weight, determination of urine volume and specific gravity, and measurement of serum electrolytes and osmolality. Inadequate replacement of evaporative water loss results in hypernatremia and hyperosmolality. Enteral fluid replacement requires 10% to 15% more fluid than when the intravenous route is used.

Most children who have sustained burns involving greater than 30% of BSA will have gained 15% to 20% over basal body weight. Diuresis of this excess retained fluid ordinarily takes 5 to 7 days, so administration of diuretics occasionally may be useful. Accumulation of excessive edema may convert an initially partial-thickness burn to a full-thickness injury, or it may accentuate pulmonary impairment. In children with extensive deep burns, hemoglobinuria may develop, in which case management should include the administration of mannitol and additional fluids to avoid acute tubular necrosis.

Blood Replacement

Thermal injury to the skin results in red blood cell loss in proportion to the size and depth of the burn. In addition to an immediate destruction of red blood cells circulating through the injured capillary bed, there is partial cellular damage that diminishes the half-life span of many of the remaining red blood cells. Because plasma loss is the predominant loss during the first 48 hours postburn, however, relative polycythemia occurs first. Consequently, administration of red blood cells is not indicated during the first 48 hours unless there has been extensive blood loss from associated injuries. After the process of burn wound excision begins, blood administration usually is required.

Nutrition

Nutritional requirements are related to body deficits and metabolic rate in all disease states. Children have increased metabolic rates compared with adults, and this is accentuated by the cellular and hormonal effects of burn injury that result in hypermetabolism, compounded by heat loss. Most patients are in a persistant catabolic state with marked negative nitrogen balance. Inadequate protein replacement not only results in impaired wound healing, but also an increased susceptibility to infection. Burn-injured patients with severe malnutrition have been shown to have a high incidence of sepsis and associated mortality. The best route for nutritional supplementation is enteral feedings because they are more effective than parenteral nutrition and carry less risk of infection. Tube feedings commonly are associated with diarrhea, however, which may complicate management. If patients are unable to take adequate food by mouth voluntarily, a small feeding tube should be used for feeding supplementation. Because of the increased rate of evaporative water loss and a natural tendency to hyperosmolality, tube feedings should be iso-osmolar with a caloric density of one half to two thirds of a calorie per milliliter. The specific aim should be to provide an intake of 100 kcal/kg/24 hours

TABLE 17-4 ■ Approaches to Nutrition in Children with Burns	
Herndon (Galveston)	1800 kcal/m²/24 hr + 1300 kcal/m² BSA/BSA burned Calorie: N₂ of 100:1
Alexander (Cincinnati)	BMR × 1.2 with 3 g of protein/kg/24 hr Calorie: N₂ of 100:1

BMR, basal metabolic rate.

and 3 g/kg/24 hours of protein equivalent (Table 17-4). The ultimate goal is to maintain body weight and to prevent excessive weight loss. Patients who lose greater than 20% of basal weight have a markedly increased mortality.

Stress ulceration is a well-known complication of shock, sepsis, and severe injury. Along with enteral feeds, patients should receive ulcer prophylaxis with antacids and proton-pump inhibitor drugs.

Pain Control

Pain is a significant problem for burn-injured children throughout the entire course of treatment. In the emergency situation, intravenous morphine is useful in small amounts, but administration should be modified according to the child's physiologic state at the time. When the patient is hemodynamically stable, pain medication should be given as indicated. When children are able to take oral fluids, oral codeine, morphine, or meperidine may be used. Analgesics should be administered before dressing changes and wound débridement. Additionally, diazepam may be useful to alleviate the many psychological stresses that the injured children may undergo. Conscious sedation is another useful technique when procedures are being performed. Diphenhydramine is extremely helpful for children with healing partial-thickness injury who develop severe itching.

WOUND CARE
Escharotomy

Circumferential full-thickness burns of the extremities may cause progressive distal ischemia, especially as edema accumulates with fluid resuscitation. This ischemia may result in vascular compromise of fingers or toes. Also, circumferential full-thickness burns of the thorax or abdomen may result in respiratory embarrassment that can be alleviated by escharotomy. Serial assessment of peripheral pulses using Doppler sonography is a useful supplement to clinical judgment. If there is any indication of impending peripheral circulatory compromise, escharotomy should be performed. This involves an incision made through eschar alone on the lateral and medial aspects of the extremity throughout the area of burn. Usually it is unnecessary to perform escharotomy for partial-thickness burns. Fasciotomy almost never is required except in patients with extensive electrical injuries. When necessary, escharotomy is performed best

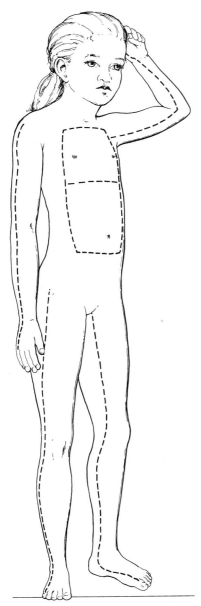

FIGURE 17-3 ■ Appropriate incisions for escharotomy, which should be performed for constricting injuries associated with full-thickness burns. Patients with partial-thickness burns rarely require escharotomy. Fasciotomy is not needed except for crush or electrical injuries or when there are associated fractures.

during the first 8 to 24 hours after burn. Figure 17-3 shows the position of incisions useful for the relief of the constricting effects of full-thickness burns.

Infection Control

Because the skin is an effective barrier to the entry of bacteria into the body, whenever skin is extensively damaged, infection is a danger. The cellular response to injury results in immunosuppression, and this response is proportional to the extent of the burn. In addition to the generalized immunosuppressive effects of the burn, defense mechanisms are compromised further by the presence of necrotic tissue, which is why early excision has been emphasized in more recent years. Patients with

inhalation injuries are particularly susceptible to bacterial pneumonia, now the leading cause of mortality in patients with extensive burn injuries, whether or not inhalation damage has occurred. For all these reasons, conventional isolation techniques are useful for protecting patients with extensive burns.

The prime advance that has improved survival in burn patients has been the introduction of effective topical antibacterial agents; 1% silver sulfadiazine is the most commonly used agent, although 10% mafenide acetate or other topical antibacterials are used occasionally as backup agents. Silver sulfadiazine or mafenide cream should be applied twice daily, and the patient should be turned regularly to expose all areas of the body. Regardless of the agent used, careful bacterial surveillance must be followed; in patients with extensive, deep injuries who develop sepsis, periodic burn wound biopsies for quantitative bacteriologic studies are helpful. If a patient's physiologic state deteriorates and infection becomes a problem, the type of agent used should be changed, and other approaches to infection control should be initiated. Blood and urine cultures and cultures of intravenous catheters and pulmonary secretions must be obtained regularly. The goal is to anticipate infection rather than treat it when it has become established. *Pseudomonas* is now less common as the cause of infection than opportunistic organisms, such as *Enterobacter cloacae*, *Providencia stuartii*, *Serratia marcescens*, *Candida*, *Phycomycetes*, and occasional viruses. More recently, methicillin-resistant *Staphylococcus aureus* infection has become more common.

Antibiotic Therapy

Systemic antibiotics generally are indicated only for specifically identified infection in the lungs, urinary tract, or elsewhere or when invasive infection is detected in the burn wound by biopsy with a quantitative bacterial count greater than 10^5 organisms per gram of tissue. Blood levels of systemic antibiotics must be monitored because of the unpredictable nature of drug metabolism in the burn-injured patient. Prophylactic antibiotic administration is effective and useful for the prevention of graft loss from infection after extensive skin-grafting procedures but does not prevent burn wound infection.

Other Approaches to Infection Control

In patients with large injuries, such as burns involving greater than 50% of BSA, it may be helpful to administer gamma globulin weekly during the first month after injury. Patients with severe invasive burn wound infection may require the administration of subeschar antibiotics. Administration of fresh-frozen plasma may be helpful in patients with ongoing burn wound infection or sepsis, and a variety of immunomodulators and immunostimulators are being investigated. Because the most effective method of infection control is to accelerate removal of necrotic tissue and to accomplish wound closure, early excision and grafting is the primary approach to wound care at this time.

Coverage of the Burn Wound

Previously the approach to wound care was daily application of topical silver sulfadiazine, a light dressing, and daily débridement. Although this approach, which usually took 3 weeks, was satisfactory for patients with partial-thickness burns, it left patients with large full-thickness burns in jeopardy of invasive burn wound infection.

Because definitive closure of the burn wound and removal of necrotic tissue are key to survival, infection control, and correction of hypermetabolism, early excision of the burn wound currently is practiced. Excision is initiated within 24 to 48 hours postburn. This timing also minimizes blood loss because some wound edema is still present. Although a variety of techniques are available, blood loss is minimized with an electrosurgical knife. Tangential excision through subcutaneous tissue is associated with significant bleeding, and it is less if excision is performed to fascia. Deep partial-thickness injuries are excised best tangentially and immediately grafted as soon as the depth of injury is clear.

Severe inhalation injury associated with inadequate oxygenation despite mechanical ventilation is a contraindication to burn wound excision. Operative burn wound excision should be performed in a heated operating room with supplemental heat devices and minimal exposure of the patient. Procedures must be performed expeditiously, preferably using two teams.

In extensive burn injuries, sequential procedures involving excision of 10% to 20% of body surface, and sometimes more, are performed carefully monitoring body temperature and extent of blood loss. Immediate autografting is performed in priority order: face and neck, hands, arms, feet, legs, and trunk. In patients with massive burn injuries it is usually best to excise the maximum amount of necrotic tissue, which is usually either on the anterior or posterior trunk. Available autograft donor sites include the scalp and other areas of the body where skin is thick so that recropping of the donor sites can be performed on a regular basis. Routine mesh expansion of autografts is performed. Many centers have extensive experience with cultured epithelial cells derived from skin biopsies performed at the time of admission. Until sufficient autograft tissue is available, the excised wound bed may be covered with allografts, xenografts, or one of a variety of biologic dressings and skin substitutes. Traditional delayed wound excision and grafting was associated with increased rates of invasive wound infection and sepsis and mortality compared with the results in current patients who have early excision within 48 hours. The goal with primary excision is to accomplish complete wound coverage within the first 5 to 7 days postburn. An important consideration in children is the careful application of an appropriate wound dressing to prevent dislodgment of crucial skin grafts.

REHABILITATION

As with all forms of major trauma, physical and occupational therapy efforts should be initiated at the outset of treatment, first to prevent excessive peripheral edema and later to prevent contracture formation and hypertrophic scarring. A successful long-term functional and psychological result depends to a great degree on the quality and intensity of rehabilitative efforts. Constant attention to maintenance of functional positions of joints is required with appropriate splinting and encouragement of active and passive motion, including the use of dynamic splints. Because pressure is an effective measure to prevent hypertrophic scarring, elastic compression dressings and garments supplemented by a good exercise program are vital. Pressure dressings should be maintained for at least 1 year at a pressure of approximately 30 mm Hg. Patients with massive burn injuries require multiple surgical procedures over several years to achieve an ideal functional and psychological result. The extent to which reconstructive procedures are required is related at least in part to how patients are cared for initially. Long-term outcome of children who survive massive burn injury may involve residual physical disability, which may be addressed through the years, but a satisfactory quality of life can be achieved. In terms of survival, current figures indicate that children with burns in the range of 40% to 59% of BSA have a mortality of 0 to 2%. Children with burns in excess of 60% of BSA have a mortality of approximately 15%, and many patients with burns more extensive than that are surviving today.

SUGGESTED READINGS

American Burn Association: Practice guidelines for burn care. J Burn Care Rehabil Suppl, 2001.

These guidelines represent the first evidence-based approach to standardizing most aspects of current burn care.

Hart DW, Wolf SE, Chinkes DL, et al: β-blockade and growth hormone after burn. Ann Surg 236:450-457, 2002.

These authors have pioneered the use of anabolic agents to combat burn-induced catabolism, which is discussed thoroughly in this article.

Robson MC, Burnett RA, Leitch IOW, et al: Prevention and treatment of postburn scars and contracture. World J Surg 16:87-96, 1992.

This is an excellent source of information regarding care during the rehabilitation phase.

Sheridan RL, Hinson MI, Liang MH, et al: Long-term outcome of children surviving massive burns. JAMA 283:69-79, 2000.

This article serves as a basis for an aggressive approach to children with extensive burn injury.

Child Abuse

18

Child abuse is addressed in a separate chapter because 5000 children die each year as a result of abuse. Poor treatment of children has been a problem since the earliest days of humanity, but because children were not believed to have any rights, maltreatment was not considered to be wrong. It is an issue of international scope. Child abuse was brought to the attention of modern society in 1946 by Caffey, who described a syndrome of multiple long bone fractures in infants associated with subdural hematoma. The battered child syndrome has many manifestations, including physical and mental abuse, nutritional and hygienic neglect, sexual abuse, delayed treatment of illnesses, and neglect of a child's safety. Homicide is a steadily increasing problem in older children.

The precise incidence of child abuse is unknown, but it is known to vary in different cultures. Violent forms of child abuse are increasing in number in a disturbing fashion. Estimates are that more than 1 million children in the United States are abused each year and that 5% or more of patients presenting with mild injuries in emergency departments have had deliberate injuries. It is estimated that 1 in every 25 children is abused.

Knowledge of the epidemiology of child abuse and the specific patterns of injury is helpful to physicians in terms of recognition and verification. Most commonly, the victims of abuse are younger than 2 years of age, when they have limited ability to communicate. More boys than girls are injured, but far more girls are sexually abused. Sexual abuse most commonly occurs at age 10 years or older but may occur earlier. In terms of life-threatening injuries related to physical abuse, most victims are younger than 1 year of age, with the greatest mortality in the 6- to 12-month age group. Premature infants, infants and children with complicated medical problems, and stepchildren are at particular risk. Although children from all levels of society are potential victims, most more recent experience related to serious and life-threatening injuries has been among low socioeconomic status populations, particularly transient groups. Increasing societal violence affects low socioeconomic status groups more than others. In most instances, children are injured at home by a party known to them. In three fourths of cases, one or both parents are involved, and more than half the time the abuser is a young single mother. Boyfriends, siblings, babysitters, and others close to the family are other common abusers.

Although it is unusual for alcohol and illicit drugs to be involved with deliberate physical abuse, it is common for these factors to be related to problems of neglect or to incidental shootings. Most individuals who injure their children are immature, young people under extreme financial and social stress. Most mothers and fathers who injure their children have abnormal personality characteristics, and many were previously victims of child abuse themselves.

DIAGNOSIS

The history offered to explain manifestations of child abuse is characteristically evasive. Parents may bring a child to the emergency department for an injury that occurred several days previously, and they may try to explain the injury as spontaneous and unwitnessed. Almost always there is a marked discrepancy between the history offered and the manifestations of injury seen on physical examination. In general, the manifestations of injury are far more severe than the simple mechanism offered as an explanation. There also may be a discrepancy in chronology or no explanation for manifestations of repeated injury over time. At other times, infants and children are said to have injured themselves in a fashion that exceeds their developmental physical abilities. Parents may make visits to many different emergency departments to avoid detection by visiting the same facility more than once; state-supported registries have been developed to detect these situations. Whatever the evasive technique used by the caregiver of the child, if the story does not match the injury pattern, child abuse should be suspected and investigated carefully. This investigation is crucial in infants younger than 6 months of age because they appear to be at the highest risk for lethal injury.

PATTERNS OF INJURY ASSOCIATED WITH PHYSICAL ABUSE

Because of a variety of causes, the battered child syndrome has multiple manifestations, and many of them mimic the clinical pictures of organic syndromes, including infection, metabolic disease, malignancy, dermatologic disease,

TABLE 18-1 ■ Patterns of Injury Characteristic of Abuse in Order of Frequency
Repetitive soft tissue injuries
Contusions, abrasions, lacerations, burns
Evidence of repetitive fractures
Solitary head injury, subdural hematomas
Visceral injuries

coagulation disorders, and central nervous system disorders. With careful initial evaluation, most of these medical illnesses are not difficult to eliminate as diagnostic possibilities so that the focus can be placed appropriately on the matter of deliberate injury. Certain patterns or combinations of injuries are characteristic so that their recognition is helpful in terms of verifying that abuse is the cause of the injury seen. Another facet of the abuse profile is that there is a predictable pattern of progressive injury in many instances. In the order of frequency as noted in Table 18-1, the types of injury encountered include soft tissue injuries, fractures, and head injuries. In emergency department populations, injuries may be solitary and generally minor, but in hospitalized patients, combined injuries and evidence of a prior injury are the rule. Patients with fractures usually have evidence of either multiple fractures or old soft tissue injuries, and patients with severe head injuries usually have evidence of old fractures and old soft tissue injuries.

Soft Tissue Injuries

In most instances, soft tissue injuries are described as related to falls or other minor events, but the physical findings belie the history and suggest greater force or a different mechanism. Children who are abused and present with bruises and abrasions have lesions on the cheeks, trunk, buttocks, genitalia, and upper legs most frequently. Fresh bruises associated with fading ecchymoses indicative of repeated injury are seen frequently. Although lacerations are generally accidental, lacerations of the lip and labial frenulum in infants are rarely accidental. Occasionally the skin lesions have a pattern of hand marks or are characteristic of whipping with a light cord, belt, belt buckle, or other object. Other marks that indicate forceful placement of a hand over the child's mouth and nose or marks on the neck that suggest choking are also typical. Pinch marks on the body or genitalia and puncture wounds are characteristic and usually related to inappropriate disciplinary measures.

Frequently a child with multiple soft tissue injuries around the face and sometimes a head injury has characteristic ocular findings. Children younger than age 3 years with retinal hemorrhages, detachment, and scarring or periorbital ecchymosis should be suspected of being abused. These injuries also may be of varying ages.

Burn injury is an extremely common form of abuse. Among the most common are contact burns produced by lighted cigarettes, irons, and radiators. Immersion burns in a pattern suggestive of lowering a child's buttocks and posterior trunk into a tub of boiling water is characteristic of deliberate abuse when associated with a history that cannot possibly explain the event. Typically the child flexes the knees so that the posterior knee areas are spared. Patients with unusual patterns of burn injury also usually have multiple old bruises and scars.

Visceral Injuries

Most patients with severe visceral injury related to abuse do not survive to reach the hospital, but 10% to 15% of children who are hospitalized for abuse show some manifestation of abdominal or thoracic injury. Almost invariably the history does not suggest that an internal injury has occurred, but a combination of multiple skin bruises, anemia, and abdominal distention, sometimes associated with pain, indicates an abdominal injury. In addition to the unexplained anemia, the clinician may be able to elicit signs of peritoneal irritation, localized tenderness, or hematuria. Routine radiographic survey, contrast-enhanced computed tomography (CT), and sometimes peritoneal lavage may be required to make the diagnosis. Common forms of intra-abdominal injury associated with child abuse include liver and renal fractures with bleeding, duodenal hematoma, duodenal and jejunal rupture, pancreatic fracture, mesenteric tears with bleeding, and rectal injuries. The most common cause of these injuries is a sharp blow to the midabdomen with a fist compressing the viscera against the vertebral column.

Similarly, deliberate thoracic trauma is related to blunt injury with manifestations of pulmonary contusion, mediastinal emphysema, and traumatic asphyxia. At least half of children who have severe abdominal and thoracic injuries related to abuse die. Late recognition is a major factor accounting for the high mortality.

Musculoskeletal Injuries

From a diagnostic point of view, the pattern of skeletal injury encountered in child abuse is the most definitive in terms of diagnosis. Also, fractures are common, occurring in approximately one fourth of children who have suffered physical abuse. The biomechanics of injury most frequently indicate that the fracture in question was related to a pulling or twisting motion rather than what might be explained by a fall. Notation of multiple fractures at various stages of healing is diagnostic and is differentiated easily from the rare congenital and metabolic bone disorders of childhood. Almost all children with multiple fractures also have a variety of soft tissue manifestations of abuse. Although bone scans and magnetic resonance imaging (MRI) may be helpful to survey the skeleton, long bone films are more specifically diagnostic. Because the epiphyseal-metaphyseal junction is one of the weakest areas in growing bone, it is extremely vulnerable to the force of pulling, twisting, or shaking an infant so that among the most common orthopedic manifestations of abuse are epiphyseal separations, metaphyseal fractures, and subperiosteal hemorrhages (Figs. 18-1 and 18-2). Small metaphyseal fragments displaced with the epiphysis and metaphyseal demineralization and periosteal elevation are characteristic findings. The so-called bucket-handle fracture of epiphyseal-metaphyseal separation is virtually pathognomonic. An additional suspicious pattern is that of a diaphyseal spiral fracture supposedly the result of a minor fall. Table 18-2 lists skeletal findings that may

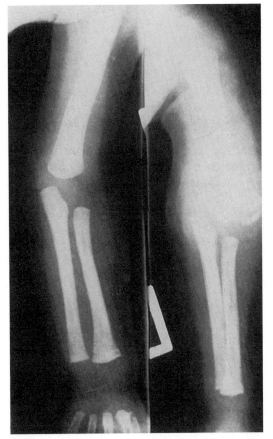

FIGURE 18-1 ■ Arm radiographs obtained in a child known to be abused shows evidence of periosteal elevation in the radius and ulna and a metaphyseal fracture of the humerus on the left that supposedly resulted from a fall. This mechanism of injury is not consistent with the radiographic findings.

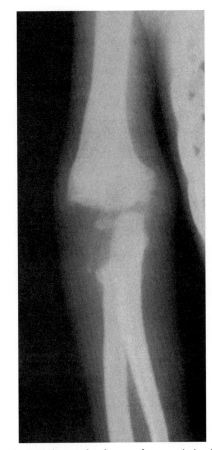

FIGURE 18-2 ■ Radiograph shows characteristic findings of epiphyseal separation and a metaphyseal fracture typically related to sudden jerking forces rather than direct injury.

verify the diagnosis of deliberate injury. Overall the larger bones of the body are involved most often and most severely. In order of frequency, fractures involve the humerus; femur; tibia; forearm bones; and, far less commonly, clavicle, facial bones, and ribs.

Intracranial Injuries

The third most common and most serious manifestation of child abuse is head injury. This injury usually is associated with soft tissue and skeletal manifestations of injury that can be determined to have occurred early and repetitively. Head injuries are frequent probably because the head is relatively large in infants compared with the rest of the body, and the face represents the child. Head injuries are the main cause of mortality in the child abuse syndrome, followed by visceral injuries. Also, head injuries are the main cause of long-term disability and retardation.

The typical child with a head injury related to deliberate abuse presents in a coma with few if any signs of external trauma because most are injured by a blow from an open hand, by severe shaking (shaken baby syndrome), or by being thrown against a wall. Occasionally a subgaleal hematoma and orbital hemorrhage may be found, but most patients have no such manifestations. The clinical

presentation is usually that of chronic subdural hematoma with symptoms that progress from irritability and lethargy to outright coma. Children who present late may have manifestations of hydrocephalus from intraventricular hemorrhage. Clinical and radiographic findings show skull fractures in less than half of patients, but because most who sustain severe head injury are infants, gradual spreading of the fontanelles may be evident (Fig. 18-3). A CT scan usually shows bilateral subdural hematomas and rarely epidural hematomas. Infants injured by severe shaking have bilateral retinal hemorrhages and clinical and CT findings that indicate marked increases in intracranial pressure. Limited areas of hemorrhage are seen around the brain and even within the cortex, and the characteristic pattern of severe diffuse axonal injury is present. The outlook for these patients is poor.

TABLE 18-2 ■ Musculoskeletal Manifestations of Abuse

Spiral fractures attributed to "falls"
Subperiosteal calcification with no history of injury
Multiple fractures in various stages of healing
Bucket-handle fractures or epiphyseal-metaphyseal separation and fragmentation from pulling or shaking forces
Unexplained fractures associated with chronic subdural hematomas

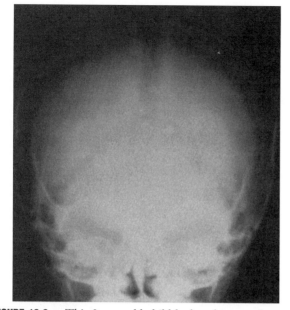

FIGURE 18-3 ■ This 2-year-old child had no history of trauma but presented with progressive lethargy. This skull radiograph shows spread fontanelles, and CT scan confirmed a massive subdural hematoma. There also were skeletal fractures and soft tissue injuries of varying ages.

Other Manifestations of Abuse

In addition to deliberate trauma, many other manifestations of abuse occur across the spectrum of childhood. Sexual abuse, which usually is found in girls 10 to 12 years old, may be manifested by rape, incest, and a variety of other bizarre presentations. This form of abuse is increasing in incidence. With the marked increase in drug use, children are now presenting with drug overdoses and addiction. Children who have sustained physical abuse usually show manifestations of serious neglect. A child may present with failure to thrive with marked nutritional deficiency or starvation. A caregiver may deny a child normal medical care either deliberately or by neglect. A lack of supervision and provision for safety may be evident in infants and toddlers; this is usually associated with hygienic neglect. Finally, constant psychological and emotional abuse and intimidation may have serious effects on a child's developmental status and reaction to others in the environment.

LEGAL CONSIDERATIONS AND OUTLOOK

Verification of the diagnosis of child abuse is key to intervention. Physicians are universally protected when reporting suspected child abuse in good faith to the appropriate civil agencies so that intensive investigations can be performed and the child isolated from the home when appropriate. Breaking the cycle is a vital factor that allows treatment to be given not only to the injured child, but also to the family. Only about 10% of children must be taken from the home permanently, whereas the remainder of the families can be rehabilitated by means of long-term psychiatric care and social service involvement. Immediate and vigorous intervention is the only method that has been found to prevent subsequent injury and mortality. Child abuse is a growing social problem, and the degree of violence and injury is increasing. As new immigrant groups are growing, new, ethnically based types of abuse are being seen as well.

SUGGESTED READINGS

Caffey J: Multiple fractures of the long bones of infants suffering from chronic subdural hematoma. AJR Am J Roentgenol 56:167, 1946.

This article not only presents information that is useful today, but also it is the first article to alert society that something should be done about child abuse. It is a classic description of the problem.

Carty HM: Fractures caused by child abuse. J Bone Joint Surg Br 75:849, 1993.

This is a thorough review of the various musculoskeletal manifestations of child abuse with an analysis of mechanism of injury as related to history. This article is important because of the frequency of these injuries.

Jones E, McCurdy K: The links between types of maltreatment and demographic characteristics of children. Child Abuse Negl 16:20, 1992.

This article presents information on current trends in society and socioeconomics as related to child abuse.

National Clearinghouse on Child Abuse and Neglect: Child Maltreatment: Reports from the States to the National Center on Child Abuse and Neglect. Washington, DC, National Clearinghouse on Child Abuse and Neglect, 1995.

Much current information is available on epidemiology and patterns of abuse in children on their website, available at: nccanch@calib.com.

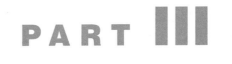

PART III

Tumors

19

Neuroblastoma

Neuroblastoma is an embryonal tumor of neural crest origin that may arise at any site in the sympathetic nervous system, including the brain, neck (3%), mediastinum (20%), para-aortic sympathetic ganglia (24%), pelvis (3%), and adrenal medulla (50%) (Fig. 19-1). This neoplasm is the second most common solid tumor of infancy and childhood, being exceeded only by brain tumors. More than 25% of cases are diagnosed before 1 year of age; 50% of cases present by age 2 years, and 90% are diagnosed by age 8 years. There are approximately 500 new cases of neuroblastoma per year in the United States. Neuroblastoma occurs more frequently in boys (1.2:1). The reported incidence is 8 to 10 cases per 1 million per year. This lesion has occurred in patients with other neural crest–related conditions (neurocristopathies), including Hirschsprung's disease, Klippel-Feil syndrome, Waardenburg's syndrome, and Ondine's curse (congenital central alveolar hypoventilation syndrome); patients with Beckwith-Weidemann syndrome; patients with fetal alcohol syndrome; and mothers taking phenylhydantoin for seizure disorders (fetal hydantoin syndrome). Alcohol has been established as a teratogen; in addition to neuroblastoma, adrenal carcinoma has been observed after maternal alcohol abuse during pregnancy. The association of neuroblastoma and adrenocortical hyperplasia (Cushing's syndrome) also has been observed. Familial instances of neuroblastoma have been reported in identical twins and a mother and daughter. Evidence of the embryonal nature of the tumor with secretion of metabolites from the tumor causing maternal hypertension, sweating, pallor, headaches, and palpitations has been documented. Further evidence of the embryonal occurrence of neuroblastoma includes cases associated with antenatal death, instances of placental invasion by the tumor, and reports of prenatal diagnosis by ultrasonography in asymptomatic fetuses.

A specific chromosomal type has not been detected in patients with neuroblastoma, although many chromosomal abnormalities are noted in many neuroblastoma cells. The most frequent are 1p36 deletions and 1p loss of heterozygosity; these are associated with advanced stages of the disease, indicating that this area of chromosome 1 may contain a tumor suppressor gene. *N-myc*, *ras*, and other oncogenes have been identified; most are poor prognosis factors.

Neuroblasts can be identified in 7-week fetuses and form neuroblastic nodules by 12 weeks' gestation. These nodules increase in size and number until 15 to 17 weeks' gestation. Examination of fetal adrenal tissues shows the presence of neuroblastoma in situ in 100% of adrenal glands studied at 17 to 20 weeks' gestation but in only 1:39 to 1:263 adrenal glands in newborns or infants younger than 3 months of age who die from other causes. These observations suggest that neuroblastoma in situ may undergo regression, or differentiation and does not present as a clinical case of neuroblastoma. Clinical tumor development may be related to defective regression or further malignant progression.

Neuroblastoma cells secrete many products, including hormones (e.g., vasoactive intestinal polypeptide [VIP]) and other vasoactive substances, including catecholamines and their byproducts (homovanillic acid [HVA], vanillylmandelic acid [VMA], 3-methoxytyramine, metanephrines, and dopamine); rarely a parasympathetic neuroblastoma may occur and secrete acetylcholine. Because it is a neural crest tumor with hormonal capacity, this neoplasm should be classified in the family of amine precursor uptake decarboxylase tumors.

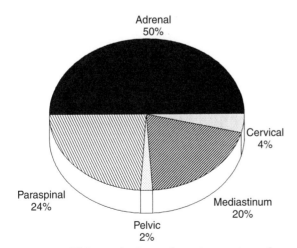

Adrenal
50%

Cervical
4%

Mediastinum
20%

Pelvic
2%

Paraspinal
24%

FIGURE 19-1 ■ This graph shows the primary sites of tumor occurrence for infants and children with neuroblastoma. Most cases occur in the adrenal medulla and the retroperitoneal paraspinal sympathetic ganglia.

CLINICAL MANIFESTATIONS

Presenting symptoms in cases of neuroblastoma vary according to the location of the primary lesion and whether or not tumor metastasis has occurred. The most common sites of hematogenous tumor metastases are the bone marrow (Fig. 19-2), bone cortex, liver, and skin; rarely lung and brain are sites. Metastases to lymph nodes are common. An abdominal mass is palpable in more than 50% of patients secondary to a primary adrenal or paraspinal tumor. The mass is often large, hard, nodular, and sometimes tender on palpation. Respiratory distress may herald the presence of a posterior mediastinal lesion, whereas Horner's syndrome (ptosis, myosis, anhidrosis, and heterochromia) may lead one to suspect a primary tumor affecting the stellate ganglion (Fig. 19-3). Proptosis or bilateral orbital ecchymosis ("panda eyes") is another presenting finding and usually indicates metastases to the orbit. Systemic manifestations, such as anemia, failure to thrive, weight loss, and malnutrition, often are noted in advanced cases. Children with bone metastases affecting the lower extremities may refuse to walk because of severe leg pain. Hypertension may accompany this lesion in 35% of cases as a result of release of catecholamines from the tumor or from pressure on the adjacent kidney. Paraplegia or cauda equina syndrome may occur as a result of tumor extension through intervertebral foramina into the extradural space causing spinal cord compression. A pelvic mass may cause bladder or vascular compression. More unusual manifestations include cerebellar ataxia and opsomyoclonus (myoclonic jerking and nystagmus, also called *dancing-eye syndrome*), which are probably caused by an antigen-antibody complex affecting the cerebellum and not from a tumor metastasis, and hypokalemic watery diarrhea syndrome, resulting from release of VIP from the tumor. Some neonates and young infants may present with hepatomegaly related to tumor infiltration and multiple subcutaneous tumor nodules (Fig. 19-4). These latter patients also may have respiratory distress secondary to

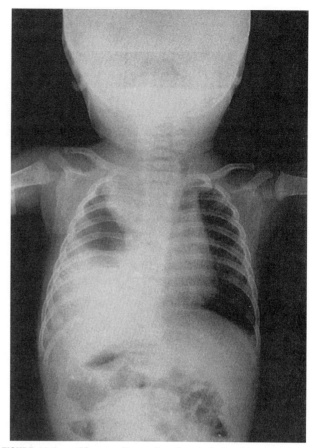

FIGURE 19-3 ■ Chest radiograph of an infant with a posterior mediastinal neuroblastoma.

diaphragmatic elevation from the enlarged liver, symptomatic gastroesophageal reflux, and a coagulopathy. Neuroblastoma may be detected serendipitously in a fetus on a prenatal ultrasound. Mass screening using a urine spot test for VMA and HVA also has been used in Japan and Quebec, Canada, to detect patients with

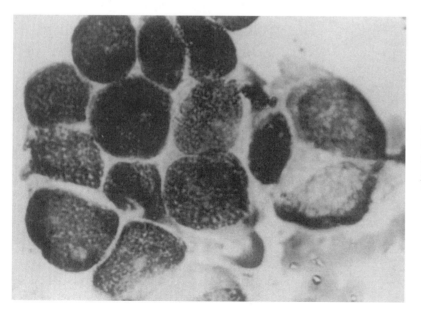

FIGURE 19-2 ■ Rosettes of neuroblasts obtained from the bone marrow from a patient with metastatic neuroblastoma. (From Welch KJ: Pediatric Surgery, 4th ed. St Louis, Mosby-Year Book, 1986.)

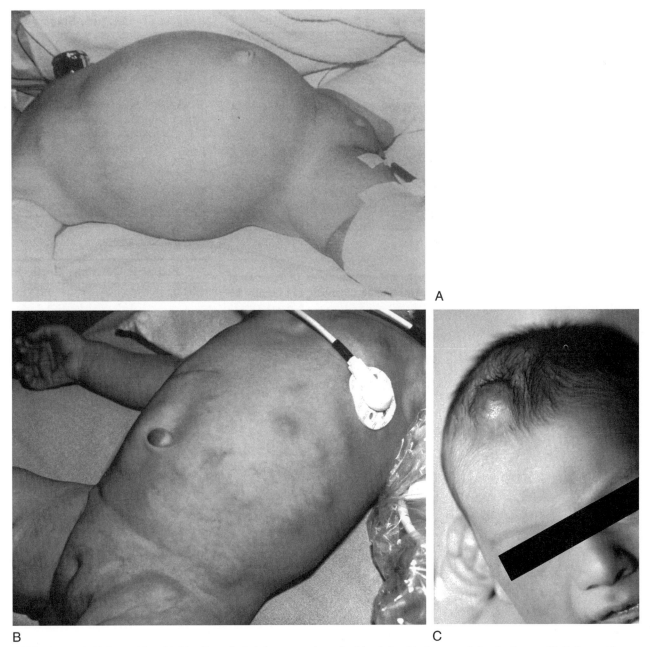

FIGURE 19-4 ■ **A,** Infant with a highly distended abdomen and a palpable right-sided upper abdominal mass. **B,** Infant with stage 4-S neuroblastoma with multiple subcutaneous tumor nodules, sometimes called the *blueberry muffin syndrome*. **C,** When isolated, this tumor metastasis can be mistaken for a hemangioma as seen in another infant with stage 4-S neuroblastoma.

asymptomatic tumors, but this screening has not been associated with improved survival compared with control populations.

The diagnosis of neuroblastoma in most cases is confirmed by obtaining a series of radiographic and chemical studies. Plain radiographs of the involved area (e.g., neck, chest, abdomen) often show stippled calcification within the tumor mass, which is highly suspicious of neuroblastoma (Fig. 19-5). Many cases that present in the first year of life may be nonadrenal. Paraspinal widening commonly is observed in tumors that arise in the lower mediastinum and close to the celiac axis. Ultrasound is often the first imaging modality for cervical or abdominal

masses. Imaging reveals a solid mass of mixed echogenicity, often lobulated. The exception is neonatal adrenal neuroblastoma, which may be cystic. Computed tomography (CT) with intravenous contrast material usually can distinguish Wilms' tumor from neuroblastoma in cases of retroperitoneal tumors because the latter usually depresses the kidney and displaces it downward (adrenal tumor) or laterally (paraspinal tumor) without intrinsic distortion of the renal collecting system (see Fig. 19-5). CT also is useful to determine the presence of liver metastasis. Magnetic resonance imaging is the most useful test to document whether extradural tumor extension has occurred and may show the presence of bone marrow

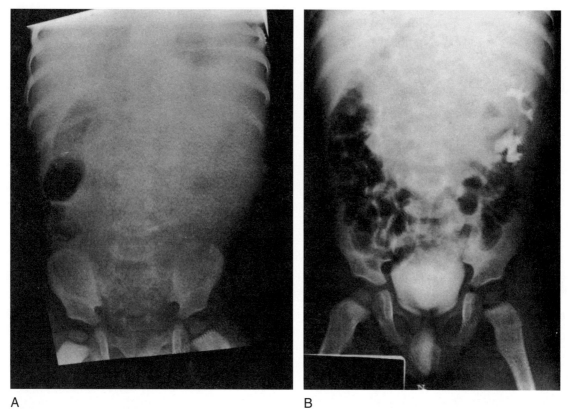

A   B

FIGURE 19-5 ■ **A,** Abdominal radiograph in an infant with a large abdominal mass that contains fine speckled calcification highly suggestive of neuroblastoma. **B,** An intravenous urogram obtained before the patient's referral to Riley Children's Hospital Cancer Center shows lateral displacement of the left kidney by a paraspinal mass. CT is the preferred imaging modality.

involvement and major blood vessel encroachment. Isotopic bone scans (technetium-99m pertechnetate pyrophospate) and long bone radiographs usually document the presence of bone cortex metastases, and the isotope is picked up by the primary tumor. Iodine-123-labeled metaiodobenzylguanidine (MIBG), which is metabolized by adrenal medullary tissue, is useful in identifying the primary tumor and metastases. Bone marrow aspirate (BMA) may show rosettes of metastatic foci of neuroblasts (see Fig. 19-2). Immunocytologic analysis of BMA may be more sensitive than conventional analysis in detecting tumor cells and may provide prognostic information. If BMA is negative, bone marrow biopsy of both iliac crests is required for adequate staging. Studies indicate that serial immunocytologic analysis of peripheral blood samples can identify circulating neuroblasts, documenting tumor dissemination. A urine aliquot is obtained from which VMA-to-creatinine and HVA-to-creatinine ratios are calculated; these are abnormal in 90% of cases. This method was found as reliable as the traditional 24-hour collection. Metanephrine and normetanephrine levels may be obtained when VMA and HVA levels are normal. When levels are elevated, all are useful as tumor markers to follow disease response to treatment or recurrence. Additional preoperative studies include obtaining blood samples for serum alanine aminotransferase, bilirubin, creatinine, lactic dehydrogenase (LDH), neuron-specific enolase (NSE), ferritin,

coagulation profile, complete blood count, and platelet count. An increased LDH is a marker for rapid cellular turnover as seen in more advanced disease, just as are increased NSE (a cytoplasmic protein associated with neural cells) and ferritin, which are produced by the tumor cells.

STAGING AND TREATMENT

Tumor staging is important to guide therapy and determine prognosis. Several staging systems have been used in the past, of which the Evans staging system was the most widely used in North America (Table 19-1). Table 19-2 depicts a variant of the latter, the international staging system, now widely used in clinical trials. This system takes into account preoperative and operative criteria and histologic assessment of lymph nodes. The importance of adequate ipsilateral and contralateral lymph node sampling is stressed for abdominal primaries, although positive nodes may be important only with unfavorable histology. The peculiar 4-S stage occurs almost exclusively in infants younger than 1 year old and represents a special group of patients with an excellent prognosis despite the presence of distant metastases, but only to the liver, skin/subcutaneous tissue, or bone marrow (see Fig. 19-4B). Large abdominal or thoracic tumors that cross the midline, encase the great vessels, and are deemed unresectable at diagnosis are automatically considered stage 3.

TABLE 19-1 ■ Evans Staging System

Stage	Description
I	Tumor confined to organ of origin
II	Tumor extends beyond organ of origin but does not cross the midline; unilateral lymph nodes may be involved
III	Tumor extends beyond midline; bilateral lymph nodes may be involved
IV	Distant metastases (skeletal, other organs, soft tissues, distant lymph nodes)
IV-S	Would be stage I or II; remote disease confined to liver, subcutaneous tissues, and bone marrow, but without evidence of bone cortex involvement

In the absence of metastases and when the tumor appears resectable, surgery is indicated with the goal of complete resection. For abdominal primaries, inspection of the liver with biopsy of any suspicious lesion and extensive sampling of lymph nodes are required, even if they appear normal. This includes para-aortic nodes from the aortic hiatus to the bifurcation and aortocaval and right paracaval nodes; even nodes along the celiac axis and superior and inferior mesenteric arteries may contain tumor. A minimum of six to nine nodes representing these areas is required for adequate staging.

For thoracic or cervical primaries, the same principles apply except that contralateral nodes are not sought, and fewer nodes are necessary for adequate staging. The main tumor is sent immediately sterile to pathology so that fresh tissue may be sampled for DNA flow cytometry, assessment of the *N-myc* oncogene, and electron microscopy before being fixed in formalin. After fixation, the tissue is processed for light microscopy with hematoxylin and eosin staining and immunohistochemistry. Typically, neuroblastomas are composed of small round blue cells that have a tendency to form rosettes. The Shimada pathologic classification system (Table 19-3) has established histologic features that have prognostic value. Neuroblastic tumors are divided into stroma-rich and stroma-poor categories. Stroma-rich tumors contain Schwann-like spindle cell stroma with the appearance of a ganglioneuroblastoma, a favorable pattern that may be diffuse, with immature cells uniformly distributed in a well-differentiated fashion or intermixed throughout the tumor in microscopic clusters. Unfavorable stroma-rich tumors have a nodular appearance. Three variables distinguish stroma-poor tumors into favorable or unfavorable categories (see Table 19-3)—age at diagnosis, neuroblast differentiation, and the mitosis-karyorrhexis index.

In some instances within the same patient, neuroblastoma is noted with varying stages of maturation and differentiation to ganglioneuroblastoma and ganglioneuroma. Sometimes undifferentiated neuroblasts appear as small, round, blue cells that may be difficult to distinguish from other tumor cell populations, including undifferentiated lymphoma, Ewing's tumor, primitive neuroectodermal tumor, and certain cases of embryonal rhabdomyosarcoma. An accurate diagnosis usually can be made by ultrastructural evaluation of the neuroblastoma cell, which shows the presence of neurosecretory granules, neurotubules, and neurofilaments. Immunohistochemistry typically stains positively for neurofilament, synaptophysin, and NSE but not for vimentin and other markers typical of the other tumors with "small blue cells."

For patients with metastatic disease and a large tumor and for patients with a tumor that appears unresectable without compromising significant structures, such as kidney, duodenum, or great vessels, the diagnosis can be made clinically by the appearance of the tumor and elevation of urinary catecholamines. Enough tumor cells still are required, however, to assess important prognostic factors, such as *N-myc* amplification, DNA ploidy, and Shimada histologic classification. This assessment ideally is accomplished by an open biopsy and requires at least 1 g of viable tumor; alternatively, percutaneous biopsies with a core needle or bone marrow biopsies may provide a sufficient amount of cells, especially if the patient is a poor operative risk. Depending on the age of the patient and other prognostic factors (Table 19-4), various chemotherapeutic regimens can be used to shrink the tumor. When the tumor is responding well, plans are made for second-look surgery (or a delayed primary surgery) after 3 months with the goal of achieving a macroscopic complete resection. This second-look surgery should be done even if the patient appears in complete remission because CT scan may miss small foci of residual disease, especially in the abdomen.

TABLE 19-2 ■ International Neuroblastoma Staging System

Stage	Description
1	Localized tumor confined to area of origin, complete excision, with or without microscopic residual disease; ipsilateral and contralateral lymph nodes negative (nodes attached to primary tumor and removed en bloc with it may be positive)
2A	Unilateral tumor with incomplete gross excision; ipsilateral and contralateral lymph nodes negative
2B	Unilateral tumor with complete or incomplete excision; positive ipsilateral nonadherent regional lymph nodes; contralateral lymph nodes negative
3	Tumor infiltrating across the midline with or without lymph node involvement; or unilateral tumor with contralateral lymph node involvement; or midline tumor with bilateral lymph node involvement or bilateral infiltration (unresectable)
4	Dissemination of tumor to distant lymph nodes, bone, bone marrow, liver, or other organs
4-S	Localized primary tumor as defined for stage 1 or 2 with dissemination limited to liver, skin, or bone marrow (limited to infants <1 year old)

TABLE 19-3 ■ Modified Shimada Pathologic Classification of Neuroblastic Tumors

	Favorable Histology	Unfavorable Histology
Stroma-rich	Well differentiated (ganglioneuroma) Ganglioneuroblastoma, intermixed	Ganglioneuroblastoma, nodular
Stroma-poor (i.e., neuroblastoma)		
Age <18 mo	MKI <4%	MKI >4% or undifferentiated
Age 18-60 mo	MKI <2% and differentiating	MKI >2% or undifferentiated/poorly differentiated
Age >5 yr	None	All

MKI, mitosis-karyorrhexis index (number of mitoses and karyorrhexis calculated per 5000 cells).

In more recent years, risk-stratification has helped to guide therapy greatly (see Table 19-4). For low-risk patients without organ-threatening or life-threatening symptoms, surgery is usually curative, and chemotherapy, which is not without risks in these young infants, is used only in patients with recurrence or progression of disease. Intermediate-risk patients are treated with combination chemotherapy. The safest, most effective agents currently seem to be cyclophosphamide, doxorubicin, carboplatin, and etoposide (VP-16); vincristine, cisplatin, and other agents also are active. Granulocyte colony-stimulating factor is used to decrease the length of periods of neutropenia, minimizing the risk of infection.

For high-risk patients, the poor prognosis justifies a much more intense regimen using a combination of multiple chemotherapy agents (cisplatin, etoposide, vincristine, doxorubicin, cyclophosphamide, ifosfamide, and carboplatin), followed by surgery to attempt to achieve a complete remission (i.e., no macroscopic disease). Local radiotherapy may be used at this point or later in the treatment for any additional unresectable tumor. Marking the edges of viable unresectable tumor with titanium clips at the time of surgery is useful for planning postoperative radiotherapy. Nephrectomy may be warranted at this stage if it would allow a complete resection. During induction chemotherapy, some protocols call for peripheral blood stem cell collection. After complete or partial remission is achieved, myeloablative doses of chemotherapy agents are used, followed by peripheral blood stem cell rescue. Some use a second similar course (with different agents), again followed by stem cell rescue. In addition, radiotherapy is given to the site of the primary tumor because of the high rate of local recurrence.

Tumors can present with special features, such as massive hepatomegaly with respiratory distress and neurologic symptoms from cord compression. Infants with stage 4-S neuroblastoma may present with such massive hepatomegaly from tumor infiltration as to cause respiratory compromise from elevation of the diaphragm, renal failure from an abdominal compartment syndrome, or gastroesophageal reflux with malnutrition and aspiration pneumonia. When these complications occur, urgent treatment is required, but these infants tolerate therapy less well than older children. Low-dose chemotherapy with or without low-dose radiation therapy is usually effective in stopping tumor growth. When gas exchange

TABLE 19-4 ■ Neuroblastoma Risk Groups

INSS Stage	Age	N-myc Status*	Shimada Histology	DNA Ploidy†	Risk Group
1	0-21 yr	Any	Any	Any	Low
2A/2B	<365 days	Any	Any	Any	Low
	≥365 days-21 yr	Nonamplified	Any	—	Low
	≥365 days-21 yr	Amplified	Favorable	—	Low
	≥365 days-21 yr	Amplified	Unfavorable	—	High
3	<365 days	Nonamplified	Any	Any	Intermediate
	<365 days	Amplified	Any	Any	High
	≥365 days-21 yr	Nonamplified	Favorable	—	Intermediate
	≥365 days-21 yr	Nonamplified	Unfavorable	—	High
	≥365 days-21 yr	Amplified	Any	—	High
4	<365 days	Nonamplified	Any	Any	Intermediate
	<365 days	Amplified	Any	Any	High
	≥365 days-21 yr	Any	Any	—	High
4S	<365 days	Nonamplified	Favorable	>1	Low
	<365 days	Nonamplified	Any	=1	Intermediate
	<365 days	Nonamplified	Unfavorable	Any	Intermediate
	<365 days	Amplified	Any	Any	High

*N-myc nonamplified = 1 copy; amplified >1 copy.
†DNA Ploidy: DNA index >1 (aneuploid) or = 1 (diploid).
INSS, international staging system.
Reproduced from the Children's Oncology Group protocols; with permission.

remains inadequate despite intubation and mechanical ventilation or oliguria stops responding to fluid administrations and diuretics, it may be necessary to enlarge the abdominal cavity with the use of Silastic or Vicryl mesh. Although there are risks of septic complications, this is the only solution in some cases. Nasojejunal tube feedings or total parenteral nutrition may be required for several days or weeks. The hepatomegaly may stabilize, but it may take months to regress completely. Although there are documented cases of complete spontaneous regression of stage 4-S disease in young infants, most clinicians currently advocate low-dose chemotherapy to prevent some of these complications in patients with unfavorable markers (see Table 19-4).

Some children may present with paraplegia, paresthesia, or gait disturbance from spinal cord compression by tumor. This happens most often with posterior mediastinal tumors, which tend to infiltrate into the foramina along sympathetic nerve trunks. In the past, posterior laminectomy allowed decompression of the spinal cord and debulking of the tumor but was associated with long-term spinal growth disturbance; the same was true for radiation therapy. Although laminotomy may be a worthwhile alternative with fewer sequelae than laminectomy, the current trend is to use chemotherapy for debulking. The fear that this might cause tumor necrosis with edema worsening neurologic sequelae has been dispelled. Surgical resection is reserved for patients who show progressive neurologic deterioration after initiation of chemotherapy. Asymptomatic children with a significant amount of tumor in the spinal canal discovered by CT or magnetic resonance imaging should be approached in the same fashion because of the risks of acute edema or bleeding into the spinal component at the time of excision of the mediastinal tumor.

After the child recovers from this emergency procedure, the primary mass is resected (if possible) by thoracotomy. During this procedure, it is often impossible to avoid leaving small amounts of residual disease along the sympathetic nerve roots as they emerge from the foramina. These areas simply are marked with titanium clips for future imaging. A small amount of residual localized disease with negative nodes results in a stage IIA, which has a good prognosis, especially in the chest.

PROGNOSIS

The two key determinants of survival in instances of neuroblastoma are the age of the patient and stage of disease at diagnosis. Although age older than 1 year is associated with more advanced stages (Fig. 19-6), at equal stage infants still have a survival advantage. An experience with 266 cases of neuroblastoma treated at the James Whitcomb Riley Hospital for Children, Indianapolis, Indiana, documented that survival in infants younger than 1 year of age is 76%, whereas it is 32% for children older than 1 year. Survival in stage I cases was 100% (14 of 14); in stage II, 81% (42 of 52), in stage III, 38% (24 of 62), in stage IV, 12%; and in stage IV-S, 81% (17 of 21). Children with primary tumors affecting the neck or pelvis had 100% survival, whereas patients with mediastinal tumors had 81% survival (35 of 43). The worst prognosis was observed in infants and children with primary tumors of the retroperitoneum (adrenal and paraspinal). A relatively improved outlook can be expected for patients who are younger than 1 year of age; with stage I, II, or IV-S disease; and with normal levels of serum NSE and ferritin. High levels of LDH, NSE, and ferritin are thought to represent large tumors with a high cellular turnover and are associated with a poorer prognosis. These markers have lost some significance in more recent years since the *N-myc* oncogene has emerged as one of the most important prognostic factors, independent of age and tumor location. Infants who unexpectedly did poorly almost universally were found to have *N-myc* amplification. This finding is reflected in the risk stratification used by the Children's Oncology Group (COG) (see Table 19-4), in which the previously mentioned serum markers have not been retained as independent prognostic variables. NSE is not required as part of preoperative testing in current COG studies. Favorable Shimada tumor histology; a nondiploid tumor (or aneuploid or hyperdiploid/hypodiploid) on DNA-flow cytometry; good nutrition; and primary tumors located in the neck, pelvis, and mediastinum have an improved survival. Children with VIP secretion–related hypokalemic watery diarrhea syndrome and children with opsomyoclonus have a greater than 90% survival and often have more mature tumors (i.e., ganglioneuroblastomas). The latter cases

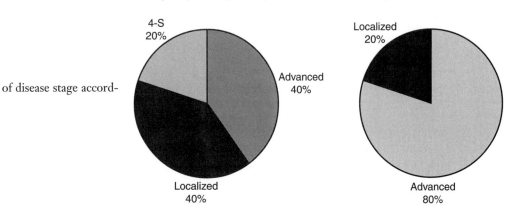

FIGURE 19-6 ■ Distribution of disease stage according to age.

usually involve low-stage (I, II) tumors with favorable markers. Despite excellent survival, patients with opsomyoclonus often have continued neurologic disturbance and learning disabilities even after tumor resection. The observation that patients who had received adjuvant chemotherapy because of their initial disease stage made a better neurologic recovery than patients who had surgery alone has led to new studies examining the usefulness of chemotherapy in this peculiar subset of patients. The use of intravenous immunoglobulins also is being explored because of the possibility that opsomyoclonus is an antibody-mediated phenomenon.

In contrast, a poor outlook can be expected for patients with stage III or IV (advanced) neuroblastoma, amplified *N-myc*, unfavorable histology, age greater than 1 year, or tumor in the abdomen. Intermediate-risk patients have an estimated 3-year survival greater than 80% with moderately intensive chemotherapy, whereas 3-year survival is less than 30% in the high-risk group despite intensive therapy; this contrasts with a greater than 90% survival for low-risk patients, most of whom are cured with surgery alone. Retroperitoneal primary tumors, an elevated HVA-to-VMA ratio, elevated serum LDH and ferritin levels, diploid DNA-flow cytometry, and malnutrition at diagnosis may be other markers of a poor prognosis.

Mass screening programs initiated in Japan evaluating urinary levels of VMA and HVA in 6-month-old infants have uncovered many cases of neuroblastoma. There is a 15% false-negative rate if VMA is screened only, and this rate is reduced to 8% if VMA and HVA are screened. The survival in these cases has been exceptionally high compared with survival of patients with neuroblastoma who present with clinical disease and are diagnosed by conventional measures. The Japanese screening effort has doubled the incidence of neuroblastoma in young infants noted before the onset of screening but has not decreased the number of cases observed in older children. These observations strongly suggest that the increased number of neuroblastic tumors detected by screening programs probably represents instances of neuroblastoma that otherwise would regress and not present clinically. Most of these tumors have favorable markers. Reports have surfaced, however, indicating the later occurrence of malignant neuroblastoma in a few infants who previously had been screened negative. A careful analysis of false-negative cases indicated that they were of a diploid nature or had *N-myc* amplification. Mass screening at 6 months of age may be too early to detect cases with a diploid mode or *N-myc* amplification, and screening should be repeated at 12 to 18 months of age.

Another mass screening program was carried out in Quebec, Canada, from 1989 to 1994. In Quebec, there was already in place an extensive infrastructure for collecting the urine of infants on filter papers for screening for inborn errors of metabolism, such as tyrosinemia and Tay-Sachs disease. Screening took place at 3 weeks and 6 months of age; the results were similar to those in Japan. Screening doubled the incidence of localized disease but did not decrease the number of patients with advanced-stage disease or the overall mortality from neuroblastoma. None of the patients detected by screening had *N-myc* amplification, whereas most patients who were negative at the time of screening and later developed neuroblastoma had at least one unfavorable factor (*N-myc*, DNA index, or histology). The cost of the screening combined with the cost and unnecessary morbidity of treatment of patients whose tumor otherwise would have regressed led to the conclusion that mass screening was not effective, and it was abandoned. A study from Germany where screening was done at 1 year of age gave the same results. The authors estimated that two thirds of all cases detected by screening would have regressed spontaneously. The potential risks were highlighted by the fact that all 3 children who died in the group of 143 detected by screening had localized disease and died from complications of treatment. Acknowledging that many neuroblastomas detected by early screening may regress spontaneously, several Japanese centers have developed criteria for simple observation of these patients. These criteria consist of small tumors that correspond to stage I, II, or IV-S by imaging and bone marrow biopsy. Tumor size and urine catecholamines are monitored closely. Because neuroblastomas also may be detected incidentally by prenatal or postnatal ultrasonography, the COG has initiated a similar prospective study of observation only. This study uses much stricter criteria in terms of tumor size (≤ 16 cm^3 if solid or ≤ 65 cm^3 if cystic), taking into account the fact that neonates with cystic neuroblastomas may have a larger tumor yet have an excellent prognosis.

The advent of new and more effective cell cycle, kinetic-oriented chemotherapy programs that recruit the neuroblastoma tumor cell from the resting phase (where it is relatively resistant to tumor kill) to a proliferative phase, where it is accessible to chemotherapy and irradiation, also may be useful. Targeting therapy with monoclonal antibodies labeled with isotopic chemotherapy agents, hyperthermia, and intraoperative radiotherapy have been used as treatment adjuncts in advanced cases but so far have been clinically ineffective. Iodine-123-labeled MIBG is picked up by the neuroblastoma cell and can be used as a method of detecting sites of metastatic tumor foci; it also has been used to target therapy but by itself is not curative. Adoptive immunotherapy using interleukin-2 with lymphokine-activated killer T cells and tumor infiltrating lymphocytes has produced a tumor response in patients with malignant melanoma (another neural crest tumor) and has been effective in reducing tumor burden in C-1300 murine neuroblastoma in the experimental setting. Other paths being explored are the use of *cis*-retinoic acid, a vitamin A derivative, which has a differentiating effect on neuroblastoma cell lines; antiangiogenic therapy; and pro-apoptotic agents.

Many more genetic and biologic factors may have prognostic value in neuroblastoma, including allelic deletion at chromosome 11 q 23, which may be the site of a neuroblastoma suppressor gene; 14 q LOH and 17 q gain; telomerase activity; survivin expression; nerve growth factor; and neurotrophin receptors of the Trk family (*Trk-A*, *Trk-B*, and *Trk-C*). Multidrug resistance protein expression and other factors also are being studied. A better understanding of the development and biologic behavior of the neural crest cell; an improved understanding of the immune aspects of neuroblastoma; a reassessment and clarification of the role of screening programs; refinements in combined therapy; and a more careful selection of patients for aggressive treatment based on age, stage, tumor histology, tumor markers, DNA flow cytometry, *N-myc* oncogene analysis, and other factors undoubtedly would prove useful in reducing the mortality and morbidity of this lethal pediatric malignancy. Although therapy is being intensified in high-risk groups, it is being lessened or modified in low-risk and intermediate-risk groups to avoid long-term complications of chemotherapy, such as cardiotoxicity (doxorubicin), nephrotoxicity and ototoxicity (cisplatin), and sterility and second malignancies such as leukemia (etoposide, topotecan, alkylating agents), and complications of radiation therapy, such as impaired or asymmetric growth and secondary solid tumors (especially sarcomas).

SUGGESTED READINGS

Brodeur GM, Maris JM: Neuroblastoma. In Pizzo PA, Poplack DG (eds): Principles and Practice of Pediatric Oncology, 4th ed. Philadelphia, Lippincott Williams & Wilkins, 2002, p 895.

This chapter in an oncology textbook provides an up-to-date review of the genetics aspects, the cellular and molecular pathogenesis of neuroblastoma, staging, and treatment (includes 572 references).

Grosfeld JL: Neuroblastoma. In O'Neill JA, Rowe MI, Grosfeld JL, et al (eds): Pediatric Surgery, 5th ed. St Louis, Mosby–Year Book, 1998.

This chapter in a major pediatric surgery textbook covers the subject in great depth.

Grosfeld JL, Rescorla FJ, West KW, et al: Neuroblastoma in the first year of life: Clinical and biologic factors influencing outcome. Semin Pediatr Surg 2:37, 1993.

This article describes the development of neural crest cells, development of neuroblasts, and regression in relation to the occurrence of neuroblastoma in the first year of life. The article describes the clinical and biologic factors that influence the relatively high survival rate of these patients compared with older children.

Haase GM, Perez C, Atkinson JB: Current aspects of biology, risk assessment, and treatment of neuroblastoma. Semin Surg Oncol 16:91, 1999.

This is an excellent review (includes 166 references).

Iwanaka T, Yamamoto K, Ogawa Y, et al: Maturation of mass-screened localized adrenal neuroblastoma. J Pediatr Surg 36:1633, 2001.

This article provides insight on the natural history of neuroblastoma detected by mass screening.

Katzenstein HM, Kent P, London WB, et al: Treatment and outcome of 83 children with intraspinal neuroblastoma: The Pediatric Oncology Group experience. J Clin Oncol 19:1047, 2002.

This report examines the various approaches available for the treatment of thoracic tumors extending into the spinal canal. It indicates that intensive chemotherapy is an effective initial approach.

Knudson AG Jr, Meadows AT: Regression of neuroblastoma IV-S: A genetic hypothesis. N Engl J Med 302:1254, 1980.

This classic report explores the cause of spontaneous regression of neuroblastoma.

Nakagawara A, Arima-Nakagawara M, Scavarda NJ, et al: Association between high levels of expression of the trk gene and favorable outcome in human neuroblastoma. N Engl J Med 328:847, 1993.

This important article documents the association of high levels of the proto-oncogene trk with improved outcome in neuroblastoma.

Shimada H, Ambros IM, Dehner LP, et al: The International Neuroblastoma Pathology Classification (the Shimada system). Cancer 86:364, 1999.

This article describes the most recent modifications to the Shimada classification.

Shimada H, Chatten J, Newton WH Jr, et al: Histopathologic prognostic factors in neuroblastoma: Definition of subtypes of ganglioneuroblastoma and an age-linked classification of neuroblastoma. J Natl Cancer Inst 73:405, 1984.

This article describes the original Shimada histologic classification of neuroblastoma, which categorizes stroma-rich and stroma-poor tumors and how they influence prognosis.

Woods WG, Gaa RN, Gao R-N, et al: Screening of infants and mortality due to neuroblastoma. N Engl J Med 346:1041, 2002.

This article describes in detail the Quebec, Canada, experience with mass screening for neuroblastoma and reviews the worldwide experience with this strategy indicating that mass screening does not improve survival.

Renal Tumors

20

WILMS' TUMOR

Background and Incidence

Since its original description by Wilms in 1899, Wilms' tumor (nephroblastoma) has been the focus of considerable interest among pediatric physicians. Wilms' tumor is an embryonal tumor of renal origin. Approximately 500 new cases of this pediatric malignancy are seen in the United States annually, representing slightly more than 10% of all cases of childhood cancer. The estimated incidence in Europe is one to two cases per 1 million. Most cases are diagnosed between the ages of 1 and 4 years. Wilms' tumor can occur in older children, however, and occasionally can be detected in adolescents or young adults. Although most Wilms' tumors occur as sporadic events, the isolation of genes associated with the development of Wilms' tumor has been reported. The first gene (*WT1*) was isolated when an association between a constellation of developmental abnormalities (aniridia, genitourinary malformations, and mental retardation [WAGR syndrome]) and an increased risk for the development of Wilms' tumor was made (Table 20-1). Subsequent investigation showed that there was a deletion of the short arm of chromosome 11 at band p13. This deletion was found to contain the gene responsible for aniridia and the *WT1* locus. *WT1* (also called *Wilms' tumor suppressor gene*) has been found to encode a DNA binding protein that is expressed primarily in the fetal kidney and in tissues that give rise to the genitourinary system. This protein is essential for normal renal and gonadal development. Inactivation of the gene may be responsible for the occurrence of Wilms' tumor. In addition to the deletion of *WT1* and its association with

Wilms' tumor in the WAGR syndrome, a dominant mutation of this gene has been identified in children with the Denys-Drash syndrome. This syndrome comprises intersex anomalies, mesangial sclerosis with progressive renal failure, and Wilms' tumor. The altered protein product in this syndrome is dysfunctional and produces phenotypic abnormalities more severe than the absence of the protein in WAGR syndrome.

Subsequently a second site for a gene associated with Wilms' tumor (*WT2*) was identified again on chromosome 11 at band 15. This site was identified in association with Beckwith-Wiedemann syndrome (an overgrowth syndrome including visceromegaly, macroglossia, and hyperinsulinemic hypoglycemia), a second syndrome associated with Wilms' tumor (see Table 20-1). Duplication of the genetic material at this site that was received from the father has been linked to the genetic syndrome, and the putative association has been made with the insulin-like growth factor-2 gene (*IGF2*), but this has not been confirmed definitively.

Clinical Presentation

The mean age at presentation for Wilms' tumor is 3 years. Wilms' tumor is relatively uncommon in the first 3 months of life; however, one third of all cases are seen between 6 and 12 months of age. Although this embryonal renal neoplasm is observed infrequently after 8 years of age, older children, adolescents, and occasionally young adults can be affected. Wilms' tumor usually presents with a large, round, smooth, and firm abdominal mass that often is detected by a parent while bathing the infant or child or on a routine well-baby examination in the pediatrician's office. The mass is usually nontender. The tumor can grow rapidly, which may result from hemorrhage into the tumor, cystic degeneration, or actual exponential tumor growth. Gross hematuria may be noted in 10% to 15% of cases, often after relatively minor trauma related to injury of an enlarged kidney involved by tumor. Evaluation leads to the unsuspected finding of a Wilms' tumor. Occasionally, bilateral flank masses are palpable in instances of bilateral Wilms' tumor. Microscopic hematuria may be noted in almost 20% of cases. Anorexia, fever, and weight loss may be observed in 10% to 15% of cases. Elevated blood pressure may be present in 20%

TABLE 20-1 ■ Wilms' Tumor: Associated Findings

Beckwith-Wiedemann syndrome
Sporadic aniridia
Hemihypertrophy
Positive family history
Genitourinary anomalies
11p13 deletion

---

of cases and is related to a renin-angiotensin–induced hypertension caused by compression of the juxtaglomerular apparatus by the tumor. The serum renin levels may be elevated in these patients. The tumor also rarely may be a site of erythropoeitin production resulting in polycythemia. The urine of patients with Wilms' tumor may contain elevated levels of hyaluronidase. Laboratory tests are usually otherwise unremarkable except in rare instances in which a screening bleeding and clotting evaluation may show pseudo–von Willebrand's disease.

Diagnostic Evaluation

Evaluation of the site and extent of tumor involvement can be accomplished expeditiously with a few carefully chosen tests. A plain abdominal radiograph often shows a mass effect with displacement of viscera and occasionally the presence of calcification (<10%). The calcification usually is located in the periphery of the tumor and has more of an eggshell appearance rather than the speckled microcalcifications seen in infants with an adrenal neuroblastoma. Abdominal ultrasound usually documents that the kidney is the site of the primary tumor; discerns whether the mass is a cystic or solid lesion (Wilms' tumor appears primarily as a solid mass); and indicates if intravascular extension of the tumor has occurred into the renal vein, inferior vena cava, or occasionally right atrium. Modern ultrasonography obviates the need for an inferior venacavogram. The next diagnostic test obtained is a computed tomography (CT) scan of the abdomen with intravenous contrast administration (Fig. 20-1). CT scan shows the extent of the tumor within the kidney, often with a rim of normal renal parenchyma around the margin and intrinsic distortion of the collecting system with medial displacement of the kidney. In contrast, a neuroblastoma rarely distorts the collecting system and generally indents or compresses the renal parenchyma rather than being surrounded by it. Neuroblastoma displaces the kidney downward (adrenal tumors) or laterally

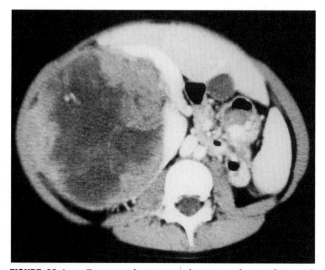

FIGURE 20-1 ■ Computed tomography scan of an infant with a large renal mass. The normal renal parenchyma is shown surrounding the Wilms' tumor arising within the kidney.

(paraspinal tumors). CT scan also defines the origin of the tumor within the kidney; identifies the presence of enlarged and suspicious pararenal, paracaval, and para-aortic lymph nodes; evaluates the possible presence of a second Wilms' tumor in the opposite kidney; assesses caval extension; and determines if the patient has hematogenous hepatic metastases. A chest radiograph is obtained to evaluate for the presence of pulmonary metastases, and a thoracic CT scan is performed for a more precise evaluation of pulmonary metastases. These studies detect the most common sites of tumor spread: local and regional lymph nodes, lung, and liver. A CT scan cannot determine the resectability of a tumor, however, because this can be assessed accurately only by surgical exploration. A metastatic bone survey is obtained only in patients with the clear cell variant of Wilms' tumor that has a propensity for osseous metastasis, which is an otherwise rare occurrence in patients with other histologic variants of Wilms' tumor. Similarly, cerebral metastases should be considered in children with the rhabdoid variant. Arteriograms are rarely helpful in the preoperative evaluation of Wilms' tumor, and for most patients this test is rarely necessary. Magnetic resonance imaging may be of help in patients with suspected caval or atrial thrombus or in patients with bilateral Wilms' tumor or diffuse nephroblastomatosis when ultrasound is unclear.

The role of screening ultrasonography to evaluate infants and children with predisposition for Wilms' tumor (Beckwith-Wiedemann syndrome, hemihypertrophy, aniridia, WAGR syndrome, Denys-Drash syndrome, and prior Wilms' tumor) in the presence of multiple nephrogenic rests has not been resolved. In the 1980s and 1990s, studies showed a shift toward identification of lower stage tumors in these cohorts, suggesting that screening is successful in identifying these children at earlier stages of disease. What has not been proved is that this identification increases overall survival rates. It does increase the proportion of children in whom renal-sparing procedures can be performed, however. Current recommendations are for ultrasound every 3 months until 6 to 8 years of age. For children with Beckwith-Wiedemann syndrome and hemihypertrophy, the adrenals and liver should be evaluated in addition to the kidney because this group is also at risk for other embryonal tumors.

Pathologic Variants

One of the most valuable lessons from the National Wilms' Tumor Study Group (NWTSG) is the significance of histology on tumor behavior. Beckwith and colleagues through a series of publications identified subgroups of renal tumors with distinct biologic behavior, including aggressiveness of the tumor, patterns of metastasis and recurrence, and response to therapy. Although in the initial NWTSG study all tumors were treated in a similar manner, now therapy is based on the histology and the stage of the tumor. The histology of Wilms' tumors is divided into favorable histology (FH) and unfavorable histology (UH). FH lesions represent 89% of the cases, whereas UH occurs in 11% of cases. FH tumors contain more differentiated epithelial cells characterized by blastemal, epithelial, mixed, cystic, and even

TABLE 20-2 ■ Wilms' Tumor: Unfavorable Histology (11%)		
Histology (%)	**Relapse (%)**	**Mortality (%)**
Anaplastic (4.4)	55	45
Clear cell (4.0)	23	77
Rhabdoid (2.3)	90	86

glomerular elements. These tumors respond to standard therapy and have a favorable prognosis. A cystic variant of Wilms' tumor has an extremely favorable prognosis.

UH tumors are subgrouped further into anaplastic (4.4%), clear cell (4%), and rhabdoid (2.3%) histology (Table 20-2). Anaplastic tumors are characterized by nuclear pleomorphism and hyperchromatic cells with enlarged atypical nuclei with an increased number of bizarre mitotic figures and extreme hyperdiploidy. Beckwith described a difference in behavior between anaplastic tumors with focal anaplasia (<10% of the microscopic fields viewed involved with anaplasia) or diffuse anaplasia (>10% of the microscopic fields studied involved with anaplasia). Anaplastic tumors are rare in children younger than age 2 years.

The final two subgroups of UH tumors have an appearance more characteristic of sarcomas than of FH Wilms' tumors. Clear cell tumors (clear cell sarcoma of the kidney [CCSK]) are composed of nests of polygonal-to-stellate cells with pale cytoplasm, small nuclei, and inconspicuous nucleoli. There is a strong male predilection for this tumor, which metastasizes to multiple bones, particularly the skull, and appears to disseminate early. The rhabdoid tumor has sheets of monomorphous cells with an acidophilic cytoplasm that contains intermediate filaments but no cross-striations. It is seen commonly in children younger than age 2 years and may occur bilaterally. This tumor may occur at extrarenal sites and sometimes is associated with a separate primary midline brain tumor of the same histology. This tumor has the worst prognosis of all of the histologic subtypes.

Staging

The treatment of patients in North America with Wilms' tumor on the NWTSG protocols is based on surgical stage and radiographic evaluation for metastatic disease. The surgical stage is determined by capsular penetration of the renal capsule, lymph node involvement, positive microscopic margins for residual tumor, preoperative or operative rupture of the tumor, and bilateral renal tumors (Table 20-3 and Fig. 20-2). In the NWTSG studies, central review of the pathology has been performed by the pathology center. The histologic classification in Wilms' tumor is more crucial in defining the prognosis and therapy of the tumor than is the stage of the disease.

Operative Technique

Operative management of Wilms' tumor includes a carefully planned, well-monitored radical resection of the affected kidney under general endotracheal anesthesia. The procedure is performed through a long transverse transabdominal incision two fingerbreadths above the umbilicus or a thoracoabdominal incision. The incision extends from the midaxillary line on the ipsilateral side to the anterior axillary line on the contralateral side. The incision must be large enough to examine both kidneys to evaluate for bilateral involvement and to remove the lesion without tumor rupture. A flank incision is not adequate to achieve these goals. It is important to avoid tumor spill because this carries an increased risk of intra-abdominal tumor recurrence. If the tumor is large and involves the upper pole of the kidney and significantly elevates the diaphragm, a thoracoabdominal incision may be helpful.

The opposite kidney and liver are evaluated first for possible tumor involvement. In children with Wilms' tumor on the right side, the hepatic flexure, right colon attachments, and mesentery are separated carefully from the surface of the tumor and retracted medially. The tumor is freed carefully from the duodenum and liver; this usually allows exposure of the infrahepatic vena cava.

TABLE 20-3 ■ Wilms' Tumor Staging	
Stage	**Description**
I	Encapsulated unilateral tumor without capsular or nodal involvement that is completely resected without tumor spill
II	Unilateral tumor with involvement of renal capsule or hilar fat, adherence to local surrounding structures including the renal vein, without lymph node involvement that is completely resected without tumor spill
III	Unilateral tumor with regional lymph node involvement, preoperative tumor rupture, significant intraoperative tumor spill, incomplete resection, or tumor biopsy only
IV	Hematogenous metastases to lung, bone, brain, and liver and distant lymph node involvement
V	Bilateral renal tumors

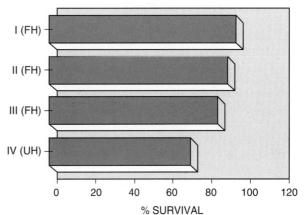

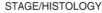
STAGE/HISTOLOGY

FIGURE 20-2 ■ Incidence of various stages and histology in 1439 patients enrolled in the third NWTSG study. Stage V cases are omitted from the graph and account for 6% of cases.

When feasible, the hilum of the right kidney is approached initially. The renal artery and vein are identified; the vein is palpated carefully for intravascular extension of tumor thrombus; and if free of tumor, the vessels are individually doubly ligated and divided. The proximal renal vein and artery also are suture ligated. Early ligation limits blood loss during the resection and theoretically reduces the risk of hematogenous and lymphatic metastases during the procedure. Early ligation may not always be possible, and mobilization of the tumor may be necessary in some instances to identify the vascular pedicle without injury to other structures. Although there is a theoretical risk of encouraging lymphatic metastases if the renal vein is tied before the artery, because of the excellent response of Wilms' tumor to chemotherapy, there is no evidence that this causes a problem in cases of this tumor. When the blood supply has been controlled, the tumor is dissected free from the aorta, taking with the tumor Gerota's fascia and the perirenal fat to minimize the risk of tumor rupture. The lymph node–bearing tissues in the renal hilum and ipsilateral para-aortic region are excised for staging purposes. Obtaining adequate lymph node biopsy specimens is crucial, because failure to do so has resulted in increased local recurrence rates, presumably from understaging the tumor and undertreatment with adjuvant therapy.

Occasionally an additional tumor vessel is seen entering the vena cava directly from the tumor. The ureter should be dissected down to a level near the bladder because Wilms' tumor also can have tumor extension within the lumen of the ureter. The renal fossa is freed, and any attachments to the diaphragm may require excision of a portion of this muscular structure en bloc with the tumor. It is better to resect a segment of the diaphragm to which the tumor is densely adherent than to rupture the tumor. The right adrenal gland can be spared if the tumor is small or is located in the inferior pole; however, this organ must be excised if the primary lesion involves the superior pole of the kidney. The main right adrenal vein enters directly into the vena cava, while the superior adrenal vein courses through the diaphragm. On the right side, direct extension of tumor into the liver also requires en bloc resection of the affected hepatic tissue (1.5% to 7%). Involvement that requires an extensive hepatic resection probably is managed best with preoperative chemotherapy after an incisional biopsy with delayed resection when the tumor and extent of involvement will be more limited. Combined resections have been associated with an increased incidence of surgical complications and morbidity. In most patients, the tumor responds to chemotherapy and has significant reduction in size and a decrease in vascularity and friability. A second-look resection of the tumor is almost always successful.

In children with Wilms' tumor arising on the left side, the splenic flexure of the colon is mobilized, and the descending colon and mesentery are separated from the tumor. The spleen and pancreas are elevated and retracted anteriorly and superiorly, exposing the entire upper retroperitoneal space and diaphragm. Medial dissection allows exposure of the aorta, and the left renal vein can be seen crossing over the aorta to enter the kidney. The renal vein is palpated and evaluated for intravascular tumor extension. The renal artery and vein are carefully doubly ligated and divided as described for the right side. The tumor is freed by dissecting the mass away from the aorta. The superior mesenteric artery is identified and preserved. In large left-sided tumors, the superior mesenteric artery is draped over the medial aspect of the tumor and kidney. In this situation, particular attention must be paid to avoid injury or inappropriate ligation of this vessel mistaking it for the left renal artery. If the tumor is centrally or superiorly located, the left adrenal gland should be excised en bloc with the tumor. The renal fossa is entered and the tumor dissected from its bed from above downward along with Gerota's fascia and the perirenal fat. The left ureter is divided near the bladder, and the dissection is completed by removing the left para-aortic lymph node–bearing tissues with the specimen to evaluate for tumor involvement.

In most patients with intravascular tumor extension into the renal vein, the vein can be opened, and the tumor thrombus can be extracted. It is important to obtain control of the vena cava above and below the renal vein before making the venotomy. If tumor extends into the vena cava, the level of involvement (subhepatic, intrahepatic, or suprahepatic or in the atrium) usually is identified preoperatively by ultrasonography. In most cases, the tumor can be extracted with the aid of a Fogarty catheter for infrahepatic extension of the thrombus. If there is extension of the tumor to the level of the intrahepatic vena cava, control of the vena cava at the level of the diaphragm is necessary. For patients with suprahepatic or atrial involvement, tumor extraction is accomplished best by a thoracoabdominal approach with cardiopulmonary bypass. Studies suggest these latter patients may be managed best by preliminary biopsy and treatment with chemotherapy before resection. Chemotherapy often diminishes the size of the tumor thrombus and decreases the need for bypass. In many cases, the tumor thrombus retracts out of its atrial or caval extension.

The management of bilateral Wilms' tumor must be individualized according to the extent of tumor present in both kidneys with a goal to preserve adequate disease-free functional renal parenchyma to avoid renal failure. The initial procedure should be bilateral biopsy to establish the histology in both kidneys. Approximately 4% of cases have discordant histology between the two sides, frequently involving anaplasia, so that bilateral biopsies are crucial. The patient is treated with chemotherapy based on the histology and stage and restudied by abdominal CT with contrast to evaluate tumor response and determine whether a second-look surgical procedure would be beneficial. If considerable bilateral tumor persists, additional chemotherapy is administered, and further surgical exploration is delayed. This failure of the tumor mass to resolve is often due to the presence of mature rhabdomyomatous tissue that does not respond to therapy. A third-look procedure may be necessary to try to resect remaining tumor and preserve renal tissue. Radiation therapy is withheld if possible in these cases to reduce the risk of radiation injury to the remaining renal parenchyma. In some instances, bench surgery may permit tumor resection; however, this requires vascular reimplantation of the remaining kidney in the pelvis in a manner similar to a renal transplant. In some patients, the tumor persists in both kidneys, and resection of the tumor with preservation of functioning renal tissue is not possible. The only remaining option for these rare patients ultimately is bilateral nephrectomy. Their subsequent care includes peritoneal dialysis or hemodialysis and chemotherapy for approximately 1 year before attempting a renal transplant, but this is rarely indicated.

Treatment and Prognosis

After surgical excision, treatment depends on tumor stage and histology. In patients with FH, "local" stage determines whether the patient receives pulse courses of two-drug (vincristine and actinomycin D) or three-drug (vincristine, actinomycin D, and doxorubicin [Adriamycin]) chemotherapy. It also determines whether the patient receives local irradiation to the tumor bed. Patients with hematogenous metastases (stage IV) receive three-drug therapy and radiotherapy to the lungs if they are involved but do not receive flank irradiation unless they have a stage III primary tumor. Response of FH tumors to this therapy has been good, with results from the most recently closed fourth NWTSG study (NWTS-4) reporting 2-year, relapse-free survival rates for the pulse intensive arm as follows: stage I/FH, 94.9%; stage I/anaplastic, 87.5%; stage II/FH 85.9%; stage III/FH 91.1%; stage IV/FH 80.6%; and stages I through IV/CCSK, 84.1% (Fig. 20-3).

Therapy for UH tumors has been intensified because of the poor response to standard therapies. On current protocols, children with anaplastic tumors receive treatment with cyclophosphamide and etoposide alternating with cyclophosphamide, vincristine, and doxorubicin. If an anaplastic tumor is completely resected and considered stage I, the outcome is similar to stage I infants with FH after treatment with two drugs. In more advanced stages, however, anaplastic tumors have a dismal outcome. Results from NWTS-3 and NWTS-4 showed that children with diffuse anaplasia had 4-year survival by stage as follows: stage II, 55%; stage III, 45%; and stage IV, 47%. CCSK has shown an improved response to intensification of therapy. The interval to relapse in CCSK is extended so that long-term follow-up is required. Results from NWTSG studies that added doxorubicin to treatment showed added benefit with a 6-year, relapse-free survival of 63.5% compared with 25% for patients treated without doxorubicin added to actinomycin D, vincristine, and irradiation. Results from NWTS-4 have not been published. Therapy of these patients includes cyclophosphamide and etoposide alternating with cyclophosphamide, vincristine, and doxorubicin. Survival at 2 years is 91% but declines to 77% at 4 years. Infants and children with rhabdoid tumors have aggressive disease, with widespread metastases, and frequently die early (within 1 to 2 years—90% relapse rate and 86% mortality) despite multidrug treatment, including cyclophosphamide and etoposide alternating with carboplatin and etoposide. Relapse in Wilms' tumor is associated with significant mortality. In FH cases, retrieval therapy achieves overall survival approximating 50%, and in UH cases, retrieval is much less frequent. The current overall survival for all patients with Wilms' tumor is 80%. If only patients with FH are considered, the survival rate is 90%.

An alternative treatment program in patients with stage III and IV tumors using preoperative chemotherapy is used routinely in Europe according to protocols developed by the International Society of Pediatric Oncology. The concept is to shrink the tumor, making the resection easier and safer to perform and to reduce significantly the

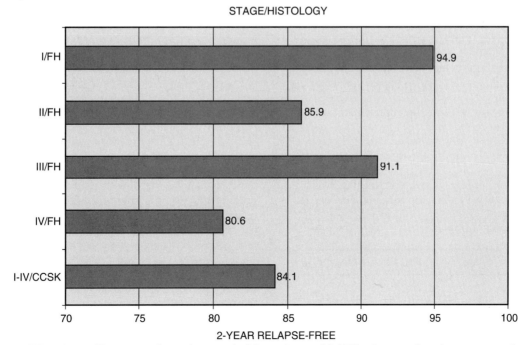

FIGURE 20-3 ■ Two-year relapse-free survival in patients with Wilms' tumor based on stage and histology (NWTS-4).

rate of operative rupture and tumor spill. Extensive tumor necrosis, low mitotic activity, and high degrees of differentiation of residual tumor limited to the kidney are FH findings for infants and children treated with preoperative chemotherapy. A major problem in evaluating the true efficacy of preoperative chemotherapy is an increased ambiguity of tumor stage. Also, there may be more tumor bed recurrence with this approach than with primary resection followed by chemotherapy.

The role of radiation therapy in patients with Wilms' tumor has changed. Because of a high incidence of late effects related to its use (i.e., cardiomyopathy, pulmonary fibrosis, and second malignant neoplasms), radiation therapy currently is employed more selectively. Stage III patients with gross or microscopic residual tumor, intraabdominal tumor spill, tumor spread to regional lymph nodes, and peritoneal involvement receive unilateral flank irradiation that crosses the midline at a dose of 1080 cGy. For patients with diffuse intraperitoneal involvement, preoperative intraperitoneal rupture, or diffuse spill, the area comprising the total abdomen and pelvis is irradiated to 1050 cGy. Stage IV cases with pulmonary involvement receive 1200 cGy to the lungs. Treatment with three-agent chemotherapy and whole-lung irradiation is as effective alone as when surgical excision of multiple metastases also is performed. The incidence of pulmonary relapse is low (7%), but 13% develop radiation pneumonitis as a complication of therapy. Only if lesions persist after therapy should consideration be given for resection. In children with anaplastic, clear cell, and rhabdoid tumors, local flank irradiation has been used in all stages (except stage I anaplastic tumors) because of their more aggressive behavior and increased local recurrence.

Another special circumstance is management of intravascular extension of tumor thrombus, which occurs in 4% of cases. Appropriate excision of the primary tumor and tumor thrombus when feasible is advised. The level of tumor thrombus is an important preoperative consideration (infrahepatic cava [61%], intrahepatic cava [14%], suprahepatic inferior vena cava [21%] or right atrium [4%]) (Table 20-4). In the last-mentioned cases, cardiopulmonary bypass should be an available surgical adjunct. Although cardiovascular bypass has been used successfully by many investigators in the field to remove tumor thrombus safely from the right atrium and pulmonary artery, more recent studies as mentioned earlier have suggested that preoperative chemotherapy can achieve regression of the tumor thrombus and simplify the tumor resection and decrease the complications and the morbidity of surgery. This approach has been recommended by the NWTSG for patients with extensive caval involvement or atrial extension. The level of thrombus involvement does not affect survival. The overall survival for infants and children with intravascular tumor extension was 88%, 89%, and 62% for stages II, III, and IV. The key indicators for survival in these cases are stage and tumor histology.

The management of bilateral Wilms' tumor must be based on two goals: first, to obtain complete resection of the tumor and, second, to preserve renal parenchyma to avoid renal failure. As mentioned earlier, current therapeutic recommendations include initial bilateral biopsy, preliminary chemotherapy, avoidance of irradiation, and delayed resection of the tumors to achieve maximal resolution of their size allowing preservation of renal tissue. In many cases, extensive involvement of at least one kidney prevents successful preservation of any kidney on that side. In a relatively large group of stage V NWTSG patients, the 3-year survival was 76% despite a conservative approach to resection and institutional variation in therapy. Most patients have FH tumors (90%) that respond well to therapy. Of bilateral tumors, 10% have UH, and 4% have discordant pathology with FH on one side and UH on the other. This latter observation supports the recommendation that biopsy specimens of both kidneys must be obtained. The best prognosis in stage V disease is in patients younger than 3 years old, with FH, negative lymph nodes, and a low stage for the most advanced of the two renal lesions. A progressive decline in the frequency of chronic renal failure has been encountered in children with bilateral Wilms' tumors in the sequence of studies by the NWTSG. The incidence in NWTS-1 and NWTS-2 was 16.47%; for NWTS-3, the incidence was 9.9%; and for NWTS-4, only 3.8% of the children developed chronic renal failure. Although the latter group may see an increase as the time interval grows, it is believed that the overall decline is related to delay in resection of the tumor and attempts at renal parenchymal preservation. The value of chemotherapy in preserving renal parenchyma has been confirmed by the United Kingdom Children's Cancer Study Group.

Based on the successful outcome in selected stage V patients after partial nephrectomy, renal salvage and partial nephrectomy has been suggested as an alternative to nephrectomy in patients with unilateral stage I tumors. The criteria for renal salvage includes a tumor involving one pole occupying less than one third of a functioning kidney; no evidence of invasion of the collecting system or renal vein; and clear margins between the tumor, kidney, and surrounding structures. In an evaluation of 43 potential cases, only 2 met these criteria. This suggests that a small proportion of patients would be candidates for this type of therapy, and it would be difficult to determine any benefit for the procedure in view of the excellent survival rate achieved for stage I cases after standard nephrectomy (95%). Reports have used preoperative chemotherapy to decrease the size of the tumor and increase the proportion of patients in whom renal-sparing procedures can be performed. The risks and benefits of this approach in the patient without a high risk for bilateral disease has not been established, and the incidence of chronic renal failure in the NWTSG cohort of patients who had unilateral nephrectomy was extremely low (0.25%).

TABLE 20-4 ■ Wilms' Tumor: Vena Caval Involvement

Caval Site	%
Infrahepatic	61
Intrahepatic	14
Suprahepatic	21
Right atrium	4

A review concerning late effects of cancer treatment seen in survivors of NWTS-1 and NWTS-2 at 5- to 10-year follow-up indicated that 1% of patients developed a second malignancy, 7% developed a benign tumor, the incidence of scoliosis was decreased in survivors that did not receive irradiation, there was no increased risk of psychological disorders in children receiving vincristine, and there was no major increase in cardiovascular disorders after treatment with doxorubicin. The incidence of renal failure has declined during the series of NWTSG protocols. Most of these cases have had bilateral tumors requiring bilateral nephrectomy or resection of most of their renal parenchyma. A smaller cohort of patients had Denys-Drash syndrome with its mesangial sclerosis. The incidence of renal failure in children from hyperfiltration glomerulonephritis after a unilateral nephrectomy is extremely rare, even doubtful.

The goal of the NWTS-5 study, which is in progress, is to identify genetic factors that would predict tumor behavior comparable with factors that have been identified in neuroblastoma. Each of the treatments is single armed by stage and histology so that after completion of the study putative prognostic factors, such as loss of genetic material from chromosomes 1p, 7p, and 16q, can be evaluated.

MESOBLASTIC NEPHROMA

Mesoblastic nephroma (renal embryoma) is a renal tumor that usually presents in infants younger than 3 to 4 months of age. The tumor is embryonic in nature and has been detected on prenatal ultrasound. The mass appears as a solid lesion with a concentric ring pattern. An abdominal CT scan with contrast enhancement shows a solid neoplasm (that occasionally contains calcium) with intrarenal distortion of the collecting system. The treatment of choice is nephrectomy with lymph node sampling because a rare case may behave in a malignant fashion. More than 95% of mesoblastic nephromas are benign and require no adjuvant therapy.

NEPHROBLASTOMATOSIS

Nephroblastomatosis (nodular renal blastema) is a benign but premalignant condition with subcapsular nests of primitive metanephric epithelial rests around the rim of the kidney. This condition may be multifocal and may involve both kidneys. The nephrogenic rests may undergo sclerosis or involution, or alternatively hyperplastic overgrowth may produce an adenomatous rest (no mitosis) or with tumor induction progress to Wilms' tumor (with mitosis). Of cases, 99% of synchronous bilateral Wilms' tumor and 94% of metachronous bilateral tumors contain areas of nephrogenic rests. The risk of a nephrogenic rest becoming malignant is estimated to be 1% to 3%.

RENAL CELL CARCINOMA

Renal cell carcinoma is a relatively rare condition in children. The disease usually presents in older children and adolescents. The most common presenting finding is an abdominal mass. Hematuria is a frequent finding.

Diagnosis is achieved by ultrasound, which shows a solid intrarenal mass. Abdominal CT with contrast enhancement confirms the presence of an intrarenal mass often with distortion of the collecting system. The most common sites of tumor metastases are the regional lymph nodes, lung, liver, and bone. The therapy of choice is radical nephrectomy and lymphadenectomy that is adequate for localized tumors. No chemotherapeutic agents are effective for this tumor. Trials of immunotherapy and bone marrow transplantation are in progress for patients with metastatic disease. Although renal cell carcinoma is less radiosensitive than Wilms' tumor, irradiation may provide palliation in patients with residual disease or inoperable tumors. The overall survival is 50%.

SUGGESTED READINGS

Aronson DC, Medary I, Finlay JL, et al: Renal cell carcinoma in childhood and adolescence: A retrospective survey for prognostic factors in 22 cases. J Pediatr Surg 31:183-186, 1996.

This excellent summary of a significant cohort of children and adolescents with renal cell carcinoma describes the risk factors for survival.

Beckwith JB: Nephrogenic rests and the pathogenesis of Wilms tumor: Developmental and clinical considerations. Am J Med Genet 79:268-273, 1998.

The author presents a succinct summary of the role of precursor lesions in the development of Wilms' tumor.

Coppes MJ, Egeler RM: Genetics of Wilms' tumor. Semin Urol Oncol 17:2-10, 1999.

This is an excellent summary of the genetic origin of Wilms' tumor.

Ebb DH, Green DM, Shamberger RC, Tarbell NJ: Solid tumors of childhood. In Devita VT Jr, Hellman S, Rosenberg SA (eds): Cancer: Principles and Practice of Oncology, 6th ed. Philadelphia, Lippincott Williams & Wilkins, 2001, pp 2169-2214.

This chapter contains a section on Wilms' tumor that gives an excellent overview of the presentation and management of affected infants and children.

Evans A, Norkool P, Evans I, et al: Late effects of treatment for Wilms' tumor: A report from the National Wilms' Tumor Study Group. Cancer 67:331-336, 1991.

This report is present information concerning the deleterious late effects of cancer therapy in patients with Wilms' tumor.

Green DM, Breslow NE, Beckwith JB, et al: Comparison between single-dose and divided-dose administration of dactinomycin and doxorubicin for patients with Wilms' tumor: A report from the National Wilms' Tumor Study Group. J Clin Oncol 16:237-245, 1998.

This important report evaluates the results of the fourth NWTSG study and provides background for the results from preceding studies.

Horwitz JR, Ritchey ML, Makeness J, et al: Renal salvage procedures in patients with synchronous bilateral Wilms' tumors: A report from the National Wilms' Tumor Study Group. J Pediatr Surg 31:1020-1025, 1996.

This article summarizes the benefits to delayed surgical intervention for children with bilateral Wilms' tumors at presentation.

Ritchey ML, Shamberger RC, Haase G, et al: Surgical complications after primary nephrectomy for Wilms' tumor: Report from the National Wilms' Tumor Study Group. J Am Coll Surg 192:62-68, 2001.

This article contains an excellent summary of the surgical complications associated with nephrectomy for Wilms' tumor and a discussion of the best methods for reducing these complications.

Shamberger RC, Guthrie KA, Ritchey ML, et al: Surgery-related factors and local recurrence of Wilms tumor in National Wilms Tumor Study 4. Ann Surg 229:292-297, 1999.

This article reaffirms the crucial role of the surgeon in minimizing the risk for local recurrence in Wilms' tumor by providing appropriate lymph node sampling and avoidance of tumor rupture during nephrectomy.

Shamberger RC, Ritchey ML, Haase GM, et al: Intravascular extension of Wilms tumor. Ann Surg 234:116-121, 2001.

This article summarizes the experience with the largest reported series of children with vascular extension of Wilms' tumor and proposes an optimal method for their management.

Tournade M-F, Lemerle J, Sarrazin D, Valayer J: Tumours of the kidney. In Voute PA, Barrett A, Bloom HJG, et al (eds): Cancer in Children: Clinical Management, 2nd ed. Berlin, Springer-Verlag, 1986, pp 252-264.

This easy-to-read monograph published by participants in the International Union Against Cancer gives the reader a European perspective in the management of Wilms' tumor with special reference to preoperative chemotherapy.

Rhabdomyosarcoma

21

Rhabdomyosarcoma is a highly malignant tumor that tends to involve local structures early and eventually to metastasize to distant sites by hematogenous and lymphatic spread. Rhabdomyosarcoma is the most common soft tissue sarcoma in children. Although the tumor occurs frequently in the trunk and extremities in adult patients, in children rhabdomyosarcoma can arise from virtually any site. Rhabdomyosarcoma has a peak incidence between the ages of 2 and 5 years, and 70% of patients are younger than 10 years of age at the time of diagnosis. There is a second peak of occurrence between 12 and 18 years of age. Rhabdomyosarcomas represent 10% to 15% of all solid tumors, 6% of all pediatric cancers, and 50% of all soft tissue sarcomas. This tumor is more common in boys (1.5:1.0) and whites. Approximately 250 newly diagnosed cases are seen in the United States annually.

GENETIC FACTORS

Many genetic syndromes are associated with rhabdomyosarcoma, including instances of the Beckwith-Wiedemann syndrome with loss of heterozygosity at the 11p15 locus; the neurofibromatosis NF-1 gene located at 17q11 (a tumor suppressor gene); and the Li-Fraumeni syndrome, a familial clustering of a spectrum of cancers including breast cancer, glioblastoma, osteosarcoma, leukemia, and rhabdomyosarcoma. Li-Fraumeni syndrome is associated with germline mutations of the p53 oncogene located on chromosome 17p3, with inactivation of this tumor suppressor gene. Other risk factors for rhabdomyosarcoma include maternal use of marijuana, maternal use of cocaine, fetal alcohol syndrome, exposure to radiation, and a history of stillbirths. Rhabdomyosarcoma also has been observed in families with the basal cell nevus syndrome.

Many children with alveolar rhabdomyosarcoma contain chromosomal translocations between chromosomes 2 and 13 associated with fusion of the PAX3 transcription factor to a forked head DNA binding protein t(2;13)(q35;q14)PAX3(FKHR). This translocation is associated with a poor prognosis. A smaller number of children with alveolar rhabdomyosarcoma contain a translocation at t(1;13)(q36;q14) associated with the PAX7(FKHR)

fusion gene. Some embryonal rhabdomyosarcomas show loss of heterozygosity on the short arm of chromosome 11p15.12 leading to an overexpression of insulin-like growth factor-2. The MDM2 oncogene is expressed by some sarcomas, including rhabdomyosarcoma, and may be responsible for multidrug resistance and reduced tumor response. Chromosomal evaluation of tumor tissue from children with rhabdomyosarcoma may help differentiate this neoplasm from other small round blue cell tumors. There are no specific tumor markers for children with rhabdomyosarcoma. In regard to DNA flow cytometry, diploid tumors have a worse prognosis than hyperdiploid tumors (usually embryonal). Alveolar tumors often show near tetraploidy.

CLINICAL FINDINGS

Before 1969, survival in rhabdomyosarcoma was 10% to 15%. Considerable improvement in survival has been achieved since then. This improvement has been influenced by the establishment of cooperative study groups (the Intergroup Rhabdomyosarcoma Study [IRS] group) and the development of combined multidisciplinary treatment programs using surgery, local and regional radiotherapy, and multiagent chemotherapy. Further improvements in survival have resulted from improved imaging techniques, an appreciation of the natural history of this tumor arising from specific primary tumor sites, the categorization of tumor histology into favorable and unfavorable types, the determination of the extent of disease at the time of diagnosis by staging criteria, and the prompt referral of patients to pediatric cancer centers.

AGE

In contrast to infants with neuroblastoma, patients younger than age 1 year with rhabdomyosarcoma do not have an improved survival rate. Most survivors are in the 1- to 5-year age group or at least younger than age 10 years. Children older than age 10 have a worse prognosis. In general, children with rhabdomyosarcoma have a better survival rate than adults with the same tumor. In IRS III, 6% of the patients were younger than age 1 year, 35% were 1 to 4 years old, 25% were 5 to 9 years old,

21% were 10 to 14 years old, and 13% were older than age 15 at the time of diagnosis. A small subset of infants with congenital rhabdomyosarcoma presents in the neonatal period with alveolar tumors and metastases to the skin (subcutaneous lesions) and brain and has an extremely high mortality.

STAGING

Careful staging of the extent of disease is important in regard to treatment and prognosis. Clinical staging of the tumor correlates closely with the length of remission and patient survival. The stage of disease is related to the pretreatment imaging assessment of the tumor; regional lymph nodes (which may require biopsy); and other imaging studies (chest radiograph), bone marrow aspirate, or radioisotopic scintiscan to evaluate for tumor at remote sites (the TNM system) (Table 21-1). Primary tumor site and size (<5.0 cm or >5.0 cm in diameter) and histology are other risk factors to consider. Clinical groups are based on the amount and extent of residual tumor noted after the initial surgical procedure (Table 21-2).

TUMOR PATHOLOGY

The pathologic classification of rhabdomyosarcoma includes many distinct histologic types, including embryonal with botryoid and spindle cell variants and alveolar, pleomorphic, and undifferentiated forms of the tumor. Embryonal rhabdomyosarcoma is the most common histologic type (60%) and has a good prognosis. The botryoid variant of embryonal rhabdomyosarcoma (5% to 6% of cases) occurs in a submucosal location and extends into the lumen of the bladder, vagina, uterus, nasopharynx, bile duct, and perineum and often presents as a polypoid mass or in grapelike clusters. The spindle cell variant of embryonal rhabdomyosarcoma often is noted in paratesticular tumors. Pleomorphic tumors are relatively uncommon in infants and children. Some tumors contain a mixture of different tumor cell types, especially alveolar and embryonal forms. The IRS

TABLE 21-2 ■ Clinical Groups

Group I: Localized disease completely removed
   a. Confined to muscle or organ of origin
   b. Infiltration outside of organ or muscle of origin; regional nodes not involved
Group II: Total gross resection with evidence of regional spread
   a. Grossly resected tumor with microscopic residual
   b. Regional disease with involved lymph nodes, completely resected with no microscopic residual tumor
   c. Regional disease with involved lymph nodes, grossly resected, but with evidence of microscopic residual tumor and/or tumor involvement in the most distal regional node in the dissection
Group III: Incomplete resection or biopsy with presence of gross disease
Group IV: Distant metastases

pathology center has modified the pathologic classification by placing specific tumors into good, intermediate, and poor prognostic categories (Table 21-3). The good prognostic types are botryoid and spindle cell, the intermediate prognostic types are embryonal and pleomorphic, and the poor prognostic tumor types are alveolar and undifferentiated.

Alveolar rhabdomyosarcoma accounts for 20% of childhood cases. This cell type grows in cords with clusters of small round tumor cells with an abundant eosinophilic cytoplasm. The most common sites of alveolar cell tumors are the extremities, trunk, and perineum. Alveolar tumors have been observed at most primary sites. They have the worst prognosis and are associated with the highest rate of regional lymph node and bone marrow involvement, tumor recurrence, and distal tumor spread. Although these tumor types are well recognized, in approximately 10% to 15% of cases, deciding on the exact cell type may be elusive. Electron microscopy, DNA flow cytometry, immunohistochemical studies, and evaluation of the specific genetic makeup of the tumor tissue may help clarify the exact cell of origin and result

TABLE 21-1 ■ Pretreatment (Site, Size, TNM) Staging

Stage	Site	T Status	Size (a or b)	Node Status	Metastases
1	Favorable	T1 or T2	< or >5.0 cm (a)	N0 or N1 or Nx	None (M0)
2	Unfavorable	T1 or T2	<5.0 cm (b)	N0 or Nx	None (M0)
3	Unfavorable	T1 or T2	>5.0 cm (a or b)	N1	None (M0)
	Unfavorable	T1 or T2	< or >5.0 cm (a or b)	N0 or N1 or Nx	None (M0)
4	Either	T1 or T2	< or >5.0 cm	N0 or N1	Yes (M1)

T1 = tumor confined to anatomic site of origin.
T2 = tumor extension and/or tumor fixed to surrounding tissues.
a = tumor size <5.0 cm diameter.
b = tumor size >5.0 cm diameter.
N0 = regional lymph nodes negative.
N1 = regional lymph node involved.
Nx = lymph node status unknown or site that precludes node evaluation.
M0 = no distant metastases.
M1 = metastases present.

TABLE 21-3 ■ Histologic Types

Good Prognosis	Intermediate Prognosis	Poor Prognosis
Botryoid	Embryonal	Alveolar
Spindle cell	Pleomorphic	Undifferentiated

in a greater understanding of the influence of the various histologic subtypes on survival. Current treatment protocols include the histologic findings as a prognostic factor that may modify the intensity of the therapy.

RADIATION THERAPY

In early IRS studies, radiation doses of 6000 cGy were employed in most children with rhabdomyosarcoma and achieved local tumor control in 85% to 90% of patients. This dose was associated with an unacceptable incidence of adverse late effects, however. Lower doses (4000 to 5500 cGy, with some patients receiving <4000 cGy) resulted in an increased rate of local and regional tumor recurrence (>30% in groups II and III and 40% in group IV). Subsequently, it was noted that infants and children with group I lesions that were completely resected experienced excellent survival with two-drug chemotherapy (vincristine and actinomycin D) alone and did not require radiation therapy, avoiding the unnecessary sequelae of treatment. In more advanced cases (groups II through IV), to reduce the incidence of local recurrence, radiation therapy is an important treatment adjunct, however, particularly in locations not amenable to wide local excision of the primary tumor. In IRS III and IV, patients with stage III tumors were managed with hyperfractionated radiation techniques with the theoretical advantage of delivering a tumor dose (5800 cGy) that would increase tumor kill while preserving normal tissues. The doses were reduced for specific sites, such as lung (1800 cGy) and abdomen (1300 cGy). Evaluation of the data showed no advantage using the hyperfractionated technique when compared with conventional radiotherapy delivery and a higher complication rate. Brachytherapy has been employed in the management of patients with soft tissue sarcoma with varying degrees of success. The insertion of interstitial beads or rods in the bladder, vagina, and other sites (skeletal muscle) has resulted in excellent survival in some cases with good local control at the primary tumor site. Newer protocols have been designed to evaluate whether intensifying chemotherapy administration to reduce the radiation dose still would maintain good local tumor control but decrease the incidence of radiation-induced complications.

CHEMOTHERAPY

Chemotherapy is administered to all patients with rhabdomyosarcoma. The major role of chemotherapy is to eradicate microscopic residual disease after resection of the primary tumor. Neoadjuvant multiagent chemotherapy also may reduce the size of initially unresectable tumors and allow subsequent surgical excision at a delayed

operative procedure. Chemotherapy is given initially in an induction treatment program, then continued as maintenance therapy, with a prolonged course given for an extended period. Vincristine, actinomycin D, and cyclophosphamide (VAC) have been the mainstay drugs for IRS I, II, III, and IV. In IRS II, chemotherapy was intensified with pulse-VAC, which was compared with pulse-VAdrC-VAC, adding doxorubicin during the induction and in repetitive courses.

Overall 5-year survival improved from 55% in IRS I to 63% in IRS II. In IRS III, cisplatin and VP-16 (etoposide) were added to the treatment regimen but showed no specific advantage over VAC. Treatment programs compared VAdrC-VAC plus cisplatin versus pulse-VAC plus VAdrC plus cisplatin and VP-16. In IRS III, doxorubicin did not improve outcome in group III or IV patients or group II patients with embryonal rhabdomyosarcoma compared with VAC alone. In group I patients with paratesticular tumors, there was no benefit observed by adding cyclophosphamide to vincristine and actinomycin D therapy because survival was 95% with the latter two drugs alone. In IRS III, cisplatin-treated patients with stage III genitourinary tumors had an improved survival (81%) compared with similar cases in IRS II (71%). In IRS IV, patients with primary tumors at good prognosis sites (vagina, vulva, orbit) that were stage 1 with favorable histology received VAC or vincristine, actinomycin D, and ifosfamide (VAI) for 1 year and no radiotherapy, whereas patients with stage 1 paratesticular tumors received vincristine and actinomycin D alone. For stage 2 tumors, in addition to three-drug chemotherapy that compared VAC versus VAI versus vincristine, ifosfamide, and VP-16 (VIE), patients also received conventional radiotherapy; patients with stage 3 tumors received a similar chemotherapy program and were randomized to hyperfractionated versus conventional radiotherapy. There was no significant difference using VAC versus the other drug regimens, and hyperfractionated radiation was not beneficial. In IRS IV, patients with embryonal tumors (stage 1, 2, or 3/groups II or III) benefited from three-drug chemotherapy with a 3-year event-free survival of 83% compared with vincristine and actinomycin D alone in IRS III. VP-16 and ifosfamide had a favorable response rate in pilot studies in patients with metastases at diagnosis. Patients with metastases treated with melphalan and vincristine did not do as well. Melphalan also was associated with a high rate of second malignancies (7.2% at 5 years) and more toxicity. Topotecan was administered to patients with newly diagnosed stage 4 alveolar rhabdomyosarcoma or undifferentiated sarcoma and achieved a complete or partial response rate in 45% when followed by VAC, surgery (when possible), and irradiation.

SURVIVAL DATA FROM INTERGROUP RHABDOMYOSARCOMA STUDY GROUP STUDIES

The overall 5-year survival rate for IRS I was 55%; for IRS II, 63%; for IRS III, 71%; and (3-year survival) for IRS IV, 74%. Survival according to clinical group in

TABLE 21-4 ■ Primary Tumor Sites	
Favorable	**Unfavorable**
Orbit	Parameningeal head and neck
Superficial head and neck	Bladder/prostate
Paratesticular, vagina, vulva	Extremities
	Others
	Gastrointestinal
	Bile duct
	Retroperitoneum
	Trunk
	Intrathoracic
	Perineum
	Perianal

IRS III was 93% for clinical group I, 81% for clinical group II, 73% for clinical group III, and 30% for clinical group IV.

Current treatment programs in IRS V are based on data acquired from the previous IRS studies I through IV and were modified in an attempt to achieve improved survival, while reducing the risk of late adverse events. Treatment depends on whether a specific patient has a favorable or an unfavorable prognosis based on primary tumor site (Table 21-4), histology, and extent of tumor characterized by clinical group and TNM evaluation at diagnosis. Guidelines for surgical management include an attempt to remove the primary tumor whenever possible; perform primary re-excision for microscopic residual disease; perform a true cancer operation with wide local excision (when possible) in patients in whom lesser procedures have been attempted before referral; and, in carefully selected stage III cases, perform a second-look procedure after radiotherapy (6 months after the onset of treatment).

SPECIFIC PRIMARY TUMOR SITES
Vaginal, Vulval, and Uterine Tumors

In IRS studies comprising 151 girls with nonbladder genitourinary tumors, 82 (54%) tumors were vaginal, 26 (17%) tumors were uterine, 23 (15%) tumors were cervical, and 20 (13%) tumors were primary lesions of the vulva. Of cases, 24 (16%) were group I tumors, 14 (9%) were group II, 97 (64%) were group III, and 16 (11%) had metastases at diagnosis and were group IV. Of the vaginal and uterine tumors, 89% were group III lesions. The mean age was 5.2 years. Patients with vaginal tumors were usually younger than age 10 years. Patients with tumors of the uterus, cervix, and vulva were older (>10 years old). Of tumors, 52% had botryoid histology, 35% were embryonal, and 3% were alveolar or undifferentiated. Of the lesions involving the vulva, 45% were alveolar or undifferentiated compared with only 5% of the vaginal cases.

Vaginal rhabdomyosarcoma often presents with discharge or bleeding from the vaginal introitus or prolapse of a polypoid mass. In more advanced cases, urinary tract symptoms (from urethral compression) and constipation may be present. The diagnosis is made by vaginoscopy and biopsy of the lesion. Bimanual rectal examination, pelvic computed tomography (CT), vaginal ultrasound, and cystoscopy clarify the extent of the lesion. The inguinal area should be evaluated for the presence of enlarged lymph nodes, which may be involved with tumor. Chest radiograph, bone marrow aspirate, and radioisotopic bone scan are obtained to rule out possible tumor spread. Vaginal rhabdomyosarcoma arises beneath the mucous membrane of the anterior vaginal wall near the vesicovaginal septum, making the posterior bladder wall and urethra vulnerable to tumor invasion. In contrast, rectal involvement is uncommon because the tumor often extends parallel to the rectovaginal septum rather than into the rectum. Most vaginal tumors occur in young infants and children. The differential diagnosis includes yolk sac tumors and neurofibromas.

Most vaginal tumors have embryonal histology (often botryoid) and are particularly sensitive to chemotherapy. Despite the dramatic response to chemotherapy, microscopic residual disease often persists, and further treatment is necessary. Treatment includes biopsy alone or limited local excision followed by courses of chemotherapy. Patients with local relapse can be salvaged successfully with more extensive surgery and radiation therapy. Tumor is found at second-look surgery or rebiopsy in 70% of the cases. Delayed tumor resection includes a simple vaginectomy or vaginectomy and hysterectomy but rarely ever requires an anterior pelvic exenteration. The rate of hysterectomy was reduced from 48% to 22% and rate of vaginectomy from 66% to 41% in IRS III and IV with more intensive chemotherapy and irradiation in advanced cases. Of patients, 62% required a surgical procedure more extensive than a biopsy. The closer the primary tumor is located to the uterine cervix, the more likely that a hysterectomy may be required, and in that event, at least one ovary should be preserved whenever possible. Of interest is the fact that lymph node involvement is rare in primary tumors of the cervix. Deaths usually are limited to girls with metastases at the time of diagnosis. More than 90% of patients have an intact bladder, and more than 70% retain their uterus. Brachytherapy using radon implants also has been used successfully as an alternative method of treatment in France in the management of vaginal rhabdomyosarcoma. Successful vaginal replacement in postvaginectomy survivors using a colon segment has been described.

Rhabdomyosarcoma of the vulva accounts for 13% of nonbladder genitourinary cases in girls. In IRS I and II, nine patients were staged as follows: three as group I, two as group II, three as group III, and one had metastases (group IV). The histology is alveolar or undifferentiated in 45% of cases. Local excision and chemotherapy was successful in five of nine cases (including three with hemivulvectomy). Positive lymph nodes were identified in one of three patients who had an inguinofemoral node dissection. Seven of nine patients remained disease-free.

Rhabdomyosarcoma of the uterus usually occurs in preadolescent and teenage girls. There are two main types of presentation. The first is a single polyp that prolapses through the cervix and may fill the vagina.

The second is an intramural infiltrative tumor that is more extensive and often penetrates into the peritoneal cavity. The diagnosis is confirmed by obtaining a trans-vaginal biopsy specimen in polypoid cases and performing cervical dilation and curettage to obtain a biopsy specimen of the intrauterine infiltrative tumors. An abdominal CT scan with intravenous contrast material often delineates the extent of tumor and may allow detection of suspicious pelvic and para-aortic lymph nodes and evaluation for urinary tract obstruction from compression of the ureters. Chest radiograph, bone marrow aspirate, and radioisotopic bone scan are obtained to screen for remote disease. Uterine tumors are often large (>5.0 cm in diameter) and more invasive. Of intermediate-risk patients with uterine tumors, 27% had regional lymph node involvement. Of uterine tumors, 80% are embryonal, and 20% present with metastases. The best prognosis is in patients with polypoid lesions. None of the girls with infiltrative tumors in IRS II survived, but none received radiation therapy. The 5-year survival was 52%. Girls with uterine rhabdomyosarcoma do not have the same favorable outcome as girls with either primary vaginal or vulval lesions (92%). A more aggressive treatment program including irradiation should be employed in these cases, especially for infiltrative submucosal tumors. In IRS V, a 36-Gy radiation dose is employed for microscopic residual disease in low-risk patients, and a 50.4-Gy radiation dose is employed for gross residual disease in intermediate-risk patients.

For all patients with nonbladder genitourinary tumors, the failure-free survival was 69%, and the overall survival for all groups was 82%. The 5-year failure-free survival rate in groups I through III was 72%, with an overall survival of 87%. This compared with a 43% failure-free survival and 43% overall survival for group IV cases. Initial treatment failures are common, with 9 of 38 in IRS I and II, 25 of 97 in IRS III, and 9 of 16 in IRS IV. There was a high salvage rate in patients with recurrent disease compared with rhabdomyosarcoma occurring at other sites (10% to 15%). Age is an important factor: Overall survival was 94% in group I through III patients age 1 to 9 years versus 76% in infants younger than 1 year and children older than 10 years. Tumor status also influenced outcome: T1 lesions isolated to the organ of origin had a 98% survival, whereas T2 tumors that extended beyond the site of origin or involved surrounding structures had a 71% survival.

Rhabdomyosarcoma of the Bladder and Prostate

Patients with rhabdomyosarcoma of the bladder commonly present with urinary frequency, dysuria, straining to void, hematuria, dribbling, acute urinary retention, and an abdominal mass. Hydronephrosis and renal deterioration may result from ureteral obstruction. Primary prostatic tumors almost always can be palpated on rectal examination. Diagnosis usually can be confirmed by transrectal ultrasound, CT scan with contrast, voiding cystourethrogram, cystoscopy, and biopsy of the tumor. Cystoscopy allows the endoscopist to evaluate the extent of bladder involvement and acquire tissue for biopsy.

Most bladder tumors occur posteriorly at the trigone. The primary tumor may involve the dome of the bladder. Most of these tumors are embryonal (71%) or botryoid (20%), and a few are alveolar. Enlarged pelvic and retroperitoneal lymph nodes can be detected by CT. Lymph node involvement occurs in 24% of bladder lesions and 41% of prostate tumors. CT also may document if liver metastases are present. A chest radiograph is obtained to evaluate for the presence of lung metastases, and bone marrow aspirate and radioisotopic bone scans are useful to detect remote disease.

In some instances, the tumor may be so large that it is difficult to determine the exact origin of the primary tumor (i.e., bladder or prostate). If the pelvic tumor is extrinsic to the bladder or prostate, it is designated a non-genitourinary pelvic rhabdomyosarcoma. The behavior of this latter group of tumors is not as favorable as bladder/prostate lesions. In IRS I, cystectomy and anterior exenteration resulted in a 91% survival, but a poor quality of life was noted in survivors. More recent treatment programs for bladder/prostate tumors were designed to avoid the need for cystectomy and anterior exenteration. Although the concept of primary chemotherapy and limited surgical resection is feasible for girls with vaginal and vulval tumors, similar survival data and improved bladder salvage rates have not been as good in boys with bladder/prostate rhabdomyosarcoma. Although early IRS II data showed a survival rate of 71% and an intact bladder in 38%, the late results of these organ-sparing programs were disappointing, with disease-free survival at 3 years noted in only 46%. Bladder relapse occurred in 38% of patients, and 23% experienced regional relapse. Bladder salvage was achieved in only 25% of patients. Similar results were observed in the United Kingdom, where the overall survival was 55%, with 30% retaining an intact bladder. Only 20% of boys with bladder neck or prostatic tumors had an intact bladder. In IRS III, when cisplatin was added to VAdrC-VAC chemotherapy and irradiation was employed, the survival rate improved to 87%, and the bladder salvage rate improved to 59%. These data also included girls with vaginal tumors, however, which have a better prognosis. In contrast, partial resection of 15% to 80% of the bladder wall for tumors arising in the dome or sides of the bladder distant from the trigone was effective therapy in 26 of 33 (78.7%) patients. Relapse occurred in six patients, all of whom died. Of the survivors, 25 had an intact bladder. A pelvic lymph node dissection was done in 14 of the patients and a retroperitoneal lymph node dissection (RPLND) in 4, with only 1 of the latter patients having involved nodes. At laparotomy, the omentum was adherent to the tumor in 20% of cases, and peritoneal implants were noted in 15%. These observations suggest that partial cystectomy is a reasonable procedure for selected tumors arising from the dome of the bladder when intraoperative assessment indicates that the resection can remove the entire tumor. Ureteral reimplantation and bladder augmentation may be necessary in some cases.

Chemotherapy and radiation therapy should be employed as adjunctive treatment. A review of the data concerning localized bladder or prostate tumors indicates that after aggressive primary chemotherapy, extensive local tumor resection followed by radiation therapy and a prolonged course of chemotherapy results in an improved survival. Early assessment of the response to initial chemotherapy and irradiation is essential to ensure improved survival and bladder salvage. In patients who require cystectomy, a nonrefluxing colon conduit or a segment with an appendiceal stoma is preferable to an ileal loop for urinary diversion.

Paratesticular Tumors

Paratesticular rhabdomyosarcoma accounts for 7% of all cases of the tumor and presents as a unilateral, firm, slightly movable mass that is usually painless. In some cases, an associated hydrocele is present, which may obscure the presence of the tumor and delay diagnosis. A similar lesion may occur in girls along the round ligament. These tumors spread by lymphatic routes to the para-aortic lymph nodes, following the course of the spermatic cord into the retroperitoneal space. Inguinal lymph node metastases may occur if the dartos muscle or scrotal skin is involved by tumor spread. Patients with paratesticular tumors have a favorable prognosis. Most present with clinical group I tumors. Most have an embryonal histology (often spindle cell type), some are mixed, and others may show an undifferentiated pattern. Alveolar histology is rare. Operative treatment is carried out through an inguinal incision. After high ligation of the spermatic cord at the level of the internal inguinal ring, the tumor and testis are mobilized, and a radical orchiectomy and excision of the entire spermatic cord are performed. If a previous scrotal biopsy was performed before referral or the scrotal skin and dartos muscle are involved by tumor, a hemiscrotectomy is added. In girls with primary rhabdomyosarcoma of the round ligament, resection of the mass at the internal ring is recommended. Retroperitoneal lymph node evaluation is necessary in boys older than age 10 years. CT is not always accurate in determining whether retroperitoneal lymph nodes are involved by tumor. In IRS III, CT alone was relied on to detect the presence of tumor in retroperitoneal lymph nodes. Although the overall survival in this study was 91%, boys younger than age 10 had a 97% survival, whereas boys older than age 10 had a 63.5% failure-free survival and an overall survival of 84%. The difference was due to down-staging and undertreatment related to the failure to detect retroperitoneal lymph node involvement by CT only. Boys older than age 10 years require an ipsilateral RPLND as part of routine staging, and boys with positive lymph nodes require intensified chemotherapy (VAC for 1 year) and nodal irradiation. Unilateral lymph node dissection with nerve-sparing techniques carries a low risk of injuring the sympathetic nerves and interference with ejaculation. At the time of the RPLND procedure, the opposite side also should be inspected, with biopsy of any suspicious lymph nodes. Temporary relocation of the normal contralateral testis to the adjacent thigh is advisable to avoid potential injury to the remaining gonad if radiotherapy is used (i.e., stages 2, 3). Boys with stage I disease are treated with vincristine and actinomycin D only and do not receive radiation therapy. In patients with a negative RPLND, radiation of the retroperitoneal space can be avoided.

Extremity Tumors

Tumors of the extremities account for 19% of all cases of rhabdomyosarcoma. Patients usually present with a localized painless mass. Many patients with extremity tumors are preteens or adolescents. Of patients, 32% present with group I tumors, 26% present with group II tumors, 19% present with group III tumors, and 23% present with group IV tumors. Lower extremity lesions are more common than lesions affecting the upper extremity. Regional lymph node involvement is observed in 12% of cases. Histology is alveolar in nearly half of cases. Of patients with localized tumors, 80% survive if the lymph nodes are negative compared with 46% of patients with positive lymph nodes. Complete tumor excision is essential and is associated with better outcomes even if it requires re-excision of margins noted to be positive on histologic study. In IRS III, boys with stage 1 tumor who underwent re-excision of the primary site had an improved disease-free survival and reduced local recurrence rate.

Radiation therapy is required in all patients with incomplete tumor resection (groups II, III). Chemotherapy is employed in all cases. Amputation rarely is performed, and limb salvage with good function can be achieved in most patients (96%) when careful muscle compartment techniques are employed. More aggressive therapy is required for patients with alveolar lesions. The 5-year survival rate is 74% for groups I through III, and the local relapse rate is 16%. Relapsing patients do poorly, with only a 10% to 15% salvage rate noted. Primary tumors larger than 5.0 cm in diameter, positive lymph nodes, local relapse, age older than 10 years at diagnosis, and distant metastases adversely affect outcome.

Head and Neck Tumors

The head and neck region is a common site for childhood rhabdomyosarcoma, accounting for 35% of cases. Tumors occurring in these locations frequently are misdiagnosed as infectious or inflammatory disorders, and treatment with antibiotic therapy may delay diagnosis. Rhabdomyosarcoma is the third most common neck malignancy in childhood after Hodgkin's disease and non-Hodgkin's lymphoma. Head and neck tumors can be divided into three categories: (1) orbital tumors (10%); (2) nonparameningeal tumors (cheek, neck, temple, scalp, parotid, oropharynx, larynx) (10%); and (3) parameningeal tumors (nasopharynx, middle ear, nasal cavity, paranasal sinuses, mastoid region, pterygopalatine, infratemporal fossa) (15%). Orbital tumors have a favorable outcome (90% survival), whereas nonparameningeal tumors have a better outcome (55% survival) than parameningeal lesions (47% survival). In IRS III, 70% of parameningeal neoplasms presented as group III tumors because of the difficulty in achieving a wide local tumor resection in confined anatomic sites of occurrence. In IRS IV, orbital tumors were considered stage 1, nonparameningeal tumors were considered stage 2 or 3 (according to pretreatment TNM characteristics), and parameningeal tumors were managed as stage 3 cases.

Presenting signs and symptoms vary according to the origin of the primary tumor. Patients with nasopharyngeal tumors usually have local pain, airway obstruction, sinusitis, epistaxis, and occasionally dysphagia. Nasal congestion or cranial nerve palsy may be observed. Children with middle ear tumors often present with a polypoid mass in the auditory canal associated with pain and a history of recurring otitis media. Earaches, aural discharge, or Bell's palsy from involvement of the facial nerve may be noted. Orbital tumors are associated with eyelid swelling, ptosis, headache, decreased visual acuity, occasional extraocular muscle disturbances, and other visual disturbances. Patients with facial lesions often present with a painful swelling associated with trismus and may have cellulitis over the mass. A painful mass in the cheek or neck in a child with trismus rarely is caused by a benign disorder, and the diagnosis of rhabdomyosarcoma should be suspected. Laryngeal tumors may present with a pertussis-like cough and hoarseness from involvement of the vocal cords or the recurrent laryngeal nerve.

Rhabdomyosarcoma of the head and neck often grows rapidly and may involve vital structures such as the skull, mandible, cervical spine, or lungs—which makes these lesions more difficult to treat. Parameningeal lesions may extend into the central nervous system, resulting in cranial nerve palsies, meningeal symptoms, and respiratory paralysis as result of brainstem involvement. The clinical evaluation of head and neck patients should include chest and skull radiographs with views of the sinuses and middle ear, complete oropharynx and nasopharynx evaluation (by nasopharyngoscopy), direct and indirect laryngoscopy, CT scan of the head and neck and vertebral bodies, magnetic resonance imaging, radioisotopic bone scan, cranial nerve examination, and lumbar puncture for cerebrospinal fluid cytology.

Orbital Tumors

Patients with orbital tumors have an excellent prognosis, making this location a favorable tumor site. In IRS IV, group I orbital tumors were treated with vincristine and actinomycin D alone and had a 91% failure-free survival and overall 100% survival. Group II patients were treated with vincristine and actinomycin D and radiation therapy. In IRS V, the dose of radiation will be reduced to 36 Gy for embryonal cases and 45 Gy for others to decrease the adverse late effects (e.g., cataracts, vision disturbance, bone hypoplasia) observed in previous studies when higher radiation doses were employed. Group III patients will receive VAC plus radiation therapy.

Nonparameningeal Tumors

Patients with nonparameningeal tumors (cheek, scalp, parotid, oral cavity, larynx, pharynx) should undergo complete excision of the primary tumor when possible; however, a clear wide tumor margin can be achieved in only a few more superficial tumors. In most cases, biopsy followed by neoadjuvant chemotherapy (VAC) results in an excellent tumor response, often shrinking the tumor to permit a second surgical procedure, at which time complete resection may be possible with less cosmetic deformity and good local control. The incidence of cervical lymph node involvement is low, making a cervical neck dissection unnecessary in most cases. If enlarged suspicious lymph nodes are observed, however, a biopsy specimen should be obtained. In IRS V, nonparameningeal tumors are considered intermediate-risk lesions and require VAC and radiation therapy. Overall survival for local/regional cases is 80%.

Parameningeal Tumors

Primary tumors at parameningeal sites are rarely amenable to complete surgical resection. In early IRS studies, 35% of cases developed meningeal extension of tumor that was not prevented by chemotherapy alone. These tumors are considered intermediate-risk tumors that need more intensive treatment. Intrathecal chemotherapy is useful if cerebrospinal fluid cytology shows the presence of tumor cells. Irradiation of the primary tumor and whole brain is employed only for patients with intracranial extension. If there is no evidence of cranial extension, involvement of the base of the skull, bone erosion, or cranial nerve abnormalities, radiation is directed at the primary tumor only. Some patients may be amenable to skull-based surgical procedures after initial chemotherapy and irradiation. In IRS V, these cases will receive high-dose cyclophosphamide and receive irradiation on day 0 plus VAC.

Tumors of the Trunk

Rhabdomyosarcoma of the trunk includes tumors occurring in the chest wall, abdominal wall, and paraspinal tissues. These tumors rapidly infiltrate the surrounding tissues by direct extension, have a low incidence of lymph node involvement, and have a high recurrence rate. Tumors of the trunk more often have alveolar histology. Children present clinically with chest pain, a mass, pleural effusion, and occasionally shortness of breath. Because of the infiltrative nature of these lesions, the exact extent of the tumor involvement may be difficult to assess accurately even with CT. The tumor may involve the diaphragm and extend into the abdominal cavity. Tumors involving the diaphragm often are considered unresectable at diagnosis. The treatment of choice is wide local excision and may include segments of the chest wall and diaphragm and full-thickness resection of portions of the abdominal wall. If resection is not possible at the time of diagnosis, neoadjuvant chemotherapy after biopsy results in local control and often permits complete resection at a second surgical procedure. The overall survival is approximately 50%. Paraspinal tumors are associated with a high relapse rate and have a 50% overall survival. Newer protocols employ intensified application of chemotherapy and adjunctive radiation therapy.

Retroperitoneal Tumors

Rhabdomyosarcoma arising in the retroperitoneum accounts for 8% of all childhood cases. The tumors usually are advanced at the time of diagnosis. Clinical presentation includes abdominal pain, abdominal mass, and occasionally hydronephrosis owing to ureteral obstruction. Extension into bony structures may occur. Despite surgical resection, chemotherapy, and irradiation, there is a high local relapse rate, and distant spread is common (liver, lung, bone). Survival in IRS I and II was 28%. More recent reports suggest that resection of bulk disease may be beneficial. Resection in conjunction with intensified chemotherapy and irradiation has improved survival to 46%.

Perianal and Perineal Tumors

Rhabdomyosarcoma may present in the perineum or perianal area and involve the external anal sphincter and pelvic floor muscles. These cases represent 2% of all cases of rhabdomyosarcoma in children. The tumor may present as a subcutaneous mass or as a verrucous-appearing tumor. Diagnosis may be delayed because a mass in this area may be misdiagnosed as a perianal abscess, and the verrucous appearance may be confused with viral condylomata. Constipation and dysuria also may be noted. In IRS I and II, the most common histologic patterns were alveolar (56%) and embryonal (30%). The median age was 6 years (range 1 to 19 years). Sexes were affected equally. Patients were classified as group I in 15 cases, group II in 4, group III in 15, and group IV in 6. Spread to regional lymph nodes was observed in six cases (pelvic and inguinal). Group I patients received chemotherapy only, whereas groups II, III, and IV received chemotherapy and irradiation. The overall disease-free 3-year survival was 42%. Group I patients had an excellent outcome (100%), and 64% of group II cases survived. Survival has been achieved after abdominoperineal resection, colostomy, chemotherapy, and irradiation and in a few cases after biopsy alone, chemotherapy, and irradiation. Radiation proctitis and pelvic skeletal hypoplasia may result from radiation doses greater than 45 Gy. Inguinal lymph node sampling is suggested because overlooking regional spread may down-stage the lesion and result in undertreatment. Because of the poor prognosis, excision of the primary tumor should be accomplished whenever possible in local/regionalized cases followed by intensified chemotherapy and perhaps reduced radiation doses.

Bile Duct Tumors

Rhabdomyosarcoma of the bile duct presents with abdominal pain, fever, and jaundice. The site of tumor origin may be the common bile duct, common hepatic duct, or ampulla of Vater. The lesion is often polypoid and obstructs the lumen of the bile duct. Occasionally, jaundice is fleeting because a portion of the tumor may break off and pass through the ampulla of Vater, temporarily relieving complete obstruction. Cholangitis and liver abscess may complicate the clinical course. The diagnosis is made by abdominal ultrasound that shows a solid mass in the bile duct that is distended proximally. Magnetic resonance cholangiopancreatography also may be useful. Endoscopic retrograde cholangiopancreatography is performed to obtain a biopsy specimen and obtain a cholangiogram. If endoscopic retrograde cholangiopancreatography is unsuccessful, a transhepatic cholangiogram is performed. A CT scan should be obtained to rule out liver metastases or identify suspicious lymph nodes in the porta hepatis. A chest radiograph, isotopic bone scan, and bone marrow aspirate should be obtained to rule out remote disease. Widespread disease at the time of diagnosis is noted frequently. Most tumors of the bile duct have an embryonal histology, often botryoid in nature. Because of the poor prognostic outlook, some clinicians have recommended a more

aggressive surgical approach, and reports document that survival in localized cases has been achieved after pancreatoduodenectomy and Roux-en-Y hepaticojejunostomy followed by chemotherapy and local irradiation. Despite the administration of adjuvant chemotherapy, however, the postoperative course in many of these patients may be characterized by local recurrence and subsequent death. In contrast, more recent studies indicate that intensified neoadjuvant chemotherapy can lead to remission, relief of jaundice, and significant and extended improvement in more than half of cases—particularly cases with favorable histology.

Other Sites

Occasionally rhabdomyosarcoma can arise in the smooth muscle of the small intestine, breast, and bronchus. Lesions of the tongue and trachea can present with airway obstruction. Rhabdomyosarcoma of the lung may arise within a previously existing congenital cystic adenomatoid malformation or other lung cyst, and it has occurred in extralobar sequestrations. These latter lesions question the wisdom of conservative management by observation of congenital lung cysts proposed by some pulmonologists. Rhabdomyosarcoma also has been reported to arise within a pancreatic cyst.

RELAPSE

Relapse at a local or regional site in a patient with previously localized disease is an ominous finding. Survival after recurrence depends on the initial tumor histology, stage and group, and occasionally the type of recurrence. Overall survival after relapse in IRS III and IV was 20% (group I, 43%; group II, 12%; group III, 11%; and group IV, 8%). A 64% survival was noted, however, after recurrence in botryoid tumors compared with 26% in alveolar tumors and 5% in undifferentiated sarcomas. Patients with group I alveolar or undifferentiated tumors had a 40% relapse rate compared with 3% for other tumor types. In stage 1/group I embryonal rhabdomyosarcomas, the relapse was local in 72% of cases, in regional lymph nodes in 50%, and in distant sites in 26%. Survival for children with embryonal tumors was 52% for stage 1/group I, 20% for stage 3/group II or III, and 12% for stage 4/group IV. Group IIc patients with alveolar or undifferentiated tumors continued to have a high relapse rate despite intensification of treatment in IRS III and IV.

METASTATIC DISEASE

Patients with metastatic disease at the time of diagnosis have a poor prognosis. The 5-year survival for stage 4/group IV patients was 21% in IRS I, 27% in IRS II, and 30% in IRS III. The 3-year survival in IRS IV is 27% despite intensification of therapy. The 10-year survival rate for early IRS studies was 10%.

Metastases occur by hematogenous and lymphatic routes and involve lymph nodes (33%), lung (50%), bone (35%), bone marrow, liver (22%), brain (20%), breast (5%), and other sites. Age and histology had an impact on survival with metastatic disease in IRS III and IV.

Children younger than age 10 years with embryonal tumors had a 50% survival at 5 years compared with a 25% survival rate noted in children with embryonal tumors who were older than 10 years and with alveolar or undifferentiated tumors who were younger than 20 years.

Resection of persistent solitary pulmonary metastasis (or a few metastases) after chemotherapy and irradiation may result in an occasional survivor. Selected patients with metastatic disease that is controlled (bone marrow and lungs cleared after chemotherapy) may be candidates for a second-look procedure to achieve local tumor control. This approach is especially applicable to all superficial sites of primary tumor, including the trunk, perineum, extremities, and certain head and neck sites.

Because of the extremely poor results in patients with relapse, refractory, and metastatic disease, more intense treatment with aggressive high-dose multimodal chemotherapy and hematopoietic stem cell rescue has been attempted. None of these efforts were found to be beneficial. Novel treatment protocols to deal with metastatic disease are urgently needed. Antiangiogenic agents, insulin-like growth factor-1 fusion transcripts, targeted immunoradiotherapy, antitumor treatments using viral vectors, interleukin-2 immunomodulation, and tumor vaccines are on the horizon and no doubt will be employed in future pilot studies.

INTERGROUP RHABDOMYOSARCOMA STUDY GROUP V

IRS V was developed from information accrued from IRS studies I through IV. In IRS IV, it became clear that protocols employing VIE and VAI chemotherapy offered no advantage over the standard VAC therapy. Similarly, hyperfractionated radiation was not beneficial compared with conventional radiotherapy. The overall 3-year failure-free survival in IRS IV was similar to IRS III (76%). At 5 years in IRS III, survival was reduced to 71%. Intensified therapy employing three drugs, surgical resection of the tumor, and radiation therapy improved survival of patients with embryonal tumors with local/regional disease (groups II and III) to 83% in IRS IV versus 74% in IRS III. This improvement was likely due to a higher dose of alkylating agent (cyclophosphamide). Patients with stage 2/group II did slightly better than group I patients (73% versus 71%), suggesting they may have benefited from radiation therapy as well. Age also became a factor, with improved outcomes noted in children younger than age 10 years with vaginal and paratesticular tumors and metastatic disease. Based on these observations, in IRS V, patients are placed into low-risk, intermediate-risk, and high-risk treatment categories according to tumor site, histology, tumor size, pretreatment TNM stage, clinical group, and in some instances age of the patient.

Low-Risk Protocols

Low-risk patients are stratified into two distinct subgroups: A and B (Box 21-1). In subgroup A, therapy includes

---

> ### BOX 21-1 Low-Risk Protocols
>
> **Subgroup A (Embryonal or Botryoid Tumors Located at Favorable Sites)**
> 1. Orbit, nonparameningeal head and neck, nonbladder prostate genitourinary (vagina, vulva, paratesticular), tumor of any size (a or b), completely resected or microscopic residual disease (lymph node–negative) (stage 1, clinical group I, II; N0, M0)
> 2. Favorable site, tumor any size (a or b), gross residual disease in orbit only (lymph node–negative) (stage 1, clinical group III; N0—orbit only)
> 3. Unfavorable site (all sites excluding those listed above), tumor size <5.0 cm (a), completely resected (lymph node N0 or Nx) (stage 2, clinical group I; N0, Nx)
>
> **Subgroup B**
> 1. Favorable tumor site, tumor size (a or b), microscopic residual disease (lymph node–positive) (stage 1, clinical group III; N1; bilateral retroperitoneal lymph nodes need staging in boys >10 years old with paratesticular tumors)
> 2. Favorable tumor site, tumor size (a or b), gross residual disease (lymph node–positive)—orbit only (stage 1, clinical group III; N1; orbit only)
> 3. Favorable site (except orbit), any size (a or b), gross residual disease (lymph node–negative, lymph node–positive, or Nx) (stage 1, clinical group III; N0, N1, or Nx)
> 4. Unfavorable site, small tumor (a) with microscopic residual disease (stage 2, clinical group II; N0, Nx)
> 5. Unfavorable site, small tumor (a) with lymph node–positive or large tumor (b) regardless of lymph node status, completely resected or microscopic residual disease (stage 3, clinical group I or II; N0, Nx, or N1)

---

vincristine and actinomycin D and no radiotherapy for clinical group I and vincristine and actinomycin D plus radiotherapy for microscopic residual tumor. In subgroup B, chemotherapy includes VAC, and radiotherapy is reduced to 36 Gy for microscopic residual disease, lymph node–negative, and to 45 Gy for gross residual disease orbit only and clinical group III after complete second-look tumor resection. If the histology on the final pathology report changes from an embryonal tumor to either alveolar or undifferentiated sarcoma, the patient gets switched to an intermediate-risk treatment program.

Intermediate-Risk Protocol

Children with intermediate-risk tumors comprise 55% of newly diagnosed patients with rhabdomyosarcoma. These cases have fared suboptimally in prior IRS studies, with a 3-year progression-free survival varying from 50% to 79%. Because dose intensification of chemotherapy has improved the overall survival in IRS III and IV, IRS V studies for intermediate-risk patients will attempt to employ dose intensification using escalating doses of

TABLE 21-5 ▪ Intermediate-Risk Protocol

Stage/Group	Site	Histology	Size	Nodes	Metastases	Age (yr)
2/III	Unfavorable	Embryonal	a	N0 or Nx	M0	
3/III	Unfavorable	Embryonal	a	N1	M0	
	Unfavorable	Embryonal	a	N0 or N1 or Nx	M0	All <21
1, 2, or 3/I, II, III	Unfavorable or favorable	Alveolar	a or b	N0 or N1 or Nx	M0	
4/I-IV	Unfavorable or favorable	Embryonal	a or b	N0 or N1	M1	<10

TABLE 21-6 ▪ High-Risk Protocol

Stage/Group	Site	Histology	Size	Nodes	Metastases	Age (yr)
4/IV	Favorable or unfavorable	Embryonal	a or b	N0 or N1	M1	>10
	Favorable or unfavorable	Alveolar or undifferentiated	a or b	N0 or N1	M1	<21

cyclophosphamide as the agent of choice. Intermediate-risk cases are defined in Table 21-5. Treatment consists of four courses of escalating cyclophosphamide plus VAC.

High-Risk Protocol

Irinotecan is a topoisomerase I inhibitor that initiates apoptosis and kills cells during the S phase of the cell cycle associated with DNA replication. Pilot studies indicate the drug results in a 45% complete or partial response rate in cases with metastatic disease; however, a 26% progression rate also was noted when irinotecan is given alone. The IRS V high-risk protocol evaluates the efficacy of irinotecan plus vincristine given as an up-front window alternating with VAC in children older than age 10 years with newly diagnosed metastatic disease (stage 4/group IV) with embryonal histology and children younger than age 21 with alveolar or undifferentiated sarcoma (Table 21-6). The IRS V study also will define and compare clinical features of subgroups of alveolar tumors that exhibit t(2;13) and t(1;13) translocations.

SUGGESTED READINGS

Arndt CAS, Donaldson SS, Anderson JR, et al: What constitutes optimal therapy for patients with rhabdomyosarcoma of the female genital tract? Cancer 91:2154-2168, 2001.

This important study reviews the results of IRS III and IV and compares outcomes of girls with vaginal, vulval, and uterine tumors with outcomes in previous studies (IRS I and II).

Crist WM, Anderson JR, Meza JL, et al: Intergroup Rhabdomyosarcoma Study IV: Results for patients with non-metastatic disease. J Clin Oncol 19:3091-3102, 2001.

This article describes the results observed in children with rhabdomyosarcoma in the IRS-IV. Improvement in survival in nonmetastatic patients with embryonal tumors was related to chemotherapy dose intensification, better staging, and improved local control.

Donaldson SS, Mesa J, Breneman JC, et al: Results from the IRS-IV randomized trial of hyperfractionated radiotherapy in children with rhabdomyosarcoma—a report from the IRSG1. Int J Radiat Oncol Biol Phys 51:718-728, 2001.

This important article documents an increased toxicity rate and no statistical benefit using hyperfractionated techniques compared with conventional radiotherapy.

Pappo AS, Anderson JR, Crist WM, et al: Survival after relapse in children and adolescents with rhabdomyosarcoma: A report from the IRSG. J Clin Oncol 17:3487-3493, 1999.

This report documents that relapse after initial therapy often carries a poor prognosis, especially in children with alveolar and undifferentiated sarcomas. Stage and clinical group at the time of diagnosis are also important factors influencing outcome after relapse.

Raney RB, Anderson JR, Barr FG, et al: Rhabdomyosarcoma and undifferentiated sarcoma in the first two decades of life: A selective review of Intergroup Rhabdomyosarcoma Study group experience and rationale for Intergroup Rhabdomyosarcoma Study V. J Pediatr Hematol Oncol 23:215-221, 2001,

This article reviews data from previous IRS studies I through IV that establish the rationale for the new IRS-V study treatment protocols.

Rodriguez-Galindo C, Hall DA, Onyekwere O, et al: Neonatal alveolar rhabdomyosarcoma with skin and brain metastases. Cancer 92:1613-1620, 2001.

This article contains an important observation of an aggressive form of alveolar rhabdomyosarcoma seen in neonates associated with subcutaneous and brain metastases and a high mortality.

Wiener E: Soft tissue sarcomas. In Carachi R, Azmy A, Grosfeld JL (eds): The Surgery of Childhood Tumors. London, Arnold Publishers, 1999, pp 210-242.

This excellent chapter concerning rhabdomyosarcoma and other soft tissue tumors in children is comprehensive and informative.

Wiener ES, Anderson JR, Ojimba JI, et al: Controversies in the management of paratesticular rhabdomyosarcoma: Is staging retroperitoneal lymph node dissection necessary for adolescents with resected paratesticular rhabdomyosarcoma? Semin Pediatr Surg 10:146-152, 2001.

This article documents the inaccuracy of CT scans in detecting retroperitoneal lymph node involvement and the increased risk of mortality in boys older than age 10 years with paratesticular tumors. Staging unilateral RPLND is necessary in this subgroup of patients.

22

Liver Tumors

Malignant liver tumors account for approximately 1% of all childhood tumors. Although relatively infrequent, liver tumors present a diagnostic and a therapeutic challenge. It is generally stated that two thirds of all liver masses in children are malignant; however, most published series do not take into account small benign asymptomatic lesions discovered incidentally, unless the child was admitted to the hospital or a biopsy was done. Advances in technology, a better understanding of segmental liver anatomy, improvements in operative technique, and development of effective chemotherapy have changed significantly the diagnostic work-up and treatment approach for children with these neoplasms.

BENIGN LIVER TUMORS

Benign tumors include vascular anomalies, mesenchymal hamartoma, focal nodular hyperplasia (FNH), hepatic adenoma, and teratoma. Vascular anomalies are the most common benign tumor of the liver and tend to present in infancy, as does mesenchymal hamartoma. FNH and adenoma usually are seen in older children.

Vascular Anomalies

There has been a lot of confusion about the nomenclature of vascular anomalies as applied to all body parts, including the liver. The classification of vascular malformations proposed by Mulliken in 1982 now is accepted internationally but is not being used by all liver specialists yet. This classification is based on the clinical behavior and the cellular characteristics of the two major categories of vascular anomalies: tumors, which grow actively then involute, and malformations, which are errors of embryonic development (Table 22-1).

Proliferative Lesions

Hemangiomas account for 80% to 90% of hepatic vascular anomalies. The term *benign infantile hemangioendothelioma* is synonymous with hemangioma. The name apparently was given by pathologists because of the hypercellular pattern of type II (seen in 20% of cases, the other 80% being type I), which has microscopic similarities to other types of hemangioendotheliomas (kaposiform, epithelioid). These latter lesions are tumors of intermediate malignant potential, between the always benign

hemangiomas and angiosarcomas. The term *hemangioma* is used here instead of the confusing *infantile hemangioendothelioma*.

More than 90% of liver hemangiomas present in the first 6 months of life, most within the first 2 months. They may be solitary or multifocal, the latter often associated with hemangiomas of the skin and other organs. Patients with three or more organs involved are labeled as having *disseminated hemangiomatosis*. The most common sites of involvement after liver and skin include the brain, gastrointestinal tract, lung, and bone. Liver hemangiomas have a 2:1 female preponderance, less than the 5:1 ratio observed for skin lesions. Although patients with small isolated lesions may be relatively asymptomatic, 80% of patients with multiple hepatic hemangiomas have the classic triad of hepatomegaly, congestive heart failure, and anemia. Other presenting signs and symptoms include respiratory distress from the enlarged liver, jaundice, and profound thrombocytopenia from platelet trapping (Kasabach-Merritt syndrome). Intraperitoneal hemorrhage, congenital hypothyroidism, and fetal anasarca also have been described. Asymptomatic solitary hemangiomas also may be discovered incidentally by prenatal or postnatal ultrasound.

Imaging studies are essential in the diagnosis of liver tumors. Ultrasound with Doppler is often the first test performed in a child presenting with an abdominal mass. Multifocal lesions appear as echolucent nodules associated with high-flow vessels. Solitary hemangiomas may be more heterogeneous. Indirect signs of increased arterial flow with shunting include an enlarged hepatic artery with tapering of the aorta below the celiac axis and dilation of

---

TABLE 22-1 ▪ Vascular Anomalies

Vascular tumors (proliferative)
  Hemangioma
  Hemangioendothelioma (kaposiform, epithelioid)
  Angiosarcoma
Vascular malformations (developmental errors)
  Slow-flow: capillary, venous, lymphatic
  Fast-flow: arterial, arteriovenous
  Complex/combined: Klippel-Trénaunay, Proteus, and other
    syndromes

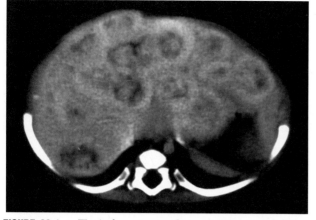

FIGURE 22-1 ■ Typical contrast-enhanced CT scan of diffuse hemangiomas in a 4-month-old boy. Because of his rapidly increasing abdominal girth and the fact that the lesions filled 75% of the liver, he was treated with steroids and had a good response. He was followed for 3 years, with persistent but regressing heterogeneous lesions on serial ultrasound examinations. He remained well 8 years after diagnosis.

the hepatic veins and right atrium. Ultrasound examination of a liver mass usually is followed by a dynamic computed tomography (CT) scan; this entails a sequence before intravenous contrast material is injected, followed by arterial and venous phases 30 and 60 seconds after contrast material injection and sometimes a delayed phase. This test is usually diagnostic in multifocal hemangiomas, which have low attenuation on the precontrast sequence, with occasional speckled calcifications; after intravenous contrast material, the lesions enhance either diffusely or more often centripetally (i.e., rim enhancement, or "target sign") followed by gradual filling in the center of the lesions (Fig. 22-1).

Magnetic resonance imaging (MRI) has gained popularity and is the most useful single imaging modality according to some authors. Multifocal hemangiomas are hypointense on T1-weighted sequences and uniformly hyperintense on T2-weighted sequences; solitary lesions are more heterogeneous because of a variable degree of central necrosis.

Radionuclide scans are occasionally helpful in the differential diagnosis of liver tumors but are rarely necessary for vascular lesions. Finally, arteriography is generally reserved for patients with congestive heart failure, who may benefit from therapeutic embolization, which must be extensive to be effective.

Asymptomatic liver hemangiomas can be observed without treatment but should be followed closely until the rapidly proliferative phase is over (6 to 8 months). As for hemangiomas elsewhere in the body, involution generally starts at 10 to 12 months of age and continues for many years. Imaging studies of the brain and chest radiographs are appropriate for patients with multiple hemangiomas. Many patients, especially patients with large lesions or with diffuse liver involvement, develop complications such as high-output cardiac failure or hepatomegaly with respiratory distress and abdominal compartment syndrome. Supportive treatment consists of

digoxin and diuretics; the first-line antiangiogenic therapy is prednisone, 2 to 3 mg/kg daily. A rapid response is expected within 1 to 2 weeks in 70% of patients. After 6 weeks, the steroids are tapered slowly over several months. If there is no clinical response after 10 to 14 days, the second-line treatment is interferon-α. The response is slow compared with the dramatic effects sometimes seen with steroids; there is no synergism, and the two agents should not be given simultaneously at therapeutic dosage. Selective embolization should be considered if a patient requires mechanical ventilation or if congestive heart failure or failure to thrive persists after a reasonable trial of pharmacologic therapy. Low-dose chemotherapy (cyclophosphamide or vincristine) and radiation therapy also have been used, the latter being abandoned because of long-term risks, especially secondary malignancies. Surgery has a limited role. In some patients with respiratory compromise or abdominal compartment syndrome, the abdominal cavity may be enlarged temporarily with the use of a resorbable mesh. With focal hemangiomas localized to one lobe, surgical resection after embolization should be considered. Liver transplantation is another option for patients with diffuse hepatic hemangiomas who fail to respond to medical therapy and embolization; these latter patients usually have either extensive intrahepatic arteriovenous fistulas or significant portal venous supply.

The mortality rate of infants with symptomatic diffuse liver hemangiomas used to be 30% to 50%. With the above-outlined treatment strategies, especially since the availability of interferon-α and the use of selective embolization in expert hands, the mortality has decreased to 10%. Interferon-α also has been useful to reverse the Kasabach-Merritt phenomenon (typical platelet count <10,000/mm³) but by itself is effective in only 50% of cases. The Kasabach-Merritt phenomenon should not be confused with disseminated intravascular coagulation, which also can occur in rare instances. Some authors caution against the use of heparin with the former because it can stimulate tumor growth and aggravate platelet trapping. Platelets should not be given unless there is active bleeding or a surgical procedure is planned. Interferon-α is not without side effects and complications, the most severe being spastic diplegia; patients require careful neurologic assessment and discontinuation of therapy at the first sign of toxicity.

Vascular Malformations

Vascular malformations account for 10% of hepatic vascular anomalies in children and affect both sexes equally, in contrast to hemangiomas. The most common are arteriovenous malformations (AVMs), which may present in newborns in the same fashion as diffuse hemangiomas with congestive heart failure. MRI can distinguish between an AVM and a large solitary hemangioma. Embolization and surgical resection are indicated. In older children, hepatic AVMs are associated most often with hereditary hemorrhagic telangiectasia (Osler-Rendu-Weber disease); in some of these patients, liver transplantation may be the only solution. Arterioportal fistulas, portovenous fistulas, and pure venous or venolymphatic malformations are other rare anomalies that require expert imaging, especially angiography, for precise diagnosis and treatment.

Mesenchymal Hamartoma

Mesenchymal hamartomas are uncommon hepatic tumors that usually present in the first 2 years of life and may be diagnosed prenatally. Most involve the right lobe of the liver, and they are almost always solitary lesions. The tumor may achieve significant size but often presents clinically as an asymptomatic abdominal mass. Laboratory tests, including those affecting liver function, are normal; α-fetoprotein (AFP) occasionally is elevated, although rarely as high as with hepatoblastoma. Abdominal ultrasound usually shows a mixed solid and cystic tumor that is well demarcated from the surrounding hepatic tissue. Hepatic scintigraphy with technetium-99m shows reduced uptake of the tracer in the tumor. CT and MRI show the fluid-filled spaces with septations, surrounded by a thick wall. Purely solid lesions are uncommon and usually are seen in young infants. The treatment for hamartomas is resection of the involved segment or lobe. The lesion is benign. Occasionally, it is difficult to separate a more solid-appearing hamartoma from a malignancy, especially when the AFP level is elevated. The prognosis is generally excellent.

Hepatic Adenoma

Most cases of hepatic adenoma occur in women who take oral contraceptive pills. Hepatic adenoma is a relatively rare neoplasm in preadolescent children but must be considered in the differential diagnosis of a liver mass in older adolescent girls. Occasionally, children with type I or IV glycogen storage disease or with congenital hepatic fibrosis develop hepatic adenomas. The clinical presentation ranges from patients presenting with an asymptomatic mass to patients presenting with abdominal pain or emergently because of hemoperitoneum from spontaneous rupture. On CT and ultrasound studies, the mass appears solid and well circumscribed. The vascularity of the lesion is variable, and heterogeneity secondary to necrosis is frequent. AFP levels and liver function tests are normal. Patients with known predisposing factors may be observed; birth control pills and other medications should be discontinued. Fine-needle biopsy may be helpful in achieving a diagnosis if there is an absence of mitotic figures or bizarre nuclei in the cells recovered. Resection is indicated in patients without an inciting cause because of the risk of bleeding and because this solid mass cannot always be differentiated from a hepatocellular carcinoma (HCC) (Fig. 22-2). The adenoma generally involves the right lobe of the liver and is often yellow-tan. If the mass is recognized as an adenoma, simple enucleation, when possible, is an acceptable procedure. If the diagnosis is not clear, partial hepatic resection or lobectomy occasionally may be necessary. Recurrence is unlikely.

Focal Nodular Hyperplasia

The cause of FNH is unknown. The use of oral contraceptive pills has been implicated in some cases; the current thought is, however, that hormones do not cause

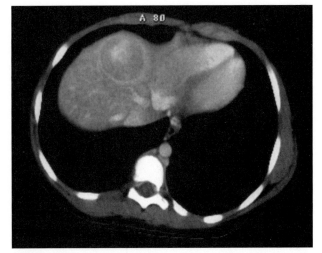

FIGURE 22-2 ■ Patient with congenital hepatic fibrosis who developed a well-circumscribed lesion in segment IV discovered during routine ultrasound at 9 years of age. This CT scan with intravenous contrast material clearly delineates a mass with central and peripheral enhancement; there was no uptake on the technetium hepatate liver/spleen scan with near-normal uptake on the gallium scan. Overall, these features are typical of an adenoma. The lesion was enucleated, and the patient remained well 5 years later, with persistent portal hypertension. (Courtesy of Dr. Hélène Flageole.)

FNH but may stimulate its growth. This tumor is four times more common in girls, and 85% of cases occur after age 15 years. There are multiple lesions in 10% to 15% of patients. The usual clinical presentation is an asymptomatic mass greater than 4 to 5 cm. The lesion appears solid on ultrasound and has a typical "central stellate scar" with peripheral hypervascularity on CT scan (Fig. 22-3). The central scar enhances during the delayed phase of the dynamic CT scan. Other tumors that may mimic FNH by having a "central scar" on CT include fibrolamellar HCC, cholangiocarcinoma, and hemangioma. Hepatic scintigraphy shows uptake of the isotope by the tumor. Angiography shows a hypervascular pattern but usually is not required for diagnosis. This is a benign condition that does not require excision. A needle biopsy may be useful in achieving a diagnosis in some patients. Microscopic examination reveals normal hepatocytes surrounded by fibrous tissue and chronic inflammatory cells. When imaging studies are inconclusive and a percutaneous biopsy cannot be obtained, a laparotomy may be necessary to separate this lesion from a malignancy. Open biopsy is advised. If the diagnosis is clear, no further surgery is necessary; if the diagnosis is still in question, tumor excision is advised.

Other Tumors and Malformations

Many other primary tumors affect the liver in infants and children; other lesions are metastatic. Regenerating nodules, as seen with cirrhosis, tyrosinemia, and other entities such as nodular regenerative hyperplasia, may mimic benign or malignant lesions. Teratomas of the liver are extremely rare neoplasms and are more often benign than malignant. The tumor may contain neuroectodermal

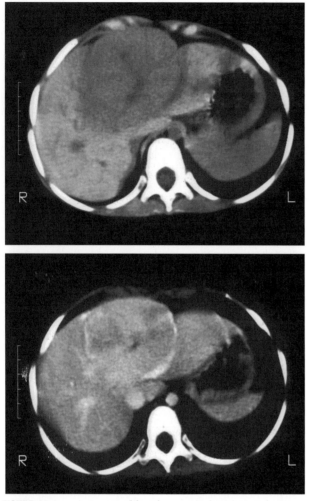

FIGURE 22-3 ■ A 5-year-old girl presented with a right upper quadrant mass, confirmed to be within the liver and hypervascular on ultrasound examination. CT scan (top), before intravenous contrast material, shows typical central stellate area of decreased attenuation. Early after contrast material infusion (bottom), there is peripheral enhancement. The diagnosis of FNH was confirmed by technetium-99m scan (heterogeneous mass with uptake of tracer equal to the normal liver tissue) and ultrasound-guided needle biopsy. The patient was observed and remains asymptomatic 6 years later. (Courtesy of Dr. Luong Nguyen.)

elements, which allows differentiation from a hepatoblastoma on pathologic study. The treatment of choice is resection (see Chapter 24).

Hepatic cysts usually are classified as congenital or parasitic. Congenital cysts may be solitary or multiple. More than 50% of patients with polycystic liver disease have polycystic renal disease. The cysts are benign structures that usually are lined with a single layer of epithelial cells. They must be differentiated from Caroli's disease, which also may be associated with polycystic kidney disease. Technetium-99m hepatoiminodiacetic acid (HIDA) scan differentiates simple cysts ("cold," without tracer uptake) from cysts communicating with the biliary tree. Most simple cysts are asymptomatic; they can be found in 3.6% of the population and usually do not require treatment. In more recent years, large solitary

hepatic cysts have been detected in utero on prenatal ultrasound (Fig. 22-4). They may be mistaken for a choledochal cyst. Infants with a large cyst may present with an asymptomatic palpable right upper quadrant mass that is cystic on ultrasound. If the cyst is large or symptomatic, it should be excised or unroofed. For large cysts and cysts more deeply embedded with clear content, unroofing and marsupialization allowing drainage into the peritoneal cavity are reasonable procedures and can be accomplished by laparoscopy. If the cyst contains bile, signifying the presence of a connection to the biliary system, a cholangiogram should be obtained through the cyst to verify the integrity of the biliary tree; a cyst Roux-en-Y jejunostomy would not be indicated for Caroli's disease because this increases the risk of recurrent cholangitis.

Various pediatric malignant neoplasms can metastasize to the liver, including neuroblastoma, Wilms' tumor, rhabdomyosarcoma, lymphoma, and germ cell tumors. A right-sided Wilms' tumor or adrenal tumor also may invade the liver. The treatment of these lesions is discussed elsewhere.

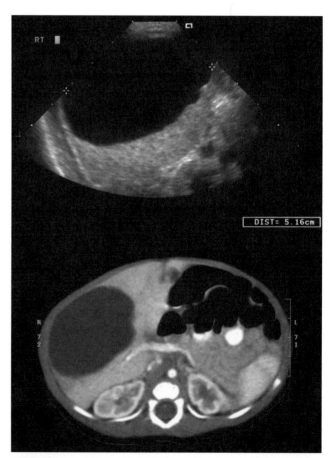

FIGURE 22-4 ■ Neonate with a large liver cyst, which had been diagnosed by prenatal ultrasound at 34 weeks' gestation. Sonogram (top) shows the anechoic content and the lack of a discernible wall, confirmed by CT scan 1 month later (bottom). There was no uptake on HIDA scan (not shown), confirming this to be a simple cyst. It increased in size in the first 6 months of life and became symptomatic. It was unroofed easily through a laparoscopic approach. (Courtesy of Dr. Hélène Flageole.)

MALIGNANT LIVER TUMORS

Incidence and Epidemiology

Malignant liver tumors constitute 1% to 2% of all pediatric malignancies; they include hepatoblastoma, HCC, and other rare tumors (mesenchymal sarcoma, rhabdomyosarcoma of the bile ducts, and cholangiocarcinoma). Hepatoblastoma is more common and is observed in children in the first 4 years of life (two thirds by 24 months of age), whereas HCC occurs in older children and adolescents. Malignant liver tumors are more frequent in boys than girls with a 2:1 ratio observed. They are noted more commonly in children with hemihypertrophy, Beckwith-Wiedemann syndrome, Fanconi's anemia, fetal alcohol syndrome, type 1 glycogen storage disease, hereditary tyrosinemia, and after cirrhosis secondary to a variety of conditions, including cholestasis from the use of total parenteral nutrition in infancy (Table 22-2). Reports have documented the occurrence of HCC 9 to 16 years after successful treatment of right-sided Wilms' tumor with chemotherapy and irradiation. In addition, hepatic sarcomas have occurred after irradiation for hepatic hemangioma in infancy. The association of total parenteral nutrition cholestasis with hepatoblastoma is being re-examined; it is becoming evident that prematurity is an important factor because 10% of hepatoblastomas occur in infants weighing less than 1 kg at birth, and 20% to 25% occur in infants born before 37 weeks' gestation. Epidemiologic studies are required to determine the role of total parenteral nutrition, caffeine, and other substances that may be toxic to the premature liver. The clear relationship between hepatoblastoma and prematurity may explain the increasing incidence of this tumor.

The occurrence of hepatoblastoma in twins has been reported in a family with familial adenomatous polyposis. The precise relationship of the familial polyposis gene located on the long arm of chromosome 5 and hepatoblastoma is not clear. Epidemiologic studies concerning liver tumors further suggest that hepatoblastoma is a malignant tumor related to maldevelopment that may be associated with 11p or 5q chromosomal mutations. DNA flow cytometry may show a hyperdiploid pattern within the tumor in association with chromosomal translocations (trisomy of chromosomes 2, 8, and 20); this may be associated with a poorer prognosis. HCC has an important association with chronic hepatitis and cirrhosis caused by hepatitis B virus, especially in Taiwan, where there is a high prevalence of hepatitis B infection. Studies of the DNA in HCC tissue indicate that hepatitis B viral sequences have been incorporated.

Pathology

Hepatoblastoma and HCC are epithelial malignancies. These tumors occur more commonly in the right lobe of the liver but also can be multicentric. Spread to other parts of the liver occurs by direct extension and by intrahepatic lymphatic and vascular channels. The tumor can extend into the hepatic veins and vena cava. The lungs, brain, and bone marrow can be the site of hematogenous spread. Extrahepatic spread may occur in the regional lymph nodes in the porta hepatis.

Hepatoblastomas are classified into epithelial lesions that are either predominantly fetal (well differentiated) or embryonal (immature and poorly differentiated), mixed epithelial and mesenchymal, or anaplastic categories. The tumor cells have a high nuclear-to-cytoplasmic ratio, a basophilic or amphophilic cytoplasm, and evidence of mitotic activity. In the fetal and embryonal variants, tumor cells frequently are arranged in cords two to three cells thick. The mixed epithelial-mesenchymal variant often has a spindle cell characteristic, whereas anaplastic hepatoblastoma may present with sheets of loosely connected cells with a high mitotic rate and scant cytoplasm.

HCC frequently has the same histologic appearance as seen in adults, often with large pleomorphic tumor cells resembling mature hepatocytes. A variant of HCC called *fibrolamellar carcinoma* has a slower growth leading to a better short-term survival rate. It represents only 15% to 20% of HCC. This relatively rare neoplasm occurs primarily in younger people between ages 5 and 25 years and is grossly nodular in appearance. The microscopic appearance of these lesions shows eosinophilic neoplastic hepatocytes containing hyaline globules and distinct pale bodies surrounded by fibrous bands that take on a lamellar configuration.

Clinical Presentation and Diagnosis

The presence of a right upper quadrant mass that moves on respiration is the most frequent presenting finding (90% of cases). Nausea and vomiting occasionally are noted from compression of the stomach or duodenum by the enlarged liver. In older children with HCC, the mass may be painful. Weight loss and anemia occasionally are observed. A few cases of hepatoblastoma present with precocious puberty (virilization) in boys that probably is caused by human chorionic gonadotropin (hCG) production by the tumor. Although the hCG serum level may be normal in some patients with virilization, immunoperoxidase staining has confirmed that the hepatoblastoma cells in these patients are the site of hCG production. Estrogen and progesterone receptors also may be present in some hepatoblastoma cells. The serum levels of liver enzymes may be slightly elevated, but the bilirubin is almost always normal except in advanced cases. Platelet counts often are increased. The serum AFP level is elevated in 90% of patients with hepatoblastoma and approximately half of children with HCC. Elevated AFP levels also can be seen in children with malignant teratomas (yolk sac tumors)

TABLE 22-2 ■ Factors Associated with Malignant Liver Tumors

Beckwith-Wiedemann syndrome
Hemihypertrophy
Prematurity
TPN cholestasis
Familial polyposis, Gardner's syndrome
Type 1 glycogen storage disease
Fanconi's anemia
Cirrhosis
Hepatitis B
Tyrosinemia

TPN, total parenteral nutrition.

and teenagers with germ cell tumors of the testes and ovaries. The serum ferritin level is elevated in most patients (97%) with HCC but also is elevated in 87% of non–tumor bearing patients with cirrhosis. The AFP and serum ferritin level may serve as tumor markers to monitor therapeutic response and tumor recurrence.

The diagnostic work-up of a liver tumor includes many radiographic studies. A plain abdominal radiograph shows a mass effect on the right upper quadrant that may contain calcification. A chest radiograph should be obtained to rule out lung metastases. Ultrasound combined with Doppler interrogation documents whether the mass is solid or cystic, identifies the kidneys as being extrinsic to the tumor, and evaluates the hepatic veins and vena cava for possible intravascular tumor extension. An abdominal CT scan with intravenous contrast material demarcates the extent of the neoplasm within the liver and usually can exclude the presence of a vascular tumor. CT outlines the site of the tumor, clarifies its relationship to the hilar structures and hepatic veins, evaluates for multicentricity and involvement of the contralateral lobe, and often can predict resectability (Fig. 22-5). Bone marrow aspirate and CT of the lungs also are obtained. Although a hepatic angiogram was obtained in most patients in the past, a greater appreciation of the segmental anatomy and vascular variations has made this test less necessary, and it has been replaced to a large extent by magnetic resonance angiography. We do not perform an arteriogram routinely and have been satisfied with the information obtained by noninvasive studies. Neither CT nor angiography is always accurate, and in some cases the true extent of the tumor can be appreciated only at the time of laparotomy.

Staging and Treatment

The treatment program for patients with liver tumors depends mainly on the extent of disease at the time of diagnosis and whether or not the tumor is resectable. The staging system has evolved over the years to reflect this fact. The Children's Oncology Group has adopted the system used in European studies by SIOPEL (*Société Internationale d'Oncologie Pédiatrique*, Epithelial Liver Group), which is detailed in Figure 22-6. This more complex grouping system allows a precise description of the pretreatment extent of disease, hence the name *PRETEXT*; it is a better tool to compare outcome between various treatment strategies. A patient may be labeled as *group III A$_p$, v, m*, meaning that three out of four "sectors" are involved by tumor, there is ingrowth into the vena cava, and metastases are present (see Fig. 22-6). The former staging system designed by the Children's Cancer Study Group often is used to report prognosis (Table 22-3). This system refers to postoperative staging, whereas the SIOPEL grouping system is applied before treatment. The treatment of choice is complete resection of the primary tumor. For localized disease in which imaging studies predict resectability by segmentectomy or lobectomy, a primary resection is indicated, followed by chemotherapy. When the tumor is large or multicentric, a safe and complete resection is more likely to be achieved with a strategy of initial biopsy, chemotherapy, and delayed primary resection (Fig. 22-7). The biopsy can be done

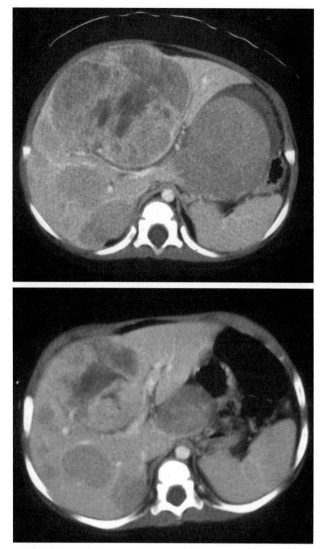

FIGURE 22-5 ■ Patient who presented at 14 months of age with multifocal hepatoblastoma (top). Despite a good response with chemotherapy (bottom, after two courses), liver transplantation is the only hope for cure for these patients.

through a small laparotomy or under laparoscopic or imaging guidance. Most hepatoblastomas show a good response to the initial cycles of chemotherapy, but eventually only patients with complete resection have an opportunity for cure even when adjunctive therapy is employed. The current availability of the Cavitron ultrasonic aspirator (CUSA) dissector (Valley Labs, Boulder, Co.), rapid transfusers, and hypothermia/controlled hypotension/hemodilution techniques has made hepatic resection a much safer and well-controlled procedure. The operative mortality for hepatic resection in children is less than 5% in most major centers.

Operative Technique

A detailed description of operative techniques is beyond the scope of this chapter, but several principles are worth highlighting. A thorough knowledge of the segmental anatomy as described by Couinaud is essential (Fig. 22-8). Appropriate blood products must be readily available;

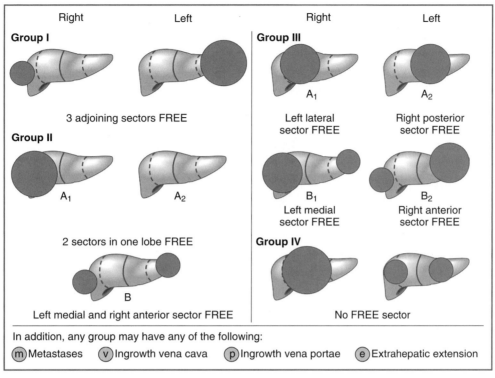

FIGURE 22-6 ■ SIOPEL pretreatment grouping system, also called *PRETEXT*.

lower extremity intravenous sites should not be used because of potential blood loss from the vena cava or the hepatic veins with the need to clamp the former. At times, total vascular isolation of the liver is needed. A right subcostal incision with left-sided extension usually provides adequate exposure, although a midline T extension or a thoracoabdominal incision may be useful in older children. On entering the abdomen, an evaluation is made of lymph nodes at the porta hepatis and other signs of tumor extension beyond the liver. Resectability is confirmed after complete mobilization of the liver; intraoperative ultrasound is a useful adjunct, especially when the tumor is close to the hepatic veins. According to the site of the tumor, the appropriate branches of the hepatic artery, portal vein, and bile duct are isolated. If excessive bleeding is encountered during transsection of the liver parenchyma, the intact vessels supplying the liver tissue to be preserved may be clamped temporarily for 10 to 15 minutes (total time ≤60 minutes). After the resection is completed, the raw surface of the remaining liver is checked carefully for bleeding sites or bile leak. Closed-suction drains are used to drain the suprahepatic and

subhepatic spaces. T-tube drainage of the bile duct is contraindicated.

Most infants and children tolerate hepatic resection well. The major cause of morbidity and mortality is intraoperative hemorrhage. Although the availability of rapid transfusion systems makes this less of a problem than in the past, minimizing blood loss is an important consideration. Because of the potential risk of circulating tumor cells, autotransfusion, a technique often used in cases with significant blood loss from a severe liver injury, is not applicable.

Postoperative Management

The three major metabolic problems encountered after an extensive hepatic resection are hypoglycemia, hypoalbuminemia, and hypoprothrombinemia. Children are given maintenance infusions containing 10% dextrose in 0.25% normal saline, and daily infusions of albumin and vitamin K for the first postoperative week when there has been an extensive resection or prolonged clamping of the hilar vessels intraoperatively. Most children are able to tolerate oral intake in 2 to 3 days. Postoperative complications include bleeding from the edge of the remaining liver, subphrenic abscess, biliary fistula, wound infection, and occasionally biliary obstruction from inadvertent ligation of the remaining bile duct. Hepatic regeneration occurs quickly in children and may be complete by the second to third postoperative week. Because of the fact that some chemotherapeutic agents (doxorubicin) interfere with hepatic regeneration, chemotherapy is withheld for 3 weeks in children whose liver function seems compromised because of the extent of resection or concomitant liver disease (i.e., cirrhosis with HCC).

TABLE 22-3 ■ Children's Cancer Study Group Staging

Stage	Description
I	Tumor localized and completely resected
II	Tumor resected with microscopic residual disease
III	Unresectable tumor or gross residual disease
IV	Metastatic disease to lungs, bone, bone marrow, brain

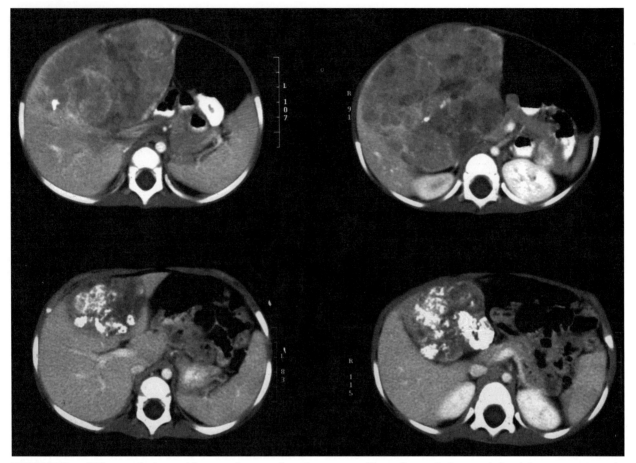

FIGURE 22-7 ■ CT scan of a hepatoblastoma that may have been resectable at diagnosis (top row), but lobectomy was made easier and safer after chemotherapy (bottom row). Prominent calcifications are seen after chemotherapy, and the right portal vein is now clearly free (bottom left).

Adjuvant Therapy and Prognosis

The best survival in children with hepatoblastoma is achieved in patients with stage I or II disease (complete macroscopic resection) who receive chemotherapy (80% to 100%); survival decreases to 40% in the presence of gross residual tumor. Survival may be 95% for stage I tumors with predominantly fetal histology; chemotherapy is not necessary in these patients. Less than 50% of patients with hepatoblastoma have completely resectable tumors at diagnosis. With the strategy of initial biopsy and preoperative chemotherapy, nearly 75% of initially unresectable tumors become resectable, with patients achieving a complete remission after surgery (stage I or II). This strategy generally consists of four courses of cisplatin, vincristine, and 5-fluorouracil. Doxorubicin, carboplatin, cyclophosphamide, etoposide, and others also have been used to treat pediatric liver cancer. Newer drugs, such as irinotecan, are being studied. Neoadjuvant chemotherapy not only increases resectability but also reduces the risk of intraoperative tumor spill and the need for blood replacement. A rapid decrease in AFP levels with chemotherapy seems to predict a better prognosis.

When hepatoblastoma remains unresectable, a cure can be achieved only with orthotopic liver transplantation (see Fig. 22-5). Five-year survival rates of 70% to 80% have been reported in combined series from several centers. Because tumor cells may become resistant to chemotherapy and because heroic attempts at resection invariably result in tumor recurrence, the current trend is to evaluate the response to chemotherapy after two courses and plan the transplantation after the fourth course in patients whose tumor appears unresectable. The availability of a living donor greatly facilitates planning; when resectability seems feasible but doubtful, the donor can be on standby and used only after intraoperative assessment of the extent of tumor. Two more courses of chemotherapy are used after transplantation. Success has been reported in patients who had lung metastases that regressed with preoperative chemotherapy; in these patients, the duration of post-transplantation chemotherapy is increased to four or more courses. Factors associated with a worse outcome include tumor recurrence before transplantation (as opposed to transplantation as the initial resection), anaplastic or undifferentiated histology, multicentricity with extrahepatic spread, vascular invasion, and the lack of response to preoperative chemotherapy.

Hepatic artery chemoembolization is a technique that has been described to improve resectability in selected patients. It results in drug levels within the tumor 50 to 400 times greater than with conventional chemotherapy,

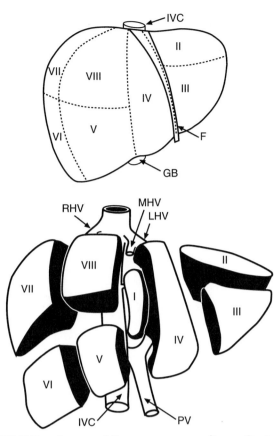

FIGURE 22-8 ▪ Segmental liver anatomy according to Couinaud.

without an increase in systemic toxicity. Other therapies, such as radiofrequency ablation; ultrasonic, microwave, or laser thermal ablation; and cryotherapy, are still at the experimental stage; some of these have been used in adult liver tumors, mostly for palliation. Although the overall survival for patients with hepatoblastoma is around 70% and improving steadily because of effective chemotherapy, the efficacy of adjuvant treatment for HCC is limited, resulting in a dismal 15% cure rate. Complete surgical resection is the only hope, but is more often achievable in the fibrolamellar variant than with the usual HCC. Liver transplantation for unresectable HCC has an extremely high failure rate and has been abandoned by most groups except for the fibrolamellar variant. This does not apply to situations in which transplantation is indicated for a metabolic disease such as tyrosinemia and the liver contains a small nodule of HCC. Because of the failure of current

chemotherapeutic agents, the addition of antiangiogenic agents is being explored; these include cyclooxygenase-2 inhibitors, anti–vascular endothelial growth factor antibodies, topotecan, thalidomide, and other substances.

SUGGESTED READINGS

Burrows PE, Dubois J, Kassarjan A: Pediatric hepatic vascular anomalies. Pediatr Radiol 31:533, 2001.

This article discusses techniques and imaging patterns of vascular anomalies of the liver.

Exelby PR, Filler RM, Grosfeld JL: Liver tumors in children in the particular reference to hepatoblastoma and hepatocellular carcinoma: American Academy of Pediatrics Surgical Section Surgery. J Pediatr Surg 10:329, 1975.

This is a classic review of many cases from the experience of members of the Surgical Section of the American Academy of Pediatrics. These results represent a good historical control with which to compare newer methods of treatment.

Han YM, Park HH, Lee JM, et al: Effectiveness of preoperative transarterial chemoembolization in presumed inoperable hepatoblastoma. J Vasc Interv Radiol 10:1275, 1999.

This article describes the successful use of hepatic arterial chemoembolization for unresectable hepatoblastoma.

Mulliken JB, Fishman SJ, Burrows PE: Vascular anomalies. Curr Probl Surg 37:517, 2002.

This excellent monograph describes the current classification and treatment of vascular anomalies.

Pimpalwar AP, Sharif K, Ramani P, et al: Strategy for hepatoblastoma management: Transplant versus nontransplant surgery. J Pediatr Surg 37:240, 2002.

This article from a busy transplant unit updates the role of liver transplant in the management of hepatoblastoma.

Pritchard J, Brown J, Shafford E, et al: Cisplatin, doxorubicin, and delayed surgery for childhood hepatoblastoma: A successful approach—results of the first prospective study of the International Society of Pediatric Oncology. J Clin Oncol 18:3819, 2000.

This article describes neoadjuvant and adjuvant therapy for hepatoblastoma.

Tomlinson GE, Finegold MJ: Tumors of the liver. In Pizzo PA, Poplack DG (eds): Principles and Practice of Pediatric Oncology, 4th ed. Philadelphia, Lippincott Williams & Wilkins, 2002, p 847.

This chapter in an oncology textbook provides a thorough review of malignant liver tumors in children.

23

Lymphomas

HODGKIN'S DISEASE

Hodgkin's disease, a malignant lymphoid disorder of unknown etiology, has a characteristic bimodal age-specific incidence. The first peak is between 15 and 40 years of age, and the second peak is between 45 and 55 years. Only 4% of patients with Hodgkin's disease are younger than 10 years of age; another 11% of patients are between 11 and 16 years old. Of all patients, 85% are older than age 17. Hodgkin's disease accounts for 5% of childhood malignancies. The incidence is approximately six cases per 1 million children. Hodgkin's disease is more common in boys in the first decade of life, but girls are affected more commonly during the teenage years. Young age is a favorable prognostic factor, with children younger than age 16 having the best prognosis and adults older than age 50 the worst prognosis. Hodgkin's disease in children has a natural history, tumor biology, and response to therapy that is similar to the disease in adults. There are, however, some unique aspects of Hodgkin's disease in children, including complications and late effects of therapy. Modern management of Hodgkin's disease has evolved since the 1980s through a better understanding of the predictability of tumor spread, development of clinical and pathologic staging criteria, and improvements in radiotherapy and chemotherapy.

Clinical Presentation

The most common cause of lymphadenopathy in children is benign lymphoid hyperplasia. This observation often delays the diagnosis of Hodgkin's disease because painless cervical lymphadenopathy is the most frequent presenting finding. Persistent and progressive lymph node enlargement eventually prompts the performance of cervical lymph node biopsy. Characteristically, lymph nodes involved by Hodgkin's disease are nontender, firm, and often rubbery. Cervical lymphadenopathy is present in almost 80% of cases of Hodgkin's disease in children. Enlarged axillary lymph nodes are noted in one third of patients, and inguinal lymph nodes are positive in only 5%. In more than 50% of patients, there is evidence of enlarged mediastinal lymph nodes in children with positive cervical nodes. Respiratory distress related to mediastinal lymph node enlargement is much less common in children with Hodgkin's disease than in children with non-Hodgkin's lymphoma (NHL) (Fig. 23-1). Facial swelling, a plethoric appearance from the neck up, and distended neck veins should alert the clinician to the possibility of superior vena caval obstruction from mediastinal involvement. Palpable lymphadenopathy may be present in the scalene lymph nodes above the clavicle in patients with mediastinal involvement. The spleen and liver are palpable on abdominal examination in only a relatively few patients with advanced disease. Malaise, anorexia, weight loss, and fever are observed in more than 30% of patients at the time of diagnosis.

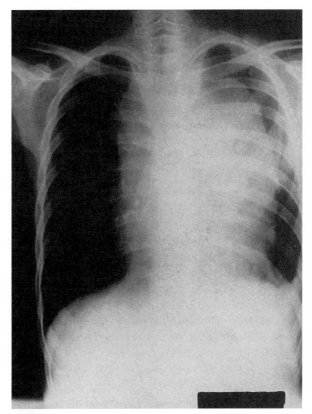

FIGURE 23-1 ■ Chest radiograph in a teenage boy with Hodgkin's disease and a mediastinal mass.

Diagnosis

The diagnosis of Hodgkin's disease is made by histologic evaluation of lymph node biopsy material. Reed-Sternberg cells, which are large mononuclear cells with abnormally basophilic nucleoli with multilobulation, must be seen to confirm the diagnosis. There are four histologic subclassifications of Hodgkin's disease: (1) lymphocyte predominance, (2) nodular sclerosing, (3) mixed cellularity, and (4) lymphocyte depletion. The most frequently observed subtype in children is nodular sclerosing (>65%), followed by mixed cellularity and lymphocyte predominance (Fig. 23-2). Lymphocyte depletion has the worst prognosis; this subtype is exceptionally uncommon in children. The best prognosis is observed in cases with lymphocyte predominance, which occurs more frequently in children younger than age 10 years than in other age groups. Occasionally, normal lymph nodes may be interspersed with nodes containing malignant cells, and a second biopsy may be necessary. In the absence of palpable peripheral lymph nodes and radiographic evidence of mediastinal disease, mediastinoscopy, thoracoscopy, and endoscopic biopsy or thoracotomy may be necessary to obtain tissue for diagnosis.

Staging

Clinical staging follows the recommendations set forth in the Ann Arbor staging classification (Table 23-1). A careful and detailed clinical history and complete physical examination are performed for each patient. Confirmation of "B" systemic symptoms, including a history of fever, night sweats, and weight loss, may be of prognostic importance. Pruritus is not a common finding in children, although it is in adults.

Baseline laboratory data include a complete blood cell count and differential smear and erythrocyte sedimentation rate. Other tests used as indicators of active disease in adults may be of less importance in children because the serum alkaline phosphatase level may be elevated as a result of bone growth, and the serum copper level can be elevated as a result of inflammation or infection. Baseline tests of liver and renal function also are obtained. Because none of these studies are specific, the diagnosis must be confirmed by a lymph node biopsy.

Many radiographic and scintigraphic tests are employed preoperatively in the clinical staging process. The most frequent site of disease is the chest. Anteroposterior and lateral chest radiographs are obtained routinely and often show most intrathoracic abnormalities.

TABLE 23-1 ■ Ann Arbor Staging Criteria for Hodgkin's Disease	
Stage*	**Definition**
I	Involvement of a single lymph node region (I) or a single extralymphatic organ or site (I_E)
II	Involvement of two or more lymph node regions on the same side of the diaphragm (II) or localized involvement of an extralymphatic organ or site and of one or more lymph node regions on the same side of the diaphragm (II_E)
III	Involvement of lymph node regions on both sides of the diaphragm (III), which also may be accompanied by involvement of the spleen (III_S) or by localized involvement of an extralymphatic organ or site (III_E) or both (III_{SE})
IV	Diffuse or disseminated involvement of one or more extralymphatic organs or tissues, with or without associated lymph node involvement

*The absence or presence of fever, night sweats, or unexplained weight loss (≥10% in the previous 6 months) also is noted in each case by adding the suffix "A" for no symptoms and "B" for symptoms.

Computed tomography (CT) of the chest provides additional information not seen on routine chest radiographs in approximately 10% of patients; CT is particularly useful in evaluating the pulmonary parenchyma. The pretreatment CT scan also serves as an excellent baseline to evaluate treatment response or subsequent relapse.

Lung involvement occurs in 5% to 10% of patients and may be related to direct extension from either a mass or paratracheal and hilar lymph nodes. The presence of pleural fluid most often reflects lymphatic or venous obstruction and resolves with treatment; it does not imply the presence of pleural disease. The presence of pericardial effusion usually suggests direct extension of disease into the pericardium. An echocardiogram may be a useful diagnostic test in these instances.

Lung and pericardial effusions are commonly staged as "E" lesions (extralymphatic extension) rather than stage IV disease. A practical working definition of an E lesion is disease outside of lymph nodes that can be encompassed in a curative radiotherapy field whether the disease is or is not in direct continuity with involved lymph nodes. Magnetic resonance imaging may be more useful than CT in differentiating residual fibrosis from tumor recurrence after initial therapy. Gallium-67 scintigraphy

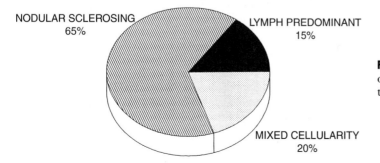

FIGURE 23-2 ■ Pie chart shows the histologic cell types of Hodgkin's disease. More than 65% of patients have the nodular sclerosing cell type.

evaluates supradiaphragmatic disease more effectively than intra-abdominal disease and may be useful in separating recurrent intrathoracic disease from a reactive fibrotic mass. A pretreatment scan helps establish if a given tumor takes up gallium and if follow-up studies would be informative.

Bipedal lymphangiography is an accurate method of evaluating pelvic and retroperitoneal lymph nodes. In centers where this test is performed routinely, the accuracy is greater than 95%. This is far greater than the accuracy observed in other centers where lymphangiography is an infrequently performed diagnostic study. Lymphangiography is technically more difficult to perform and interpret in children. The procedure requires heavy sedation or in some instances a general anesthetic. Lymphangiography is negative in 70% of pediatric patients and positive in 19%. Lymphangiography also shows abnormalities of reactive hyperplasia in 11% to 12% of children. The sensitivity of lymphangiography is 80% (e.g., disease was documented in four out of every five patients thought to have positive lymph nodes on the study). Complications of lymphangiography include allergic reactions, infection (lymphangitis), and, rarely, pulmonary (oil) embolism. Lymphangiography does not opacify the mesenteric lymph nodes in the porta hepatis, splenic hilum, or celiac axis—areas that may be involved in 15% to 20% of patients.

Many centers use abdominal CT to evaluate the retroperitoneum for enlarged lymph nodes. The criteria of involvement of lymph nodes by CT examination are based entirely on the size of the lymph nodes. The sensitivity of this test in children with Hodgkin's disease is only 40%. It is difficult to separate enlarged lymph nodes caused by reactive hyperplasia from lymph nodes containing tumor by size alone. CT cannot detect the structural changes noted in early involvement of small retroperitoneal lymph nodes and is accurate in assessing splenic involvement in only 19% of patients. A relative paucity of retroperitoneal fat makes it more difficult to evaluate lymph nodes by CT in most children than in adults. The spleen is involved in approximately 30% to 40% of patients and the liver in 5% of patients with Hodgkin's disease at the time of diagnosis. Visceral involvement does not always result in visceromegaly, and the lesions are often less than 1 cm in size, making them difficult to detect on CT, ultrasound, or scintigraphy. Bone involvement occurs in 5% of pediatric patients at diagnosis, a much lower incidence of involvement than in adults (10% to 20%). Bone marrow biopsy is performed as part of the surgical staging process. Magnetic resonance imaging visualizes the bone marrow cavity well and may provide a guide for sampling sites.

Surgical staging involves a staging laparotomy with splenectomy, multiple (×4) liver biopsy specimens (one wedge and one deep-needle biopsy from each lobe), and sampling of multiple lymph nodes from the splenic hilum; celiac axis; porta hepatis; right and left, high and low para-aortic areas; right and left, common and external iliac areas; and a mesenteric lymph node (see Table 23-2). This procedure must be carried out in a concise manner, carefully separating each sample for the pathologist to examine. Although partial splenectomy and selective

TABLE 23-2 ■ Staging Laparotomy for Hodgkin's Disease
Midline incision
Splenectomy
Partial splenectomy misses 13%
Liver biopsy ×4
Needle from each lobe—2
Wedge from each lobe—2
Multiple lymph node sites
Splenic hilum, porta hepatis, suprapancreatic, bilateral para-aortic, bilateral iliac, mesenteric
Oophoropexy in girls

splenectomy (based on the presence of visual or palpable splenic nodules or large splenic hilar nodes at laparotomy) have been advocated by some investigators, these procedures have a significant risk of false-negative assessment (12% to 15%) of the extent of disease. Accurate staging requires a complete splenectomy. The splenic hilar node area and the other biopsy sites are marked with titanium clips. Titanium avoids the scatter of the CT beam on follow-up studies seen when stainless steel clips are used. Para-aortic lymph node biopsies should coincide with enlarged lymph nodes seen on CT or identified by lymphangiography. These studies should be available for viewing in the operating room at the time of laparotomy. An intraoperative abdominal radiograph may be useful to confirm proper biopsy. The use of staging laparotomy is controversial at present. Some argue that the main purpose of staging laparotomy is to identify patients who should be treated with chemotherapy, and because current protocols are mostly chemotherapy-based, laparotomy is unnecessary. Staging laparotomy is used less frequently now.

In girls, a bilateral oophoropexy should be performed by mobilizing and tacking the ovaries in the midline behind the uterus to protect them from possible radiation therapy delivered in an inverted-Y port, which may be necessary in approximately 20% of patients. A titanium clip can be placed on the ovarian tacking sutures for visualization by the radiation oncologist on an abdominal scout radiograph obtained before marking the prospective radiation port. Bone marrow biopsy specimens should be obtained at the conclusion of the staging laparotomy under the same anesthetic.

Results of Laparotomy

Staging laparotomy documented that inaccurate clinical staging was a frequent occurrence. Many patients were either understaged or overstaged (35% to 40%). After laparotomy, an increase in the stage was seen more commonly because of unsuspected splenic (26%), splenic hilar node, celiac node, or porta hepatis involvement. Of cases, 3% had unsuspected liver involvement. The most common site of lymph node involvement in clinical stage I and II cases is the splenic hilar node (10%), and this is almost always in association with splenic involvement. Para-aortic lymph nodes are positive in 5% of clinical stage I and II cases. Porta hepatis and mesenteric lymph nodes are positive in 1% and less than 1% of patients respectively. Liver (2%) and bone marrow (<1%) involvement is detected infrequently in clinical stage I and II patients. In most cases, liver and bone marrow involvement is detected only after the presence of splenic involvement. Of interest are the results of staging laparotomy in patients with cervical lymph node involvement. Subdiaphragmatic involvement is seen in 11% of patients with suprahyoid cervical lesions and 38% of patients with infrahyoid cervical disease.

Favorable groups of patients with clinical stage I disease that have less than a 10% chance of having subdiaphragmatic disease include (1) patients with mediastinal disease only, (2) males with lymphocyte predominance histologic subtype, and (3) females with clinical stage I disease. In children with clinical stage III disease, the role of laparotomy is to down-stage the patient by proving there is no subdiaphragmatic involvement. Approximately 28% of clinical stage III patients are down-staged by a staging laparotomy. The results of staging show that stage I disease is more common in the youngest patients: 18% of children younger than age 10 years have stage I tumors compared with 7% of children 11 to 16 years old and 11% of older patients. Stage IV disease is uncommon in the young children. Only 3% of children younger than age 10 years have stage IV disease compared with 13% of children 11 to 16 years old and 11% of older patients. Stages II and III comprise 75% of the patients in all age groups.

Despite the benefits of staging laparotomy, many complications are related to the procedure, although surgical mortality is rare. Atelectasis, wound infection, intestinal obstruction, left-sided pleural effusion, retroperitoneal hematoma, subdiaphragmatic abscess, transient pancreatitis, and thrombotic episodes have been observed in 6% to 7% of patients. The most common complication is intestinal obstruction (2% to 4% of patients), which is usually a late event that often occurs more than 6 months postoperatively. There is an increased risk of intestinal obstruction in children receiving abdominal irradiation with an inverted-Y field. Most patients are managed by simple lysis of adhesions, and bowel resection is usually not necessary.

Long-term complications of staging laparotomy are related to the asplenic state. The incidence of postsplenectomy sepsis in patients with Hodgkin's disease was 11% to 13% before the development of polyvalent pneumococcal, hemophilus, and meningococcal vaccines and use of perioperative and prophylactic antibiotics. Most postsplenectomy infections are caused by encapsulated organisms with cell walls, including pneumococci and *Haemophilus influenzae*, as well as by *Streptococcus* and *Neisseria* species. Even before splenectomy, some patients with advanced Hodgkin's disease show evidence of immunologic dysfunction characterized by anergy to skin-test antigen challenge and an increased susceptibility to bacterial, fungal, and viral infections. Herpes zoster may occur in 33% of patients with Hodgkin's disease. Routine use of vaccines for the three most commonly involved encapsulated organisms should decrease the frequency of sepsis after splenectomy. Vaccines also have been shown to be effective in children with sickle cell disease who are functionally asplenic. The more recently developed conjugated pneumococcal vaccine should be used in sequence with the older pure polysaccharide vaccine to achieve the broadest coverage and duration of immunity along with the HIB-conjugate and meningococcal vaccines. Recommendations for revaccination from the Centers for Disease Control are evolving, but currently are for every 3 years for children younger than age 10 years and every 5 to 6 years for individuals older than age 10. The required interval for the conjugate pneumococcal vaccine has not been established. It is preferable to administer the vaccines before splenectomy to achieve the highest levels of antibody production, but if this opportunity is lost, patients still should be vaccinated. It has been shown that immunization in the midst of therapy (chemotherapy or radiotherapy or both) is often ineffective, so vaccination 6 to 12 months after completion of treatment should be considered if not done preoperatively. Perioperative parenteral antibiotics are started 30 minutes before the operation and continued for 24 hours. Most pediatric oncologists favor the postoperative use of long-term prophylactic penicillin (or erythromycin if the patient is allergic to penicillin), although their efficacy in conjunction with current immunizations has not been established with randomized studies. Antibiotics and immunization have significantly reduced the incidence of postsplenectomy sepsis in children with Hodgkin's disease but have not eliminated it completely. Combined programs of chemotherapy and irradiation are employed in the treatment of many of these patients, which reduces their immunity and increases the risk of opportunistic infection despite precautions.

Therapy

The early treatment of Hodgkin's disease was predicated on the concept of spread of the disease from the primary area of occurrence to the next contiguous lymph node site. Radiotherapy was administered according to the extent of tumor detected by clinical staging and the results of staging laparotomy. Irradiation was applied to the area initially involved by disease (involved field irradiation) and contiguous lymphoid spread (extended field). If the mediastinal lymphatics were involved (stage II) and the results of laparotomy were negative, mantle radiation was given to include the lymphatics of the lower mediastinum and the splenic hilum and para-aortic lymph nodes to the L-4 level. Patients with stage III disease received total nodal irradiation with an inverted-Y field. The effectiveness of chemotherapy in the management of stage IV patients with combinations of drugs, including nitrogen mustard, vincristine, procarbazine, and prednisone (MOPP) and more recently doxorubicin (Adriamycin), bleomycin, vinblastine, and dacarbazide (ABVD), significantly changed the overall treatment plan for this disorder. The combination of chemotherapy and radiation was used to control stage III disease and was found to be more effective than extended field irradiation alone. This was also true in children with relapse. Combination therapy allowed the dose for each modality to be reduced and made it possible to lessen early toxicity and adverse late effects. This was especially important in the management of Hodgkin's disease in growing children.

This combined therapy also has diminished the role of staging laparotomy, which was crucial to define the

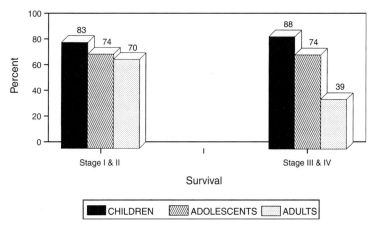

FIGURE 23-3 ■ Long-term survival in Hodgkin's disease in children is higher than in adults in all stages. The best results are achieved in children younger than 10 years of age at the time of diagnosis.

anatomic extent of tumor when irradiation was used as a single modality. The results of these newer protocols were dramatic, with the overall 5-year survival of children with Hodgkin's disease reaching 90%. The youngest patients have the best prognosis. Data concerning 2163 patients with Hodgkin's disease from Stanford University indicate that the overall relapse-free survival is 80% in children younger than 10 years of age compared with 74% in children 11 to 16 years old, and 64% in adults. Long-term projected survival at 20 years is 74% for children and adolescents versus only 37% for adults. For patients with stages I and II disease, the projected 26-year freedom from relapse rate is 83% for children, 73% for adolescents, and 70% for adults with localized disease. The projected 26-year survival rates were statistically similar for children (67%) and adolescents (78%); however, both were much better than the 39% predicted survival in adults. In patients with advanced disease (stages III and IV), relapse-free survival for children was 77%, for adolescents was 75%, and for adults was only 57%. Of the children, 88% are alive at 26 years compared with only 39% of adults (Fig. 23-3).

The 1990s produced changes in treatment and controversies in management in an effort to refine care, maintain a high survival rate, reduce the relapse rate, and limit adverse late effects. Although new drug protocols have been used, there is no clear advantage to alternating courses of MOPP and ABVD compared with either given alone. ABVD seems to have less toxicity and fewer adverse late effects than MOPP. Other combinations of drugs have been employed with the addition of cyclophosphamide and chlorambucil to the previously used agents; however, long-term data concerning any improved effectiveness are not available.

Complications of Therapy

There are significant complications of treatment related to chemotherapy and radiation. Complications of chemotherapy depend on the use of specific agents and include myelosuppression, cardiovascular deterioration (anthracyclines), pulmonary impairment (bleomycin), gonadal dysfunction (alkylating agents), and neurologic impairment (*Vinca* alkyloids). Therapy-related infertility is a major concern because long-term survival is

anticipated in more than 90% of patients. Since the development of testicular-shielding techniques in boys and oophoropexy during laparotomy in girls, radiation-induced gonadal dysfunction has been reduced considerably. Most cases of testicular azoospermia are caused by treatment with six cycles of MOPP or MOPP analogues and are often irreversible. Recovery of spermatogenesis is possible with only three courses of MOPP, and the use of ABVD carries a low risk of sterility.

Other adverse effects of treatment include tissue injury related to irradiation, including hypothyroidism (two thirds of cases), myelosuppression, pericarditis, pneumonitis, nephritis, skeletal hypoplasia, growth retardation, bone osteonecrosis, breast hypoplasia, and gonadal dysfunction. Growth impairment is more common in children younger than 13 years of age receiving doses greater than 35 Gy to large areas of the body. The thyroid gland in children is more sensitive to radiation exposure, and the incidence of hypothyroidism is dose related. The risk of thyroid dysfunction in children receiving less than 25 Gy to the neck is 17% but is 78% for children receiving more than 25 Gy. Reversal of thyroid dysfunction may occur in 36% of children. Second neoplasms, including thyroid carcinoma, parathyroid adenoma, soft tissue sarcoma, osteogenic sarcoma, breast cancer, and basal cell carcinoma, usually occur in the radiation portal and are probably radiation induced.

There is also an increased risk of acute nonlymphoblastic leukemia and non-Hodgkin's lymphoma (NHL). For the survivors of Hodgkin's disease who develop leukemia, prior splenectomy carried a twofold risk, whereas the use of nitrogen mustard and procarbazine carried a ninefold risk of this second malignancy. Cyclophosphamide and chlorambucil also have been implicated in the development of leukemia after treatment of Hodgkin's disease. The risk of leukemia as a second tumor is related to chemotherapy or combined treatment with chemotherapy and irradiation and is highest in the group of patients that relapse and receive salvage chemotherapy after failing radiation therapy (6% to 16% of patients). The occurrence of leukemia as a second neoplasm is observed between 3 and 9 years posttherapy (mean 5 years). The risk of leukemia is less after ABVD therapy than with MOPP. The lowest incidence of leukemia is observed in patients who remain in remission after treatment with radiation therapy alone (0.2%). New cases of leukemia are not seen after 10 years. The risk of developing aggressive NHL approaches that of leukemia with time and appears cumulative: 2% at 5 years, 5% at 10 years, 9% at 15 years, and 18% at 20 years. These data indicate that long-term follow-up is essential.

Future Directions

Now that cure can be achieved in most cases of Hodgkin's disease, the goal of future therapy is to refine treatment programs to maintain the current cure rate, reduce complications and adverse late effects, and assure affected children an optimal quality of life. Current trends suggest that therapy should be tailored according to the patient's age and the stage and extent of disease. For older teenagers who have achieved growth, with localized (stage I or II) disease, radiation therapy alone may be appropriate treatment. For young children in whom growth and development is a major consideration and children with advanced (stage III) or bulky disease (especially in the mediastinum or upper abdomen), combined-modality treatment programs using lower doses of chemotherapy and limiting irradiation to less than 25 Gy yield the highest cure rate with the least morbidity. Systemic chemotherapy alone for early-stage disease is being evaluated. The current role of staging laparotomy with splenectomy is controversial, and its indications may need to be redefined. Although surgical staging is essential if radiation therapy alone is to be employed, when systemic chemotherapy is used, either alone or in combination with radiation therapy, many centers rely on clinical staging alone.

NON-HODGKIN'S LYMPHOMA

NHL in childhood comprises a heterogeneous group of diseases that represent 7% to 10% of all pediatric malignancies. NHL is the third most common pediatric malignancy, exceeded only by leukemia and brain tumors. There is a male predominance with a boy-to-girl ratio of 3:1. Although there are more than 15 different types of adult NHL, more than 90% of children with NHL fit into three histologic subtypes: lymphoblastic lymphoma (LBL), small noncleaved cell (Burkitt's and non-Burkitt's) lymphoma,

TABLE 23-4 ■ Immunodeficiency States Associated with an Increased Risk of Non-Hodgkin's Lymphoma
HIV
Wiskott-Aldrich syndrome
Bloom's syndrome
Ataxia-telangiectasia
Combined immunodeficiency syndrome
X-linked lymphoproliferative syndrome
Organ transplantation

and large cell (histiocytic) lymphoma (Table 23-3). All of these tumors are rapidly growing, aggressive neoplasms with a propensity for widespread systemic dissemination. Although the cause of NHL is unknown, many factors, including viral infections and immunodeficiency, have been implicated. Endemic forms of Burkitt's lymphoma have been observed in Africa and New Guinea and may represent 50% of all childhood cancers in those regions. Epstein-Barr virus (EBV) DNA and nuclear antigens have been identified in 95% of African Burkitt's lymphoma cells. The sporadic form of Burkitt's lymphoma occurs in Europe and North and South America. Although these tumors appear histologically similar to African Burkitt's tumor, EBV DNA is identified in only 10% to 20% of these cases. The occurrence of EBV-related NHL in patients with a variety of congenital and acquired immunodeficiency syndromes is well documented (Table 23-4), including human immunodeficiency virus (HIV), Wiskott-Aldrich syndrome, Bloom's syndrome, ataxia telangiectasia, severe combined immunodeficiency disease, and X-linked lymphoproliferative syndrome; it also is seen in organ transplant recipients who are chronically immunosuppressed. EBV-induced NHL occurring in immunodeficient patients results from disturbances of the immune defenses of the host. Most cases of endemic and sporadic Burkitt's lymphoma contain a translocation of a segment of the long arm of chromosome 8 containing the c-*myc* proto-oncogene to the long arm of chromosome 14 (8q–;14q+). Translocation of the c-*myc* proto-oncogene produces an abnormal expression of its gene product, resulting in a cell capable of unlimited proliferation, leading to neoplastic transformation.

TABLE 23-3 ■ Non-Hodgkin's Lymphoma: Histologic Correlation with Biologic Factors			
Histology	**Phenotype**	**Cytogenetic**	**Clinical**
Lymphoblastic (28.3%)	T cell	14q11t (11;14),t(1;14), (8;14),t(10;14)	Mediastinal mass, effusion, SVCS
	Early pre-B cell	7q34	Adenopathy
Small cell, noncleaved (38.6%)	B cell	8q24	Abdominal mass, tumor lysis, jaw
	Burkitt's	t(8;14)t(8;22)	
	Non-Burkitt's	t(2;8)	
Large cell, histiocytic (26.1%)	B cell	t(2;5)	Extranodal sites
	T cell	(p23;q35)	Lung, face, skin, bone

Tumor Classification

Lymphoid malignancies may be classified according to morphology, immunophenotype, histochemical staining, cytogenetic markers, and molecular analyses. In NHL, the tumor cells retain certain functional and surface features of the cell lines from which they are derived: either B cells or T cells. B cells are distinguished by showing a rearrangement of the immunoglobulin genes and expression of the product of these genes in the cytoplasm or on the cell surface or by B cell–specific cell surface antigens shown by reactivity with a panel of anti–B cell antibodies. T cells can be identified by demonstration of expression of T cell–specific surface antigens or the presence of rearrangement of T-cell receptor genes.

Most NHL cases can be classified by histologic subtype (see Table 23-3) into three major groups: (1) LBL (28.1%), (2) small noncleaved cell (Burkitt's and non-Burkitt's) lymphoma (38.8%), and (3) large cell (histiocytic) lymphoma (26.3%). Most LBLs express T-cell surface antigens. Small noncleaved cell lymphomas have a mature B-cell surface antigen (mainly immunoglobulin M), and large cell lymphomas can be divided into two histopathologic subtypes: an immunoblastic B-cell tumor and a large cell anaplastic tumor derived from T cells.

Clinical Presentation

NHL in children frequently presents with generalized lymphoid and extranodal involvement. The disease often has an abrupt onset with rapid growth and widespread progression. All lymph nodes, including Peyer's patches in the bowel, mediastinum, thymus, Waldeyer's ring, pelvic organs, liver, and spleen, may be involved. Extralymphoid involvement is observed in the skin, testis, bone, bone marrow, and central nervous system. The general pattern of clinical presentation correlates well with the histologic subtype of the tumor.

LBL usually presents above the diaphragm with 50% to 75% of patients having an anterior mediastinal mass (Fig. 23-4). Supradiaphragmatic lymphadenopathy is also present. Large, bulky mediastinal masses may be associated with pleural effusions and often respiratory symptoms because of compression of the trachea (wheezing, dyspnea, cough, tachypnea, and respiratory distress). Occasionally, dysphagia is observed from compression of the esophagus. Superior vena caval obstruction and cardiac constriction may be encountered and are characterized by distended neck veins; neck, upper extremity, and facial edema; and plethoric appearance of the neck and face. Mental confusion related to hypoxia also may be noted. In patients with generalized lymphadenopathy or hepatosplenomegaly, bone marrow involvement and central nervous system spread should be suspected. If more than 25% of the bone marrow is replaced by lymphoblasts, the child probably has T-cell lymphoblastic leukemia.

Small noncleaved cell (Burkitt's or non-Burkitt's) lymphoma is a B-cell tumor that usually presents in the abdomen. This is a fast-growing tumor with doubling times observed within 24 hours in some cases. Although the endemic (African) and sporadic forms have a similar histologic appearance, they differ in their clinical presentation. The endemic form first appears in the eye, orbit, or jaw (72%), and the sporadic form is almost always abdominal. The endemic form occurs in more tropical environments and peaks in children 4 to 9 years old. The sporadic form has a wider geographic distribution and a broader age distribution. Of sporadic cases, 95% occur in nonblacks. Most endemic cases occur in native populations indigenous to Africa. There is a 3:1 boy-to-girl ratio seen in endemic Burkitt's lymphoma. Male involvement in abdominal lymphoma (Burkitt's and non-Burkitt's) in the 5- to 8-year age group may be 5:1 to 10:1; however, in teenagers with sporadic B-cell lymphoma, the sexes are affected more equally.

In abdominal lymphoma, more than 60% of cases involve the small bowel, especially the ileum, and probably arise in Peyer's patches. Other reported sites of

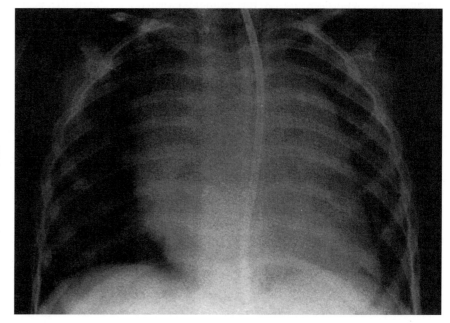

FIGURE 23-4 ■ Large mediastinal mass in a child with T-cell NHL who presented with respiratory distress.

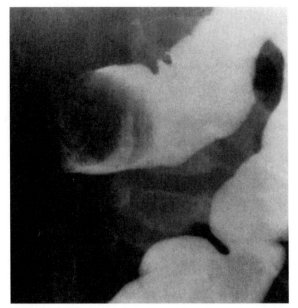

FIGURE 23-5 ■ Barium enema study shows an ileocolic intussusception in a 5-year-old boy. The lead point was a B-cell NHL.

intra-abdominal involvement include the colon, appendix, Meckel's diverticulum, ovaries, kidneys, liver, and lymph nodes in the mesentery and retroperitoneal space. Clinical presentation may vary and includes abdominal pain, anorexia, and right lower quadrant tenderness that may be mistaken for appendicitis; the presence of an abdominal mass, acute cramping pain, bilious vomiting, and evidence of intestinal obstruction associated with an intussusception occurring in children older than age 5 years has a high likelihood of being caused by a pathologic lead point (Fig. 23-5). A chronic nonstrangulating intussusception in the cecum of preadolescents and teenagers most often is caused by lymphoma. Children with massive abdominal involvement by bulky disease associated with ascites have an increased risk of developing tumor lysis syndrome. In cases that are not associated with acute symptoms or intestinal obstruction, a bone marrow aspirate and biopsy may avoid the need for laparotomy in 20% of patients. The presence of L-3 lymphoblasts involving 6% to 25% of the marrow is sufficient to make the diagnosis of Burkitt's or B-cell lymphoma. Children with more than 25% L-3 lymphoblasts in the marrow have B-cell leukemia. If there is an acute abdominal picture or intussusception, laparotomy is performed; if the tumor is localized, it should be resected when possible, but attempts at resection of extensive lesions should be discouraged because they only delay the onset of chemotherapy, which is the curative modality.

Large cell lymphomas (histiocytic) often occur in extranodal sites and are widely disseminated. Primary sites may include the skin, testis, eye, tonsils, soft tissues, and occasionally mediastinum but almost never the abdomen. Most of the tumors are of B-cell origin; however, they are occasionally T cell and sometimes null cell (non–T cell, non–B cell) in origin. Large cell lymphomas occur more often in older children 10 to 15 years old.

Diagnosis

Because NHL is such a heterogeneous group of diseases, each of which is treated differently, it is essential to perform a diagnostic biopsy in a facility that is fully capable of performing the important histopathology studies, immunophenotyping, and cytogenetic studies essential to establishing the diagnosis of NHL. Palpable cervical and supraclavicular lymph nodes are easily accessible masses.

In patients with respiratory distress as a result of a large mediastinal mass, a general anesthetic carries significant morbidity. A biopsy of a cervical lymph node using a local anesthetic with the patient sitting upright is often useful in these situations. Occasionally, short-term, low-dose radiation therapy to the chest results in prompt relief of respiratory embarrassment, but radiotherapy makes diagnosis difficult if part of the mass is not shielded for future biopsy. A similar problem occurs with the systemic administration of steroids. Of patients, 20% have bone marrow involvement at the time of diagnosis. Bilateral bone marrow biopsy specimens result in a higher yield than a single biopsy specimen. If the patient has a pleural effusion or ascites, cytologic studies and immunophenotyping from aspirates often can be diagnostic without a tissue biopsy. Other pretreatment tests include a complete blood cell count and differential smear, liver and renal function tests, values for serum uric acid, calcium, phosphorus, lactate dehydrogenase, and serum electrolyte levels. Also needed are a chest radiograph, chest or abdominal CT scan (according to the presenting findings on physical examination), scintigraphic bone scan and gallium scan, and lumbar puncture to evaluate cerebrospinal fluid for cytologic study. In contrast to patients with Hodgkin's disease, lymphangiography and staging laparotomy are not required in children with NHL.

Staging

Although the Ann Arbor staging system used for Hodgkin's disease was tested in NHL, it provided poor prognostic discrimination. The most frequently used staging system is based on the Murphy staging criteria. This system characterizes patients with localized disease (stage I and II), who have a better prognosis than patients with primary tumors in unfavorable sites (mediastinum, thymus, epidural, paraspinal, or primary central nervous system) or patients with more advanced disease (stage III with disease on both sides of the diaphragm and stage IV with disseminated disease). The staging system used for endemic Burkitt's lymphoma uses tumor location and tumor burden to identify the five stages.

Treatment

The treatment of NHL depends on histology, stage, and immunophenotype. Current multiagent protocols use intensive therapy often for much shorter intervals than were historically used. Survival rates in the 90% range are achieved for small noncleaved cell tumors and large cell immunoblastic tumors and in the 80% to 90% range for LBLs and anaplastic large cell tumors. Most tumors require prophylactic therapy for central nervous system involvement generally using intrathecal administration of methotrexate or ara-C. These agents generally have supplanted the use of craniospinal irradiation, which is less effective and associated with more adverse effects, including growth and intellectual impairment.

Tumors currently are treated based on their cell markers and not their less precise histologic classification. The B-cell tumors, including Burkitt's and Burkitt's-like (small noncleaved cell) lymphoma and large cell immunoblastic B-cell tumors, are treated with short-duration but intensive therapy, which has proved more effective than less intense but prolonged therapy. Current regimens include high-dose methotrexate and ara-C in conjunction with additional agents such as ifosfamide or etoposide.

Therapeutic trials for (T-cell) LBL employ modifications of standard acute lymphocytic leukemia (ALL) therapy with a goal to increase survival. Results suggest that the addition of multiple courses of high-dose methotrexate may increase survival significantly. Another successful modification has been the addition of high-dose L-asparaginase to the therapeutic regimen. Both alterations have increased survival rates significantly. Optimal therapy for large cell anaplastic tumors has not been established. Modifications of several B-cell lymphoma protocols have been used with relative success.

All childhood NHLs respond to a wide range of agents probably because of their high growth fraction. Radiotherapy is used rarely except for some patients with residual local disease after induction therapy. Patients with refractory or relapsed NHL have been treated with high-dose chemotherapy programs followed by autologous or allogeneic bone marrow transplantation. Patients treated by bone marrow transplantation after the first relapse (early) have a better survival following the transplant (50% at 2 years) than patients with refractory disease (5% to 20%) treated later. Recurrent tumor is the major cause of bone marrow transplantation failure.

Tumor Lysis Syndrome

A major complication of treatment of NHL is tumor lysis syndrome. This complication may be anticipated in any patient with disseminated disease or excessively bulky disease with a large tumor burden. Tumor lysis syndrome is related to hyperuricemia as a result of rapid destruction of the tumor cells when treatment is initiated. This problem is compounded in some cases by compromise of renal function as a result of bilateral kidney infiltration by lymphoma. Administration of allopurinol and hyperhydration with 3 to 4 L/m^2 of intravenous fluids may prevent the adverse effects of rapid tumor lysis. Alkalinization of the urine is helpful in improving the solubility of uric acid. If hyperphosphatemia occurs, however, alkalinization must be stopped because calcium phosphate precipitates may occur in an alkaline environment. Diuretics must be used with caution because they may lower the urine pH and enhance hyperuricemia. Renal dialysis may be necessary as a life-saving intervention if metabolic complications, such as hyperkalemia, acidosis, and hyperphosphatemia, cannot be controlled otherwise.

SUGGESTED READINGS

Glick RD, LaQuaglia MP: Lymphomas of the anterior mediastinum. Semin Pediatr Surg 8:69-77, 1999.

The diagnostic strategies for children presenting with an anterior mediastinal mass are discussed.

Hudson MM, Donaldson SS: Hodgkin's disease. In Pizzo PA, Poplack DG (eds): Principles and Practice of Pediatric Oncology, 4th ed. Philadelphia, Lippincott Williams & Wilkins, 2002.

A comprehensive, contemporary summary of therapy for pediatric Hodgkin's disease is presented.

Jenkins D, Doyle J, Berry M, et al: Hodgkin's disease in children: Treatment with MOPP and low dose, extended field irradiation without laparotomy. Med Pediatr Oncol 18:265, 1990.

This article documents the use of clinical staging without a staging laparotomy when combined therapy (irradiation and chemotherapy) is employed in the management of children with advanced Hodgkin's disease.

Kurtzberg J, Graham ML: Non-Hodgkin's lymphoma: Biologic classification and implication for therapy. Pediatr Clin North Am 38:443, 1991.

This report concerning children with NHL presents an updated review of the current concepts of management of this heterogeneous group of malignant tumors.

Link MP, Donaldson SS, Berard CW, et al: Results of treatment of childhood localized non-Hodgkin's lymphoma with combination chemotherapy with or without radiography. N Engl J Med 322:1169, 1990.

Radiotherapy is probably not indicated in children with localized NHL treated with combination chemotherapy.

Magrath IT: Malignant non-Hodgkin's lymphomas in children. In Pizzo PA, Poplack DG (eds): Principles and Practice of Pediatric Oncology, 4th ed. Philadelphia, Lippincott Williams & Wilkins, 2002.

This chapter presents a comprehensive, current summary of therapy for NHL in children and adolescents.

Raney RB: Hodgkin's disease in childhood: A review. J Pediatr Hematol Oncol 19:502-509, 1997.

Current therapy of Hodgkin's disease in children and the occurrence of secondary tumors are reviewed.

Whalen TV, La Quaglia MP: The lymphomas: An update for surgeons. Semin Pediatr Surg 6:50-55, 1997.

This article is a succinct summary of the lymphomas with particular emphasis on the factors most crucial to surgeons.

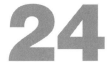

Teratomas and Germ Cell Tumors

Teratomas are embryonal neoplasms derived from totipotential cells that contain tissue from at least two and more often three germ layers (ectoderm, endoderm, and mesoderm). The exact cause of teratomas is obscure and may vary according to the site of origin. Totipotential cells are found in close proximity to Hensen's node in the early embryo. Some of these primitive cells rest in the coccygeal region and may develop abnormally, resulting in the formation of a sacrococcygeal teratoma. An excessive rate of twinning has been observed in families with sacrococcygeal teratoma (10% of cases) and has led to a theory that the tumor may be the result of an abortive attempt of twinning. Teratomas neither go through a primitive streak phase of development nor have evidence of systemic organogenesis, however. Totipotential cells arising from the urogenital ridge are thought to be the origin of gonadal teratomas. Genetic studies and nuclear sex determination of these neoplasms indicate that ovarian teratomas invariably have female sex markers, whereas testicular tumors may have male or female markers. Other theories suggest that ovarian teratomas also may be caused by parthenogenesis (development from a single unfertilized gamete).

Teratomas can occur in almost any organ but tend to develop more commonly in midline or paraxial locations and can be observed from the brain (cephalad) to the coccyx (caudad). These tumors can be solid or cystic (and sometimes mixed); can be benign (80%) or malignant (20%); and are observed more commonly in the neck, oropharynx, anterior mediastinum, retroperitoneum, and gonadal, presacral, and sacrococcygeal regions. Teratomas occurring in infancy and early childhood are usually extragonadal, whereas teratomas in older patients and young adults frequently arise in the ovaries and testes. This difference in presentation accounts for the fact that in most reports from children's centers concerning teratomas, the tumors occur more frequently in the neonatal age group, and the most common site of tumor occurrence is the sacrococcygeal area (Fig. 24-1 and Table 24-1). There is a strong female predominance, with 75% to 80% of cases occurring in girls (excluding testis tumors).

HISTOLOGY

The histologic appearance of teratomas may vary considerably. Even within the same tumor, there may be areas of variable differentiation (Fig. 24-2). The tumor may contain differentiated tissues derived from each of the germ cell layers, including epidermis, brain and glial

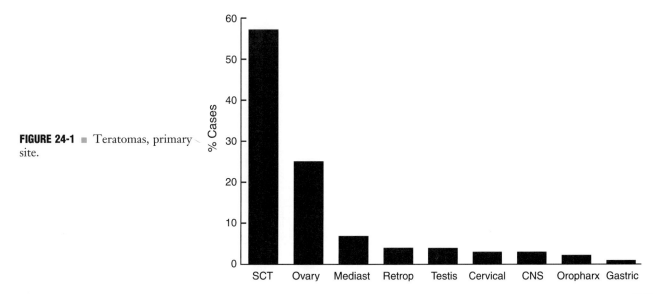

FIGURE 24-1 ■ Teratomas, primary site.

TABLE 24-1 ■ Site of Tumor Occurrence (Based on Information from Various Centers)

Site	Incidence (%)
Sacrococcygeal region	45-65
Anterior mediastinum	10-12
Gonadal (ovary and testis)	10-35
Retroperitoneum	3-5
Cervical area	3-6
Presacral area	3-5
Central nervous system	2-4
Other rare sites (e.g., liver, kidney, vagina, stomach)	<1

tissue, cartilage, connective tissue, respiratory mucosa, bone, fat, striated muscle, lymph tissue, peripheral nerve, choroid plexus, intestinal mucosa, and, less commonly, many other tissues not mentioned here.

The germ cell (totipotential cell) may be the precursor of various tumors, including benign teratomas, embryonal carcinoma, endodermal (yolk sac) sinus tumors, and choriocarcinoma. The benign-appearing teratomas (particularly teratomas that arise in the ovaries) often have immature elements that have been the topic of some controversy. Grading the degree of immaturity from I to IV, teratomas with a greater degree of immaturity (grades III and IV) tend to be larger, more aggressive lesions with a higher risk of recurrence and malignant change. Endodermal sinus tumors (yolk sac tumors) have the appearance of extraembryonic tissues, including yolk sac, chorion, amnion, and allantois. These tumors contain small cavities lined by cuboidal or columnar epithelium with a capillary loop in the center, resulting in a glomerular-like appearance (Schiller-Duval bodies) that closely resembles the endodermal sinus of the rat placenta. The tumor also contains cells with intracellular droplets that stain positive for periodic acid–Schiff testing and are composed of α-fetoprotein (AFP) and other proteins. Patients with endodermal sinus tumors have elevated serum levels of AFP. The chorion is another extraembryonic source of malignant teratoma, the choriocarcinoma. This tumor contains multinucleated syncytial trophoblasts and vacuolated cytotrophoblasts and produces human chorionic gonadotropin (hCG). In addition, malignancy may arise

from any of the differentiated tissues that compose a teratoma, including variants of adenocarcinoma, rhabdomyosarcoma, and neuroblastoma. Extrarenal Wilms' tumor also may arise from the renal elements within a teratoma.

TUMOR MARKERS

The major fetal serum protein is AFP, which is an α-globulin. The fetal liver is the main source of AFP, although early in intrauterine life some AFP is produced in the yolk sac and the fetal intestine. Binding with concanavalin A can differentiate between AFP derived from liver and that from yolk sac. AFP levels frequently are elevated in normal newborns and reach adult levels by 9 months of age. A log curve of 95% predictability of normal versus tumor-affected infants based on the half-life decay of AFP in vivo has been developed. Within 4 or 5 days after a complete resection of an AFP-producing tumor, the AFP level returns to near-normal levels that persist because of liver synthesis. Postoperative monitoring of AFP levels is useful in detecting early tumor recurrence.

The placenta is the normal site of hCG production. This glycoprotein hormone is composed of an α and β subunit. The immunoassay for hCG measures the β subunit, which is more specific to this hormone. hCG most commonly is secreted by testicular tumors and gestational trophoblastic lesions. Chorionic syncytiotrophoblasts and primitive embryonal cells in the testis are the source of β-hCG production. In addition to teratomas, other tumors that secrete β-hCG include hepatoma, hepatoblastoma, and germinomas of the pineal gland. Approximately 4% of boys with precocious puberty have a β-hCG-producing tumor.

CLINICAL PRESENTATION AND TREATMENT

Because the clinical presentation and management of teratomas vary considerably according to tumor site, each is discussed separately.

Sacrococcygeal Teratoma

Sacrococcygeal teratoma is the most common neonatal tumor and the most frequently occurring teratoma. Of all

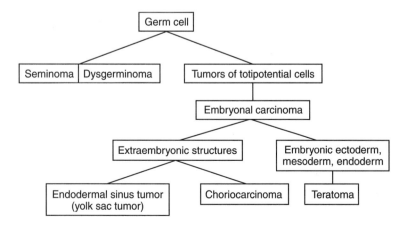

FIGURE 24-2 ■ Diagram of the histogenetic relationship and degree of differentiation among the various tumors of germ cell origin.

teratomas, 50% to 70% arise in the sacrococcygeal region. Of cases, 80% occur in girls and 10% in families with a history of twinning.

Most cases are seen in the newborn period (first month of life), and the remaining cases usually present by age 4 years. An increasing number of teratomas are being detected antenatally by prenatal ultrasound studies. The presence of a teratoma in the fetus may be accompanied by polyhydramnios and a uterine size larger than might be expected for the gestational age.

Findings associated with mortality are fetal hydrops and placentomegaly. These are manifestations of high-output cardiac failure produced by arteriovenous shunting within the tumor. When hydrops occurs, it is associated with dilated cardiac ventricles, increased aortic flow, and a dilated inferior vena cava. Often fetal sonography also reveals high-velocity blood flow within the tumor. Although placental blood flow is increased, its proportion of flow in the descending aorta is decreased, confirming the "steal" of blood flow to the sacral tumor. All of these findings support the hypothesis that the hydrops and congestive heart failure result from high-output failure produced by the tumor vascular steal. Additionally, prematurity from polyhydramnios or cesarean section performed before 30 to 32 weeks' gestation results in

increased mortality. Intralesional hemorrhage or rupture of the tumor during delivery or the rapid onset of respiratory insufficiency may lead to rapid demise of the patient shortly after delivery and before transport and referral for surgical treatment. These observations suggest that when a teratoma is detected antenatally, the mother should be referred to a high-risk obstetric center with immediately available up-to-date neonatal intensive care, qualified pediatric surgical expertise, and well-trained pediatric anesthesiologists. Evidence supports the concept of delivery by planned cesarean section at a high-risk center in selected cases involving large sacrococcygeal tumors (>5 cm) after 32 weeks' gestation. In some cases at greatest risk for fetal demise in utero, intervention may be appropriate.

Tumors are classified according to the system developed by Altman and colleagues, representing 405 patients treated by the members of the Surgical Section of the American Academy of Pediatrics (Figs. 24-3 and 24-4). Type I tumors are predominantly external, are attached to the coccyx, and may have a small presacral component (45.8%) (Fig. 24-3A). Type II lesions have an external mass and a significant presacral pelvic extension (34%) (Fig. 24-3B). Type III tumors are visible externally, but the predominant mass is pelvic and intra-abdominal

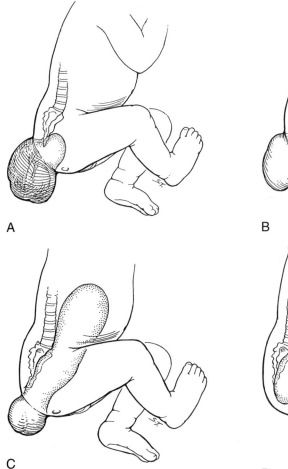
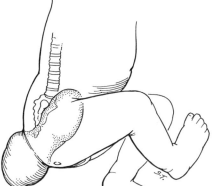
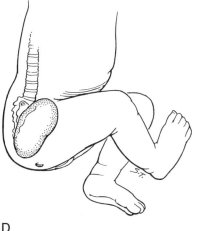

A

B

C

D

FIGURE 24-3 ■ Classification system developed by Altman for sacrococcygeal teratomas based on the degree of pelvic and abdominal extension. **A,** Type I. **B,** Type II. **C,** Type III. **D,** Type IV.

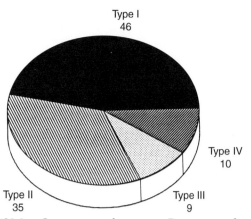

Type I
46

Type IV
10

Type III
9

Type II
35

FIGURE 24-4 ■ Sacrococcygeal teratoma. Percentage of patients in various stages.

(8.6%) (Fig. 24-3C). Type IV lesions are not visible externally but are entirely presacral (9.6%) (Fig. 24-3D).

Symptoms

Most external tumors are asymptomatic, with the exception of the presence of a visible large mass. As previously noted, rupture of the tumor and hemorrhage may occur as a result of a difficult delivery. Pelvic tumors or tumors that extend into the abdominal cavity may present with compression of the rectum or rectosigmoid and urinary tract obstruction. Symptoms of neurologic dysfunction generally indicate intraspinal extension of the tumor or the presence of malignancy. Associated congenital anomalies are observed in 12% to 15% of cases and occur more frequently with presacral tumors. The most commonly observed defects are anorectal malformations, including imperforate anus and anorectal stenosis, anorectal agenesis (with an occasional rectovaginal fistula), and spinal abnormalities (the Currarino triad). Spinal defects observed include a central sacral defect, sacral hemivertebrae, and, less commonly, absence of the sacrum and coccyx or an anterior meningocele. These latter cases are familial, have an autosomal dominant inheritance, and may be caused by a variant of the split notocord syndrome. Delay in diagnosis of the presacral lesion is common because a rectal examination may not be possible in many cases with anorectal stenosis. Presenting symptoms in some of these unusual cases include perirectal abscess or fistula in ano.

Diagnostic Tests

The diagnosis usually is determined by the clinical findings on physical examination, sera for AFP and β-hCG, and a variety of radiographic studies. Plain radiographs of the tumor may show the presence of calcification within the tumor and on the lateral view may show anterior displacement of the rectum by the tumor. The sacrum may appear abnormal (e.g., hemivertebrae, agenesis). Computed tomography (CT) of the pelvis with intravenous and rectal contrast material documents urinary tract displacement or obstruction and outlines the extent of the tumor more accurately. CT also can evaluate for periaortic lymph node enlargement and shows whether liver metastases are present. Magnetic resonance imaging is a useful diagnostic

test in instances of sacral vertebral abnormalities or spinal cord extension of tumor. A chest radiograph is obtained to rule out the presence of pulmonary metastases.

The differential diagnosis of sacrococcygeal tumor includes lipomeningocele, lipoma, chordoma, rectal duplication, and epidermoid cyst. Neuroblastoma also can occur in the presacral area.

Treatment

The treatment of choice for infants with sacrococcygeal teratoma is complete surgical resection. The operative approach varies according to the extent of the tumor (Fig. 24-5). A posterior sacral approach is required for type I and II lesions, whereas a combined abdominosacral procedure is necessary for type III and IV tumors. Except for rare emergencies related to tumor rupture, external hemorrhage, or intratumor shunting or hemorrhage that adversely affects the neonate's hemodynamic status, the tumor can be resected on an elective basis within the first week of life.

In patients with external tumors, the procedure is performed in the prone (knee-chest) position with the hips and shoulders supported to allow adequate anterior chest expansion during anesthesia (see Fig. 24-5C). The procedure is performed using an inverted chevron incision with its apex located above the base of the teratoma. This incision provides excellent exposure and keeps the subsequent wound closure at a distance from the anal orifice. A rectal pack or Hegar dilator may be placed in the anal canal to aid in identification of the rectal wall during the dissection. After raising skin flaps off the tumor, the attenuated retrorectal muscles must be identified carefully and preserved. The mass is mobilized close to its capsule, and hemostasis is effected with electrocautery. The main blood supply to the tumor usually arises from a primitive midsacral artery or from branches of the hypogastric artery. After division of the coccyx from the sacrum, the vessels can be observed exiting the presacral space anterior to the coccyx. In lesions that are particularly vascular with high blood flow, preliminary transabdominal ligation of these vessels or temporary vascular occlusion of the lower aorta has been described to decrease the bleeding during the presacral and pelvic dissection. The use of extracorporeal membrane oxygenation also has been described for the extremely large or vascular lesions in which excessive fluid shifts or hemorrhage may result in operative mortality. Hypothermia with hypoperfusion has been used. The coccyx always is excised in continuity with the tumor because failure to remove the coccyx is associated with a 35% recurrence rate. The tumor can be carefully dissected free from the rectal wall. The retrorectal muscles are reconstituted, and the levator muscles are attached superiorly to elevate and support the rectum. A small suction catheter may be placed in the retrorectal and presacral space and brought out a lateral stab wound. The wound is closed in layers with interrupted absorbable sutures. An occlusive dressing is placed over the wound to protect it from contamination by stool. The patient is kept prone for a few days postoperatively to maintain cleanliness of the wound.

In infants with type III and IV sacrococcygeal tumors, a combined abdominal and perineal procedure is performed,

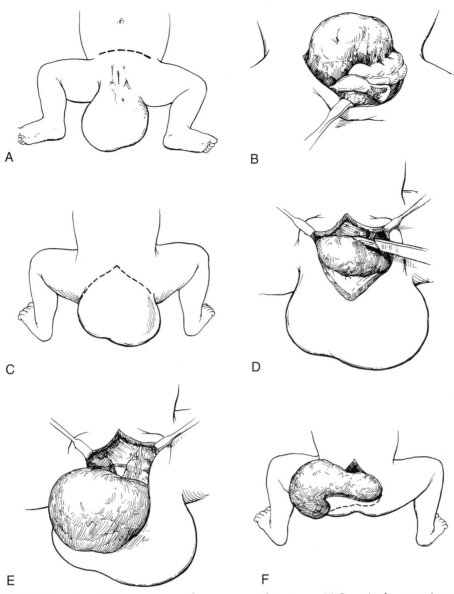

FIGURE 24-5 ■ Surgical management of sacrococcygeal teratoma. (1) Steps in the operative removal of a sacrococcygeal teratoma growing upward into the pelvis and lower abdomen and downward in the more usual fashion. **A,** Initial incision. **B,** Mobilization of the mass from the pelvic viscera. (2) **C,** Prone position with the cutdown in the arm and inverted V incision over the lower sacrum and buttocks. **D,** Transection of the lower sacrum and further mobilization of the pelvic mass up to the point of the previous dissection from above. **E,** Delivery of the pelvic component of the mass and separation of the lower part of the mass from the rectum anteriorly, the gluteus muscles, and the levator ani muscles. The dissection is facilitated if a petrolatum (Vaseline) pack is within the rectum to distend it. **F,** Final separation of the tumor by incising the skin at an appropriate point adjacent to the anus.

starting with a lower abdominal transverse laparotomy incision to mobilize the entire abdominal portion of the tumor and to control the blood supply. The abdominal wound is closed and the patient turned and placed in the prone position for the sacral portion of the procedure, as previously described.

The most frequent complications of excision of a sacrococcygeal teratoma are intraoperative hemorrhage and wound infection. Resection of teratomas with significant intrapelvic and intraperitoneal extension may be associated with temporary or persistent urinary retention in the postoperative period and with difficulty with fecal continence. The major cause of mortality is hemorrhagic shock. Most infants have normal anal continence.

Adjunctive Therapy

Most sacrococcygeal teratomas in newborns are benign (97%) and require no other therapy after complete resection. Presently the survival rate is greater than 95%. Patients are followed periodically by monitoring the AFP level, chest radiograph, and careful physical examination with special emphasis on the rectal examination, which may detect a presacral recurrence. Recurrent tumor may be benign and should be re-excised to minimize its long-term risks for malignant transformation.

In rare instances, a previously resected benign tumor may be associated with a malignant recurrence. In infants who present after age 1 month (38%) and infants having tumors with many immature elements, the risk of malignant change is greater. Older children who present with neurologic symptoms, obstipation, or appearance of a new external mass should be considered to have a malignant lesion until proved otherwise. In these cases, initial percutaneous biopsy and chemotherapy facilitate subsequent dissection and decrease the risks of complications. The overall incidence of malignancy in sacrococcygeal lesions is 20% and includes cases of embryonal carcinoma, endodermal sinus tumor, germ cell tumors, and choriocarcinoma. Occasionally a pure malignant tumor with a single cell type may be observed.

Malignant tumors are treated with adjunctive chemotherapy. The most active antineoplastic drugs are cisplatin, bleomycin, and vinblastine. Etoposide (VP-16) and doxorubicin (Adriamycin) also have been used. Although malignant sacrococcygeal teratomas had a poor prognosis in the past, more recent reports indicate an improved survival after administration of intensive courses of chemotherapy. In some instances, the primary malignant tumor may be unresectable. After obtaining a biopsy specimen to confirm the presence of malignancy, the patient is treated with multiagent chemotherapy. AFP level, CT scan, and chest radiograph are followed closely, and if a good tumor response is observed, a second-look resection of the tumor is attempted. A complete resection is often possible. After chemotherapy, the histologic appearance of the tumor is often that of a benign teratoma, suggesting that treatment results in destruction of the malignant component.

Chemotherapy also has been effective in the treatment of metastatic foci in the lungs and liver. Surgical resection of residual areas of metastases is reasonable in patients who have a good response to chemotherapy. Currently, radiation therapy rarely is used in the management of this tumor. Reported results of North American cooperative group trials of therapy with etoposide, bleomycin, and cisplatin have shown dramatic results. In 74 cases with malignant sacrococcygeal lesions (59% with metastatic disease), an overall 4-year survival rate of 90% was achieved with an event-free survival of 84%. Of the 45 cases initially treated with biopsy, 42 were successfully resected after induction therapy. No survival benefit was seen to primary resection. A German cooperative group trial of cisplatin-based therapy also documented excellent outcome in this cohort. Although survival was not linked closely to initial local stage or distant metastases, the completeness of resection was the strongest prognostic indicator. This group also favored initial preoperative chemotherapy after biopsy with delayed resection because a higher frequency of complete resections were achieved following this strategy.

Mediastinal Teratomas

Mediastinal teratomas account for approximately 20% of all mediastinal neoplasms in pediatric patients.

Mediastinal tumors occur at any age from newborn to adolescent. Most tumors arise in the anterior mediastinum with boys and girls equally affected. Symptoms range from acute respiratory distress to a chronic cough, chest pain, or wheezing. Occasionally, rupture of the tumor into a bronchus may result in hemoptysis or expectoration of hair. Some boys with mediastinal teratomas may present with precocious puberty related to secretion of β-hCG by either a benign or a malignant tumor. These β-hCG-producing neoplasms are associated with Klinefelter's syndrome. Boys with anterior mediastinal mass and β-hCG production should have chromosomal karyotyping performed.

The chest radiograph shows an anterior mediastinal mass on the lateral view. In 35% of cases, the tumor is calcified. An anterior mediastinal mass with calcification must be considered a teratoma until proved otherwise. Ultrasound examination of the chest shows a mass with cystic and solid components and may help separate the mass from the pericardium and heart. CT often clarifies the extent of the tumor and its relationship to surrounding structures.

The differential diagnosis includes thymoma, lymphatic malformation, thymic cyst, mediastinal non-Hodgkin's lymphoma, esophageal duplication, and bronchogenic cyst. Approximately 15% to 20% of mediastinal teratomas are malignant. Sera should be obtained from AFP and β-hCG levels. In a review, the pathology in malignant mediastinal lesions in girls was entirely yolk sac tumor, whereas in boys, yolk sac tumor, germinoma, choriocarcinoma, and a predominance of mixed malignant elements were seen.

The treatment of choice is a right-sided thoracotomy or median sternotomy and resection of the tumor. Resection may not be possible in malignant lesions that infiltrate vital intrathoracic structures. In these cases, preoperative treatment with chemotherapy may facilitate resection. Survival in malignant cases is predicated on complete resection of the primary tumor followed by administration of postoperative chemotherapy because cure is unusual with resection alone. Almost 20% of cases have immature cellular elements on histologic study. This carries almost no increased risk of malignancy in young children but is associated with a high mortality from progressive tumor in older teenagers and young adults.

Primary intrapericardial teratomas are rare, with most cases occurring in the first year of life (25% in the newborn period). The sexes are affected equally. Presenting findings include symptoms of congestive heart failure and evidence of cardiac tamponade. The diagnosis is confirmed by obtaining an echocardiogram that documents a mass compressing the cardiac chambers and a pericardial effusion. The tumor usually arises from the base of the ascending aorta and compresses the atria. The treatment of choice is excision, which may be a hazardous procedure because aortic disruption can occur during the dissection. Most pericardial teratomas are benign.

Results from cooperative group trials have shown excellent results from a regimen of etoposide, bleomycin, and cisplatin, although not as favorable as the results for children with sacrococcygeal lesions. The 4-year survival rate was 71% with an event-free survival rate of 69%.

Of patients, 18 received chemotherapy after initial biopsy; the tumor remained stable or increased in size in 6 and decreased a mean of 57% in 12 patients. Aggressive attempts at resection were deemed appropriate to maximize the survival rate in this cohort.

Rarely a teratoma may arise in the heart. Cardiac teratomas occur almost exclusively in girls, present with signs and symptoms of congestive heart failure, and are located in the right side of the heart. Of cardiac teratomas, 25% are malignant. The chest radiograph usually shows nonspecific cardiomegaly. The electrocardiogram may show an intraventricular block because of tumor involvement of the conduction system. Other arrhythmias also may be observed. The diagnosis is suspected on echocardiography, which shows the presence of a multicystic intracardiac mass. Associated congenital heart defects are common (atrial septal defect, ventricular septal defect). The treatment of choice is prompt resection, when possible, before the occurrence of complete outflow obstruction or a fatal arrhythmia. Malignant teratomas should be treated with chemotherapy. Cardiac transplantation may be a reasonable alternative in cases of benign teratomas that are unresectable.

Retroperitoneal Tumors

Teratomas arise in the retroperitoneum relatively infrequently and represent only 4% of all teratomas. Although retroperitoneal teratomas may present throughout childhood, most are observed during infancy, with 50% of the cases occurring in the first year of life and 75% of cases by 5 years of age. Girls are affected more commonly than boys (2:1). Patients usually present with a large, easily palpable abdominal mass (6 to 15 cm) that may cause symptoms of alimentary tract compression. Plain abdominal radiographs often show displacement of bowel and calcification within the tumor. The pattern of calcification is more distinct and appears different from the diffuse stippled calcification seen in neuroblastoma. Occasionally, bony elements can be seen. Abdominal ultrasound may show the tumor as cystic and solid. CT of the abdomen separates the tumor from the adrenal gland and kidney, indicating that the lesion is not a neuroblastoma or Wilms' tumor, which are much more common retroperitoneal tumors than teratomas in children. Occasionally a retroperitoneal teratoma may be the site of origin of a nonrenal Wilms' tumor, however.

The differential diagnosis also includes retroperitoneal lymphatic malformation, omental or mesenteric cyst, and fetus in fetu. The last-mentioned is a rare abnormality that probably represents an abortive attempt of identical twinning in which one fetus (the parasite) is drawn into the abdominal cavity of the host fetus (the autosite) in early intrauterine life and is attached retroperitoneally, with the blood supply to the former supplied by the host's superior mesenteric artery. These unusual cases show true organogenesis and an axial skeleton, separating them from teratomas, which never undergo organogenesis.

The therapy of choice for retroperitoneal teratoma is laparotomy and complete resection of the tumor. This approach is often successful because most cases are benign. Although 20% of cases are malignant at diagnosis, another 12% to 42% of cases may show the presence of immature

tissues, and glial implants occasionally have been observed. Malignant recurrence has been reported in patients with benign teratomas containing immature components.

Teratomas of the Head and Neck

Teratomas may occur in the brain, eye, orbit, oropharynx, nasopharynx, and neck. *Intracranial teratomas* account for nearly 50% of all brain tumors in the first 2 months of life. A second cluster of tumors occurs in the teenage years (12 to 16 years). The pineal gland is the most common site of origin. Teratomas also may occur in the hypothalamus, the ventricles, the suprasellar region, and the cerebellum. Most teratomas in newborns are benign; however, most intracranial teratomas in older children and young adults are malignant. Almost 50% of cases are classified as germinomas, although all histologic types have been observed, including benign mature and immature teratoma, yolk sac tumor, embryonal carcinoma, and choriocarcinoma. In many instances, the tumor shows a mixed histologic pattern. The most common presenting finding in newborns is increased intracranial pressure related to obstructive hydrocephalus. Most of these tumors are benign and occur equally among boys and girls. In older children and teenagers, intracranial teratomas are more common in boys (2:1) and frequently present with severe headaches in 50% of patients. Other presenting findings include lethargy, visual disturbances, seizures, and vomiting. Boys with tumors that produce β-hCG may present with precocious puberty.

The diagnosis is achieved by obtaining skull radiographs, CT, or magnetic resonance imaging. Teratomas are midline or paraxial supratentorial tumors that are often calcified. The treatment of intracranial teratomas is difficult and often unrewarding. Many neonatal tumors are not resectable. Palliative shunting to reduce intracranial pressure and relieve hydrocephalus is of little long-term benefit if the tumor cannot be excised. In addition, shunting may spread the tumor to extracranial sites. Chemotherapy may be of value in patients who require shunting procedures. The only long-term survivors had complete resection. For older children with germinomas, a better outlook can be expected, with 66% of patients responding to a combination protocol of biopsy, radiation, and chemotherapy. Survival with intracranial endodermal sinus tumor is less than 20%. This poor survival may be related to a penchant for this lesion to seed the intraspinal canal in more than 20% of cases.

Teratomas occurring in the *oropharynx* represent approximately 2% of all teratomas. The tumors most commonly present in neonates or infants and occur equally among boys and girls. The primary site of tumor origin may be the tongue, nasopharynx, palate, sinus, mandible, or tonsil. On rare occasions, multicentric tumors have been noted in more than one site. The tumor may be diagnosed in utero by prenatal ultrasound. Maternal polyhydramnios may be observed as a result of the inability of the affected fetus to swallow because of tumor obstructing the oropharynx. At birth, the tumor may be large and protrude from the mouth and may cause severe respiratory distress requiring immediate intubation. In some instances, large tumors cause no distress at all. Plain radiographs of the neck and chest and CT of the head and neck usually show calcification within the lesion and delineate the extent of the tumor. Sera for AFP also is obtained. The treatment of choice is early excision because continued growth of the tumor results in respiratory embarrassment and feeding difficulties. Most tumors are benign, and recurrence is uncommon after complete resection.

Cervical teratomas are relatively rare lesions and represent 1.5% to 5.5% of all teratomas. These cases are associated with an increased incidence of prematurity and stillbirth, related to polyhydramnios resulting from obstruction of fetal swallowing. The diagnosis can be suspected on prenatal ultrasound, and polyhydramnios is noted in more than 20% of cases in which the tumor is greater than 10 cm. In some instances, this tumor is associated with pulmonary hypoplasia. The lesion appears cystic and solid, and calcification is observed in 50% of cases. At birth, infants may have severe respiratory distress and often require immediate endotracheal intubation. Large cervical teratomas also may require early cesarean section and prompt intervention by endotracheal intubation to avoid severe life-threatening respiratory distress after delivery. In selected cases, endotracheal intubation or tracheostomy may be required while the infant is still oxygenated by the intact uteroplacental circulation to avoid asphyxiation if the trachea is completely occluded. The differential diagnosis includes an infiltrating or cystic lymphatic malformation, branchial cleft cyst, or congenital thyroid goiter. Plain radiographs of the neck may show calcification highly suggestive of teratoma. CT delineates the extent of the tumor and shows mixed cystic and solid components. The treatment of choice is excision, which is performed through a collar incision. The tumors lie deep to the strap muscles, often are well encapsulated, and usually are attached to the pretracheal fascia. If the tumor arises from the thyroid gland, the tumor should be excised with a thyroid lobectomy. Any enlarged lymph nodes should be excised with the tumor because glial metastasis may be present. After excision, a drain is left in place for 24 to 48 hours.

Cervical teratomas are almost always benign in infants even though an occasional infant may have a regional lymph node that contains glial tissue that does not require adjunctive therapy. More than 35% of cervical teratomas contain thyroid tissue. On rare occasions, the thyroid gland may be the site of origin of the tumor. In contrast, cervical teratomas in adults may have a high incidence of malignancy (>60%). Thyroid function should be evaluated after resection of a cervical teratoma because hypothyroidism has been reported.

Gastric Teratomas

Gastric teratomas are rare lesions that present in the first year of life and are more common in boys than girls. The tumors present clinically with symptoms of gastric outlet obstruction or upper gastrointestinal bleeding with a palpable epigastric mass. These tumors are usually large (averaging 10 to 15 cm), are often multicystic, and are frequently calcified on plain radiographs of the abdomen. An upper gastrointestinal contrast study defines the relationship of the tumor to the stomach. Upper endoscopy may show compression of the gastric lumen by an extrinsic mass or evidence of erosion by the tumor. Resection of the tumor is the procedure of choice and often requires resection of a portion of the stomach and the tumor (wedge excision, partial gastrectomy).

Vaginal Teratomas

Teratomas of the vagina are rare and occur in the first year of life, often presenting in the neonatal period. The presenting findings include an easily visible vaginal mass or bleeding. The differential diagnosis includes embryonal rhabdomyosarcoma. Most of these lesions are endodermal sinus tumors. Sera for AFP and β-hCG are obtained for preoperative evaluation, and a chest radiograph is obtained to rule out lung metastases. CT delineates the extent of the lesion. If the tumor is isolated to the vagina, the operative treatment includes local resection of the tumor by vaginectomy and multiagent chemotherapy tailored to lower doses (one half dose) in neonates and infants. If the uterus is involved by tumor, a hysterectomy is required. Preliminary adjuvant chemotherapy may limit the extent of required resection.

Ovarian Teratomas

The most common ovarian tumor in childhood is teratoma. Teratomas account for 50% of all ovarian neoplasms in the pediatric age group. Most ovarian teratomas present in children 6 to 15 years old and are unusual in the first 2 to 3 years of life. The most common presenting symptom is abdominal pain, observed in 50% to 90% of reported cases. Acute abdominal pain results from torsion of the tumor in approximately 25% of cases. Most teratomas are large, averaging 10 to 15 cm. Plain abdominal radiographs show calcification in 50% of cases, often resembling a tooth. Tumors are distributed equally between the left and right ovaries and are bilateral in 5% to 10% of cases. Abdominal ultrasound shows a mass composed of cystic and solid components.

The treatment of choice is oophorectomy for benign tumors with an intact capsule and mature elements on histologic studies. At the time of surgery, any ascitic fluid should be collected for evaluation of the presence of tumor cells. In the absence of peritoneal fluid, appropriate peritoneal washings should be obtained for cytologic evaluation. The peritoneal surfaces, including the undersurface of the diaphragm, should be examined carefully for peritoneal implants, and biopsy specimens should be obtained, although involvement is much less common than in epithelial tumors seen in adults. Omentectomy also is recommended only if gross involvement is present.

Treatment for tumors with immature tissues and instances of extraovarian peritoneal glial implants is controversial. Immature tissues have malignant potential and can be graded from 0 to III. Results have confirmed the safety of surgery alone for immature teratomas, but also have shown a significant incidence of yolk sac tumor or primitive neuroectodermal tumor being identified on central pathology review (almost one third of the cases). The overall 3-year, event-free survival was 93%, but this varied significantly by site: ovarian, 97.8%; testicular, 100%; and extragonadal, 80%. Most girls with glial implants have a benign course, although malignant transformation has been recorded rarely. Grading of glial implants is probably advisable, with administration of chemotherapy limited to patients with grade II and III tumors. Elevated serum AFP levels also indicate the malignant potential of these histologically immature tumors because most patients with benign ovarian teratomas have normal AFP levels. Using cisplatin-based multiagent regimens, the survival with localized malignant germ cell tumors of the ovary is 95% to 100% for stage I and II and 94% to 96% for stage III and IV. This exceeds the survival achieved with the same chemotherapy program in non-gonadal germ cell tumors. The occurrence of malignant transformation in mature ovarian teratomas in middle age with the development of squamous cell carcinoma or other tumors has been reported and is a reason not to ignore these lesions.

Testicular Teratomas

Teratomas are the most common tumors affecting the testis in children. Tumors tend to occur in two age groups: during the first 2 years of life and in teenagers and young adults. Infants most often present with a nontender asymptomatic scrotal mass. In 15% of these cases, a hydrocele may be present. Preoperative serum AFP and β-hCG levels are measured. A chest radiograph and abdominal CT are obtained to rule out spread of disease to the retroperitoneal lymph nodes, liver, and lungs.

Surgery is performed through an inguinal incision. The external oblique fascia is incised, and the cremasteric fascia is opened. The spermatic cord is identified at the internal ring, and a tourniquet or vascular clamp is applied to reduce the risk of vascular and lymphatic tumor spread. The testis is mobilized, inspected, and palpated. If a solid lesion is observed, a radical orchiectomy with excision of the spermatic cord to the level of the internal ring is performed. If the tumor is a clearly benign teratoma, no other therapy is required. Radical orchiectomy alone in stage I disease (80% of cases) in infants younger than 1 year old is associated with a 78% survival. Most malignant tumors in infants are endodermal sinus tumors, which rarely metastasize to the retroperitoneal lymph nodes. Retroperitoneal lymph node dissection is not necessary in infants with stage I disease younger than 2 years of age if preoperative abdominal CT is normal. If the tumor markers (AFP and β-hCG) return to normal postoperatively, this confirms stage I disease. If the tumor markers remain elevated, stage II or III disease (20% of cases) is present, and the child requires retroperitoneal staging and chemotherapy. In stage III disease, retroperitoneal node dissection is performed for enlarged lymph nodes on CT scan, and chemotherapy is administered. Current data indicate that radical orchiectomy alone in stage I disease results in an excellent survival (92%), as good or better than orchiectomy and retroperitoneal lymph node dissection (85%). When the retroperitoneal lymph nodes are involved with metastatic disease (stage II), retroperitoneal lymphadenectomy and chemotherapy increase the survival rate. A unilateral retroperitoneal lymph node dissection is as effective as a bilateral dissection. Children with metastatic disease benefit from chemotherapy, and the combination of cisplatin and etoposide avoids the pulmonary complications associated with use of bleomycin. Further information concerning testis tumors can be found in Chapter 27.

SUGGESTED READINGS

Altman RP, Randolph JG, Lilly JR: Sacrococcygeal teratoma: American Academy of Pediatrics Surgical Section Survey—1973. J Pediatr Surg 9:389, 1974.

This classic article reports 405 cases of sacrococcygeal teratoma treated by members of the Surgical Section of the American Academy of Pediatrics. The staging system described in this important article is still in place today.

Billmire D, Vinocur C, Rescorla F, et al: Malignant mediastinal germ cell tumors: An intergroup study: J Pediatr Surg 36:18-24, 2001.

This is a nice summary of mediastinal lesions treated in a cooperative group trial highlighting the difficulties of tumors in this area.

Currarino G, Coln D, Votteler T: Triad of anorectal, sacral, and presacral anomalies. AJR Am J Roentgenol 137:395, 1981.

This radiologic report describes the association of sacrococcygeal and presacral tumors with anorectal anomalies, sacral defects, and anterior meningoceles.

Englund AT, Geffner ME, Nagel G, et al: Pediatric germ cell and human chorionic gonadotropin–producing tumors. Am J Dis Child 145:1294, 1991.

This article documents the association of precocious puberty and hCG in children with mediastinal germ cell tumors.

Flake AW, Harrison MR, Adzick NS: Fetal sacrococcygeal teratoma, J Pediatr Surg 21:563, 1986.

This seminal report indicates that high-output cardiac failure may be present in the fetus with a sacrococcygeal teratoma resulting in polyhydramnios and premature delivery.

Grosfeld JL, Billmire DF: Teratomas in infancy and childhood. Curr Probl Cancer 11:3, 1985.

This monograph concerning teratomas in the pediatric age group offers an extensive overview of the topic.

Ikeda H, Okumura H, Nagashima K, et al: The management of prenatally diagnosed sacrococcygeal teratoma. Pediatr Surg Int 5:192, 1990.

This article describes an increased mortality associated with cesarean section before 32 weeks' gestation in infants with prenatal ultrasound diagnosis of sacrococcygeal teratoma.

Marina NM, Cushing B, Giller R, et al: Complete surgical excision is effective treatment for children with immature teratomas with or without malignant elements: A Pediatric Oncology Group/Children's Cancer Group intergroup study. J Clin Oncol 17:2137, 1999.

Immature teratomas do not require adjuvant therapy even when microscopic foci of malignant elements are identified.

Nakayama DK, Killian A, Hill LM, et al: The newborn with hydrops and sacrococcygeal teratoma. J Pediatr Surg 26:1435, 1991.

Infants with large sacrococcygeal teratomas and hydrops also may have severe respiratory insufficiency and renal failure, which resolve after removal of the tumor.

Rescorla F, Billmire D, Stolar C, et al: The effect of cisplatin dose and surgical resection in children with malignant germ cell tumors at the sacrococcygeal region: A pediatric intergroup trial (POG/CCG 8882). J Pediatr Surg 36:12, 2001.

This report of more recent cooperative group trials shows the remarkable results achieved from modern chemotherapy.

Schneider DT, Calaminus G, Reinhard H, et al: Primary mediastinal germ cell tumors in children and adolescents: Results
of the German cooperative protocols MAKEI 83/86, 89,
and 96. J Clin Oncol 18:832, 2000.

*This cooperative group trial strongly supports the use of initial
chemotherapy for mediastinal lesions to enhance the chances of
complete resection and cure.*

Tsuchida Y, Watanasupt W, Nakajo T: Anorectal malformations associated with a presacral tumor and sacral defects.
Pediatr Surg Int 4:398, 1989.

*This article reviews 51 cases with Currarino syndrome, depicting
the variable factors seen in this anomaly.*

Mediastinal Masses

Mediastinal masses are classified according to the compartment in which they arise. A convenient way of evaluating these lesions is to divide the mediastinum into three major compartments in the lateral view: anterosuperior, middle, and posterior mediastinum (Fig. 25-1). Each of the three compartments extends from the thoracic inlet to the diaphragm and is bounded laterally by mediastinal parietal pleura. The anterior mediastinum extends from the inner table of the sternum to the anterior aspect of the trachea and pericardium and the pericardial reflection onto the great vessels (Table 25-1). The anterosuperior compartment contains the thymus, lymph nodes and lymphatic vessels, connective and adipose tissue, and occasionally ectopic thyroid and parathyroid tissues. The boundaries of the middle mediastinum (sometimes called the *visceral compartment*) extend from the pericardium anteriorly to the prevertebral fascia

TABLE 25-1 ■ Mediastinal Masses in Children		
Superoanterior	**Middle**	**Posterior**
Thymus	Lymphoma (T and B cell)	Neurogenic tumors
Hyperplasia Cyst	Hodgkin's disease	Neuroblastoma Ganglioneuroma
Lipoma Thymoma	Inflammatory granuloma	Neurofibroma Neurilemoma
Carcinoma Lymphoma		
Hodgkin's disease	Bronchogenic cyst	Pheochromocytoma
Dermoid Teratoma	Enterogenous cyst	Neurenteric cyst
Germ cell tumor Seminoma	Hemangioma	PNET Hamartoma
Cystic hygroma Lipoblastoma	Pericardial teratoma	Cystic hygroma Lipoma, lipoblastoma
	Cardiac tumor	Anterior thoracic meningocele
	Rhabdomyoma Myxoma Fibroma Lipoblastoma Hemangioma	

PNET, primitive neuroectodermal tumor.

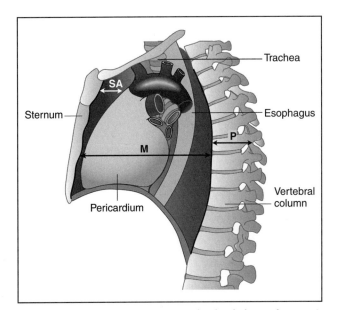

FIGURE 25-1 ■ The mediastinum can be divided into three main anatomic compartments in the lateral view. SA, superoanterior mediastinum; M, middle mediastinum (the visceral compartment); P, posterior mediastinum (paravertebral sulcus).

posteriorly. The middle mediastinum contains the trachea, major bronchi, paratracheal spaces, and esophagus (primitive foregut structures). The heart and great vessels are included in the middle mediastinum. The posterior mediastinum is a bilateral compartment that extends from the posterior aspect of the trachea to the spine. Paravertebral tissues are included in the posterior mediastinum (also called the *paravertebral sulcus*). The posterior mediastinum contains thoracic spinal ganglia, the sympathetic chain proximal portion of the intercostal nerves, connective tissue, and lymphatics. The location of the mediastinal mass and the age of the patient are often useful factors to consider in arriving at a correct preoperative diagnosis because there is a predilection for lesions to arise in certain compartments. In solid lesions, the presence of calcification in the tumor and the presence of tumor markers are helpful in achieving an accurate preoperative diagnosis. Although the chest radiograph remains a useful diagnostic study, the availability of ultrasonography, computed tomography (CT), and magnetic resonance imaging has enhanced significantly diagnostic accuracy for mediastinal masses in the pediatric age group.

MEDIASTINAL CYSTS

Mediastinal cysts and tumors are relatively common in infants and children. Mediastinal cysts may be congenital and present as a complex *variant* of normal anatomic tissue. Although cysts of the mediastinum are often asymptomatic, they usually require removal. If cysts are symptomatic, they may present with chest pain, cough, respiratory distress, hemoptysis, and dysphagia. The various cysts encountered include bronchogenic cysts, thymic cysts, enterogenous cysts, neurenteric cysts, dermoid cysts, cystic hygroma, and pericardial cysts.

Diagnostic studies include anteroposterior and lateral chest radiographs, CT scan, contrast barium swallow, and occasionally ultrasonography. Esophagoscopy, bronchoscopy, and arteriography may be useful in selected cases. The exact preoperative diagnosis is often not possible without either a biopsy or histologic examination after excision.

Thymic Cysts

Thymic cysts occur in the anterior mediastinum and are usually asymptomatic. These cysts may be associated with cervical components. Thymic cysts are lined by ciliated epithelium and contain lymphocytes and cholesterol crystals in the lining. They may undergo malignant degeneration or may be the site of lymphoid tumor growth. Thymic cysts may present with symptoms including wheezing and upper respiratory infection. They can expand rapidly as a result of either hemorrhage or infection. In general, when recognized, thymic cysts should be removed because of these potential complications.

Enterogenous Cysts

Enterogenous cysts or esophageal duplications are of foregut origin and are found in the middle mediastinum. Enterogenous cysts consist of a smooth muscle–walled structure containing mucosal epithelium including ectopic gastric tissue. They share a common smooth muscular wall with the normal esophagus. These cysts communicate with the lumen of the esophagus in 20% of cases. Cervical or upper thoracic vertebral anomalies (particularly hemivertebrae) often are associated with enterogenous duplication cysts. In some instances, these cysts may attach to or communicate with the spinal canal or occasionally to the dura and are referred to as *neurenteric cysts.* Neurenteric cysts form when the foregut and primitive notochord are in close approximation and may be due to failure of complete separation or herniation of the

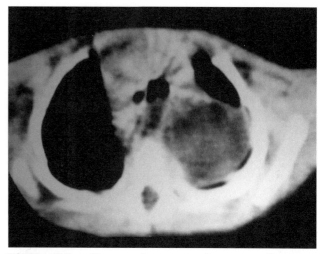

FIGURE 25-2 ■ Computed tomography scan shows an esophageal duplication extending into the right chest from the mediastinum.

foregut endoderm into the notochord ectoderm. This type of cyst resides in the middle and posterior mediastinum. Patients with neurenteric cysts may present with pain or neurologic findings. They are at risk for developing complications such as paraplegia and meningitis. In addition, it is common (10% to 15%) for a patient with a mediastinal enterogenous cyst to have an associated intra-abdominal intestinal duplication (Fig. 25-2). Mediastinal enterogenous cysts may extend inferiorly and penetrate the diaphragm to end blindly in the abdomen or may communicate with the lumen of the jejunum or ileum (Fig. 25-3). Rarely, multiple esophageal duplication cysts have been observed. The presence of ectopic gastric mucosa within the cyst wall can result in peptic ulceration, bleeding, or perforation. Duplication cysts may

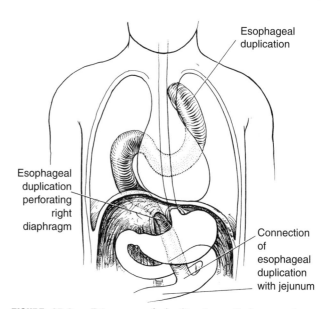

Esophageal duplication

Esophageal duplication perforating right diaphragm

Connection of esophageal duplication with jejunum

FIGURE 25-3 ■ Diagram of duplication of the esophagus communicating with the jejunum.

enlarge significantly and act as a space-occupying lesion that compresses the lungs or normal esophagus causing respiratory distress or dysphagia. For these reasons, excision of the cyst is recommended. Patients with neurenteric cysts may require cyst excision and a laminectomy to excise completely the communication to the spinal canal.

Cystic Hygromas

Cystic hygromas are multilocular, thin-walled, endothelial-lined cysts containing lymphatic fluid in dilated lymphatic channels (see Chapter 28). They are congenital in nature and most commonly arise in the posterior triangle of the neck. The cysts are derived from the primitive jugular lymphovenous sacs. In 10% to 15% of cases, the cyst extends into the mediastinum, descending between the subclavian vessels. Rarely, they may arise primarily within the mediastinum. Intracystic hemorrhage or infection may cause the cysts to enlarge rapidly and result in tracheal compression and sudden onset of respiratory distress, warranting urgent operative, intervention.

Pericardial Cysts

Pericardial cysts are almost always asymptomatic and most often appear as an incidental finding at the cardiophrenic angle on a routine chest radiograph usually on the right side. These cysts are thin walled, are lined by flattened mesothelium, contain clear fluid, and may be removed easily to verify their benign nature.

Dermoid Cysts

Dermoid cysts and teratomas are some of the largest mediastinal tumors seen in children. The term *dermoid cyst* applies to a lesion composed entirely of ectodermal derivatives. The typical dermoid cyst is a thick-walled, fibrous sac lined by squamous epithelium. The cyst may contain various skin appendages, hair, occasionally teeth, and typical caseous detritus. The tumors almost invariably are found in the anterior mediastinum but rarely are located within the pericardiurn. Dermoid cysts rarely may undergo malignant degeneration. The malignant tissues usually are consistent with carcinoma rather than sarcoma. Removal of dermoid cysts is warranted because of the risk of infection and subsequent rupture into the pleura, pericardium, or a bronchus. In the latter cases, the patient occasionally may present clinically by coughing up hair.

Bronchogenic Cysts

Bronchogenic cysts are located in the middle mediastinum. Embryologically, these cysts originate before the bronchi are formed in the fetus and persist after birth close to the bifurcation of the main stem bronchi at the carina (Fig. 25-4). Hilar and carinal bronchogenic cysts represent groups of epithelial cells from the developing trachea and lung buds that are pinched off and become separated from the tracheobronchial tree. The earliest separation is usually dorsal from the presumptive esophageal portion of the foregut, whereas the later separations are from the ventral or tracheal portion of the foregut. The rarely observed paratracheal or paraesophageal cyst probably is derived from tracheal

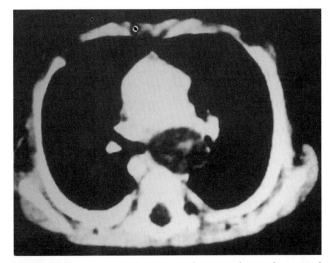

FIGURE 25-4 ▪ Computed tomography scan shows the typical finding of a bronchogenic cyst located in the region of the carina partially narrowing the right main stem bronchus.

diverticula and subsequently pinched off from the parent organ. Bronchogenic cysts are usually but not exclusively extrapulmonary masses (Fig. 25-5). They do not communicate with the normal tracheobronchial tree, and they do not have a unique blood supply. In addition, bronchogenic cysts do not contain distal lung structures (alveoli).

On microscopic examination, bronchogenic cysts are thin walled and lined by ciliated columnar epithelium and have a fibrous tissue wall that often contains cartilage and sometimes bronchial glands. These cysts are often

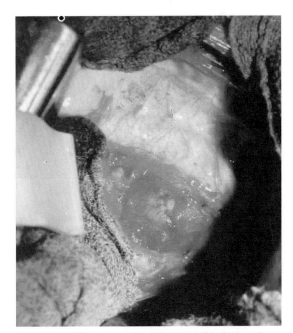

FIGURE 25-5 ▪ This operative photograph shows the same patient as in Figure 25-4. The bronchogenic cyst lies just below the right main stem bronchus and the carina. Symptoms of cough and wheezing were relieved after removal.

asymptomatic and may be noted incidentally as an unexpected finding on a chest radiograph. Parabronchial bronchogenic cysts (particularly those in the subcarinal area) often compress the trachea, however, resulting in air trapping and respiratory distress in newborns. They may be detected on chest radiograph or CT scan of the chest. Symptomatic cysts should be excised, and asymptomatic cysts should be removed for definitive pathologic diagnosis and because of the risk of infection. A rare case of adenocarcinoma in a bronchogenic cyst occurring in an 8-year-old girl has been reported. Most bronchogenic cysts can be excised safely by thoracoscopic resection. Thoracoscopy may be contraindicated in children with subcarinal compressive cysts associated with left lung distention and a mediastinal shift. In some cases, it is extremely difficult to separate the posterior wall of the cyst from the normal bronchus. Near-complete excision and leaving the attached portion of the cyst wall on the bronchus is reasonable treatment and has not been associated with recurrence.

SOLID MEDIASTINAL TUMORS

Mediastinal tumors are fairly common in children and can be either benign or malignant. Approximately 60% are malignant. These tumors include Hodgkin's disease, non-Hodgkin's lymphoma, neurogenic tumors, thymomas, teratomas, lipomas, lipoblastoma, germ cell tumors, and other rare lesions. Lymphoid tumors (Hodgkin's disease and non-Hodgkin's lymphoma) are the most frequently observed mediastinal tumors (Table 25-2).

About 40% to 60% of children with Hodgkin's disease present with an anterior mediastinal mass. The mass may be manifested by coughing, wheezing, or severe respiratory distress. In general, the surgeon's involvement with these patients is to provide tissue for diagnosis. Treatment is nonsurgical and involves multimodal chemotherapy and irradiation. Children with non-Hodgkin's lymphoma, usually T-cell lymphoblastic lesions, may present with a bulky anterior mediastinal mass in 25% to 30% of cases. They present with respiratory distress, pleural effusion, and occasionally superior vena caval syndrome (5% to 6%). It is preferable to obtain a biopsy specimen from nonmediastinal sources, such as bone marrow aspirate, pleural fluid, or lymph node tissue, to make a diagnosis and avoid a general anesthetic. That may not always be possible, and open biopsy of the mediastinum under general anesthesia may be required. In patients with a large mediastinal mass, a CT scan of the chest documenting a tracheal area of greater than 50% of normal and pulmonary function tests that show a peak expiratory flow rate greater than 50% of predicted are preoperative indicators that anesthesia may be tolerated. In patients with mediastinal lymphomas, echocardiography is the best tool for evaluation to rule out restriction of cardiac output. If output is restricted, these patients should be treated without biopsy. Biopsy of the tumor using an anterior parasternal approach (Chamberlain procedure)

TABLE 25-2 ■ Incidence of Mediastinal Tumors in Children in the 1990s[*,†]

Tumor Type	Number of Cases				
	Simpson (1991)	Saenz et al (1993)	Cohen et al (1991)	Grosfeld et al (1994)	Total
Neuroblastoma	16	32	13	50	111
Ganglioneuroma	9	14	8	14	45
Neurofibroma	4	3	—	2	9
Neurilemoma	1	3	1	5	10
Pheochromocytoma	—	2	—	—	2
PNET	—	2	—	2	4
Hodgkin's disease	29	34	1	49	113
NHL	34	6	3	38	81
Teratoma (benign)	7	2	4	18	31
Germ cell tumor	—	—	—	3	3
Thymoma	—	—	2	3	5
Thymic carcinoma	1	—	1	1	3
Cystic hygroma	3	1	3	11	18
Lipoma	—	3	1	3	7
Lipoblastoma	—	—	—	2	2
Rhabdomyosarcoma	—	—	—	1	1
Fibroma	—	—	—	1	1
Hemangioma	—	—	—	1	1
Hamartoma	—	—	—	1	1
Total	104	102	37	205‡	448

[*]Lymphoid tumors are the most common mediastinal tumor in the pediatric age group (194/448 = 43.3%). Posterior mediastinal neurogenic tumors are the second most common group of tumors (181/448 = 40.4%), whereas teratomas and germ cell tumors are the third most frequently observed neoplasms (34/448 = 7.5%).
[†]Data from Simpson I, Campbell PE: Prog Pediatr Surg 27:92, 1991; Saenz N, et al: J Pediatr Surg 28:172, 1993; Cohen AJ, et al: Ann Thorac Surg 51:378, 1991; Grosfeld JL, et al: Ann Surg Oncol 1:121, 1994.
‡Nine additional cases added to this review.
PNET, primitive neuroectodermal tumor; NHL, non-Hodgkin's lymphoma.

is an effective method of obtaining a tissue diagnosis. Therapy includes multiple-agent chemotherapy and occasionally bone marrow transplantation. Hodgkin's disease and non-Hodgkin's lymphoma are discussed in more detail in Chapter 23.

As a group, neurogenic tumors are the second most common thoracic tumors of infancy and childhood (see Table 25-2). The benign tumors—ganglioneuromas, schwannomas, and neurofibromas—may enlarge without producing any symptoms until Horner's syndrome (ptosis and meiosis on the affected side) resulting from involvement of the stellate ganglion is observed, or significant tracheal displacement produces respiratory symptoms. Neuroblastoma (see later) is a highly malignant embryonal tumor of neurogenic origin with approximately 20% occurring in the posterior mediastinum. In a third of cases, the tumor may be asymptomatic and is identified by its presence on a chest radiograph. In some instances, the tumor causes lung compression and respiratory distress. Pain may occur because of involvement of nerve trunks or symptoms from distant metastases (particularly bone metastases). Occasionally the neuroblastoma may erode the ribs and extend through the chest wall, producing a visible mass. Extension of tumor into the spinal canal may occur through the spinal foramina causing neurologic deficits (10% to 15%).

Ganglioneuroma

Ganglioneuromas are the most common neurogenic mediastinal tumors of childhood. Most cases have been reported in infants and children. These tumors can become large and are usually well encapsulated. Histologically the tumor cells have the appearance of a typical ganglion cell, indicating their origin from the sympathetic chain. These tumors frequently widen the intercostal spaces and can extend into the spinal canal. Because they are well encapsulated, they usually can be excised. In rare cases, ganglioneuromas are the result of maturation of a neuroblastoma from a malignant to a benign tumor.

Neurofibroma and Neurilemoma

Neurofibromas arise from the nerves in the posterior mediastinum, such as intercostal nerves, the phrenic nerve, the vagus nerve, or the sympathetic chain. They may be isolated tumors or present with multiple neoplasms related to neurofibromatosis (von Recklinghausen's disease). Scoliosis is often an associated finding, and widening of the intervertebral foramina is common. The isolated tumors are well encapsulated and usually readily removed; however, the tumors associated with neurofibromatosis tend to extend along nerve sheaths so that total removal is often impossible. Malignant degeneration can occur but usually takes place in large tumors and in older patients. Neurilemoma (schwannoma) also arises from nerve sheaths and similarly can be benign or malignant.

Neuroblastomas

Neuroblastomas are malignant tumors of sympathetic origin, arising from the precursor neural crest cell. Most neuroblastornas in infancy and childhood are found in the retroperitoneum (adrenal [50%], paraspinal [20%]).

Tumors can arise primarily in the posterior mediastinum in 20% of cases and the neck and pelvis in the remaining 10%. Measuring 24-hour urinary catecholamines and byproducts such as vanillylmandelic acid and homovanillic acid (usually elevated) can suggest the diagnosis. The tumor appearance on plain radiographs is usually characteristic, showing a sharply circumscribed posterior mediastinal lesion in a paravertebral location containing fine calcifications. The tumor extent can be clarified by a contrast-enhanced CT scan. The metaiodobenzylguanidine radionuclide (MIBG) scan also has been used to diagnose this tumor and evaluate for the presence of bone metastases. Neuroblastomas can be dumbbell-shaped and extend into the spinal canal. Magnetic resonance imaging is useful in detecting intraspinal extension. Complete resection is often not possible; however, even with an incomplete resection leaving small amounts of tumor in the intraspinal foramina, the prognosis for lesions arising in the mediastinum is much better than that observed in patients with primary intra-abdominal neuroblastomas. The overall survival for children with a mediastinal primary is 80%. The findings at operation and evaluation of tumor tissue for important biologic and genetic characteristics often determines outcome. Diploidy, unfavorable Shimada histology, amplification of the N-*myc* oncogene, absent or low *trk*-A proto-oncogene levels, loss of heterozygosity of chromosome 1p36, advanced stage disease (stages 3 and 4), and age greater than 1 year at diagnosis adversely influence the prognosis. More in-depth information concerning this unusual pediatric neoplasm can be found in Chapter 19.

Teratoma

Teratoma is the third most common mediastinal tumor (Fig. 25-6). Teratomas almost always are located in the anterior mediastinum. They can be benign or malignant (20%), can be solid or cystic, and contain derivatives of all three embryonic germ layers. Teratomas also may involve the pericardium. On a chest radiograph or CT scan of the chest, calcifications (occasionally teeth) noted in an anterior mediastinal tumor are consistent with a diagnosis of teratoma until proved otherwise. Benign lesions almost always can be resected, whereas malignant

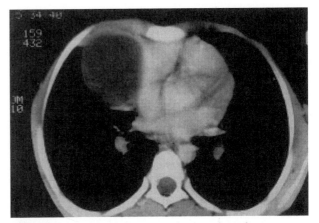

FIGURE 25-6 ■ Computed tomography scan shows large teratoma of the left cardiophrenic angle.

lesions are often unresectable because of local invasion of surrounding intrathoracic tissues. In the neonatal period, benign teratomas occasionally may be the cause of acute life-threatening respiratory distress. Malignant teratomas are often sensitive to cisplatin-based chemotherapy programs that can shrink a previously unresectable tumor and occasionally allow for a subsequent second-look resection. Delayed attempts at resection after primary chemotherapy administration is also effective treatment. Occasionally a germ cell tumor of the anterior mediastinum may present with precocious puberty in boys with Klinefelter's syndrome. Patients with malignant teratomas or germ cell tumors often have elevated serum α-fetoprotein levels and may have an elevated serum β-human chorionic gonadotropin level. The final completeness of tumor resection is the strongest prognostic indicator of event-free survival. The current survival for mediastinal germ cell tumors is greater than 85%. An in-depth discussion of teratomas can be found in Chapter 24.

Thymoma

Thymomas are extremely rare in children and are managed in the same manner as they are in adults. A significantly enlarged thymus in early infancy can mimic a tumor and result in respiratory distress. The fact that enlargement of the thymus gland in this age group is almost never due to a malignant process should encourage either continued observation or a brief course of steroids to shrink the size of the gland. Thymolipoma is a benign thymic neoplasm that can be diagnosed in infants and children.

Other Tumors

A wide variety of other rare tumors of the mediastinum have been reported in children, including hemangioma, lipoma, lipoblastoma, rhabdomyosarcoma, peripheral neuroectodermal tumors, osteogenic sarcoma, fibromas, pheochromocytoma, and a group of anaplastic carcinomas and sarcomas. Many additional conditions can mimic a mediastinal mass and must be considered in the differential diagnosis, such as intrathoracic extension of thyroid goiter, pulmonary artery aneurysm, aneurysms of the great arteries of the mediastinum, and occasionally an unusual presentation of a congenital diaphragmatic hernia. The most common cardiac tumors of infancy in decreasing order of frequency include rhabdomyoma, myxoma, fibroma, and lipoblastoma. Most of these lesions arise in the right atrium. Cardiac tumors can be detected on prenatal ultrasound studies. The diagnosis usually is made before age 1 year. Patients present with a heart murmur or cardiac arrhythmias. Most patients survive tumor resection.

SUGGESTED READINGS

Grosfeld JL, Skinner MA, Rescorla FJ, et al: Mediastinal tumors in children: Experience with 196 cases. Ann Surg Oncol 1:121-127, 1994.

A large series of mediastinal tumors in children from a single institution is described.

Michel JR, Revillon Y, Montupet P, et al: Thoracoscopic treatment of mediastinal cysts in children. J Pediatr Surg 33:1745-1748, 1998.

This excellent article describes the efficacy of thoracoscopic excision of mediastinal cysts and its contraindications.

Patrick DA, Rothenberg SS: Thoracoscopic resection of mediastinal masses in infants and children: An evaluation of technique and results. J Pediatr Surg 36:1165-1167, 2001.

This article describes experience with minimal access resection of mediastinal tumors.

Philippart AI, Farmer DL: Benign mediastinal cysts and tumors. In O'Neill JA Jr, Rowe MI, Grosfeld JL, et al (eds): Pediatric Surgery, 5th ed. St Louis, Mosby, 1998, pp 839-851.

This chapter presents an up-to-date, in-depth review of all of the various considerations related to mediastinal masses.

Sbragia L, Paek BW, Feldstein VA, et al: Outcome of prenatally diagnosed tumors. J Pediatr Surg 36:1244-1247, 2001.

This article concerning a large number of prenatally diagnosed fetal tumors documents a worse prognosis for tumors that arise in the mediastinum.

26

Endocrine Tumors

Tumors of the endocrine system are relatively uncommon in children. If neuroblastoma is excluded, endocrine tumors account for approximately 1% of all pediatric malignancies. Endocrine tumors may manifest in the form of a mass or more commonly by signs and symptoms related to either overproduction or deficiency of hormonal secretion.

CENTRAL NERVOUS SYSTEM TUMORS

Endocrine-related tumors may arise in the pineal, pituitary, and hypothalamic areas of the brain. Pineal and suprasellar germinomas are usually of germ cell origin and secrete β-human chorionic gonadotropin (hCG), causing precocious puberty. The behavior and management of germ cell tumors are discussed extensively in Chapters 24 and 27.

Gliomas of the hypothalamus cause two distinct clinical presentations: (1) diencephalic syndrome and (2) precocious puberty. The former clinical pattern is seen with tumors that arise in the anterior hypothalamus and third ventricle and is manifested by wasting, vomiting, pallor, and nystagmus. Precocious puberty may be associated with tumors of the hypothalamus, especially gliomas and astrocytomas that release an excess of gonadotropin-releasing hormone.

Craniopharyngioma is the most common tumor involving the hypothalamic-pituitary area in children. It is a nonsecretory tumor that accounts for 5% of all intracranial tumors in childhood and 90% of neoplasms arising in the pituitary region. These tumors usually are located in the sella, are calcified, and commonly result in a deficient secretion of growth hormone, causing short stature and hypogonadism. Deficiencies of adrenocorticotropic hormone (ACTH) and thyroid-stimulating hormone and diabetes insipidus are observed less commonly. Treatment includes surgical removal when possible and administration of hCG for gonadotropin deficiency, thyroxine for thyroid-stimulating hormone deficiency, hydrocortisone for ACTH deficiency, and desmopressin for diabetes insipidus.

Although pituitary adenomas are uncommon in children, when present, 75% of adenomas are functional.

The most prominent findings include gigantism from overproduction of growth hormone, prolactinomas with excess release of prolactin, and Cushing's syndrome as a result of excessive ACTH secretion. Transsphenoidal tumor resection and radiotherapy are usually therapeutic modalities for patients with gigantism, whereas bromocriptine administration reduces the size and rate of secretion from prolactinomas. If shrinkage of the tumor does not occur with medical therapy, surgical intervention is required with radiation therapy as backup for residual disease. Pituitary adenomas may be associated with the multiple endocrine neoplasia type I (MEN-I, formerly called *Werner's syndrome*), which is discussed later in this chapter.

In children with Cushing's syndrome, the site of the lesion must be determined (e.g., pituitary, adrenal, or an ectopic site of excessive cortisol or ACTH production; Table 26-1). Older children are more likely to have pituitary-induced Cushing's syndrome. The treatment of choice is pituitary transsphenoidal microsurgery (microadenectomy). In inoperable cases or instances of incomplete resection, low-dose pituitary irradiation or direct implantation of yttrium 90 or gold (Au 198) may be curative.

TABLE 26-1 ■ Etiology of Cushing's Syndrome

Exogenous corticosteroid administration
ACTH-dependent causes
   Cushing's disease (pituitary adenoma)
   Ectopic ACTH production
      Carcinoid tumors (especially bronchial)
      Pancreatic islet cell carcinoma
      Thymoma
      Medullary thyroid carcinoma
      Pheochromocytoma
      Neuroblastoma
      Small cell bronchogenic carconoma
ACTH-independent causes
   Adrenal adenoma
   Adrenocortical carcinoma
   Adrenal hyperplasia

Modified from Skinner MA, Mayforth RD: Endocrine disorders and tumors. In Ashcraft KW (ed): Pediatric Surgery, 3rd ed. Philadelphia, WB Saunders, 2000, p 1033.

ADRENAL TUMORS

More than 90% of adrenal tumors arise in the medulla. Adrenocortical tumors in children are relatively rare (only 0.2% of all cases of pediatric cancer), but they are potentially fatal neoplasms. Most are hormonally functional and produce symptoms of virilization (most commonly), Cushing's syndrome, aldosteronism, or feminization. Most cases present during the first decade of life, are frequently malignant, and occur more commonly in girls. The nonfunctional type is more common in boys. Mean age at onset is approximately 4.5 years of age. In 2% to 10% of cases, tumors are bilateral.

There is a relationship between the appearance of adrenocortical tumors and the occurrence of brain tumors (medulloblastoma and astrocytoma), fetal alcohol syndrome, Beckwith-Wiedemann syndrome, and hemihypertrophy. Although the cause of these tumors is unknown, adrenocortical tumors have been reported in siblings, suggesting that there may be an inherited predisposition. They also have been described in association with congenital adrenal hyperplasia. A mutation of the *p53* tumor suppressor gene has been found in many adrenocortical carcinomas. The Li-Fraumeni syndrome, caused by a germline mutation of *p53*, is an autosomal dominant disorder that predisposes to adrenocortical carcinomas and many other neoplasms. The clinical presentation of adrenocortical tumors varies, with approximately 50% presenting with a palpable mass and 95% with manifestations of hormonal secretion.

Conn's Syndrome (Primary Hyperaldosteronism)

Conn's syndrome is rare in childhood. About 12 case reports exist, and all of the patients had a benign adrenal adenoma. The presenting findings include hypertension, polyuria, and hypokalemia. Most of the symptoms are caused by hypertension. The mass may be small but can be detected by computed tomography (CT). The serum and urinary levels for aldosterone are usually elevated. The treatment of choice is surgical excision, which may be achieved through a limited retroperitoneal approach or by laparoscopy because these tumors are often small.

Virilizing Adrenal Neoplasm

Virilization is caused by excessive production of androgenic steroids, including testosterone, androstenedione, and dihydroepiandrosterone (DHEA). The diagnosis is made by measuring levels of plasma testosterone, urinary and plasma DHEA, and 17-ketosteroid (KS). The 17-KS is a nonspecific measure of androgenic metabolites and is elevated significantly in instances of adrenocortical carcinoma but usually not in benign cases. Two thirds of the 17-KS is produced in the adrenal gland, and one third is gonadal.

Adrenal hyperplasia is the most common cause of virilization if noted at birth or during early infancy. After infancy, a tumor must be suspected. Symptoms and signs in prepubertal girls include accelerated growth, advanced bone age, the presence of pubic hair, deepening of the voice, and clitoromegaly (Fig. 26-1). The differential diagnosis includes a Sertoli-Leydig cell tumor of the

ovary, which would be associated with a normal 17-KS level. Ultrasonography or CT of the abdomen and pelvis establishes the origin of the tumor. In boys, precocious puberty with early virilization may be caused by Leydig cell tumors of the testis (unilateral enlarged testis with tumor), isosexual precocity, or an ectopic hCG-producing tumor. These patients have bilateral testicular enlargement, whereas tumors with an adrenal cause result in normal-sized or small testes.

All virilizing adrenal tumors are potentially malignant, and one cannot rely solely on microscopic appearance. Criteria associated with a malignant behavior are listed in Table 26-2. A bimodal distribution of adrenocortical tumors in children often is noted, with a cluster younger than 5 years of age and the other between 9 and 16 years old.

Cushing's Syndrome

Cushing's syndrome may be related to adrenocortical tumor, adrenal hyperplasia, pituitary adenoma, or an ectopic tumor producing ACTH as previously discussed (see Table 26-1). Of young children with Cushing's syndrome, 80% have an adrenal neoplasm, whereas in older children a pituitary adenoma is more common. Cushing's syndrome as a result of adrenal pathologic conditions is associated with hypertension and hypercortisolism, with loss of diurnal variation. Clinical presentation includes growth retardation, obesity (90%), moon facies (25%), and buffalo hump (25%) (Fig. 26-2). The obesity is typically truncal in adults but often generalized in children, and muscle wasting may be masked. Violaceous skin striae may be observed on the abdominal wall, flank, and upper thighs. Facial acne, hirsutism, and premature appearance of axillary and pubic hair also are noted. Hypercortisolism suppresses growth hormone release and somatomedin synthesis and release.

Cortisol excess is detected by measuring levels of plasma cortisol, urinary 17-hydroxycorticosteroid (17-OH), and urinary free cortisol. The last measurement is a more sensitive indicator of cortisol excess. The 17-OH levels are significantly elevated with increased cortisol secretion and in cases of adrenocortical carcinoma with virilization. The highest 17-OH corticosteroid levels are observed in cases of malignancy. In patients with nonfunctioning adrenocortical carcinoma, 17-KS and 17-OH levels may be normal. Precursors such as pregnenolone may be elevated, however, and act as a marker for tumor recurrence. Although dexamethasone suppression has been used to separate benign from malignant lesions, the test is not always accurate. Plasma ACTH is undetectable because of pituitary suppression by the elevated cortisol.

Tumor Localization

In addition to the previously noted chemical determinations, identification of adrenal neoplasms requires a series of radiographic and scintigraphic studies. Plain abdominal radiographs may show a calcified suprarenal mass. Chest radiographs are obtained to search for the presence of lung metastases. A bone scan or skeletal survey may show the presence of bone metastases. Abdominal ultrasound studies are good screening tests to confirm the presence of a solid suprarenal mass and to evaluate

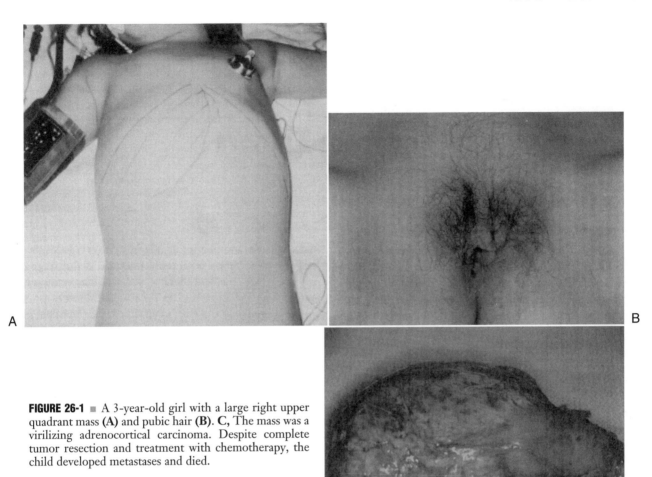

FIGURE 26-1 ■ A 3-year-old girl with a large right upper quadrant mass **(A)** and pubic hair **(B)**. **C,** The mass was a virilizing adrenocortical carcinoma. Despite complete tumor resection and treatment with chemotherapy, the child developed metastases and died.

for the presence of tumor extension into the adrenal vein or vena cava. Detection of small adrenal tumors by ultrasound may be more difficult. Abdominal CT is a more accurate diagnostic test and clearly delineates the extent of the tumor, detects liver metastases, identifies enlarged para-aortic lymph nodes, and rules out a contralateral

TABLE 26-2 ■ Factors Associated with Prognosis in Adrenocortical Tumors		
	Good Prognosis	**Poor Prognosis**
Age (yr)	<5	>10
Tumor weight (g)	<100 (or <50)	>500 g (or >100)
Size (cm)	<5	>5
Mitoses (per 50 high-power fields)	<20	>20
Local invasion	Absent	Present
Metastases (nodes, lungs, liver)	Absent	Present
Duration of symptoms (mo)	<6	>6
Necrosis ≥25% of the tumor	No	Yes

tumor. Magnetic resonance imaging (MRI) can detect 1-cm adrenal lesions on coronal slices and gradually may supplant CT because it avoids radiation. Adrenal scintigraphy uses radiolabeled cholesterol compounds that localize in tissues that produce steroid hormones to detect the presence of adrenocortical tumors. Incorporation of the radioisotope may be enhanced by ACTH stimulation and dexamethasone suppression. Iodocholesterol analogues, such as ^{131}I-6β-iodomethyl norcholesterol (NP 59) may distinguish between benign and malignant adrenal tumors because carcinomas do not concentrate the isotope as readily as normal tissues. Bilateral symmetric images in a patient with elevated 17-hydroxycortisol levels usually reflect bilateral adrenal hyperplasia. Unilateral uptake of the isotope is consistent with adenoma, whereas bilateral nonvisualization is consistent with carcinoma. Disadvantages include the limited availability of these isotopes and exposure to radiation.

Therapy

The treatment of choice for children with adrenocortical tumors is complete surgical excision. Perioperative and postoperative steroid support is important because the contralateral gland usually has atrophied from chronic

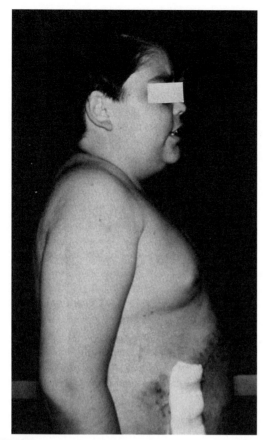

FIGURE 26-2 ■ An obese 14-year-old boy with moon facies and buffalo hump characteristic of Cushing's syndrome. The boy had an adrenocortical adenoma.

suppression. Small adenomas can be removed by laparoscopy, whereas for large tumors, the operative procedure is performed through an anterior transverse transperitoneal incision so that the tumor, liver, and periaortic lymph nodes can be evaluated carefully. Intraoperative contralateral adrenal assessment has become less necessary with current diagnostic imaging. In children with large primary tumors, a thoracoabdominal incision may provide excellent operative exposure. Radical adrenalectomy gives patients the best chance for survival. Patients with large tumors should undergo radical periaortic node dissection (from diaphragm to aortic bifurcation) because complete tumor excision gives the best hope for cure. Local recurrences and solitary metastases should be excised because long-term survival has been described after resection of liver, lung, or brain metastases. The use of radiofrequency ablation has been described for unresectable lesions.

Although adrenocortical tumors usually are considered radioresistant, an occasional survivor has been observed after 1500 to 3000 cGy. Radiotherapy can shrink an unresectable tumor, allowing subsequent second-look resection. The most effective chemotherapeutic agent is mitotane (ortho-para DDD), an isomer of the insecticide DDT. Although mitotane therapy results in tumor regression in 34% to 61% of cases in adults with adrenocortical tumors, this treatment has not improved the survival rate. The response rate is better when mitotane is administered prophylactically before the appearance of metastases. Sporadic case reports document an occasional survivor despite residual disease after mitotane therapy. Mitotane also has been used in combination with 5-fluorouracil, cisplatin, etoposide, and streptozocin without significant improvement in survival. Poor results also have been noted in patients with adrenocortical carcinoma treated with other multidrug chemotherapy. Mitotane therapy is associated with significant toxicity in most patients (91%); gastrointestinal complications were noted in 83%, neurotoxicity in 41%, and a skin rash in 12% of patients. Several other side effects are possible, and adrenal insufficiency is expected to develop. Toxicity is reduced by administration of mitotane with cellulose, which decreases gastric absorption. Other agents useful in patients with adrenocortical lesions include an aminoglutethimide, a desmolase inhibitor, and metyrapone, an 11-β-hydroxylase inhibitor that helps suppress steroid production and minimize some of the adverse effects of excessive steroid production. Radiotherapy also has been used for palliation of metastases.

Prognosis

Given the difficulties in differentiating adrenocortical adenomas from carcinomas, prognosis is difficult to determine. Patients with adenomas generally are cured by surgical resection. Even with a histologic diagnosis of carcinoma, children younger than 5 years old have a better prognosis than older children (70% survival versus <13%). Complete resection of carcinomas results in a 67% chance of survival, whereas survival is virtually zero when gross tumor is left in place. Aggressive resection is indicated, including involved adjacent organs if necessary. Secondary complete resection of local recurrence or distant metastasis was useful in one adult series, with a 57% versus 0% 5-year survival when complete resection was not possible. Duration of symptoms of less than 6 months also correlates with an improved survival (70% versus <10%), highlighting the malignant potential of adrenocortical tumors.

PHEOCHROMOCYTOMA

Pheochromocytomas arise from chromaffin cells in the adrenal medulla; extra-adrenal pheochromocytomas, also called *paragangliomas*, can occur in sympathetic ganglia anywhere from the neck to the pelvis (organ of Zuckerkandl). These lesions are the cause of hypertension in 0.1% of all hypertensive patients as a result of excessive catecholamine production. In 80% to 90% of cases, the tumor is benign. It is difficult to discern between benign and malignant tumors histologically; the clinical course of the patient is the most accurate method of determining the final diagnosis and eventual outcome. Pheochromocytoma may occur as a sporadic lesion (usually in the adrenal gland) or as part of a familial syndrome (10%). Extra-adrenal tumors and multiple pheochromocytomas are observed more frequently in children and tend to have an increased risk of malignancy (40%) (Fig. 26-3).

Pheochromocytoma is classified as an APUD tumor (amine precursor uptake and decarboxylation). Familial

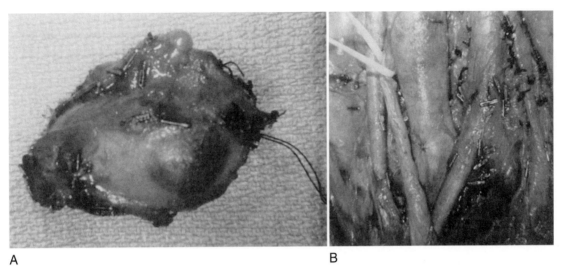

A B

FIGURE 26-3 ■ **A,** A relatively small extra-adrenal pheochromocytoma that arose from a paraspinal sympathetic ganglia in a 13-year-old girl who experienced paroxysmal hypertension, tachycardia, and severe headache while horseback riding. **B,** The operative field after tumor excision shows the bifurcation of the aorta and vena cava. The vascular tape is around the right ureter.

cases of APUD tumors may occur as a solitary lesion or in combination with other manifestations of MEN (MEN-IIA and MEN-IIB). These syndromes are related to mutations in the *RET* proto-oncogene, located on chromosome 10q11.2. Approximately 50% of patients with MEN develop pheochromocytoma, whereas virtually all patients develop medullary carcinoma of the thyroid. The latter usually occurs at a younger age, whereas pheochromocytoma usually develops later, in the teens or 20s. MEN-IIA also is called *Sipple's syndrome* and is characterized by the occurrence of pheochromocytoma, medullary carcinoma of the thyroid, and parathyroid adenoma or hyperplasia. MEN-IIB also is called *mucocutaneous neuroma syndrome* and is characterized by the association of pheochromocytoma, medullary carcinoma of the thyroid, submucosal neuromas, and ganglioneuromas of the visceral plexus. von Hippel–Lindau disease, von Recklinghausen's disease (neurofibromatosis 1), tuberous sclerosis, and Sturge-Weber disease all have an increased incidence of pheochromocytoma. Pheochromocytoma occurs in 2% of patients with neurofibromatosis 1. In patients with neurofibromatosis who present with hypertension, the incidence of pheochromocytoma may be 55%. Familial extra-adrenal pheochromocytomas may occur in unusual sites, such as the renal hilum and lower urinary tract (within the bladder). Approximately 2% of cases arise in the neck and mediastinum. Neck lesions are called *chemodectomas* when they arise from chemoreceptors, such as the carotid body or vagal body.

Signs and Symptoms

Symptoms in patients with pheochromocytoma include episodic headache, facial pallor, diaphoresis, palpitations, tremors, apprehension, anxiety, epigastric pain, chest pain, weakness, exhaustion, and light-headedness. Occasionally, older patients experience syncope, and some have a myocardial infarction, Prinzmetal's syndrome (coronary spasm), or cardiomyopathy. Some children have abdominal discomfort, constipation, and rarely adynamic ileus. Greater than 80% of patients have hypertension, but only 25% to 45% have paroxysmal episodes. An abdominal mass can be palpated in approximately 15% of patients. Atypical symptoms can occur in one third of patients. Psychiatric symptoms, such as impending doom, overanxiety, and hyperventilation, also may be observed. Patients with bladder tumors may experience syncope with micturition. Orthostatism is characteristically the hallmark of hypertension associated with pheochromocytoma.

Tumor Secretion

Pheochromocytomas can produce either epinephrine or norepinephrine. Epinephrine is produced more commonly in adrenal tumors, and norepinephrine is more frequent in extra-adrenal tumors. Lesions that exclusively produce dopamine are often malignant. Some pheochromocytomas produce somatostatin, ACTH, vasoactive intestinal polypeptide (VIP), and substance P. There is also an increased incidence of malignancy in tumors with intestinal polypeptide production. These peptides can be detected on immunohistochemical staining of the tumor tissues.

A 24-hour urinary collection to determine levels of catecholamines, vanillylmandelic acid, dopamine, and metanephrines is obtained to make a diagnosis. Metanephrines are chemically more stable and are altered less commonly by stressful events than either epinephrine or norepinephrine. Chemical stimulation tests with glucagon to stimulate a pressor effect and produce hypertension with phentolamine backup to modify the pressor response are now rarely necessary. Clonidine (an antihypertensive drug) has been used to suppress blood pressure, but it does not reduce plasma catecholamine levels in patients with pheochromocytoma. The plasma catecholamine level is lowered in normal patients.

Tumor Localization

Localization of the primary tumor is influenced by whether the tumor is sporadic or familial. In children, 20% to 30% of tumors are extra-adrenal compared with 10% to 15% in adults. Bilateral adrenal pheochromocytomas may be present in 7% of adults, 24% of children, and in almost 50% of patients with familial tumors. Although angiography and selective venography were popular diagnostic studies in the past, they now are used rarely.

The most useful tests employed for tumor localization are the ^{131}I-metaiodobenzylguanidine (MIBG) scintiscan, MRI, and CT with contrast material. Although there is less experience with MRI, the current tendency is to avoid any radiation because of the long-term risks of inducing a malignancy, especially in young children. MIBG is concentrated in adrenergic tissues and is highly useful in documenting the presence of primary adrenal and extra-adrenal tumors and recurrent and metastatic disease in more than 90% of cases. Because it is more expensive, it usually is reserved for patients in whom CT or MRI fails to identify a tumor. Scanning with indium In[111] pentetreotide (OctreoScan) and positron emission tomography (PET) also have been used when other imaging modalities have failed.

Treatment

After diagnosis, the medical management of patients with pheochromocytoma involves the use of phenoxybenzamine (1 to 2 mg/kg/24 hours in four divided doses) as an α-adrenergic blocking agent to control blood pressure. This agent has a more selective effect at α-adrenergic receptors and is associated with a lesser blood pressure rebound effect than phentolamine. It should be initiated under careful monitoring and with vigorous fluid resuscitation. β-Blockade with propranolol is especially useful in the prevention of arrhythmias but should never be given before α-blockade to avoid rebound hypertension. Angiotensin inhibitors (captopril) and calcium channel blockers (nifedipine, verapamil) may be useful in controlling blood pressure in an urgent situation.

After medical therapy is established, blood pressure is controlled, and blood volume is re-expanded (this usually takes 2 to 3 weeks), the treatment of choice is a well-monitored and controlled surgical excision of the tumor under a general endotracheal anesthetic using enflurane with a nondepolarizing muscle relaxant (pancuronium). Atropine is not used to avoid tachycardia. Central venous catheter, arterial catheter, pulse oximeter, and electrocardiographic leads should be in place before starting the operation. Phentolamine, propranolol, and nitroprusside should be available to control fluctuations in blood pressure during the procedure. Crossmatched blood also should be available for transfusion because of the contracted plasma volume and red blood cell mass.

Abdominal exploration classically is performed through a long transverse or chevron-shaped upper abdominal transperitoneal incision. Tumors of the right adrenal gland are exposed by mobilizing the hepatic flexure of the colon and the duodenum. The peritoneum at the base of the liver overlying the kidney and adrenal is incised to allow further exposure of the gland. On the left side, the splenic flexure is mobilized, and the spleen and pancreas are elevated anteromedially to expose the upper portion of the kidney and the adrenal gland. The tumor should be mobilized with as little handling as possible to avoid stimulating catecholamine production during the procedure. When possible, careful identification and ligation of the adrenal veins before mobilizing the tumor is advisable. The adrenal veins are fairly constant, with the right adrenal vein entering the vena cava directly and the left adrenal vein entering the left renal vein. A small vein draining superiorly to the diaphragm (inferior phrenic vessels) may be noted on both sides. The arterial supply to the adrenal glands is derived from multiple small vessels directly from the aorta and inferior phrenic and renal arteries. The contralateral adrenal gland, paraspinal areas, base of the mesentery, and pelvis are examined carefully for possible second tumors, especially in familial cases and children. Bilateral adrenalectomy is recommended in patients with pheochromocytoma associated with MEN-II because 90% have either bilateral tumors or adrenal medullary hyperplasia. More recently, a laparoscopic approach to small pheochromocytomas has been used. This approach may allow more gentle tissue handling, decreasing the amount of catecholamine release during operation. This approach is reserved for surgeons familiar with laparoscopic adrenalectomy and other retroperitoneal procedures.

Prognosis

Children with benign tumors should be cured after complete surgical resection. It is often difficult, however, to distinguish a benign from a malignant pheochromocytoma on light microscopy. The finding of direct involvement of surrounding structures at laparotomy, the presence of metastases, the detection of tumor in a lymph node excised with the specimen, and the patient's clinical course (i.e., recurrence of tumor) are the best indicators of malignancy. Even when a malignant tumor is encountered, tumor growth is often slow, and prolonged survival commonly is observed. Recurrence of tumor after resection ranges from 12% to 46% in adult studies. Malignant tumors are encountered less frequently in young children. Recurrence may be related to failure to detect a second tumor at the initial operation, the development of a second primary tumor in the opposite adrenal gland, intraoperative tumor spill at the initial procedure, or true metastases. Sites of metastatic disease include the lymph nodes, liver, and lungs. Most cases of tumor recurrence occur within 5 years, although occasional late recurrences at greater than 10 years have been observed. MIBG scintiscans and PET are useful in detecting recurrent intra-abdominal disease or distant metastases (pulmonary nodules). If metastases are hormonally active, recurrence of symptoms may occur. These patients may be treated with resection of the metastatic focus if feasible, α-blocking and β-blocking agents, and chemotherapy. Combined treatment with streptozocin, 5-fluorouracil, vincristine, dacarbazine, and cyclophosphamide results in a greater than 50% response rate. High-dose ^{131}I-MIBG, octreotide, and tumor chemoembolization also have been used. The 5-year survival in malignant cases is 44%.

PANCREATIC TUMORS

Pancreatic neoplasms (see also Chapter 68) can be cystic or solid, benign or malignant, and endocrine or exocrine. Endocrine tumors of the pancreas originate mainly in the islet cells (Table 26-3). Diagnosis of these tumors depends on the recognition of clinical syndromes associated with autonomous secretion of a variety of endocrine substances elaborated by different secretory granules within the islet cells. Some pancreatic adenomas are seen as part of MEN-I. This autosomal dominant condition also includes adenomas of the anterior pituitary gland (20% of patients), parathyroid adenomas or hyperplasia (90%), and occasionally adrenal cortical adenomas or hyperplasia and carcinoids. It is related to a defective tumor suppressor gene located on chromosome 11q13; patients without a family history represent de novo mutations of the gene.

Insulinomas are the most common islet cell tumors. Of tumors, 80% are solitary, and 90% are benign. Malignant insulinomas account for 10% of lesions and usually are documented at the initial presentation. Malignant insulinomas in childhood are exceptionally rare. Most cases have been identified in children older than age 4 years, although reports of islet cell adenomas occurring in neonates have been documented. These latter cases may be heralded by seizure activity related to hypoglycemia and must be distinguished from the more commonly occurring instances of diffuse nesidioblastosis noted in newborns.

Most older children present with Whipple's triad, characterized by documenting hypoglycemia with fasting associated with irrational behavior or neurologic sequelae relieved by the administration of glucose. The diagnosis is confirmed by reproducible hypoglycemia in a controlled environment (fasting) and by showing simultaneous hyperinsulinemia. A plasma insulin-to-glucose ratio greater than 1.0 is diagnostic (<0.4 being normal). Measuring the C peptide level is useful in ruling out an exogenous source of insulin. Proinsulin levels also should be measured and may indicate malignancy if elevated. The tumor is rarely palpable on physical examination. Preoperative tumor localization occasionally may be difficult, and a small percentage may be ectopic (2%). CT is diagnostic in more than 50% of cases but is not always sensitive because of the presence of small tumors (<1 cm). Octreotide scintigraphy, endoscopic ultrasound, and MRI may be useful. Selective celiac and superior

mesenteric arteriography is diagnostic in 60% to 70% of cases; however, this test has a higher false-positive rate. Transhepatic portal venous sampling has been employed with an 86% rate of tumor localization. In institutions where rapid insulin assay is available (e.g., within 30 minutes), this technique can be used during the operation. Intraoperative ultrasonography has been used with increasing frequency to localize islet cell tumors of the pancreas and seems useful in selected cases in which the tumor is not palpable.

At operation, the islet cell tumor is often pink and firmer than the surrounding gland. The tumor is usually discrete and well encapsulated. Most tumors simply can be enucleated. This is a reasonable procedure in children because most of the lesions are benign (>90%). If all methods of tumor localization have been unsuccessful, distal pancreatectomy with careful sectioning of the gland is advisable, with resection of greater than 80% of the gland rarely indicated. Intraoperative insulin monitoring may be useful in these latter instances. The exception to this rule is in patients with MEN-I, who tend to have multiple microadenomas and may require a 95% resection for cure of the hyperinsulinism. Most infants and children with insulinomas are cured by appropriate surgical excision; however, some may have varying degrees of mental retardation if hypoglycemic episodes before resection resulted in severe seizures. Streptozocin is an effective chemotherapeutic agent for patients with malignant insulinomas. Octreotide, a long-acting analogue of somatostatin, is also useful in suppressing the hormonal secretion in all types of pancreatic endocrine tumors.

In contrast to adults, VIP secretion in children more often is associated with a neurogenic tumor (neuroblastoma, ganglioneuroma) than a primary lesion of the pancreas. Of the 56 reported cases of VIP-producing tumors in children, only 2 cases were related to primary pancreatic islet cell lesions. In one patient, the lesion was a non-beta islet cell tumor, and in the other, islet cell hyperplasia was noted. The other 54 cases all were related to secretion of VIP from neurogenic tumors. In cases of pancreatic VIPoma, VIP probably is produced in cells of neural origin in the islet cells. VIP secretion results in a syndrome consisting of profuse watery diarrhea, hypokalemia, and achlorhydria (referred to as *WDHA syndrome*, *Verner-Morrison syndrome*, and *pancreatic cholera*). The diarrhea usually is unassociated with crampy abdominal pain. Patients often develop a metabolic acidosis and a prerenal azotemia as a result of dehydration. The pathophysiology of the disease is thought to be caused by endocrine stimulation of cyclic adenosine monophosphate in the exocrine cells of the gut, which results in active secretion of electrolytes and water into the intestinal lumen.

Glucagonoma and somatostatinoma are tumors that occur primarily in adults. We are unaware of their occurrence in early childhood.

Gastrinoma is associated with G-cell production of gastrin resulting in gastric hypersecretion and severe peptic ulcer diathesis (Zollinger-Ellison [Z-E] syndrome). Diarrhea commonly is associated. Gastrinoma is part of

TABLE 26-3 ■ Islet Cell Tumors		
Cell Type	**Hormone**	**Tumor**
Alpha cell	Glucagon	Glucagonoma
Beta cell	Insulin	Insulinoma
G cell	Gastrin	Gastrinoma
Delta cell	Somatostatin	Somatostatinoma
Delta$_1$ cell	VIP	VIPoma

MEN-I in 10% to 25% of cases overall. It is the most common functioning pancreatic lesion associated with MEN-I in adults, but this association appears less common in children and even nonexistent according to some authors. A total of 44 cases of childhood Z-E tumors were registered in the Childhood Disease Registry, Bismarck, North Dakota, until 1992 (the registry no longer exists). There were 38 cases in boys. The youngest patient was a 5-year-old girl who also had Marden-Walker syndrome (generalized connective tissue syndrome). The mean age was 11.7 years. Forty one children, had tumors, and hyperplasia was observed in 3. Of the 41 tumors, 27 were malignant (65%). This is similar to the findings in adults, in whom 60% of the tumors are malignant, with many showing liver metastases at the time of diagnosis. The diagnosis rests on a radioimmunoassay study documenting an elevated gastrin level (usually >500 pg/mL; normal <200 pg/mL).

A CT scan generally is used to locate the tumor and document the presence of liver metastases preoperatively. As for insulinomas, octreotide scintiscan, MRI, and endoscopic ultrasound also can be valuable. The medical treatment of gastrinoma was facilitated greatly with the advent of H_2-blockers and improved further with proton-pump inhibitors. Medical treatment alone has been useful in controlling the disease in most adults, but more recent evidence suggests an improved survival when the tumor is resected. Currently, surgery is offered for possible cure to all patients with the Z-E syndrome who do not have metastatic disease or MEN-I; the latter tend to have multiple lesions and rarely are rendered disease-free by surgery. Children with gastrinoma would require lifelong medical therapy, and concerns with compliance support a more aggressive surgical approach to this tumor in the pediatric age group. In 30% of patients, the lesions can be multiple and involve more than one anatomic area. If the tumor is a solitary lesion, however, and there is no evidence of metastases, resection of the primary tumor is a reasonable procedure. When preoperative studies have failed, intraoperative ultrasound is useful to localize the lesion. Intraoperative endoscopy with transillumination also is helpful because 70% occur in the head of the pancreas or the duodenum. The latter may be visible only after duodenotomy. Total gastrectomy ultimately may be required for patients who fail medical therapy and have unresectable residual tumor or metastases. Resection of lymph node and liver metastases is useful because the tumor is often slow growing, and even patients with metastases may have extended survival if the stomach also has been removed. In the 1990s, the reported 1-year and 10-year survival rates were 75% and 42% and slightly less for patients with metastases. Currently, patients with resected disease have a better than 90% survival. Patients with metastatic or unresectable islet cell tumors may experience symptomatic relief with octreotide; chemotherapy with streptozocin, 5-fluorouracil, and doxorubicin also has increased survival. Other chemotherapeutic agents and interferon have been used. Hepatic artery chemoembolization has been employed for liver metastases.

SUGGESTED READINGS

Ciftci AO, Senocak ME, Tanyel FC, et al: Adrenocortical tumors in children. J Pediatr Surg 36:549-554, 2001.

This article describes a series of 30 children with adrenocortical tumors from a single center. In Turkey, children often present late (mean time from symptoms to diagnosis of >8 months), resulting in poor outcome.

Fraker DL, Jensen RT: Pancreatic endocrine tumors. In DeVita VT Jr, Hellman S, Rosenberg SA (eds): Cancer: Principles and Practice of Oncology, 5th ed. Philadelphia, Lippincott-Raven Publishers, 1997, pp 1678-1704.

This is an extensive review of endocrine malignancies by leaders in the field of endocrine surgery.

Hack HA: The perioperative management of children with phaeochromocytoma. Paediatr Anaesth 10:463-476, 2000.

This article reviews the pharmacology and pathophysiology of pheochromocytoma, highlighting differences between children and adults.

Honigschnabl S, Gallo S, Niederle B, et al: How accurate is MR imaging in characterization of adrenal masses: Update of a long-term study. Eur J Radiol 41:113-122, 2002.

A more recent report of the role of MRI in adrenal tumors is presented.

Koch CA, Pacak K, Chrousos GP: Endocrine Tumors. In Pizzo PA, Poplack DG (eds): Principles and Practice of Pediatric Oncology, 4th ed. Philadelphia, Lippincott Williams & Wilkins, 2002, pp 1115-1148.

This is an excellent chapter in a more recent pediatric oncology textbook.

Lack EE: Tumors of the adrenal gland and extra-adrenal paraganglia. In Rosai J, Sobin LH (eds): Atlas of Tumor Pathology, Third Series, Fascicle 19. Washington, DC, Armed Forces Institutes of Pathology, 1997.

An important reference for pathologists, this atlas discusses the difficulties in differentiating between adrenocortical adenomas and carcinomas in children.

Miller KA, Albanese C, Harrison M, et al: Experience with laparoscopic adrenalectomy in pediatric patients. J Pediatr Surg 37:979-982, 2002.

The authors report their experience in 17 patients; a mean length of hospitalization of 35 hours makes this approach attractive for benign adrenal pathology.

Norton JA, Fraker DL, Alexander HR, et al: Surgery to cure the Zollinger-Ellison syndrome. N Engl J Med 341:635-644, 1999.

This important article reports the results of a National Institutes of Health prospective study from 1981 until 1998; 151 patients participated in the study. It provides details about the surgical protocols and documents excellent cure rates in patients with sporadic gastrinomas.

Ribeiro RC, Michalkiewicz EL, Figueiredo BC, et al: Adrenocortical tumors in children. Braz J Med Biol Res 33:1225-1234, 2000.

The first author is one of the world experts in this field. The higher incidence of adrenocortical tumors in Brazilian children (10 times normal) is noted, the cause of which is unknown. The diagnosis, management, and prognosis are reviewed.

Ross JH: Pheochromocytoma: Special considerations in children. Urol Clin North Am 27:393-402, 2000.

This article reviews pheochromocytoma in children.

Schulick RD, Brennan MF: Long-term survival after complete resection and repeat resection in patients with adrenocortical carcinoma. Ann Surg Oncol 6:719-726, 1999.

The benefits of aggressive surgery are highlighted in this article.

Teinturier C, Pauchard MS, Brugieres L, et al: Clinical and prognostic aspects of adrenocortical neoplasms in childhood. Med Pediatr Oncol 32:106-111, 1999.

This excellent article describes 54 children with adrenocortical tumors.

Gonadal Tumors

27

Gonadal tumors represent approximately 2% of all pediatric malignancies and are distributed evenly between ovarian and testicular tumors. The most common types of gonadal tumors are listed in Table 27-1.

OVARIAN CYSTS AND TUMORS

The ovary has an abdominal location in most infants and children and descends into the pelvis as it enlarges at puberty. Most ovarian lesions in young patients present with an abdominal mass. The ovary has an infundibular pedicle so that when involved by a mass, the lesion is often mobile.

TABLE 27-1 ■ Most Common Types of Primary Gonadal Tumors in Children	
Ovary	**Testis**
Germ cell	
Teratoma	Teratoma
Mature (cystic, solid or mixed)	
Immature (grade 1 to 3)	
Associated with malignant GCT component	
Associated with malignant somatic component	
Yolk sac tumor	Yolk sac tumor
Dysgerminoma	Seminoma
Embryonal carcinoma	Embryonal carcinoma
Mixed malignant GCT	Mixed malignant GCT (teratocarcinoma)
Choriocarcinoma	Choriocarcinoma
Gonadoblastoma	Gonadoblastoma
Polyembryoma	
Non–germ cell	
Epithelial	—
Serous, mucinous, others (benign or malignant)	
Sex cord–stromal	Sex cord–stromal
Granulosa-theca	Sertoli cell
Sertoli-Leydig	Leydig cell
Mixed	Mixed

GCT, germ cell tumor.

TABLE 27-2 ■ Ultrasound Characterization of Ovarian Cysts	
Simple	**Complex**
Anechoic content	Mixed cystic/solid
	Echogenic debris, fluid-fluid level
Thin wall	Septations
	Thick wall

Ovarian Cysts

Ovarian cysts frequently are detected in utero by prenatal ultrasound. About 30% of fetuses have follicular ovarian cysts greater than 1 mm. Stimulation by maternal and placental hormones has been implicated in their occurrence. The fetal incidence of ovarian cysts is disproportionately high when considering that the neonatal incidence classically is only 1 per 100,000 births. This strongly suggests that fetal ovarian cysts undergo spontaneous involution or silent torsion and resorption either late in pregnancy or shortly after birth (this is the cause of most cases of unilateral absent ovary diagnosed later in life). After birth, ovarian cysts usually present as a palpable mobile mass. The mass is rarely symptomatic and has almost no risk of malignancy.

The current indications for intervention include simple cysts greater than 5 cm and complex cysts of any size (Table 27-2). Large simple cysts (>5 cm) are associated with an increased risk of torsion of the ovary. Prenatal puncture of the cyst has been advocated, but the risks probably outweigh the benefits except for huge cysts that could lead to abdominal dystocia during vaginal delivery. The safest postnatal management of large simple cysts is probably aspiration or unroofing under laparoscopic guidance, although some authors recommend observation alone. Complex cysts are often ovarian cysts that have undergone torsion, causing bleeding within the cyst, but may represent duplications or other types of cysts (Fig. 27-1). Laparoscopy is indicated to establish the diagnosis.

Beyond the newborn period, ovarian cysts in prepubertal children are unusual. A benign cystic teratoma (discussed further) may be discovered during ultrasound

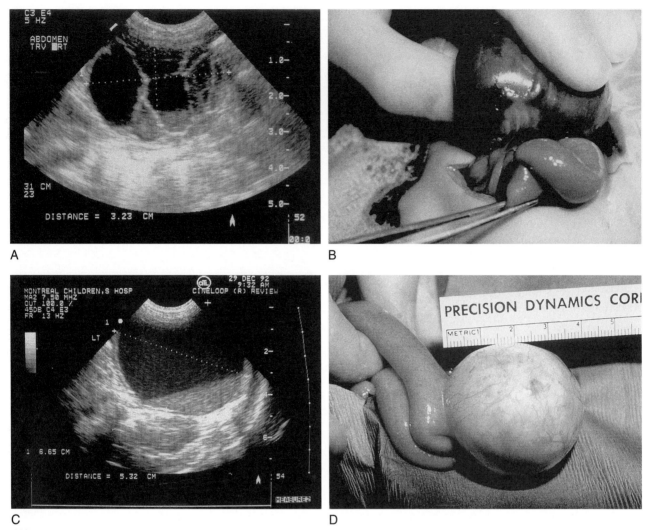

FIGURE 27-1 ■ Example of complex neonatal cysts discovered on antenatal ultrasound. **A,** Cyst with septations and debris. **B,** At operation, the twisted ovarian cyst was found adherent to small intestine, with a potential for internal hernia. **C,** Another patient, with a unilocular cyst with layering debris. **D,** At operation, this turned out to be a cystic small bowel duplication.

obtained for complaints of abdominal pain or unrelated reasons. A palpable ovarian mass in this age group should be evaluated carefully and treated as a potentially malignant lesion. In postmenarchal girls, the presence of a cyst is common, and surgical intervention is unnecessary for unilocular cysts less than 5 cm.

Most non-neoplastic ovarian cysts result from the natural cycle of ovarian follicles; these are the follicular and corpus luteum cysts. Physiologic follicles should not exceed 2 cm in diameter. Follicular cysts are the most common type of cyst and occur in neonates and older children. Occasionally, precocious puberty may be observed as a result of a follicle cyst that produces a significant excess of estrogenic hormones. For large (>5 cm) unilocular cysts that do not regress on repeat ultrasound examinations, careful excision or unroofing of the cyst with retention of the remaining normal ovary is advised. Corpus luteum cysts are seen in teenagers and develop after ovulation begins. These cysts are lined by luteinized theca and granulosa cells and may appear hemorrhagic. They may present with signs of peritoneal

irritation and can be confused with acute appendicitis. The diagnosis is made on ultrasound or at the time of laparoscopy or laparotomy. These cysts do not require treatment and usually resolve on follow-up ultrasound 6 weeks later.

Other non-neoplastic cysts are seen less frequently. Polycystic ovaries may be observed as part of the Stein-Leventhal syndrome. Paraovarian cysts are usually small, are usually benign, may be multiple, and require no special treatment. Paratubal cysts may reach large proportions and may be difficult to distinguish from ovarian cysts preoperatively. The treatment is excision (Fig. 27-2).

Ovarian Tumors

Ovarian tumors are the most common gynecologic malignancy in childhood. The peak incidence is between 10 and 14 years of age. Germ cell tumors account for 60% to 65% of ovarian tumors in children. Sex cord and stromal tumors (granulosa-theca cell tumors, Sertoli-Leydig cell tumors) and epithelial cell tumors comprise

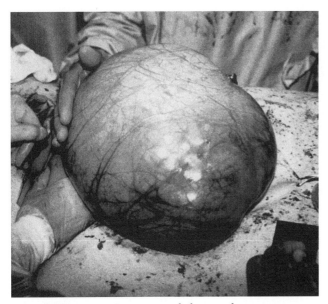

FIGURE 27-2 ■ Large paratubal cyst at laparotomy.

the remainder of the tumors (see Table 27-1). In girls older than age 15 to 17, epithelial tumors comprise almost 33% of cases.

Teratomas

Mature teratomas may be cystic, solid, or mixed tumors. In 50% of cases, calcification is observed on plain abdominal radiographs (Fig. 27-3). This benign neoplasm is the most common ovarian tumor and represents approximately 40% of all ovarian tumors. Of patients, 10% may have bilateral ovarian involvement. The clinical presentation includes abdominal pain, the presence of a mass, and occasionally an acute abdomen as a result of torsion or rupture of the tumor. Some are discovered incidentally with imaging. Tumors that are predominantly cystic, the so-called dermoid cysts, may be excised safely, preserving a rim of normal ovarian tissue near the infundibulum (see Fig. 27-3C). Controversy exists about the safety of laparoscopic excision because rupture of the cyst often occurs, leading to potential peritoneal implantation of cells. Solid teratomas are more often immature, and the treatment of choice is salpingo-oophorectomy. Immature teratomas are composed of incompletely differentiated germ cell elements with varying histologic grade (I to III). Patients with grade II or III immature teratoma were given postoperative chemotherapy in the past, but this was shown not to be necessary in more recent years. Serum α-fetoprotein levels (AFP) may be elevated preoperatively and should be monitored after operation. In these cases, careful sectioning of the specimen may reveal microscopic foci of yolk sac tumor; this does not alter management as long as AFP levels return to normal.

Malignant Germ Cell Tumors

Malignant germ cell tumors include yolk sac tumor, dysgerminoma, embryonal cell carcinoma, and choriocarcinoma.

Yolk Sac Tumors

Yolk sac tumors (also called *endodermal sinus tumors**) are characterized by rapid growth and early metastases. This aggressive, malignant germ cell tumor usually occurs in teenage girls and young adults. It is the most common malignant component to develop in teratomas. The tumor produces AFP, which serves as a diagnostic tumor marker and a method to evaluate response to treatment and monitor postoperative recurrence (see Chapter 24). The most widely used staging system for ovarian tumors is the one developed by the International Federation of Gynecology and Obstetrics (FIGO), in which stages I and II are considered localized and stages III and IV are considered advanced or disseminated disease (Table 27-3). It was developed mostly for adult tumors, most of which are epithelial tumors. A different staging system is used by the Children's Oncology Group for germ cell tumors, which takes into account tumor markers (Table 27-4). New intraoperative management guidelines are now more specific to children with germ cell tumors. Peritoneal fluid (ascites or washings) is obtained for cytology as in adults, but routine omentectomy, peritoneal biopsies, retroperitoneal lymph node biopsies, and bivalving of the contralateral ovary are no longer recommended. Instead, these areas are inspected carefully (including all peritoneal surfaces, subphrenic areas, and iliac and para-aortic nodes up to the diaphragm), and biopsy specimens are obtained only if the areas appear suspicious. When extensive involvement of the omentum is present, omentectomy is indicated. Survival for malignant germ cell tumors increased from less than 20% to 60% or more with combination chemotherapy; the advent of platinum-based chemotherapy in the 1990s has increased the disease-free survival rate further; it now exceeds 90%. Cisplatin or carboplatin usually is combined with etoposide and bleomycin (PEB). Because this combination is effective yet has significant toxicity, patients with stage I disease now simply are observed after surgery as long as the elevated serum AFP returns to normal postoperatively. With this approach, survival is close to 100%, and chemotherapy is reserved for patients who have tumor recurrence or persistently elevated AFP levels. Patients with more advanced disease often respond well to chemotherapy; after three or four cycles of PEB, second-look surgery is indicated to resect any gross disease remaining in the abdominal cavity or retroperitoneal or mediastinal nodes. Amifostine has been added to decrease the toxicity of chemotherapy, especially when using high-dose platinum.

Dysgerminomas

Dysgerminomas are derived from undifferentiated primordial germ cells. They are the counterpart to testicular seminomas. Dysgerminomas represent 16% of germ cell tumors and occur most commonly in prepubertal and adolescent girls. More than half of all dysgerminomas occur before 20 years of age. These lesions are hormonally and biologically inactive and of low-grade malignancy.

---

*The endodermal sinus is a structure that exists in fetal rats, not humans. The term *yolk sac tumor* is more appropriate.

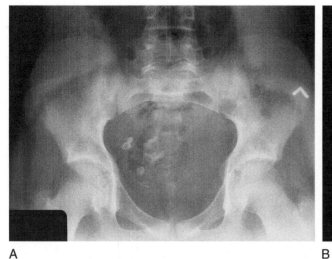

A

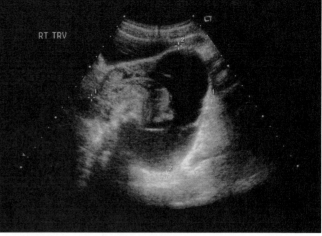

B

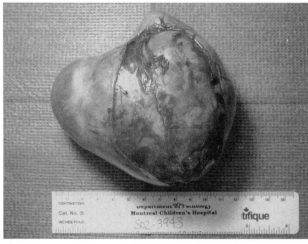

C

FIGURE 27-3 ■ **A,** This 12-year-old girl had radiographs done to investigate a scoliosis. Right pelvic calcifications were seen, some suggestive of teeth. She complained of lower abdominal pain during physical exercise. **B,** Ultrasound showed a 10.5 × 9.7 cm mixed solid/cystic mass in the right ovary, with a normal contralateral ovary. Serum α-fetoprotein and β-human chorionic gonadotropin were normal. **C,** At operation, the ovarian capsule was opened to leave a rim of normal ovarian tissue around the infundibulum, while keeping the tumor capsule intact. Microscopic examination revealed a mature teratoma containing teeth, hair, and mature brain tissue. (Courtesy of Dr. Hélène Flageole.)

TABLE 27-3 ■ FIGO Staging System for Primary Carcinoma of the Ovary	
Stage	**Description**
I	Growth limited to ovaries
IA	Growth limited to one ovary; no ascites; no tumor on the external surface: capsule intact
IB	Growth limited to both ovaries; no ascites; no tumor on the external surfaces: capsule intact
IC	Either stage IA or IB, with tumor on surface of one or both ovaries; or with capsule ruptured; or with ascites present containing malignant cells; or with positive peritoneal washings
II	Growth involving one or both ovaries with pelvic extension
IIA	Extension and/or metastases to the uterus and/or tubes
IIB	Extension to the pelvic tissues
IIC	Either stage IIA or IIB, but with tumor on surface of one or both ovaries; or with capsule(s) ruptured; or with ascites present containing malignant cells; or with positive peritoneal washings
III	Tumor involving one or both ovaries with peritoneal implants outside the pelvis and/or positive retroperitoneal or inguinal nodes; superficial liver metastasis equals stage III; tumor limited to the true pelvis but with histologically proven malignant extension to small bowel or omentum
IIIA	Tumor grossly limited to the true pelvis with negative nodes but with histologically confirmed microscopic seeding of abdominal peritoneal surfaces
IIIB	Tumor of one or both ovaries with histologically confirmed implants of abdominal peritoneal surfaces, none >2 cm; nodes negative
IIIC	Abdominal implants >2 cm and/or positive retroperitoneal or inguinal nodes
IV	Growth involving one or both ovaries with distant metastasis; if pleural effusion present, positive cytologic study required to allot a case to stage IV; parenchymal liver metastasis equals stage IV

FIGO, Fédération Internationale de Gynécologie et Obstétrique.

TABLE 27-4 ■ Children's Oncology Group Staging System for Germ Cell Tumors (Gonadal and Extragonadal)

Stage	Extent of Disease
I	Tumor limited to ovary, testis, or extragonadal site; negative tumor margins. Markers normalize after appropriate half-life decline
II	Microscopic residual disease after resection, preoperative rupture, or tumor markers remain elevated
III	Gross residual disease or biopsy only or retroperitoneal nodes positive
IV	Distant metastases including liver

Tumor spread may occur by hematogenous, lymphatic, and peritoneal routes. Patients commonly present with an abdominal mass or pain. The diagnosis is made by ultrasound, which shows a solid ovarian tumor, and computed tomography scan, which more clearly delineates the tumor margins and may detect other possible sites of intra-abdominal spread (e.g., lymph nodes, omentum).

The treatment of dysgerminoma is surgical resection. Salpingo-oophorectomy alone is adequate for tumors isolated to the ovary. Tumors may be bilateral in 5% to 10% of patients. Past recommendations to obtain a biopsy specimen of the opposite ovary at laparotomy are probably not warranted with current imaging techniques. If tumor has penetrated the ovarian capsule, peritoneal washings should be obtained, and a biopsy of the para-aortic lymph nodes and infracolic omentectomy should be performed. If the uterus is involved by direct tumor extension, hysterectomy (preferably with preservation of the contralateral ovary) may be necessary. Because dysgerminomas are highly sensitive to radiation therapy, hemipelvic irradiation with shielding of the contralateral ovary usually was employed in the past with total abdominal irradiation in cases of intra-abdominal extension. Because of the late sequelae of radiotherapy in children, including infertility, platinum-based chemotherapy has been used as the sole adjuvant treatment in more recent years. Controversy remains as to whether patients with stage I disease require any adjuvant therapy at all. The prognosis of dysgerminoma is excellent. Survival has been achieved in 90% of cases.

Embryonal Carcinoma

Embryonal cell carcinoma is less common than the yolk sac tumor and represents 6% to 8% of malignant ovarian tumors. Embryonal tumors produce AFP and β-human chorionic gonadotropin (β-hCG). Both tumor markers are useful in monitoring response to therapy and possible recurrence after surgical resection. β-hCG is responsible for the hormonal manifestations of the tumor, including abnormal vaginal bleeding, hirsutism, and precocious puberty, which may be observed in 60% of patients. Staging, surgical treatment, and chemotherapy are similar to those described for yolk sac tumors.

Choriocarcinoma

Choriocarcinoma is the least common germ cell tumor. Most of these highly malignant neoplasms produce β-hCG and are hormonally active. This hormonal activity is manifested by precocious puberty in premenarchal girls and menstrual irregularity in postmenarchal teenagers in association with a mass that may mimic a pregnancy. This tumor is significantly less responsive to chemotherapy and irradiation than other germ cell tumors. Surgical guidelines suggest that a unilateral salpingo-oophorectomy is reasonable therapy for tumors localized to the ovary. Most choriocarcinomas have extended beyond the ovary at the time of diagnosis, however, and require a more extensive tumor resection. In most patients with advanced pelvic disease, the procedure of choice is a panhysterectomy with preservation of the contralateral ovary when possible.

Gonadoblastoma

Gonadoblastomas are neoplasms that arise exclusively in dysgenetic gonads; these consist of the streak "ovaries" and dysgenetic testes seen in patients with pure gonadal dysgenesis (XY type), mixed gonadal dysgenesis (most commonly 45XO/46XY mosaicism), Turner's syndrome, and some types of male pseudohermaphroditism. Children with mixed gonadal dysgenesis have a 25% risk of developing a gonadoblastoma. Gonadoblastomas behave as benign tumors but may be associated with a malignant germ cell element, such as dysgerminoma. They are usually encapsulated and easily resectable. The tumor consists of proliferation of germ cells and sex cord cells. Because of the high risk of a second tumor, the contralateral dysgenetic gonad should be removed at the same operation. No adjunctive therapy is required unless a malignant germ cell element is present.

Sex Cord–Stromal Tumors

Approximately 13% to 18% of ovarian tumors in children are of mesenchymal sex cord or stromal origin. The most common of these tumors is the granulosa-theca cell tumor (84% of cases). Clinical presentation in premenarchal girls includes an abdominal mass and peripheral precocious puberty as a result of excessive secretion of estradiol by the tumor. Breast enlargement, early development of pubic hair, genital enlargement, and vaginal bleeding occur. In postmenarchal girls, the clinical pattern is one of menstrual irregularities or virilization. The peptide growth factor, inhibin, is elevated in patients with granulosa cell tumors and may be a tumor marker for this condition. These tumors are slow growing and usually have a benign course (>90%) in children. They can be treated effectively by unilateral salpingo-oophorectomy without adjunctive therapy in most cases. Although granulosa-theca cell tumors may be bilateral in 30% of adults, bilateral presentation in children is rare. Patients with advanced disease have a worse prognosis and require multimodal therapy.

Girls with Sertoli-Leydig cell tumors present with evidence of an abdominal pelvic mass usually in association with masculinization because of excess testosterone production. This tumor, previously termed *androblastoma* or *arrhenoblastoma*, is relatively uncommon (10% of sex cord–stromal tumors). The affected patient is usually a teenager who presents with hirsutism, clitoral hypertrophy, increased somatic growth, advanced bone age, and a gruff deepening voice. Some tumors may be hormonally inactive, and a few cases with feminization have been described. Surgical management of these patients is identical to that described for patients with granulosa-theca cell tumors.

Epithelial Ovarian Tumors

Epithelial tumors are the most common ovarian tumors in adults but are relatively infrequent in children, representing 15% of all ovarian tumors in children. After age 16 years, approximately 30% to 35% of ovarian tumors are epithelial. These tumors can be described as benign, of low malignant potential, or overtly malignant. Only 15% are malignant in children, and 30% are borderline. Epithelial tumors have been classified as mucinous, serous, clear cell, endometrioid, mixed, and undifferentiated. The staging for ovarian epithelial tumors follows the FIGO staging system for ovarian carcinoma (see Table 27-3). Most ovarian carcinomas occur in women older than age 50. Some cases are familial, and first-degree relatives have a 50% risk of developing a malignant ovarian tumor but usually not during childhood. Ca-125 is a tumor marker that is elevated in 80% of nonmucinous epithelial malignant tumors of the ovary in adults. Serum inhibin, carcinoembryonic antigen, and other markers sometimes are elevated in cases of mucinous carcinoma of the ovary. Little information is available concerning these tumor markers in children with epithelial ovarian tumors.

Epithelial ovarian tumors in children can become large, with tumors weighing more than 10 kg observed in 12-year-olds. This type of ovarian cancer spreads mainly by contiguous growth and intraperitoneal implantation. Tumor extension may involve the surface of bowel, bladder, omentum, and adjacent peritoneum, including the undersurface of the right diaphragm. In advanced cases, ascites and right-sided pleural effusion commonly are observed. Lymphatic extension occurs into the retroperitoneum in the para-aortic lymph node chain and through the broad ligament to the iliac and hypogastric pelvic lymph nodes.

Surgical staging of ovarian carcinoma includes a midline incision, obtaining peritoneal washings for cytologic study, inspection of all peritoneal surfaces and liver for tumor implants, obtaining biopsy specimens of the undersurface of the diaphragm and peritoneum, infracolic omentectomy, and sampling of para-aortic and pelvic lymph nodes. If the tumor is stage IA, a unilateral salpingo-oophorectomy is adequate, especially in young women who desire future childbearing. More advanced stages are managed by bilateral salpingo-oophorectomy and total abdominal hysterectomy. Optimal surgical debulking has been useful in reducing tumor burden in anticipation of adjunctive treatment. Stage I patients with well-differentiated tumors have a 90% 5-year survival with or without chemotherapy. Stage I patients with grade II or III tumors (undifferentiated), ruptured capsule, extracystic spread, or positive peritoneal washings or ascites and stage II patients have an 80% survival after melphalan, platinum-based chemotherapy, or intraperitoneal radioactive phosphorus (^{32}P). Patients with advanced-stage tumors (stage III and IV) are managed by debulking and three-drug chemotherapy including cisplatin, cyclophosphamide, and doxorubicin. The combination of carboplatin and paclitaxel (Taxol) has shown effectiveness, but an ideal first-line effective treatment has not been identified for advanced ovarian carcinoma. Intraperitoneal therapy with cisplatin and etoposide with thiosulfate rescue also has been used in advanced-stage disease. Second-look procedures are reasonable after treatment of advanced-stage tumors but are unnecessary in most early-stage (I and II) lesions. Biologic response modifiers, such as intraperitoneal interferon-alfa with and without added cisplatin, are being studied currently in patients with minimal residual disease after treatment. DNA-flow cytometry in patients with stage III ovarian cancer indicates that aneuploidy is associated with a poor prognosis. A poor prognosis also has been noted in ovarian tumors that express the *c-fms* oncogene.

TESTICULAR TUMORS

Tumors of the testes are relatively uncommon lesions, representing approximately 1% of all malignancies in children. Of testicular tumors seen in children, 75% are of germ cell origin. The ratio between benign and malignant varies among series. Testicular tumors are classified as germ cell tumors, gonadal stromal lesions, gonadoblastoma, tumors of supporting tissues (hemangioma, fibroma, leiomyoma), leukemic and lymphomatous infiltrates, and secondary tumors of the adnexa.

Germ Cell Tumors

The most common malignant testicular germ cell tumor is the yolk sac tumor. These represent 60% of all prepubertal testicular tumors. Most patients present before age 3 years. Most boys with a testicular tumor have a nontender mass on physical examination. Occasionally a hydrocele may be noted in association with the tumor and may be a cause of delay in diagnosis. Yolk sac tumors usually secrete AFP, which is a good tumor marker for diagnosis and to monitor recurrence. These lesions also may secrete β-hCG. Approximately 80% of boys have stage I disease, and 20% have stage II through IV tumors (Table 27-4). For boys with stage I lesions, a radical orchiectomy is the only therapy required, provided that tumor markers return to normal postoperatively. The operation is performed through a groin incision. The external inguinal ring is identified and incised in the long axis of its fibers. The cremasteric bundle is opened, and the spermatic cord is mobilized carefully at the internal inguinal ring and controlled by an occlusive vascular clamp. This prevents lymphatic and hematogenous spread of the tumor during manipulation. The testis is delivered into the wound, and if the mass is solid, a radical orchiectomy is completed with ligation of the spermatic cord at the level of the internal ring. If the tumor was biopsied through the scrotum before referral, a hemiscrotectomy generally is performed, although more recent evidence suggests that chemotherapy could treat tumor seeding adequately. Routine retroperitoneal lymph node dissection has been abandoned. In infants and children younger than age 3 years, the incidence of para-aortic lymph node involvement is relatively low (4% to 14%). Although most children with yolk sac tumors of the testes are treated with chemotherapy, in boys younger than 3 years of age with stage I tumors, current guidelines call for radical orchiectomy alone and administration of chemotherapy only if the postoperative serum AFP levels remain elevated or recurrent disease occurs. In these latter cases, the patient usually can be salvaged by chemotherapy. Radiation therapy is unwarranted in boys with stage I tumors.

A close postoperative surveillance program is an important component of follow-up care. The patient should be evaluated on a monthly basis for the first year, then every other month for 2 more years. Physical examination, chest radiograph, and serum AFP levels are evaluated. Abdominal computed tomography is performed periodically (every 3 months). In instances of tumor recurrence localized to the retroperitoneal lymph nodes, a retroperitoneal lymph node dissection is needed. The procedure usually is limited to a unilateral dissection using nerve-sparing techniques to minimize the risk of loss of ejaculation. If there is a suspicious contralateral lymph node observed at the time of the unilateral dissection, this should be biopsied, followed by the administration of chemotherapy using PEB. Combination chemotherapy also is used if AFP levels fail to normalize.

In boys with stage III disease, a retroperitoneal lymph node dissection is advisable followed by chemotherapy. If bulky disease is present, primary cytoreductive treatment with chemotherapy (three or four cycles of PEB) is followed by imaging to evaluate whether any residual disease remains. If there is persistent retroperitoneal or mediastinal disease, exploration of the thorax and retroperitoneum is needed with radical excision of all nodes. Resection of persistent distant disease (liver, lungs) also is warranted. Radiation therapy is withheld initially but may be useful in selected instances of residual disease. Survival is close to 100% for stage I and greater than 80% for advanced stages.

Teratomas of the testes are the most common type of benign neoplasms and usually occur in boys younger than 3 years of age. These tumors can be managed successfully with radical orchiectomy and do not require any adjunctive treatment (Fig. 27-4). Small encapsulated cystic teratomas also may be enucleated similar to their ovarian counterpart; the cord should be occluded atraumatically until a frozen section confirms the benign nature of the lesion.

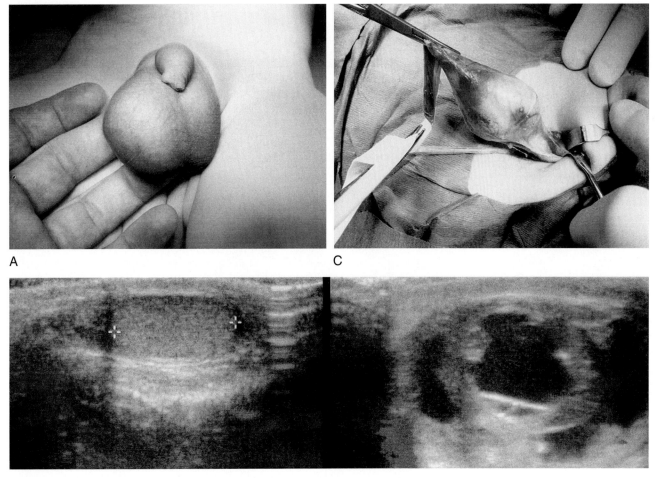

FIGURE 27-4 ■ **A,** This 1-year-old boy was referred for a right hydrocele since birth. The mass was firm on examination and appeared mixed cystic/solid by transillumination. **B,** The mixed cystic/solid mass was confirmed by ultrasound. Note the homogeneous left testis compared with the right one. Tumor markers were not elevated. **C,** A radical inguinal orchiectomy was performed. The tumor was a benign teratoma.

Teratocarcinomas or mixed germ cell tumors of the testes are observed much less frequently. They may contain a mixture of yolk sac tumor, seminoma, and choriocarcinoma. Choriocarcinoma confers a poorer prognosis. These tumors affect older teenage boys and behave in a manner similar to germ cell tumors in adults (Fig. 27-5). In the past, after radical orchiectomy (as previously described), a retroperitoneal lymphadenectomy was always performed. For stage I disease, some now reserve this procedure for patients whose tumor markers do not normalize postoperatively or were not elevated preoperatively.

Unilateral lymphadenectomy is associated with minimal morbidity, especially when nerve-sparing techniques are employed. Although relapse may occur in 10% to 15% of patients after retroperitoneal lymphadenectomy, it almost always occurs in the chest (pulmonary parenchyma), almost never in the retroperitoneum, and salvage often can be achieved by chemotherapy. Radiation therapy and second-look surgery are useful to eliminate persistent disease after chemotherapy.

Seminomas are relatively uncommon tumors in childhood. They occur more frequently in cryptorchid

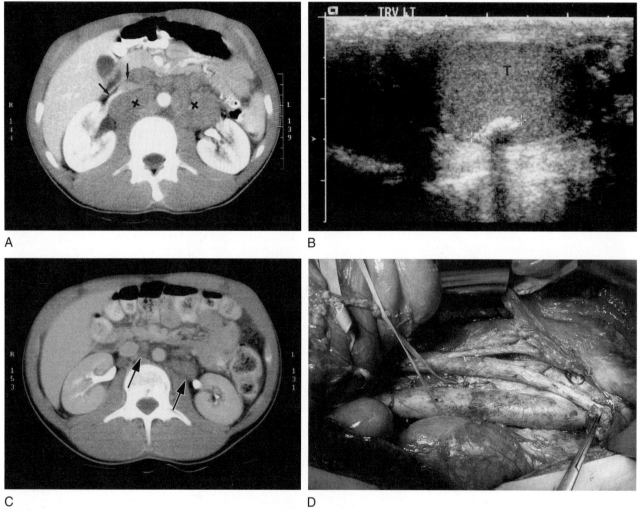

FIGURE 27-5 ■ A 17-year-old boy was referred for possible lymphoma, presenting with enlarged cervical and abdominal lymph nodes. **A,** On computed tomography, massive bilateral periaortic adenopathy can be observed (*) with anterior displacement of the right renal vein, seen joining the inferior vena cava (IVC) (arrows). **B,** Testicular examination was normal but ultrasound was requested because metastatic germ cell tumors may present in such fashion. A tiny area of calcification (with shadowing) was seen within the left testis (T). Radical orchiectomy confirmed a "burned-out" tumor with fibrosis and calcification, diffuse intratubular germ cell neoplasia (unclassified type), focal areas of seminoma, and mature teratoma. β-Human chorionic gonadotropin levels were high, and a biopsy specimen of a cervical node obtained at the time of insertion of a Port-a-Cath confirmed metastatic mixed germ cell tumor with a predominance of embryonal carcinoma and areas of choriocarcinoma. **C,** The patient had an excellent response after four courses of cisplatinum, etoposide, and bleomycin; β-human chorionic gonadotropin levels returned to normal, cervical and mediastinal adenopathies completely disappeared, but periaortic and aortocaval nodes remained enlarged (arrows). **D,** A radical retroperitoneal lymph node dissection was performed from the diaphragm to the bifurcation of the common iliac arteries. The right kidney and gallstones are recognized easily at the bottom of the picture; the IVC (encircled with an umbilical tape), aorta, inferior mesenteric artery, and both common iliac arteries are totally stripped from lymph nodes. On microscopic examination, there was no viable tumor and rare areas of mature teratoma. The patient received no further treatment and remains well 18 months postoperatively. This radical operation leads to abnormal ejaculation but was necessary in this patient because of the massive adenopathies; otherwise, tumor recurrence may be observed.

testes, however. The risk of malignancy in a cryptorchid testis is highest for gonads that remain in an intra-abdominal position. The classic statement that the increased risk of tumor occurrence in an undescended testis persists after orchiopexy is being challenged because earlier orchidopexy (before 2 years of age) seems to decrease the incidence of histologic abnormalities. Orchidopexy also allows easier palpation of the testis. In pubertal boys with undescended testis, orchiectomy is recommended if there is a normally placed contralateral testis. Seminomas are exquisitely sensitive to radiation therapy but respond to platinum-based combination chemotherapy as well.

Gonadal stromal and sex cord tumors (Sertoli cell and Leydig cell neoplasms) are rare in childhood. Leydig cell tumors secrete excessive testosterone, resulting in precocious puberty and irregular asymmetric enlargement of the testis. The few reported cases occur during infancy and are amenable to cure by orchiectomy.

The testis can be a sanctuary site for acute lymphocytic leukemia in relapse and lymphoma. These lesions can be treated successfully with either chemotherapy or scrotal irradiation with protective shielding of the contralateral testis if biopsy negative. Bilateral involvement probably is treated best by irradiation. In contrast to the procedure for most testicular tumors, testis biopsy for patients with leukemia in relapse can be performed via a transscrotal approach. Biopsy can be performed for both gonads through a single midline incision in the scrotal raphe.

Gonadoblastoma occurs in dysgenetic gonads. As mentioned earlier under ovarian tumors, these tumors occur in male pseudohermaphrodites and patients with mixed or pure gonadal dysgenesis. Gonadoblastomas are well encapsulated, slow-growing tumors that respond well to simple gonadectomy.

SUGGESTED READINGS

Andrassy RJ, Corpron C, Ritchey M: Testicular tumors. In O'Neill JA, Rowe MI, Grosfeld JL, et al (eds): Pediatric Surgery, 5th ed. St Louis, Mosby–Year Book, 1998.

This concise chapter in a major textbook is well written by experts in the field and is worthwhile reading.

Cushing B, Perlman EJ, Marina NM, et al: Germ cell tumors. In Pizzo PA, Poplack DG (eds): Principles and Practice of Pediatric Oncology, 4th ed. Philadelphia, Lippincott Williams & Wilkins, 2002.

This detailed chapter on ovarian and testicular germ cell tumors, in a more recent oncology textbook, includes the embryology, genetics, and treatment.

Giller R, Cushing B, Lauer S, et al: Comparison of high-dose or standard dose cisplatin with etoposide and bleomycin (HDPEB vs. PEB) in children with stage III and IV malignant germ cell tumors (MGCT) at gonadal primary sites: A pediatric intergroup trial (POG 9049/CCC 8882). Proc Am Soc Clin Oncol 17:525, 1998.

This paper serves as one of the bases for modern platinum-based treatment of germ cell tumors.

Haase GM, Vinocur CD: Ovarian tumors. In O'Neill JA, Rowe MI, Grosfeld JL, et al. (eds): Pediatric Surgery, 5th ed. St Louis, Mosby-Year Book, 1998.

This textbook chapter covers ovarian cysts and neoplasms in depth.

Herbst AL: Neoplastic diseases of the ovary. In Stenchever MA, Droegemueller W, Herbst AL, et al (eds): Comprehensive Gynecology, 4th ed. Mosby, St Louis, 2001, pp 955-998.

This chapter is a comprehensive reference related to both childhood and adult ovarian tumors. How treatment differs and how it is similar are discussed.

Marina NM, Cushing B, Giller R, et al: Complete surgical excision is effective treatment for children with immature teratomas with or without malignant elements: A POG/CCG intergroup study. J Clin Oncol 17:2137-2143, 1999.

Rowland RG, Herman JR: Tumors and infectious diseases of the testis, epididymis and scrotum. In Gillenwater JY, Grayhack JT, Howards SS, et al (eds): Adult and Pediatric Urology, 4th ed. Philadelphia, Lippincott Williams & Wilkins, 2002, pp 1897-1934.

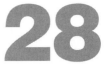

Cervical Cysts, Sinuses, and Other Neck Lesions

Cysts, lumps, and sinuses found about the head and neck often are residual embryonic structures that have failed to resorb completely or mature or may be caused by acute or chronic inflammation or neoplasms affecting the cervical lymph nodes.

CYSTIC HYGROMA (LYMPHANGIOMA)

Cystic hygromas (see Chapter 81) are multilocular cystic malformations of the lymphatic system occurring in approximately 1 in 12,000 births. The word *hygroma*, derived from Greek, means a "moist" or "watery" tumor. These lesions occur with approximately equal frequency in boys and girls. Of lesions, 50% to 65% are present at birth, and 80% to 90% are detected before the end of the second year of life.

The cause likely is related to events that occur during the development of the lymphatic system in which the primitive lymphatic buds fail to establish communication with developing veins, which results in isolated lymphatic sacs. Segments of the lymphatic system can become isolated by sequestration yet retain their ability to produce lymph and form endothelial cells. These lymphatic cysts slowly enlarge and may infiltrate into the surounding tissues by pushing other structures aside. Cystic hygromas have been detected on prenatal ultrasound as either nonseptated or septated lesions most commonly observed in the nuchal region. When associated with hydrops fetalis, chromosomal abnormalities, or structural abnormalities, early fetal death frequently is noted by 22 weeks' gestation. Karyotyping of affected fetuses may show chromosomal aneuploidy, including trisomy 18 and Turner's syndrome among others. Even when hydrops is an isolated prenatal ultrasound finding, the overall prognosis is poor. This is in contrast to the recognition of cystic hygroma after birth, when, in general, the outlook is favorable.

Clinical Features

Cystic hygroma presents as a multicystic mass with a thin wall that is lined by endothelial cells with occasional lymphocytes and varying amounts of fibrous stroma. Areas of thrombosis may be present. If there has been prior infection or hemorrhage, the cyst wall is usually thickened, and the fluid may be hemorrhagic, brown, or purulent. Although internal hemorrhage is uncommon, it may occur during delivery, particularly in large lesions of the neck.

Although cystic hygromas may appear clinically different from cavernous lymphangiomas, there is no clear distinction between the two except that hygromas tend to have much larger cystic spaces. Hygromas usually reside in close proximity to large veins and lymphatic ducts, in the neck, axilla, abdomen, and groin, whereas lymphangiomas more commonly are located peripherally on the trunk or extremities.

Hygromas present as soft, cystic, discrete, nontender masses that transilluminate and are often compressible. The cysts may vary in size from a few millimeters to several centimeters (Fig. 28-1). Of hygromas, 75% occur in the lateral neck; 20% occur in the axilla; and 5% occur in the mediastinum, retroperitoneum, pelvis, or groin. In some cases, a hygroma involves two or more areas by

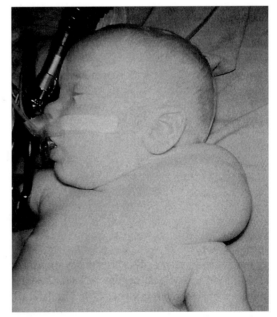

FIGURE 28-1 ■ Characteristic large cervical cystic hygroma present since birth in a 3-month-old boy.

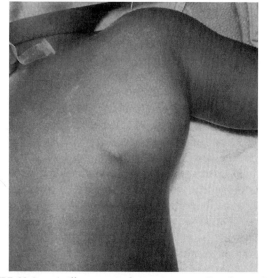

FIGURE 28-2 ■ Axillary cystic hygroma extending beneath the clavicle from a smaller cystic lesion in the neck.

direct extension. Hygromas occur on the left side of the neck approximately twice as often as on the right, presumably because the thoracic duct enters the confluence of the internal jugular vein and subclavian vein on the left side. Hygromas in the neck occasionally extend beneath the clavicle to the axilla (Fig. 28-2) or between the subclavian vessels into the mediastinum. Most hygromas are noted shortly after birth, then gradually enlarge. Approximately one third expand as a result of infection or hemorrhage, in which case tenderness may occur, and the overlying skin may have a bluish or inflamed appearance. Sudden enlargement of the hygroma may cause compression or stretching of vital structures: The spinal accessory and facial nerves are particularly vulnerable. These cysts extend downward through the thoracic inlet in approximately 15% of cases and on rare occasions produce stridor, cyanosis, apnea, or dysphagia with failure to thrive, particularly in infants.

Infection in a cystic hygroma can cause rapid enlargement with cellulitis, pain, and slow response to antibiotic therapy. Infection may result in fibrosis in the tissues adjacent to the lesion, which makes it difficult to identify the planes of dissection at the time of attempted excision. This fibrosis may result in adherence of the facial, vagus, and phrenic nerves to the wall of the cyst. Other conditions to be considered in the differential diagnosis of a cystic mass in the neck or axilla in children include hemangioma; branchial cleft cyst; jugular vein ectasia; lymphoma; teratoma; and occasionally solid neoplasms such as cervical rhabdomyosarcoma, neuroblastoma, or fibromatosis or tumors metastatic to cervical lymph nodes. Radiographs of the adjacent area rarely show bony erosion or involvement. Diagnostic ultrasonography and computed tomography are helpful in distinguishing cystic hygromas from solid lesions, although hemorrhage into a hygroma may resemble a hemangioma.

Treatment

Spontaneous remission of cystic hygroma can occur but is relatively rare. Radiation therapy is not helpful,

and percutaneous aspiration is followed by prompt reaccumulation of fluid in the cyst or by development of infection. Injection of sclerosing agents into the cysts subsequent to aspiration has been effective in controlling macrocystic lesions, but attempts to sclerose multiloculated or microcystic infiltrative hygromas have been less reliable. Injection of sclerosing solutions causes induration of the cyst wall and may make subsequent attempts at resection technically more difficult. Nonetheless, reports have indicated favorable outcome in several patients with complex hygromas after repeated injections of OK-432, a lyophilized incubation mixture of group A *Streptococcus pyogenes* of human origin. The material causes a localized, intense inflammatory reaction within the hygroma. No systemic infection or generalized inflammation has been observed. Approximately 50% of patients have had a good response to treatment. Other agents that have been employed include bleomycin fat emulsion, and pure dehydrated alcohol. Bleomycin-A5 injection has resulted in a 44% complete response, 44% partial response, and 12% failure rate. Percutaneous sclerotherapy with a dehydrated alcohol solution acts by causing cell membrane lysis, protein denaturation, and vascular occlusion.

Incision and drainage of the cyst has no place in the management of uncomplicated hygromas because recurrence, hemorrhage, and subsequent infection are frequent sequelae. Nonetheless, in occasional infants with large hygromas causing respiratory distress from extrinsic compression, aspiration or drainage may relieve the acute symptoms temporarily and make the patient a better surgical risk for complete excision at a later time.

Excision offers the best opportunity for permanent cure of cystic hygroma. Most pediatric surgeons defer excision of hygromas until 2 to 6 months of age if the rate of enlargement does not exceed general body growth. Nonetheless, some infants with large cervical hygromas that cause tracheal compression and respiratory distress require resection shortly after birth. Some infants have been treated by an EXIT (ex utero intrapartum treatment) procedure after identification of a large hygroma on prenatal ultrasound. A transverse incision in a skin crease provides optimal exposure. Care should be taken not to rupture the cyst because excision of the wall and its many extensions into adjacent tissues is more difficult and is likely to be incomplete after cyst decompression. The best dissection plane for these benign lesions is on the cyst wall because this facilitates resection and avoids unnecessary injury to any surrounding or adherent structures. Complete resection can be challenging, and recurrence of the lesion may occur in 5% to 10% of even the favorable cases. Every effort should be made to remove all remnants of the cyst; however, because of the benign nature of this anomaly, no major nerves or other important structures should be sacrificed, and an en bloc dissection is not indicated. The recurrence rate for hygromas in suprahyoid locations that are microcystic and infiltrative in nature (i.e., affecting the tongue, pharynx, and floor of the mouth) is significantly higher.

After excision of a cystic hygroma in the neck, transient postoperative palsy of the mandibular branch of the facial or the spinal accessory nerves is common.

Retraction and electrocautery should be used cautiously. Because of the dead space left behind after resection of a large hygroma, small sump catheters attached to suction are recommended after resection to prevent fluid collection in the operative field. If a small segment of the cyst wall is not excised because of adherence to a vital structure, cauterizing the surface with silver nitrate or electrocautery may reduce the incidence of postoperative fluid accumulation. If fluid should reaccumulate, it is likely at first to be unilocular; early aspiration with instillation of 1 to 3 mL of a sclerosing solution followed by compression may be curative. Most recurrences develop within a few weeks, although some may not become apparent for several months.

Mediastinal Hygroma

Some cystic hygromas that extend into the mediastinum may be retracted gently upward into the neck during the dissection without requiring a separate thoracotomy. In instances in which the intrathoracic extension is extensive, a separate thoracotomy or inverted hockey-stick extension of the cervical incision with a sternal split may be necessary to acquire adequate exposure to remove the tumor completely. In some cases, particularly in infants, the lesion may extend inferiorly to the pericardium and around the trachea and esophagus. The phrenic and vagus nerves may be adherent to the wall of the cyst, making the dissection difficult. Injury to the recurrent laryngeal nerve and the phrenic nerve should be avoided if possible to prevent the occurrence of vocal cord paralysis and diaphragmatic eventration. Occasionally the hygroma arises primarily in the mediastinum without associated neck involvement. Rapid enlargement of a mediastinal lesion can result in sudden airway obstruction and require urgent endotracheal intubation.

Although a chest radiograph can identify the presence of a mediastinal tumor, computed tomography is more accurate in delineating the exact extent of hygroma and its relationship to the surrounding structures. Removal of a mediastinal hygroma often interrupts normal lymphatic pathways and may be followed by the occurrence of postoperative chylothorax. It is important to attempt to identify the main thoracic duct and ligate all lymphatic channels that are apparent at the time of the procedure. If a thoracotomy is needed for resection, chest tubes should be placed at the time of chest closure for drainage.

Axillary Hygroma

Axillary hygromas can be excised through an incision in the axillary skin crease with retraction of the pectoralis major muscle. If a cervical hygroma extends into the axilla, the cervical portion of the tumor is dissected free to the level of the clavicle. The axillary portion may be mobilized superiorly through a generous axillary incision up to the clavicle. Using alternate traction and dissection from above and below, the entire specimen usually can be removed. Cystic hygromas communicating from the neck to the axilla may be attached intimately to the brachial plexus and subclavian vessels, making dissection tedious. Closed suction wound drainage is advised at the conclusion of the procedure to avoid fluid collection under the skin flaps.

BRANCHIAL CYSTS, SINUSES, AND REMNANTS

Embryology

The branchial arches develop early in the fourth gestational week as paired ridges on either side of the head and neck. In the 2.5-mm embryo, paired endodermal pouches evaginate laterally on the pharyngeal wall. Externally the branchial apparatus is marked by paired ectodermal clefts. Between each pair of clefts and pouches is a layer of mesodermal arches that contains skeletal muscle tissue, nerves, and connective tissue. By the fifth week, four branchial clefts are visible externally. Continued proliferation of the mesodermal tissues results in obliteration of the epithelial outpouchings. The dorsal portion of the first cleft remains as the external auditory canal; the other external clefts are obliterated. The first, third, and fourth pharyngeal pouches persist as adult organs. The first pouch becomes the eustachian tube, the middle-ear cavity, and the mastoid air cells. All that remains of the second pouch is the palatine tonsil and the supratonsillar fossa. The third pouch forms the inferior parathyroid, and the fourth pouch forms the superior parathyroid glands and the thymus. Branchial cleft anomalies are the result of incomplete resorption.

Of branchial cleft anomalies, 75% arise from the second cleft, 20% arise from the first cleft, and the few remaining cases arise from the third and fourth branchial clefts. Cysts developing from branchial structures usually present later in childhood than do sinuses, fistulas, and cartilaginous remnants, which usually are found in infancy. When complete, a fistula of the second pouch opens in the lower third of the neck along the anterior border of the sternocleidomastoid muscle presenting as a minute skin dimple (Fig. 28-3). Mucus may be noted coming from the opening. The fistula tract ascends from the skin opening through the subcutaneous tissue beneath the platysma muscle. Just above the level of the hyoid bone,

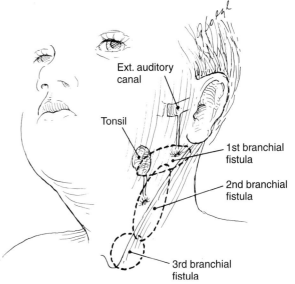

FIGURE 28-3 ■ Diagram shows the characteristic location for the external opening and internal drainage for each of the first three branchial cleft sinuses.

the tract turns medially and passes over the hypoglossal and glossopharyngeal nerves and between the bifurcation of the carotid artery. It turns medially and enters the lateral wall of the pharynx at the tonsillar fossa. These lesions are lined by squamous, columnar, or ciliated epithelium and are surrounded by a fairly thick muscular wall. The tract may be complete or incomplete. Sinuses extend a short distance from the skin opening. Bilateral branchial cleft sinuses can be observed in 10% to 15% of cases. Cysts can be located along the anterior border of the sternocleidomastoid muscle from just below the level of the hyoid bone lateral to the carotid artery. A small fistulous tract may coexist with a more proximal cyst. Cyst formation may be related to obstruction of the distal tract. Branchial cleft cysts can attain considerable size and may be complicated by infection and abscess formation.

An anomaly of the first branchial cleft may present as a small cyst lying close to the posterior border of the parotid gland and may not cause symptoms until adulthood or may present as a draining sinus located anterior to the ear, usually identified in infancy. Bilateral sinuses are noted occasionally. The fistulous tract extends to the external auditory canal and is in close proximity to the branches of the facial nerve. The facial nerve is usually lateral to the fistula.

Cartilaginous remnants of the second branchial cleft are more common than remnants of the first cleft and usually are found in the mid or lower neck. Cartilaginous remnants may be attached to the skin, located subcutaneously, or embedded in the anterior border of the muscle and usually do not have an associated sinus tract. Excision is indicated.

Cysts and sinuses that arise from the third branchial cleft are uncommon. They occur in the same areas as those of second cleft origin, but sinus tracts from the third cleft pass between the hypoglossal and glossopharyngeal nerves, course posterior to the carotid vessels (rather than between the bifurcation), and penetrate the thyrohyoid membrane to enter the pyriform sinus. Fourth branchial cleft sinuses are rare and often present as a recurring abscess in the left side of the neck. This abscess may be associated with an intrathyroid branchial cyst or suppurative thyroiditis. The epithelial tract enters the pyriform sinus.

Diagnosis

The diagnosis most frequently is based on physical findings. A branchial cleft sinus is a small painless opening located along the lower anterior border of the sternocleidomastoid muscle. Clear mucoid fluid may drain periodically and usually can be expressed with gentle manipulation. Injection of water-soluble radiographic contrast medium through a small Silastic catheter (24-gauge) placed in the orifice shows the course of the tract extending cephalad into the pharynx, but these studies are rarely needed. A small cyst may be noted along the tract. Incomplete sinus tracts are mere dimples in the skin, which often are associated with a small segment of ectopic cartilage. In older children who present with a mass, ultrasound distinguishes a cystic lesion from a solid mass, which more frequently is associated with a tumor.

Treatment

Almost all branchial cleft sinuses should be excised early in life because repeated infection is common, and resultant scarring and inflammation make resection more difficult. When infection occurs, antibiotic administration and, if necessary, incision and drainage should precede definitive excision.

Gentle instillation of 0.1 to 0.2 mL of methylene blue dye through a small 24-gauge catheter delivered from a 1.0-mL tuberculin syringe into the sinus tract at the time of operation may facilitate identification of the sinus along its entire course. Great care must be taken using this technique because excessive dye injection may result in extravasation, staining of the tissues, and confusion. Some surgeons insert a fine lacrimal duct probe or a length of stiff suture material into the tract to facilitate dissection, but this must be done delicately because rough handling of the probe or suture may result in perforation of the tract wall. A small elliptical incision is made around the cutaneous opening, excising a small ellipse of skin without dividing the attachment to the sinus tract. Dissection is carried out parallel to the tract. The tract is mobilized as far superiorly as is feasible. A second counterincision is made higher in the neck above the initial incision. The distal tract and skin ellipse are transposed cephalad through the more proximal incision and placed on gentle downward traction. The "stepladder" incision provides sufficient exposure to visualize the passage of the entire tract superiorly and its relation to the aforementioned cranial nerves and carotid bifurcation up to its termination of the tonsillar fossa. The upper end of the tract should be suture ligated with fine absorbable suture. If a cyst is present along the course of the tract, a slightly more extensive dissection may be necessary. Occasionally the tract ends blindly before reaching the tonsillar fossa. Every effort should be made to excise the entire tract because recurrence and infection are common with incomplete removal. The recurrence rate in most children's centers is less than 5%. Excision of the first branchial cleft anomalies requires a clear understanding of the anatomy of the facial nerve, parotid gland, and ear structures. Resection of third branchial cleft defects may be facilitated by endoscopic identity of the pyriform sinus at the time of neck exploration to permit complete excision of the fistulous tract. In children with fourth branchial cleft anomalies, excision of the sinus tract and left hemithyroidectomy may be required for cure.

PREAURICULAR PITS, SINUSES, AND CYSTS

Preauricular pits anterior to the tragus of the ear are usually unrelated to a branchial cleft but represent aberrant development of the auditory tubercles. These pits are lined with squamous epithelium, may contain hair and other skin appendages, and may form cysts. They extend from the skin surface down through the subcutaneous tissue in close proximity to the superficial temporal artery. The tract is deep and tortuous, leading to the cartilage of the external auditory canal. These lesions are often familial and frequently bilateral. They are usually asymptomatic, and excision is not routinely needed, but when drainage or infection occurs, it often persists or can recur so that excision is indicated. Sinuses that drain or become infected may consist of a chain of several small cysts linked together and to the skin by the sinus tract. These squamous cysts contain keratinaceous material.

An uninfected sinus is excised electively whenever the diagnosis is established; the tract usually can be identified readily and traced down to the cartilage. There is often considerable adherence to the cartilage, and a small portion of the cartilage must be removed to effect a cure. Recurrence of uninfected sinuses or cysts is uncommon.

MIDLINE NECK MASSES

Midline neck masses in newborns are rare, and although most are benign, they may produce airway problems by compressing the trachea. These lesions include cystic hygroma, hemangioma, teratoma, goiter, and midline ectopic thyroid tissue. In patients older than 6 months, swellings in the midline usually are caused by thyroglossal duct remnants, dermoid inclusion cysts, or enlarged lymph nodes.

DERMOID INCLUSION CYSTS

Where embryonic lines of fusion occur, ectodermal elements may become buried beneath the skin surface, leading to the formation of cysts. Dermoids are differentiated from epidermoid cysts by the presence of deeper dermal elements within the wall of the former, such as sebaceous glands, hair follicles, connective tissue, and papillae. Both contain keratinaceous material within the cyst cavity. The most common location on the head or neck for dermoid cysts in children is on the supraorbital ridge. Dermoid cysts also are located in the midline suprasternal area of the neck or in the upper neck in the pretracheal fascia, where they must be differentiated from the thyroglossal duct cysts. This differentiation may not be possible until attempted excision reveals keratinaceous material rather than mucus within the cyst and the absence of a sinus tract or fistula. Epidermoid lesions in the neck are attached to the skin. Malignant degeneration of dermoid cysts is rare, and removal is justified to confirm the diagnosis and to avoid infection.

MIDLINE CERVICAL CLEFTS

Midline cervical clefts are unusual anomalies that present as vertically oriented patches of thinly epithelialized tissue in the low anterior midline of the neck. They are usually several centimeters long and 4 to 6 mm wide. They may weep from a raw surface or appear pale and shiny. The cleft occasionally is accompanied by skin tags, a short sinus that ends blindly, or cartilaginous remnants. Occasional patients have an associated sternal cleft. Midline clefts occur because of imperfect fusion of the paired branchial arch tissues during the third and fourth gestational weeks. The abnormality is treated electively by excision with a Z-plasty closure to avoid scar contracture.

THYROGLOSSAL DUCT CYSTS AND SINUSES

Thyroglossal duct cysts are more common than branchial remnants and rank second only to goiter as a cause for anterior neck mass in children. Most thyroglossal duct cysts are observed in childhood, and more than half of the cases are recognized before age 5 years. The sex incidence is approximately equal, in contrast to thyroid disorders, in which girls are predominately affected. Occasional familial cases occur in girls with an autosomal dominant distribution.

Embryology

During the fourth gestational week, the tongue develops from several buds in the floor of the primitive pharynx, the initial one being the central tuberculum impar. Immediately caudal, the foramen cecum is the site of development of the thyroid diverticulum, which begins as a median endodermal thickening. As the embryo and tongue develop, the thyroid is connected to the tongue at the foramen cecum by the thyroglossal duct cyst. During this time, the branchial arches evolve, with the ventral cartilages of the second and third arches forming the hyoid bone. This development occurs from the fourth through the seventh week as the thyroid gland continues its descent to its normal pretracheal position. The thyroglossal duct may pass in front of, behind, or through the developing hyoid bone. Normally the duct disappears by the time the thyroid reaches its final position. Its lowermost aspect persists in half the population as the pyramidal lobe of the thyroid, and its origin is represented by the foramen cecum, a pit at the base of the tongue. Complete failure of this migration leads to lingual thyroid, with the thyroid developing beneath the foramen cecum within the tongue itself or just beneath it. In these cases, no other thyroid tissue is present in the neck, and although the lingual thyroid may be normal and provide adequate hormonal function, it is frequently dysgenetic, and the patient is hypothyroid. The thyroid tissue may enlarge and present as a lingual goiter as a result of inadequate feedback control of pituitary thyroid-stimulating hormone owing to deficient thyroxine production from the dysgenetic gland. Partial descent may occur, leading to sublingual thyroid or to a thyroid mass along the course of the thyroglossal duct, as in median ectopic thyroid.

When the thyroid descends fully but elements of the duct persist, a thyroglossal duct cyst may develop. Ectopic thyroid tissue may be found in the wall of the cyst or along the sinus tract from the foramen cecum. All follicular tissue is derived from the median descending thyroid diverticulum. Portions of the fourth pharyngeal pouches form the ultimobranchial bodies, which contribute cells that migrate to the thyroid and produce thyrocalcitonin. The cyst usually connects to the foramen cecum as a ductal structure, with intimate relations to the hyoid bone, although accessory ducts are common. The duct lining is a stratified squamous or ciliated, pseudostratified columnar epithelium with associated mucus-secreting glands. The incidence of ectopic thyroid tissue in or near the duct is 25% to 35%. Rarely a thyroglossal duct cyst may present in a location between the hyoid bone and the foramen cecum.

Diagnosis

Approximately 75% of thyroglossal duct anomalies present as cysts, and 25% present as draining sinuses associated with infection. In most cases, a thyroglossal duct cyst presents as an asymptomatic mass. Because of the persistent communication with the foramen cecum, however, infection caused by oral cavity bacteria occurs. An infected cyst may drain spontaneously or require surgical incision and drainage. In these cases, the external draining sinus commonly seals over but intermittently begins to drain again as reinfection occurs. Thyroglossal cysts never have primary external openings because the embryologic thyroglossal duct cysts are located in the midline at or immediately adjacent to the hyoid bone. Approximately 3% are in a lingual position, and another 7% are in a suprasternal position, where they may be mistaken for a thyroid mass or dermoid cyst (Fig. 28-4). Approximately one fourth of the thyroglossal duct cysts may be located slightly to the side of the midline.

Thyroglossal duct cysts are smooth and solitary and usually measure 1.0 to 3.0 cm in size and move when the patient swallows or protrudes the tongue, confirming the attachment to the foramen cecum and the hyoid bone. The differential diagnosis includes ectopic midline thyroid, pyramidal lobe of the thyroid gland, thyroid adenoma arising in the isthmus of the gland, metastatic thyroid cancer to a Delphian lymph node just above the thyroid isthmus, dermoid cyst, lipoma, and submental lymphadenitis. Routine thyroid scanning has been recommended to avoid the potential risk of removing the child's only thyroid tissue. Others have suggested that this ectopic thyroid tissue is usually dysgenetic and is best removed regardless of the presence of thyroid tissue. We usually reserve scintigraphy for patients in whom the thyroid cannot be palpated or identified in its usual location by ultrasound, especially if the neck mass is not cystic. Thyroid function tests should be obtained when solid ectopic thyroid tissue is found or when thyroid tissue is present in the excised cyst. This approach identifies hypothyroid children who require lifelong therapy.

Treatment

The treatment of choice for thyroglossal duct cyst is complete excision of the cyst and tract to the base of the tongue with en bloc removal of the central portion of the hyoid bone in most cases (Sistrunk procedure). Delay in treatment often results in chronic infection, in which case drainage for a few months may be necessary to permit resolution of the inflammation before undertaking excision. Administration of perioperative antibiotics 30 minutes before the procedure is useful in patients with recent infection. Excision is performed under general endotracheal anesthesia with the neck extended by placing a roll between the shoulder blades. A small transverse incision over the mass at the level of the hyoid bone in clean cases or an elliptical incision to excise a sinus tract or inflamed tissue is employed. The cyst carefully is dissected free down to the hyoid bone. The sternohyoid and thyrohyoid muscle attachments are divided. Approximately 1 cm of the central part of the hyoid bone is excised carefully, and the lateral segments on each side of the hyoid bone are left in place. The mylohyoid and the geniohyoid attachments are divided, and a wide dissection is carried up to the base of the tongue where the duct enters the foramen cecum (see Fig. 28-4). This dissection avoids leaving behind microscopic branchings of the duct that may lead to recurrence. The duct is doubly suture ligated with absorbable suture and divided. No attempt is made to reapproximate the hyoid bone. Although some surgeons favor the anesthesiologist pushing down on the floor of the mouth from above during the procedure to aid in identifying the foramen cecum, we have not found this maneuver necessary. After ensuring hemostasis, the wound is closed in layers with interrupted absorbable suture. The skin is apposed with subcuticular suture and Steri-strips. In clean cases, the patient can be sent home

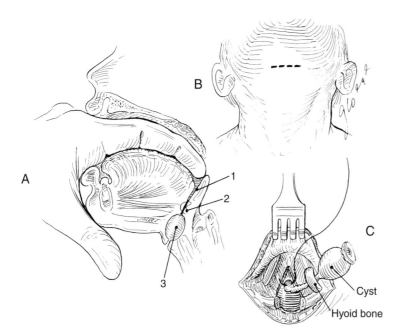

FIGURE 28-4 ■ Thyroglossal cyst. **A,** Diagram of locations: (1) lingual (rare), (2) above the hyoid bone (uncommon), (3) below the hyoid bone (common). **B,** Incision for removing a thyroglossal duct cyst or sinus. **C,** Excision of the thyroglossal cyst by the Sistrunk procedure, with dissection of the cyst to the hyoid bone, excising a 1-cm segment of bone. The sinus tract is mobilized up to the base of the tongue. An assistant's finger inserted over the tongue facilitates precise location of the end of the sinus tract. The sinus tract is ligated and divided at the base of the tongue.

Cyst

Hyoid bone

later on the day of surgery. A drain may be useful in instances of recent infection or spill of cloudy or overly purulent intracystic content; the patient is observed overnight, the drain removed in 24 hours, and the patient discharged.

The recurrence rate is 9%, and recurrence is more common in patients with infected or previously drained thyroglossal duct cysts. The risk of recurrence is greatest when the hyoid bone is not removed. Adenocarcinoma in thyroglossal duct cysts has been reported in 10% of patients in whom the lesion was not excised until adulthood. The malignancy may occur in the associated ectopic thyroid tissue and is commonly papillary thyroid carcinoma. The thyroid gland itself is usually normal. The mean age of patients with adenocarcinoma arising in thyroglossal duct cysts is older than 50 years; however, malignancy has been observed occasionally in 6-year-olds.

RANULA

Ranula is an uncommon cystic mass related to a sublingual gland and occurs in the floor of the mouth near the frenulum of the tongue. Mucous cysts can arise from any of the minor salivary glands of the oral mucous membranes and occur as small cystic lesions in the mucosa. Simple ranula is believed to be a result of partial obstruction of the sublingual salivary duct, leading to dilation of the more proximal duct. The cyst is lined with epithelium and contains fluid with an elevated salivary amylase content. Rarely the cyst may present in the anterior neck, where it may be confused with a thyroglossal duct cyst. Simple marsupialization (unroofing) of the ranula without excision provides cure in most patients.

CERVICAL THYMIC CYST

A mediastinal thymic cyst occasionally emerges through the thoracic inlet to present as a mass in the base of the neck. In this ectopic location, it is often mistaken for cystic hygroma, a branchial cleft cyst, or thyroglossal duct cyst. Chest radiographs help distinguish instances with mediastinal components. Thymic cysts most often lie anterior to the trachea, in contrast to cystic hygroma, which usually passes through the inlet on the left or occasionally the right side. Because of their embryologic derivation from the third pharyngeal pouch, thymic neck cysts may have tracts that extend caudad to enter the anterior mediastinum.

Cervical thymic cysts usually can be excised completely through a transverse cervical incision centered over the palpable mass. In cases with mediastinal extension or tracts that cannot be excised safely from the cervical approach, it may be necessary to divide the upper sternum for adequate exposure. Thymic tissue is almost invariably present in the wall of the cyst.

TORTICOLLIS

Neonatal torticollis results from fibrosis of the sternocleidomastoid muscle, producing a fibrous mass or "tumor" that shortens the muscle (Fig. 28-5). The cause is unclear, with explanations ranging from a true fibroma (a neoplasm)

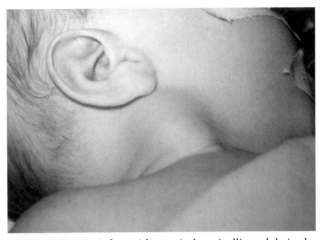

FIGURE 28-5 ■ An infant with a typical torticollis nodule in the right sternocleidomastoid muscle causing muscle shortening, a tilt of the head toward the right shoulder, and turning of the head to the left.

to that of injury to the muscle during delivery with subsequent hemorrhage and fibrous replacement. The high incidence of associated breech presentation and other abnormal obstetric positions has been used to support the injury and the tumor etiologies. Because of the tumor-like presentation, torticollis also has been called *pseudotumor of infancy* and *fibromatosis colli*. Histologically, there is little support for the neoplasm concept. The usual findings show fibrous replacement of muscle, varying degrees of muscle atrophy, minimal edema and infiltrates, and no abnormal vasculature. Some observers suggest that the mature fibrous tissue present in neonates indicates that the condition begins before birth and probably is the cause, not the result, of obstetric difficulties. Degenerating muscle fibers can be found in infants of all ages, a form of disuse atrophy produced by limitation of movement caused by the fibrosis.

Clinical Features

In most infants, a mass in the sternocleidomastoid muscle is noted first between 2 and 8 weeks of age. The delayed onset of identification supports the etiologic concept of injury in the perinatal period. The supposed injury is followed by muscle fibrosis, shortening, and positional abnormalities of the head. The face is rotated away from the affected side. The head is tilted toward the ipsilateral shoulder. Increasing facial and cranial asymmetry may result from this abnormal position over the ensuing months.

Torticollis is suspected by the physician observing the infant's abnormal head position and acquiring a history of refusal to turn to the affected side, particularly with feedings. Palpation of the neck usually shows a tumor in the central portion of the sternocleidomastoid muscle, with normal surrounding tissue and without lymphadenopathy. Radiographs of the neck and spine should be obtained to exclude associated cervical spinal abnormalities. Scoliosis also has been observed. Hip dysplasia has been noted in 10% of infants with torticollis. Although the literature is replete with articles suggesting acquisition of other tests, including fine needle aspiration, magnetic resonance imaging, computed tomography, and ultrasonography, there is little evidence to support their use in young infants because the clinical picture is so clear cut. In instances in which the parents voice concern about recommendations for conservative management in the presence of a neck mass in their infant, an ultrasound study usually calms their fears. This study documents the lesion is intramuscular (usually echogenic) and the adjacent soft tissues are normal. Torticollis or a solid neck mass presenting in an older child demands careful evaluation and often requires sophisticated diagnostic tests to rule out the presence of a neoplasm of the spinal cord or neck area.

Treatment

In most infants with torticollis, the fibrosis is insufficient to require initial operative treatment. Passive stretching exercise with daily manipulation of the head and neck usually are recommended. The parents are given physiotherapy instructions to carry out at home. When passive rotation still is limited by age 7 months, the prognosis is guarded. Parents should be encouraged to feed the infant with the head turned to the contralateral side. Massage may be of limited benefit. Early range-of-motion stretching exercises are often helpful. Improvement is noted in a few weeks to months, and the mass effect lessens and resolves. In some cases, the muscle remains taut and foreshortened, however. The criteria for operation, regardless of age, are the development of facial hemihypoplasia and persistent wryneck, which may result in permanent disfigurement and even diplopia. Approximately 12% to 15% of patients fail to respond to physiotherapy and require operative intervention.

Operative treatment involves transection between the lower and middle third of the muscle through a collar incision. The spinal accessory nerve innervates the sternocleidomastoid muscle and should be preserved. This is a relatively simple procedure and provides an esthetically acceptable scar. The neck fascia is often tight and should be divided anteriorly as far as the midline and posteriorly to the anterior border of the trapezius muscle. The sternocleidomastoid muscle is divided where the sternal and clavicular heads converge, with attention given to dividing any residual bands beneath the muscle. Excision of a short segment of the muscle ensures that reattachment of the two ends of the muscle is prevented. Attempts to reconstruct the sternocleidomastoid muscle may result in recurrent torticollis and a more difficult technical secondary operation. Postoperatively, intensive physical therapy, including full rotation of the neck in both directions and full extension of the cervical spine, is initiated as soon as it is feasible. Temporary use of a neck collar keeps the head in a straight position. In most patients, the remaining sternocleidomastoid muscle atrophies, and the facial and cranial asymmetry gradually returns to normal. Delaying the operation beyond the first year of life leads to a much slower return to normal appearance and motion.

CERVICAL LYMPHADENOPATHY

The anterior cervical lymph nodes drain the mouth and pharynx so that almost all upper respiratory and pharyngeal infections have some effect on anterior cervical nodes. Small lymph nodes are palpable in 80% to 90% of children 4 to 8 years old. Palpable lymph nodes are uncommon in infants and are more likely to be significant. Cervical lymphadenopathy is a frequent finding in various infections or inflammatory diseases and may be the first clinical manifestation of various tumors, especially lymphomas.

SUPPURATIVE CERVICAL LYMPHADENITIS

The most frequent inflammatory lesion of the cervical lymph nodes is suppurative lymphadenitis secondary to infection in the pharynx or tonsils. Most infections are caused by penicillin-resistant *Staphylococcus aureus*. The typical patient is the preschool child older than 1 year of age. Characteristically the child has a prodromal upper respiratory illness or pharyngitis. Rapid unilateral enlargement of one or more cervical lymph nodes occurs with tenderness, swelling, and erythema of the surrounding soft tissues. Fever is variable. Leukocytosis is common, with an increased number of band forms noted on differential smear. Without treatment, the lymph node usually continues to enlarge and becomes fluctuant, with the inflammatory reaction eventually extending to the overlying skin. Spontaneous drainage may occur.

With the acute onset of bilateral lymphadenitis, a nonspecific viral infection is often the cause, and this usually remits spontaneously within a few weeks. A neoplasm must be considered in the differential diagnosis of persistent lymphadenopathy even in young children. Early antibiotic therapy may abort abscess formation and resolve the process. When fluctuation is present, drainage of the abscess is necessary. Needle aspiration provides fluid for culture and in some instances allows complete resolution of the process when combined with antibiotic therapy. Occasionally, large, fluctuant, abscessed lymph nodes must be incised and drained with the patient under general anesthesia. Delay until the lymph node is clearly fluctuant results in more satisfactory drainage. Cultures are obtained at the time of drainage of the abscess. The parents are taught how to change the dressings and appropriate drain and wound care, and the child can be discharged in 24 to 48 hours.

MYCOBACTERIAL LYMPHADENITIS

Persistent unilateral enlargement of one or more cervical lymph nodes with minimal systemic symptoms suggests nonbacterial lymphadenitis. Atypical mycobacterial lymphadenitis is caused by one of the strains of atypical mycobacteria and may be primary infection entering through the pharynx and tonsils. Mycobacteria may be the cause of approximately 5% of the cases of chronic lymphadenitis in young children. Infection with atypical strains usually involves higher cervical nodes, most often in the submandibular area. Occasionally the lymph nodes in the parotid gland and preauricular area are involved. Atypical mycobacteria may enter from the environment and are not considered contagious. Infection with atypical mycobacteria usually is limited to the lymph nodes with only occasional cases showing extranodal involvement.

Lymphadenitis caused by *Mycobacterium tuberculosis* may be an extension of a primary pulmonary infection with the supraclavicular lymph nodes most often being involved. The enlarged lymph nodes in a child with *M. tuberculosis* scrofula are minimally symptomatic and usually painless. Less than 20% of patients have pulmonary tuberculosis when diagnosed, and none seem to progress from cervical adenopathy to pulmonary disease. Caseous necrosis of the lymph nodes with external drainage is common. External drainage is more likely to occur and be persistent if the lymph nodes are aspirated, biopsied, or incompletely excised. Antituberculous chemotherapy often produces a marked resolution of the lymphadenopathy within a few months.

Children with mycobacterial lymphadenitis (atypical and due to *M. tuberculosis*) must be differentiated from children with lymph node hyperplasia after viral infections, cat-scratch disease, chronic pyogenic adenitis, fungal infections, mumps, infectious mononucleosis, lymphoma, and other tumors. Tuberculin skin testing may identify the rare patient with *M. tuberculosis* infection; however, response with atypical mycobacterial infection is variable and tends to become less reactive with time. Specific skin tests for atypical mycobacteria are generally positive, although the antigens are not always available. The final diagnosis may depend on culture results after excision of the involved nodes.

When *M. tuberculosis* lymphadenitis is confirmed by positive skin test, family history, or evidence of pulmonary disease, antituberculous chemotherapy is likely to produce regression within 3 months. Chemotherapy should be continued for 2 years. The recognition of chemoresistant strains of *M. tuberculosis* in children of recent immigrants to the United States indicates the importance of involving pediatric infectious disease specialists and pulmonologists in the care of these patients.

When atypical mycobacterial infection is confirmed by old tuberculin or specific skin tests, complete surgical excision is required (Fig. 28-6). Standard tuberculous chemotherapy is of little value in the treatment of atypical infections. Children with atypical mycobacterial infection respond to complete surgical excision without drug therapy in most cases. Because the involved lymph nodes frequently are matted together in a mass-like effect, a modified neck dissection of involved lymphatic tissue is advised. After adequate resection, recurrent infection is uncommon.

CAT-SCRATCH DISEASE

Cat-scratch disease is one of the most common causes of nonbacterial chronic lymphadenopathy. Although chlamydial organisms once were considered the most likely cause, more recent findings show that the small bacillus, *Bartonella henselae*, is likely the causative agent. A scratch from a kitten usually transmits the disease. The kitten is unaffected by the disease and does not react to the cat-scratch antigen. Other animal species have been implicated only rarely.

The disorder presents with a primary papule at the inoculation site followed by development of tender regional lymphadenopathy within 2 weeks of the inoculation. Often one major lymph node is involved, but occasionally

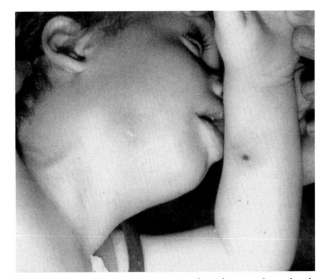

FIGURE 28-6 ■ This patient presented with an enlarged submandibular lymph node, which drained spontaneously and was associated with a positive skin test on the forearm to old tuberculin, characteristic of atypical mycobacterial infection.

a few nodes may be enlarged. The inoculation sites are commonly on the upper or lower extremities, the face, and the neck. Lymph node involvement is axillary in more than 60% of patients, with cervical, preauricular, submandibular, and epitrochlear lymph nodes less often involved. Diagnosis is confirmed by identification of cat-scratch DNA by polymerase chain reaction on purulent aspirate. Cultures of the aspirate and the nodes themselves are consistently negative for fungal and mycobacterial organisms. There is no specific treatment for cat-scratch disease because it is usually a mild, self-limited process. Most children are asymptomatic, although some may experience transient malaise, headache, vomiting, lethargy, and low-grade fever. Surgical excision is not recommended if only lymphadenopathy is present. In some instances, necrosis of the lymph node may occur, requiring complete excision.

SUGGESTED READINGS

Altman RP, Hechtman DH: Congenital lesions: Thyroglossal duct cysts and branchial cleft anomalies. In Baker RJ, Fischer JE (eds): Mastery of Surgery, 4th ed. Philadelphia, Lippincott Williams & Wilkins, 2001, pp 382-388.

A good description of operative techniques employed for thyroglossal duct cyst excision and branchial cleft procedures is provided with good illustrations.

Burstin PP, Briggs RJ: Fourth branchial sinus causing recurrent cervical abscess. Aust N Z Surg 67:119-122, 1997.

This report documents the unusual presentation of fourth branchial cleft anomalies and the relationship to the left lobe of the thyroid gland.

Charabi B, Bretlau P, Bille M, Holmelund M: Cystic hygroma of the head and neck—a long-term follow up of 44 cases. Acta Otolaryngol Suppl 543:248-250, 2000.

This study with long-term follow-up of patients with cystic hygroma documents a 50% residual or recurrence rate. Suprahyoid level lesions have a higher recurrence rate.

Dubois J, Garel L, Abila A, et al: Lymphangiomas in children: Percutaneous sclerotherapy with an alcohol solution of zein. Radiology 204:651-654, 1997.

This article describes the treatment of cystic hygroma using pure dehydrated alcohol as a sclerosing agent (zein or Ethiblock).

Edmonds JL, Girod DE, Woodroof JM, Bruegger DE: Third branchial cleft anomalies: Avoiding recurrence. Arch Otolaryngol Head Neck Surg 123:438-444, 1997.

This report documents the importance of endoscopy in identifying the pyriform sinus during the operative procedure.

Kennedy TL, Whitaker M, Pellitteri P, Wood W: Cystic hygroma/lymphangioma: A rational approach to management. Laryngoscope 111:1929-1937, 2001.

This report documents spontaneous resolution of some cases of cystic hygroma.

Ogita S, Tsuto T, Nakamura K, et al: OK-432 therapy in 64 patients with lymphangioma. J Pediatr Surg 30:1159-1160, 1995.

This seminal report describes the injection of a lyophilized mixture of group A streptococcus into the lymphatic cysts to cause an intense inflammatory response and resolution in a significant number of cases.

Smith CD: Cysts and sinuses of the neck. In O'Neill JA Jr, Rowe MI, Grosfeld JL, et al (eds): Pediatric Surgery, 5th ed. St. Louis, Mosby, 1998, pp 757-771.

This textbook chapter presents a detailed description of these lesions and an excellent overview of the subject.

Tanriverdi HA, Hendrik HJ, Ertan AK, et al: Hygroma colli cysticum: Prenatal diagnosis and prognosis. Am J Perinatol 18:415-420, 2001.

The presence of hydrops fetalis, large cyst size, septated cysts, and chromosomal and structural abnormalities is associated with a poor prognosis and high rate of intrauterine fetal death.

Triglia JM, Nicollas R, Ducroz V, et al: First branchial cleft anomalies: A study of 39 cases and a review of the literature. Arch Otolaryngol Head Neck Surg 124:291-295, 1999.

This excellent review discusses first branchial cleft defects.

Zhong PA, Zhi FX, Li R, et al: Long term results of intratumorous bleomycin-A5 injection for head and neck lymphangioma. Oral Surg Oral Med Oral Pathol Oral Radiol Endod 86:139-144, 1998.

This article documents the successful use of bleomycin-A5 in treating lymphangiomas.

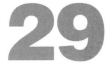

Thyroid and Parathyroid Tumors

THYROID NODULES

Solitary nodules within an otherwise normal thyroid gland occur in children and adults. Because 20% to 33% of solitary thyroid nodules in children 15 years old or younger are malignant, they are of concern, as this proportion of malignancies is much higher than that in adult series. Discrete solitary nodules of the thyroid in children are uncommon, and many who initially are suspected of having one are shown to have asymmetric enlargement of one lobe, multiple nodules, or Hashimoto's thyroiditis with prominent lobulations. An enlarged pyramidal lobe from nontoxic goiter, Hashimoto's thyroiditis, or hyperthyroidism occasionally may be misinterpreted as a nodule in children with diffuse thyroid enlargement. A solitary "cold" nodule in a child may be caused by papillary carcinoma, follicular adenoma or carcinoma, or a colloid nodule. It is rare for children to have autonomous hyperfunctioning nodules that are "hot" on thyroid scan. Purely cystic lesions may occur without other associated thyroid abnormalities but are less common in children.

Papillary carcinoma in children may be detected as a discrete solitary solid nodule, by diffuse involvement of one lobe, or by involvement of the entire gland accompanied by lymphadenopathy. Occasionally the primary thyroid carcinoma and the lymph node metastasis may be cystic with solid components in the wall. Lymph node metastases are frequently present and usually are palpable in children younger than age 15 years, although occult papillary carcinoma occurs more frequently in children than in adults. When enlarged lymph nodes are present in the paratracheal or jugular area, even though the thyroid appears normal, one should suspect papillary carcinoma.

Routine thyroid function studies are performed, although they are rarely helpful in establishing the diagnosis in a child with a solitary nodule in an otherwise normal thyroid. Detection of circulating antimicrosomal antibodies is helpful in identifying Hashimoto's thyroiditis.

Thyroid scans are helpful in identifying hyperfunctioning nodules, which are generally benign. Almost all other nodules, whether benign or malignant, are hypofunctioning, or cold. Technetium-99m or iodine-123 scans have replaced iodine-131 scans because of the lower thyroid radiation involved.

Fine-needle aspiration is helpful in evaluating most thyroid nodules in which the diagnosis is unclear, especially in adolescents. If the nodule is cystic, aspiration may eliminate the lesion; if the nodule is solid, the aspirated tissue often establishes the definitive diagnosis. Many papillary and medullary carcinomas can be diagnosed by fine-needle aspiration. Fine-needle aspiration biopsy of thyroid nodules in children usually can be performed with low risk and a high degree of accuracy with use of a local anesthetic.

Treatment of a well-defined nodule by thyroid suppression rarely is indicated in childhood. Although diffuse enlargement of a lobe may be reduced in children with an elevated thyroid-stimulating hormone (TSH) level, discrete solid nodules rarely decrease in size with thyroid suppression. Thyroid suppression should be limited to children with diffuse enlargement caused by thyroiditis or goiter in whom there is no evidence of hyperthyroidism. Thyroid hormone may be helpful after lobectomy for benign disease to prevent recurrence of nodules or goiters of the remaining thyroid gland, but this has not been well established. Another approach is to wait to give thyroid hormones until nodules appear in the remaining gland.

THYROID CANCER

The incidence of thyroid cancer in children has increased appreciably since the 1960s, and it is now one of the most common carcinomas in the pediatric age group. In past years, approximately 80% of children with thyroid carcinoma had received previous irradiation to the head or neck, but this is no longer the case because the risk of external irradiation has been known since the 1980s. Prior treatment for childhood malignancy also is related to the occurrence of thyroid carcinomas; although part of this is related to the use of irradiation, it also correlates with other factors, such as alkylating agents. Therapy for Hodgkin's disease produces most secondary tumors of the thyroid gland among cancer survivors. The mean interval from therapy is around 20 years. No other etiologic factors have been identified. In large reviews of children with thyroid carcinoma, it has been found that most have papillary tumors, with less than 10% having follicular tumors and only a few having medullary carcinoma of the thyroid (MCT).

Papillary Carcinoma

Papillary thyroid carcinoma in children almost invariably metastasizes to regional lymph nodes rather than through the systemic circulation, similar to the tumor's behavior in adults. Almost all thyroid neoplasms associated with radiation exposure are of the papillary type.

Clinical Features

Cervical lymphadenopathy and a palpable nodule in the thyroid are the most common initial manifestations of thyroid carcinoma in pediatric patients. Enlarged lymph nodes may be present for months or years before the diagnosis of cancer is established. Less than 50% of children have a palpable thyroid nodule as the first evidence of thyroid cancer. Of children with papillary thyroid carcinoma, 20% have pulmonary metastases at the time of diagnosis, and 30% have invasion of the trachea, esophagus, or neck muscles. Of children, 80% to 90% have positive lymph nodes at the time of operation, although only 60% have clinical lymphadenopathy. Paratracheal, superior mediastinal, and lower jugular lymph node regions are involved most frequently.

Treatment

Although the presumptive diagnosis of carcinoma can be established by fine-needle aspiration of the thyroid nodule or biopsy of a lymph node (Fig. 29-1), the definitive biopsy is complete lobectomy for any discrete thyroid nodule. If papillary carcinoma is identified, total thyroidectomy generally is recommended when lymph node involvement is established. Thyroid carcinoma can be diagnosed by frozen section in many children. When permanent sections are necessary to show papillary carcinoma or lymph node involvement, total thyroidectomy is deferred for a few days. Longer delay in performing total thyroidectomy can result in the development of extensive scar tissue, making the operation more difficult technically. A lesser operation with retention of a portion of the thyroid may impair accuracy of radioisotope scanning; the

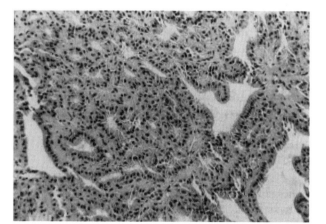

FIGURE 29-1 ■ Papillary thyroid adenocarcinoma in a 16-year-old boy.

risk of developing tumors in the contralateral side while on thyroid suppression therapy has not been established in children but is probably low. Many children have positive lymph nodes, and in these children, thyroidectomy facilitates administration of radioactive iodine. The long life span in children, even with metastasis, encourages nonaggressive surgical resection; two large studies in children failed to establish increased survival with total thyroidectomy in children with unilateral disease over lobectomy and isthmectomy alone, and both studies documented an increased frequency of complications with more extensive procedures. In these studies, factors that were correlated with decreased survival were a lower age at diagnosis and residual carcinoma in the neck after resection.

Because of the high incidence of lymph node involvement, resection of nodes in the central compartment (from the hyoid bone to the sternal notch and laterally between the jugular veins), with preservation of all four parathyroid glands, is recommended by some authorities. If the parathyroids are removed with the thyroid gland, at least one parathyroid should be implanted into the forearm as a free graft. Unilateral or, on rare occasions, bilateral modified cervical lymph node resection through an extended collar incision is advisable in patients with extensive disease. Because papillary carcinoma in children rarely invades vital structures in the neck, the jugular vein, inferior thyroid artery, thyrocervical trunk, sternomastoid muscle, and spinal accessory nerve usually can be preserved. Gross residual disease after resection is associated with a fivefold increase in recurrence.

The only indication for resecting the recurrent laryngeal nerve is direct invasion by the primary tumor in patients in whom vocal cord palsy has been shown preoperatively. If the nerve functions preoperatively, every effort should be made to preserve its integrity, even if it is surrounded by involved lymph nodes. Preoperative laryngoscopic examination of vocal cord function is advisable before undertaking extensive surgical resection of thyroid carcinoma in children.

After total thyroidectomy and lymph node resection, thyroid hormone is withheld for 6 weeks, after which a tracer dose of iodine-131 is administered, and a scan is obtained 24 hours later. A therapeutic dose of radioactive iodine ranging from 100 to 200 mCi is administered if there is evidence of uptake in the neck, mediastinum, lungs, or other areas of the body. Isotope uptake outside the immediate thyroid area or mediastinum indicates metastatic disease. If uptake is present in areas where normal thyroid tissue should not remain, most patients should receive a therapeutic course of iodine-131. Repeated smaller doses of iodine-131 in an attempt to ablate residual normal thyroid or metastases are less likely to be successful. Because of the high incidence of metastatic disease in children with papillary carcinoma, approximately 60% require iodine-131 therapy after surgery.

The prognosis with papillary carcinoma in children is usually excellent despite metastatic disease, provided that therapy has been appropriate. The combination of surgical resection followed by iodine-131 usually can eradicate the disease. Occasionally a second or third therapeutic dose of iodine-131 may be necessary to treat pulmonary metastases. The total dosage of iodine-131 should rarely exceed 600 mCi in children; complications from irradiation are unusual within this dosage limit. Children younger than age 7 years occasionally have more extensive involvement from papillary carcinoma that may not be cured by the combination of extirpative surgery and radionuclide therapy. In one series, the only deaths reported (6 of 72 patients) all occurred in children who initially presented younger than age 10 years. After therapy with radioactive iodine or after lobectomy for children without metastatic disease, children should be treated with adequate thyroxine (T_4) to suppress TSH levels.

Follicular Carcinoma

Follicular carcinomas are uncommon, are slow growing, and can be difficult to differentiate from follicular adenomas. Needle aspiration is associated with a false-negative diagnosis in 10% of cases, and it may be difficult to distinguish between a well-differentiated follicular carcinoma and a highly cellular benign follicular adenoma. The prognosis is variable and depends most on the degree of capsular invasion. Vascular invasion with this carcinoma is common, and 30% to 40% of patients have metastatic disease to the lungs and bone. This carcinoma is "functional" such that the most logical approach to it is total thyroidectomy with iodine-131 scanning and with therapeutic iodine-131 for ablation of residual disease in the neck and for metastatic disease.

Medullary Carcinoma

MCT originating from parafollicular cells (C cells) of the thyroid first was recognized in 1951. Subsequently, Sipple described the syndrome of MCT occurring in association with pheochromocytoma. Immunofluorescent studies have shown that the C cells contain the peptide hormone calcitonin, which can be assayed in the serum and thyroid tissue of patients with MCT.

Genetic screening for germline *RET* proto-oncogene mutations on chromosome 10 now identifies individuals in multiple endocrine neoplasia (MEN) IIA and IIB and familial MCT kindreds who are affected. This screening allows the performance of prophylactic total thyroidectomy before clinical or biochemical evidence of MCT has developed. This early intervention provides the greatest chance for cure. It also obviates the need for unaffected individuals in a kindred to have annual provocative testing performed. Of sporadic cases of MCT, 40% have *RET* mutation as well, but in this situation screening is of no assistance.

Clinical Features

MCT occurs in children as the major component in MEN type II and less frequently as an isolated tumor in adolescence. MEN type II syndromes are classified as MEN type IIA, which includes MCT, pheochromocytoma, and hyperparathyroidism, with normal phenotype, and MEN type IIB, which combines MCT, pheochromocytoma, marfanoid habitus, and ganglioneuroma phenotype. MEN IIA is approximately four times more frequent than MEN IIB. MCT seems to be particularly aggressive in children with MEN IIB, with metastases occurring

in 4-year-olds. Approximately 75% of children with MCT and MEN are girls. Family members at risk for MCT in the past were evaluated annually for basal calcitonin levels and after stimulation with pentagastrin and calcium, beginning at the preschool age. With current genetic testing, family members now should be evaluated for *RET* mutations.

When a palpable thyroid nodule is identified in a member of a MEN kindred, metastases are usually present, and the prognosis is unfavorable. Accurate identification of affected individuals is needed early before C-cell hyperplasia can progress to MCT with the risk of dissemination. MCT is always bilateral and multicentric, arising in areas of C-cell hyperplasia, which always precedes the development of MCT in familial syndromes. Metastatic spread to cervical lymph nodes, the central compartment, and the superior mediastinum usually occurs early, and cure, regardless of the extent of the surgical resection, is uncommon.

Total thyroidectomy is recommended for all children with MCT because any residual thyroid tissue is at high risk for recurrent neoplasm. Resection of all lymph nodes in the central compartment is recommended, preserving the blood supply to the parathyroid glands. Nodules of ectopic thymus may occur in close proximity to the thyroid gland of patients with MCT. Parathyroid hyperplasia may occur in association with MCT in MEN II kindreds.

In contrast to children with MEN II and familial MCT, both of which are familial, children with sporadic MCT usually have involvement of only one lobe of the gland. Nonetheless, total thyroidectomy is recommended to evaluate for possible C-cell hyperplasia or multicentric MCT in the contralateral lobe. In the absence of C-cell hyperplasia, an extensive evaluation of other family members is not necessary.

The prognosis of children with MCT depends on the extent of the disease at the time of the initial operation. If the tumor is confined to the thyroid and the central compartment lymph nodes, a cure is possible if postoperative stimulated calcitonin testing is negative. If the lateral lymph nodes are involved, cure is unlikely, and the prognosis is poor. The overall mortality from MCT is approximately 50% at 10 years with extensive therapy; however, more recent reports indicate a slight improvement in survival. A consensus statement from an international group on MEN syndromes recommended thyroidectomy within the first 6 months of life for infants with MEN IIB and before 5 years of age for children with MEN IIA.

HYPERTHYROIDISM

Graves' disease (hyperthyroidism) accounts for approximately 15% of all thyroid disorders in childhood, although greater than 95% of patients with this condition are diagnosed in adulthood. Almost one third of all goiters in children are associated with hyperthyroidism. Graves' disease is uncommon before age 3 years and rare in neonates; in infants, the mortality approximates 25%. Infants born to mothers with Graves' disease are at increased risk of having the condition. Hyperthyroidism in neonates usually responds within 24 to 48 hours to administration of Lugol's solution and propylthiouracil.

Children with hyperthyroidism often manifest symptoms of nervousness, irritability, diarrhea, weight loss, insomnia, and poor performance in school. Physical features often include exophthalmos, systolic hypertension, tachycardia, and weight loss. The thyroid characteristically is diffusely enlarged and often more than four times normal size. When present before the age of 10 years, acceleration in growth and bone maturation may occur.

The diagnosis of Graves' disease can be established by measurement of serum T_4 and triiodothyronine (T_3) levels by radioimmunoassay. Although usually unnecessary, thyroid scintiscans show diffuse uptake in an enlarged gland with either technetium-99m or iodine-123. Graves' disease can be differentiated from Hashimoto's thyroiditis with transient thyrotoxicosis by an iodine-123 scan, which shows minimum uptake in the latter condition. Measurement of TSH is usually of minimal benefit because it almost always is suppressed except in the rare patient with a TSH-secreting pituitary adenoma.

Treatment of hyperthyroidism in children is controversial. The antithyroid medications propylthiouracil or methimazole are preferred for initial treatment. Concomitant administration of the β-adrenergic blocker propranolol assists in controlling the acute symptoms of hyperthyroidism. If therapy produces a euthyroid state within 2 months, long-term treatment generally is recommended. Although it initially was believed that long periods of antithyroid medication eventually would produce permanent remission, more recent studies indicate that almost 75% of patients remain hyperthyroid after 2 years of therapy; more than 90% of children younger than 16 years old remain hyperthyroid. It is generally recommended that iodine-131 therapy or surgical resection should be initiated if medical therapy fails to produce persisting remission within 1 to 2 years (Fig. 29-2).

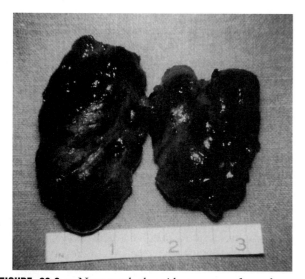

FIGURE 29-2 ■ Near-total thyroidectomy performed on a 14-year-old girl with Graves' disease, which did not respond to medical therapy.

Most children with hyperthyroidism can be made euthyroid with medications within 6 to 8 weeks. Toxicity or allergic reactions to propylthiouracil or methimazole may necessitate cessation of medical treatment. For these patients, iodine-131 therapy or surgery at an early stage may be necessary as definitive treatment. Failure of remission after antithyroid therapy usually is related to drug toxicity, resistant disease, noncompliance by the patient, or recurrence after an initial remission. Boys older than 11 years of age and all patients who develop recurrent thyromegaly after a sustained period of control of thyrotoxicosis are unlikely to obtain permanent remission. Most children with Graves' disease who do not develop permanent remission should undergo thyroidectomy or iodine-131 therapy.

For children with Graves' disease who are scheduled for thyroidectomy, preoperative preparation with propranolol neutralizes the symptoms of autonomic hyperactivity, including tremor, sweating, tachycardia, fever, and excitation, without appreciably affecting thyroid function. Propranolol should be continued for approximately 1 week postoperatively to reduce the risk of developing thyroid storm. Sufficient thyroid tissue should be removed to ensure that the child does not have persistent hyperthyroidism or develop a later recurrence. It is safer to err on the side of removing too much rather than too little thyroid tissue to minimize the likelihood of recurrent hyperthyroidism. Optimally, approximately 2 to 4 g of thyroid tissue and both parathyroid glands should be left on each side. Reoperation for recurrent hyperthyroidism is difficult technically and is associated with a moderate risk of injury to the parathyroid glands and recurrent laryngeal nerves. Hypothyroidism can be managed readily with oral thyroid replacement.

Although some surgeons recommend total thyroidectomy for Graves' disease in children and adults, this procedure carries a higher complication rate than does a lesser resection. If the ophthalmic symptoms do not improve after thyroidectomy, orbital decompression may be necessary; steroid therapy also may be beneficial.

Radioactive iodine has been used as definitive therapy for most adults with Graves' disease; however, there is concern about giving iodine-131 therapy to preadolescents because of the high incidence of hypothyroidism, the possible risk of genetic damage, and the increased risk of thyroid carcinoma. Advantages of iodine-131 therapy include ease of administration, low cost, and relative safety. It is currently believed that iodine-131 therapy for hyperthyroidism does not increase the risk for leukemia, infertility, or frequency of congenital malformations in progeny. Hypothyroidism should be treated early to minimize the risk of growth retardation.

ECTOPIC THYROID TISSUE

The thyroid originates from the foramen cecum at the base of the tongue and maintains a ductal remnant. The duct usually closes by the sixth week of life, following which the thyroid descends to its normal position on both sides of the trachea. Abnormal thyroid descent may produce a lingual thyroid inferior to the foramen cecum or in the suprahyoid area between the geniohyoid and mylohyoid muscles. In more than 60% of these unusual patients, there may be no other normal thyroid tissue in the neck. The aberrant thyroid tissue is often functionally insufficient and may produce juvenile myxedema.

Ectopic thyroid occasionally may extend into the superior mediastinum or pericardium owing to the close relationship of the developing thyroid primordium and the aortic arch. In these rare cases, it is common to have functioning thyroid tissue in the normal position. If thyroid tissue is present in the wall of the trachea, chronic cough, hemoptysis, or airway obstruction may occur. Extension of thyroid into the tracheal wall is more likely to result, however, from local invasion by a well-differentiated carcinoma or MCT than from ectopic thyroid tissue. Aberrant thyroid tissue in the midportion of the neck, although uncommon, may account for failure of total thyroidectomy to remove all functioning thyroid tissue. Thyroid tissue in lymph nodes lateral to the jugular veins, previously considered as "lateral aberrant thyroid," is clearly metastatic thyroid carcinoma, however, and not ectopic thyroid tissue.

Aberrant, or ectopic, thyroid tissue in the mediastinum or central neck can be identified by scintiscans using technetium-99m or iodine-123. These studies are particularly helpful if surgical excision is contemplated because the scan may identify the ectopic tissue as the only thyroid tissue present. In most cases, neither biopsy nor surgical excision is necessary. Compression symptoms caused by aberrant thyroid tissue usually can be relieved by thyroid suppression.

THYROIDITIS

Hashimoto's thyroiditis, or autoimmune chronic lymphocytic thyroiditis, is approximately 10 times more frequent in females and is most common in middle age. It is the primary cause of thyromegaly during childhood in nonendemic regions, and its pathogenesis is that of a genetically linked deficiency in antigen-specific suppressor T lymphocytes. The clinical disease is triggered by some form of stress, either physical or emotional, and the chronic inflammatory reaction is one that is probably a result of cytotoxic mechanisms.

Cell damage in this disease may be mediated by an antithyroid antibody–dependent, cell-mediated form of cytotoxicity or direct cytotoxicity itself by the sensitized effector T lymphocytes or an element of both. Hashimoto's thyroiditis is classified by the amount of fibrosis, with the most common form being lymphocytic infiltration with follicular cell hyperplasia, and by lymphoid follicles noted within the thyroid gland and the presence of minimal fibrosis. A fibrous variant of this condition shows much epithelial cell destruction and fibrosis on microscopic examination.

The presentation in children is usually of asymptomatic enlargement of the thyroid gland that only occasionally is found to be painful. A granular-feeling gland is often noted with nontender adjacent lymph nodes. Children rarely present as thyrotoxic, which is an important distinguishing feature between Hashimoto's thyroiditis and Graves' disease. The diagnosis generally is established by finding an elevated titer of thyroid antibodies. The most commonly obtained studies are those of thyroid peroxides (microsomal) and thyroid hemagglutinating antibodies. Titers of 1:4 could represent chronic thyroiditis in children. Should Hashimoto's thyroiditis be suspected and thyroid antibodies are negative, they should be rechecked in 3 to 6 months.

These children are rarely thyrotoxic but commonly are noted to have a transient phase of hyperthyroidism if autoimmune thyroiditis is detected early. This phase is called *toxic thyroiditis* and is distinguished from Graves' disease by the fact that it is usually mild and there is no exophthalmos. Graves' disease results from an overproduction and oversecretion of thyroid hormones because of stimulation of TSH receptors by thyrotropin receptor antibodies, whereas toxic thyroiditis is caused by the release of excessive amounts of thyroid hormones resulting from the inflammatory destruction of thyroid follicular cells. One generally can distinguish between the two disease processes, and if this is difficult, measurement of thyrotropin receptor antibodies and the performance of a iodine-123 scan usually can help to establish the diagnosis. If a child has slight elevations of T_3 and T_4 and positive antibody titers, nothing further needs to be done. These children commonly are clinically euthyroid at the time of evaluation. The diagnosis also can be made after children have been evaluated for the onset of symptomatic hypothyroidism.

Children with Hashimoto's thyroiditis usually develop diffuse, firm, and painless enlargement of the entire thyroid. The gland is often much larger than normal and occasionally may compress the trachea and produce dyspnea, hoarseness, or dysphagia.

Children with symptomatic Hashimoto's thyroiditis usually can be treated effectively with thyroid hormone suppression. At least 75% of children experience regression of the thyroid gland to less than 50% of the original size. Patients who fail to respond to suppression therapy and continue with symptomatic goiters may benefit from subtotal thyroidectomy. If the child has some manifestations of being hyperthyroid, propranolol is used. About 10% of children develop symptomatic hypothyroidism, in which case, treatment with levothyroxine is initiated. After 1 or 2 months of levothyroxine treatment, children are re-evaluated to determine if permanent hypothyroidism is present; commonly the levothyroxine can be discontinued at that time. There has been no apparent increase in the incidence of thyroid carcinoma in children with Hashimoto's thyroiditis, although a solitary nodule may be one of the early manifestations of the condition. Less than 2% of patients with Hashimoto's thyroiditis have associated malignancy.

Granulomatous subacute thyroiditis (de Quervain's disease and Riedel's chronic thyroiditis) is rare in childhood. When present, treatment with thyroid hormone may be beneficial; operative management is usually unnecessary.

Acute thyroiditis is a relatively rare disease that is recognized easily because the child generally presents with acute onset of pain within the region of the thyroid gland and often associated fever, chills, dysphagia, hoarseness, and sore throat. An upper respiratory tract infection commonly precedes the symptoms, and on examination there may be warmth and erythema of the overlying skin and some regional lymphadenopathy. The thyroid gland is enlarged but also tender. These children are not thyrotoxic, although they may appear to be "toxic" from the underlying infectious process. Laboratory tests usually show leukocytosis and an elevated erythrocyte sedimentation rate. Thyroid function studies are normal, and a thyroid aspirate generally can guide the appropriate antimicrobial therapy. Occasionally, abscess formation occurs, and ultrasound is helpful to diagnose this. Many reported cases of acute thyroiditis have been associated with an internal fistula between the left pyriform sinus and left thyroid lobe. It may be shown on a barium esophagogram when the child has recovered from the acute infectious process.

Subacute thyroiditis rarely occurs during childhood. This is believed to result from a viral infection of the thyroid gland, and these patients usually have a recent history of upper respiratory tract infection. There is pain within the region of the thyroid gland that radiates toward the jaw and ears. Although they are usually euthyroid, children may have some symptoms suggestive of hyperthyroidism. Almost uniformly, patients with subacute thyroiditis have concurrent systemic symptoms of inflammatory disease, such as fever, weakness, fatigue, and malaise, distinguishing the condition from Hashimoto's thyroiditis. Mild evidence of hyperthyroidism may be reflected in the T_3 and T_4 levels, but the thyroid antibodies are negative, and erythrocyte sedimentation rate is elevated. Children can progress through a phase of toxic thyroiditis followed by euthyroid goiter and later hypothyroidism before resuming normal thyroid function. Children with subacute thyroiditis rarely have permanent hypothyroidism. Management during the acute phase includes propranolol if necessary; salicylates, acetaminophen, and nonsteroidal anti-inflammatory agents are helpful adjuncts. Steroids are rarely used. The incidence of hypothyroidism in children and adolescents is low, identified in one study at 0.135% with a male-to-female ratio of 1:2.8; approximately two thirds of these cases had an autoimmune basis.

CONGENITAL GOITERS

Several types of congenital goiter are caused by inborn errors of metabolism based on genetic, clinical, and biochemical criteria. Each type represents a specific genetic defect that interferes with a step in thyroid hormone synthesis. Regardless of the cause, the gland is unable to produce adequate thyroid hormone, resulting in compensatory hypertrophy. Most children are hypothyroid, although occasional patients are euthyroid. Genetic defects causing congenital goiter may relate to any of the following mechanisms: (1) an iodine transport defect, (2) an iodine organification defect, (3) a partial iodine organification defect associated with deaf-mutism (Pendred's syndrome), (4) an iodotyrosine coupling defect, (5) an iodotyrosine deiodinization defect, (6) a thyroglobulin-iodinated polypeptide defect, and (7) a resistance to thyroid hormone because of receptor inadequacies. Although the diagnosis can be established in most patients by a combination of physical findings and family history, tissue culture studies may be necessary to identify the specific biochemical defect.

Long-term thyroid replacement therapy corrects the metabolic deficiency but does not always cause regression of a large goiter. An occasional child may benefit from thyroidectomy for cosmetic reasons or for relief of symptoms caused by compression (Fig. 29-3). In the uncommon Pendred's syndrome, the goiter may be composed of large nodules with histologic papillary configuration, which is benign and should be distinguished from papillary carcinoma.

Although the almost universal use of iodine in food processing has largely eliminated the occurrence of endemic goiter, occasional sporadic goiters still occur in children. Most affected children have normal thyroid function and TSH values and have no apparent dietary or drug history that might relate to the disorder. The response to thyroid hormone is usually good, with regression of the nodular goiter within a few months of therapy.

PARATHYROID

Hyperparathyroidism is the most frequent disorder of the parathyroids in children and may be primary, secondary, or tertiary. Primary hyperparathyroidism in childhood is uncommon, although many adults with the condition date the origin of their symptoms to late adolescence.

Neonatal Hyperparathyroidism

Neonatal hyperparathyroidism is a rare condition. It is accompanied by high mortality if not identified and treated early. Critical levels of hypercalcemia may develop within the first several days of life, although occasional infants have a more insidious onset with gradual elevation of calcium levels over several months. The infants often manifest symptoms of lethargy, hypotonia, dehydration, mild-to-moderate respiratory distress, slow feeding, and failure to thrive.

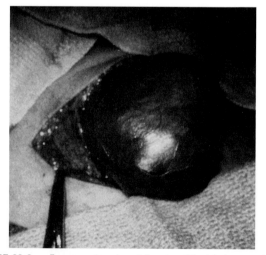

FIGURE 29-3 ■ Large goiter in a 17-year-old girl that persisted despite a long course of thyroid replacement therapy, causing compression of the trachea and disfigurement.

When initially diagnosed, serum calcium levels may be markedly elevated. Total parathyroidectomy with autotransplant of one gland to the forearm is recommended because lesser procedures have resulted in rapid recurrence of symptoms. The abnormal hyperplastic glands in infants with this disorder show features typical of chief cell hyperplasia. Neonatal hyperparathyroidism may be inherited as an autosomal recessive trait.

A few cases of familial hypocalciuric hypercalcemia have been reported that cause a benign form of hypercalcemia, usually diagnosed after age 10 years. This disorder may be transmitted as an autosomal dominant trait. Children with this disorder do not excrete normal amounts of calcium in the urine because of the abnormal renal response to parathyroid hormone. Total parathyroidectomy is usually necessary to achieve normocalcemia, with autotransplant of one gland to the forearm.

Familial Hyperparathyroidism

In familial hyperparathyroidism, which is more frequent in children than adults, diffuse chief cell hyperplasia involves all parathyroid glands. Children with the condition often have associated syndrome complexes including MEN I, MEN IIA, and familial hypocalciuric hypercalcemia. Most children are recognized during screening of family members at risk for these syndromes. Lethargy, malaise, and occasionally renal stones may develop, particularly in children with MEN I. Hyperparathyroidism is often the earliest manifestation of MEN I, although pituitary and pancreatic islet cells also may be abnormal.

All children with MEN I have chief cell hyperplasia and enlargement of the parathyroid glands. When one parathyroid gland is larger than the others, the condition may be confused with parathyroid adenoma. In these patients, it is helpful to obtain a biopsy specimen of one of the normal-appearing glands to determine the extent of parathyroid resection necessary. For children with MEN I and children with familial hypocalciuric hypercalcemia, all but 40 to 50 mg of parathyroid tissue should be removed. A lesser resection usually results in recurrence. Thompson and coworkers recommended excision of the cervical thymus for this condition because of the high incidence of supernumerary parathyroid glands in children with genetically induced hyperplasias. Many experts recommend total parathyroidectomy with autotransplantation of parathyroid tissue into a forearm muscle. Although this procedure ensures a low recurrence of hyperparathyroidism compared with subtotal parathyroidectomy, approximately 5% to 10% of patients become permanently hypoparathyroid.

Children with MEN IIA also have chief cell hyperplasia, although it is less severe than in patients with MEN I. Because all these patients have MCT, resection of parathyroid tissue usually is performed at the time of total thyroidectomy. In children with MEN IIA, parathyroidectomy should be limited to excision of only one or two enlarged glands because more extensive resection produces a higher incidence of permanent hypoparathyroidism. In contrast, children with MEN IIB do not develop hyperparathyroidism, and all parathyroid glands should be preserved at the time of total thyroidectomy.

Parathyroid Adenoma

A single adenoma is the most common cause of hyperparathyroidism in adolescent children and is more frequent in boys. Adenomas are more likely to produce hyperparathyroidism in this age group than is diffuse hyperplasia. The most common symptoms include renal stones, hypertension, headaches, constipation, weakness, and fatigue. In rare cases, children present with acute pancreatitis. Few patients are asymptomatic, although occasional children may be identified because of routine biochemical screening of family members. When the diagnosis of primary hyperparathyroidism has been established, neck exploration should be performed. Traditionally all four parathyroid glands were biopsied and the adenoma excised. Information from radiographic evaluation by ultrasonography and technetium-99m sestamibi radionuclide scans permits focused exploration of the neck if both studies identify a single lesion. Hyperplastic parathyroid glands have a decrease in intracellular fat that may be noted on histologic examination. When there is a positive family history of parathyroid disease increasing the frequency of diffuse hyperplasia, subtotal parathyroidectomy usually is indicated.

Sporadic parathyroid adenomas may result from head and neck radiation given more than 20 years earlier. An increasing number of patients who have undergone iodine-131 thyroid ablation for Graves' disease subsequently have been found to have parathyroid adenomas. Parathyroid carcinoma is a rare cause of hypercalcemia in children, but it should be considered in children with extremely high serum calcium levels.

Secondary Hyperparathyroidism

Children receiving long-term peritoneal dialysis for renal failure can develop secondary hyperparathyroidism similar to that which occurs in adults. Even with careful medical management, including attempts to reduce phosphorus absorption, a few children develop progressive renal osteodystrophy with objective bone changes, bone pain, and pruritus. If the symptoms persist or progress despite medical management, subtotal parathyroidectomy usually is recommended. These patients have an elevated alkaline phosphatase and N-terminal thyroid hormone assay levels. An attempt should be made to preserve at least one normal well-vascularized parathyroid gland, particularly in a prospective renal transplant recipient. If total parathyroidectomy is performed, one parathyroid gland should be implanted into the forearm.

In occasional children with chronic renal failure, the first manifestation of secondary hyperthyroidism may not appear until after a successful renal transplant. Hypercalcemia may become evident when the serum phosphorus level returns to normal. For these patients, if the serum calcium level does not decrease to 12 mg/dL or less within several months, parathyroidectomy should be considered. An increased level of C-terminal parathyroid hormone suggests the presence of autonomous function from localized hyperplastic parathyroid tissue (tertiary hyperparathyroidism). In these patients, all parathyroid glands may be enlarged, and subtotal parathyroidectomy should be performed.

Tertiary Hyperparathyroidism

This condition is seen mainly following renal transplantation. It results when hyperfunctioning parathyroid glands no longer respond to elevated ionized calcium levels.

SUGGESTED READINGS

Allo M, Thompson NW, Nishiyama R: Primary hyperparathyroidism in children, adolescents, and young adults. World J Surg 6:771, 1982.

This excellent review of hyperparathyroidism in children is based on a large clinical experience.

Brandi ML, Gagel RF, Angeli A, et al: Consensus: Guidelines for diagnosis and therapy of MEN type 1 and type 2. J Clin Endocrinol Metab 86:5658-5671, 2001.

A consensus report on the management of MEN syndromes is presented.

Graham SM, Genel M, Touloukian RJ, et al: Provocative testing for occult medullary carcinoma of the thyroid: Findings in seven children with multiple endocrine neoplasia type A. J Pediatr Surg 22:501, 1987.

This is one of the best reviews of this technique in the surgical literature. Although the technique is employed less frequently today to identify affected individuals, it is important in the identification of children with residual or recurrent disease.

Harness JK, Thompson NW, McLeod MK, et al: Differentiated thyroid carcinoma in children and adolescents, World J Surg 16:547, 1992.

An up-to-date extensive review of the surgical management of thyroid carcinoma in childhood is presented.

La Quaglia MP, Corbally MT, Heller G, et al: Recurrence and morbidity in differentiated thyroid carcinoma in children. Surgery 104:1149-1156, 1988.

A large institutional report of pediatric thyroid carcinoma (patients <17 years old) showed an overall excellent survival (no deaths) with a median follow-up of 20 years and a high incidence of nodal metastases (71%). Only young age and histologic subtype affected time to recurrence. Use of total or subtotal thyroidectomy or radical neck dissection was associated with increased risk of complications but did not prevent recurrence.

Newman KD, Black T, Heller G, et al: Differentiated thyroid cancer: Determinants of disease progression in patients <21 years of age at diagnosis: A report from the Surgical Discipline Committee of the Children's Cancer Group. Ann Surg 227:533-541, 1998.

A multi-institutional study of 329 patients (<21 years old) with differentiated thyroid carcinoma showed overall long-term survival of 90% and regional and distant metastases in 74% and 25% of patients. Progression-free survival was lower in younger patients and patients with residual cervical disease after surgery.

Raab SS, Silverman JF, Elsheikh RM, et al: Pediatric thyroid nodules: Disease demographics and clinical management as determined by fine needle aspiration biopsy. Pediatrics 95:46-49, 1995.

This study of fine-needle aspiration for diagnosis in patients younger than 18 years old showed an 18% incidence of malignancy and reasonable accuracy, although a false-negative misdiagnosis did occur.

Telander RL, Zimmerman D, van Heerden JA, et al: Results of early thyroidectomy for medullary thyroid carcinoma in children with multiple endocrine neoplasia type 2. J Pediatr Surg 21:1190, 1986.

One of the largest reported clinical experiences with this condition is presented, indicating the results after surgical management.

30

Bone Tumors

MALIGNANT BONE TUMORS

Primary malignant bone tumors are uncommon and constitute less than 2% of all malignant tumors in childhood. Osteogenic sarcomas and Ewing's tumors are the most frequent skeletal malignancies in children. Advances in surgical management including limb-salvage procedures, improved diagnostic imaging, and the availability of new chemotherapeutic agents for neoadjuvant therapy have improved the course of children with skeletal tumors.

Diagnostic Evaluation

Recognizing the presence of a tumor and determining the extent of disease should be accomplished as rapidly as possible. For most skeletal tumors, a fairly accurate estimate of the nature and extent of the lesion can be obtained from a thorough history, physical examination, and plain radiographs. Common bone tumors are listed in Table 30-1. Most children seek attention because of pain, which is the most common symptom. Pain is often constant, is unrelated to activity, and is worse at night. Delay in diagnosis is common because pain in some cases is thought to be related to trauma or a sports injury. The second most frequent complaint is swelling. Occasionally a pathologic fracture may be the presenting finding. The history of pain or swelling before the fracture is important. Weight loss and fever are worrisome observations and are often consistent with advanced disease. Plain radiographs should be taken in two views at right angles to each other. These radiographs detail anatomic site, effect on the bone (destruction, moth-eaten appearance), bone reaction to the lesion (i.e., endosteal, periosteal, "sunburst" or "onionskin" appearance), and findings characteristic of a specific lesion (i.e., new bone formation, calcification, ground-glass appearance). Technetium-99m bone scans may show lesions extending beyond the limits noted on plain radiographs. Radioisotopic total-body bone scans may be helpful in identifying unsuspected bone metastases (Fig. 30-1). Many investigators prefer gallium-67 or thallium-201 scans as a baseline study before therapy and 1 month after the administration of chemotherapy. Gallium-67 and thallium-201 measure the viability of tumor cells themselves rather than osteoid calcification. With the exception of myeloma and histiocytosis, lesions that show no increase in radioisotope activity are usually benign.

Computed tomography (CT) or magnetic resonance imaging (MRI) is helpful in defining the extent and nature of a bone lesion preoperatively, particularly intramedullary involvement, extraosseous extension, and degree of cortical destruction, and identifying postoperative recurrences.

TABLE 30-1 ■ Common Primary Bone Tumors

Bone-forming tumors
  Benign
    Osteoma
    Osteoid osteoma
    Osteoblastoma
  Intermediate
    Malignant osteoblastoma
  Malignant
    Osteosarcoma
      Central (medullary)
      Surface (peripheral)
      Parosteal osteosarcoma
      Periosteal osteosarcoma
      High-grade surface
Cartilage-forming tumors
  Benign
    Chondroma
      Enchondroma
      Periosteal (juxtacortical)
    Osteochondroma (osteocartilaginous exostosis)
      Solitary
      Multiple hereditary
    Chondroblastoma
      Chondromyxoid fibroma
  Malignant
    Chondrosarcoma
      Dedifferentiated chondrosarcoma
      Mesenchymal chondrosarcoma
      Clear cell chondrosarcoma
Giant cell tumor (osteoclastoma)
Marrow tumors (round cell tumors)
  Ewing's sarcoma of bone
  Neuroectodermal tumor of bone
  Malignant lymphoma of bone
  Myeloma

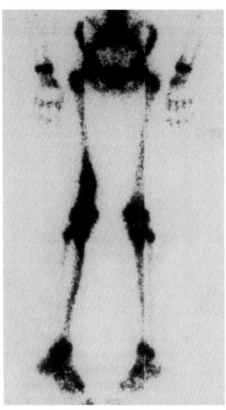

FIGURE 30-1 ■ Technetium-99m phosphonate bone scan from a 12-year-old boy with osteogenic sarcoma of the distal right femur shows increased isotope uptake in this area.

MRI is more accurate in assessing intramedullary involvement. CT is particularly useful for evaluating musculoskeletal lesions around the pelvis and spine and for identifying pulmonary metastases. Peritumor edema may be difficult to distinguish from the tumor itself. MRI provides greater detail for defining extraosseous soft tissue extension. Approximately 60% of patients with osteosarcomas and 100% of patients with predominately osteoblastic osteogenic sarcomas have an elevated serum alkaline phosphatase level. This test can be used as a tumor marker to assess the response of the patient's tumor to preoperative chemotherapy.

Adjuvant Therapy

Preoperative neoadjuvant systemic chemotherapy with high-dose methotrexate and other chemotherapeutic agents has increased survival for children with osteogenic sarcoma from less than 15% to more than 65%. Effective chemotherapy as an adjunct to surgery for osteosarcoma includes methotrexate, doxorubicin, and cisplatin. Careful monitoring of urine output, kidney function, and frequency of treatment is necessary to avoid complications from high-dose chemotherapy. Approximately half of osteosarcoma patients who receive preoperative chemotherapy show total tumor necrosis and no residual viable tumor. Tumor necrosis is often predictive of survival. Chemotherapy has produced an overall disease-free survival greater than 65%, whereas less than 11% achieve this result with surgery alone. The current treatment of choice for localized osteosarcoma is neoadjuvant

chemotherapy combined with surgery, which increases the cure rate to approximately 70%. Postoperative adjuvant chemotherapy apparently does not increase survival.

Intra-arterial infusion of doxorubicin produces considerable tumor cell necrosis; however, there is often subcutaneous exudation into the soft tissues that may cause slough of subcutaneous tissue and skin, reducing the opportunity to resect the primary tumor. After arterial infusion of doxorubicin, destruction of soft tissues with fibrosis about the joints may occur. Although arterial infusion of chemotherapy currently is used infrequently, there has been interest in the use of local infusions of cisplatin for osteosarcoma because of reduced local tissue injury.

There is little evidence to indicate that preoperative or postoperative radiotherapy reduces the incidence of local tumor recurrence after resection of limb osteosarcomas. Preoperative radiation may cause stiffness in adjacent joints. Irradiation to the entire lung in an attempt to reduce the likelihood of spread of osteogenic sarcomas has not increased survival (in contrast to Ewing's sarcoma) but has caused pulmonary fibrosis in several patients. Systemic immunotherapy has been of interest for the treatment of bone tumors, particularly osteosarcomas. The initial attempt to use adoptive immune transfer and subsequently transfer factor has not proved effective.

Surgical Considerations

The initial biopsy of a bone tumor is an important factor in determining the overall management, including subsequent operation. Biopsy material should be obtained by either large-core needle tissue biopsy or, preferably, open biopsy. Fine-needle aspiration for the diagnosis of a malignant bone tumor may lead to underdiagnosis or incorrect diagnosis and is not recommended. The biopsy incision should be placed so that the wound can be excised en bloc with the specimen when definitive resection is performed. A longitudinal biopsy incision is preferred because subsequent resection usually requires extensive longitudinal exposure. Dissection should be minimized and neurovascular structures avoided. When biopsies are required through bone and radiotherapy is planned, pathologic fracture through radiated bone is a frequent occurrence, especially when chemotherapy is added. If tumor extends through the bone cortex, an adequate specimen can be obtained from the external soft tissue mass without violating the cortex. If the cortex of the bone is entered, the cortical hole should be a small circular porthole rather than a rectangular "window" to minimize the risk of pathologic fracture.

Because the consequences of misdiagnosis are serious, needle biopsy is best reserved for areas that are difficult to expose, such as the vertebral bodies. Approximately 20% of patients with skeletal tumors require a second biopsy because the original specimen was unsatisfactory. The pathologist should examine the biopsy tissue with frozen section if necessary, to establish that the specimen contains tumor. Because a suspected tumor occasionally proves to be an infection, a portion of the biopsy specimen should be sent for culture in all suspicious lesions, especially intramedullary tumors that appear to be Ewing's sarcoma.

Amputation of an extremity or wide resection at the time of biopsy has not improved survival and may limit the options for reconstruction. In the past, it was believed that the entire bone must be removed because of the possibility of skip lesions, and that amputation should include the joint above where the original primary tumor was located. In patients who receive postamputation chemotherapy, transosseous amputations were not a source of local recurrence, provided that the level within the bone was properly selected. Skip metastases occur in less than 10% of patients, and with neoadjuvant preoperative chemotherapy the incidence of occult skip metastases is almost zero. Scanning with a bone-seeking radioisotope is a fairly precise technique for determining the extent of a bone tumor.

The standard techniques of amputation are altered for children who receive chemotherapy. High-dose methotrexate may inhibit healing of the fascia, soft tissues, and bone. Neoadjuvant preoperative chemotherapy can shrink the primary tumor, better define the surgical margins, and decrease tumor vascularity. After amputation, most children are treated with plaster dressing and an immediate postoperative prosthetic fitting. Most children are discharged within 1.5 weeks, walking with partial weight bearing on the temporary prosthesis using crutches. If postoperative chemotherapy with high-dose methotrexate is used, this alters the stump volume, increasing its size during each course of therapy. This fact should be taken into consideration when fitting for a prosthesis. Children thrive on the athletic programs available to amputees, and active participation should be encouraged.

Limb-Salvage Procedures

Since the 1980s, limb-sparing resection of osteogenic sarcomas combined with neoadjuvant preoperative chemotherapy has been used with increasing frequency. Currently, limb-salvage procedures are standard for children with osteosarcoma of the extremity. Improved surgical technique, contemporary imaging to document tumor extent accurately, and neoadjuvant chemotherapy have made limb salvage a safer alternative to amputation, provided that wide surgical margins are achieved. Adequate resection for osteosarcoma of the femur requires removal of the bone and adjacent muscles for at least 6 cm proximal to the upper level of bone reactivity on bone scan. Transmedullary resections or amputations for distal femur lesions have not resulted in an increased local recurrence rate. Few lesions of the distal femur or proximal tibia invade through the synovial lining of the joint space. This natural barrier to tumor spread permits patella salvage and preservation of the extensor mechanism in most patients. Intra-articular resection for children with osteogenic sarcoma results in excellent function.

A complication of limb-salvage surgery in younger children has been the unacceptable leg-length discrepancy when they survive through their adolescent growth spurt to adulthood. This problem has been overcome to a great extent by the development of an expandable endoprosthesis that can be lengthened every 6 months to keep up with growth. For the distal femur, many surgeons prefer an articulated metal or metal-plastic implant that leaves a movable knee joint. These implants permit early mobilization but may not always tolerate the wear and tear that teenagers and young adults place on their musculoskeletal system.

The use of allografts has been promising, although there is a delay in incorporation of allografts and a need to protect the extremity from excessive weight bearing for protracted periods. High-dose chemotherapy may inhibit bone healing, and when allografts are used to replace a joint segment of only one bone, the host ligaments must be retained for stability. For midshaft femoral tumors, reconstruction has been highly effective using allograft bone supported by an intramedullary prosthesis. Allografts fare better in the upper extremity, in which there is no risk of weight bearing. Many problems remain when dealing with cadaver allografts, including sizing, stability, fracture (16% in the lower extremity), rejection, and degeneration from long-term poor vascularity. Reconstruction of muscle defects using microsurgical techniques to permit muscle transfer adds another dimension to extremity rehabilitation after adequate resection.

Radiation Effects

In treating primary tumors of nonskeletal origin, radiation may deform the underlying osseous tissues in the field. This is particularly true in children with Wilms' tumor and neuroblastoma. Even if the entire width of the spine has been included in the radiation portal, prominent scoliosis can result, and patients should be re-examined periodically throughout their growing years. If a paraspinal or intraspinal neuroblastoma is managed by laminectomy, additional radiation treatment may result in severe kyphosis. Radiation-induced osteosarcoma may occur as a second tumor in the radiation portal in children treated for other neoplasms. The median time to occurrence is 8 years post–radiation treatment. The extremities, girdle bones, and craniofacial bones are the most common sites of occurrence. Patients with radiation-related osteosarcoma and resectable lesions can be cured after intensive chemotherapy and operative excision. The overall survival and event-free survival at 8 years are 50% and 41% respectively. Radiation to the extremities can cause considerable fibrosis and loss of range of motion. Postradiation fractures can occur in 60% of children with lesions of the long bones. Appropriate exercises initiated when radiation is started can decrease the deformities and muscle weakness.

Osteogenic Sarcoma

Less than 500 new cases of osteogenic sarcoma are diagnosed in children in the United States each year. It is the most common malignant bone tumor in childhood. This tumor occurs most often during the growth-spurt years and in locations of rapid bone growth, such as the distal femur, proximal tibia, and proximal humerus. Osteosarcoma is twice as frequent in boys. This tumor often is identified first on a plain radiograph obtained because of persistent pain noted after minor trauma. Localized swelling often is present. Most of these tumors involve the medullary cavity and are located at the metaphysis or near the ends of long bones. Plain radiographs usually show an aggressive lesion with poorly defined borders, varying degrees of osteolysis, and tumor bone formation. The periosteum frequently is elevated from the cortex. This periosteal new bone growth may appear as spicules at right angles to the shaft, giving a sunburst appearance (Fig. 30-2). The metaphysis is usually enlarged.

Osteogenic sarcoma occurs in various histologic forms—osteoblastic, chondroblastic, fibroblastic, telangiectatic, giant cell type, malignant fibrous histiocytoma–like, rosette-forming epithelioid, and others. These terms refer to the matrix, degree of vascularity, and simulation of other primary bone tumors (e.g., giant cell tumor). In osteoblastic osteosarcoma, most of the tumor matrix is composed of malignant osteoid. Spindle cells are characteristic of osteosarcoma, in contrast to the small round cells of Ewing's sarcoma. Rosette-forming epithelioid tumors have a poor prognosis, whereas telangiectatic osteosarcoma has a good prognosis.

Most osteogenic sarcomas have a high-grade malignant appearance histologically and are aggressive in nature. Poor prognostic factors include femur lesions, tumors occurring in children younger than 10 years of age, tumor in boys, metastases at the time of diagnosis, relapse after initial treatment, and a lack of tumor necrosis after neoadjuvant chemotherapy. The usual spread of osteosarcoma is via the circulation to the lung. Direct invasion of lymph nodes occurs in less than 15% of children. Metastases to other bones occasionally occur, usually when the disease is widespread and after pulmonary

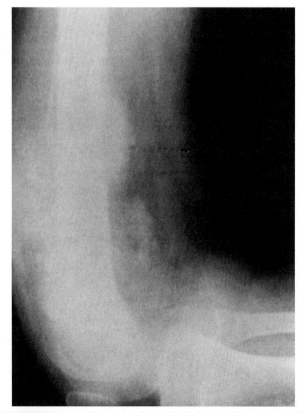

FIGURE 30-2 ■ Radiograph of the distal femur of a 12-year-old with osteogenic sarcoma. Note the periosteal elevation, "sunburst" soft tissue calcifications, and soft tissue mass.

nodules develop. Approximately 50% of patients with osteosarcoma and lung metastases have pulmonary lesions noted within 6 months and 80% by 2 years. Occasional patients develop pulmonary metastases 2 to 4 years after initial diagnosis. Most patients who die of their disease have pulmonary metastases. About 50% of patients with lung metastases also have bone metastases.

Cisplatin has been particularly helpful in reducing the incidence of pulmonary metastases. With the use of high-dose methotrexate with citrovorum rescue plus doxorubicin, approximately 65% of children have not developed pulmonary metastases and have achieved long-term survival. Newer protocols adding ifosfamide and etoposide to the chemotherapy program have improved the tumor response rate as judged by the degree of tumor necrosis in the subsequent resected specimen. Neoadjuvant chemotherapy controls subclinical metastatic disease and may shrink the primary tumor. Despite the improved tumor response to neoadjuvant treatment, it is essential to achieve complete surgical removal of the primary tumor. In some patients for whom complete surgical resection is impossible, radiation therapy may allow local tumor control. In children with pulmonary metastases, several studies have shown that one third or more can be rendered disease-free by one or more thoracotomies for removal of metastatic deposits after resection of the primary tumor and before discontinuing chemotherapy. Many surgeons recommend that even if lung nodules shown on CT disappear completely after therapy, thoracotomy with wedge resections should be performed because microscopic deposits of tumor can exist and often recur. The number of tumor nodules noted at the time of thoracotomy often exceeds the number seen on CT. Thoracoscopic removal of lung metastases is possible; however, the inability to palpate small tumor nodules not visible in a subpleural location is a limitation of this technique. Although the mainstay of operative treatment for primary osteogenic sarcoma for children in the past had been amputation, currently more than 75% of tumors can be resected with limb-salvage techniques that provide a safe and functional extremity. The advances in the surgical treatment of pediatric bone malignancies during the 1980s and 1990s have been related to the use of neoadjuvant chemotherapy programs and tumor resection with limb-salvage techniques.

Most relapses occur in patients in whom significant residual viable tumor (minimal tumor necrosis) is identified after neoadjuvant therapy when the tumor is analyzed postoperatively. Patients with localized disease who are complete responders to neoadjuvant preoperative chemotherapy (compete tumor necrosis) with complete tumor excision may not require postoperative chemotherapy. Patients with metastases at diagnosis (especially bone metastases) and patients who relapse continue to have a poor prognosis. Intratumoral neovascularization at diagnosis does not correlate with outcome in nonmetastatic osteosarcoma. High-dose chemotherapy and hematopoietic stem cell transplantation have not proved to be effective therapy after relapse. Alternative chemotherapy programs using carboplatin, methotrexate, ifosfamide, doxorubicin, and cisplatin for newly diagnosed metastatic or unresectable osteosarcoma have been disappointing. Future therapy with biologic modifiers, antiangiogenic agents, tumor vaccines, and growth receptor modulators may provide hope for high-risk patients with metastases and unresectable tumors.

Osteosarcoma Variants

Multifocal Osteosarcoma

Multifocal osteosarcoma most likely represents an osteogenic sarcoma that has metastasized directly to bone without first spreading to the lung. This form of the neoplasm has not experienced as great an improvement in prognosis as the usual type of osteogenic sarcoma. Treatment requires resection of the largest lesion to prevent fungation, with preoperative and postoperative chemotherapy. Radiation of the secondary and tertiary sites of bone involvement may provide occasional palliation.

Parosteal Osteosarcoma

Parosteal osteosarcoma is a less malignant form of osteogenic sarcoma that usually arises on the outer surface of the bone and does not involve the medullary canal. The tumor is a low-grade histologic malignancy and grows slowly, with metastases occurring several years later, if they appear at all. Adequate treatment often can be provided by local resection without chemotherapy.

Ewing's Sarcoma

Ewing's sarcoma develops within the bone marrow and consists primarily of sheets of small round cells, which distinguishes it from the spindle cells of the more common osteogenic sarcoma. Almost all bones in the body can be the site of the primary tumor; however, approximately 65% occur in the femur, tibia, humerus, or ribs, most commonly in the diaphysis or midshaft rather than the ends. Flat bones (e.g., the scapula) are often involved, which is rare for osteosarcoma. Primary tumors of the pelvis also are observed. Adolescents are affected most frequently, and the tumor is seen rarely in children before age 5 years. Boys are affected approximately twice as often as girls. Bone pain is often the first symptom, followed by swelling. Fever, elevated white blood cell count, and increased erythrocyte sedimentation rate may lead to a misdiagnosis of osteomyelitis. The serum lactate dehydrogenase level may be elevated and is associated with a poor prognosis. The tumor grows rapidly, frequently producing considerable necrosis within the tumor itself and causing fever. Characteristically, several months usually pass before the patient seeks medical advice.

Genetic evaluation of tumor tissue from patients with Ewing's tumor may show an *EWS-FLII* fusion gene associated with chromosomal translocation of t(11;22)(q24;12) or a variant *EWS* fusion gene (*EWS-ERG*) created by t(21;22) or t(7;22) translocations. Ewing's tumors rely on signaling through the insulin-like growth factor-1 receptor. Insulin-like growth factor-1 levels are higher in patients with metastases to bones or the bone marrow. Overexpression of the p53 protein is also an independent poor prognostic factor. These genetic alterations may permit Ewing's sarcoma to be distinguished from other small round blue cell tumors, including lymphoma, small cell sarcoma, neuroblastoma, rhabdomyosarcoma, and primitive neuroectodermal tumors. Immunoperoxidase stains can distinguish between a primary Ewing's sarcoma and metastatic rhabdomyosarcoma. Lymphoma often causes pain for a longer period without soft tissue swelling. Ewing's sarcoma tends to be more of a lytic destructive lesion than lymphoma.

Plain radiographs often show extensive involvement of the involved bone cortex with layers of periosteal new bone formation pushing outward and resulting in an onionskin appearance (Fig. 30-3). A radioisotopic bone scan should be performed to rule out bone metastases. Often a large soft tissue mass may be seen. CT or MRI shows extensive marrow involvement. Whole-body positron emission tomography may be useful in detecting bone marrow metastases. The most common spread of the tumor is to the lung, followed by spread to the skull, pelvis, and long bones. CT of the chest should be obtained before starting therapy because pulmonary metastases are highly sensitive to chemotherapy and may not have been seen on the chest radiograph. Because lung metastases are highly likely to recur after therapy, bilateral pulmonary radiation has improved survival. Extraosseous Ewing's sarcoma metastasizes to regional lymph nodes 25% of the time, and lymph node biopsy specimens should be obtained before treatment. Nodal metastasis is rare for Ewing's sarcoma of bone. Pelvic tumor location, high serum lactate dehydrogenase, fever, interval of onset of symptoms and diagnosis of less than 3 months, and age

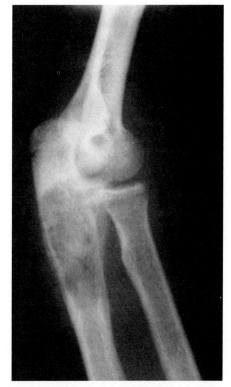

FIGURE 30-3 ■ Radiograph shows lytic lesion of the proximal ulna from a 13-year-old boy with Ewing's sarcoma. Cortical destruction has been surrounded by new periosteal bone in irregular layers (onionskin appearance). (From Welch KJ, Ravitch MM, Aberdeen E, et al [eds]: Pediatric Surgery, 4th ed. St. Louis, Mosby-Year Book, 1986.)

older than 12 years are risk factors for clinically evident metastatic disease. Before the use of chemotherapy, the prognosis for Ewing's sarcoma was poor, with only 10% of patients surviving long-term.

Radiation therapy alone to the involved bone results in a high recurrence rate of greater than 30%; however, when combined with preoperative chemotherapy, it helps prevent the emergence of tumor cells resistant to chemotherapy. A radiation dose of 4500 Gy to the entire involved bone, including a margin of a few centimeters proximally and distally but avoiding the growing epiphyseal ends, has been highly effective. Radiation is particularly helpful in treating rib lesions. In this dose range, there is a low rate of late secondary malignancies, and fibrosis and problems with surgical healing have not been encountered.

Surgical excision of the tumor plays an important role in survival. Patients with primary tumors of the ribs, clavicle, and fibula have the best prognosis because the tumor is often completely resectable. Pelvic tumors are often bulky and more difficult to remove completely with a wide tumor-free margin. After neoadjuvant chemotherapy, the size of the primary tumor often diminishes, however, permitting resection. This is especially true for primary tumors of the chest wall. Shrinkage of the tumor after adjuvant chemotherapy more clearly delineates the margins of surrounding soft tissue for adequate tumor resection. Current chemotherapy includes vincristine, doxorubicin, cyclophosphamide, and actinomycin-D alternating with ifosfamide and etoposide. The current overall 5-year survival is 64%, and the disease-free survival is 58%. Patients with a good histologic response to adjuvant chemotherapy had an improved survival (75%) compared with a 20% survival for poor responders. Tumor site, older age (>15 years old) and metastases at diagnosis are important prognostic factors. Patients who relapse within 2 years of diagnosis and initial treatment have a worse prognosis than patients who relapse later (>5 years) (4% versus 23% survival). With improved results using neoadjuvant chemotherapy, attempts to limit radiation therapy are under evaluation. Radiation therapy may be useful in patients with gross or microscopic residual disease after surgical resection and perhaps to supplement surgical treatment in high-risk areas (i.e., axial skeleton). Long-term follow-up is essential because patients with Ewing's tumor seem to have a greater risk of developing second tumors than patients with other pediatric malignancies.

Chondrosarcoma

Malignant chondrosarcoma may arise in normal bone (primary tumor) or as a secondary tumor that arises in a preexisting benign cartilaginous lesion (usually an exostosis or enchondroma). Primary lesions are more common (2:1) but rarely occur in children. Both sexes are equally affected. Most tumors occur in the axial skeleton, but 10% are located in the humerus. The radiographic appearance is a thick-walled radiolucent lesion with irregular areas of calcification. The medullary surface of the affected bone cortex may be scalloped, with cortical penetration a late occurrence. The only effective treatment is total excision of the tumor. Complete resection, site, and tumor grade are predictors of outcome. Survival in extremity tumors is far better than primary tumors arising in the pelvis. Low-grade chondrosarcomas have a better prognosis than high-grade tumors. Mesenchymal and dedifferentiated variants of chondrosarcoma are relatively rare but highly malignant tumors that may respond to neoadjuvant treatment using cisplatin, ifosfamide, and doxorubicin.

BENIGN BONE TUMORS AND TUMOR-LIKE LESIONS IN CHILDREN

Benign bone lesions in children may present a diagnostic and therapeutic challenge. A thorough understanding of the natural progression of the lesion, the growth potential of the child's extremity, and the methods of preserving motion and stability of the limb simplifies treatment. The most common benign bone lesions in childhood can be diagnosed by their clinical presentation and radiographic appearance (Figs. 30-4 and 30-5).

Osteocartilaginous Exostosis

Osteocartilaginous exostosis is the most commonly occurring benign tumor. The tumor can be sessile or pedunculated and arise near the physis. The involved bone is covered by a thin cartilage cap that appears similar to a physeal plate and undergoes endochondral ossification. Most are asymptomatic; however, simple excision of the lesion may be necessary for pain, cosmetically unacceptable mass or deformity, and limitation of range of motion. Multiple exostoses may occur as a hereditary condition and have a 1% to 2% risk of undergoing malignant degeneration (chondrosarcoma). When multiple exostoses are associated with subcutaneous hemangiomas, the condition is called *Maffucci's syndrome.*

Osteoma

Osteomas are small, painless, slowly enlarging lesions. They present as small lumps most commonly occurring

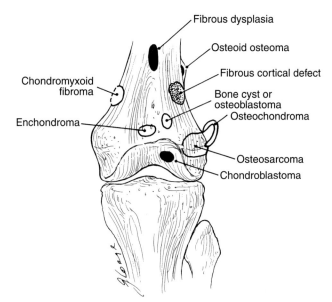

FIGURE 30-4 ■ Various types of benign bone lesions, shown in specific bone locations in which they most commonly occur.

Geographic   Permeated   Motheaten   Expansile

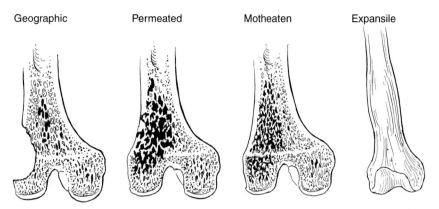

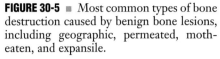

FIGURE 30-5 ■ Most common types of bone destruction caused by benign bone lesions, including geographic, permeated, motheaten, and expansile.

around the skull, although any bone may be affected. Osteomas appear as a small dense circumscribed lesion. Treatment is surgical excision if the patient is symptomatic. These lesions are benign and often simply can be observed.

Osteoid Osteoma

The peak incidence of osteoid osteoma is the second decade of life. This condition usually presents with vague pain, often nocturnal, that characteristically is relieved by aspirin or other nonsteroidal anti-inflammatory drugs. The pain may be associated with tenderness and vasomotor disturbance. Local swelling and erythema occasionally may be present. The tibia and femur are the most common locations. Lesions are small—usually less than 1 cm in size. The matrix consists of a central sclerotic area surrounded by a lucent outer zone with an intense reactive bone response. Histologically, osteoid osteoma has a central nidus of immature bone formation in association with vascularized osteogenic tissue. Surrounding the central nidus is a 1- to 3-mm lucent zone composed of loose fibrovascular tissue. A dense reactive rim of irregular mature trabecular osseous tissue surrounds the entire lesion. Plain radiographs may or may not reveal the characteristic nidus. CT, when applied in close 2-mm cuts, often accurately identifies the location of the nidus. The treatment of choice is local excision that results in immediate relief of pain. Recurrence is rare.

Osteoblastoma

Osteoblastoma usually presents in the second decade of life with focal pain that may be associated with local swelling and erythema. The tumor is more common in boys, and the most frequent site of occurrence is the spine, although this lesion also may occur in the proximal femur and tibia.

Osteoblastomas are usually metaphyseal or diaphyseal and geographic (see Fig. 30-5). The bone matrix is solid with associated radiolucent areas, and the bone reaction is generally minimal in the osseous or periosteal response about the lesion. Histologically the lesion contains osteoblasts and osteoid, woven bone with vascular components. and osteoclasts. It may be difficult to distinguish from osteoid osteoma. The larger size, ovoid shape, and presence of osteoblasts characterize osteoblastomas.

Radiographs may show an expansile radiolucent lesion with a thin shell of peripheral new bone.

Treatment is by local excision and curettage with or without bone grafting. This is successful in approximately 95% of patients. The recurrence rate after curettage alone may be 20%. Recurrence requires a more extensive resection.

Chondroblastoma

The onset of chondroblastoma is usually in the second decade and often is associated with focal pain. The tumor is more common in boys. Frequent sites of involvement include the epiphysis of the femur, humerus, tibia, and tarsal bones, Radiographs show that chondroblastoma is a geographic (oval), epiphyseal lesion; there is a flecked matrix of opaque calcification and an endosteal response of border sclerosis. The texture is gritty with small chondroid nodules. CT may illustrate better the local invasive properties of the tumor and intralesional calcification. Histologically the cells are polyhedral and separated by small scanty matrix comprising chondroid hyaline cartilage with associated osteoplastic giant cells, "chicken wire" calcification, and calcific nodules in the stroma and the chondroid.

Treatment by curettage, bone grafting, and excision of any adjacent soft tissue extension is associated with a low recurrence rate (<10%). Radiation has been used for lesions that are unresectable.

Unicameral Bone Cyst

Unicameral bone cysts develop during the first two decades of life and occur twice as frequently in boys than girls. The cyst is generally asymptomatic until a pathologic fracture occurs, although occasionally local pain or swelling may be observed. Unicameral bone cysts occur most frequently in the metaphysis of the humerus, the femur, or the tibia and occasionally in the fibula, ribs, calcaneus, talus, and ilium.

The lesion is centrally located in the metaphyseal area of the bone and is oval, with a longitudinal axis parallel to that of the bone. The lesion is lytic, with an appearance of septa produced by scalloping of the bone. The borders are smooth or scalloped, and the lesion is expansile, with thinning of the cortical bone. The wall of the cyst has a fleshy connective tissue varying in thickness up to 1 cm. Histologically the lesion is surrounded by a thin border of reactive trabecular bone. The fibrous tissue layer varies in thickness up to 1 cm and consists of spindle-shaped fibroblasts, benign reactive giant cells, loose connective tissue, lipophages, cholesterol slits, and hemosiderin.

Plain radiographs usually show a lesion with a central medullary location with its length greater than its width. There is no soft tissue component. Treatment includes percutaneous drainage of the cyst with injection of a bone matrix protein substrate through two trochars, one proximally and one distally in the cyst. This treatment results in resolution of the cyst in two thirds of cases. Nonresponders who are symptomatic may require complete curettage of the cyst, followed by bone grafting. Incomplete removal of the cyst lining may lead to recurrence. These cysts also may respond to intracystic injection of methylprednisolone acetate (40 to 80 mg).

Aneurysmal Bone Cysts

The cause of aneurysmal bone cysts is unknown, but the lesions frequently occur following other bone lesions, such as chondroblastoma, giant cell tumor, chondromyxoid fibroma, xanthoma, or osteosarcoma. All aneurysmal bone cysts should be considered as possibly having an underlying tumor. This lesion occurs 1 to 1.5 times more frequently in girls and often appears during the second decade of life. These blood-filled expansile bone cysts have been observed after a fracture and are known to enlarge rapidly during pregnancy. In long bones, the aneurysmal bone cyst may present with pain, swelling, heat, and tenderness. Of cases, 80% occur in the upper limb. Lesions in the vertebral bodies may present with signs and symptoms of spinal cord compression. The lesion often rapidly progresses in size, ballooning in 6 to 12 weeks.

Aneurysmal bone cysts are geographic and metaphyseal. Two types exist: cysts beginning within a bone and expanding out into the soft tissues and cysts beginning on the bone surface and eroding into the marrow cavity. A well-circumscribed eccentric zone of rarefaction is associated with soft tissue extension of the cyst, showing trabeculation. Soft tissue extension is produced by bulging of the periosteum, with resultant layering of new bone, which delineates the periphery of the tumor.

The lesion contains an anastomosing cavernous space filled with unclotted blood that wells up, but does not spurt, when unroofed. Histologically, there are cavernomatous spaces with septa having an unusual endothelial lining and lacking the features of normal blood vessels. Benign giant cells may be present in large numbers. Mitotic figures with anaplastic nuclei may be numerous in spindle cell areas. The microscopic appearance of this lesion is similar to that of a unicameral bone cyst, and microscopic differentiation may be difficult. Radiographs show a purely lytic expansile lesion usually arising in the metaphyses. CT may show multiple fluid levels, which is characteristic of an aneurysmal bone cyst. Treatment for accessible aneurysmal bone cysts is complete evacuation (curettage) with bone grafting. In inaccessible locations, such as the vertebral bodies, radiation therapy may be helpful.

Fibrous Cortical Dysplasia

Fibrous cortical dysplasia occurs most frequently in patients 10 to 15 years old. Boys are affected more frequently than girls. The lesion is usually asymptomatic and occurs in the large bones of the lower extremity and the proximal humerus, ribs, and skull. The lesion is expansile and erodes the cortex, extending into the cancellous tissue and sometimes occupying the entire diameter of the bone, which may lead to a pathologic fracture. Fibrous cortical defects are geographic, eccentrically located lesions that occur in the metaphysis of long bones near the epiphyseal plate. The bone matrix has a multilocalized central lucent zone with an endosteal neutral bone response.

Grossly the lesion is well defined and composed of dense fibrous tissue, with small, embedded osteoid trabeculae and a gritty quality. Microscopically, there is a proliferation of fibroblasts that produce a collagenous matrix that may contain trabeculae of osteoid and bone. In areas of degeneration, only relatively acellular fibrous or myxoid tissue may be present. No treatment is required for most asymptomatic lesions, and these may regress spontaneously. Large lesions situated in crucial weight-bearing areas may require curettage with bone grafting.

Nonossifying Fibroma

Nonossifying fibroma is believed to be the end product of an expanding fibrous cortical dysplasia. The lesion occurs most often in the second decade of life and only rarely before age 8 years. It is seldom painful and usually occurs in long bones, especially the femur and tibia. Occasionally, it is found incidentally on a plain radiograph of the femur or tibia. The lesion is a 2- to 7-cm geographic, eccentrically placed metaphyseal osteolytic lesion. Its cortical margins are thin, and the endosteal reaction is a dense bone response.

The gross and microscopic appearances of a nonossifying fibroma are the same as those of fibrous cortical dysplasia. Treatment is not necessary unless the lesion is symptomatic or located in a crucial weight-bearing area of bone. In most cases, the lesion involutes and ossifies with skeletal maturity.

SUGGESTED READINGS

Berend KR, Pietrobon R, Moore JO, et al: Adjuvant chemotherapy for osteosarcoma may not increase survival after neoadjuvant chemotherapy and surgical resection. J Surg Oncol 78:162-170, 2001.

In patients with localized disease, neoadjuvant chemotherapy and complete tumor resection may be the only treatment required.

Cannon SR: Bone tumors: Limb salvage. In Carachi R, Azmy A, Grosfeld JL (eds): The Surgery of Childhood Tumors. London, Arnold, 1999, pp 267-297.

This excellent overview concerns benign and malignant bone tumors and limb-salvage techniques.

Chansky HA, O'Donnell RJ, Howlett AT, Conrad EU III: Common bone tumors. In O'Neill JA Jr, Rowe MI, Grosfeld JL, et al (eds): Pediatric Surgery, 5th ed. St Louis, Mosby, 1998, pp 483-498.

This textbook chapter presents information concerning common bone tumors with a well-organized approach.

Cotterill SJ, Ahrens S, Paulussen M, et al: Prognostic factors in Ewing's tumor of bone: Analysis of 975 patients from the

European Intergroup Cooperative Ewing's Sarcoma Study Group. J Clin Oncol 18:3108-3114, 2000.

This review from Europe evaluates prognostic factors in 975 children with Ewing's tumor in all stages.

Ferguson WS, Goorin AM: Current treatment of osteosarcoma. Cancer Invest 19:292-315, 2001.

The current methods of managing osteosarcoma are reviewed.

Givens SS, Woo SY, Huang LY, et al: Non-metastatic Ewing's sarcoma: 20 years of experience suggests that surgery is a prime factor for successful multimodal therapy. Int J Oncol 14:1039-1043, 1999.

Patients with Ewing's sarcoma who had their tumor resected had better local control and disease-free survival.

Oberlin O, Deley MC, Bui BN, et al: Prognostic factors in localized Ewing's tumours and peripheral neuroectodermal tumours: The third study of the French Society of Paediatric Oncology (EW88 study). Br J Cancer 85:1646-1654, 2001.

This study of 141 children with Ewing's tumor and primitive neuroectodermal tumor describes the prognostic factors observed in patients with localized tumors.

Saenz NC, Hass DJ, Meyers P, et al: Pediatric chest wall Ewing's sarcoma. J Pediatr Surg 35:550-555, 2000.

This is an excellent review of a series of patients with Ewing's sarcoma involving the chest wall.

Tabone MD, Terrier P, Pacquement H, et al: Outcome of radiation related osteosarcoma after treatment of childhood and adolescent cancer: A study of 23 cases. J Clin Oncol 17:2789-2795, 1999.

This is an excellent review of patients with a previous cancer who developed osteosarcoma as a second tumor in a radiation portal.

PART IV

Airway, Lung, and Thoracic Cavity

31

Disorders of the Upper Airway

Obstruction of the upper airway is an acute emergency, requiring immediate and accurate diagnosis and treatment. Cyanosis caused by obstruction of the respiratory tract must be differentiated from disorders of the cardiovascular system, gastrointestinal system, and central nervous system (CNS) (Table 31-1). Cardiovascular and CNS disorders can be excluded if the cyanotic infant makes a rigorous effort to breathe. Lesions such as subdural hematoma from birth injury or cerebral agenesis may result in decreased respiratory drive and apnea because of an abnormality of the respiratory center. In these cases, infants are flaccid and unresponsive, and reflexes are severely impaired or absent. Cardiac malformations cause cyanosis because of right-to-left shunts or cardiac

TABLE 31-1 ■ Conditions Causing Cyanosis or Respiratory Distress

Congenital heart disease
Gastrointestinal disorders
    Tracheoesophageal fistula
    Gastroesophageal fistula
CNS disorders causing apnea
    Maternal anesthesia
    Birth trauma
    CNS malformations
Airway malformations and obstructions
    Choanal atresia
    Pierre Robin syndrome (micrognathia)
    Nasopharyngeal mass (teratoma, encephalocele)
    Hypertrophy of tonsils, adenoids
    Craniofacial anomalies
    Subglottic stenosis
    Laryngomalacia, tracheomalacia, bronchomalacia
    Vocal cord paralysis
    Laryngeal neoplasms (hemangiomas, lymphangiomas)
    Laryngeal webs, atresia
    Laryngeal papillomatosis
    Croup, epiglottitis
    Laryngeal clefts
    Laryngeal cysts and laryngocele
    Tracheal stenosis, webs
    Tracheoesophageal fistula
    Vascular rings
    Mediastinal masses

decompensation, but respiratory distress is uncommon. Only with respiratory obstruction does the cyanotic infant make strenuous respiratory effort with labored respirations. Agitation, wheezing, stridor, dyspnea, and a respiratory rate greater than 70 breaths/min are common symptoms.

Upper airway obstruction in newborns must be distinguished from other conditions that cause respiratory distress, such as spontaneous pneumothorax, posterolateral or other diaphragmatic hernias, hyaline membrane disease, idiopathic lobar emphysema, and agenesis of a lung. Newborns experiencing respiratory obstruction should have immediate suctioning and have the tongue pulled forward; this ensures a patent airway above the larynx. If the obstruction persists, a laryngoscope should be used to view the base of the tongue and epiglottis to visualize the larynx. If the larynx is patent, an endotracheal tube is placed carefully between the vocal cords into the midtrachea.

If respiratory distress continues after suctioning, the problem usually is related to the lungs or pleural activities, and a chest radiograph is obtained. Appropriate treatment can be provided based on the radiographic findings. When the obstruction is less severe and time permits a planned approach, the infant is monitored carefully. Malformations such as choanal atresia, micrognathia (Pierre Robin syndrome), cleft lip and palate, or a mass in the neck that may compress the airway are identified. A gloved index finger may be used to palpate for a mass at the base of the tongue or in the nasopharynx. If placing the infant prone or pulling the tongue forward relieves the obstruction, small catheters may be placed through each of the nares to evaluate the patency of the posterior choanae. Lateral soft tissue radiographs of the head and neck and standard chest radiographs help identify abnormalities of the chest, abdomen, and nasopharynx. Lesions in the nasopharynx, base of the tongue, and larynx often can be identified, and compression of the trachea may be observed. Passage of a small radiopaque catheter through the mouth into the stomach documents the patency of the esophagus and rules out esophageal atresia. If more than 20 mL of fluid is present in the stomach in the neonate or if the gastric aspirate contains bile, intestinal obstruction must be suspected. A contrast barium swallow may show esophageal stenosis, tracheoesophageal fistula, vascular rings compressing the trachea or esophagus, or swallowing dysfunction and aspiration owing to neurologic lesions that affect cranial nerves IX and X. Gastroesophageal reflux also must be considered even in small infants because it may be the cause of symptoms such as coughing, choking, aspiration pneumonia, apneic episodes, and respiratory arrest.

CLINICAL FEATURES

The most frequent sign of laryngeal and tracheal obstruction is stridor caused by abnormal patterns of airflow. Stridor may or may not be associated with labored breathing, increased respiratory rate, sternal and intercostal retractions, and cyanosis. The quality and type of stridor give some indication of the location of the airway abnormality. High-pitched inspiratory stridor usually indicates an abnormality in the subglottic or glottic area. Biphasic stridor with a high pitch on inspiration coupled with a low-pitched, prolonged expiratory phase usually indicates an obstruction below the larynx. Pure expiratory wheezing generally indicates bronchial involvement. Problems involving the glottis or the vocal cords primarily are usually associated with hoarseness, a weak or feeble cry, or aphonia.

CHOANAL ATRESIA

Bilateral choanal atresia may cause serious upper airway obstruction in neonates (Fig. 31-1). Neonates are obligatory nasal breathers, and suffocation occurs if an oral airway is not maintained. Within 5 to 6 weeks, the infant may learn to breathe without an oral device in place. The diagnosis of choanal atresia may be confirmed by contrast nasopharyngography but usually is made by unsuccessful attempts at passage of a suction catheter through both sides of the nares into the pharynx. Unilateral choanal atresia often is tolerated by a neonate, but bilateral obstruction causes immediate distress. Definitive treatment usually requires resection of bone to allow passage of nasopharyngeal tubes used to stent the opening, while the choanae epithelialize around the airway.

PIERRE ROBIN SYNDROME

Micrognathia, occasionally associated with cleft palate and relative glossoptosis, is a cause of marked respiratory distress in neonates (Fig. 31-2). When infants are in the supine position, the tongue can occlude the posterior pharynx resulting in acute respiratory distress. Placing the infant prone alleviates the obstruction in most cases. For infants with repeated severe episodes of airway obstruction, a nasopharyngeal tube prevents the posterior tongue from being drawn downward into the pharynx. Occasionally, tracheostomy is required and sometimes gastrostomy. The mandible grows relatively faster than does the child, allowing the oral cavity to accommodate the tongue without causing obstruction, usually by the age of 3 months. Reconstructive surgical procedures on the mandible are rarely necessary. Attempts to hold the tongue forward with sutures placed through the tip are rarely required.

SUBGLOTTIC STENOSIS

Stenosis of the airway at the level of the cricoid ring may be either congenital or acquired. Congenital subglottic stenosis is rare and consists of a soft tissue thickening of the subglottic area, occasionally involving the true vocal cords. Inspiratory and expiratory stridor are common. Minimal laryngeal inflammation precipitates airway obstruction because the cricoid is a fixed, complete ring. Most infants with congenital subglottic stenosis improve as laryngeal growth occurs; a less vigorous approach is required in the congenital cases than in the acquired form. Acquired subglottic stenosis is usually the result of prolonged endotracheal intubation. Although the exact duration of endotracheal intubation is not related clearly to subglottic stenosis, infection and trauma secondary to movement of the tube are causative factors. The incidence

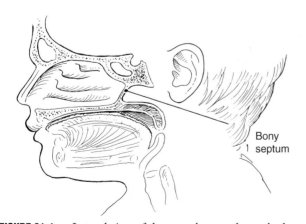

FIGURE 31-1 ■ Lateral view of the nasopharynx shows the bony septum obstructing the posterior region, characteristic of choanal atresia.

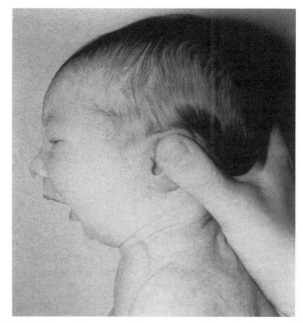

FIGURE 31-2 ■ Neonate with micrognathia and characteristic appearance of Pierre Robin syndrome.

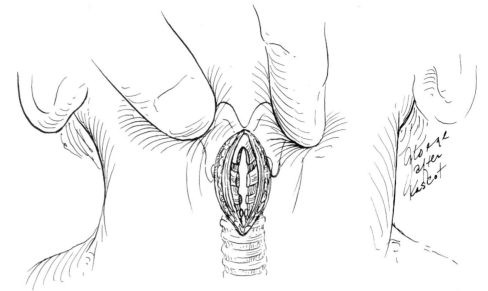

FIGURE 31-3 ■ Anterior cricoid split incision through the lower two thirds of the thyroid cartilage, the cricoid cartilage, and the first two tracheal rings. This incision with an endotracheal tube stent shows improvement in most infants with fibrous subglottic stenosis.

of subglottic stenosis occurring in neonates who require endotracheal intubation in the current era is approximately 2% to 3%.

In normal infants, the glottis is the most narrow part of the airway, and the subglottic region is usually large. Degrees of subglottic stenosis are common, and in many children, some recognizable narrowing in this area can be seen endoscopically. Severe airway obstruction may necessitate tracheostomy followed by subsequent laryngotracheoplasty when appropriate. In mild cases of fibrous stenosis (grade 1 and 2), an anterior cricoid split using an indwelling endotracheal tube as a stent for approximately 2 weeks may be effective therapy (Fig. 31-3). Anterior laryngotracheoplasty with cartilage grafting may be necessary after failure to achieve decannulation following either a cricoid split or a tracheostomy in infants with grade 2 and selected grade 3 subglottic stenosis. Cricotracheal (segmental) resection and anastomosis may be preferable in instances of more severe (grade 3 and 4) subglottic stenosis.

LARYNGEAL WEBS AND ATRESIA

Laryngeal webs and atresia are rare anomalies that may be located at a supraglottic or subglottic level. Symptoms often noted at birth are airway obstruction and weak cry. Most webs are located at the glottic level, and diagnosis can be made easily with a laryngoscope or bronchoscope. Thick webs require tracheostomy and subsequent reconstruction, whereas thin webs usually can be lysed endoscopically with electrocautery or a carbon dioxide laser, which can vaporize a web with minimal thermal damage to surrounding tissues. The latter is difficult to use safely in small infants without a tracheostomy because airway control techniques may interfere with surgical exposure. Complete atresia of the larynx is usually incompatible with life, unless there is an associated tracheoesophageal fistula large enough to sustain ventilation. Bui and colleagues described a fetus with hyperechogenic lungs, depressed diaphragm, and tracheal dilation recognized

on prenatal ultrasound consistent with the diagnosis of laryngeal atresia. The infant was delivered by cesarean section with a planned EXIT (ex utero intrapartum treatment) procedure at the same time and underwent emergency tracheostomy and survived. Definitive correction was planned at age 2 years. The EXIT procedure is described later.

CROUP (ACUTE LARYNGOTRACHEOBRONCHITIS)

Infectious croup is a viral illness caused primarily by type A or B parainfluenza viruses. It has a seasonal occurrence in the late autumn and winter and is more common than acute epiglottitis. Respiratory syncytial virus, adenovirus, coxsackievirus A, echoviruses, and measles all contribute to the spectrum of this condition. Croup is observed most commonly between ages 3 months and 3 years. The primary lesion is subglottic edema with a variable amount of tracheobronchial inflammation. A barking cough, hoarse inspiratory and expiratory stridor, and substernal retractions are typical. Radiographs of the neck can confirm the clinical impression of subglottic narrowing and can assist in ruling out other causes of airway obstruction, such as foreign bodies or lesions that might cause extrinsic compression or displacement of the airway. The white blood cell count usually is elevated with a relative lymphocytosis. Treatment includes humidification, and dramatic relief of the stridor and airway obstruction can be obtained with nebulized racemic epinephrine (2.25% solution of epinephrine hydrochloride) with intermittent positive-pressure breathing. Although this treatment may alleviate the acute condition, rebound swelling may occur within a few hours, requiring additional treatment. Dexamethasone administration occasionally may induce rapid improvement. Occasionally, endotracheal intubation is needed for 1 or 2 days, in which case, one must be prepared to do tracheostomy, although it is rarely necessary. For patients who fail to respond within 48 hours, antibiotic therapy should be instituted.

SUPRAGLOTTITIS (EPIGLOTTITIS)

Supraglottitis (formerly called *epiglottitis*) is inflammation of the supraglottic larynx that may affect the epiglottis, aryepiglottic folds, arytenoids, and ventricular bands. The condition is most common between ages 2 and 6 years. The causative organism is almost always *Haemophilus influenzae* type 13, although staphylococci and group A β-hemolytic streptococci occasionally may be present. An upper respiratory infection precedes the onset of symptoms in more than 50% of patients. The condition progresses rapidly to respiratory collapse with most children becoming toxic with an elevated temperature, tachycardia, and tachypnea. Prolonged inspiratory stridor is characteristic and is worse in the supine position. The child sits erect, is exhausted, and is hungry for air with the chin thrust forward and the tongue protruding. A symptomatic child may experience sudden airway occlusion with aspiration of secretions and cardiac arrest. A moderate leukocytosis with a shift to the left on differential smear commonly is observed. No attempt should be made to visualize the larynx or the back of the throat outside the operating room. Endotracheal intubation with the child under light general anesthesia provides the safest course of management. Tracheostomy is rarely indicated. The inflammatory process generally responds rapidly to intravenous antibiotics (cefotaxime, 100–200 mg/kg/24 hours every 8 hours in three divided doses, or ceftriaxone 75 mg/kg/day every 12 hours in two divided doses in life-threatening situations). Of *H. influenzae* cases, 15% are resistant to ampicillin. Intubation seldom is required beyond 3 days. Although tracheostomy was standard treatment for acute supraglottitis in previous years, short-term endotracheal intubation with intubation and extubation performed in the operating room is associated with a low morbidity and few complications.

LARYNGOMALACIA AND TRACHEOMALACIA

Laryngomalacia is one of the most common congenital anomalies affecting the infant larynx. Inspiratory stridor occurs when infants are active or agitated and improves when they are placed in a prone position with the neck extended. Symptoms are caused by inspiratory collapse of the supraglottic structures of the larynx. Although radiographs of the neck are helpful in ruling out other causes of stridor, the definitive diagnosis is made by direct inspection of the larynx. Direct laryngoscopy shows an elongated epiglottis bowed convexly, so-called omega-shaped epiglottis, because the arytenoids collapse medially. The aryepiglottic folds are redundant and prolapse into the glottis on inspiration. Airway obstruction usually is relieved by elevating the epiglottis with a laryngoscope. With typical laryngomalacia, the cords, subglottic larynx, and tracheobronchial tree are all normal.

No special cause for this condition has been identified other than delayed development of the structural rigidity of the supraglottic larynx. Usually no therapy is required, and the symptoms disappear by 2 years of age as the larynx grows. Laser excision of some of the floppy tissue may be curative. Rarely a tracheostomy may be needed in infants who do not improve or who experience profound carbon dioxide retention during sleep.

Tracheomalacia is due to a deficiency of the supporting cartilages of the trachea, which also may involve the main stem bronchi. The condition is believed to arise from external compression of the tracheal cartilages during development. The most common anomalies causing external compression are esophageal atresia, when the proximal esophageal pouch compresses the trachea posteriorly, and vascular ring malformations, in which the aorta or pulmonary artery compress the trachea. Symptoms are caused by collapse of the trachea during the positive-pressure phase of expiration. Symptoms depend on the severity of tracheal collapse. Infants with esophageal atresia may have a coarse barking cough. With more severe degrees of tracheal collapse, infants may develop respiratory distress and cyanosis when agitated or with forced expiration.

Lateral chest radiographs or fluoroscopy show tracheal collapse well when tracheomalacia is extensive. Bronchoscopy is the definitive study. Some clinicians favor dynamic contrast bronchography as a diagnostic procedure. For localized lesions caused by vascular rings, an angiogram or magnetic resonance angiogram may be necessary. Endoscopically the trachea is flattened in its anteroposterior diameter, and the site of collapse has a characteristic fish-mouth appearance. The primary treatment of tracheomalacia is surgical correction of the extrinsic compression, such as a vascular ring, followed by supportive management until rigidity of the cartilage is established. For milder forms, observation is in order. Growth of the trachea usually relieves symptoms by age 2 years. Anterior suspension of the aorta or innominate artery to the posterior aspect of the sternum with traction sutures has provided excellent relief for more symptomatic patients. Anterior aortopexy and occasionally tracheopexy are accomplished easily through an anterior third intercostal space incision. Adequate tracheal patency can be ascertained by intraoperative tracheobronchoscopy. Internal stenting with an expandable metallic tracheobronchial stent (Palmaz) may avoid tracheostomy in some cases. Placement of the stent requires bronchoscopic guidance. Occasionally, obstructing granulation tissue may grow over the stent requiring resection. These stents also are extremely difficult to remove. In rare instances, airway obstruction is related to isolated primary bronchomalacia. This condition can be identified by computed tomography or bronchoscopy that shows narrowing of a main stem bronchus (usually on the left side). Thoracotomy and bronchoplasty also have been effective.

VOCAL CORD PARALYSIS

Congenital paralysis of one or both vocal cords accounts for approximately 10% of congenital laryngeal anomalies. Acquired unilateral paralysis is common and occurs with moderate frequency after ligation of a patent ductus arteriosus in premature infants. Increased intracranial pressure as a result of myelomeningocele, encephalocele,

Arnold-Chiari malformations, or intracranial hemorrhage has been associated with vocal cord paralysis. Birth trauma with stretching of the neck and the recurrent laryngeal nerve may be a causative factor in some patients. In most infants, however, a cause cannot be identified. Unilateral paralysis is more frequent than bilateral paralysis and often is missed because of minimal symptoms. Laryngoscopy or flexible endoscopy with the child awake or with light anesthesia allows for observation of maximal vocal effort. Unilateral palsy usually requires no specific therapy, whereas bilateral palsy often requires tracheostomy. The paralysis is often temporary, lasting 4 to 6 weeks; however, if there is no recovery, arytenoidectomy and lateral fixation of the cord may be required.

LARYNGEAL HEMANGIOMAS

Laryngeal hemangiomas usually occur immediately below the glottis and may produce airway obstruction. With crying or straining, engorgement of the lesion may cause respiratory obstruction. Inspiratory stridor is the initial symptom, although the infant periodically may be completely free of symptoms. Most symptoms are apparent before age 3 months. Approximately 50% of patients have associated cutaneous hemangiomas. Direct endoscopic examination is required to confirm the diagnosis, although a biopsy is unnecessary and may produce severe hemorrhage. The lesion may be difficult to identify with the patient asleep in the supine position. Lowering the head of the operating room table during the examination causes engorgement and usually permits identification of the lesion.

Subglottic hemangiomas commonly involute spontaneously by 18 months of age and may not require specific therapy. For symptomatic lesions, systemic or intralesional corticosteroids may hasten involution. Tracheostomy occasionally is necessary to relieve acute airway obstruction. Resection of resistant hemangiomas with carbon dioxide laser vaporization or cryotherapy has been moderately successful. Open excision via a laryngofissure is also effective. Interferon alfa-2 has been used in cases with residual tumor in an effort to control growth and reduce the need for tracheostomy.

RECURRENT RESPIRATORY PAPILLOMATOSIS

Recurrent respiratory papillomatosis is a benign neoplastic disorder caused by human papillomavirus. Although the larynx most commonly is involved, the tracheobronchial tree also may be affected. The condition may cause stridor, hoarseness, wheezing, and upper airway obstruction at any age, but it is most common in children 18 months old to 5 years old. Approximately 60% of affected patients have mothers with condyloma acuminatum at parturition. Although occasional lesions regress spontaneously, most patients require surgical intervention using carbon dioxide or potassium titanyl phosphate (KTP) laser or cryosurgical freezing techniques to ablate the papillomas. There is a tendency for recurrence of the lesions. Treatment with autogenous vaccines, intralesional citofovir, subcutaneous interferon therapy, and more recently oral ribavirin and indole-3-carbinol currently is under evaluation.

LARYNGEAL AND LARYNGOTRACHEAL CLEFTS

Incomplete midline separation of the developing trachea and esophagus results in a common channel of variable length, usually beginning at the larynx and often extending inside the thorax. The anomaly is seen in some families and is reported with the G syndrome. Clefts are more common in boys than girls. Esophageal atresia with tracheoesophageal fistula coexists in 20% to 30% of cases. Cardiac, urinary tract, and gastrointestinal anomalies also commonly are observed. There are four types of clefts: (1) laryngeal (involving all or part of the cricoid plate), (2) extending to the cervical trachea, (3) involving the entire trachea to the level of the carina, and (4) extending beyond the carina to involve one or both main stem bronchi. Patients often present with respiratory distress associated with feeding. A hoarse cry, cyanosis, choking, and aspiration pneumonia may be observed. Endoscopic examination is the definitive method of diagnosis; however, the defect may be difficult to identify on routine bronchoscopic examination and is shown best with an endotracheal tube in the airway while observing from the esophageal side. Gastroesophageal reflux is a common occurrence and may lead to fatal aspiration pneumonitis. Tracheal intubation and early gastrostomy permit better control of the patient and should be carried out before attempting repair of the cleft. Type 1 minor clefts can be repaired by endolaryngeal microsurgical techniques; however, repair of longer clefts (type 2) is more complex and requires exposure through a lateral pharyngotomy incision with subsequent interposition of a strap muscle between the suture lines in the esophagus and trachea. The lateral neck approach allows for good exposure and construction of asymmetric suture lines to reduce the risk of leak and recurrent fistula. There is a risk of injury to the recurrent laryngeal nerve, so some surgeons prefer the anterior approach for exposure of the larynx and upper trachea. More extensive clefts (types 3 and 4) require a combined right cervical and right thoracic approach to achieve repair followed by a tracheostomy. These defects are associated with significant morbidity and mortality often exceeding 15% to 20%.

LARYNGEAL CYST AND LARYNGOCELE

A laryngocele arises as a dilation of the saccule of the laryngeal ventricle and occasionally appears in response to a sudden increase in intralaryngeal pressure. The laryngocele may be external or internal and air or liquid filled. Stridor and severe airway obstruction are noted commonly in the neonatal period. Laryngoscopy usually shows a large liquid-filled cyst involving the laryngeal ventricle and the supraglottic structures. Emergency management involves placement of an endotracheal tube and needle aspiration of the cyst. Because the cyst refills, it is important to unroof the lesion with a Bugbee electrode or a laser.

TRACHEAL STENOSIS

As with subglottic stenosis, the most common cause of tracheal stenosis in infants and children is endotracheal intubation (see Subglottic Stenosis). Although infants are affected more by subglottic stenosis, in older children and adolescents, the site of trauma to the tracheal mucosa and cartilage more often occurs below the cricoid ring at the level of an endotracheal tube balloon cuff. The incidence of postintubation subglottic stenosis in infants requiring ventilatory support was 7.5% in the 1990s; however, in more recent years, the incidence has been reduced to approximately 2% to 3%. Premature and newborn infants tolerate long-term intubation better than older children. Endoscopy provides the most helpful method of assessment to evaluate patients for the presence of subglottic and tracheal stenosis.

Dilation of the stenotic site combined with systemic steroid and intraluminal stenting has been effective in milder cases of stricture. For resistant stricture, carbon dioxide laser, electrosurgical resection with a loop or Bugbee electrode, or freezing with a miniaturized cryoprobe has been used successfully to alleviate the obstruction. Endoscopic scar resection should be applied in two or more separate stages and, when supplemented by a soft Silastic stent, is usually successful in approximately 80% of patients. More recently, the use of topical mitomycin as an adjunct has allowed for better endoscopic control of moderate subglottic scars.

For more complex stenoses, laryngotracheoplasty with submucosal resection of fibrous scar supplemented with a split-thickness skin graft over a stent has been used successfully in some patients. For severe defects, vertical incision through the stricture followed by augmentation of the luminal circumference with a free costal cartilage graft (anterior or posterior laryngotracheoplasty) has produced satisfactory results.

Tracheal stenosis below the cricoid ring often may require tracheal resection and end-to-end anastomosis. The slide tracheoplasty technique and an anterior wall pericardial patch or costal cartilage graft are alternative techniques used to repair long-segment tracheal stenosis.

VASCULAR COMPRESSION ANOMALIES

Congenital anomalies of the great vessels arising from the aorta and pulmonary artery may cause compression of the esophagus and trachea, resulting in dysphagia or airway obstruction with stridor. The anatomy and treatment of these anomalies are discussed in Chapter 87. The double aortic arch forms a tight complete ring about the trachea producing compression. All of the other vascular ring anomalies are incomplete and less likely to cause severe symptoms. The most common and yet least symptomatic vascular malformation is the aberrant right subclavian artery that arises from the descending left-sided thoracic aorta and crosses behind the esophagus to the right arm. The vessel usually produces only minimal obstruction of the esophagus with little or no airway obstruction. These patients more often complain of dysphagia.

Double aortic arch results from failure of normal resorption and remodeling of the primitive dorsal fourth right arch. The persistent right-sided aortic arch is usually the dominant of the two and crosses behind the esophagus to descend on the left side of the chest. The diagnosis is made by contrast barium swallow that shows a marked posterior indentation of the esophagus in the lateral view. In comparison, aberrant subclavian arteries produce oblique posterior esophageal indentation. At times, either conventional or magnetic resonance angiography may be needed to confirm the exact nature of the vascular anatomy. Treatment of double aortic arch consists of division of the minor arch with modest mobilization of the vessels away from the trachea and esophagus. A left-sided thoracotomy provides the best exposure and access.

Incomplete but constricting vascular rings can be caused by a persistent right-sided aortic arch in conjunction with a left descending aorta. The aorta crosses behind the esophagus, forming the right and the posterior aspects of the vascular ring; the ligamentum arteriosum or ductus arteriosus forms the left side, and the pulmonary artery forms the anterior portion of the ring. This ring is less tight and may enlarge with the patient's growth. If the right-sided arch persists with a right descending aorta, a left aberrant subclavian vessel crosses the mediastinum behind the esophagus. Compression of the airway occurs because of a patent ductus arteriosus or ligamentum arteriosus on the left side. Both of these malformations are less common and less severe than the double aortic arch. Division of the ligamentum or patent ductus arteriosus is the only treatment necessary for these incomplete vascular rings. Innominate artery compression of the trachea can produce a high degree of airway obstruction with stridor. There is no esophageal compression, and the barium swallow is normal. Bronchoscopy reveals anterior compression of the distal trachea, however, which appears pulsatile in nature and usually has flattened cartilage rings. Treatment consists of left-sided thoracotomy with suture of the innominate artery to the underside of the sternum. The pericardial reflection at the innominate artery provides the most secure tissue to place the suspension sutures.

The least common of the vascular ring anomalies, and perhaps the most severe, is pulmonary artery sling. This anomaly results when the left pulmonary artery does not branch immediately from the main pulmonary artery but arises as a branch from the right pulmonary artery passing between the trachea and esophagus to reach the left lung. Distortion of the distal trachea and bronchi are impressive. In addition, small complete cartilaginous rings surround the narrow trachea, extending occasionally throughout its entire length. The reconstruction is more complex. The left pulmonary artery is divided from the right with reanastomosis to the main pulmonary artery. The mortality is high with this condition, in part related to the presence of malformed tracheal cartilages and a high risk of persistent postoperative tracheomalacia.

EXIT (EX UTERO INTRAPARTUM TREATMENT) PROCEDURE

Fetal upper airway obstruction may be noted on prenatal ultrasound and may include large neck masses (e.g., teratomas, hemangiomas, cystic hygromas) causing intrauterine tracheal compression or distortion. These cases are referred to as instances of *CHAOS* (congenital high-airway obstruction syndrome). In these highly selected cases, a planned procedure (EXIT procedure) is done at the time of cesarean section (not before 36 weeks' gestation if possible) that ensures a successful transition to the postnatal environment. After the fetal head and shoulders are delivered from the uterus, laryngoscopy is performed, and endotracheal intubation is attempted. In approximately 15% of cases, this is not possible, and a tracheostomy is required. When the airway is controlled and the infant is stabilized, the cord is clamped, and resection of the offending lesion can be performed.

LARYNGOSCOPY AND BRONCHOSCOPY

Before the early 1970s, pediatric endoscopy was limited by the size of the available instruments. Before that time, the open-tube bronchoscope and esophagoscope provided a field of view that was too small with the light too dim to provide optimal conditions for orientation, diagnosis, or management. As a result, many indicated bronchoscopic and esophagoscopic procedures in infants and children were not carried out. In addition, because only the individual who performed the procedure had the opportunity to view the less than adequate field, the teaching of this art was limited.

The development of the Hopkins rod-lens optical system for telescopes and the establishment of fiberoptic principles in the early 1970s opened up a new era of pediatric endoscopy. The Hopkins rod-lens optical system made the development of miniature rigid endoscopes that provided clear, magnified, wide-angle images possible. The availability of fiberoptic light sources resulted in brilliant, dependable illumination for these miniature endoscopes. Now flexible equipment is available with television monitoring, which facilitates teaching.

PRINCIPLES OF PEDIATRIC ENDOSCOPY

The Hopkins rod-lens optical system provides a much larger viewing angle with significantly more light transmission and better resolution than old systems. This optical system has been adapted to fit into the relatively tiny airways of newborns with rigid and flexible scopes.

LARYNGOSCOPY

In infants and children, the most common indication for laryngoscopy is stridor. Less common indications are the presence of an abnormal cry, weak voice, and hoarseness. Laryngoscopy always is performed with the infant under general anesthesia in a fully equipped operating room with a range of pediatric endotracheal tubes available. Rigid pediatric laryngoscopes generally are used and are available in different sizes (8.5, 9.3, and 11.0 cm). The fiberoptic light source uses flexible cables. The infant anterior commissure laryngoscope is most useful for viewing the anterior commissure and larynx,

which are difficult to visualize in infants using a standard laryngoscope.

The infant larynx differs in appearance and structure from its adult counterpart. It is located higher at birth at the level of the fourth cervical vertebrae and descends to C5 by age 6 years and C6 or C7 by adolescence. The infant larynx is smaller in size and proportion to the rest of the body than the adult larynx. It is also softer than the adult larynx and tends to be located just under the base of the tongue. The diameter of the infant larynx is smaller in the subglottic region than at the glottic opening.

Laryngoscopy initially is performed without a telescope, and the various anatomic areas are visualized directly, including the base of the tongue, valleculae, piriform fossae, epiglottis, arytenoids, false cords, ventricles, vocal cords including the anterior and posterior commissures, subglottic region, and upper trachea. A good light source is essential. Then the telescope is introduced, and these structures are examined in more detail.

The lesions typically seen in infants and children during laryngoscopy are laryngomalacia, subglottic hemangioma, laryngeal papillomatosis, congenital glottic web, foreign body, and laryngeal cyst. The most common complication of laryngoscopy is postprocedure laryngeal edema, which can be managed safely with humidification and occasionally racemic epinephrine and steroids.

BRONCHOSCOPY

The area in which the miniature pediatric endoscope has had the greatest impact is bronchoscopy in neonates and small infants. In general, rigid bronchoscopes are preferred by most pediatric surgeons because visualization and the field of view are better; the infant can be ventilated continuously through a separate channel; and a third channel is available for insertion of a biopsy or foreign body–grasping forceps, a coagulating electrode, dilating balloon, or a long needle for tissue injection under direct vision. Miniature flexible bronchoscopes also are available, however. Occasionally, flexible bronchoscopes are useful in an intubated patient by passing a small flexible bronchoscope (2.5 mm) through the endotracheal tube without the need for general anesthesia. Small 2.5-mm flexible nasopharyngoscopes also are available to evaluate the nasopharynx and posterior pharynx. A laryngeal mask airway (LMA) has been used as an alternative to endotracheal intubation for flexible fiberoptic bronchoscopy in children.

Diagnostic and Therapeutic Uses

Bronchoscopy seldom is indicated in the management of acute inflammation of the larynx and upper trachea. The diagnosis of acute conditions such as croup and acute epiglottitis can be made by clinical findings and radiography. Tracheal narrowing resulting from external compression, tracheomalacia, or intrinsic tracheal stenosis usually is associated with inspiratory stridor and significant cough. Extrinsic compression can be caused by bronchogenic cysts, esophageal duplications, vascular rings, and occasionally a pharyngeal or paratracheal abscess. Bronchoscopy often is useful in evaluating external compression, and tracheomalacia is best diagnosed this way.

At bronchoscopy, a severe narrowing of the trachea as a result of anterior collapse at the level of the aortic arch is seen. This condition commonly is observed after repair of esophageal atresia and tracheoesophageal fistula in 10% to 15% of cases.

Bronchoscopy usually is required to make a definitive diagnosis of tracheal stenosis. Bronchoscopy is extremely helpful in the diagnosis of isolated tracheoesophageal fistula and in instances of recurrent tracheoesophageal fistula after initial repair. In either case, the fistula can be identified during bronchoscopy. The fistula site can be cannulated under direct vision with a small Fogarty catheter, which aids in subsequent identification of the fistula site at the time of operation through a cervical or thoracic incision. In patients with chronic recurring infection, bronchoscopy is useful in ruling out intrinsic causes of obstruction and can aid in the performance of bronchography, which may show instances of severe bronchiectasis.

Bronchoscopy is often helpful for removal of viscid tracheobronchial secretions and in the management of atelectasis in infants after major surgical procedures when more conservative methods have failed. Many times right upper lobe collapse in infants follows a major thoracic or abdominal procedure and persists for many days despite prone positioning, endotracheal suctioning, and pulmonary physiotherapy. In these situations, bronchoscopy is often effective in re-expanding the lobe and improving oxygenation. Flexible fiberoptic bronchoscopy has become a more practical tool in children since the development of flexible bronchoscopes with an external diameter of 3.5 mm and internal channel 1.2 mm. Examination can be done with topical anesthesia and sedation. It is effective in treating atelectasis, clearing secretions, and performing bronchoalveolar lavage and may be useful in obtaining bronchial biopsy specimens, localizing foreign bodies, and performing bronchography. Flexible bronchoscopy is contraindicated in instances of airway stenosis and obstruction because ventilation is precluded.

Aspirated Foreign Bodies

One of the most important therapeutic uses of bronchoscopy in infants and children is the removal of aspirated foreign bodies. Rarely, these episodes are life-threatening. In most instances, the child is usually younger than 5 years of age (80% <3 years old) and presents with a history of sudden onset of choking or coughing. The family may describe that the child was eating peanuts or playing with a small object or toy when the symptoms began. In some instances, the family is unaware that the child choked on an object. Wheezing and rhonchi may be heard on auscultation of the chest. Breath sounds may be diminished on the side of the foreign body. Findings on the chest radiograph may range from normal to showing hyperinflation (owing to air trapping) on the side of the aspiration. The chest radiograph also may show areas of atelectasis with a shift of the mediastinum toward the side of the foreign body, or if there is a long delay in diagnosis, secondary pneumonia may be observed. Occasionally a radiopaque object can be observed on the chest radiograph. The indication to perform bronchoscopy is often a history highly suggestive of aspiration or a high index of suspicion in a child with unexplained fever, wheezing, and prolonged respiratory symptoms. Bronchoscopic extraction of an aspirated foreign body can be a difficult and demanding procedure that requires significant skill and experience to perform safely; it is best to use a rigid scope for this.

Retrieval of aspirated foreign bodies should be performed in the operating room under well-monitored general anesthesia, particularly oxygen saturation. An intravenous catheter should be inserted. A full set of rigid fiberoptic endoscopic equipment must be available along with suction. A laryngoscope is used to expose the epiglottis and vocal cords. At the time of laryngoscopy, a foreign body may be noted at or just below the cords. This object can be grasped directly with a McGill forceps. If the larynx is clear, one proceeds with bronchoscopy. The Storz rigid telescopic bronchoscope is preferred and is passed gently into the trachea. The laryngoscope is removed. Approximately 10% of foreign bodies are located in the trachea. Most are located in the bronchi, with the right bronchus being the most common location. A grasping forceps may be inserted through the working port of the bronchoscope under direct visualization in smaller infants when a 3.0-mm or 3.5-mm bronchoscope is required. For older patients who tolerate a 4.5-mm or larger bronchoscope, foreign body–grasping forceps with an attached light source and telescope can be passed through the bronchoscope tube for extraction of the foreign body under direct vision. Occasionally, extraction is facilitated by breaking up the foreign body (food particle) into fragments with subsequent piecemeal removal. In some instances, a round object may be difficult to grasp. Insertion of a Fogarty balloon catheter may facilitate its retrograde removal. After the foreign body has been removed, the bronchoscope should be reinserted to ensure all the foreign-body fragments have been removed and the tracheobronchial tree is clear. The patient should be admitted for overnight observation. Children with secondary pneumonia benefit from antibiotic administration. Rarely, inability to extract a foreign body that has migrated distally requires thoracotomy and bronchotomy.

TRACHEAL ACCESS

Three primary means exist for accessing the airway in infants and children: the laryngeal mask airway (LMA), endotracheal intubation, and tracheostomy tube placement. The LMA is a simple, less invasive, effective means for providing airway access. Formed of an inflatable miniature "mask" placed at the end of a ventilating tube, the deflated or partially inflated LMA is inserted with the mask opening facing the tongue while the device is slid along the palate into the posterior pharynx until resistance is felt in the area of the cricopharyngeus (Fig. 31-4). As the cuff is fully inflated, the tube protrudes slightly farther from the mouth if in proper position. The mask partially obstructs the esophagus and provides a seal around the larynx, which allows effective ventilation at low pressures. The presence of bilateral breath sounds and appropriate levels of carbon dioxide on capnography

TABLE 31-2 ■ Airway Access Device Size and Distance from the Lips to the Midtrachea by Age			
Age	Endotracheal Tube I.D. (mm)	Lips to Midtrachea (cm)	LMA Size
Premature	2.5	10	—
Full-term newborn	3.0	11	1
1-6 mo	3.5	11	1.5
6-12 mo	4.0	12	1.5
1-2 yr	4.5	13	2
2-10 yr	4.5-6.0	14-18	2.5-3.0
10-20 yr	6.0-8.0	18-24	4

TABLE 31-3 ■ Drugs Used for Endotracheal Intubation in Children	
Drug	Dose
Sedatives	
Etomidate	0.2-0.3 mg/kg IV
Thiopental	3-5 mg/kg IV
Ketamine	1-2 mg/kg IV
Propofol	1-2 mg/kg IV
Midazolam	0.1-0.3 mg/kg IV
Neuromuscular blocking agents	
Succinylcholine	1.5-2.0 mg/kg IV
Pancuronium/vecuronium	0.1-0.2 mg/kg IV
Other drugs	
Atropine (before succinylcholine)	0.02 mg/kg IV
Lidocaine (for head injury)	1.5 mg/kg IV
Fentanyl (for head injury)	3-5 μg/kg IV

IV, intravenously.

shows proper placement. LMA devices are available in a variety of sizes ranging from those appropriate for newborns to adults (Table 31-2). The LMA can be used for accessing the airway, especially under emergency circumstances, in patients in whom endotracheal intubation cannot be performed. Endotracheal intubation can be performed through the LMA. The LMA also can be used to access the trachea during bronchoscopy because the device provides a guide for the flexible bronchoscope down to the larynx. Although excellent for providing airway access under many circumstances, the LMA is tolerated only by patients who are fully anesthetized. Because it does not provide protection of the airway, the LMA should not be used in patients who are at risk for airway aspiration, such as acute trauma patients with uncertain history of recent oral intake or patients with bowel obstruction. Likewise, the LMA should be used only for short-term airway access. LMA use is relatively contraindicated in patients undergoing intra-abdominal procedures or laparoscopy because of the risk of aspiration and bowel insufflation during ventilation via the LMA. The LMA usually cannot provide adequate ventilation for patients with respiratory insufficiency because of the relatively high ventilatory pressures required and associated leaks.

Endotracheal Intubation

Endotracheal intubation usually is performed for one of three reasons: (1) failure of ventilation or oxygenation, (2) need for airway protection, or (3) concern for deterioration that warrants prophylactic intubation. Nasotracheal and orotracheal intubation can be performed.

Although the nasotracheal tube is better stabilized than the orotracheal tube, performance of nasotracheal intubation is more difficult and is associated with complications such as epistaxis, sinusitis, and nasal alar erosion. Another disadvantage of the nasotracheal tube is that it is longer than an orotracheal tube, making it easier to occlude with mucus and secretions. For these reasons, orotracheal intubation is used almost exclusively in infants and children.

In the setting of a moribund patient or one who is in cardiac arrest, immediate intubation without sedation may be indicated. Most other infants and children who require airway access should receive anesthesia or the combination of a sedative and a neuromuscular blocking agent to facilitate laryngoscopy (Table 31-3). Etomidate is a quick-onset (<1 minute), ultrashort-acting (<10 minutes), nonbarbiturate hypnotic agent with minimal cardiodepressant effects. The recommended dose is 0.3 mg/kg intravenously. Succinylcholine is a short-acting depolarizing neuromuscular blocking agent that allows return of spontaneous respiration within approximately 5 minutes. The short-acting nature of these drugs makes them optimal for intubation under most circumstances. Patients with increased intracranial pressure, such as after head trauma, should be well sedated during intubation with agents such as thiopental or etomidate to prevent increases in intracranial pressure during laryngoscopy. Children who are hemodynamically unstable

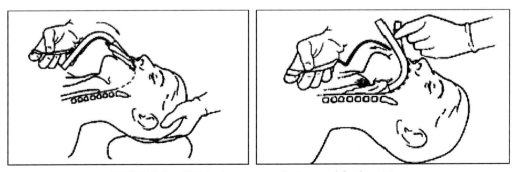

FIGURE 31-4 ■ LMA placement technique and final position.

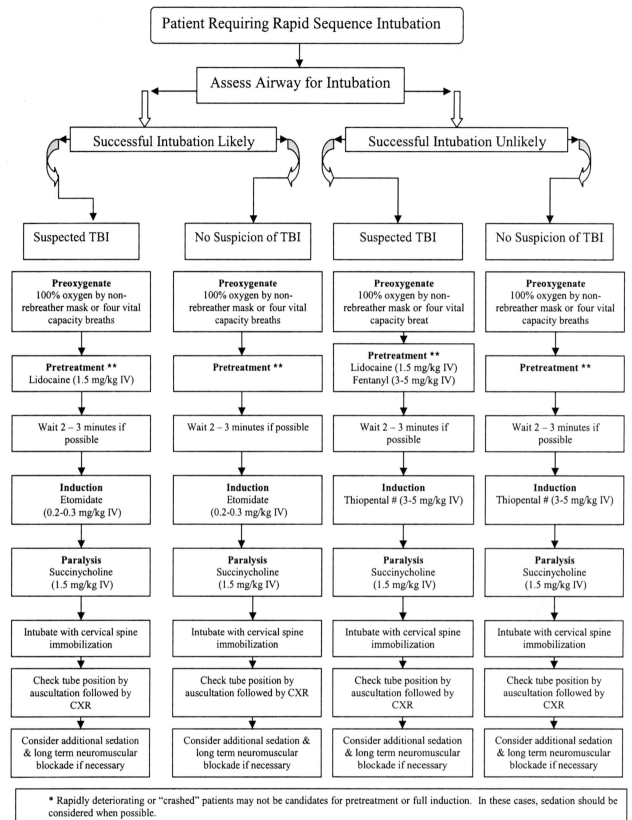

FIGURE 31-5 ■ Pathway for rapid-sequence intubation. TBI, traumatic brain injury; IV, intravenous; CXR, chest x-ray.

TABLE 31-4 ■ Indications for Use of Rapid-Sequence Induction During Intubation in Children

Uncertain status of oral intake
Trauma
Pregnancy
GI obstruction
Disorders of GI motility
Gastroesophageal reflux

GI, gastrointestinal.

can be sedated with ketamine during laryngoscopy because of its limited effect on the circulatory system. Patients with unknown oral intake status should have airway access performed by rapid-sequence intubation. This technique can be used to achieve intubation safely under most circumstances (Table 31-4 and Fig. 31-5). With rapid-sequence intubation, cricoid pressure is applied to occlude the esophagus to reduce the risk of aspiration of gastric contents. Before intubation, patients should undergo airway assessment to identify a difficult airway, such as micrognathia, retrognathia, limited mouth opening, limited spine mobility, or high Mallampati classification (Table 31-5).

Preoxygenation typically is performed via mask ventilation before endotracheal intubation. An oral airway may be used to retract the tongue in a heavily sedated patient, enhancing mask ventilation. The larynx is viewed via an end-lit laryngoscope. Typical blades on the laryngoscope include the curved MacIntosh, the straight Miller with a curve at the end, and the straight Wisconsin. The appropriate blade for a newborn or infant is size 0 or 1. The larynx is more anterior in infants and children, which may make the technical aspects of intubation in the pediatric patient more difficult. If intubation is unsuccessful after three attempts, another team member should attempt endotracheal intubation, or another means of airway access should be sought. Options when emergent airway access is required and endotracheal intubation has failed include cricothyroidotomy, which should not be performed in patients younger than 10 years old because of the risk of tracheal injury; transtracheal jet ventilation; and tracheostomy placement (see later).

Table 31-2 provides guidelines for selecting a proper tube size according to age. A rule of thumb is that uncuffed tube size = (16 + age)/4 and is approximately the size of the little fingernail. Cuffed tube size = 3 + (age/4). The proper tube size must be chosen to prevent significant

TABLE 31-5 ■ Mallampati Classification for Examination of the Oropharynx with the Mouth Wide Open*

Class I	Complete view of uvula, tonsillar pillars, soft palate
Class II	Partial view of uvula and tonsillar pillars, complete view of soft palate
Class III	View of soft palate only

*As the Mallampati class increases, the potential for difficult intubation increases.

air leak around it, especially if mechanical ventilation is used; to protect the lungs from aspirated secretions or gastric contents; and to prevent damage to the trachea and larynx. Tube fit can be tested by ensuring that there is a small air leak with sustained 15 to 20 cm H_2O airway pressure. Cuffed tubes are almost never necessary in patients younger than 8 years old because of the narrow subglottic region.

Because of the short length of the trachea in children, especially neonates and infants, it is easy to perform an inadvertent endobronchial intubation. One technique to avoid this complication is to have an assistant place the tip of the index finger in the suprasternal notch (see Fig. 31-6A). The tip of the endotracheal tube can be palpated as it passes the finger so that advancement of the tube beyond this point is prevented. Another method is to advance the tube until breath sounds become diminished on one side, typically on the left. The tube can be withdrawn 1 to 2 cm beyond the point where breath sounds return. The distance to the midtrachea from the lips can be estimated roughly at 12 + (age/2) and is approximately 11 cm in a full-term newborn, 23 cm in a man, and 21 cm in a woman. Adequate fixation of the endotracheal tube is accomplished by placing tincture of benzoin on the skin and adhesive tape to the maxillary area of the jaw to limit tube mobility.

Tracheostomy

Although occasionally performed under emergent circumstances, tracheostomy usually is performed in infants and children to provide a means of long-term ventilatory support postoperatively, in patients with primary pulmonary insufficiency, in patients with a severe upper airway malformation, or in patients with CNS malfunction. The operation is performed less frequently than previously because of increased success with prolonged orotracheal and nasotracheal intubation.

Preparation for Operation

In general, no child should undergo tracheostomy without prior endotracheal intubation; an exception would be rare patients with mechanical obstruction of the upper airway that precludes intubation or patients in whom emergent airway access via endotracheal intubation has failed. Unless in emergent situations, tracheostomy tube placement in infants and young children should never be attempted outside the operating room. Performance of tracheostomy airway access in adolescents, usually intubated, and in the intensive care unit may be an acceptable alternative. Percutaneous dilational tracheostomy tube access can be performed relatively safely in full-grown adolescents older than 15 years of age under bronchoscopic guidance.

Operative Technique

The child is placed in the supine position with the neck maximally extended over a shoulder roll (Fig. 31-6A). This position not only provides exposure of the neck, but also tenses the trachea and draws its upper portion out of the mediastinum. A transverse skin incision is made one fingerbreadth above the sternal notch. The incision is

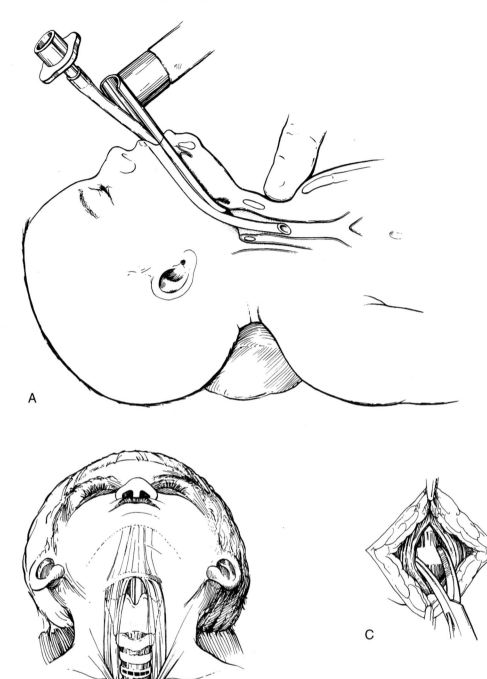

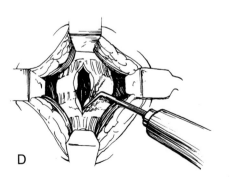

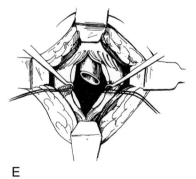

FIGURE 31-6 ■ **A-H,** Intubation and tracheostomy (see text).

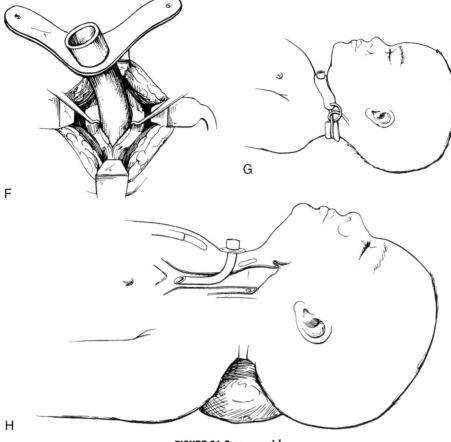

F

G

H

FIGURE 31-6 ■ cont'd.

deepened through the subcutaneous tissues with needle-point cautery. Small, self-retaining retractors are a great help in obtaining satisfactory exposure. The strap muscles are teased apart, and any blood vessels are cauterized. The thyroid isthmus usually can be retracted superiorly to expose the trachea. The second tracheal ring is identified and marked with the cautery. Before incising the trachea, the surgeon must ensure that the necessary tracheostomy tubes are at hand and that any adapters needed to make a connection to the anesthesia tubing are available. If a cuffed tube is being used, the endotracheal tube is advanced down to the carina while the tracheal incision is being made, then withdrawn under direct vision to just below the incision, where the balloon is reinflated. This avoids inadvertent puncture of the balloon and compromise of the ability to ventilate. A longitudinal incision through the second and third rings is made preferably with a knife, and hemostasis at the cut edges of the trachea is obtained. If cautery is used on the trachea, one must ensure that minimal fraction of inspired oxygen is being administered into the airway. The incision must be long enough to allow easy insertion of the tracheostomy tube. Tracheal cartilage never is excised in infants or young children; excision leads to loss of tracheal support, with subsequent stricture. Two 3-0 polypropylene (Prolene) sutures are placed through the edges of the second or third tracheal ring to aid in placing the tube during the operation and postoperatively

in case of accidental dislodgment. Under direct vision, the anesthesiologist withdraws the endotracheal tube until its tip is just proximal to the tracheostomy. This tube should not be removed until the tracheostomy tube is fixed in position and proves to be satisfactory. The tracheostomy tube is inserted into the trachea. Ventilation via the tracheostomy tube is initiated, and assessment for end-tidal carbon dioxide performed. The tube chosen should be just large enough to fit into the trachea with minimal force. Typically the tracheostomy tube size outer diameter is equivalent to that of the endotracheal tube. While the retractors are still in place, the anesthesiologist administers a sustained inflation to approximately 20 cm H_2O to determine whether the tracheostomy tube is airtight. If there is a large air leak, the tube is removed, and the next larger size is inserted (cuffed tracheostomy tubes are never used in infants unless there are high ventilator pressure requirements). If the tracheostomy site is substantially larger than the tube, the skin on either side of the tube can be approximated loosely with absorbable sutures.

Finally, while an assistant holds the tube in place, the tube is tied securely with tapes encircling the neck. No one except the surgeon is permitted to loosen these ties until the stoma is well established in 5 to 7 days, at which point the tracheostomy is changed. Both sides of the chest are auscultated, and a chest film is obtained to verify the proper position of the tip of the tube just above the carina. In small infants, the tip of the tube may extend

TABLE 31-6 ▪ Short-Term and Long-Term Complications of Tracheostomy Tube Placement
Infection: wound or pneumonia
Obstruction of tracheostomy from mucus plugs or blood
Tracheal ulceration or perforation from tracheostomy tube
Erosion of tracheostomy tube into innominate artery
Hemorrhage from trachea
Cannulation of bronchus (usually right)
Accidental decannulation
Granuloma formation at tracheostomy site
Stricture of trachea at tracheostomy site
Pneumothorax during performance of tracheostomy

accidentally into the right bronchus. This extension can be corrected by placing padding under the flange of the tube to lift it out of the neck slightly. Adjustable neck flange tracheostomy tubes that allow variation in length are available and work well in circumstances where tracheal anatomy is nonstandard. Custom tracheostomy tubes are relatively easy to obtain when the necessary size and length are determined. The length of the tracheostomy tube typically is determined by the outer diameter.

Postoperative Care

Proper nursing care of the child with a fresh tracheostomy is essential to success and initially includes suctioning every 2 hours, peristomal cleansing with 0.25% acetic acid every 4 hours, proper use of tie pads, and hydrocolloid gel (DuoDerm) around the site if excoriation occurs. Parents must be taught routine and emergent tracheostomy care and cardiopulmonary resuscitation. Home monitoring of patients with critical airways should be considered.

At the time of anticipated decannulation, the tracheostomy tube can be plugged during the day at home. Tracheostomy plugging during the day and night is appropriate while an inpatient in a monitored bed. After the tube has been removed, the stoma should be occluded to ensure that ventilation through the larynx is unobstructed. If there is any hint of stridor, an elective bronchoscopy should be performed. Occasionally a mass of granulation tissue from the stoma protrudes into the trachea, occluding it; this tissue must be removed. Complications of tracheostomies are listed in Table 31-6.

SUGGESTED READINGS

Black RE, Johnson DG, Matlak ME: Bronchoscopic removal of aspirated foreign bodies in children. J Pediatr Surg 29:682-684, 1994.

This excellent review focuses on a high index of suspicion for the presence of an aspirated foreign body as an indication for bronchoscopy.

Bouchard S, Johnson MP, Flake AW, et al: The EXIT procedure: Experience and outcome in 31 cases. J Pediatr Surg 37:418-427, 2002.

This is the largest single series of cases in which the EXIT procedure has been performed. Indications and outcomes are reviewed.

Bui TH, Grunewald C, Frenckner B, et al: Successful EXIT (ex-utero intrapartum treatment) procedure in a fetus diagnosed prenatally with congenital high-airway obstruction syndrome due to laryngeal atresia. Eur J Pediatr Surg 10:328-333, 2000.

This article describes survival of an infant with laryngeal atresia detected prenatally after tracheostomy at an EXIT procedure.

Evans KL, Courteney-Harris R, Bailey CM, et al: Management of posterior laryngeal and laryngotracheoesophageal clefts. Arch Otolaryngol Head Neck Surg 121:1380-1385, 1995.

This article reviews the clinical features, associated anomalies, management, and morbidity and mortality associated with laryngotracheal clefts.

Filler RM, Forte V: Lesions of the larynx and trachea. In O'Neill JA Jr, Rowe MI, Grosfeld JL, et al (eds): Pediatric Surgery, 5th ed. St Louis, CV Mosby, 1998, pp 863-872.

This chapter provides an extensive overview of the various disorders affecting the upper airway in infants and children.

Filler RM, Forte V, Fraga JC, et al: The use of expandable airway stents for tracheobronchial obstruction in children. J Pediatr Surg 30:1050-1056, 1995.

Experience with tracheal stents is described.

Hartley BE, Cotton RT: Pediatric airway stenosis: Laryngotracheal reconstruction or cricotracheal resection? Clin Otolaryngol 25:342-349, 2000.

This study suggests that selection of the correct procedure is related to severity of stenosis by grade.

Inwald DP, Roebuck D, Elliott MJ, Mok Q: Current management and outcome of tracheobronchial malacia and stenosis presenting to the pediatric intensive care unit. Intensive Care Med 27:722-729, 2000.

This study evaluates factors leading to mortality in children with tracheobronchomalacia. Only complex cardiac defects and syndromic conditions contributed to mortality.

Matute JA, Villafruela MA, Delgaso MD, et al: Surgery of subglottic stenosis in neonates and children. Eur J Pediatr Surg 10:286-290, 2000.

An evaluation of a large series of patients with subglottic stenosis and outcomes of therapy based on severity is presented.

Nussbaum E, Zagnoev M: Pediatric fiberoptic bronchoscopy with a laryngeal mask airway. Chest 120:614-616, 2001.

This article describes the efficacy of LMA in avoiding general endotracheal anesthesia in children requiring flexible fiberoptic bronchoscopy.

Walner DL, Loewen MS, Kimura RE: Neonatal subglottic stenosis—incidence and trends. Laryngoscope 111:48-51, 2001.

This report updates and reassesses the current incidence of subglottic stenosis in the neonatal unit.

Warren WH, Faber LP: Bronchoscopic evaluation of the lungs and tracheobronchial tree. In Shields TW, LoCicero J, Ponn RB (eds): General Thoracic Surgery, 5th ed. Philadelphia, Lippincott Williams & Wilkins, 2000, pp 259-271.

Bronchoscopic principles and general comparisons between rigid and flexible bronchoscopy are reviewed.

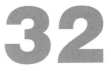

Congenital Anomalies of the Lung

Inadequate lung development may present as agenesis, aplasia, or hypoplasia of the lung or as a vascular malformation. Cystic adenomatoid malformation (CAM), congenital lobar emphysema (CLE) or overinflation, and pulmonary sequestration are the three congenital lesions of the lung that may present as abnormal cystic areas in early life. These three malformations, which share similar clinical and embryologic characteristics, frequently are difficult to diagnose; all require surgical treatment.

EMBRYOLOGY OF THE TRACHEOBRONCHIAL TREE AND LUNG

By the end of the third week of gestation, the first indication of the laryngotracheal groove can be seen in the upper end of the foregut. While the laryngotracheal groove is forming, there is a proliferation of the mesenchyme of the primitive mesentery (mediastinum) by division of cells lining the coelomic cavity. From this mesenchyme, the cartilage, muscle, and connective tissue of the lungs develop. In the 8-mm embryo, the buds of the secondary bronchi are present, and separation of the trachea and esophagus is well under way. Separation is complete by the time the embryo is 11 to 14 mm, by which time three to five orders of bronchi have been generated.

At the start, the level of the tracheal bifurcation is high in the cervical region; during the next month, it descends to the level of the first thoracic vertebra; and at birth, it is at the level of the fourth or fifth thoracic vertebra. At the same time, the lungs, which are at first dorsal to the heart, grow laterally and ventrally to surround it. All major bronchial buds are present before closure of the pleuroperitoneal canals. Until about the third month of gestation, the right lung grows faster than the left, becoming larger and having more generations of bronchial branching. This difference persists throughout life.

Cartilage appears in the trachea and primary bronchi at about 10 weeks' gestation and in the segmental bronchi at 16 weeks' gestation. Glands appear during the 11th week and reach their full extent by the 30th week.

The alveoli develop during the latter portion of gestation and the first few years of life. There is a rapid increase in the number of alveoli until 6 months of age and a slower rate of proliferation until 12 years. The mean size of alveoli in the newborn infant is 150 μm and in the adult is 280 μm. Alveolar ducts with a few alveoli are the only respiratory portions of the tree present at birth, and most of the alveoli are formed from them subsequently. The most distal bronchioles in the newborn are converted into alveolar ducts by centripetal formation of new alveoli during the first 2 months of postnatal life. Alveolization of the terminal bronchioles themselves occurs until the fourth year. The number of generations of branching of the respiratory tree does not increase, however, and may decrease with age. At birth, the infant has 24×10^6 alveoli; the adult has 296×10^6 alveoli. The number of generations of airways increases only from 21 to 23, and most of this is achieved by age 8 years.

CLINICAL FEATURES AND PATHOLOGY

The degree of lung development and the amount of encroachment on the thoracic space determine the symptoms or lack of symptoms in the neonate with a pulmonary malformation.

Pulmonary Agenesis, Aplasia, and Hypoplasia

Pulmonary agenesis refers to complete absence of one or both main stem bronchi. In the absence of bronchial development, the lung also fails to form. In aplasia of the bronchus, there is one normal bronchus and a small, blind-ending nub of the opposite bronchus and no lung on the affected side. Agenesis of bronchi and lungs has been described in eight cases. More than 200 instances of unilateral pulmonary agenesis and aplasia have been described.

Multiple anomalies are reported in more than 50% of cases. Cardiac anomalies predominate, followed by complex skeletal abnormalities (e.g., hemivertebrae and absent ribs), esophageal atresia with tracheoesophageal fistula, and genitourinary abnormalities.

The chest appears symmetric in most instances at birth. The trachea deviates to the affected side. Because of expansion of the solitary lung into the opposite thoracic space, breath sounds may be heard equally well on both sides of the chest except for the axilla on the affected side. The heart usually is shifted against the lateral chest wall on the side of the agenesis (Fig. 32-1). In the past, one third of these patients died within 5 years. The prognosis is much better now because of more effective antibiotic treatment of pulmonary infection.

Pulmonary hypoplasia is characterized by small lung size, a low ratio of lung weight to body weight, and a decreased number of bronchial generations and alveoli. The main stem bronchi and proximal bronchial branches are normal. The small lungs are believed to result from crowding in utero associated with congenital diaphragmatic hernia or eventration, diaphragmatic paralysis, anencephaly, congenital thoracic dystrophy, or oligohydramnios. Lung growth depends on secretion of lung fluid, distention of air spaces by the glottic closing mechanism, and space to expand. One or both lungs may be hypoplastic. Diaphragmatic hernia, eventration, and phrenic nerve paralysis compress the lung against a normal-sized chest wall. Phrenic nerve paralysis occurs in association with Werdnig-Hoffmann disease or phrenic nerve agenesis. Pulmonary hypoplasia also occurs with anencephaly; presumably the fetus does not develop chest wall excursions that allow the lung to expand.

Infants born with pulmonary agenesis or aplasia may have few symptoms at birth, but if the normally developed

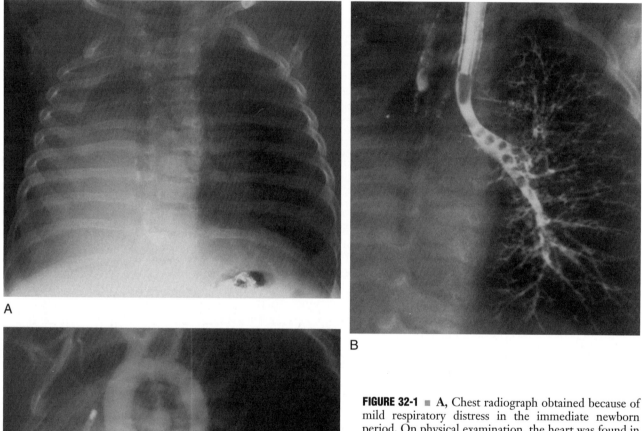

A

B

C

FIGURE 32-1 ■ **A,** Chest radiograph obtained because of mild respiratory distress in the immediate newborn period. On physical examination, the heart was found in the right chest, and no breath sounds were audible on that side. The chest radiograph revealed a shift of the mediastinum into the right chest, which was believed to be consistent with pulmonary agenesis. **B,** At 3 months of age, a bronchogram was performed, which revealed complete absence of the right bronchus. **C,** An arteriogram subsequently was obtained after the child had had multiple pulmonary infections. The arteriogram showed the heart occupying the right hemithorax and a single pulmonary artery to the left lung.

lung is impaired by atelectasis, infection, or immaturity, severe respiratory distress may be evident with or without manifestations of persistent fetal circulation. In cases of pulmonary hypoplasia, few manifestations may be evident unless the infant decompensates from an associated congenital heart defect. Infection may cause problems later in childhood because of poor pulmonary dynamics.

Anomalies of the Pulmonary Vessels and Parenchyma

A variety of anomalies of pulmonary vasculature are of significance. Anomalous systemic arteries supplying the lung are discussed under Pulmonary Sequestration. In addition, some cases of hypoplastic lung with anomalous systemic arteries have been reported. There are also reported instances of absence of the pulmonary artery to one lung. Patients with this anomaly show some reduction in the volume of the abnormal lung. The normal hilar vascular radiograph shadows are reduced. There is usually overdistention of the contralateral lung in patients who have absence of one pulmonary artery.

Congenital Pulmonary Arteriovenous Malformation

Congenital pulmonary arteriovenous malformation (AVM) is uncommon. The lesion may be small and insignificant, or there may be a large, direct communication within the lung between the pulmonary artery and vein. The connection is usually in the form of an aneurysmal sac.

The lesions may be multiple and may occur in more than one lobe or in both lungs. They may be associated with obvious telangiectases of the lung. Most reported patients with pulmonary AVM have had hereditary Osler-Weber-Rendu syndrome.

Most AVMs of the lungs suggest cavernous vascular malformations, but others resemble true arteriovenous connections. The walls of these vessels are characteristically thin, and the arterial and venous branches supplying and draining the AVM may be large and obvious on a plain radiograph.

Most patients do not have clinical symptoms with pulmonary AVM, but when the lesions are large and the shunt of unoxygenated blood into the peripheral circulation is sufficient, desaturation is evident. Cardiac enlargement may be associated with large arteriovenous connections. Dyspnea on exertion is the most common presenting symptom, but on rare occasions, brain abscesses may occur from pulmonary vascular shunting. Hemoptysis is a common occurrence and may be severe to the point of exsanguination. Fatal hemorrhage has been known to occur from rupture of peripheral AVMs on the surface of the lung.

Cystic Adenomatoid Malformation

CAMs are cystic, solid, or mixed intrapulmonary masses that communicate with the normal tracheobronchial tree and rarely have an anomalous arterial blood supply arising from the aorta rather than the pulmonary artery (Fig. 32-2). In the past, CAMs have been called *congenital lung cysts*. There are three types classified by histologic

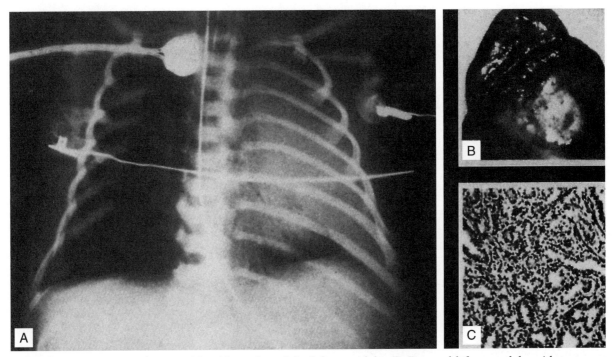

FIGURE 32-2 ■ **A,** Cystic adenomatoid malformation of the left upper lobe. **B,** Resected left upper lobe with cyst open. **C,** Cystic adenomatoid malformation type III has no normal lung tissue. Closely packed gland-like structures lined by cuboidal epithelium suggest immature lung. (H&E, × 200.) (From Wesley JR, Heidelberger KP, DiPietro MA, et al: Diagnosis and management of congenital cystic disease of the lung in children. J Pediatr Surg 21:202, 1986.)

appearance according to size, shape, and spacing of the cysts. Type I cysts have large, irregular, and widely spaced cysts with lining cells of cuboidal or low columnar epithelium and occasional foci of mucus-containing cells. Type II cysts are smaller, closer together, and more numerous. Histologically, type II cysts resemble closely packed dilated bronchioles. Type III cysts may be so small that they are not recognizable. They are closely packed, curved channels lined by cuboidal epithelium, resembling late fetal lung in appearance. Types II and III also may be found in sections of extralobar sequestrations. Cartilage is essentially lacking in all three types. Embryologically, CAMs arise from excessive proliferation of bronchial structures without alveoli.

Infants born with CAMs display early respiratory distress when lesions are large, but if lesions are small, several years may pass before the cystic areas become evident. Many infants with CAM die in utero or present at birth with hydrops and inadequate pulmonary function. Experimental studies have shown that the hydrops results from increased intrathoracic pressure from the expanding lesion, which impairs venous return to the heart producing central venous hypertension. Relief of the elevated pressures resolves the hydrops. Prenatal ultrasound has identified many CAMs. Some of these lesions diminish in size on serial examinations, some resolve completely, and some enlarge progressively.

Congenital Lobar Emphysema

Infants with CLE have overdistention of one lobe, which produces compression and atelectasis of adjacent lobes and, if severe, can shift the mediastinum (Fig. 32-3). Respiratory symptoms appear as the lobe progressively overinflates; half of patients present within the first 2 days of life. Other patients may not present with symptoms for several days or weeks depending on how long it takes for critical overexpansion to occur. Many infants present with mild-to-moderate tachypnea associated with limited degrees of emphysema. On close observation, some of these patients improve, and the lesions gradually resolve, but two thirds of this subset of patients with CLE fail to gain weight and eventually require surgical management.

In CLE, the grossly large, overdistended lobe characteristically "pops out" at the time of thoracotomy. The vascular supply is normal. A normally placed, although partially obstructed, bronchus is identified in less than 50% of patients. The lesion is one of air trapping, with histologic examination showing a normally formed acinus with greatly overexpanded alveoli. There is no tissue destruction. Embryologically the cartilage of the involved bronchus fails to develop, leading to collapse and air trapping on expiration. The polyalveolar lobe syndrome has been shown to be another cause of lobar emphysema. Infants with this condition have normal airways and arteries, but the resected lobe shows a threefold

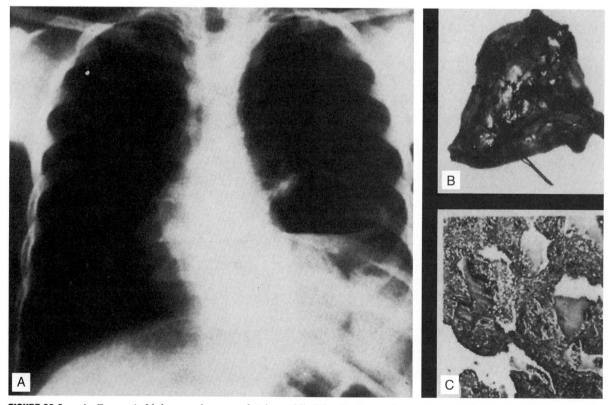

FIGURE 32-3 ■ **A,** Congenital lobar emphysema of right middle lobe. **B,** Overinflated right middle lobe herniating from the thorax at surgery. **C,** Lobar emphysema showing greatly distended alveoli and some operative hemorrhage. (H&E, × 83.) (From Wesley JR, Heidelberger KP, DiPietro MA, et al: Diagnosis and management of congenital cystic disease of the lung in children. J Pediatr Surg 21:202, 1986.)

to fivefold increase in the number of alveoli, representing a gigantic alveolar unit. If other congenital lesions are present, they usually involve the heart.

Pulmonary Sequestration

Pulmonary sequestrations are masses of abnormal lung tissue that receive an anomalous arterial blood supply and do not communicate with the tracheobronchial tree by normally related bronchi (Figs. 32-4 and 32-5). They are intralobar in 90% and extralobar in 10% of cases.

An intralobular sequestration lies within a lobe of the lung, almost always the lower lobe, invested by its visceral pleura. The arterial supply is usually systemic and either comes from the abdominal aorta and penetrates the diaphragm to supply the sequestration or is from multiple arteries from the adjacent thoracic aorta (85% to 90% of cases). Cases also have been reported with the arterial supply arising from a coronary artery. In this situation, the patient may present with secondary cardiac symptoms of ischemia. Venous drainage from an intralobar type can be pulmonary or systemic (azygos vein). Microscopically, in rare instances, the intralobar sequestration is normal lung parenchyma intersected by many large blood vessels in a random fashion. In the usual case,

there is extensive acute and chronic organizing inflammation, often so severe that little normal tissue remains. Infection is usually present. The remainder of the lobe around the sequestration is sharply demarcated and normal.

An extralobar sequestration is a spongy mass of lung tissue with its own investing pleura outside the normal lung parenchyma, which may occur at varying levels in the chest or beneath the diaphragm, but most frequently at the costophrenic sulcus in the posterior mediastinum. They are present on the left side in two thirds of affected patients. Sequestrations frequently occur in association with posterolateral diaphragmatic hernia. The parenchyma may be normal, dysplastic, or immature with areas of interstitial edema and dilated lymphatics. The immature or dysplastic areas may resemble CAM types II and III in 50% of extralobular lesions. In contrast to intralobar types, infection is rarely a problem with extralobar sequestration. Arterial supply and venous drainage have either systemic or pulmonary origins.

There is no agreement as to the embryologic origin of pulmonary sequestration. Many theories have been advanced; the most plausible is failure of the pulmonary artery to develop fast enough to supply the whole of the

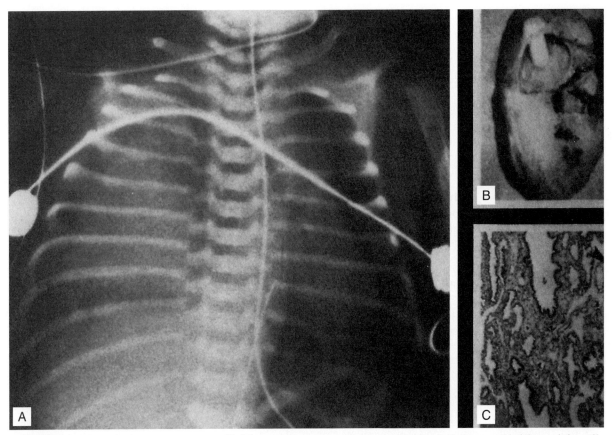

FIGURE 32-4 ▪ **A,** Intralobar sequestration of left lower lobe; infected, with air-fluid level. **B,** Resected left lower lobe; silk tie-on aberrant vascular pedicle. **C,** Intralobar sequestration with distended air spaces, fibrosed alveoli septa, and edema fluid. Acute and chronic inflammatory cells are seen in air spaces in interstitium. (H&E, × 83.) (From Wesley JR, Heidelberger KP, DiPietro MA, et al: Diagnosis and management of congenital cystic disease of the lung in children. J Pediatr Surg 21:202, 1986.)

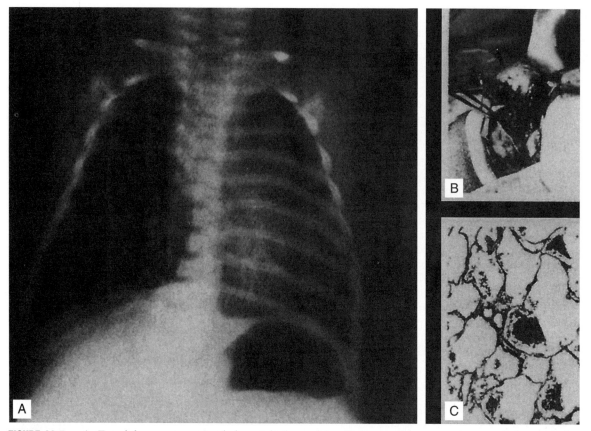

FIGURE 32-5 ■ **A,** Extralobar sequestration below right lower lobe. **B,** Resected sequestration; anomalous vascular pedicle; large cyst has been cut and propped open. **C,** Extralobar sequestration with dysplastic alveolar ducts and bronchioles. Dilated lymphatics are prominent at lower right; aberrant elastic artery. (H&E, × 83.) (From Wesley JR, Heidelberger KP, DiPietro MA, et al: Diagnosis and management of congenital cystic disease of the lung in children. J Pediatr Surg 21:202, 1986.)

growing lung, leading to formation (or persistence) of systemic arterial supply from the aorta. The distribution of arterial supply within these lesions is dysplastic so that these vessels undergo cystic or fibrous degeneration after birth. Whether they become intralobar or extralobar depends on their distance from the normal lung.

Infants born with sequestration are generally not symptomatic at birth because these abnormalities are small in relation to the normal lung. Extralobar sequestration may be discovered incidentally at the time of repair of a congenital diaphragmatic hernia, but otherwise may take several years to become clinically manifest. Intralobar sequestration is characterized by recurrent bouts of pneumonia occurring in the same location, usually a lower lobe, after 2 years of age. The systemic arterial supply to the segment can result, however, in high-output cardiac failure from shunting through the sequestration.

DIAGNOSIS

Plain film radiography is the first imaging study performed and remains the cornerstone for diagnosis and follow-up. The selective use of additional imaging studies may help to arrive at an accurate differential diagnosis and to plan a surgical approach. Computed tomography (CT) can separate cystic from solid components in a radiopaque lung mass. Intravenous contrast administration enhances a cyst wall or solid parenchyma and differentiates it from fluid (Fig. 32-6).

Pulmonary Agenesis, Aplasia, and Hypoplasia

Chest radiographs show opacification of the side of deficient development that represents the heart and great vessels. The solitary lung fills the contralateral chest and extends across the midline to a varying extent but does not appear hypolucent or emphysematous (see Fig. 32-1). Bronchoscopy, bronchography, echocardiography, CT, and pulmonary angiography confirm that there is only one bronchus and one pulmonary artery, although CT alone is probably adequate to make the diagnosis.

Anomalies of the Pulmonary Vessels

Angiography is the most accurate imaging study available for precise definition of anatomic detail of abnormal or absent pulmonary vessels. Although angiography is the most definitive imaging procedure, plain radiography may suggest the presence of an AVM or the absence of a pulmonary artery, showing an appearance of increased or diminished vascular markings. At times, CT with

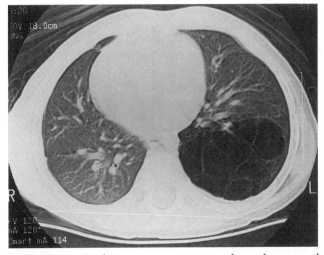

FIGURE 32-6 ■ Axial, intravenous contrast–enhanced computed tomography of the chest of a patient with cystic adenomatoid malformation shows the cystic air-filled mass with absence of pulmonary vessels.

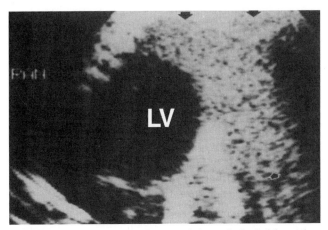

FIGURE 32-7 ■ Transverse ultrasound through the left hemithorax of a patient with cystic adenomatoid malformation shows a solid echogenic mass (arrows) adjacent to the heart. LV, left ventricle. (From Wesley JR, Heidelberger KP, DiPietro MA, et al: Diagnosis and management of congenital cystic disease of the lung in children. J Pediatr Surg 21:202, 1986.)

intravenous contrast injection and duplex ultrasound studies are capable of showing the vascular abnormality.

Cystic Adenomatoid Malformation

Although plain radiographs are frequently all that is required for diagnosis in emergent circumstances, CT can show lung markings or septations within a hyperlucent portion of the lung. In cases in which a soft tissue, water-dense mass is adjacent to the chest wall, ultrasound is a less costly alternative and more readily performed than CT and, in selected cases, may be as sensitive (Fig. 32-7). Ultrasound has the added advantage in that it does not require sedation in an infant who may have respiratory compromise. These latter studies also may help to differentiate CAM from anomalies that may have a similar appearance on plain chest radiography,

such as thoracic duplications. In the spectrum of pulmonary anomalies, some cystic abnormalities also have an aberrant systemic arterial supply.

Congenital Lobar Emphysema

Plain films of the chest are ordinarily sufficient to make the diagnosis of CLE and for serial follow-up in patients with few symptoms. Upper and middle lobes are most commonly involved, and rarely does this entity affect the lower lobes. CT with and without intravenous contrast administration not only shows the extent and nature of the abnormally overinflated portion of the lung, but also that of the compressed normal lung. Special rapid-sequence CT techniques with three-dimensional reconstruction may show areas of bronchial narrowing. Bronchoscopy is capable of identifying a site of cartilage deficiency in a major bronchus or an unsuspected obstructing lesion, as can bronchography, although the latter study is rarely required. CLE can be diagnosed in the fetus effectively by ultrasound and magnetic resonance imaging. Sequential studies have revealed that these lesions may decrease in size in the growing fetus but still can present with air trapping and respiratory distress after birth.

Pulmonary Sequestration

When patients have recurrent infections, plain chest radiographs usually show areas of scarring or active pneumonia in the same area. The lower lobes are involved most often, usually on the left. Dynamic CT scans during bolus injection of intravenous contrast material sometimes may show a systemic artery feeding a sequestration, but if not, arteriography is in order. Occasionally, ultrasound also may show a large vessel traversing the diaphragm going to a lower lobe abnormality that may be suspected to be a sequestration. Magnetic resonance imaging often clearly delineates the lesion and the systemic artery.

Thoracic and upper abdominal aortography are most useful in identifying anomalous systemic arterial supply in cases in which a cystic lesion is located adjacent to the diaphragm. Such an artery usually originates from the descending thoracic aorta or upper abdominal aorta below the diaphragm. The digital computer-enhanced subtraction technique allows anomalous arterial blood supply to be outlined by injecting contrast material via a peripheral vein (Fig. 32-8). This technique reduces the morbidity associated with an arterial puncture and catheterization, especially in infants. Angiography is not always required when operation is indicated, provided that the surgeon is aware of the possible presence and location of anomalous vessels.

TREATMENT

Indications for Operation

The exact diagnosis is not as important as the decision to resect the lesion. The decision as to whether or not a cystic pulmonary mass should be resected is based on its appearance on serial chest radiographs in conjunction with the patient's clinical symptoms. Most children with congenital cystic disease of the lung tend to develop symptoms from

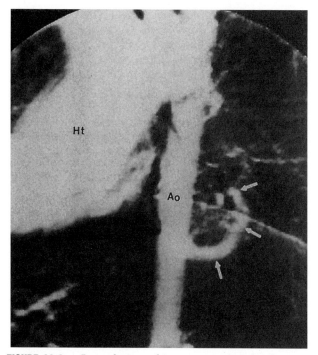

FIGURE 32-8 ■ Lateral view of intravenous digital subtraction angiogram after intravenous contrast administration shows an extralobar pulmonary sequestration with a large anomalous systemic artery (arrows) arising from the aorta (Ao) at the level of the diaphragm. Ht, heart. (From Wesley JR, Heidelberger KP, DiPietro MA, et al: Diagnosis and management of congenital disease of the lung in children. J Pediatr Surg 21:202, 1986.)

recurrent infections in the cyst. This is especially true of intralobar sequestration and CAM. These cysts also can cause compression and collapse of adjacent bronchi and lung tissue with resultant respiratory distress. Extralobar sequestrations are generally asymptomatic, as are most bronchogenic cysts. The rare parabronchial bronchogenic cyst can cause bronchial obstruction and air trapping in the newborn, resulting in severe respiratory distress. CLE usually causes marked air trapping and respiratory distress in the first 48 hours of life.

With improved safety of pediatric anesthesia and the development of sophisticated noninvasive diagnostic techniques, there should be no delay in operating on a symptomatic infant with congenital cystic disease of the lung. Asymptomatic pulmonary cysts generally require removal because of the tendency of these lesions to become infected over time. Another reason for resection is the rare association of congenital pulmonary cysts and a malignant neoplasm. One case report described an embryonal rhabdomyosarcoma arising within a bronchogenic cyst in a 2.5-year-old girl, and a second case of embryonal rhabdomyosarcoma arising from an asymptomatic CAM was reported in a 3-year-old girl. CAMs also have been associated with the development of pulmonary blastoma. Any cyst that is enlarging on serial chest radiographs should be resected owing to the respiratory compromise that will ensue and the propensity for infection to occur in the cyst or in the adjacent compressed lung tissue. If a congenital cyst is infected at the time of diagnosis, it can be removed safely when tissue levels of broad-spectrum antibiotics have been established. Unless the patient is a poor surgical risk, the only reason for following a lesion long-term would be if serial films showed progressive resolution, indicating the possibility of an acquired infectious cyst that has the potential for complete resolution. In utero resection for a fetus with hydrops has been shown to prevent fetal demise, which occurs in almost all cases in which hydrops occurs. This intervention should be restricted to use for well-defined indications and at specialized centers.

Surgical Management

Surgical management should include complete lobectomy for patients with CAM, CLE, and intralobar pulmonary sequestration. In the case of children with CLE who are symptomatic, the surgeon should be present at the time of anesthetic induction because patients with CLE may not tolerate positive-pressure ventilation well, and rapid thoracotomy may be necessary to relieve the compression of the remaining normal lung tissue. Segmental resection carries a prohibitively high complication rate with prolonged air leaks or recurrent infection or both, frequently requiring reoperation for completion of the lobectomy. Infants and children tolerate lobectomy extremely well with growth and expansion of the remaining lung tissue so that total lung volume and pulmonary function return toward normal. This response is most vigorous in the very young because new acini and alveoli can form until age 5 years. After this period, lung growth is achieved principally by enlargement of existing alveoli. Extralobar pulmonary sequestration may be associated with a diaphragmatic hernia, and the surgeon should keep this in mind when operating for either condition. In 15% of sequestrations, there are multiple arteries perfusing the segment, and these can arise from the abdominal aorta and perforate the diaphragm to enter the lung and arise directly from the thoracic aorta.

In the case of pulmonary AVMs, as little pulmonary tissue as possible should be removed. This is particularly the case in patients who have multiple vascular malformations of the lung. It is occasionally feasible to excise the aneurysmal sac of an AVM and its vessels without excising any lung tissue at all, but usually segmental resection is required.

SUGGESTED READINGS

Adzick NS, Harrison MR, Crombleholme TM, et al: Fetal lung lesions: Management and outcome. Am J Obstet Gynecol 4:884-889, 1998.

This article describes successful intervention for CAM in the fetus.

Buntain WL, Isaacs H, Payne VC, et al: Lobar emphysema, cystic adenomatoid malformation, pulmonary sequestration, and bronchogenic cysts in infancy and children: A clinical group. J Pediatr Surg 9:85, 1974.

This is the largest reported series of congenital cystic diseases of the lung.

Cass DL, Crombleholme TM, Howell LJ, et al: Cystic lung lesions with systemic arterial blood supply: A hybrid of congenital cystic adenomatoid malformation and bronchopulmonary sequestration. J Pediatr Surg 32:986-990, 1997.

This article provides some understanding of the common origin of various types of congenital cystic lesions of the lung. It documents that both CAM and pulmonary sequestration can have a systemic arterial blood supply.

Conran RM, Stocker JT: Extralobular sequestration with frequently associated congenital cystic adenomatoid malformation, type 2: Report of 50 cases. Pediatr Dev Pathol 2:454-463, 1999.

This series documented a 50% incidence of pathologic CAMs in extralobular sequestrations.

Olutoye OO, Coleman BG, Hubbard AM, et al: Prenatal diagnosis and management of congenital lobar emphysema. J Pediatr Surg 35:792-795, 2000.

The efficacy of prenatal diagnosis of CLE is shown, as is the natural history of this entity.

Papagiannopoulos KA, Sheppard M, Bush AP, Goldstraw P: Pleuropulmonary blastoma: Is prophylactic resection of congenital lung cysts effective? Ann Thorac Surg 72:604-605, 2001.

A link between CAM and pulmonary blastoma is shown.

Rice HE, Estes JM, Hedrick MH, et al: Congenital cystic adenomatoid malformation: A sheep model of fetal hydrops. J Pediatr Surg 29:692-696, 1994.

The mechanism for fetal hydrops in CAM was established in this experimental study.

Wesley JR, Heidelberger KP, DiPietro MA, et al: Diagnosis and management of congenital cystic disease of the lung in children. J Pediatr Surg 21:202, 1986.

This series of congenital cystic diseases of the lung provides an excellent discussion of the diagnostic modalities and the various entities.

Infections of the Lung and Airway

33

Pulmonary infections affect children of all ages. Although most mild-to-moderate infections can be treated effectively on an outpatient basis, some patients still require hospitalization. The availability of vaccines and a wide spectrum of antibiotics has decreased the incidence of severe lung infections and their complications, including empyema, bronchiectasis, and lung abscess. There has been an increase, however, in the use of immunosuppressive medications and intensive chemotherapy that predisposes immunocompromised patients to an increased risk of infection. Adjunctive techniques, including bronchoalveolar lavage and lung biopsy, may be required in immunocompromised patients to achieve diagnosis and guide therapy.

EPIDEMIOLOGY

Data indicate that the rate of respiratory infection is highest in younger children (6 months to 5 years old) and decreases with age. The incidence of respiratory infections for children younger than 5 years old is approximately 3.0 to 3.6 per 100. From an etiologic standpoint, *Streptococcus pneumoniae* and viral agents are the most common causes of respiratory infections. Respiratory syncytial virus (RSV) prevails in young children (<2 years old) with a larger proportion of community-acquired pneumonia caused by *S. pneumoniae* in children older than 2 years of age. In 40% to 60% of community-acquired pneumonia cases, no causative agent may be identified.

COMMUNITY-ACQUIRED BACTERIAL PNEUMONIA

Streptococcus pneumoniae

S. pneumoniae or pneumococcus is a major cause of morbidity and mortality. It is the most common pathogen observed in infants and children and is responsible for approximately 500,000 cases of pneumonia per year in the United States. Pneumococcus is a gram-positive coccus that is part of the normal flora in children and adults. Colonization rates, particularly of the nasopharynx, decrease with age, but colonization is an important factor in the development of infection. Symptoms include fever,

cough, tachypnea, malaise, and occasional emesis. Clinically, patients may have decreased breath sounds and rales on auscultation of the chest. Chest radiographs show lobar, multilobar, or sometimes segmental infiltrates (Fig. 33-1), and 40% of these patients also present with pleural effusion. Outpatient treatment often is carried out and may be complicated by bacterial resistance to antibiotic therapy. For patients infected with pneumococcal strains showing low-to-intermediate resistance, penicillin and other β-lactam antibiotics are still effective. Cephalosporins may be used in cases with strains showing high levels of resistance or if there is no clinical improvement observed with conventional therapy. The incidence of resistant strains to penicillin increased from 8.6% in 1996 to 21% to 26% in 2002. The introduction of new heptavalent conjugate pneumococcal vaccines reduced the severity of disease. These vaccines are safe and effective and are recommended for all children age 2 to 23 months. Pneumococcal polysaccharide vaccine is recommended in addition to conjugate pneumococcal vaccines for high-risk patients.

Haemophilus influenzae

This small, encapsulated, gram-negative bacillus is a common cause of community-acquired pneumonia. Greater than 95% of invasive cases of *Haemophilus* are caused by the type B strain. *Haemophilus* infections are seasonal, occurring more frequently in the winter and spring. The clinical presentation includes fever, tachypnea, elevated white blood cell count, and the presence of unilateral consolidation with pleural effusion on chest radiographs. Extrapulmonary manifestations, such as meningitis and epiglottitis, are observed commonly with this organism. Treatment depends on the sensitivity to β-lactam antibiotics. Cephalosporins are employed for strains producing β-lactamase. The overall incidence of *Haemophilus* infection has been reduced dramatically following the introduction of the *Haemophilus influenzae* type B conjugate vaccine. Immunization is recommended at 2 and 4 months of age using PedvaxHIB or Comvax. Secondary transmission of invasive *Haemophilus* still may be significant in the household or day care setting. In theses cases, prophylaxis with rifampin may be required for children at risk and for elimination of nasopharyngeal carriage of the organism.

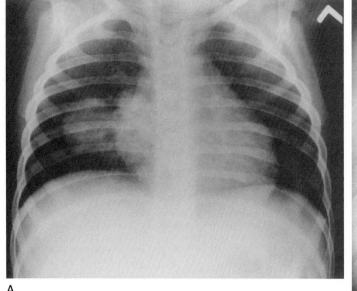

A

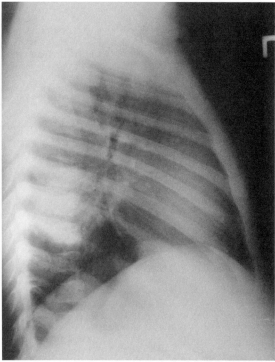

B

FIGURE 33-1 ■ Chest radiograph of a 1.5-year-old boy with fever and dyspnea shows a typical round pneumonia of the superior segment of the lower lobe; an air bronchogram can be seen within the opacity. **A,** Anteroposterior view. **B,** Lateral.

Staphylococcus aureus

These ubiquitous gram-positive cocci are found commonly on the skin and nasal mucosa, with 20% to 30% of the population being normal carriers of this bacterium. *S. aureus* produces toxins and enzymes responsible for the production of a pyogenic exudate or an abscess. Staphylococcal infections usually occur in infancy and early childhood. Primary pneumonias often occur during the winter and spring. Patients present with fever and the rapid onset of respiratory symptoms with progressive clinical and radiographic deterioration if left untreated. Primary pneumonias display unilateral lobar consolidation on chest radiographs. Secondary infection/pneumonia usually follows a prolonged febrile illness and often is accompanied by septicemia documented by positive blood cultures. These infections usually present as diffuse bilateral infiltrates on chest radiographs. Staphylococcal pneumonia often is associated with a pleural effusion, empyema, lung abscess, or pneumatoceles during the healing phase. These lesions require follow-up until complete resolution is observed. Initial treatment involves the use of appropriate antistaphylococcal antibiotic agents. If penicillin allergy exists, other agents, including vancomycin, clindamycin, and macrolides, may be used. The duration of treatment is usually 3 to 4 weeks. Fever may persist for 1 to 2 weeks after the institution of therapy.

Mycoplasma and Chlamydia

Mycoplasma pneumoniae and *Chlamydia pneumoniae* are unique pathogens that can cause respiratory infections in children of all ages. Most infections occur in school-age children or adolescents. These organisms may present as an atypical pneumonia. *M. pneumoniae* and *C. pneumoniae*

have similar seroepidemiologic characteristics. Infection is spread by person-to-person contact and usually involves a 1- to 2-week incubation period. The clinical presentation of atypical pneumonia is similar to that of an RSV infection. There is gradual onset of symptoms, including sore throat, hoarseness, and rhinitis, with or without fever. These upper respiratory tract symptoms progress to the lower respiratory tract over several days and include cough, pleuritic chest pain, rales, and rhonchi. *Mycoplasma* also can be associated with fever, chills, headache, and myalgias. These infections display interstitial infiltrates with unilateral subsegmental distribution on the chest radiograph, but this can be variable. The diagnosis usually is achieved on clinical grounds based on the history and physical examination. Other adjunctive tests, including polymerase chain reaction (PCR) studies, culture, and serology, confirm the diagnosis. Macrolides, erythromycin, and clarithromycin are the mainstays of therapy. Azalide (azithromycin) medications may be as effective as standard macrolide antibiotics with a much shorter course of therapy (5 days).

Mycobacterium tuberculosis

Tuberculosis (TB) in childhood almost invariably results from infection spread by an adult with active pulmonary disease. Aggressive treatment of infection during the early stages of disease has a major impact on reducing morbidity and disseminated infection. In North America, surgical complications of TB have been reduced dramatically as a result of effective medical therapy and careful follow-up. More recent reports concerning the epidemiology of TB in developed nations have common themes: (1) Immigrants and their children have the highest incidence of TB,

(2) more serious disease occurs in young children, and (3) screening tests play an important role in identifying children with TB. The emergence of antibiotic-resistant strains of TB may represent a problem in the future.

Primary pulmonary TB is a disease of the lymphatic system, the "primary complex." Primary TB results in secondary damage to the lungs through obstruction or damage to the large airways leading to atelectasis, chronic infection, and bronchiectasis. Most primary infections heal without leaving any lesions in the lung other than the Ghon complex (calcium deposit in a mediastinal or hilar lymph node). The healing of the primary lesion is believed to be associated with a positive host-organism balance, attributed either to a strong natural host resistance or a small initial inoculating dose. If the natural defense mechanisms are unable to control the primary infection, tuberculous pneumonia progresses with caseation, often accompanied by pleural effusion. Clinical manifestations include fever, dyspnea, and cough. Suspicion for TB should be raised in any child with chronic cough, history of contact with an adult with TB, failure to thrive, or inability to recover from infection despite adequate treatment.

The diagnosis of TB is established by culturing *Mycobacterium tuberculosis*, obtained from sputum, bronchial washings, gastric aspirates, or other infected material. A reliable urine test for TB using polymerase chaine reaction (PCR) has been introduced. In children, a positive tuberculin skin test indicates active disease requiring antituberculous therapy. The tuberculin test may be negative in immunosuppressed children or children with disseminated TB that may be anergic. Antituberculous therapy may be indicated when the disease is suspected in these patients because the organism may take several weeks to grow in culture. It is now evident that the absorption of antituberculous drugs in adults may be impaired by many factors, including food consumption, regardless of the immune status of the patient. There is a paucity of this type of data for children, but drug monitoring may be indicated to ensure that proper tissue levels are being delivered. Standard medications, such as rifampin, isoniazid, ethionamide, ethambutol, and pyrazinamide, can cause hepatotoxicity.

Operative intervention is required only in cases with significant lung damage. In contrast to adults, this often involves the lower lobes in children. The operation should be conservative in nature, usually consisting of a wedge resection, segmental resection, or lobectomy. The general indications for surgical intervention in childhood TB include (1) major airway obstruction by extraluminal lymph nodes, (2) chronic airway compromise, (3) airway obstruction by intraluminal material, (4) post-TB pulmonary destruction with or without fungal superinfection, (5) chronic cavitary lesions, and (6) TB-induced bronchiectasis.

Atypical Mycobacteria

Atypical mycobacteria (AMB) species first were identified in the 1950s. The incidence of AMB infections was relatively stable until the 1980s, when an increase in incidence was noted concurrently with the human immunodeficiency virus (HIV) epidemic. The most common presentation of AMB infections is cervical lymphadenitis. It is important to distinguish AMB infection from tubercular infection because the latter mandates vigorous treatment and tracking of the infection by public health authorities. The incidence of pulmonary infections with AMB is low. These infections may be seen in patients with cystic fibrosis (CF). Differential diagnosis includes staphylococcal abscess, cat-scratch fever, and lymphoma. These patients should undergo investigation for AMB and tubercular infection with sputum samples using PCR, high-performance liquid chromatography, or DNA probe techniques. Clarithromycin, rifampin, ethambutol, ciprofloxacin, and sulfonamides have been used in the treatment of cervical TB. AMB cervical lymphadenitis is treated by complete surgical excision of the affected lymph nodes, with antibiotic treatment reserved for unresectable lesions. Conversely, pulmonary AMB infection is treated primarily with antibiotics.

VIRAL INFECTIONS

Bronchiolitis

The most common cause of bronchiolitis in infants is RSV, accounting for 125,000 hospital admissions per year and 200 to 500 deaths per year in the United States. Other pathogens have been implicated with bronchiolitis, including parainfluenza, influenza, and adenoviruses. Peak times for infection are early winter through the spring, with the mode of transmission being direct contact. The peak incidence of infection occurs between the ages of 2 and 6 months. The illness starts as an upper respiratory infection with rhinorrhea, cough, and low-grade fever. Lower respiratory symptoms rapidly progress over the next 24 to 48 hours. At this time, patients may have tachypnea, alar flaring, retractions, and wheezing but no rales. High fever subsequently may be observed. Oxygen saturations may decrease to less than 95% but do not correlate with clinical findings. Patients exhibit hyperinflation, interstitial pneumonitis, and occasionally pleural thickening on chest radiographs.

Several patient populations are at increased risk for RSV, including premature infants, infants younger than 6 weeks old, children with chronic lung impairment or congenital heart disease, and aboriginal populations. Symptomatic and asymptomatic children shed RSV. The rate of shedding decreases with age. Immunocompromised patients can shed virus for longer periods, however, regardless of age. The overall mortality from RSV is 1% but can be 4% in patients at risk. A presumptive diagnosis of bronchiolitis often can be made on the clinical presentation and lack of rales on auscultation supported by radiographic appearance. Confirmation of infection requires a nasopharyngeal aspirate. Treatment for bronchiolitis is generally supportive with supplemental oxygen, maintenance of hydration, and close monitoring. Interruption of viral transmission is pamount to prevent hospital epidemics; strict hand-washing precautions and isolation of affected patients are important. Bronchodilators and inhaled steroid medications have a limited role in the overall treatment plan but may provide temporary symptomatic relief. Vaccination against RSV should be provided to high-risk children.

PARASITIC INFECTIONS

Echinococcus

Echinococcus hydatid disease is a parasitic tapeworm infection of sheep and dogs that is transmissible to humans. Hydatid disease is common in Egypt, Turkey, Greece, the Middle East, South Africa, and Australia. Previously rare in the United States, hydatid disease has been diagnosed in several patients living in the southwestern and mountain states. Cysts may occur in the liver, spleen, and lungs. Most patients with pulmonary disease are children. These cysts should be removed because 30% of these lesions eventually may rupture, producing pleural or bronchial seeding sometimes associated with acute anaphylaxis. Some children are asymptomatic, but others have a nonproductive cough. Chest radiographs typically show a single large pulmonary cyst. The most useful confirmatory test is the serum indirect hemagglutination titer. Gentle manipulation with wedge resection of the involved segment of the lung using a stapling device is recommended.

IMMUNOCOMPROMISED PATIENTS

Cancer Patients

The overall cure rates for all types of childhood cancers currently exceed 75%. This improvement has been the result of cooperative studies and multidisciplinary care programs; improved chemotherapy regimens, often with increased intensity of therapy; and the availability of pediatric intensive care facilities. A persistent problem is the threat of serious opportunistic infections. The most important factor contributing to the risk of infection is the degree of neutropenia. Neutrophil counts less than $1.0 \times 10^9/L$ place patients at significant risk for bacterial infection. If the duration of neutropenia is prolonged, the incidence of fungal infections also is increased.

The lung is the most common site of opportunistic infection in the immunocompromised patient. The incidence of pneumonia in this population ranges from 0.5% to 10%. The mechanism of infection is either from aspiration of pathogens from the upper airway or by hematogenous spread. The immune system can be affected adversely in different ways depending on the type, duration, and intensity of chemotherapy employed. Combination chemotherapy can impair different facets of the immune response as a result of the variable mechanisms of action of these agents.

Bacterial Infections

Bacterial infections are the most common cause of pulmonary infection noted early in the course of chemotherapy. Bacteremia, aspiration, ciliary dysfunction, decreased pulmonary toilet, impaired mucosal barriers, and endotracheal intubation all can predispose to infection. Deficiencies in immunoglobulins, which are necessary for proper opsonization, place these patients at risk of infection by encapsulated bacteria, such as *S. pneumoniae* and *H. influenzae*. With the advent of more intensive chemotherapy regimes, gram-negative bacilli are the most common pathogens identified. The risk of infection in bone marrow transplant (BMT) patients has been reported to be 10% to 15% within the first 100 days after transplantation. The most common gram-negative species causing infection include *Pseudomonas, Klebsiella,* and *Enterobacter*. These patients present with early pulmonary infiltrates that can be treated successfully with β-lactams and aminoglycosides. Infiltrates that persist longer than 7 days on treatment usually are due to these same organisms that have intrinsic resistance, requiring an alternative treatment protocol. Gram-positive infections usually are caused by *Staphylococcus, S. pneumoniae,* and group A streptococcus. β-Lactams and vancomycin are usually effective drugs in these cases. *Listeria* may produce late and refractory infiltrates. *Nocardia asteroides* infections are uncommon but can be severe, can mimic TB, and may be associated with central nervous system spread. Sulfonamides are the treatment of choice for this organism. Rarely the occurrence of empyema or a chest wall abscess requires drainage.

Fungal Infections

Fungal infections are a common cause of mortality in immunocompromised patients. An increased incidence of invasive fungal infections is noted in patients with prolonged neutropenia who are receiving steroids or antibiotics. There are two major patterns to fungal infection: (1) opportunistic infections with *Aspergillus* and *Candida* species, the two most common mycoses in immunocompromised patients, and (2) reactivation of latent infections with *Histoplasma, Coccidioides,* and *Blastomyces*.

The lung is the most common site of infection with *Aspergillus*. The upper airway is the usual portal of entry. This exposure can be reduced in an environment using laminar flow and high-efficiency filters. *Aspergillus* infections are rapidly invasive and cause tissue necrosis with hemorrhage resulting from the thrombosis of pulmonary arteries and veins. This leads to the development of a cavitary lesion seen on chest radiograph. Plain chest radiographs are not as sensitive as computed tomography (CT) scans in diagnosis of *Aspergillus* that may present with either diffuse infiltrates or nodular disease (Fig. 33-2). Intravenous amphotericin B is the treatment of choice, and response may be gauged by the recovery of white blood cells and granulocytes. The response of pulmonary aspergillosis to amphotericin B treatment alone is 5%. Surgical resection, usually lobectomy, of localized disease may be required to achieve survival if no clinical improvement is observed. Lipophilic amphotericin may have improved efficacy over the standard preparation. In BMT patients, the incidence of aspergillus infection can be 10%. These patients may have other problems, such as graft-versus-host disease, that make the diagnosis more difficult. In these cases, a lung biopsy may be required, although 40% of patients have positive sputum samples.

Candida is the most common fungal organism responsible for infection in immunocompromised patients, with the oral cavity being the major site. Lung infections are uncommon with this organism except with disseminated candidiasis. Radiographs may be nonspecific. Bronchoalveolar lavage (BAL) can be useful, but a lung biopsy usually is required. If left untreated, the prognosis is

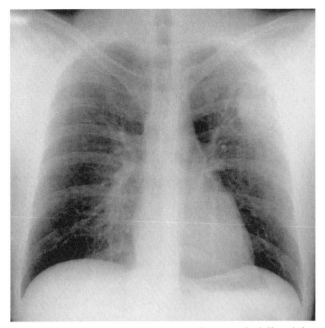

FIGURE 33-2 ■ Left upper lobe aspergilloma with diffuse bilateral lung infiltrates in a 17-year-old patient with acute lymphoblastic leukemia undergoing intensive chemotherapy.

uniformly poor. *Candida* may arise from overgrowth in the intestine in patients treated with antibiotics.

Viral Infections

Viral infections are relatively uncommon in cancer patients except if they are severely immunocompromised. Intact humoral immunity is important to protect against enteroviral infections, whereas cellular immunity is required to fight infections by the herpesviruses. The incidence of cytomegalovirus (CMV) infection varies with the underlying disease process. It is more prevalent in patients with allogeneic rather than autogenous BMT. This infection is usually the result of reactivation of a latent infection and presents with fever, headache, malaise, and myalgias. Radiographs are nonspecific, showing diffuse, nodular, or atelectatic changes within the lung. The diagnosis may be confirmed by BAL with cytology or PCR on recovered specimens. Treatment includes the use of gancyclovir and immunoglobulins. In BMT patients, interstitial pneumonias are caused by CMV infection in 50% of instances. The risk of CMV infection seems to be increased in patients who have concurrent graft-versus-host disease, receive frequent transfusions, or receive methotrexate or antithymocyte medications. Varicella is rare in immunocompetent patients. Of patients having visceral involvement, 30% may develop pneumonia. This can increase to 80% if patients are receiving concurrent chemotherapy. These patients present with diffuse bilateral fluffy infiltrates on chest radiographs. If the patient has been exposed to varicella, chemotherapy should be stopped for the period of incubation. Passive immunization with immunoglobulins should be administered at this time. Treatment of active infection includes acyclovir. Herpes infections are usually rare, unless there is concomitant gingivostomatitis. RSV infection can be problematic in

BMT patients because of their decreased T cell–mediated immunity. In immunocompromised patients, RSV infections can be life-threatening. Only supportive treatment can be offered; preventive immunization is recommended for high-risk patients.

Pneumocystis carinii

This unusual organism has properties of protozoa (susceptible to trimethoprim) and fungi (based on RNA studies). It is encountered rarely unless the patient is immunocompromised. Routine prophylaxis has reduced dramatically the incidence of this infection. Infection is usually the result of reactivation of latent disease. BMT patients and patients receiving steroids are at particular risk. Patients usually present with fever, dry cough, and dyspnea. The infection can follow a fulminant course with bilateral hilar infiltrates that progress to the periphery noted on the chest radiograph. The diagnosis is confirmed by histology and cytology that identifies trophozoite cysts recovered by BAL. Lung biopsy is occasionally necessary to achieve diagnosis. Trimethoprim/sulfamethoxazole (TMP/SMX) is the mainstay of treatment. If no response occurs within 72 hours, a lung biopsy is indicated. Aerosolized or intramuscular pentamidine may be used if myelosuppression or rash occurs as a result of TMP/SMX administration.

HIV/AIDS Patients

Early diagnosis and treatment of HIV is associated with prolonged survival. Acute pneumonia is the most common severe infection in HIV-infected children in the United States. The most common organisms are *S. pneumoniae*, *S. aureus*, group A streptococcus, *H. influenzae*, and *Pseudomonas*. The clinical features of respiratory infections in children with HIV/acquired immunodeficiency syndrome (AIDS) are similar to those with normal immune systems. The diagnosis is based on clinical information and radiographic findings. Opportunistic and atypical infections need to be excluded. The differential diagnosis of pulmonary infiltrates in this population also includes noninfectious causes, such as non-Hodgkin's lymphoma. Prevention plays a key role for these patients, including routine immunization against *Haemophilus*, pneumococcus, and TMP/SMX prophylaxis for *P. carinii*. Treatment should be initiated against the specific pathogen as soon as possible, although 30% of patients may not have an identifiable pathogen and are treated empirically.

Pneumocystis carinii

P. carinii infection is the most common AIDS-defining illness in children younger than 1 year old. The mortality with this infection is higher in children despite their having higher CD4 levels compared with adults. The incidence of *P. carinii* pneumonia has decreased, however, with the introduction of prophylactic therapy. The clinical presentation and treatment were described earlier.

Lymphoid Interstitial Pneumonitis

Lymphoid interstitial pneumonitis is a chronic lymphocytic infiltrative process seen in older children with HIV and is another AIDS-defining illness. Patients usually present with the insidious onset of respiratory symptoms. Fever and clubbing may be observed. The clinical course is benign but may predispose patients to subsequent bronchiectasis or cystic disease. Plain radiographs can show persistent reticulonodular infiltrates and hilar adenopathy that can be appreciated better by CT scan. Lung biopsy is necessary to confirm the diagnosis. Systemic steroid administration over 4 to 6 weeks usually leads to resolution of the infiltrates.

Tuberculosis

An increase in the incidence of TB in children in developed countries has been related to the increase in TB in HIV-infected adults, who serve as the primary source of transmission to children. Children at risk are those exposed to adults with active TB, to institutionalized patients, and to intravenous drug abusers. The clinical features are similar to those noted in immunocompetent patients but with a greater predilection for disseminated disease or unusual presentation. Chest radiographs show lobar or diffuse infiltrates and atelectasis resulting from bronchi being compressed by hilar lymphadenopathy. Children with TB require HIV testing. The diagnosis is based on the clinical, epidemiologic, and radiographic data available. The best noninvasive culture technique is acquiring an early morning gastric aspirate sample of retained overnight secretions (30% to 40% positive yield). The yield is higher with BAL or bronchoscopy, but these procedures are more invasive. HIV-infected children should undergo frequent skin testing for TB every 9 to 12 months. Prevention is key, and determining the TB status of all adults in the affected household is essential. In patients with significant exposure, isoniazid, regardless of skin test result, is indicated. If a repeat purified protein derivative in 3 months is negative, the medication can be stopped. Treatment of active infections includes multiagent therapy. Patients must be monitored for potential untoward interactions between antiretroviral medications and TB medications.

Atypical Mycobacterial Infections

There are several species of AMB that are clinically significant in patients with HIV. These include *M. avium intracellulare*, *M. lepraemurium*, and *M. scrofulaceum*. These bacteria are a major source of morbidity for HIV-infected children and usually cause systemic infection later in the course of AIDS. In the past, HIV patients infected with AMB had a 7-month life expectancy. With the advent of more effective HIV and AMB treatment, however, the disease is less common, and the prognosis is improved. These organisms commonly colonize in the respiratory and gastrointestinal tracts. The clinical presentation usually includes failure to thrive, abdominal pain, and fatigue rather than respiratory symptoms. Patients also may have leukopenia, thrombocytopenia, and an increased serum lactate dehydrogenase level. The diagnosis is achieved with a blood culture or biopsy of a normally sterile site, including bone marrow and lymph nodes. TB must be ruled out. Prevention is achieved with effective antiretroviral therapy. Primary prophylaxis with clarithromycin or azithromycin is based on the CD4 counts. Treatment of active infections includes administration of clarithromycin, ethambutol, ciprofloxacin, or azithromycin. Macrolides inhibit the metabolism of many antiretroviral medications.

Viral Infections

CMV infection can present as chronic interstitial pneumonitis and usually is accompanied by retinitis, hepatitis, or colitis. Respiratory symptoms include nonproductive cough, dyspnea, and hypoxemia. Chest radiographs often show diffuse interstitial infiltrates. The diagnosis is achieved by identifying viral inclusions in specimens, including urine samples or biopsy specimens of the lung or liver.

Fungal Infections

Systemic fungal infections are relatively uncommon because most infections involve the skin or mucosal surfaces. Pulmonary mycoses are being identified with increasing frequency, however, in patients with HIV. Histoplasmosis also has been reported in immunocompromised HIV patients. A primary fungal focus may progress rapidly to disseminated disease that can be fatal if left untreated. Severe disease presents with fever and reticulonodular lobar infiltrates on chest radiographs. *Cryptococcus* and coccidiomycosis usually are associated with disseminated infection. Of these patients, 50% have concurrent pulmonary infection. Fever, headache, and confusion may be observed. Aspergillosis is another relatively uncommon infection that usually presents with pulmonary disease and sinusitis. Patients may experience fever, cough, dyspnea, and pleuritic chest pain. For most mycoses, sputum analysis, BAL, and occasionally open-lung biopsy are required to confirm the diagnosis. Systemic amphotericin B is the treatment of choice. In the case of aspergillosis, itraconazole can be used for suppressive therapy.

The immunocompromised child requires constant surveillance and aggressive management strategies. In patients with pulmonary infiltrates, broad-spectrum antibiotics should be started promptly. If no response if observed over the next 48 to 72 hours, a change in the antibiotic regimen and possibly the addition of amphotericin B and TMP/SMX may be indicated. For persistent lung infiltrates, either BAL or lung biopsy should be performed. The results of lung biopsy for patients with persistent lung infiltrates have influenced the management of these patients in 90% of the cases.

CYSTIC FIBROSIS

CF is the most common autosomal recessive disease in whites and affects all of the body's exocrine gland secretions. Almost 30,000 people are affected in the United States (1 in 2500 births). The prognosis for this disease has improved since the 1970s but has plateaued since the mid-1990s, with a current life expectancy of older than 30 years of age. CF (mucoviscidosis) is characterized by thick, inspissated mucus, chronic infection, and neutrophil-dominated inflammation of the airways. The CF transmembrane conductance regulator (*CFTR*) gene is a cyclic adenosine phosphate–dependent chloride channel located on chromosome 7q21-31. The delta F508 mutation at this locus is responsible for 70% of the abnormal genes. One hypothesis suggests that the loss of CFTR as an ion channel in CF decreases fluid production and enhances sodium absorption. This leads to impaired ciliary function and mucus transport. Others suggest increased sodium in the air-surface layer inactivates antimicrobial defense and impairs lung defenses, including intraluminal killing of ingested bacteria. Homozygous patients also have increased bacterial binding to the airway epithelia, especially *Pseudomonas*. There also seems to be dysregulation of the inflammatory cascade in CF patients, leading to chronic inflammatory changes.

Patients with CF usually present within the first 4 years of life with acute or persistent signs and symptoms of recurring pulmonary infections and failure to thrive. A nonproductive cough usually progresses to a loose productive cough with copious purulent secretions. Classic physical characteristics include a barrel chest, digital clubbing, and occasional cyanosis. Initial pulmonary function tests show an obstructive pattern; however, a restrictive pattern may develop later in the disease process.

In the first decade of life, the most common organism isolated from CF patients is *S. aureus* (40%), followed by *H. influenzae* (15%) and *Burkholderia cepacia* (3.5%). Clinically, *Pseudomonas* is the most important pathogen in CF. *Pseudomonas* is usually the first pathogen isolated in children younger than 1 year old, and more than 80% of CF children are infected with this organism by 18 years of age. These bacteria secrete biofilms that enable them to avoid normal clearance mechanisms and resist penetration of antibiotics. *Pseudomonas* also produces exotoxins that contribute to its virulence, increasing the viscosity of secretions and further impairing ciliary transport. *B. cepacia* is an organism with intrinsic antibiotic resistance. Patients infected with this organism present with high fever, rapid pulmonary deterioration, and increased mortality. Viral infections may pose a special problem, particularly in young children with CF in whom they may predispose to secondary bacterial infection. RSV in this population can be particularly severe and may require respiratory support.

Medical treatment for CF patients includes the aggressive use of intravenous, oral, and nebulized antibiotics. The increased life span of CF patients can be attributed directly to the development of effective antipseudomonal medications. Maintenance therapy is designed to prolong the duration of time between pulmonary infections with *Pseudomonas*. Phase III clinical trials have shown the effectiveness of nebulized tobramycin. Macrolides are also effective because they possess anti-inflammatory properties and prevent biofilm formation. The clearance of the abnormal viscid secretions is paramount and includes regular chest physiotherapy and postural drainage. The efficacy of mucolytic agents such as acetylcysteine (Mucomyst) and Dnase is still not clear. Attempts to reduce the inflammatory response with steroids or other anti-inflammatory medications have been complicated by side effects. Adequate nutritional support and early treatment of pancreatic insufficiency has resulted in improved growth with gains in height and weight noted. Lung transplantation remains the final resort for patients with end-stage pulmonary disease. Approximately 1200 patients from the United States, Canada, England, and France have undergone lung transplantation for CF. The optimal time to provide the maximal benefit from lung transplantation is still unclear. Gene therapy has not progressed beyond phase I trials despite the gene being identified in the 1990s but is a future consideration.

CHRONIC AND RECURRENT PNEUMONIA

Pneumonias are a common cause of illness and hospitalization in children. Differentiating between recurrent or persistent pneumonia may be difficult. There is no uniform definition for these types of pneumonias, and radiographic abnormalities may persist for several weeks to months before true resolution. Optimally the diagnosis of recurrent pneumonia should be made only after complete resolution of the index infection. From a practical standpoint, recurrent pneumonias may be defined as those occurring twice in 1 year or as three separate episodes over any time frame. In contrast to episodes of acute pneumonia, an underlying cause may be identified in chronic or recurrent pneumonia in 92% of the cases. Asthma is the most common cause of recurrent pneumonia followed by aspiration.

Pneumonias may be classified into those that affect a single region of the lung and those that affect multiple areas. Abnormalities associated with an infection of a single segment of the lung include instances of intraluminal obstruction (owing to a foreign body or bronchial tumor), extraluminal compression (TB and fungal lymphadenopathy, tumors, and vascular rings), and structural abnormalities of the airway or lung (tracheal bronchus, localized bronchiectasis, congenital cystic adenomatoid malformation, and sequestration). Abnormalities causing pneumonia in several regions of the lung include recurrent microaspiration, asthma, immunodeficiency syndromes, mucociliary dysfunction (CF), structural abnormalities (bronchomalacia, Williams-Campbell syndrome), bronchopulmonary dysplasia, and other more uncommon causes such as Wegener's granulomatosis and idiopathic pulmonary fibrosis. Recurrent lung infiltrates also may occur in the acute chest syndrome in patients with sickle cell disease (Fig. 33-3).

Clinical evaluation of patients with chronic or recurrent pneumonias requires a thorough history and physical examination. The frequency; duration and severity of previous infections; and associated symptoms, such as fever, wheezing, and weight loss, are important historical details. The timing of the onset of symptoms, especially in the context of congenital malformations or a family history of genetic diseases such as CF, can help narrow the differential diagnosis. A thorough assessment of the child's growth and developmental pattern is necessary. Comparison of a recent chest radiograph and radiographs of previous episodes of pneumonia may provide important findings that may direct management and further investigations. The clinical status of the child dictates the urgency of subsequent examinations. The need for supplemental oxygen or respiratory support often can be assessed by the physical examination in conjunction with pulse oximetry and arterial blood gas analysis. Patients with a localized pneumonia may require bronchoscopy

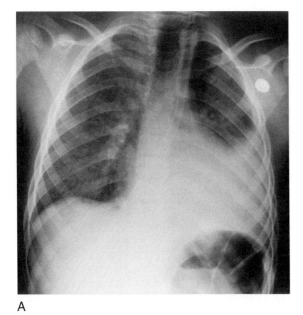

A

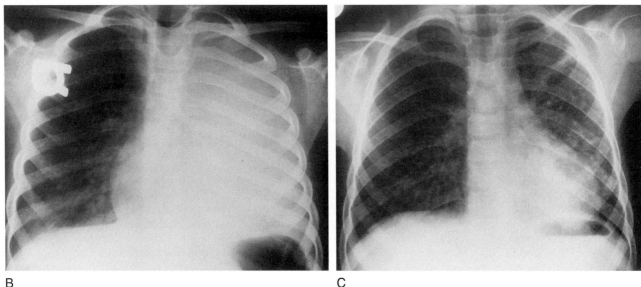

B

C

FIGURE 33-3 ■ Acute chest syndrome in sickle cell disease. A 5-year-old girl known to have hemoglobin S/β-thalassemia presented with nasal congestion, cough, and chest pain. The initial chest radiograph was normal (not shown); she was admitted for intravenous hydration and analgesia. Antibiotics were started when she became febrile, increasingly tachypneic, and hypoxic. **A,** Two days after admission, the chest radiograph shows airspace disease mostly in the left lower lobe. **B,** On day 5 of admission, there is a complete opacification of the left hemithorax, with increased airspace disease in the right base. **C,** Four days later, after exchange transfusion, there is marked improvement.

for foreign-body removal or to assess for structural abnormalities or CT of the chest to identify parenchymal lung lesions. Patients with multifocal pneumonias may require an upper gastrointestinal series, radiolabeled milk scan, or pH study to rule out aspiration owing to gastroesophageal reflux disease or swallowing coordination disorders. Pulmonary function tests to evaluate for asthma and evaluation to rule out immunodeficiency syndromes or other systemic diseases may be indicated.

COMPLICATIONS OF PNEUMONIA
Pneumatocele

Pneumatoceles are small, thin-walled structures consisting of single or multiple cysts within an air-lined cavity resulting from alveolar and bronchiolar necrosis. Pneumatoceles often follow infection by *S. aureus*, group A streptococcus, and occasionally *H. influenzae.*

With *S. aureus* infections, pneumatoceles may be identified early in the disease process and may be present in 80% of patients; pneumothorax and pyopneumothorax are complications resulting from rupture. These lesions may be difficult to distinguish from congenital cysts of the lung. Pneumatoceles often resolve spontaneously, whereas congenital abnormalities of the lung rarely involve. Follow-up chest radiographs are required until resolution, and a CT scan may be useful in suspicious instances (Fig. 33-4).

Lung Abscess

A pulmonary abscess develops when a localized infection in the parenchyma becomes necrotic and cavitates. When appropriate systemic antibiotic therapy is administered early, the frequency of primary lung abscess decreases considerably. Secondary abscesses developing in immunocompromised, severely ill, or occasionally very

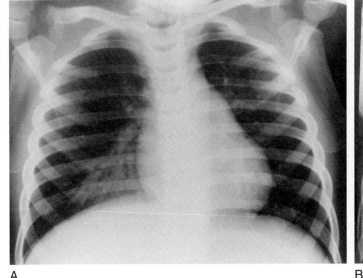

A

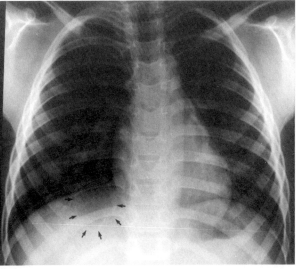

B

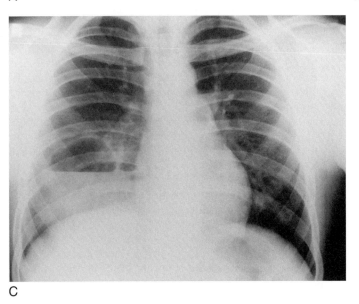

C

FIGURE 33-4 ■ **A,** A 5-year-old child presented with a right lower lobe pneumonia that responded to intravenous antibiotics. **B,** During outpatient monitoring, small cysts were noted 6 weeks later and appeared to coalesce in a larger pneumatocele on this radiograph, taken 11 weeks after the initial study. Follow-up was recommended. **C,** At 14 years of age, the same patient presented with a new episode of infection with a large air-fluid level and some smaller ones. Intravenous antibiotics were required for more than 2 weeks. CT confirmed the presence of three cysts. Six weeks later, a right lower lobectomy was performed, and microscopic examination confirmed a type I congenital cystic adenomatoid malformation.

young patients have become a more frequent problem. Occasionally, congenital bronchogenic or pulmonary cysts may become secondarily infected. These lesions may be indistinguishable from lung abscess on a chest radiograph (see Fig. 33-4).

Pathogenesis

Aspiration of gastric contents is a leading cause of chronic pneumonia and lung abscess in children, particularly children with neurologic impairment (Fig. 33-5). Aspiration may occur acutely during induction of anesthesia, during epileptic seizures, after trauma, and in children with severe gastroesophageal reflux disease. Aspiration of foreign bodies, including blood or foreign material after tonsillectomy, was previously a common antecedent of lung abscess. These events are now relatively infrequent because they often can be prevented by performing prompt bronchoscopy and endoscopic extraction of foreign bodies and by endotracheal intubation, which protects against aspiration during operations on the oropharynx.

Lung abscess occasionally may follow bacterial pneumonia. The most common causative organisms are *S. aureus*, *Streptococcus viridans*, group A hemolytic streptococcus, and occasionally *Pneumococcus* and *H. influenzae*. Other bacteria implicated in lung abscess include *Klebsiella*; *Escherichia coli*; *Pseudomonas*; and the anaerobic bacteria *Bacteroides*, *Peptostreptococcus*, and *Peptococcus*. Children with cellular or humoral immune deficiencies (congenital or acquired) occasionally are unable to eradicate a pulmonary infection despite administration of antibiotics. Progression of the pneumonic process may lead to necrosis of pulmonary parenchyma with eventual abscess formation. When lung abscess occurs in infants, an underlying congenital anomaly, such as bronchogenic cyst or congenital cystic adenomatoid malformation, should be suspected (see Fig. 33-4). In older children, an intralobar sequestration may be the site of recurring pneumonias and abscess formation and require excision.

The position of the child at the moment of aspiration often determines the location of the lung abscess.

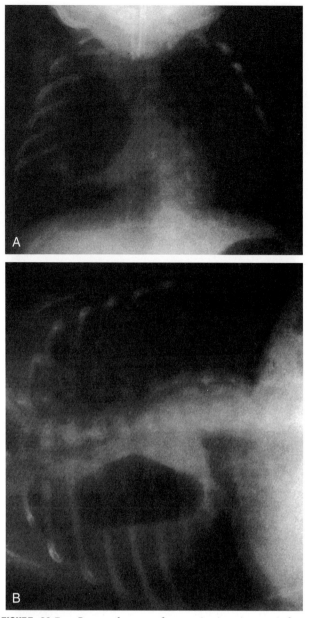

FIGURE 33-5 ■ Lung abscess after aspiration in an infant. **A,** A thick-walled cavity is present on the anteroposterior supine view. **B,** An air-fluid level is visible on the lateral decubitus view.

In supine patients, the superior segments of the lower lobes are most often involved. If the child is lying on the right side, the right upper lobe is at risk; if the child is lying on the left side, the apical posterior segment of the left upper lobe may be the vulnerable site. An upright child often aspirates into the basilar segments of lower lobes.

Diagnosis

The most common symptoms caused by lung abscess include productive cough, chest pain, hemoptysis, weight loss, fever, chills, general malaise, and anorexia. Purulent sputum may be produced by older children; younger patients usually swallow their secretions. Putrid sputum

is characteristic of an anaerobic abscess. The affected area of the chest may be dull to percussion and have decreased breath sounds on auscultation. Leukocytosis commonly is observed.

The diagnosis may be achieved by obtaining a chest radiograph that shows a cavity, commonly with an air-fluid level (see Fig. 33-5B). Abscess should be distinguished from pneumatocele, a localized collection of intrapulmonary air that usually does not have an air-fluid level, and from empyema with an air-fluid level. When chest radiographs are nondiagnostic, thoracic ultrasound or CT may be useful.

Treatment

A specific bacteriologic diagnosis should be established before treatment whenever possible. Diagnostic bronchoscopy with direct aspiration of purulent fluid from the bronchus on the affected side should be performed except in older children who are able to cough up a satisfactory sputum sample. Needle aspiration of a peripheral abscess cavity under fluoroscopic control has been used to obtain culture material with moderate success.

The preferred treatment of lung abscess is administration of appropriate intravenous antibiotics and drainage. Satisfactory drainage usually can be accomplished by chest physiotherapy with postural drainage and percussion and by occasional bronchoscopic aspiration. For children who are unable to cough adequately, therapeutic bronchoscopy or transbronchial drainage may be necessary. Intravenous antibiotics are recommended for 2 to 4 weeks, followed by oral antibiotics for a total treatment period of 6 to 8 weeks. Antibiotics are discontinued when the child is symptom-free and the chest radiograph is clear. The most effective antibiotics are penicillin V and clindamycin. Gentamicin usually is recommended for coliform bacteria.

Medical therapy is frequently unsuccessful in neonates and immunosuppressed children, in whom the mortality approaches 20%. Percutaneous catheter drainage of the abscess may be helpful in acutely ill children, particularly for children who experience rapid progression of the disease despite maximal antibiotic therapy.

Surgical resection of the abscess by segmental resection or occasionally lobectomy is recommended for chronic large and thick-walled abscess or for the few patients who do not respond to intensive antibiotic therapy or drainage. Other indications for operation include chronic abscesses lasting longer than 3 months, persistent hemoptysis, bronchial stenosis, severe bronchiectasis, and extensive pulmonary necrosis. The mortality associated with primary lung abscess should be negligible. In patients having secondary pulmonary abscesses, the mortality is high (60% to 75%).

Bronchiectasis

Bronchiectasis is a progressive condition leading to irreversible dilation of the airways associated with recurring bacterial infection and inflammatory destruction of bronchial and peribronchial tissue (Fig. 33-6). The morbidity and mortality have decreased significantly as a result of improvement in antibiotic therapy and vaccinations against common pathogens. The pathogenesis of

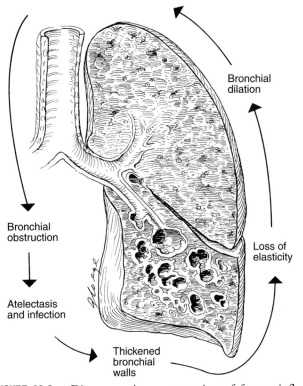

FIGURE 33-6 ■ Diagrammatic representation of factors influencing the pathogenesis of bronchiectasis.

Labels in figure:
Bronchial dilation
Bronchial obstruction
Atelectasis and infection
Thickened bronchial walls
Loss of elasticity

bronchiectasis has three stages. Initially, there is destruction of the ciliary epithelium that is replaced with cuboidal squamous epithelium. In the early stages of disease (cylindrical bronchiectasis), there is localized damage to the elastic tissue of the airway associated with edema and inflammation. Later in the disease (saccular bronchiectasis), the damage extends to the muscle layers and cartilage of the airways with anastomoses forming between pulmonary and bronchial arteries in the areas of saccular dilation. There is also evidence to support a host-mediated component to local tissue damage.

There are many causes of bronchiectasis. Infection is the most common, especially in patients with TB and histoplasmosis. Bronchiectasis may not result from the index infection but is usually the result of concomitant or subsequent infection with other agents, especially viruses, certain fungi, and occasionally *Mycoplasma*. CF is the most common genetic cause of bronchiectasis, resulting from infection and bronchial obstruction with inspissated mucus. Other causes include congenital absence of supportive airway cartilage (Williams-Campbell syndrome), tracheomegaly, Marfan's syndrome, α_1-antitrypsin deficiency, foreign-body aspiration, ciliary abnormalities (Kartagener's syndrome), immunodeficiencies (IgA), asthma, and right middle lobe syndrome.

Patients with bronchiectasis usually present during the preschool years with cough, profuse sputum production, wheezing, and chest pain. Of patients, 50% may have clubbing of the fingertips, which is reversible. The diagnosis is suggested on plain radiographs of the chest that show bronchial dilation, bronchial thickening, and a signet ring sign. CT of the chest has replaced bronchography as a method to document the severity of disease. The distribution of bronchiectasis may shed some light on the underlying cause. Patients with TB have unilateral involvement, whereas patients with CF and viral-induced disease have involvement of the upper and lower lobes. Treatment focuses on identifying and treating the underlying cause in addition to postural drainage techniques and chest physiotherapy. Antibiotic therapy is required for acute exacerbations. Adequate nutritional support is needed to prevent failure to thrive as a result of recurrent infections. Segmental resection or lobectomy may be indicated for patients with localized disease who have recurrent infections and hemoptysis.

Empyema

Empyema refers to the accumulation of purulent material in the pleural cavity. In children, empyema is generally the result of underlying pneumonia and less often due to lung abscess or bronchiectasis. It also may occur after chest trauma, intrathoracic esophageal perforation, or thoracic surgical procedures.

Pathology

Normally the pleural membranes are permeable to liquid, and a small amount of fluid exists between the visceral and parietal pleura to minimize friction during respiration. When the adjacent lung is healthy, the pleural cavity generally is resistant to infection. When established, empyema exhibits three stages: (1) an exudative or early stage, when the fluid is thin and of low cellular content; (2) a fibrinopurulent stage with large numbers of polymorphonuclear cells and fibrin deposition that progressively impairs lung expansion and can lead to the formation of fluid loculations; and (3) a final stage or organizing empyema with a thick exudate and fibroblasts that invade the fibrinous peel. The empyema may be diffuse and involve the entire pleural space, or it may be localized and encapsulated in an interlobar, diaphragmatic, or paramediastinal location.

Pneumococci, streptococci, and mixed bacteria from the oropharynx were previously the most common organisms in childhood empyema. Currently the most common organisms are *S. aureus*, *H. influenzae*, and *S. pneumoniae*, probably because of changing antibiotic resistance patterns. In addition, anaerobic bacteria have been reported with increasing frequency in instances of empyema in children.

Diagnosis

Symptoms of empyema in children usually include a short history of pulmonary infection followed by respiratory distress, fever, and cough. Abdominal, chest, or shoulder pain; abdominal distention; and adynamic ileus may intensify the respiratory difficulty. The chest radiograph often shows bilateral pulmonary involvement with pneumatoceles. Haziness of the hemithorax may represent either pulmonary consolidation or pleural fluid. In the early exudative phase, the pleural fluid flows freely along the lateral chest wall on decubitus views (Fig. 33-7). In advanced empyema, the exudate is a solid mass of fibrin, which does not move with changes in the

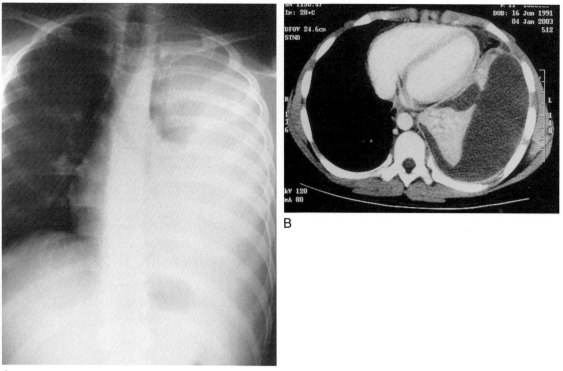

FIGURE 33-7 ■ An 11-year-old boy presented with left-sided pleuritic pain and fever. **A,** Chest radiograph shows a large left-sided effusion with mediastinal shift. **B,** Because of concern about an underlying malignancy, a CT scan was obtained. This shows a large nonloculated fluid collection, with a collapsed lower lobe; fluid can be seen in the fissure. A chest tube was inserted and drained 400 mL of serous fluid, with a lactate dehydrogenase of 4000 U/L. There were no bacteria on Gram stain, but cultures grew *Streptococcus*. The patient improved with intravenous antibiotics, and the chest tube was removed 8 days later.

child's position. In the intermediate fibrinopurulent stage, loculations are characteristic. Air-fluid levels within the loculations suggest the presence of anaerobic organisms.

Treatment

Primary therapy for empyema is the administration of high-dose intravenous antibiotics. Effective drainage of the pleural space also speeds the resolution of the empyema. Fluid that layers in the decubitus position may be amenable to chest tube drainage alone (see Fig. 33-7). Loculated fluid collections may not be drained sufficiently by tube thoracostomy, and the optimal management of these patients is still debated. One clinical pathway uses ultrasound to evaluate empyema identified on a chest radiograph for the presence of loculations. If loculations are identified, early video-assisted thoracoscopic surgery (VATS) is advocated. With VATS, the length of hospital stay and cost are reduced significantly compared with the national children's database (National Association of Children's Hospitals and Related Institutions [NACHRI]). Others have recommended chest tube insertion after diagnostic thoracentesis, however, particularly if the fluid has any of the following characteristics: (1) gross pus, (2) pH less than 7.0, (3) lactate dehydrogenase greater than 1000 U/mL, (4) glucose less than 40 mg/dL, and (5) positive Gram stain. If resolution and clinical improvement do not occur within the first few days after chest tube insertion, VATS is performed. The use of fibrinolytics

is controversial. Urokinase is currently not available, and recombinant streptokinase has had inconsistent results in two adult trials and some small pediatric series.

INTRATHORACIC ACCESS AND PROCEDURES

Spontaneous Pneumothorax

Spontaneous pneumothorax usually results from rupture of an apical pulmonary bleb or bulla without evidence of other lung pathology. In contrast, secondary spontaneous pneumothoraces occur in the context of underlying lung disease, such as CF or *P. carinii* pneumonia. The incidence of pediatric spontaneous pneumothorax (PSP) in the United States is estimated to be 7.4 to 18 per 100,000 boys and 1.2 to 6 per 100,000 girls. Typically the patient is a thin, lean adolescent who presents with the acute onset of ipsilateral pleuritic chest pain and a nonproductive cough. Most patients with PSP are clinically stable when initially evaluated. A few patients may present with symptoms, however, including respiratory distress and hypotension secondary to a tension pneumothorax. Other clinical findings in patients with PSP include tachypnea and tachycardia. Chest radiographs confirm the diagnosis and may identify secondary pathology within the lung. Expiratory films may be helpful to identify small pneumothoraces.

Most patients who present with an acute PSP require supplemental oxygen and intravenous access. For the few patients presenting with a tension pneumothorax, immediate needle decompression in the second intercostal space (in the midclavicular line) is necessary even before chest radiograph confirmation, followed by the prompt placement of a chest tube in the axilla. PSP of less than 15% often can be managed by observation and supplemental oxygen alone. Heimlich valves connected to the pleural drain allow for outpatient management of small spontaneous pneumothorax in compliant patients. Large spontaneous pneumothoraces require the placement of a chest tube attached to an underwater seal and drainage. After confirming that the chest tube is located and functioning properly, an air leak that persists for more than 5 to 7 days may require further intervention. For most young children (<8 years old), chest tube drainage is sufficient for treatment. Adolescents tend to have a high recurrence rate, however, of 40% to 60%. CT scans are more sensitive in detecting blebs and bullae than chest radiographs, but it is unclear whether their routine use for PSP changes management.

The indications for surgical management of PSP include recurrence, persistent air leak, bilateral disease, and possibly the presence of large bullae. VATS seems to be superior to standard thoracotomy with less postoperative pain and fewer complications noted in several series. Transaxillary minithoracotomy (TAMT) is a viable alternative to VATS and has certain advantages, particularly in instances of poor visualization and the presence of dense adhesions. For pleurodesis, thoracoscopic pleural abrasion and talc poudrage are effective techniques. Apical pleurectomy is more effective and can be performed easily through a TAMT incision. For bilateral disease, VATS and TAMT are effective. Despite similar results, VATS has become more popular among surgeons for the treatment of PSP. The recurrence rate after VATS ranges from 2% to 14%, although this rate decreases with increasing experience. For TAMT, the reported recurrence rate is 2%.

Chest Tube Insertion in the Newborn for Pneumothorax

In preparation of chest tube insertion, the infant is placed in an oxygen hood or, if intubated, maintained on ventilator support, restrained, and monitored using pulse oximetry and an electrocardiogram. The procedure is performed with adequate light, sterile technique, and appropriate instruments and supplies. After local anesthesia, a 3- to 4-mm incision is made over the fourth interspace in the midaxillary line behind the pectoralis fold. A mosquito clamp is placed through the incision and used to spread the subcutaneous tissues and advanced upward just over the rib to enter the chest cavity. An appropriate-sized tube, usually 8F or 10F, is advanced into the pleural cavity (Fig. 33-8). The tube is advanced superiorly and anteriorly 3.0 to 4.0 cm, being certain that all of the holes in the tube are intrapleural, yet avoiding a tube that is inserted too far and kinks after reaching the mediastinum. The tube is sutured in place, and an occlusive dressing is applied. The tube is attached to an underwater seal at 10 to 15 cm of negative pressure, remembering that a high negative pressure would add to the positive pressure applied by a ventilator, possibly leading to barotrauma.

A chest radiograph is obtained to determine appropriate placement of the tube and expansion of the lung. Excessive bubbling indicates a continued source of air leak from the injured lung, a bronchopulmonary fistula, or perhaps a leak in the drainage system.

The most frequent complications related to chest tube insertion are (1) injury to the intercostal vessels during insertion and (2) lung perforation during tube insertion. If there is excessive bleeding and continued significant air leak, operative correction is required.

Chest Tube Insertion in Older Children

Pneumothorax in older children is usually encountered in patients with CF, spontaneous rupture of an emphysematous bleb, asthma, and blunt trauma. A tube thoracostomy is required in symptomatic patients. Chest tube insertion in older infants and children also may be required to drain large pleural effusions from a variety of causes, including chylothorax, traumatic hemothorax, lymphoma, pneumonia, empyema, and other causes.

Conscious sedation with intravenous fentanyl (1 mg/kg) and midazolam (0.1 mg/kg) may be useful in toddlers and older children. Alternatively, ketamine (1 mg/kg) with or without midazolam provides excellent analgesia and sedation, while preserving respiratory reflexes and cardiac parameters. Children are kept in a supine elevated position with a small roll placed under the affected hemithorax. The ipsilateral arm is positioned superiorly and laterally. The chest tube size is determined by the child's weight and whether the problem is a pneumothorax, a transudate, or an exudate (Table 33-1). Tube placement is similar to that for infants. If the patient has a pleural effusion, the location of the tube placement is determined by correlating the physical examination with the findings on chest radiograph, ultrasound, or chest CT. The chest tube should not be inserted below the level of the seventh rib to avoid injury to the spleen, liver, or diaphragm.

Bronchoscopy and Bronchoalveolar Lavage

Bronchoscopy is described in detail in Chapter 31. It is essential for the performance of BAL. The amount of saline used for BAL in children is usually 10 to 20 mL or 1 to 2 mL/kg divided into 4 aliquots; 80% of the fluid may be recovered. The first aspirate is sent for culture and Gram stain, whereas cytology is better performed on latter samples to ensure the presence of alveolar cells.

TABLE 33-1 ■ Guide for Chest Tube Selection

Patient weight (kg)	Size (F)		
	Pneumothorax	Transudate	Exudate
<3	8-10	8-10	10-12
3-8	10-12	10-12	12-16
8-15	12-16	12-16	16-20
16-40	16-20	16-20	20-28
>40	20-24	24-28	28-36

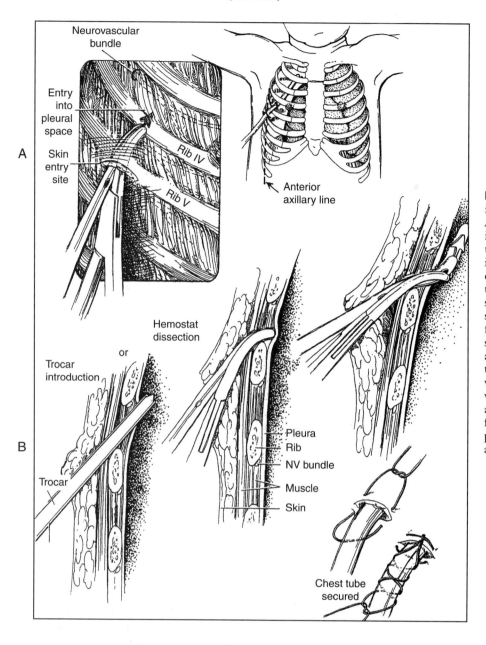

FIGURE 33-8 ■ Chest tube insertion in the newborn for pneumothorax. **A,** Preferably a small hemostat is inserted through a small incision in the anterior or midaxillary line and is tunneled upward, entering the chest above the next rib. The chest tube is inserted and secured with a suture ligature. Several knots should be placed after each circumferential pass of the thread to avoid slippage. **B,** A trocar can be used as an alternative method of tube insertion, as long as the trocar is withdrawn by a few millimeters within the tube; this technique allows easier guidance of the tube, for example, if it has to be placed posteriorly and inferiorly to drain an effusion.

Although there are no absolute contraindications to BAL, there is a risk of hemorrhage and hypoxemia during the procedure. Patients also may have transient pulmonary infiltrates after BAL, which resolve over the ensuing 12 hours. An alternative way to perform BAL in patients with diffuse disease is to pass a small catheter directly into the endotracheal tube and "wedge" it as distally as possible before lavage and aspiration. Fluoroscopy also may be a useful adjunct for such techniques if samples from a specific lobe or segment is sought. Greater than 100,000 organisms per high-power field usually indicates infection. The role of BAL in patients with CF and asthma remains to be determined. BAL does play a role, however, in providing diagnoses in cases of interstitial pneumonia in immunocompromised patients and lung diseases such as alveolar proteinosis or pulmonary hemorrhage.

Lung Biopsy

Open-lung biopsy should be done early in the diagnostic evaluation of diffuse pulmonary disorders in children and is generally the preferred method for establishing a diagnosis. Needle lung biopsies are fairly reliable and accurate; however, pneumothorax or hemothorax occurs in approximately one third of patients. Larger specimens are obtained by open-lung biopsy for cultures, histologic study, special staining and occasionally electron microscopy. It is easier to avoid air leaks and to secure complete hemostasis with an open wedge biopsy and routine use of a chest tube. Mortality after open-lung biopsy is rarely a result of the procedure; death, when it occurs, almost always is caused by the patient's underlying disease. A tissue diagnosis is established in most patients after open-lung biopsy and influences subsequent therapy in more than 90% of patients. The preoperative diagnosis is confirmed in approximately 60% of patients and corrected in more than 35%.

Children requiring open-lung biopsy are often immunosuppressed and have spreading pulmonary infiltrates and impending respiratory failure. Biopsy should be performed early to prevent air leak. Careful preoperative review of chest radiograph is essential to identify the optimal site for biopsy (i.e., an area of heavy infiltrate). A small anterior thoracotomy incision is performed, and the biopsy specimen is obtained using a stapling device. The procedure is safe and expeditious; in smaller children, a Lahey clamp allows an adequate biopsy specimen through a smaller incision, especially if the lung parenchyma is stiff and cannot be brought out through the incision (Fig. 33-9). Alternatively a transaxillary incision may provide adequate access to lung tissue desired for lung biopsy. Lung biopsy also can be performed by thoracoscopy. This technique allows visualization of the entire lung and biopsy of different lobes if necessary. In the presence of severely diseased and noncompliant lungs or in patients requiring high ventilatory pressures, a small anterior thoracotomy may be less invasive.

Thoracoscopic Procedures

Advances in technology have enabled thoracoscopy to become a standard technique for children. The development of high-resolution cameras and fine instruments has permitted thoracic procedures to be performed using minimal access techniques even in small infants. At present, there are many indications for thoracoscopy, including lung biopsy, pleurodesis, lung resection, biopsy and resection of mediastinal masses, and esophageal myotomy for achalasia.

Anesthetic Considerations

The ability to obtain near or complete collapse of the ipsilateral lung during thoracoscopic procedures helps with visibility and maneuverability, especially in young infants and children. Limitations exist, however, with regard to single-lung ventilation. The smallest double-lumen tube is 26F and cannot be used in patients weighing less than 30 kg. Even the use of a bronchial blocker requires the use of a 6.0 endotracheal tube (minimum size). In neonates and small children, simple endotracheal intubation allows excellent visualization. The addition of low-flow (1 L/min) and low-pressure (4 to 5 mm Hg) carbon dioxide insufflation at the beginning of the procedure keeps the lung totally collapsed. Hypercarbia may be corrected by increasing the minute ventilation.

Procedures

Lung biopsies are performed to diagnose chronic infiltrates, interstitial lung diseases, or masses of unknown etiology, often in patients who are immunosuppressed. Patient position and trocar placement vary with the location of the intended biopsy. Three to four ports may be used, often using the "baseball diamond" configuration to maximize visibility and maneuverability (Fig. 33-10). Small children may accommodate only 2.5- to 5-mm ports; biopsies are performed by placing endo-loop devices doubly at the base of the biopsy site with the specimen excised distal to the loops. Slippage of the

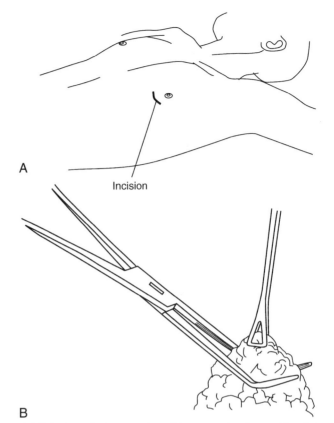

FIGURE 33-9 ■ **A,** An open-lung biopsy can be done with minimal morbidity using a small anterior thoracotomy. **B,** The lingula can be grasped easily and provides an adequate specimen in patients with diffuse lung infiltrate; in small children (or when a stiff lung cannot be brought outside the chest wall), a Lahey clamp is used to obtain the biopsy specimen instead of a linear stapler. After the lung tissue above the Lahey clamp is cut sharply with a scalpel, a continuous U suture is passed underneath the clamp, the clamp is released, and the suture is tightened and brought back as a simple continuous stitch. This provides excellent hemostasis and prevents air leaks.

loop has been noted to occur in some patients, indicating our preference for the anterior open thoracotomy for young children. The Ligasure (Valley Labs, Boulder, Co.) device also may prove useful for lung biopsy, but experience with this instrument is limited. Larger children accommodate a 12-mm endoscopic vascular stapler that can be placed directly through the chest wall, without the use of a port. Enough space is required inside the chest to open the jaws of the stapler (Fig. 33-11). Careful evaluation of preoperative CT scans allows for proper placement of ports in the event that a single lesion or region of the lung requires biopsy. Chest tube placement at the completion of the procedure depends on the underlying disease and the procedure accomplished. Needle-localization procedures also may be performed to help locate specific lesions. In this case, blood taken from the patient is injected over the intended site of biopsy after being localized by preoperative CT. These areas are identified and excised easily. Mediastinal masses may be biopsied or excised using thoracoscopic techniques. Placing the patient in the prone position may be more advantageous for lesions located in the posterior

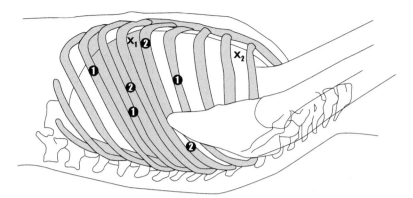

FIGURE 33-10 ■ Patient position and trocar placement for thoracoscopic procedures varies according to the "target." For a biopsy of the lingula, the patient is supine with elevation of the left side, and the ports could be placed as in (1). For upper lobe or superior mediastinal lesions, the patient is positioned more lateral, with a roll under the right side to open the intercostal spaces as in (2); the most posterior port also could be placed in front of the scapula. The operating table can be tilted further up, down, or sideways to allow the lung to fall away from the target. The telescope is placed initially at "home base" of the "baseball diamond." The position of the instruments and telescope can be modified, taking into account that the stapler requires a larger incision and should be placed where a chest tube would be left at the end of the procedure.

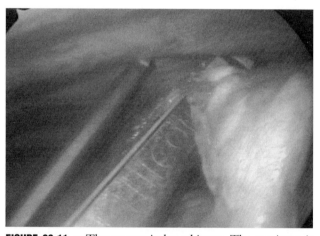

FIGURE 33-11 ■ Thoracoscopic lung biopsy. The specimen is seen on the right side as the stapler is opened. A small remaining bridge of tissue is cut with scissors because it already is stapled.

mediastinum, such as foregut duplication cysts, because the lung falls anteriorly. Three or four port sites may be required for these procedures.

Pleurodesis and decortication also are performed easily using thoracoscopy. For the treatment of persistent pneumothorax in patients with CF or for the palliative treatment of refractory malignant pleural effusions, pleurodesis by talc poudrage can be achieved by attaching a suction trap containing sterile talc directly in-line with the carbon dioxide–insufflation tubing. When insufflation begins, the talc is dispersed into the field as a "snowstorm." This technique allows for even, accurate distribution of the talc to all pleural surfaces. Usually less than 5 g of talc is required. For the treatment of empyema, complete evacuation and irrigation of the

pleural cavity and even decortication can be performed without the morbidity of a thoracotomy incision. Similar to lung biopsies, port sites are placed in a triangular fashion with or without low-pressure and low-flow insufflation. Formal ports usually are required only for the telescope, whereas the instruments may be placed directly into the thoracic cavity for easier manipulation of tissues. This technique is less advantageous and effective for more advanced empyemas, in which the fibrinopurulent "peel" is quite dense and adherent to the visceral pleura.

The advantage of thoracoscopic procedures is clear. The morbidity and wound pain associated with formal thoracotomy can be reduced significantly by thoracoscopy.

ACKNOWLEDGMENT

The author would like to acknowledge the contributions of Pramod S. Puligandla, MD, MSc, FRCSC, in the preparation of this chapter. His participation was greatly appreciated.

SUGGESTED READINGS

Chernick V, Boat TF, Kendig EL: Disorders of the Respiratory Tract in Children, 6th ed. Philadelphia, WB Saunders, 1998.

This chapter provides an in-depth description of the various congenital and acquired disorders of the respiratory system.

Finck C, Wagner C, Jackson R, et al: Empyema: Development of a critical pathway. Semin Pediatr Surg 11:25-28, 2002.

This article provides a more recent description of current management options in children with acute and chronic empyema.

Heath PT: Epidemiology and bacteriology of bacterial pneumonias. Pediatr Respir Rev 1:4-7, 2000.

This article is an excellent source of information on current patterns of bacterial pneumonias and their treatment.

Hewitson JP, Von Oppell UO: Role of thoracic surgery for childhood tuberculosis. World J Surg 21:468-474, 1997.

This is a description of where surgery fits in the management of childhood TB, especially in the setting of HIV/AIDS.

Neville K, Renbarger J, Dreyer Z: Pneumonia in the immunocompromised pediatric cancer patient. Semin Respir Infect 17:21-32, 2002.

Patient care protocols are provided for prevention and management of the various types of pneumonia that occur in immunocompromised oncology patients.

34

Chest Wall Deformities

Various malformations of the chest wall may appear at birth or be identified in infancy, early childhood, or early adolescence. The most common are the pectus excavatum and pectus carinatum anomalies. Developmental abnormalities may involve ribs, costal cartilages, or the sternum alone.

SKELETAL ANOMALIES

A variety of deviations from the normal pattern of 12 symmetric ribs occasionally may occur. One or more ribs may be completely absent or only partially developed. A rib may bifurcate and one component articulate with a hypoplastic adjacent rib or fuse with it. If the costal defects are extensive, they may cause moderate-to-severe functional impairment or abnormalities in appearance. Severe fusion can lead to progressive kyphoscoliosis or may cause serious compression of the lungs with resultant ventilatory disturbance (Fig. 34-1). An extreme form of narrow, rigid thorax with multiple cartilaginous anomalies, in which the patient progresses to death through respiratory insufficiency, has been termed *asphyxiating thoracic dystrophy of the newborn*, or Jeune's syndrome. Infants with severe fusion anomalies may require prolonged respiratory assistance. Spinal defects, such as hemivertebrae, often are associated with costal abnormalities. Attempts at surgical correction generally have been unrewarding because volume increase provided by surgical reconstruction does not improve respiratory insufficiency. These infants experience recurrent pneumonias, leading to interstitial fibrosis and eventually pulmonary hypertension, which causes death in infancy or early childhood. They also frequently have associated cardiac anomalies and other systemic malformations that result in high mortality.

In Poland's syndrome, a variant of the pectus abnormalities, there is a variable combination of absence of the pectoralis major and minor muscles, ipsilateral breast hypoplasia, absence or hypoplasia of the nipple, and absence or posterior displacement of the segments of two to four ribs in association with shortened or webbed fingers of the ipsilateral hand (Fig. 34-2). Patients with this syndrome may undergo reconstruction with rib grafts from the contralateral thorax to stabilize the chest wall, followed by muscle-flap transfer, and eventually breast reconstruction during adolescence for females. Absence of the pectoralis muscle also may occur as an isolated defect. Anomalies of the ribs and sternum, particularly the pectus defects often in their most severe form, commonly occur in patients with Marfan syndrome and in association with certain congenital heart defects.

Supernumerary ribs are located most frequently in the cervical region and rarely cause symptoms. In rare cases, an extra rib may arise in the midthoracic level and cause

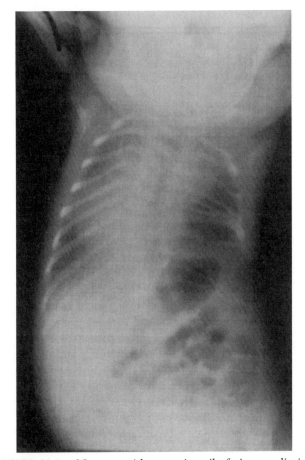

FIGURE 34-1 ■ Neonate with extensive rib fusion, scoliosis, displacement of mediastinal structures, and severe respiratory distress.

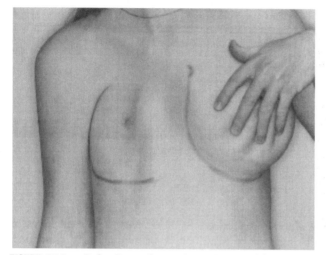

FIGURE 34-2 ■ Poland's syndrome in a 17-year-old girl. This figure shows absence of segments of four ribs of the right side of the chest, breast hypoplasia, and absence of the pectoralis major and minor muscles.

discomfort by pressure on adjacent intercostal nerves; rib resection is curative.

STERNAL DEFECTS

The literature contains numerous case reports describing varieties of cleft sternum under various names. Analysis of the clinical and experimental literature suggests a continuous spectrum of deformities of the sternum, the heart, the pericardium, the diaphragm, and the abdominal wall—which may exist in a variety of combinations, presumably depending on the time, duration, and nature of the injury to the fetus. These defects can be classified in most cases, however, into one of four major categories. First, the *cleft or bifid sternum* is characterized by separation of the sternum but with intact skin overlying the bony defect and with the heart in a normal anatomic position within the thorax. The sternum most frequently is split from the superior aspect but may be divided entirely between the two halves. Second, in *thoracoabdominal ectopia cordis*, the sternum is split, generally from the inferior aspect but with intact skin or an omphalocele membrane overlying the heart, which is displaced in most cases inferiorly into the abdominal cavity through a defect in the diaphragm and pericardium (historically called *Cantrell's pentalogy*, although the entity was well described previously). Third, in *thoracic ectopia cordis*, the heart protrudes through the chest wall with an obvious defect in the sternum and the thoracic soft tissues. Repair of this lesion and the fourth and rarest entity, *cervical ectopia cordis*, in which the heart is displaced superiorly into the neck, is complicated by the severe displacement of the heart out of the chest cavity, which is extremely difficult to cover at the time of repair and closure. The heart does not tolerate being returned into the thoracic cavity because of torsion of the great vessels and pressure on the right ventricle. Intrinsic cardiac anomalies are seen with the latter three lesions. In thoracoabdominal ectopia cordis, the most frequent associated lesions are

tetralogy of Fallot and diverticulum of the left ventricle, which often extends through the defect in the diaphragm into the abdominal cavity. In thoracic ectopia cordis, the most frequent cardiac anomaly is tetralogy of Fallot followed by transposition of the great vessels.

CLEFT STERNUM

Failure of the embryonic sternal bars to meet and fuse in the midline leads to the development of a sternal cleft, also called *bifid sternum* or *congenital sternal fissure*. A simple cleft of the sternum occurs in most cases without other major anomalies. An unexplained association exists between bifid sternum and hemangiomas of the airway.

Most sternal clefts involve the manubrium and extend inferiorly to encompass varying amounts of the sternum. Approximately half of all isolated sternal clefts extend inferiorly to the level of the fourth or fifth rib, one fourth go down to the xiphoid, and the remaining one fourth are complete clefts. Partial isolated clefts are usually superior in location. When inferior clefts occur, they usually are associated with thoracoabdominal ectopia cordis (pentalogy of Cantrell). The configuration of the superior defect varies from that of a broad U shape, occasionally 3 to 6 cm across, which is usually seen in partial clefts, to a narrow U shape, which most often occurs when the cleft extends to the xiphoid. When the sternal cleft is broad, the heart often can be seen to pulsate through the skin.

In bifid sternum, in which the defect is confined to the sternum and is covered with skin, surgical repair may be elective. Repair almost always is performed because of concern about the visibly pulsating heart and the possibility of cardiac injury. These patients are asymptomatic, and except for vulnerability to local injury, the lesion presents no handicap to normal activity. Repair in infancy, when the chest wall is most flexible, has the greatest chance of achieving primary closure. A satisfactory closure of the cleft sternum usually can be obtained without cartilage or bone grafts, by completing the cleft or excising a wedge from its inferior margin, freshening the edges of the defect, and approximating the two sternal halves with interrupted nonabsorbable suture. Undue tension on the suture line and underlying heart may be avoided by making oblique relaxing incisions in the upper three costal cartilages bilaterally.

THORACOABDOMINAL ECTOPIA CORDIS

In thoracoabdominal ectopia cordis, a flat omphalocele may be present on the abdominal wall, and in these infants, repair of the abdominal defect is preferred before infectious complications occur. In these cases, complete repair includes repair of the diaphragmatic defect and closure of the sternal defect and the abdominal wall.

Repair in early infancy is generally recommended if the patient is healthy. Increase in the size of the defect can occur during the first few months of life. With age, the chest wall becomes more rigid and loses the flexibility necessary for repair. Several patients have survived into adulthood with or without surgical repair of the sternal defect but with correction of the associated omphalocele.

Although thoracic and cervical ectopia cordis are generally incompatible with life, thoracoabdominal ectopia with a distal sternal cleft has a much better prognosis.

PECTUS EXCAVATUM

Pectus excavatum, or funnel chest, is a congenital malformation of the anterior thorax characterized by a prominent depression of the body of the sternum, usually involving its lower half to two thirds, with its deepest point just above the junction with the xiphoid (Fig. 34-3). The lower costal cartilages bend posteriorly to form a depression, the lateral borders of which usually are angled more sharply than the superior and inferior portions of the deformity. The first and second ribs, corresponding costal cartilages, and manubrium are essentially normal. Asymmetric deformities are common, with the concavity usually being deeper on the right side and the sternum rotated posteriorly slightly to the right. The most common configuration is a symmetric depression involving the lower half of the sternum extending laterally almost to the costochondral junctions. The chest wall characteristically has a decreased anteroposterior diameter.

Pathology

The pathogenesis of pectus excavatum is unclear, but it has no relation to the formation of rickets. A band of tissue may retract the sternum posteriorly; however, this concept is not supported by operative findings or by the therapeutic ineffectiveness of simple retrosternal dissection. It has been suggested that the musculature in the anterior half of the diaphragm is deficient and that its fibrous contracture causes the defect. A more recent theory is that the deformity results from unbalanced overgrowth in the costochondral regions, further explaining the occasional asymmetric appearance; frequent association with other defects of osteogenesis and chondrogenesis; and existence of a completely opposite type of deformity, pectus carinatum, in family members. The involved cartilages are often fused, bizarrely deformed, or rotated. Resected cartilage segments occasionally show a disorderly arrangement of cartilage cells, perichondritis, and areas of aseptic necrosis.

Clinical Features

Pectus excavatum is inherited through either parent, although not clearly as a recessive trait. The anomaly is believed to occur in 1 in 400 births but is uncommon in blacks and Hispanics. Other malformations may coexist, especially musculoskeletal anomalies, including scoliosis (approximately 20%), clubfoot, syndactylism, Marfan syndrome, and Klippel-Feil syndrome. The deformity is usually apparent soon after birth, progresses during childhood, and becomes even more pronounced in early adolescence. Deep inspiration tends to accentuate the deformity. Regression rarely occurs spontaneously.

Symptoms are infrequent during early childhood, apart from a shy awareness of the abnormality and a typical unwillingness to expose the chest while swimming or taking part in other social or athletic activities. Easy fatigability and decreased stamina and endurance often become apparent during early adolescence when children become involved in competitive sports. When the deformity is moderate to severe, the heart is considerably displaced into the left side of the chest, and pulmonary expansion during inspiration is moderately confined, resulting

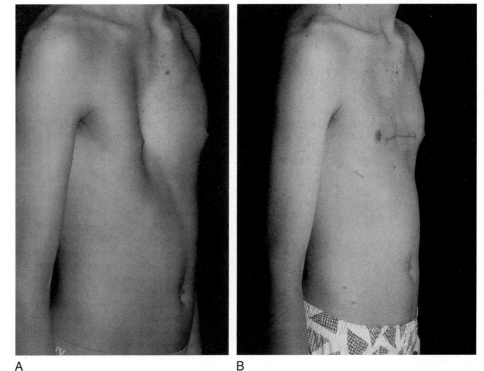

FIGURE 34-3 ■ **A,** Moderately severe pectus excavatum deformity in a 14-year-old boy. **B,** Same patient after repair of the pectus deformity with a retrosternal strut.

A

B

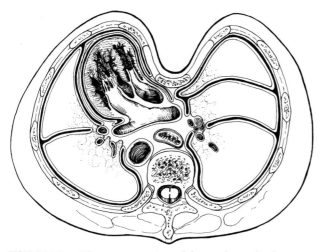

FIGURE 34-4 ■ Transverse section of thorax shows displacement of the heart into the left side of the chest by the lower sternum in a child with moderate pectus excavatum deformity.

in a "restrictive defect" on pulmonary function tests (Fig. 34-4). Many of these patients have an asthenic habitus, poor posture, and a relaxed protuberant abdomen. The xiphoid may be bifid, twisted, elongated, or displaced to one side.

A few methods of grading anterior thoracic deformities have been proposed, although none has been widely accepted. Most include some measurement of the distance between the sternum and the spine as a primary factor. Transverse and anteroposterior measurements obtained from computed tomography of the chest, as used by Haller, are accurate; however, this method is costly, and in our experience is rarely necessary because similar measurements can be obtained from standard chest radiographs. One alternative technique for objective assessment of the deformity, which can be applied to children of all ages, is based on a deformity grade obtained from several measurements taken from posterior-anterior and lateral chest radiographs. Surgical repair was recommended for patients beyond infancy with an inflexible deformity and a severity rating of approximately 5 on a scale of 1 to 10 in a series reported by Welch. Commonly the deformity worsens with the growth spurt that occurs in early adolescence.

Standard chest radiographs usually show the heart to be displaced into the left side of the chest. Electrocardiographic abnormalities are common, consisting primarily of right-axis deviation and depressed ST segments caused by rotation of the heart within the thorax and not an intrinsic abnormality of the heart. Echocardiograms may show mitral valve prolapse, especially in patients with Marfan syndrome; mitral valve prolapse is rarely of clinical concern. A functional systolic cardiac murmur is often present along the upper left sternal border, in most cases caused by the close proximity between the sternum and the aorta and pulmonary artery.

Conventional pulmonary function tests are almost always normal or show mild restrictive defect in children with pectus excavatum. It is difficult to obtain reliable measurements in patients younger than 7 years old.

Derveaux and colleagues evaluated 88 patients with pectus excavatum and carinatum with pulmonary funtion tests before and 1 to 20 years after repair (mean 8 years) by a method that involved fairly extensive chest wall dissection.

Preoperative studies were normal (>80% of predicted) except in subjects with scoliosis and pectus excavatum. The postoperative values for forced expiratory volume in 1 second and vital capacity were decreased in all groups when expressed as a percentage of predicted, although the absolute values at follow-up may have been greater than at preoperative evaluation. Radiographic evaluation of these individuals confirmed improved chest wall configuration, suggesting that the relative deterioration in pulmonary function was not the result of recurrence of the pectus deformity. An inverse relationship was found between preoperative and postoperative function. Individuals with less than 75% of predicted function had improved function after operation, whereas results were worse after operation if the preoperative values were greater than 75% of predicted. Almost identical results were found in a study by Morshuis and colleagues, who evaluated 152 patients before and at a mean follow-up of 8 years after operation for pectus excavatum. These physiologic results were in contrast to the subjective improvement in symptoms from the subjects and the improved chest wall configuration. The decline in pulmonary function in the postoperative studies was attributed to the operation because the preoperative defect seemed to be stable regardless of the age at initial repair. Both of these studies were limited by the lack of an age-matched and severity-matched control group without surgery. Kaguraoka and colleagues evaluated pulmonary function in 138 individuals before and after operation for pectus excavatum. A decrease in the vital capacity occurred during the initial 2 months after operation, with recovery to preoperative levels by 1 year after surgery. At 42 months, the values were maintained at baseline despite a significant improvement in the chest wall configuration. These studies and many more performed since the 1960s have failed to document consistent improvement in pulmonary function resulting from surgical repair despite reported symptomatic improvement. Several of the more recent studies have shown deterioration in pulmonary function at long-term evaluation attributable to increased chest wall rigidity after operation. Despite this finding, workload studies have shown improvement in exercise tolerance after repair and are probably the best studies to identify preoperative cardiopulmonary deficits. The latter statement suggests that cardiac restriction may be more the issue than pulmonary functional impairment.

Measurements of cardiac output using right ventricular catheterization have shown diminished cardiac output in preoperative patients during upright exercise. These findings are not demonstrable in patients tested supine without exercise and account for the erroneous reports of no physiologic impairment in these patients. Routine stress testing in a few hospitals has shown abnormal cardiovascular or respiratory parameters in more than 20% of patients. Angiocardiograms may show compression of the right ventricular outflow tract and right ventricle. In occasional patients, this compression is reflected physiologically in right ventricular catheterization measurements and pressure waves similar to those of constrictive pericarditis. In these selective cases, after surgical repair, cardiac output during intensive upright exercise has increased by an average of 38%, and the hemodynamic response to mild exercise has changed toward normal.

Studies by Cahill and associates using the cycle ergometer to evaluate exercise performance in children of various ages, before and after pectus repair, have shown a significant improvement in maximal voluntary ventilation. Exercise performance was improved as measured by total exercise time and by maximal oxygen consumption. After repair, the patient showed a slower heart rate and higher minute ventilation compared with preoperative values. These observations support the hypothesis that a restricted cardiac stroke volume and the increased work of breathing described in several pectus excavatum patients may be ameliorated by operative repair of the anomaly, improving exercise tolerance in some patients, but postoperative testing in many cases fails to establish which parameter has improved the level of symptomatic function.

Treatment

Because almost all young children with pectus excavatum deformities are asymptomatic, the selection of patients for surgical correction requires good clinical judgment. In the past, many pediatric surgeons recommended that children with moderate-to-severe depression of the sternum should undergo surgical repair between ages 2 and 4 years. This decision was based on the fact that the repair can be performed far more readily at this age than in adolescence or later life. Mild-to-moderate deformities unlikely ever to require repair are not treated during this period. Although it may be difficult to determine the severity of a depression anomaly shortly after birth, many chest wall defects are well defined after age 1 year. Early repair of pectus excavatum by techniques that resect the costal cartilage is discouraged now, however, since the report by Haller that described children developing an acquired thoracic constricting deformity of the chest after repair in early childhood. Most surgeons performing surgery using a technique that involves resection of the costal cartilages currently wait until the children are older, at least 6 to 8 years old, or into their adolescent growth spurt. Some surgeons prefer to delay repair until the chest has achieved full growth. Older children and young adults are still candidates for operative correction.

Surgical repair for pectus excavatum involves various modifications of the original procedure described by Brown and modified by Ravitch and Welch or by a more recent innovation by Nuss of minimally invasive correction of the deformity without costal cartilage resection. Maintenance of the elevated sternum in the corrected position by external traction almost universally has been abandoned in favor of various methods of internal fixation. Internal sternal support after repair of excavatum deformities minimizes the occurrence of postoperative respiratory distress caused by paradoxical chest wall motion and maximizes the extent to which the defect is corrected.

The standard operative technique requires general endotracheal anesthesia with the patient supine. A transverse incision in the inframammary crease provides adequate exposure to the upper sternum (Fig. 34-5). Cutaneous and pectoralis muscle flaps are elevated with electrocautery to expose the depressed portion of the sternum and the abnormal costal cartilages. The lower five costal cartilages are resected, with preservation of the perichondrial sheaths (Figs. 34-6 and 34-7). The xiphoid is divided from its attachment to the sternum if it is angled anteriorly and would protrude when the position of the sternum is corrected. In most cases, the attachments of the inferior costal cartilages and intercostal muscles to the sternum can be preserved, and this avoids a defect at the base of the sternum (see Fig. 34-7). A transverse wedge osteotomy is performed through the anterior table of the sternum with an osteotome or a Hall air drill at the level of the cephalad transition from the normal to the depressed sternum, usually at the level of insertion of the second or third costal cartilages (Fig. 34-8). The posterior table of the sternum is fractured by upward traction on the sternum, and the lower sternum is elevated

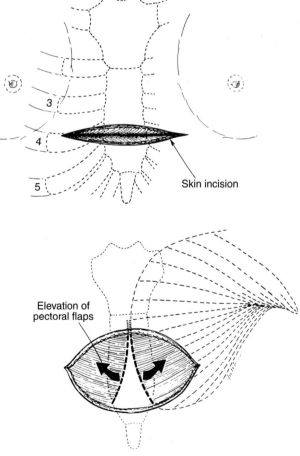

FIGURE 34-5 ■ Surgical technique for repair of pectus excavatum. A transverse incision is placed below and well within the nipple lines and, in females, at the site of the future inframammary crease. The pectoralis major muscle is elevated from the sternum along with portions of the pectoralis minor and serratus anterior bundles.

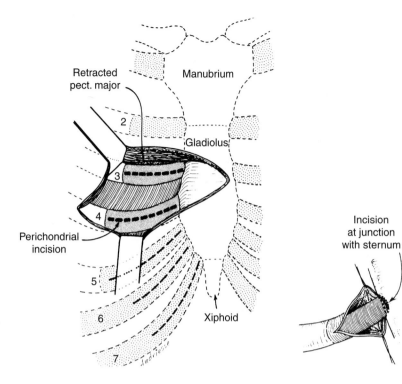

Retracted
pect. major

Manubrium

2

Gladiolus

3

4

Perichondrial
incision

5

6

Xiphoid

7

Andriesse

Incision
at junction
with sternum

FIGURE 34-6 ■ Subperichondrial resection of the costal cartilages is achieved by incising the perichondrium anteriorly. It is dissected away from the costal cartilages in the bloodless plane between perichondrium and costal cartilage. Cutting back the perichondrium 90 degrees in each direction at its junction with the sternum (inset) facilitates visualization of the back wall of the costal cartilage.

to the desired position where it is secured (Fig. 34-9). In the past, many surgeons used only sutures through the osteotomy site to hold the sternum anteriorly, but currently, most surgeons use a retrosternal bar to fix the body of the sternum securely in its corrected position (Figs. 34-10 and 34-11). A stainless steel Adkins support bar is placed transversely under the sternum across the anterior chest, where it is attached on each side to the rib just lateral to the costochondral junction at such a level that the inferiormost portion of the sternum is given maximal support. Patients in whom extensive cartilage resection has been performed and a long segment of sternum mobilized inferior to the transverse osteotomy experience considerable posterior leverage on the bar, and suture fixation is inadequate in these cases. The support bar generally is removed 6 months postoperatively,

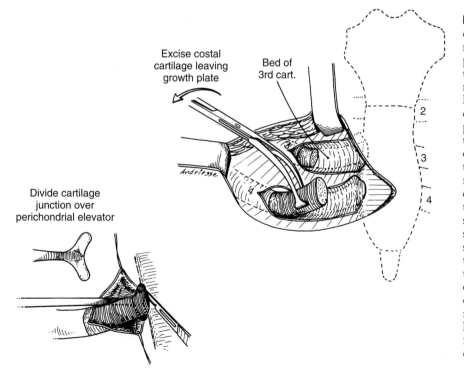

Excise costal
cartilage leaving
growth plate

Bed of
3rd cart.

2

3

4

Andriesse

Divide cartilage
junction over
perichondrial elevator

FIGURE 34-7 ■ The cartilages (cart.) are divided at their junction with the sternum with a knife having a Welch perichondrial elevator held posteriorly to elevate the cartilage and protect the mediastinum (inset). The divided cartilage can be held with an Allis clamp and elevated. The costochondral junction is preserved with a segment of costal cartilage on the osseous ribs by incising the cartilage with a scalpel. Costal cartilages three through seven generally are resected, but occasionally the second costal cartilages must be removed if posterior displacement or funneling of the sternum extends to this level, as may be seen in older patients. Segments of the sixth and seventh cartilages are resected to the point where they flatten to join the costal arch. Familiarity with the cross-sectional shape of the medial ends of the costal cartilages facilitates their removal. The second and third cartilages are broad and flat, the fourth and fifth are circular, and the sixth and seventh are narrow and deep.

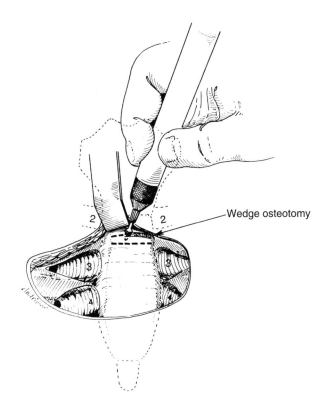

FIGURE 34-8 ■ The sternal osteotomy is created above the level of the last deformed cartilage and the posterior angulation of the sternum, generally the third cartilage but occasionally the second. Two transverse sternal osteotomies are created through the anterior cortex with a Hall air drill (ConMed Corp, Utica, NY) 2 to 4 mm apart.

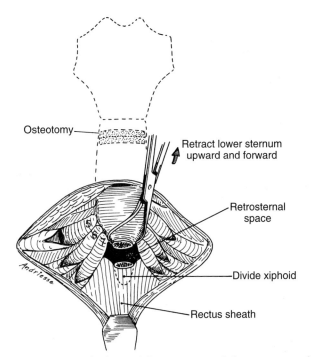

FIGURE 34-9 ■ The base of the sternum and the rectus muscle flap are elevated with two towel clips, and the posterior plate of the sternum is fractured. The xiphoid can be divided from the sternum with electrocautery, allowing entry into the retrosternal space. This step is not necessary with the use of a retrosternal strut. Preservation of the attachment of the perichondrial sheaths and xiphoid avoids an unsightly depression that can occur below the sternum.

FIGURE 34-10 ■ Use of retrosternal struts and Rehbein struts. Rehbein struts are inserted into the marrow cavity (inset) of the third or fourth rib, and the struts are joined medially to create an arch anterior to the sternum. The sternum is sewn to the arch to secure it in its new anterior position. The retrosternal strut is placed behind the sternum and is secured to the rib ends laterally to prevent migration.

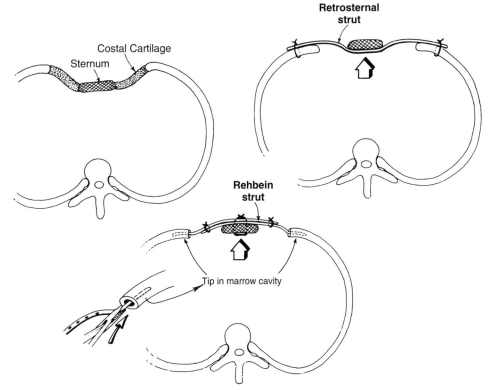

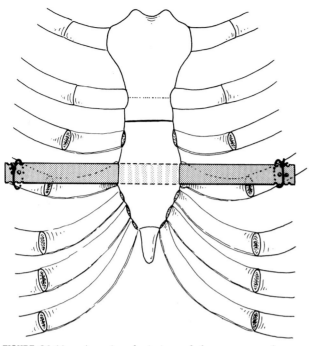

FIGURE 34-11 ■ Anterior depiction of the retrosternal struts. The perichondrial sheath to either the third or the fourth rib is divided from its junction with the sternum, and the retrosternal space is bluntly dissected to allow passage of the strut behind the sternum. It is secured with two pericostal sutures laterally to prevent migration. The wound is flooded with warm saline and cefazolin solution to remove clots and inspect for a pleural entry. A single-limb medium Hemovac drain (Snyder Laboratories, Inc, New Philadelphia, OH) is brought through the inferior skin flap to the left of the sternum and placed in a parasternal position to the level of the highest resected costal cartilage.

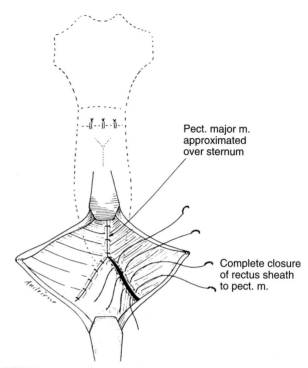

FIGURE 34-12 ■ The pectoral muscle (pect. m.) flaps are secured to the midline of the sternum, advancing the flaps to obtain coverage of the entire sternum. The rectus muscle is joined to the pectoral muscle flaps, closing the mediastinum. (From Shamberger RC, Welch KJ: Surgical repair of pectus excavatum. J Pediatr Surg 23:615, 1988.)

using a general anesthetic, on an outpatient basis. Various malleable metallic wires, metal strips, and segments of autologous rib have been used successfully by other workers to provide sternal support.

Care is taken to maintain a good blood supply to the lower sternum and to avoid complete transection at the site of the transverse osteotomy to prevent necrosis of the distal segment. The wound is drained by a Silastic drain placed below the muscle flaps (Fig. 34-12). Using this technique, correction of the deformity can be achieved, transfusion is rarely required, and postoperative complications are limited.

Frequent deep inspirations and incentive spirometry are encouraged during the early postoperative period to minimize the occurrence of atelectasis. Hospitalization, regardless of the patient's age, is usually 2 to 3 days and rarely longer than 4 to 5 days postoperatively. The chest should be protected from direct trauma for 4 to 6 weeks, after which it becomes a solid structure.

Patients may return to full physical activity, including body contact sports, after the strut is removed. Periosteal regeneration of new cartilage and healing of the sternal fracture is usually complete within 2 months after surgery and provides a rigid support for the chest wall. Because the pectoralis muscles are reconstructed after elevation from the anterior chest wall during the repair, extensive physical activity using the pectoralis muscles should be deferred for at least 2 to 3 months postoperatively.

There is virtually no mortality associated with repair of pectus excavatum or pectus carinatum deformities. Pneumothorax occurs in less than 10% of patients and is often so minimal that it requires no treatment. The substernal support bar may migrate slightly and become visible in the subcutaneous tissues but is rarely problematic.

Although there is a slight tendency for pectus excavatum deformities to recur during adolescence, this happens in less than 5% to 10% of patients when autogenous or prosthetic sternal supports are used during the repair. Repair during the adolescent growth spurt also may decrease the opportunity in which recurrence can occur. There is a propensity for older children to develop hypertrophic scar in these repairs, but these scars can be treated with intralesional triamcinolone.

A method of elevation of the sternum with a retrosternal bar without resection or division of the costal cartilages has been reported by Nuss and associates. These authors repaired pectus excavatum in 42 patients younger than 15 years of age (median age 4 years) by placing a convex steel bar under the sternum and anterior to the heart through small bilateral thoracic incisions on the lateral aspect of the chest. As initially described, a long clamp was passed blindly behind the sternum and out the contralateral opening. A tape was drawn across and used to pull the bar through the chest. The bar initially is placed with the concave side anteriorly, then it is rotated once in position (Fig. 34-13).

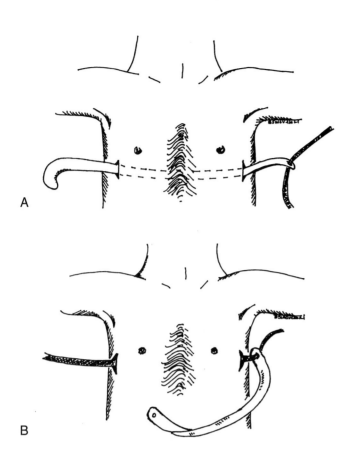

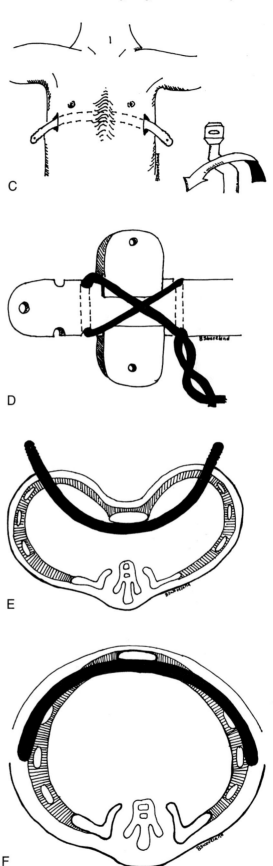

FIGURE 34-13 ■ Nuss procedure for elevation of the sternum. **A,** A long Lorenz (Walter Lorenz Surgical, Inc, Jacksonville, FL) tunneler is passed across the chest behind the sternum and anterior to the heart. **B,** An umbilical tape is drawn back across the chest with the device, and to it is secured the convex steel Lorenz bar, which is guided into the substernal tunnel using the umbilical tape to keep it on track. **C,** The Lorenz bar is shown with its convex aspect directed posteriorly. It is rotated 180 degrees with a special device, the Lorenz Flipper, compressing the sternum anteriorly. **D,** A stainless steel cross-piece is secured to each end of the bar with a heavy No. 3 wire. When it is wired together, the whole apparatus is sutured to the soft tissues of the chest with multiple sutures to achieve secure fixation to the chest wall to prevent rotation of the bar and loss of correction of the deformity or side-to-side movement of the bar. The entrance of the bar under the rib is at the inner aspect of the pectus ridge. **E,** Schematic depiction of the Lorenz bar after placement. **F,** Depiction after rotation 180 degrees producing anterior displacement of the sternum and costal cartilages. (Reproduced with permission from Donald Nuss, MD, Children's Hospital of the King's Daughters, Norfolk, VA.)

The bar is left in position for 2 years before removal when presumed permanent remodeling of the cartilages has occurred. Although Nuss in his initial report warned that the "upper limits of age for this procedure require further evaluation," the technique has been used widely in older patients; long-term results from this population have not been reported yet, however.

A modification adopted by many surgeons as reported by Hebra and associates involves the use of thoracoscopy to visualize passage of the clamp behind the sternum. This change followed an instance of cardiac perforation occurring during blind passage of the clamp. Other surgeons elevate the sternum with a bone hook during passage of the clamp to open the retrosternal space anterior to the heart.

Molik and associates reported a series of 35 patients treated with the Nuss technique compared with 68 patients treated with a standard open technique. Although the length of the operative procedure was shortened, a significant amount of pain occurred in older patients undergoing the Nuss procedure compared with patients receiving an open repair. The patients had an average hospital stay of 4.0 days for the standard repair and 4.8 days for the Nuss repair. Complications encountered in the series were more frequent in the cohort receiving the Nuss repair and included rotation of the bar, production of a marked pectus carinatum deformity in one instance, persistent chest wall asymmetry, and chronic pain requiring removal of the bar. Bar rotation is avoided using lateral stabilizers. After a procedural learning period, complications will lessen. These authors concluded, "long-term follow-up also will be required to assure both health professionals and the public which is the procedure of choice for patients with pectus excavatum." Children should be followed long-term after repair by any technique until they reach full stature, at which time recurrence should be a rare event.

PECTUS CARINATUM

Protrusion deformities of the anterior chest wall are approximately 10 times less frequent than depression deformities. Associated disorders, including congenital heart disease, marfanoid habitus, scoliosis, kyphosis, and musculoskeletal defects, are as frequent as in patients with pectus excavatum. The deformity typically is mild or almost imperceptible in early childhood and becomes increasingly prominent during the rapid growth in early adolescence.

Pathology

Pectus carinatum is believed to stem from an overgrowth of costal cartilages, with forward buckling and secondary deforming pressure on the gladiolus or body of the sternum (Fig. 34-14). Carinatum deformities are more variable than excavatum anomalies, with two principal forms. One form is termed *chondromanubrial*, in which the protuberance is maximal in the upper portion of the sternum, and the gladiolus is directed posteriorly so that an apparent saucerization type of compression is evident. The second and more common form, termed *chondrogladiolar*, shows the greatest prominence in the lower portion or body

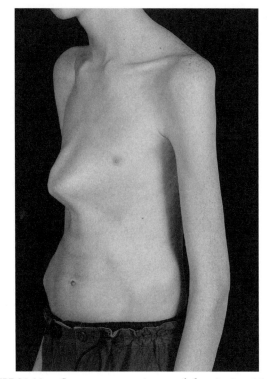

FIGURE 34-14 ■ Severe pectus carinatum deformity in a 15-year-old boy.

of the sternum. Minor forms of the anomaly may be more frequent, in which one, or occasionally two, costal cartilages may buckle outward, usually at the level of the manubrium but without sternal deformity. Persistent discomfort in the protruding cartilage may warrant local subperiosteal resection.

Clinical Features

In most cases, pectus carinatum produces no symptoms beyond local tenderness or pain in the protruding portion of the chest. No studies have shown a pulmonary or cardiac abnormality resulting from this deformity, in contrast to pectus excavatum. In some case, its association with scoliosis or kyphosis results in pulmonary abnormalities, however. Various chest deformities occur in other family members in approximately one quarter of these patients, and other musculoskeletal abnormalities are seen in 20% of patients.

Treatment

Considerable variation in surgical treatment is necessary because of the diversity of carinatum deformities. The same exposure is used as for the excavatum deformities, with resection of the more severely involved costal cartilages while preserving the perichondrium intact. The transverse osteotomy across the anterior table of the upper sternum is filled with a wedge of costal cartilage to secure it in a more downward position with transsternal sutures that cover the deformity. The remainder of the repair is similar to that used for excavatum deformities. Asymmetric protrusion deformities may require unilateral costal cartilage resection with resection of the anterior table of one side of the sternum. Some surgeons prefer the Ravitch repair, in which the involved cartilages are resected, but sternal osteotomy is not performed. The perichondrial sheaths are reefed up by a series of sutures pulling the sternum down and correcting the protrusion.

Complications after surgical repair of carinatum deformities are uncommon and resemble complications in patients with depression anomalies. The long-term results after surgery are more dramatic than results after excavatum repair.

COMMENT

This chapter presents several approaches to the management of chest wall deformities. Careful testing generally reveals that most patients with pectus excavatum have cardiopulmonary deficits and that surgery is indicated to improve physiologic function.

Treatment philosophies vary widely. Many believe that in most instances chest wall abnormalities produce cosmetic rather than physiologic problems. These surgeons operate to improve the appearance of the chest because the deformity interferes with the child's self-image and psychosocial development. They further believe that in a smaller number of cases there is severe compression and displacement of cardiac and pulmonary tissue resulting in significant physiologic abnormalities. Only in these cases, they believe, is surgery necessary to improve cardiopulmonary function. In some patients with Marfan syndrome, cardiac surgeons have requested repair of the defects before cardiac surgery. In a few cases, combined cardiac procedures and concomitant repair of the chest wall deformity have been performed successfully.

SUGGESTED READINGS

Beiser GD, Epstein SE, Stampfer M, et al: Impairment of cardiac function in patients with pectus excavatum with improvement after operative correction. N Engl J Med 287:267-272, 1972.

This is a well-documented review of the physiologic changes in cardiac function caused by pectus excavatum and the improvement resulting from repair.

Derveaux L, Clarysse I, Ivanoff I, et al: Preoperative and postoperative abnormalities in chest x-ray indices and in lung function in pectus deformities. Chest 95:850-856, 1989.

This is one of several reports that provides less than convincing evidence of pulmonary improvement after surgical correction of pectus excavatum.

Haller JA Jr, Colombani PM, Humphries CT, et al: Chest wall constriction after too extensive and too early operations for pectus excavatum. Ann Thorac Surg 61:1618-1624, 1996.

This is the seminal article that raised concerns regarding early repair for pectus excavatum and delayed impairment in chest wall growth.

Kaguraoka H, Ohnuki T, Itaoka T, et al: Degree of severity of pectus excavatum and pulmonary function in preoperative and postoperative periods. J Thorac Cardiovasc Surg 104:1483-1488, 1992.

The authors showed an inverse relationship between improvement in pulmonary abnormalities and initial impairment in pulmonary function.

Molik KA, Engum SA, Rescorla FJ, et al: Pectus excavatum repair: Experience with standard and minimal invasive techniques. J Pediatr Surg 36:324-328, 2001.

This is one of the first reports to compare the minimally invasive technique with the standard open technique in older children and adolescents and identifies some of the problems with its use in older patients.

Morshuis WJ, Folgering HT, Barentsz JO, et al: Exercise cardiorespiratory function before and one year after operation for pectus excavatum. J Thorac Cardiovasc Surg 107:1403-1409, 1994.

This excellent study evaluates cardiopulmonary function in pectus excavatum.

Nuss D, Kelly RE Jr, Croitoru DP, et al: A 10-year review of a minimally invasive technique for the correction of pectus excavatum. J Pediatr Surg 33:545-552, 1998.

This is the first description of a "minimally invasive technique" for repair of pectus excavatum in young children.

Shamberger RC: Congenital chest wall deformities. Curr Probl Surg 33:469-552, 1996.

A comprehensive discussion of chest wall deformities is presented.

Shamberger RC, Welch KJ: Sternal defects. Pediatr Surg Int 5:156-164, 1990.

This article presents a compilation of the world's experience in sternal defects and ectopia cordis.

35

Chylothorax

Effusion of chylous fluid into the thorax may occur spontaneously in newborns and usually is attributed to congenital abnormalities of the thoracic ducts or trauma from delivery. The occurrence of chylothorax in most cases cannot be related to the type of labor or delivery, and lymphatic effusions may be discovered prenatally.

Chylothorax in older children is rarely spontaneous and occurs almost invariably after trauma or cardiothoracic surgery; however, some patients with thoracic lymphangioma may present in this older age group. Operative injury may be in part a result of anatomic variations of the thoracic duct. Neoplasms, particularly lymphomas and neuroblastomas, occasionally have been noted to cause obstruction of the thoracic duct. Lymphangiomatosis or diffuse lymphangiectasia may produce chylous effusion in the pleural space and peritoneal cavity. Extensive bouts of coughing have been reported to cause rupture of the thoracic duct, which is particularly vulnerable when full after a fatty meal. Other causes include mediastinal inflammation, subclavian vein or superior vena caval thrombosis, and misplaced central venous catheters.

PATHOPHYSIOLOGY

The thoracic duct develops from outgrowths of the jugular lymphatic sacs and the cisterna chyli. During embryonic life, bilateral thoracic lymphatic channels are present, each attached in the neck to the corresponding jugular sac. As development progresses, the upper third of the right duct and the lower two thirds of the left duct involute and close. The wide variation in the final anatomic structure of the main ductal system attests to the multiple communications of the small vessels comprising the lymphatic system. The thoracic duct originates in the abdomen at the cisterna chyli located over L2 (Fig. 35-1). The duct extends into the thorax through the aortic hiatus, then passes upward into the posterior mediastinum on the right before shifting toward the left at the level of T5. It then ascends posterior to the aortic arch and into the posterior neck to the junction of the subclavian and internal jugular veins.

Many variations are present in the entire ductal system, and the typical course of the thoracic duct is present in only approximately 50% of individuals. The most common variations are a double system originating from the cisterna or a multiple ductal pattern at the level of the diaphragm. In the chest, a rich collateral system originates from intercostal spaces, the posterior mediastinum, and visceral lymphatics, which communicate freely with the main duct via collecting trunks.

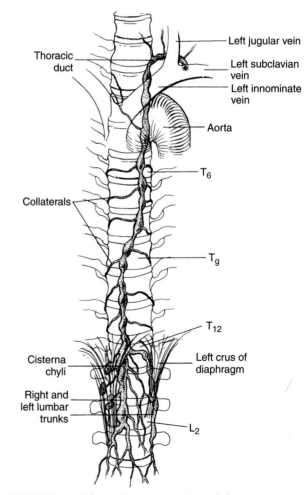

FIGURE 35-1 ■ Schematic representation of the most common anatomic arrangement of the thoracic duct.

The thoracic duct contains smooth muscle in the wall that is capable of contracting with sufficient force to propel lymph upward toward the jugular venous junction at a rate of 50 to 200 mL/hr in the fasting state. The rate of lymph flow in the thoracic duct varies widely and relates to the volume of fat ingestion, scar tissue in the mediastinum, presence of portal hypertension, and other factors. The flow of chyle superiorly into the subclavian vein is enhanced by the presence of valves in the thoracic duct, the portal pressure, and the differential gradient between the negative intrapleural pressure and the positive intra-abdominal pressure.

The chyle contained in the thoracic duct conveys approximately three fourths of the ingested fat from the intestine to the systemic circulation. The fat content of chyle varies from 0.4 to 4.0 g/dL. The large fat molecules absorbed from the intestinal lacteals flow through the cisterna chyli and superiorly through the thoracic duct. Total protein content of thoracic duct lymph is also high. When chyle leaks through a thoracic duct fistula, considerable fat and lymphocytes may be lost. The thoracic duct also carries white blood cells, primarily lymphocytes (T cells)—approximately 2000 to 20,000 cells per milliliter. Eosinophils also are present in higher proportion than in circulating blood. Loss of lymphocytes through a thoracic duct fistula may lead to an immunocompromised state; external drainage of the thoracic duct was used as an adjunct to immunosuppression in the early era of organ transplantation. Chyle seems to have a bacteriostatic property, which accounts for the rare occurrence of infection complicating chylothorax.

CLINICAL MANIFESTATIONS

Birth trauma formerly was thought to be the cause of many neonatal chylothoraces, but the increasing use of prenatal ultrasonography has changed this perspective. Noniatrogenic chylothorax occurring in young children usually is related to congenital anomalies of the chyliferous vessels, cisterna chyli, or the thoracic duct itself. Most of these chylothoraces result from intrapleural leakage from dilated and thin-walled intercostal, diaphragmatic, or accessory mediastinal lymphatics. When there is lymphatic overload, these alternate lymphatics may dilate considerably eventually to become transudative lymphatic varices. In other cases, subpleural lymphatics may rupture into the pleural cavity, as in certain cardiac anomalies (e.g., total anomalous pulmonary venous return).

The accumulation of chyle in the pleural space from a thoracic duct leak may occur rapidly and produce pressure on other structures in the chest, causing acute respiratory distress, dyspnea, and cyanosis with tachypnea. In the fetus, a pleural effusion may be secondary to generalized hydrops, but a primary lymphatic effusion (idiopathic; secondary to subpleural lymphangiectasia or pulmonary sequestration; or associated with Down syndrome, Turner's syndrome, and Noonan's syndrome) can cause mediastinal shift and result in hydrops or lead to pulmonary hypoplasia. Postnatally the effects of chylothorax and the prolonged loss of chyle may include malnutrition, hypoproteinemia, fluid and electrolyte imbalance, metabolic acidosis, and immunodeficiency.

In a neonate, symptoms of respiratory embarrassment observed in combination with a pleural effusion strongly suggest chylothorax. The involved side presents characteristic findings of intrapleural fluid with respiratory lag, flatness on percussion, diminished breath sounds, and shift of the mediastinum. Fever is uncommon. Chest radiographs typically show massive fluid effusion in the ipsilateral chest with pulmonary compression and mediastinal shift. Bilateral effusions also may occur. Aspiration of the pleural effusion reveals clear straw-colored fluid in the fasting patient, which becomes milky after feedings. Analysis of the chyle generally reveals a total fat content of more than 400 mg/dL and a protein content of more than 5 g/dL. In a fetus or a fasting neonate, the most useful and simple test is to perform a complete cell count and differential on the fluid; when lymphocytes exceed 80% or 90% of the white blood cells, a lymphatic effusion is confirmed. The differential can be compared with that obtained from the peripheral blood count, in which lymphocytes rarely represent more than 70% of white blood cells.

Most cases of traumatic chylothorax develop after thoracic operations, in particular, repair of patent ductus arteriosus, coarctation of the aorta, Fontan procedure, and Blalock-Taussig shunt. Injury to the thoracic duct in the left chest is particularly common during secondary thoracotomies for correction of lesions in the descending aorta or esophagus just inferior to the arch. If lymphatic drainage is noted at operation, the proximal and distal ends of the thoracic duct should be ligated.

As chyle accumulates in the pleural space from a thoracic duct leak, progressively more pronounced respiratory symptoms develop as pulmonary compression becomes more severe. Dyspnea, tachypnea, and eventually arterial desaturation with cyanosis can develop. Nutritional deficiency is a late manifestation of chyle depletion and occurs when dietary intake is insufficient to replace the thoracic duct fluid loss.

THERAPY

Thoracentesis may be sufficient to relieve spontaneous chylothorax in some infants; however, chest tube drainage is necessary for most infants. Tube drainage allows quantification of the daily chyle leak and promotes pulmonary re-expansion, which may enhance healing. Chylothorax in newborns usually ceases spontaneously. Because identifying the site of the fluid leak is difficult, surgery often is deferred for several weeks. Similarly, most cases of traumatic injury to the thoracic duct can be managed successfully by chest tube drainage and replacement of the protein and fat loss. If drainage persists in quantities beyond the tolerance of the infant or child and shows no evidence of diminishing, or if it persists after 2 to 3 weeks without decreasing, thoracotomy and ligation of the thoracic duct on the side of the effusion may be necessary. Standard contrast lymphangiography or isotope lymphangiography using technetium-99m colloid may be helpful in identifying the site of the fistula.

Occasionally the chylous fluid may enter the pericardial sac and cause chylopericardial tamponade, in which case pericardiocentesis should provide immediate relief; then a pericardial window can be made. Although bilateral spontaneous chylothorax in newborns is rare, it can produce fatal respiratory distress unless recognized and drained promptly.

Although small quantities of short-chain fatty acids are absorbed through the portal venous circulation, 80% to 90% of all fat absorbed from the gut is transported by way of the thoracic duct in the form of chylomicrons. Feedings restricted to medium-chain or short-chain triglycerides theoretically result in reduced lymph flow in the thoracic duct and may enhance spontaneous healing of a thoracic duct fistula. It has been shown, however, that any enteral feeding, even with clear fluids, greatly increases thoracic duct flow. For patients who experience large chylous fluid losses, withholding oral feedings and providing total parenteral nutrition is preferred. Cultures of chylous fluid are rarely positive; providing long-term antibiotics during the full course of chest tube drainage is not necessary.

When chylothorax remains resistant despite prolonged chest tube drainage, total parenteral nutrition, and somatostatin therapy, thoracotomy on the ipsilateral side may be necessary. The decision whether to continue with conservative management or to undertake surgical intervention should be based on the nature of the underlying disorder, the duration of the fistula, the daily volume of fluid drainage, and the severity of nutritional depletion or immunologic depletion or both. Ingestion of cream before surgery may facilitate identification of the thoracic duct and the fistula. When identified, the draining lymphatic vessel should be suture ligated above and below the leak with reinforcement by a pleural or intercostal muscle flap. The repair can be assessed by 30 seconds of lung hyperinflation. Meticulous dissection of the thoracic duct with isolation of the fistula is rarely feasible. When a leak cannot be identified with certainty or when multiple leaks originate from the mediastinum, ligation of all the tissues surrounding the aorta at the level of the hiatus provides the best results. Fibrin glue and argon-beam coagulation also have been used for ill-defined areas of leakage or incompletely resected lymphangiomas.

Thoracoscopy may be used occasionally to avoid thoracotomy. The leak, if visualized, can be ligated, cauterized, or sealed with fibrin glue. If the leak cannot be identified, pleurodesis can be done with talc or other sclerotic agents under direct vision through the thoracoscope, but this technique probably should be avoided in infants because of the consequences on lung and chest wall growth. If there is concomitant chylopericardium, a pericardial window can be fashioned. Because thoracoscopy is less invasive, some surgeons advocate early intervention (5 to 10 days). This approach may be indicated in conditions in which the failure rate of conservative management is higher, such as superior vena cava thrombosis or problems associated with increased right heart pressures.

Pleural peritoneal shunts have been used for refractory chylothorax in which a leak has not been identified and in patients who do not respond to initial nonoperative management. This approach has been used with occasional success in patients with congenital anomalies of the thoracic duct or lymphangiomas and in patients who have persistent drainage after cardiac surgery. A Denver double-valve shunt system is the type most commonly employed; it is totally implanted and allows the patient or parent to pump the valve to achieve decompression of the pleural fluid into the abdominal cavity, where it is reabsorbed.

SUGGESTED READINGS

Farmer DL, Albanese CT: Fetal hydrothorax. In Harrison MR, Evans MI, Adzick NS, et al (eds): The Unborn Patient, 3rd ed. Philadelphia, WB Saunders, 2001.

Longaker MT, Laberge J-M, Dansereau J, et al: Primary fetal hydrothorax: Natural history and management. J Pediatr Surg 24:573-576, 1989.

The above two references discuss the embryology, physiology, and pathology of fetal lymphatic drainage. The authors describe when and how to treat fetal chylothorax and related indications.

Merrigan BA, Winter DC, O'Sullivan GC: Chylothorax. Br J Surg 84:15-20, 1997.

This article presents a thorough discussion of primary and secondary chylothorax and treatment and expected results.

Nguyen DM, Shum-Tim D, Dobell AR, et al: The management of chylothorax/chylopericardium following pediatric cardiac surgery: A 10-year experience. J Card Surg 10:302, 1995.

Chylothorax is being seen increasingly with staged cardiac repairs in neonates. Information on incidence and recommendations for timing of operative treatment are provided based on the authors' analysis of cases.

Reynolds M: Disorders of the thoracic cavity and pleura and infections of the lung, pleura and mediastinum. In O'Neill JA, Rowe MI, Grosfeld JL, et al (eds): Pediatric Surgery, 5th ed. St. Louis, Mosby, 1998, p 899.

This chapter discusses acquired causes of chylothorax and infectious complications of chylothorax.

Tieheuban KS, Kron IL, Carpenter MA, et al: Pleuroperitoneal shunts for refractory chylothorax after operation for congenital heart disease. Ann Thorac Surg 53:85, 1992.

The indications and results of pleuroperitoneal shunts, a last resort treatment of chylothorax, and the conditions that have the highest incidence of this problem are described.

Van Straaten HL, Gerards LJ, Krediet TG: Chylothorax in the neonatal period. Eur J Pediatr 152:2-5, 1993.

This article describes the various causes of chylothorax and how to treat them in the neonate. A progressive approach is outlined.

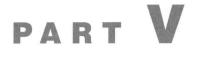

Esophagus

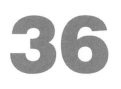

Congenital Abnormalities of the Esophagus

VARIANTS OF ESOPHAGEAL ATRESIA

The most life-threatening congenital anomalies of the esophagus are the variants of esophageal atresia (EA) and tracheoesophageal fistula (TEF). The incidence of the various forms of EA in the general population is approximately 1 in 4000 live births.

EMBRYOLOGY

The structure that develops into the trachea and the esophagus first appears as a ventral diverticulum of the foregut at 22 to 23 days' gestation. As the diverticulum elongates, masses of endodermal cells form ridges of tissue on each side that ultimately divide the foregut into tracheal and esophageal channels. The process begins at the carina and extends in a cephalad direction. By 26 days' gestation, the trachea and esophagus have become completely separated to the level of the larynx.

Interruption of the septation process is the traditional explanation of the development of TEF, but it does not explain why EA forms. Rats exposed to doxorubicin (Adriamycin) during gestation have provided more recent insights into the pathogenesis of EA and TEF. The notochord likely has a role in the development of axial organs such as the esophagus and trachea. Initially adherent, the foregut and notochord in normal embryos become progressively separate over gestation. The two structures remain adherent in doxorubicin-treated embryos, interfering with tracheoesophageal septation and development. A potential explanation of the vertebral anomalies that so often accompany EA is that the notochord itself is abnormal in this model.

Although nearly all EA variants seem to be sporadic, familial EA has been reported. Preliminary genetic studies have identified a defect at the 2p23-p24 chromosomal locus.

CLASSIFICATION

Figure 36-1 depicts the anatomic classification of tracheoesophageal anomalies. Proximal EA with distal TEF is the most common type, accounting for 85% to 90% of all cases. Isolated EA is the second most common form, seen in 5% to 7%. TEF without EA (so-called H-fistula) is third, present in 2% to 6%. Rare forms exist, including EA with proximal TEF and EA with proximal and distal TEF, each form accounting for less than 1% of cases.

ASSOCIATED ANOMALIES

The incidence of recognizable congenital defects associated with EA is about 55%. Table 36-1 lists the incidence of various organ system anomalies. The presence of a cardiac malformation is particularly important and is often the major determinant of mortality. Presence of cardiac malformation also predicts the presence of abnormalities in other organ systems, with more than half of

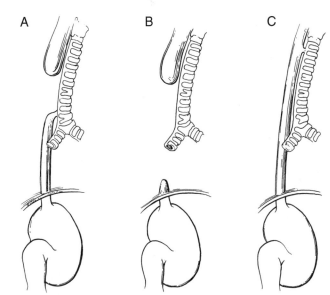

FIGURE 36-1 ■ Three most common types of EA. **A,** Proximal atresia and TEF. **B,** EA without fistula. **C,** TEF without EA. (Adapted from Coran AG, Behrendt DM, Weintraub WH, Lee DC: Surgery of the Neonate. Boston, Little, Brown, 1978.)

TABLE 36-1 ■ Incidence of Associated Anomalies

Anomalies	%
Cardiac	23
Musculoskeletal	18
Anointestinal	16
Genitourinary	15
Head and neck	10
Mediastinal	8
Chromosomal	6
Pulmonary	2
Overall	52
Single system	27
Two systems	13
Three or more systems	12

From Rokitansky A, Kolankaya A, Bichler B, et al: Analysis of 309 cases of esophageal atresia for associated congenital malformations. Am J Perinatol 11:123-128, 1994.

pulmonary, head and neck, chromosomal, and mediastinal malformations being found in association with congenital heart disease. Ventricular septal defects are the most common associated heart defect. Tetralogy of Fallot, transposition of the great vessels, dextrocardia, and, in Down syndrome, atrioventricular endocardial cushion defects are common. Because the heart defect may require palliative or corrective surgery, early evaluation with echocardiography is mandatory, and this study also shows whether the aortic arch is left-sided or right-sided to guide which side to select for thoracotomy. In 5% of cases, a right-sided arch is present, indicating that a left thoracotomy is in order.

Imperforate anus complicates EA in approximately 9% of cases; duodenal atresia, in 5%; and malrotation, in 4%. Data suggest that malrotation may be associated with a higher proportion of other associated anomalies and may have a correspondingly worse prognosis. Rarely an infant has atresias at multiple levels (e.g., EA and distal TEF, duodenal atresia, and imperforate anus). In such cases, it is usually best to deal with the intestinal obstruction first, but the infant with respiratory distress sufficient to require positive-pressure ventilation should undergo division of the fistula initially.

Two or more anomalies occur in nearly half of infants with EA. Tracheoesophageal anomalies are part of the VATER complex (vertebral, anorectal, tracheoesophageal, radial limb, and renal anomalies). The term VACTERL includes cardiac defects, gives separate emphasis to other limb anomalies, and guides the search for associated defects. Hydrocephalus has been recognized as a part of the spectrum, hence the new acronym, VACTERL-H. An increased association exists between tracheoesophageal anomalies and aneuploidies, specifically trisomies 13, 18, and 21. Other syndromes include CHARGE (coloboma, heart defect, choanal atresia, growth and mental retardation, genital hypoplasia, ear anomalies), Potter's syndrome, and "schisis" syndrome (cleft lip and palate, omphalocele, and hypogenitalism).

DIAGNOSIS AND CLINICAL FINDINGS

More than 90% of fetuses with EA (with or without TEF) have polyhydramnios. On prenatal ultrasound, a blind-ending proximal esophageal pouch may be seen. A small or absent stomach bubble also may be present, but in one report, among fetuses with only an absent stomach bubble and polyhydramnios, only 44% had EA. When it is thought that an accurate prenatal diagnosis is required, magnetic resonance imaging may improve diagnostic accuracy, giving images of an intact esophagus from mouth to stomach in normal cases and a blind-ending esophageal pouch in affected fetuses.

The infant with EA, unable to swallow, drools saliva and spits up undigested formula. As liquid pooling in the blind proximal esophageal pouch spills into the airway, the infant may cough or choke. It is impossible to pass a nasogastric tube into the stomach because it meets resistance part way down the esophagus.

Symptoms from TEF are primarily those of aspiration. The infant coughs, chokes, and may become cyanotic. Aspiration may induce wheezing, and aspiration of gastric juice through the distal TEF may result in aspiration pneumonia. An H-type TEF with an intact esophagus may be difficult to diagnose. The infant can swallow, and a nasogastric tube passes easily into the stomach. Recurrent aspiration suggests the presence of a fistula.

The diagnosis of EA can be made by chest radiography after placement of a soft nasogastric tube as far as possible in the esophagus. The chest radiograph shows the tube coiled in the esophagus with the loop in the upper mediastinum, but the air-filled proximal esophageal pouch generally is dilated in any case (Fig. 36-2A). A relatively narrow proximal pouch suggests the presence of a proximal TEF that has decompressed the esophagus. Films should include the abdomen to show whether gas fills the stomach and loops of small intestine. The presence of gas-filled intestinal loops establishes the presence of a distal TEF. If the radiograph fails to show any gas in the abdomen, presumably no fistula exists, and the infant has an isolated EA (Fig. 36-2B). In a few cases, however, a distal fistula may exist but is occluded by mucus or other material.

A contrast study is no longer necessary to make the diagnosis of EA and distal TEF or isolated EA. Some recommend a contrast study to detect an isolated H-type TEF. Contrast swallow may not opacify the fistula, however, because of the slanted orientation of the TEF from a proximal orifice in the trachea down to a more distal lumen in the esophagus. This configuration resembles an "N" rather than an "H." A single swallow may not flow retrograde up the fistula. If a fistula is suspected, a tube may be passed just past the cricopharyngeus, and contrast material may be injected into the proximal esophagus under pressure during fluoroscopy. Care must be taken not to flood the airway with isotonic soluble contrast material because it is important to exclude pharyngeal aspiration of barium into the tracheobronchial tree.

The preferred and most accurate approach for direct identification of a fistula is bronchoscopy, either flexible

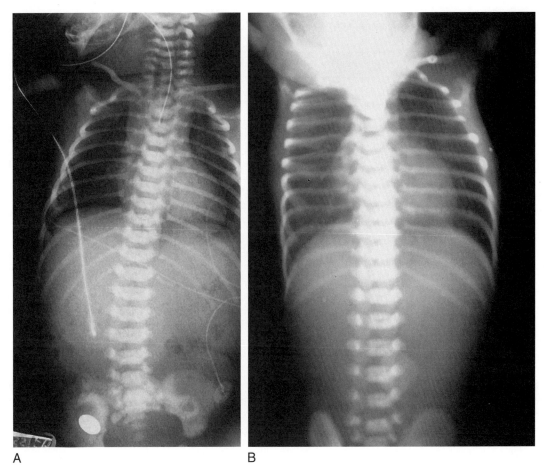

FIGURE 36-2 ■ **A,** Plain radiograph shows the orogastric tube hung up in the upper esophagus and gas in the abdomen, indicating the presence of a proximal EA and a distal TEF. **B,** The blind upper pouch is outlined by 0.5 mL of contrast material in a patient with isolated EA as indicated by a gasless abdomen.

or rigid. The fistula orifice may be obscure, appearing as only a dimple in the posterior tracheal membrane. A fine Fogarty catheter can be used to probe irregularities in the posterior tracheal membrane that might enter a fistula. When a TEF is identified, the catheter can be left in place with the balloon inflated on the esophageal side to serve as a guide when undertaking division of the fistula. If a TEF is not found, dilute methylene blue can be injected into the trachea and the esophageal lumen carefully observed by concomitant esophagoscopy for the appearance of dye. The distal esophagus eventually should be evaluated for an associated distal stenosis in cases of EA with TEF or H-type fistula.

Some advocate routine bronchoscopy for any infant with a tracheoesophageal anomaly. Findings that influence subsequent therapy are present in about one fourth of cases. Findings of immediate surgical significance are rare, however. Examples include the discovery of unexpected proximal TEF (which has an incidence of only 0.2%), or an unsuspected distal TEF in an infant with an apparent isolated EA and a gasless abdomen. Most argue that routine bronchoscopy is not needed, but all agree that the procedure is mandatory in any infant with a tracheoesophageal anomaly who has postoperative complications involving the respiratory system.

PREOPERATIVE TREATMENT

Pneumonitis is the most critical problem in the immediate preoperative period, resulting from aspiration of pharyngeal contents and from reflux of gastric juice into the trachea. Preoperative treatment involves the prevention of further aspiration and reflux and treatment of any pneumonitis that may be present. Keeping the infant supine and elevated 30 to 45 degrees decreases the risk of aspiration. A sump catheter keeps the proximal pouch clear of saliva. In theory, a gastrostomy further decreases the likelihood of aspiration by decompressing the stomach, but, in fact, gastrostomy usually is not needed. Broad-spectrum antibiotics and vitamin K_1 should be administered preoperatively.

TREATMENT

Esophageal Atresia with Distal Tracheoesophageal Fistula

The goal is to divide the TEF and repair the EA at a single operation. In a healthy infant without major associated anomalies, pneumonia, or significant prematurity, repair can be done within 1 day of birth and without a gastrostomy. Occasionally a gastrostomy is in order

TABLE 36-2 ■ **Waterston Risk Groups and Current Survival Figures**

Group	Survival (%)	Description
Low risk		
A	100	Birth weight >2500 g and otherwise well and free from complications
B	100	Birth weight 2000-2500 g and well, or higher weight with moderate associated anomalies (noncardiac anomalies, patent ductus arteriosus, ventricular septal defect, atrial septal defect)
High risk		
C	42	Birthweight <2000 g and well, or higher weight with severe associated anomalies, including complex congenital heart disease

From Dunn JC, Fonkalsud EW, Atkinson JB: Simplifying the Waterston's stratification of infants with tracheoesophageal fistula. Am Surg 65:908-910, 1999.

after a repair if the anastomosis is under a great deal of tension.

Extreme prematurity, significant pneumonia, or severe associated congenital anomalies all increase the risk of surgery and postoperative morbidity. Table 36-2 lists the risk groups as classified by Waterston in 1962. The classification assigns risk of mortality based on size, the presence of respiratory distress, and the presence of associated anomalies. At the time of Waterston's original report, infants in the highest risk group (group C) underwent a staged operation with initial placement of a gastrostomy, division of the TEF, then later anastomosis of the esophagus after treatment or resolution of pneumonia, prematurity, and other severe anomalies. With improvements in neonatal surgery and critical care, this staged approach is rarely needed. Infants weighing less than 1000 g have undergone primary repair successfully. Currently, survival of Waterston groups A and B patients (low risk) approaches 100%, leaving the preponderance of deaths among group C patients (high risk). Birth weight no longer independently predicts mortality.

The presence of severe respiratory distress complicates management. The need for ventilatory support to overcome increased pulmonary resistance increases mortality severalfold. Aspiration pneumonia and respiratory distress syndrome strongly influence the choice, order, and timing of operations. Because further respiratory compromise may occur from continued aspiration or the natural progression of respiratory distress syndrome, affected infants may benefit from early fistula ligation with primary anastomosis, if feasible. This is because with severe intrinsic lung disease, positive-pressure ventilatory support may escape through the TEF instead of filling the lungs. Under the circumstances, loss of ventilating volume via a gastrostomy may lead to sudden deterioration. If a gastrostomy is done before fistula ligation and respiratory collapse occurs, placing the gastrostomy under a water seal or clamping it completely may permit inflation of the lungs, at least temporarily until the fistula can be ligated.

Additional measures that may help are as follows: Surfactant therapy may improve respiratory distress syndrome sufficiently in newborns with EA and distal TEF to prevent this complication. Oscillatory ventilation may restore ventilation to the lungs despite the fistula. Occlusion of the fistula with a Fogarty balloon placed via bronchoscopy may prevent loss of ventilation through a distal TEF. Deliberate right main stem intubation and one-lung ventilation, bypassing the site of fistula, may be life-saving.

Because pulmonary compliance may deteriorate, particularly in low-birth-weight infants, the most opportune time to ligate the fistula in infants with respiratory complications may be immediately after the diagnosis of EA and TEF. The patient's condition may not permit ligation of the fistula and anastomosis of the esophagus. In this circumstance, the end of the fistula is closed and is sutured to the prevertebral fascia; this preserves its length for later anastomosis. Marking it with a surgical clip facilitates x-ray identification of the distal esophagus.

A right-sided posterolateral extrapleural thoracotomy via the fourth interspace provides good exposure for repair. If a right-sided aortic arch is present, a left thoracotomy is used. Most surgeons prefer the extrapleural approach because an anastomotic leak does not result in an empyema, but instead an esophagocutaneous fistula that generally undergoes spontaneous closure. Keeping the pleural space pristine also facilitates later surgical access to the area should a second procedure be required. Others contend that current results using a transpleural approach are the same as with the extrapleural approach, and the former is simpler and quicker. The essential features of the repair are shown in Figures 36-3 and 36-4.

If anastomosis is difficult after complete dissection of the proximal esophagus because of a long gap, a proximal esophagomyotomy can be carried out by incising the muscularis (Lividitis procedure), either in the chest or occasionally in the neck through a separate cervical incision (Fig. 36-3C). This procedure usually gives an additional 1.0 to 1.5 cm of length. This maneuver is possible in the upper esophagus, where the blood supply extends longitudinally in the submucosa. In contrast, the distal esophagus has a segmental blood supply that has been thought not to tolerate extensive dissection. It has been shown, however, that mobilization of the distal esophageal segment down to the level of the esophageal hiatus as part of the repair of a long-gap EA can be accomplished without complication.

A single-layer anastomosis is employed most commonly to connect the two esophageal segments. Occasionally the Haight two-layer, telescoping anastomosis is used when there is a great deal of tension (see Fig. 36-4). An 8F or 10F catheter is passed from the nose, past the anastomosis, and into the stomach. If the tube fails to pass completely into the stomach, the infant likely has an associated distal esophageal stenosis. The nasogastric tube allows postoperative gastric decompression in the immediate postoperative period and feedings later if

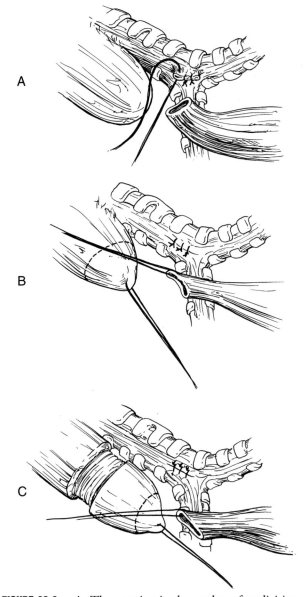

FIGURE 36-3 ■ **A,** The opening in the trachea after division of the TEF is being closed with 5-0 and 6-0 nonabsorbable suture. **B,** The feasibility of a primary anastomosis between the two esophageal segments is assessed. **C,** This diagram shows a proximal esophagomyotomy being used to gain additional length.

anastomotic complications preclude oral feedings. A chest tube is left near the anastomosis.

Postoperative Care

After operation, the infant should be kept elevated. A premeasured nasogastric tube, measured from the nose to 1 cm above the anastomosis during operation, is taped to the infant's bedside. Suction catheters should be measured against this tube so that when passed into the upper esophagus, which initially may collect secretions, they do not disturb the anastomosis. Antibiotics are continued until the chest tube is removed. If there is no evidence of saliva leaking through the chest tube, tube or gastrostomy feedings may begin by the 4th postoperative day. On the 7th to 10th postoperative day, a water-soluble contrast swallow

is performed. If no leak is seen, oral formula feedings may begin, and the chest tube may be removed.

Complications

Three types of complications are related to the esophageal anastomosis: leak, stricture, and recurrent fistula. The incidence of leak varies from 5% to 10%, depending on the type of anastomosis and the degree of tension at the anastomosis. In general, incidence of leak is lower with a Haight two-layer anastomosis (5%) than with a single-layer one (10%). Conversely, the stricture rate, defined as a requirement for at least two dilations for symptoms, is higher with a Haight anastomosis (10% to 15%) than a single-layer one (5% to 10%). Essentially all leaks except for a complete anastomotic disruption can be managed expectantly with parenteral nutrition and withholding oral feedings until spontaneous closure in 1 to 3 weeks. Complete disruption of the anastomosis (complicating <2% of cases) requires immediate cervical esophagostomy and closure of the distal esophagus.

Most strictures respond to periodic dilations every 3 to 6 weeks over a 3- to 6-month period. Strictures that do not respond to this regimen usually are associated with severe gastroesophageal reflux disease (GERD). The incidence of recurrent TEF is hard to determine because few series have been recorded. The rate seems to be 2% to 5%, however, regardless of the type of anastomosis used. Most recurrent fistulas are the result of a leak and do not close spontaneously once established. Rarely a small recurrent TEF closes spontaneously within 3 to 4 weeks. If the recurrent TEF is still present after 4 weeks, surgery is required. Recurrent TEFs are difficult to repair, and they have a 20% recurrence rate. Some type of autogenous tissue, such as pleura, muscle, pericardium, or azygos vein segment, must be placed between the esophageal and tracheal suture lines to decrease the risk of recurrent TEF.

Two other significant complications seen postoperatively are GERD and tracheomalacia. The incidence of GERD in various series ranges from 20% to 40% and is probably secondary to extensive mobilization of the distal esophagus. Physiologic studies document disturbed motility of the distal esophagus and the stomach that may contribute to symptoms associated with GERD. Simple maneuvers, such as upright positioning, thickened feedings, and administration of the prokinetic agent metoclopramide and an H_2-blocker, are effective in most cases. Of patients with postoperative reflux, 30% continue to have significant GERD, however. Significant reflux-related complications include anastomotic stricture that resists dilation and pulmonary aspiration, which mandate fundoplication. The Nissen fundoplication, which involves a 360-degree wrap, may obstruct the esophagus, however, regardless of how loosely it is constructed because of the esophageal dysmotility present in so many infants with EA. Some surgeons prefer to use a partial wrap technique.

Tracheomalacia of a severe degree has been reported with increasing frequency as a complication of EA itself, not of the repair. Symptomatic tracheomalacia occurs in 25% of patients with EA with TEF. The diagnosis of tracheomalacia is best made at bronchoscopy; the typical finding is "fish-mouthing" or tracheal collapse during

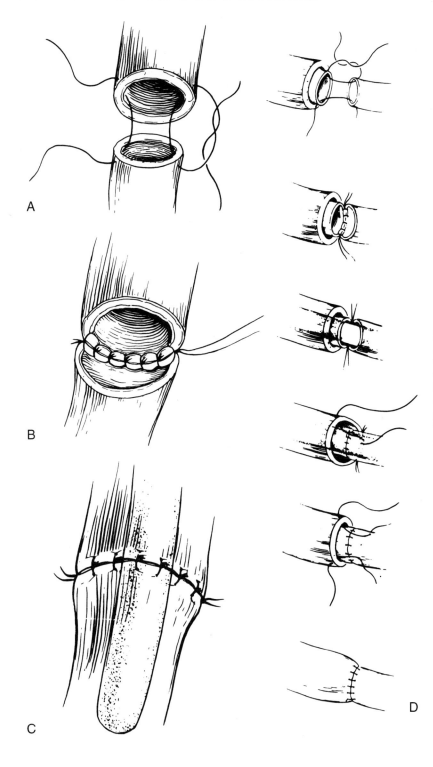

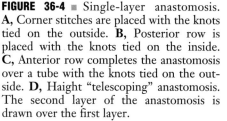

FIGURE 36-4 ■ Single-layer anastomosis. **A,** Corner stitches are placed with the knots tied on the outside. **B,** Posterior row is placed with the knots tied on the inside. **C,** Anterior row completes the anastomosis over a tube with the knots tied on the outside. **D,** Haight "telescoping" anastomosis. The second layer of the anastomosis is drawn over the first layer.

inspiration at the level of the aortic arch. The diagnosis requires an experienced endoscopist who can pass a thin endoscope into a spontaneously breathing infant. Most infants with tracheomalacia improve with time. A few develop chronic severe respiratory difficulty, however, that can result in respiratory arrest. Some surgeons have treated these patients with aortopexy to the undersurface of the sternum, which opens the trachea by pulling its anterior wall forward. Aortopexy is best reserved for infants who cannot be extubated or have had a well-documented respiratory arrest.

Results of Operation

As summarized earlier, surgical survival rates approach 100% among infants with EA and distal TEF free of associated malformations and ventilator dependence. Severe congenital heart disease is the major cause of early mortality (see Table 36-2).

Among older children and adults who have recovered from EA repair as infants, persistent respiratory symptoms are common. Of children, 40% wheeze, of whom half require hospitalization before the age of 5 years from bronchitis and pneumonia. This situation improves over time. A nonproductive cough is encountered frequently. When studied later in life, pulmonary function testing often reveals a restrictive lung defect. Bronchodilators fail to improve airflow in two thirds of patients, despite the fact that many post-EA patients have asthma.

Some degree of dysphagia occurs in 30% over the long-term. GERD is a significant problem in 46%. Barrett's esophagus is present in 7%, reflecting long-standing GERD. Esophageal squamous cell carcinoma was reported in a 38-year-old who formerly had EA with distal TEF. As a high-risk group of children with major congenital anomalies who had been ventilated as newborns, children with EA have more learning, emotional, and behavioral problems than children in the general population. For all these reasons, long-term follow-up is indicated.

Isolated Esophageal Atresia

Suction of the upper pouch should be initiated immediately at birth to prevent aspiration. A gastrostomy is used for feeding in all instances and usually can be carried out electively in the first 24 to 48 hours of life. Gastrostomy may be difficult because the stomach is diminutive and is confused easily with the transverse colon. Care must be taken to preserve the epiploic arcade if a gastric tube or pull-up esophagoplasty is planned. When the gastrostomy is in place, feedings provide nutritional support and enlargement of the gastric pouch so that it can be used for later definitive repair.

The ideal goal in EA with a long gap is primary anastomosis of the native esophagus. Dilation with a weighted bougie passed into the upper pouch daily and a Bakes dilator through the gastrostomy into the lower segment every few days using fluoroscopy permits one to measure the length of the gap between the upper and lower pouches as they lengthen over time. A gap of longer than 3 cm, roughly three vertebral bodies on a chest film, is considered a *long gap* EA. Elongation of the upper esophageal pouch, and possibly the lower segment, over a period of weeks is the simplest maneuver to bring the ends of a long gap EA together. Many surgeons do not think the lower segment can or needs to be lengthened using this technique because gastroesophageal reflux accomplishes this. Maximal growth usually is achieved over 6 weeks to 3 months.

Delayed primary esophageal anastomosis is attempted when it is estimated that maximal length has been achieved and the two ends are nearly approximated. Extensive mobilization of proximal and distal esophagus to the thoracic inlet via the right chest is required to provide the necessary length for anastomosis. Sometimes myotomy is required. Even with these maneuvers, the anastomosis is usually under tension. If anastomosis is impossible (i.e., >4 cm gap between the two esophageal segments after all the preceding maneuvers have been done), two options are available. First, the more traditional approach is to perform a cervical esophagostomy (preferably on the left side of the neck to make esophageal replacement at a later date easier) and to perform an esophageal replacement with colon or stomach at 12 to 18 months of age. Second, more recently, some centers have elected to carry out esophageal replacement with a gastric transposition at the time of the initial thoracotomy. The surgeon should be prepared to do this at the time of thoracotomy by preparing the abdomen for laparotomy to mobilize the stomach into the chest.

Postoperative Care

Postoperative care is the same as with EA and distal TEF except for the fact that the risk of postoperative GERD is higher. The small stomach, combined with GERD, may make oral and gastrostomy feeding difficult. Feeding after an esophageal replacement proceeds in the same manner as after primary anastomosis. Close follow-up is necessary to monitor the anastomotic sites between the native esophagus and stomach with the esophageal substitute for leak or stricture. A cervical esophagostomy requires scrupulous skin care, with frequent changes of dry cloth dressings or collection in a stoma bag and protective ointments and skin barriers around the margin of the stoma.

Complications

The rates of leak (31%), stricture (44%), and GERD (56%) are correspondingly higher among long gap patients than patients in whom the gaps measure less than 1 cm (leak, 6%; stricture, 17%; and GERD, 36%). Still, it is better to preserve the esophagus and tolerate the complications than to resort to esophageal replacement. The success rate for delayed primary repair in most reported series of long gap EA is 70%. The management of leak, stricture, and GERD is the same as that for EA with distal TEF. Strictures are aggravated in all cases by the presence of GERD, and a correspondingly higher proportion of isolated EA patients requires surgical fundoplication.

Results

As noted, the complication rates are related to the length of the gap. As a group, isolated EA has an overall higher rate of complications than EA with distal TEF. Mortality of the two groups is essentially the same and is related to the presence of associated severe cardiac anomalies.

Isolated or H-Type Tracheoesophageal Fistula without Atresia

Repair should proceed when the diagnosis is made unless active pneumonia is present. Perioperative antibiotics are used for 24 hours. Nearly all isolated TEFs lie at the junction of the cervical and thoracic trachea. The connection joins the esophagus a short distance distally, forming an "N" instead of an "H" as noted earlier. Under general anesthesia, bronchoscopy allows passage of a Fogarty balloon catheter through the fistula into the esophagus. The inflated balloon holds the catheter in place, controls escape of positive-pressure breaths into the esophagus, and helps identify the fistula during exploration.

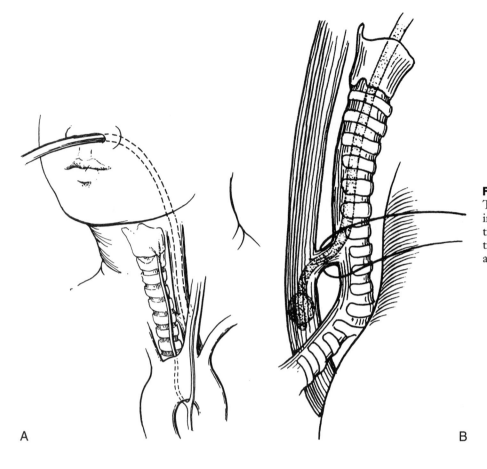

A   B

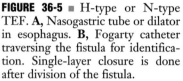

FIGURE 36-5 ■ H-type or N-type TEF. **A,** Nasogastric tube or dilator in esophagus. **B,** Fogarty catheter traversing the fistula for identification. Single-layer closure is done after division of the fistula.

The standard approach is through the lower right side of the neck to avoid damage to the thoracic duct. A right transthoracic approach through the third intercostal space is necessary for the rare intrathoracic TEF. Figure 36-5 shows the general principles of the operative approach and repair.

Postoperative Care

Care is straightforward for patients in good condition preoperatively. Antibiotics are discontinued after 24 hours, and feedings are introduced after 48 hours.

Results and Complications

The results are generally excellent. Mortality is rare. Infants generally swallow normally and are free from pneumonia. Recurrent fistulas are rare, much less common than in cases of EA with distal TEF. Lymphatic leaks, development of lymphocele, and chylous fistulas are more likely to occur in cases approached through a left cervical incision. Occasionally, temporary vocal cord paralysis occurs.

Laryngotracheoesophageal Cleft

Laryngotracheoesophageal cleft is a rare anomaly that most likely represents the extreme form of isolated TEF. Three forms of cleft are recognized: type I, limited to the posterior larynx; type II, partial cleft of the esophagus and trachea; and type III, a complete cleft extending from the larynx to carina.

Clinical Findings and Diagnosis

Symptoms can vary depending on the extent of the cleft. Most patients have respiratory distress aggravated by feeding beginning immediately after birth. Other findings commonly seen are hoarseness, absent or weak cry, stridor, cyanosis, recurrent aspiration, and choking with feedings.

Radiographic contrast studies show the cleft in most situations, but sometimes it is difficult to differentiate a cleft from simple spillover from the esophagus and pharynx into the airway. The definitive study is direct laryngoscopy and bronchoscopy. Careful examination of the posterior wall of the larynx and subglottic area is necessary because folds of mucosa may obscure the defect. Using the endoscope to press on the posterior wall of the larynx is sometimes necessary to visualize the defect. Even experienced endoscopists sometimes miss the lesion.

Operative Procedure

Anterior exposure of the larynx and upper trachea is used to close the clefts involving the upper airway (type I) without risking injury to either recurrent nerve. Postoperative laryngeal instability is common, requiring prolonged intubation. For this reason, some authorities recommend a lateral approach through the cricopharyngeus muscle and the lateral pharyngeal wall.

The best operative approach to a lower cleft (type II) is through a right thoracotomy. An incision in the

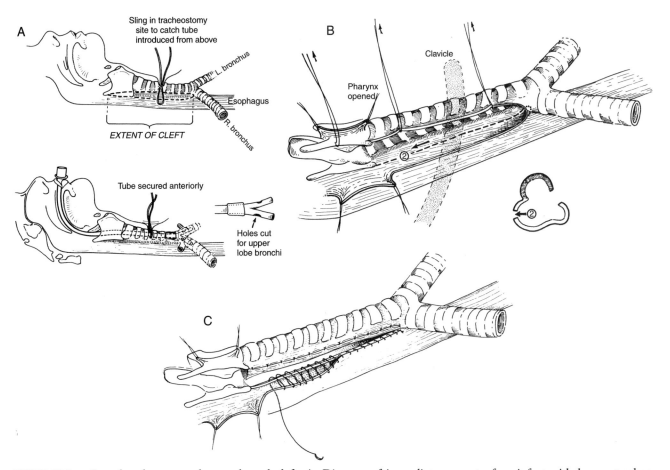

FIGURE 36-6 ▪ Complete laryngotracheoesophageal cleft. **A,** Diagram of immediate support of an infant with laryngotracheo-esophageal cleft. A special tube as shown with distal bifurcation and flanged ends is inserted into the main stem bronchi. As shown in the first and second drawings, a loop is passed into the tracheostomy, which serves to draw the tube forward into the trachea. **B,** A longitudinal incision is made in the tracheoesophageal groove upward from the level of the cleft at the carina. A second incision is made on the opposite wall of the trachea and esophagus, freeing these two structures. A small bit of esophagus is left all along the back wall of the trachea to allow adequate tissue for closure of the trachea. **C,** The trachea has been closed, and the esophagus is being closed as a separate unit. Closure of the laryngeal portion of the cleft and lateral pharyngeal wall have not yet been accomplished. (From Donahoe PK, Gee PE: Complete laryngotracheoesophageal cleft: management and repair. J Pediatr Surg 19:143, 1984.)

tracheoesophageal groove opens both structures longitudinally (Fig. 36-6). Separation of the two structures leaves a strip of esophageal wall on the trachea to allow closure of the airway without stenosis. Complete laryngotracheal repair (type III) using thoracic and anterior laryngofissure approaches is used for the repair of complete clefts (see Fig. 36-6).

Results and Complications

Postoperative survival is still relatively poor, averaging 75%. The cleft is common (30%), as are laryngeal and tracheal instability, both of which can lead to recurrent pneumonia and inability to wean infants from the ventilator.

SUGGESTED READINGS

Celli J, van Beusekom E, Hennekam RCM, et al: Familial syndromic esophageal atresia maps to 2p23-p24. Am J Hum Genet 66:436-444, 2000.

This is the first genetic study identifying a potential genetic marker for EA.

Dunn JC, Fonkalsud EW, Atkinson JB: Simplifying the Waterston's stratification of infants with tracheoesophageal fistula. Am Surg 65:908-910, 1999.

This is one of many reports that documents greatly improved survival among infants of any birth weight free from severe anomalies and respiratory complications.

Engum SA, Grosfeld JL, West KW, et al: Analysis of morbidity and mortality in 227 cases of esophageal atresia and/or tracheoesophageal fistula over two decades. Arch Surg 130:502-509, 1995.

This large review provides data that reflect the present management of tracheoesophageal anomalies, including the improvement in survival and the management of the varied complications that can occur.

Orford J, Maglick P, Cass DT, et al: Mechanisms for the development of esophageal atresia. J Pediatr Surg 36:985-994, 2001.

The authors review the histologic and biochemical events associated with development of EA and TEF in the doxorubicin rat model. Notochord-foregut separation, a feature of normal development, fails to occur in doxorubicin-exposed embryos and disturbs tracheoesophageal separation. Further work using this model promises to provide valuable insights into the embryogenesis of EA and TEF.

Rokitansky A, Kolankaya A, Bichler B, et al: Analysis of 309 cases of esophageal atresia for associated congenital malformations. Am J Perinatol 11:123-128, 1994.

Of 309 cases of EA from the University of Vienna, 162 (52.4%) had associated congenital malformations. In the last 5 years of the study, the survival rate of the group free from anomalies was 100%, whereas the survival rate among patients with major anomalies was 63%.

Schier F, Korn S, Michel E: Experiences of a parent support group with the long-term consequences of esophageal atresia. J Pediatr Surg 36:605-610, 2001.

The authors summarize the valuable experiences of a group of former EA patients, aged 10 to 34 years. They report high incidences of respiratory (80%) and esophageal complications, including dysphagia (30%) and GERD (46%).

Templeton JM, Templeton JJ, Schnaufer L, et al: Management of esophageal atresia and tracheoesophageal atresia in the neonate with severe respiratory distress syndrome. J Pediatr Surg 20:394-397, 1985.

This report showed the potential deleterious effect of gastrostomy in this group of patients and the importance of early control of TEF.

Esophageal Stenosis, Stricture, and Replacement

Stenosis of the esophagus may be either congenital or acquired with most acquired lesions being related to gastroesophageal reflux followed by corrosive strictures. Gastroesophageal reflux and its complications are discussed in detail in Chapter 39.

CONGENITAL STENOSIS

Congenital stenosis of the esophagus is relatively rare, and despite the congenital nature of the disorder, many children are not symptomatic until they are 4 to 6 years of age. Congenital stenoses are of two general types. The first is congenital diaphragm or web, and the second is associated with a persistent cartilaginous remnant within the wall of the esophagus (Fig. 37-1). The lesions usually are differentiated easily because congenital webs normally are seen in the upper third of the esophagus, whereas stenoses associated with tracheobronchial remnants, which constitute an obstructing ring, ordinarily are located near the distal end of the esophagus. The latter lesions are seen occasionally in patients with proximal esophageal atresia and distal tracheoesophageal fistula, which is why it generally is advised that patients who are having repair of esophageal atresia with tracheoesophageal fistula have a catheter passed into the stomach at the time of operation to rule out such an association. Other more unusual types of congenital esophageal stenosis include variants of tracheoesophageal fistulas from the upper and lower segments of the esophagus associated with a narrow central segment, distal esophageal stenosis associated with isolated esophageal atresia, and esophageal stenosis associated with intramural duplications (see Chapter 36).

It is thought that all forms of congenital esophageal stenosis may have their origin during the period of formation and separation of the trachea and esophagus. Although these lesions are thought to have their origin early in gestation, other associated anomalies, such as cardiac malformations, are uncommon, perhaps because these lesions are isolated and intrinsic only to the esophagus.

Diagnosis

Esophageal stenosis related to persistent tracheobronchial remnants is usually of sufficient degree to cause vomiting early in infancy. When this occurs in the neonate who recently has had repair of esophageal atresia with tracheoesophageal fistula, the symptoms of dysphagia and vomiting may be difficult to distinguish from anastomotic stricture above the congenital stenosis or gastroesophageal reflux (see Fig. 37-1). Patients with esophageal webs or diaphragms may present with symptoms at any time, but the most common presentation is when solid food is introduced to the diet. For a variety of reasons, diagnosis may be delayed for some time so that infants or children who present with chronic dysphagia and postprandial vomiting should be investigated for the possibility of a congenital stenosis.

There are no distinctive physical or laboratory findings related to making the diagnosis of congenital stenosis of the esophagus. In patients who have had persistent vomiting related to congenital stenoses of the esophagus that have gone undiagnosed and untreated, weight loss, malnutrition, and dehydration may be evident. In infants, aspiration pneumonia may be the first sign encountered.

The mainstays of diagnosis are esophagoscopy and x-ray imaging. Either barium or soluble contrast swallow must be performed under careful fluoroscopic control. Imaging may show a tapered narrowing, but frequently the finding is fleeting as the contrast material passes downward so that precise definition of a stenosis may be difficult. These patients frequently may show a lack of coordination of swallowing in the upper esophagus and abnormal transmission of peristaltic waves, which makes imaging difficult and which highlights the importance of esophagoscopy. In the distal esophagus, gastroesophageal reflux is a common association, particularly in infants. At times, it is helpful to pass a small Foley balloon catheter into the distal esophagus with or without placement of contrast material above. Then the balloon is inflated slightly and pulled gently upward until the stricture is encountered. The latter is an important technique when resection is planned to identify the location of the stenosis accurately. In an esophageal web, contrast swallow may show a sharp cutoff with a small central opening. At other times, a blind esophageal pouch may be noted just below a stenosis, particularly when located in the lower third of the esophagus. The most helpful diagnostic tool is esophagoscopy. A rigid esophagoscope of sufficient size

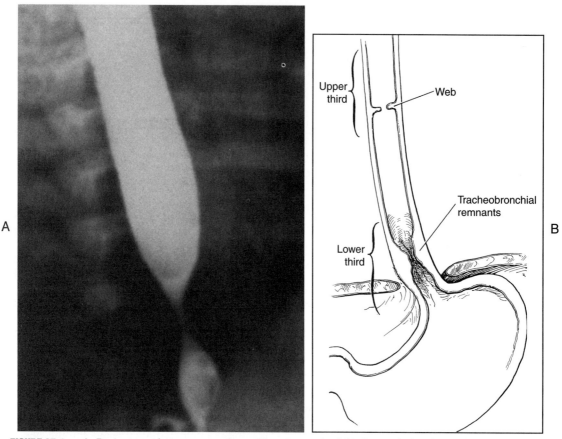

FIGURE 37-1 ■ **A,** Barium esophagogram performed in a 1-month-old infant with dysphagia shows congenital esophageal stenosis that could not be dilated. This is characteristic of a persistent cartilaginous remnant. Resection with end-to-end anastomosis was curative. **B,** The usual locations of the two most common forms of congenital esophageal stenosis: esophageal web, which usually occurs in the upper third of the esophagus, and persistent cartilaginous tracheobronchial remnants, which usually are encountered in the lower third of the esophagus.

and with good optics should be used so that the upper esophagus is distended above the level of the stricture, making it more evident.

Treatment and Results

Depending on the pathologic condition encountered, it may be possible to treat a stenosis at the time of esophagoscopy. In the case of thin webs or diaphragms in the upper third of the esophagus, it is often possible to dilate them at the time of esophagoscopy or to open them up with a laser or electrocautery probe applied through the scope under direct vision. At other times, passage of a bougie or dilation with a balloon catheter on one or more occasions may be all that is necessary. An older but still useful technique is passing string through the esophagus and bringing it out via a gastrostomy, which permits guided dilation with Tucker tapered dilators. This and balloon dilation are probably the safest approaches to dilation.

In instances in which upper esophageal webs are too thick to be dilated or when rigid persistent tracheobronchial rings are present in the lower esophagus, resection and anastomosis via right thoracotomy is the best approach. As mentioned, it is important at the time of

operation to pass a catheter into the esophagus from above that can be palpated or to pass a small Foley balloon catheter distally, then pull it upward to engage the stenosis so that it can be identified. This is because congenital stenoses are related to lesions within the esophageal wall that do not distort the wall of the esophagus itself. Generally, a short, sleeve resection is best with end-to-end anastomosis between what appears to be normal esophagus on either end. Although Heineke-Mikulicz esophagoplasty is occasionally successful, most clinicians believe that it is a less desirable technique because it leaves the pathologic conditions in place, and it is not useful in cases of persistent cartilaginous remnants.

Similar to esophageal atresia with tracheoesophageal fistula, gastrostomy is used less often than previously after repair of an esophageal stenosis. Gastrostomy is sometimes a helpful procedure, however, to protect an anastomosis under tension or when esophageal motility is deranged. Whether gastrostomy is used or not, all patients with esophageal anastomoses probably should be evaluated for postoperative stricture by calibration or other means and dilation if necessary to avoid a secondary anastomotic stricture. Scar tissue at the level of an esophageal anastomosis tends to constrict during maturation over approximately 6 months, so it is generally best to anticipate that postoperative stricture may occur and to avoid it. Postoperative leaks are uncommon in repaired esophageal stenoses, and long-term results are excellent, provided that anastomotic stricture is avoided.

With regard to congenital esophageal stenoses, those related to persistent tracheobronchial remnants are treated best by resection and anastomosis. With regard to fibromuscular stenoses, repeated dilations may be attempted, but some patients require either myotomy or resection and anastomosis. Most instances of web or membranous stenosis may be treated by either endoscopic or balloon dilation or partial resection with carbon dioxide laser or electrocautery. In rare instances of multiple stenoses, the lesions are managed best as noted earlier according to the individual site.

ACQUIRED STRICTURES

The most common cause of an acquired stricture of the esophagus is reflux esophagitis with or without Barrett's changes. This subject is discussed in detail in Chapter 39.

At times, inflammatory esophagitis, particularly eosinophilic esophagitis, may result in the formation of a stricture of unclear etiology. Dilation, an elimination diet, and steroids are usually effective treatment.

Corrosive injuries of the esophagus are generally the result of accidental ingestion of strong alkali in young children or as a result of a suicide attempt in older children and adolescents. Most corrosive injuries occur in children younger than age 5 with 90% the result of alkali burns and 10% related to acid ingestions. The most common agents involved are sodium or potassium hydroxide and sulfuric acid. These ingestions still constitute a significant problem in childhood despite federal packaging and labeling laws and a variety of preventive measures. Of young children who swallow caustic agents accidentally, 60% are boys, whereas girls predominate in the older age group in which suicide is more common. Solid granular forms of caustic cleansers for household or industrial use are highly irritating and difficult to swallow, so severe injuries are usually associated with ingestion of liquid agents. Accidental ingestion of Clinitest tablets, which contain sodium hydroxide, or tiny watch batteries containing potassium hydroxide may cause significant local injury or even perforation. Certain vaginal douche solutions that contain strong acids not only may cause significant esophageal damage, but also damage to the gastric antrum and outlet. Frequently ingested liquid agents such as bleach and washing detergents rarely cause esophageal injury of any significance. With all substances, however, the volume ingested and the duration of time the mucosa is exposed to the agent determine the extent and depth of the injury. Potassium and sodium hydroxide produce the most severe form of injury because they produce damage by liquefaction necrosis that progresses through the esophageal wall until the alkali is neutralized. Strong acids produce coagulation necrosis, in effect sealing the esophageal wall, so that continued penetration is unusual, although the damage may extend into the stomach as well, sometimes sparing the esophagus.

With alkali, at times the degree of damage is so severe that tracheoesophageal fistulas are produced, and if aspiration of the agent occurs, laryngeal and tracheal damage may result.

Diagnosis

A child may be witnessed to have swallowed a caustic agent, but frequently it is suspected only on the basis of finding a child playing with a container that holds a caustic substance. Every effort should be made to document the possible agent, its physical and chemical characteristics, and its volume, so the parents should always bring the container to the emergency department so that this information may be gathered.

Initially, there may be few symptoms with small-volume ingestions, but with larger volume ingestions, there is generally severe edema and esophageal spasm resulting in vomiting, dysphagia, drooling, fever, and anterior chest pain. If there has been an injury to the larynx or trachea, laryngospasm or severe wheezing with respiratory distress may be present. Burns of the lips, mouth, and tongue strongly suggest esophageal injury because approximately one fourth of patients with oral burns have associated esophageal injury. Approximately 5% of patients with esophageal burns do not have any demonstrable oropharyngeal injury. If the stomach or lower esophagus has been injured, abdominal pain and tenderness may be present.

Although there are no specific laboratory tests that are reliable indicators of either the presence or the severity of esophageal damage, the white blood cell count tends to be elevated, with a shift to the left of the differential count. In severe cases, edema of the soft tissues of the neck and mediastinum may be evident on plain chest film and mediastinal emphysema or free air in the abdomen if perforation has occurred.

Esophagoscopy is mandatory in all instances of suspected ingestion of a corrosive agent to determine whether the esophagus has been injured regardless of whether oropharyngeal burns are present. It is best to defer esophagoscopy if the child has a full stomach, but it should be performed within the first 24 hours to make a diagnosis. In mild injuries, only redness may be noted; superficial and widely scattered ulcerations are seen with moderate injuries; and in severe injuries, the ulcerations are deep and circumferential with extreme friability of the mucosa. A flexible scope is useful because the stomach and the esophagus can be visualized.

Contrast esophagogram should be performed within the first 48 hours after injury even if extensive injury has been shown on esophagoscopy (Fig. 37-2). Esophagogram is capable of showing the nature of esophageal motility, which has predictive value because the presence of a rigid noncontracting esophagus correlates with severe esophageal injury and the potential for extensive stricture formation. Serial studies may be performed to monitor the extent of progressive scarring and whether mucosal bands are forming. Contrast studies also are useful to assess the status of the antrum and pylorus. The prime time for esophageal stricture formation is 3 to 4 weeks after injury. Follow-up at this interval is important even for patients thought to have only mild injuries.

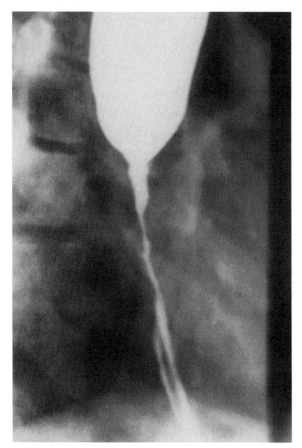

FIGURE 37-2 ■ Esophagogram shows a significant lye stricture 1 month after ingestion. This stricture did not respond to bougienage after 1 year and required resection and partial replacement with a segment of left colon.

Treatment

The goal of initial treatment is to avoid stricture formation and to prevent systemic sepsis, which may result from mediastinitis. There is good evidence that administration of systemic antibiotics, usually ampicillin and gentamicin for 7 to 14 days depending on the severity of the injury, is helpful in preventing the extension of injury. Although prednisone steroid treatment for 3 weeks was thought to be a useful preventive measure in the past, randomized studies have failed to confirm any benefit from its use.

In addition to the measures mentioned earlier, during the acute healing phase it is crucial to maintain good nutrition either with a feeding tube or parenterally. In children with mild injuries in whom there is no disturbance of motility, a clear liquid diet followed 3 or 4 days later with modified solids may be satisfactory. Close follow-up is important even in patients thought to have mild injuries.

In severe injuries, it is best to pass a feeding tube to provide enteral nutrition and to maintain access so that bougienage can be performed. In some patients with particularly severe injuries, it is best to perform a gastrostomy initially to provide nutrition. If stricture is not present after 3 to 4 weeks, patients may be followed monthly for 1 year. If a stricture is encountered,

esophageal dilations are performed best with string guidance, although endoscopically guided balloon dilation is also an option.

Results and Complications

Approximately one third of patients who sustain caustic esophageal injury develop strictures, but only 5% or less eventually develop resistant strictures unresponsive to treatment. It is generally accepted that if aggressive and frequent esophageal dilation does not produce resolution of the stricture within 1 year, further options may be needed. Reports have suggested that for patients with resistant strictures, esophageal replacement is not the only option. Rivosecchi and others used removable Silastic stents fixed to a nasogastric tube for this purpose. After dilation, stents are placed under general anesthesia using fluoroscopic control and left in place an average of 6 weeks. Antibiotics, dexamethasone, and antacids have been administered simultaneously. This method is not useful for patients who have sustained perforations or developed acquired tracheoesophageal fistulas. Under these circumstances, esophageal replacement is the best option.

ESOPHAGEAL REPLACEMENT

Modern esophageal replacement procedures were devised primarily to treat patients with esophageal carcinoma, but they have been applied to children with a variety of congenital and acquired disorders. Transposition of the stomach into the right side of the chest initially was employed in adults, but use of these procedures in children was complicated by gastric distention and respiratory distress, so this led to the development of other replacement procedures in which the volume of the substitute and the risk of distention were less. In more recent years, use of the entire stomach as a substitute brought through the esophageal bed in the posterior mediastinum has been successful. Four approaches to esophageal substitution are in use at present: (1) some form of colon interposition, (2) total gastric pull-up through the posterior mediastinum, (3) gastric tube interposition, and (4) substitution with jejunum. Each of these methods has utility in specific clinical situations with which the surgeon must be familiar, but each surgeon should develop competency with at least one method to produce reliable results.

Indications

The most common indication for total or partial esophageal replacement is acquired esophageal stricture. Replacement should be considered for patients with corrosive strictures that are resistant to dilation or stenting after about 1 year. At the time of the replacement procedure, transhiatal esophagectomy can be performed and the replacement placed in the esophageal bed, or the damaged esophagus can be resected electively at a later date through a right thoracotomy.

The second most common indication for esophageal replacement is in patients with long-gap esophageal atresia with or without fistula. Although many these patients can be treated by esophageal stretching and delayed anastomosis with or without circular myotomy of the upper pouch, many of these patients still require esophageal substitution.

In this group of patients, gastric pull-up procedures are used most frequently at present.

Resistant strictures resulting from chronic gastroesophageal reflux may require only limited esophageal resection to the level of the midesophagus, usually with a short segment of colon. Patients with advanced Barrett's changes associated with anaplasia also may require esophagectomy and substitution.

At times, patients with severe immunodeficiency disorders may develop *Candida* or other fungal infections of the esophagus and lengthy resistant strictures. Rarely, children with extrahepatic portal hypertension and severe esophagogastric varices may develop intractable bleeding unresponsive to sclerotherapy and other conservative measures. If they are not candidates for portosystemic shunt procedures because of widespread portal phlebitis, total esophagectomy and esophageal replacement may be the only option. Colon interposition also has been used primarily in these patients.

Timing of Operation

For the most part, it has been considered best to perform esophageal replacement procedures after 1 year of age when children are sitting upright most of the time because all methods of esophageal substitution are associated with some degree of gastric reflux. Because total gastric transposition has been performed much earlier in infants with long-gap esophageal atresia, they have required nursing in the upright position, which seems to be effective in most instances. Gastrostomy with or without cervical esophagostomy otherwise may be used to maintain infants until they are 1 year old. If substitution procedures are delayed until a child is 1 year old, it is important that when gastrostomy feedings are given, simultaneous sham feedings also should be given by mouth so that children become conditioned to enjoy tasting and eating. Although with sham feedings infants will be more likely to take feedings by mouth when a substitution procedure has been performed, significant feeding problems are usually present in infants for several months.

Other Considerations Common to All Methods of Substitution

Because acid reflux occurs in all patients, regardless of the method of substitution used, vagotomy and pyloroplasty are useful adjuncts. Although there is not universal agreement with the latter, numerous cases of ulceration in colonic and gastric tubes and stricture related to ulceration at cologastric anastomoses have been reported. There also have been numerous reports of Barrett's metaplasia at the level of the cervical anastomosis, so there is support for using these acid-lowering procedures. Either gastrostomy or feeding jejunostomy probably is indicated in all cases to provide a method of gastric decompression to protect anastomotic suture lines and to provide a reliable method of nutrition, because these patients usually do not eat well for several months after esophageal substitution.

There is probably no ideal esophageal substitute compared with the patient's own esophagus in the long run. At present, most individuals use colon as a replacement, most likely because more options are available using different portions of the colon, and the techniques have been worked out to a greater degree than with other approaches. The second most commonly used technique at present is total gastric transposition through the esophageal bed; this method seems to be gaining popularity. Use of a reverse gastric tube constructed from the greater curvature of the stomach and jejunal interposition either with in-continuity vascular supply or as a free graft are options when the aforementioned options are not available or have failed.

Esophageal Replacement with Colon

For esophageal replacement with colon (Fig. 37-3), either the right or the left side of the colon may be used and placed substernally, behind the hilum of the lung in either side of the chest, although the left side of the chest is used most commonly, or it may be placed in the posterior mediastinum. The proximal anastomosis can be made either within the thorax when only portions of the esophagus need to be replaced or in the neck when a cervical esophagostomy is present. The distal anastomosis may be made either to the stomach or to a short stump of distal esophagus. Although the right-sided colonic replacement is isoperistaltic and the left is antiperistaltic, both types of replacement seem to function equally well, provided that the conduit is straight. On long-term follow-up, many colon replacements have become tortuous and redundant within the thorax to the point where transmission of food is delayed and difficult. The latter problem may not become evident for many years after the original operation, emphasizing the importance of long-term observation. A contrast study of the colon should be obtained preoperatively to ascertain that no anomalies or disease is present that would preclude use of the colon as a replacement. The only absolute contraindication to colonic interposition is inadequate arterial supply or venous drainage when tested before division of the bowel. Other relative contraindications include associated anomalies, such as high imperforate anus, short colon, or failure of a previous colon replacement procedure in which the colon would be foreshortened excessively if colon were selected for a second bypass procedure. An appropriate bowel preparation and preoperative antibiotics are indicated.

The right side of the colon with a short length of terminal ileum is taken out of continuity after testing that the right colic and ileocolic vessels can be interrupted and that there is adequate arterial supply and venous return via the middle colic vessels. If these are determined to be adequate, it is possible to take this portion of the colon and terminal ileum out of continuity and to divide the mesenteric tissues up to the arcades to straighten the colon out as much as possible. After ileotransverse colon anastomosis, the terminal ileal end of the proximal right side of the colon is brought upward behind the stomach so that it can be passed upward to reach the neck. When the right side of the colon is used, it accommodates to either the retrosternal or the posterior mediastinal position. Although it can be passed through the right side of the chest, long-term follow-up of patients who have had right retrohilar positioning of the right side of the colon has shown an unacceptable incidence of tortuosity.

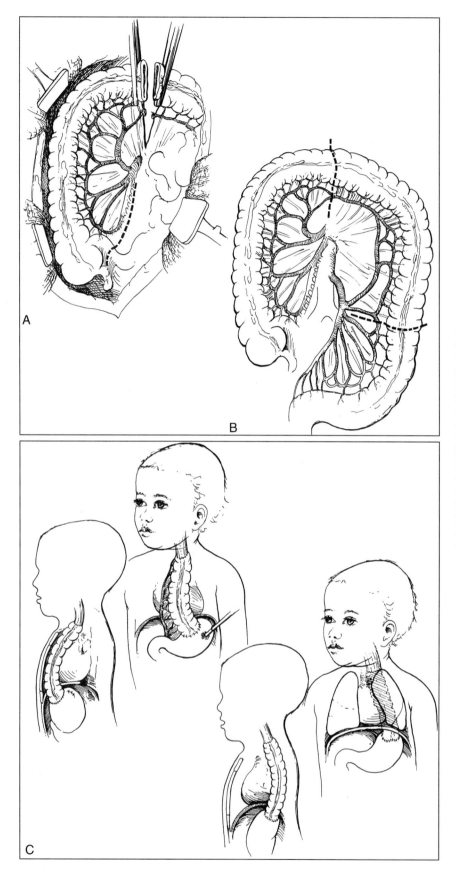

FIGURE 37-3 ■ **A,** Isolation of the right colon for esophageal substitution basing the blood supply on the middle colic artery and vein. The terminal ileum is included so that either it or the cecum can be used for the proximal anastomosis. **B,** Extent of left transverse and descending colon ordinarily used for esophageal substitution, particularly via the left chest. The left colon is placed in antiperistaltic fashion based on the blood supply of the left colic artery and vein. **C,** Series of four drawings shows the positioning of the right colon in a substernal location and the left colon in the left retrohilar space. It is not usually a problem to obtain adequate length using these methods.

Tortuosity occurs less when right-sided colon segments are placed retrosternally and rarely when segments are placed in the posterior mediastinum.

Another option is use of the left transverse and descending colon segment with blood supply based on a pedicle of the left colic artery and vein. As with other procedures, the blood supply is tested with bulldog clamps first to see that the segment will be able to survive when its communications to the middle colic vessels have been divided. The distal end of the colon is brought upward, usually behind the stomach and pancreas, either through a lateral incision in the diaphragm or through the esophageal hiatus. Generally, it has been considered to be easier to bring the left side of the colon upward behind the hilus of the left lung rather than through the bed of the normal esophagus, but either is possible. Replacement with left-sided colon is ideal when only portions of the esophagus require replacement, but the procedure also is quite satisfactory for replacement of the entire esophagus with anastomosis in the neck because few such patients develop tortuosity through the years.

It is probably wise to perform vagotomy and pyloroplasty, regardless of whether the right or left side of the colon is being used, to avoid the long-term potential of anastomotic ulceration and stricture, which occurs most commonly at the cologastric anastomosis. This also may be an effective way to avoid delayed occurrence of Barrett's metaplasia in the cervical esophagus. Approximately 7 to 10 days after colon replacement, the anastomosis is imaged with soluble contrast material before initiating oral feeds because the incidence of proximal anastomotic leak after any form of colon interposition is 30% to 50%. Most of these leaks close promptly and require nothing more than drainage. Of patients who do develop anastomotic leaks, approximately half develop strictures that require revision, which is usually successful. Although necrosis of the colon segment within the mediastinum has been reported, it is an uncommon complication.

Gastric Transposition

With gastric transposition (Fig. 37-4A and B), a preoperative bowel preparation is performed in case the stomach

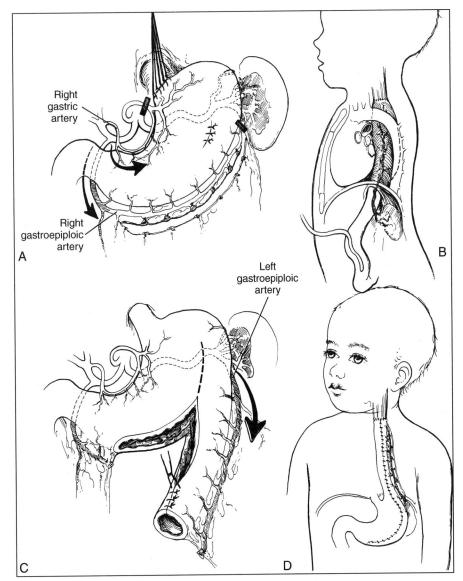

FIGURE 37-4 ■ Gastric transposition. **A,** Complete dissection of the stomach preserving the gastroepiploic and right gastric vessels sufficiently to permit the entire stomach to be brought upward in the natural bed of the esophagus. The gastroesophageal junction is sutured closed. **B,** The apex of the fundus is used for the anastomosis to the proximal esophagus in the neck. **C** and **D,** Technique used to prepare a reversed gastric tube, which may be brought upward to the proximal esophagus by whatever route chosen. Vagotomy and pyloroplasty are added to this procedure to avoid acid-peptic complications within the gastric tube. Vagotomy and pyloroplasty also are part of the gastric transposition procedure.

Right gastric artery

Right gastroepiploic artery

Left gastroepiploic artery

proves to be an unacceptable substitute because of inadequate blood supply or other considerations. Because the transposed stomach will be dependent on right gastric arterial supply, the left gastric artery is test occluded with a bulldog clamp before division. The gastroepiploic vessels are preserved, and an extensive Kocher maneuver is performed to mobilize the duodenum thoroughly. Pyloroplasty or pyloromyotomy is performed. The esophageal hiatus is opened widely, and the initial dissection of the lower esophagus is performed bluntly to the extent necessary. Gastric transposition without thoracotomy has distinct advantages, particularly in infants. If an esophagostomy is present, it is incorporated into a cervical incision, and the sternocleidomastoid muscle is retracted laterally along with the carotid artery, internal jugular vein, and vagus nerve. The proximal esophagus is identified and mobilized with great care taken to preserve the recurrent laryngeal nerve on both sides. This approach permits complete mobilization of the esophagus from above and below within the mediastinum. After complete mobilization of the stomach and duodenum, the gastroesophageal junction is divided and inverted with a two-layer closure. This permits the highest point of the fundus to be used for the anastomosis, and this site can be sutured to a tube that can be used to bring the stomach through the hiatus and mediastinum to the level of the cervical esophagus. Care must be taken to prevent torsion of the gastric segment as it is brought upward, and the apex of the stomach should be under minimal tension. Division of the left triangular ligament of the liver may help to relieve the tension to shorten the route through which the stomach passes. The apex of the stomach can be sutured to the proximal esophagus in either one or two layers, and it is useful to suture the esophagus near the anastomosis to the adjacent cervical muscles to maintain the anastomosis in the neck should leakage occur.

As with all anastomoses between substitute and proximal esophagus, it is probably best to use a Penrose drain in the neck postoperatively. As with colon replacement, a contrast study of the conduit is performed postoperatively. Construction of a feeding jejunostomy is best performed routinely in these patients for the reasons mentioned earlier. Postprandial gastric distention is little or no problem when gastric conduits have been placed in the posterior mediastinum. Some patients require gastric transposition via thoracotomy primarily because of complications of previous surgical procedures.

The incidence of proximal anastomotic leak after gastric transposition ranges from 6% to 38% in various reports. Most close, and fewer of these patients who have leaks seem to develop strictures compared with patients who have leaks after colon or reversed gastric tube replacement.

Reversed Gastric Tube Replacement

The third most common form of esophageal replacement used in children at present is with a reversed gastric tube (see Fig. 37-4C and D). Although an antegrade gastric tube attached to the antrum and supplied by the right gastroepiploic vessels has been used in the past, the reversed gastric tube based on the left gastroepiploic vessels is the more established procedure. If a gastrostomy is being performed in a patient in whom it is planned to perform a reversed gastric tube later, the gastrostomy should be placed in a location that would not compromise the later construction of a gastric tube.

For the construction of a reversed gastric tube, the right gastroepiploic vessels are divided close to the pylorus, and construction of the tube begins approximately 2 cm proximal to it. A stapler is used to construct the tube approximately 2 cm from the greater curvature extending high on the fundus, taking care to preserve the origin of the left gastroepiploic artery from the splenic artery. The latter is particularly a consideration when dividing the short gastric vessels during construction of the tube and mobilization of the stomach. The end of the tube may be brought upward in reverse fashion through the substernal space up to the neck, in a left retrohilar position, or even through the posterior mediastinum, although the latter is rarely used. Vagotomy, pyloroplasty, and gastrostomy generally are added to the procedure.

As with the other replacement procedures, a postoperative contrast study is performed 7 to 10 days after the procedure. Feedings are begun gradually either by mouth or by gastrostomy. Most patients take frequent small feedings until the gastric remnant enlarges. The incidence and types of complications that occur after reverse gastric tube replacement procedures are identical to complications following colon replacement. Although long-term follow-up is necessary for these patients, reverse gastric tubes do not develop tortuosity over the long-term.

Jejunal Replacement

Replacement of the esophagus with a segment of jejunum (Fig. 37-5) generally is performed only as a last resort when the other methods are not available for some reason. The other procedures are more reliable, technically easier to perform, and associated with fewer complications because of their better blood supply.

The technique for creating a jejunal conduit is essentially that of constructing a long Roux-en-Y limb. A point is selected distal to the first vasa recta jejunalis, at which point the jejunum and its mesentery are divided, leaving the arcades intact. One of the problems in constructing a jejunal limb is that excess length ordinarily is required to prevent the mesenteric vessels from being on too much tension. Basically the same technique is used as that described for the construction of a Hunt-Lawrence pouch for replacement of the stomach after total gastrectomy. Vagotomy and pyloroplasty ordinarily are added to avoid peptic ulceration at the point of anastomosis with the stomach, as with colon interposition. The jejunum is less resistant to peptic ulceration than the stomach when interposed between the pharynx and the stomach.

Another approach used to improve the blood supply to transposed jejunal segments has been microvascular anastomosis between the inferior thyroid vessels and the distal arcade vessels at the proximal end of the transplant, providing blood supply at both ends of the conduit. In the case of replacement of short portions of the upper esophagus, occasionally free jejunal grafts have been used, again using microvascular anastomotic techniques.

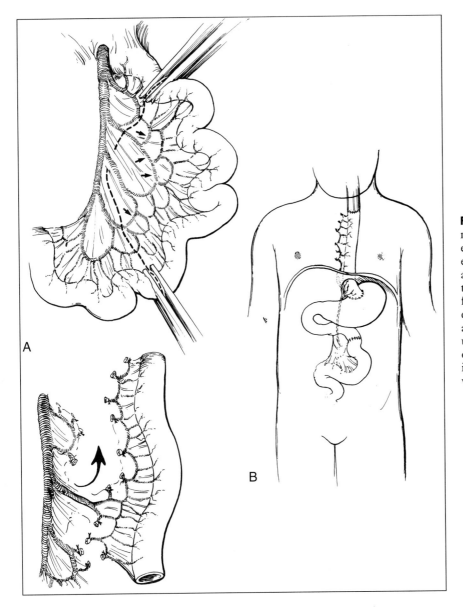

FIGURE 37-5 ■ **A** and **B**, In rare instances, neither colon nor stomach is available for esophageal reconstruction, and it is necessary to consider use of a jejunal segment as a last resort. As shown in the drawing, the jejunum is divided just beyond the first vasa recta jejunalis artery, and a sufficient length is prepared based on the arcade vessels. The segment is brought upward either in the substernal location or via the chest. Vascularity of jejunal interpositions is more unreliable than with either colon or stomach.

SUGGESTED READINGS

DePeppo F, Zaccara A, Dall'Oglio L, et al: Stenting for caustic strictures: Esophageal replacement replaced. J Pediatr Surg 33:54-57, 1998.

This follow-up study of 31 children with caustic strictures of the esophagus presents a convincing argument for stenting rather than replacement, and the method is presented in detail.

Hirschl RB, Yardeni D, Oldham K, et al: Gastric transposition for esophageal replacement in children. Ann Surg 236:531-541, 2002.

This study of 41 children who had gastric transposition procedures in several institutions discusses all the details that promote success with this operation.

Spitz L, Kiely E, Spamon T: Gastric transposition for esophageal replacement in children. Ann Surg 206:69, 1987.

The authors describe an innovative approach to esophageal replacement in very young patients. This is an alternative to gastric tube interposition.

Takamizawa S, Tsugawa C, Mouri N, et al: Congenital esophageal stenosis: Therapeutic strategy based on etiology. J Pediatr Surg 37:197-201, 2002.

This study of 36 patients categorizes various types of congenital esophageal stenosis and describes the best approaches to diagnosis and treatment.

Waterston DJ: Colonic replacement of esophagus (intrathoracic). Surg Clin North Am 44:1441, 1964.

The Waterston approach to esophageal replacement with left colon has stood the test of time. This is a classic article.

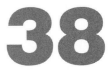

Esophageal Rupture and Perforation

Although esophageal perforation has been well described in adults since 1900, the first case of a successful repair of a spontaneous perforation in a neonate was not reported until 1952. Since then, numerous reports have pointed out that some patients may be treated nonoperatively or only with simple drainage. Operative and nonoperative approaches to treatment and ways to determine when each is appropriate are discussed in this chapter.

CLASSIFICATION

Esophageal perforation can be spontaneous or traumatic; the latter is more common. Spontaneous perforation of the esophagus associated with vomiting in neonates and infants accounts for less than 45% of all reported cases. Traumatic perforation can be secondary to ingested foreign objects; diagnostic or therapeutic manipulations of the esophagus, such as esophagoscopy with or without dilation; ingestion of caustic substances, such as lye; and blunt or penetrating trauma to the chest. Iatrogenic perforation of the esophagus secondary to esophageal dilation is the most common clinical situation. Blunt, mercury-weighted bougies are more often the cause of perforation with dilation procedures than are string-guided or balloon dilators.

CLINICAL FINDINGS AND DIAGNOSIS

Respiratory distress is often the first clinical sign of esophageal rupture in newborns and infants. If the perforation remains undiagnosed and feedings are continued, the respiratory distress worsens. The perforation often causes diffuse esophageal spasm so that dysphagia follows. This condition is manifested by drooling and increased oral secretions. Subcutaneous emphysema can appear fairly quickly after rupture, particularly with large perforations, although this is more common in older children than in infants. Older children often complain of substernal chest pain in these instances. Fever and progression to septic shock can occur within hours after the rupture if the perforation has ruptured into the free pleural cavity or has caused mediastinitis.

When a perforation is suspected, a chest film should be obtained immediately to determine if pneumothorax and pneumomediastinum are present. In newborns and infants, spontaneous perforation of the distal esophagus usually occurs into the right side of the chest, whereas in older children and adults, perforation is usually into the left side of the chest. A chest film may show malposition of the nasogastric tube or a foreign body in the esophagus (Fig. 38-1). If the perforation is submucosal, a pneumothorax is not seen, and pneumomediastinum is the only finding on the lateral plain film of the chest which shows pneumomediastinum best (Fig. 38-2). No matter what the cause of the perforation, a soluble contrast, not barium, study of the esophagus is required to establish the diagnosis and to localize the perforation (Fig. 38-3). If the contrast esophagogram does not adequately show a highly suspected perforation, diagnostic esophagoscopy may be required.

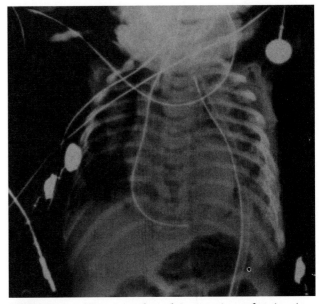

FIGURE 38-1 ■ Upper esophageal iatrogenic perforation in a premature infant. Note the position of the presumed nasogastric tube in the right side of the chest. The tube was withdrawn, and nonoperative therapy resulted in complete recovery.

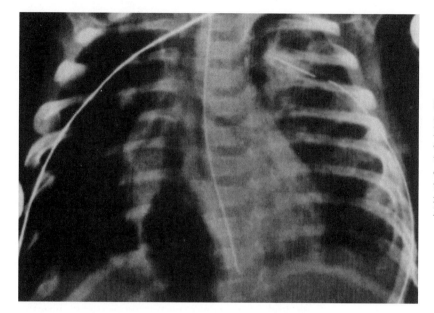

FIGURE 38-2 ■ Spontaneous rupture of the esophagus in a newborn. There is a large collection of gas in the mediastinum to the right of the esophagus. The nasogastric tube within the esophagus was placed after the perforation occurred, and contrast studies performed through the tube confirmed a lower esophageal rupture, which was repaired successfully at 24 hours by direct suture.

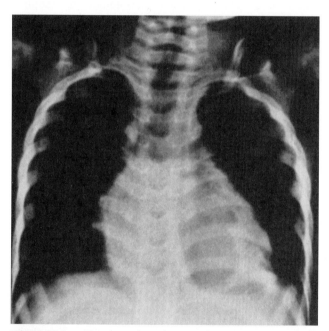

FIGURE 38-3 ■ Esophageal perforation from dilation for longstanding peptic esophagitis. This collection of gas in the mediastinum behind the heart was found 1 hour after esophageal dilation. Subsequent esophagram showed distal esophageal perforation.

TREATMENT

The appropriate treatment of an esophageal perforation depends on the site and cause of the perforation. Some iatrogenic perforations, if recognized early, can be managed nonoperatively. An example may be iatrogenic perforation in the neck, especially in newborns or infants secondary to pharyngeal suctioning or from passage of an endotracheal or nasogastric tube. In this situation, it is imperative to position a nasogastric tube into the true lumen of the esophagus and institute broad-spectrum antibiotics and total parenteral nutrition. Often, esophagoscopy is required to pass the tube into the true lumen. Similar management may be possible for iatrogenic thoracic injuries when these injuries are detected less than 24 hours after their occurrence. Intraluminal penetrations from foreign bodies, such as coins, may respond to nonoperative therapy when the foreign body is removed. Exploration usually is required, however, for iatrogenic perforations, which are noticed late after their occurrence, especially in the toxic patient.

Penetrating and blunt injuries to the esophagus require mandatory exploration. This is especially true in the cervical region because other structures also can be injured. These cervical perforations can be approached through a collar incision, which provides optimal exposure to each side of the neck. The usual approach to the injured thoracic esophagus is through a right thoracotomy for lesions in the upper and mid thorax and a left thoracotomy for lesions in the lower esophagus. Some injuries to the lower esophagus in the neonate also can be explored through a right thoracotomy. The role of thoracoscopy for these injuries is unclear. In the stable, nontoxic patient who requires simple drainage and débridement, thoracoscopy may play a role in selected patients. Most patients requiring operative intervention generally require thoracotomy, however, with attempted closure or patch of the esophageal perforation, débridement and drainage of the mediastinum, and, perhaps, reinforcement with a pericardial or intercostal muscle flap around the area of injury. In cases with gross contamination of the thoracic cavity and severe mediastinitis, cervical esophagostomy may be required. In this instance, the esophageal perforation should be closed and a gastrostomy performed. The divided distal cervical esophagus should be tacked to the cervical prevertebral fascia for subsequent reanastomosis to the esophagostomy. There have been scattered reports of ligation of the esophagus with absorbable suture coupled with a gastrostomy and feeding jejunostomy and nasogastric suction of the blind esophageal pouch for severe injuries. In these few cases, spontaneous recanalization of the esophagus at the site of the cervical suture ligation has been found on subsequent esophagrams. For injuries requiring reinforcement of the suture line, various tissues have been used, including omentum, diaphragm, pleura, pericardium, and intercostal muscle. Creation of a pleural flap reinforced by intercostal muscle proved effective in one adult series.

After primary repair, a water-soluble contrast study is performed 7 to 10 days later to determine whether the perforation has sealed and to evaluate the esophagus for the presence of a stricture. If the perforation is closed and there is no evidence of stricture formation, the patient is begun on oral feedings, and the chest tube is removed. Late strictures can develop and usually respond to esophageal dilation. If perforation occurs during dilation for a long, rigid stricture, esophageal resection and replacement may be required. Mortality depends on prompt detection of the injury, especially if iatrogenic in nature, and early intervention along with broad-spectrum antibiotics, gastric decompression, and nutritional supplementation either with total parenteral nutrition or a feeding jejunostomy.

SUGGESTED READINGS

Engum SA, Grosfeld JL, West KW, et al: Improved survival in children with esophageal perforation. Arch Surg 131:604-610, 1996.

The authors describe their experience with 24 children with esophageal perforation who were treated over a 20-year period. They found that most esophageal perforations can be closed primarily and that the esophagus can be salvaged despite late presentation.

Kerschner JE, Beste DJ, Conley SF, et al: Mediastinitis associated with foreign body erosion of the esophagus in children. Int J Pediatr Otorhinolaryngol 7:89-97, 2001.

Over a 10-year period, four patients developed esophageal perforation and associated mediastinitis secondary to retained esophageal foreign bodies. Three of these patients were managed conservatively with foreign body removal, intravenous antibiotics, and cessation of oral nutrition.

Panieri E, Millar AJ, Rode H, et al: Iatrogenic esophageal perforation in children: Patterns of injury, presentation, management, and outcome. J Pediatr Surg 31:890-895, 1996.

In their experience over 25 years, the authors found most children with iatrogenic injuries could be managed successfully by conservative measures, and pleural drainage with surgical procedures could be reserved for large disruptions of the esophagus, intra-abdominal perforation, and cases that did not respond to appropriate conservative measures.

Sartorelli KH, McBride WJ, Vane DW: Perforation of the intrathoracic esophagus from blunt trauma in a child: Case report and review of the literature. J Pediatr Surg 34:495-497, 1999

This case report discusses management of esophageal injuries in children and reviews the pediatric literature.

Zumbro GL, Anstadt MP, Mawulawde K, et al: Surgical management of esophageal perforation: Role of esophageal conservation in delayed perforation. Am Surg 68:36-40, 2002.

The authors reviewed 22 adult patients with delayed presentation of esophageal perforation over a 15-year period. Most of the perforations occurred in the lower third of the esophagus. This article provides an excellent discussion of various options available for treatment of esophageal injuries.

Gastroesophageal Reflux and Other Disorders of Esophageal Function

39

Fundoplication is currently either the first or the second most commonly performed intra-abdominal procedure in infants and children in most pediatric surgical centers. In 1943, Allison first described an operative method of hiatus repair for correction of symptoms related to gastroesophageal reflux (GER). Four years later, Neuhauser and Berenberg described "chalasia" as a benign condition that was treated effectively with upright positioning and thickened feedings. In the 1960s, the popular Allison repair was replaced with procedures described by Nissen, Hill, and Belsey for surgical management of GER.

Since the 1970s, surgical correction for GER has been performed primarily with either a partial (Thal, Boix-Ochoa, Dor, Toupet) or complete (Nissen) fundoplication. In general, it seems that the Nissen fundoplication is more effective in preventing GER, but it may lead to dysphagia and troublesome bloating in some patients compared with a partial fundoplication, which seems not as effective in preventing reflux but does not lead to postoperative obstructive symptoms. These symptoms after the Nissen procedure seem to be minimized with use of an appropriate-sized bougie and ligation and division of the short gastric vessels for sufficient mobilization of the stomach.

PATHOPHYSIOLOGY

Chalasia is a benign variant of vomiting and is seen early in life, usually after burping or feeding or when the infant is placed in a recumbent position. Chalasia in infancy does not interfere with normal growth or development and rarely leads to other complications. It is a self-limited process with symptoms resolving by 18 to 24 months of age in most patients. Usually, there is no treatment indicated for these symptoms, and diagnostic evaluation rarely is required.

In contrast to physiologic vomiting (chalasia), GER can present as a single or as multiple clinical conditions resulting in significant morbidity or near-fatal events. Many barriers exist to protect the patient against reflux of gastric juice into the esophagus (Table 39-1). The two most important anatomic factors inhibiting GER appear to be the length of the intra-abdominal esophagus and the angle of His. Although no absolute effective intra-abdominal esophageal length that prevents GER has been identified, there is correlation between increased intra-abdominal esophageal length and lack of GER. It seems that an intra-abdominal length of 3 to 4.5 cm in adults with normal intra-abdominal pressure provides competency of the lower esophageal sphincter (LES) most of the time. A length of 3 cm seems sufficient in preventing reflux in approximately half of adult patients, whereas a length of less than 1 cm results in reflux in most patients. When the usual acute angle of His becomes more obtuse, GER is more prone to develop. Conversely, accentuation of this angle seems to inhibit reflux. The ability of the angle of His to participate in prevention of GER may be diminished as a result of abnormal development or may be iatrogenic, as occurs after gastrostomy placement.

Physiologic components to this barrier against reflux include the LES; the difference between intra-abdominal and intrathoracic pressures; and various mediators, such as gastrin, prostaglandins, and catecholamines. The LES arises from the inner circular muscle layer of the esophagus, which is asymmetrically thickened in the distal esophagus. This thickened muscle layer creates a high-pressure zone that can be measured manometrically. This muscular thickening extends onto the stomach more prominently on the greater than the lesser curve. The LES is an imperfect valve that creates a pressure gradient in the distal esophagus. The ability to prevent GER is directly proportional to the LES pressure and its length, provided

TABLE 39-1 ■ Barriers to Gastroesophageal Reflux and Mechanism of Failure	
BARRIERS TO GER	**MECHANISM OF FAILURE**
LES	Inappropriate relaxation
	Reduced LES length and pressure
	Intrathoracic location
	Abnormal smooth muscle function
Angle of His	More obtuse angle (gastrostomy)
	Abnormal development
Length of intra-abdominal esophagus	Length <3 cm (adults)

that LES relaxation is normal. Malposition of the LES, which can occur with a hiatal hernia or with abnormal development, results in loss of the protective function of the LES and contributes to development of GER. LES relaxation occurs with esophageal peristalsis, which is initiated by the swallowing mechanism. If this normal relaxation is exaggerated and is unassociated with swallowing, GER results. There is growing support for identifying these inappropriate LES relaxations as the primary mechanism for GER. Although the barrier function of the LES is sometimes imperfect, it is usually highly effective. Short LES length, abnormal smooth muscle function, increased frequency of transient LES relaxation, and LES location within the chest can contribute individually or in combination to LES failure and GER. Disruption of the LES from a hiatal hernia, abnormal LES function, or previous esophageal surgery all can lead to poor function and subsequent GER.

CLINICAL MANIFESTATIONS

There is a great deal of variability in the clinical presentation of GER in infants and children. Persistent regurgitation is the most common clinical symptom of GER, especially in young children and in neurologically impaired patients. This excessive vomiting can result in inadequate nutritional intake and can lead to growth failure. Respiratory symptoms also are seen commonly in infants and children secondary to GER and associated aspiration. Delineating the role of GER as the etiologic agent for ongoing respiratory symptoms can be difficult because of the commonality of the symptoms that often are seen with other pulmonary diseases. Chronic cough, wheezing, choking, apnea, or near sudden infant death syndrome (SIDS) all can be attributed to GER, however. Acid stimulation within the esophagus causes vaguely mediated laryngospasm and bronchospasm, which clinically presents as apnea or choking or can present mistakenly as asthma. Esophageal inflammation, as seen with esophagitis, likely enhances this mechanism. Although major hemorrhage is a rare presenting symptom, occult blood loss with iron deficiency anemia can occur occasionally.

In pediatric patients, another presenting symptom is irritability owing to pain. This discomfort can lead to crying in infants despite consoling measures. Although small volumes of feedings in infants can alleviate this discomfort briefly, it is not a lasting benefit. Pain is a presenting symptom often in older children as well. As in adults, the pain is usually retrosternal in location and is described as heartburn. Whether in infants or older children, long-standing GER with esophagitis can lead to chronic inflammation with eventual scarring and stricture formation. When a stricture develops, pain and dysphagia are the two most commonly associated symptoms. Barrett's esophagitis is a premalignant condition in which metaplasia occurs in the distal esophageal squamous epithelium leading to replacement with columnar epithelium. In adults, it is believed to be the result of chronic esophageal injury from gastric acid reflux. This condition is rare in infants and children. When it does develop, however, serious complications often result. In addition

to the increased risk for adenocarcinoma in adults, approximately 50% of these patients develop an esophageal stricture, and many develop ulcerations. Barrett's esophagitis can be seen in the older child and teenager as a result of long-standing GER. For this reason, endoscopy and biopsy may be more appropriate in the evaluation of the older patient when compared with the infant. When Barrett's esophagitis is documented in the child, it usually can be managed successfully with fundoplication.

Sandifer's syndrome is seen rarely today in children with GER. These children present with an unusual lateral and posterior posturing of the head and neck that is a result of reflux of gastric juice into the posterior pharynx. These children often present with a clinical picture of opisthotonos.

DIAGNOSTIC EVALUATION

When GER has been entertained as the cause of the patient's symptoms, diagnostic evaluation should be initiated. Among the possible studies used for evaluation of GER are the upper gastrointestinal (GI) series, 24-hour pH monitoring, esophageal manometry, upper GI endoscopy, and gastric emptying studies. The use of these studies varies according to the medical center in which the patient is seen. Most pediatric centers use the 24-hour pH study as the gold standard for evaluating GER. Some centers use upper GI radiography and upper GI endoscopy, however. The preoperative evaluation of gastric emptying also varies from center to center. Although some surgeons and gastroenterologists believe that all patients should undergo a radionuclide gastric emptying study preoperatively, many do not because gastric emptying is thought to improve with fundoplication owing to a decrease in the capacity of the stomach. For this reason, it can be difficult to interpret which patient with delayed gastric emptying on a preoperative study is benefited by a gastric emptying operation at the time of fundoplication. Esophageal manometry is not used routinely in children but is beneficial when there is concern that achalasia may be the cause for the patient's symptoms or there is concern about an esophageal motility disorder.

The 24-hour pH monitoring test is an objective way to document the presence or absence of GER. This test can be particularly helpful in patients in whom the history is unclear or confusing, such as a patient presenting with respiratory symptoms only. For an accurate result, it is important to cease all antireflux medication before the study. Proton-pump inhibitors should be withheld for 7 days, and histamine receptor blockers should not be given for 48 hours before the examination. The final score is calculated on the percentage of total time that the pH of the distal esophagus is less than 4, the total number of reflux episodes, the number of episodes lasting longer than 5 minutes, and the longest reflux episode.

An upper GI series is the most frequently used study for initial evaluation of GER. Although not as sensitive as 24-hour pH monitoring, it can be performed on an outpatient basis. In addition, if reflux is documented on this study, and if the patient's symptoms are consistent with this diagnosis, 24-hour pH monitoring may not be necessary in all circumstances. If the upper GI series is normal, however, and the suspicion of reflux persists, 24-hour pH monitoring is recommended. In centers in which the upper GI series and 24-hour pH monitoring are employed routinely for diagnosis, the upper GI series is used primarily to document anatomic abnormalities or gastric outlet obstruction that might be contributing to the patient's symptoms. The upper GI series provides a crude evaluation of whether or not there is normal or delayed gastric emptying.

Endoscopic evaluation of the esophagus and stomach is used in some centers for the routine evaluation of infants and children with suspected GER. When endoscopy is used, biopsy is performed to document the presence or absence of esophagitis and to exclude histologically malignancy in Barrett's esophagus in older children. Symptoms of hematemesis or irritability in infants or dysphagia with or without heartburn in infants and children should prompt esophagogastroscopy to determine if esophagitis is present.

The presence of delayed gastric emptying is assessed best preoperatively using a technetium 99m pertechnetate scan. Neurologically impaired children with GER have been shown to have delayed gastric emptying more often than neurologically normal children. Conflicting studies regarding the benefit and complication rates for these patients undergoing emptying procedures at the time of fundoplication have been reported. In addition to assessing delayed gastric emptying, the technetium scan is able to help evaluate possible pulmonary aspiration.

TREATMENT

Medical Management

Initial treatment for GER is usually medical, although older children with the diagnosis of Barrett's esophagitis may be managed best initially with fundoplication. Initial nonoperative treatment in infants includes upright positioning and thickened feedings with or without the addition of prokinetic agents (e.g., metoclopramide, erythromycin). Most infants respond to medical treatment and do not require a surgical procedure. H_2-blockers, such as cimetidine or ranitidine, also may improve the success of nonoperative therapy. A proton-pump inhibitor (e.g., omeprazole) has revolutionized medical therapy and is the most effective agent for nonoperative treatment of this disorder. The prokinetic agent cisapride has been used widely for medical management of symptoms of GER in the past, but is not currently routinely available in the United States because of its arrhythmogenic side effects.

Indications for operation without initially attempting medical therapy include the presence of severe esophagitis, Barrett's metaplasia, stricture, a near-SIDS event, and, in some centers, apnea and bradycardia in infants. If medical therapy is employed for other symptoms, failure of medical therapy constitutes an indication for surgical intervention. It is unclear what is the appropriate time between initiation of medical therapy and consideration of surgical intervention for failure of medical therapy. Although in infants, it seems reasonable to use medical therapy for several months before operation, in older children, the risk of esophagitis and stricture is greater,

and medical therapy probably should not be employed more than 6 to 8 weeks.

Surgical Procedures

As previously mentioned, many operations have been used in the surgical management of infants and children with GER, including the Nissen fundoplication and the Nissen-Rossetti modification, the anterior (Thal) fundoplication, the Hill posterior gastropexy, the Boerema gastropexy, the Boix-Ochoa procedure, the Belsey Mark IV operation, and the posterior (Toupet) fundoplication. The Nissen procedure is the most commonly used fundoplication in the United States, whereas the Nissen-Rosetti operation is popular in Europe. The primary difference between the Nissen-Rosetti operation and the Nissen operation is that the short gastric vessels are not ligated and divided in the Rosetti modification. This modification is beginning to fall into disfavor, however, because there is insufficient mobilization of the fundus, and complications such as wrap disruption and dysphagia are being documented in long-term follow-up studies.

The Nissen fundoplication is a full 360-degree wrap, whereas the Thal fundoplication is an anterior 270-degree partial wrap. Cited disadvantages of the Nissen procedure are the inability to vomit, dysphagia, and the development of gas bloat syndrome. When an appropriate esophageal bougie is used during the operation, however, dysphagia should not be a significant clinical problem, and the inability to vomit also usually is not significant. Gas bloat syndrome seems to occur less frequently in children than in adults. Although the Thal fundoplication has a higher incidence of recurrent reflux compared with the Nissen fundoplication, it does not have these associated postoperative problems. The Nissen fundoplication lends itself best to the laparoscopic approach and is the most commonly performed laparoscopic fundoplication in the world.

When either the Nissen or the Thal operation is performed open or laparoscopically, the results are good, especially in the short-term. Because the laparoscopic approach for either operation has not been used extensively for more than 5 years as of this writing, long-term results with the laparoscopic approach are not known. A recurrence rate of 10% for the Nissen procedure and 15% to 20% for the Thal operation has been found in most large series performed in the open fashion. The most common cause for recurrence with the Nissen fundoplication is transmigration of the wrap through the crura followed by breakdown of the wrap. Symptoms of recurrent reflux are more common in patients with neurologic impairment than in patients who are neurologically normal. Postoperative intestinal obstruction, which may occur in 15% to 25% of cases after an open fundoplication, is rare following the laparoscopic operation.

A common scenario for pediatric surgeons is a child, usually neurologically impaired, in need of a gastrostomy for enteral alimentation. Decisions of whether or not to perform an evaluation for GER and how to perform this evaluation vary from surgeon to surgeon. At the least, most surgeons obtain an upper GI series to evaluate for the presence or absence of GER. In a patient without clinical symptoms of reflux and a normal upper GI series, gastrostomy alone may be acceptable. In neurologically impaired children without evidence of GER on studies, the incidence of GER after gastrostomy alone is 10% to 15%. In a patient with symptoms of reflux but a normal upper GI study, however, a pH study is recommended. If reflux is noted on either the upper GI series or the pH study, and especially if the patient is neurologically impaired, a fundoplication in addition to the gastrostomy is recommended. In neurologically impaired patients, some surgeons also routinely order a gastric emptying study to evaluate whether or not delayed gastric emptying is present and, if so, perform a gastric emptying procedure. Commonly performed gastric emptying procedures include pyloroplasty, pyloromyotomy, and antroplasty. Each of these operations can be performed in association with an open or laparoscopic fundoplication. If performed appropriately, each seems to be equally effective.

Some neurologically impaired patients with GER are managed initially by radiographic placement of a nasojejunal tube for enteral alimentation. If a gastrostomy has been created previously, and GER has developed, a gastrojejunal tube placed via the gastrostomy stoma also can be used. The main disadvantage of this approach is the frequent dislodgment of these tubes and recurrent trips to the fluoroscopy suite for reinsertion. In addition, underlying reflux and the basic pathologic conditions remain untreated.

Two special circumstances that merit thoughtful evaluation before fundoplication are the patient who previously has required repair of esophageal atresia and the patient, usually neurologically impaired, who has failed two or three prior fundoplications. In the former clinical condition, there is underlying esophageal dysmotility, and this dysmotility may be aggravated by a 360-degree fundoplication. For this reason, a partial fundoplication usually is recommended in these patients. In the latter circumstance, the patient who already has failed two or three previous fundoplications, esophagogastric dissociation is an attractive alternative approach. With this procedure, a Roux-en-Y esophagojejunostomy is performed. Enteral feeding is accomplished usually through a gastrostomy.

Technique

Nissen Fundoplication

The Nissen fundoplication can be performed either laparoscopically or open. The laparoscopic approach is being used more frequently because of its perceived advantages of reduced discomfort and hospitalization and earlier return to routine activities, such as school or sports in older children. Whether performed laparoscopically or open, the operation is done in a similar fashion. In the open operation, either an upper midline incision or a left subcostal incision is used for access to the abdominal cavity. With the laparoscopic operation, five small (3 or 5 mm) incisions are employed. In most children, a 5-mm incision can be made in the umbilicus with the incision hidden in the umbilical scar. Through this incision, a 5-mm cannula is introduced into the abdominal cavity, a pneumoperitoneum is created, and the telescope with the attached camera is introduced through this cannula. In most infants and young children,

the remainder of the operation can be performed with 3-mm instruments. Older children may require 5-mm instruments. Some surgeons use cannulas through these incisions, whereas others are beginning to place the instruments directly through the skin without cannulas because an adequate pneumoperitoneum is maintained easily in infants and children without cannulas. In the patient's right upper abdomen, a grasping forceps is introduced through one of the small incisions and situated under the left lobe of the liver. The jaws of this instrument are secured to the diaphragm, and the left lobe of the liver is elevated anteriorly to allow visualization of the gastroesophageal junction. The two primary working ports for the laparoscopic procedure are in the left and right midepigastrium. Through a small incision in the patient's right midepigastrium, a grasping forceps is inserted, which is used in the surgeon's left hand for retraction purposes. The left midepigastric incision is the main working site for the surgeon, and this is the incision through which dissecting instruments and needle holders are inserted. The final incision is situated in the patient's left subcostal region. An atraumatic grasping forceps is placed through this incision for the assistant's use (Fig. 39-1). For the laparoscopic procedure, patients are positioned at the foot of the bed, and the surgeon stands there in the so-called French position. Monitors are located usually on either side of the patient at the head of the table.

Whether performed in an open or laparoscopic fashion, the short gastric vessels are ligated and divided. With the laparoscopic approach, these vessels usually are divided using cautery in the young child or the ultrasonic scalpel in older patients. After division of the short gastric vessels, the esophageal hiatus is skeletonized, and an adequate length of intra-abdominal esophagus is obtained. Usually a hiatal hernia is present that requires one or two

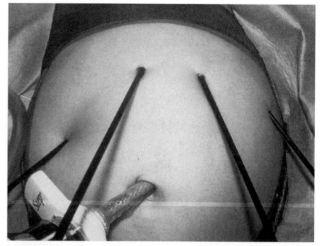

FIGURE 39-1 ■ Incisions for a laparoscopic fundoplication in an infant. The main working sites for the surgeon are in the two incisions in the central portion of the epigastrium. Under the patient's right subcostal margin is an incision through which an instrument is placed for elevation of the left lobe of the liver. Through the incision in the left subcostal region, grasping forceps have been used by the assistant for retraction. The only cannula used in this patient is in the umbilicus, through which a 5-mm telescope is inserted.

silk sutures for closure. With the laparoscopic approach, these sutures can be tied either intracorporeally or extracorporeally. After crural repair, an appropriate-sized dilator is directed through the mouth and into the stomach to ensure that the esophagus has not been narrowed with the crural repair (Fig. 39-2A). The fundus of the stomach is brought through the retroesophageal space, and the 360-degree wrap is completed using silk sutures (Fig. 39-2B). The sutures are tied intracorporeally or extracorporeally with the laparoscopic approach. The fundoplication is performed over the same bougie to ensure that the esophagus is not narrowed significantly with creation of the 360-degree wrap. If required, a gastrostomy can be placed at the time of the fundoplication. When the laparoscopic approach is employed, there are a variety of techniques for placement of the gastrostomy, but the U-stitch technique created by Georgeson seems to be the most effective. With this technique, a gastrostomy button is placed primarily at the time of the fundoplication (Fig. 39-3).

Thal Fundoplication

This fundoplication also can be performed using a left transverse incision or the laparoscopic technique. The left lobe of the liver is detached from the diaphragm and retracted downward and to the right with the open procedure or elevated anteriorly with the laparoscopic approach. A nasogastric tube passed into the stomach provides decompression, allows easy identification of the lower esophagus, and provides some stability for the stomach during creation of the anterior fundoplication. A Dacron tape is passed around the lower esophagus (including both vagal branches) for traction purposes. As the esophagus is retracted to the left, the crura are identified and approximated to create a hiatus of reasonable size, using a permanent, figure-8 suture. This suture is used to fix the posterior esophagus to the hiatus repair. With the open approach, the anterior fundoplication is accomplished

using a continuous polypropylene suture beginning at the greater curvature gastroesophageal junction. The suture line approximates the upper, anterior gastric wall to the lower, anterior esophagus and extends up the left side of the esophagus to the hiatus. The suture line is continued across the anterior esophagus toward the right incorporating gastric wall, esophagus, and hiatus. When the right side of the esophagus is reached, the suture line is turned caudally to approximate the gastric wall and the esophagus down to the lesser curvature gastroesophageal junction (Fig. 39-4). With the laparoscopic operation,

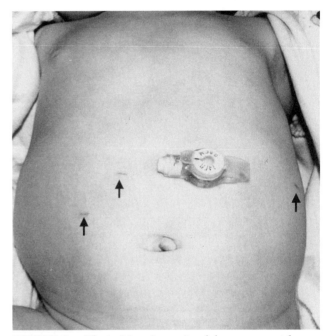

FIGURE 39-3 ■ The incisions (arrows) and the gastrostomy button that was placed at the time of the laparoscopic fundoplication in this infant. The incisions were closed only with Steri-strips.

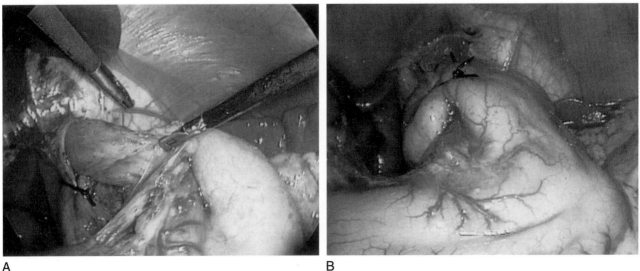

A   B

FIGURE 39-2 ■ **A,** The stomach is retracted caudally to straighten the esophagus as an esophageal bougie is directed into the stomach. Note the suture that was used to approximate the crura posteriorly. **B,** A completed laparoscopic Nissen fundoplication. Three sutures were used to perform the fundoplication, and the length of the fundoplication measures 1.8 cm.

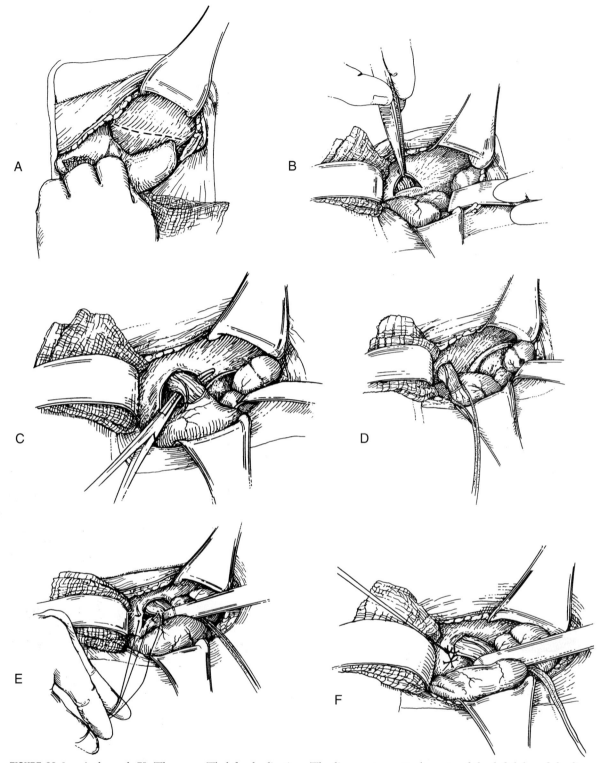

FIGURE 39-4 ■ A through **K,** The open Thal fundoplication. The ligamentous attachments of the left lobe of the liver are taken down from the underside of the diaphragm, beginning from the free margin near the spleen. The liver can be turned downward and to the right, exposing the hiatus. An incision is made over the gastroesophageal junction in a transverse manner. The hiatus is lifted to allow dissection of the esophagus on either side. A blunt dissector is passed behind the esophagus, attempting to incorporate the posterior vagus nerve segment with the esophageal muscle. Dacron tape is passed about the esophagus when the dissector is withdrawn, allowing the esophagus to be pulled downward, while the hiatus is pushed upward to free an appropriate length of esophagus for placement in the intra-abdominal position. A figure-8 suture of 2-0 silk on a cardiovascular needle is used to approximate the crura behind the esophagus. This same suture affixes the esophagus posteriorly to the hiatus. Placement of this limiting stitch not only reduces the incidence of postoperative hiatus hernia, but also allows better fixation of an intra-abdominal esophagus.

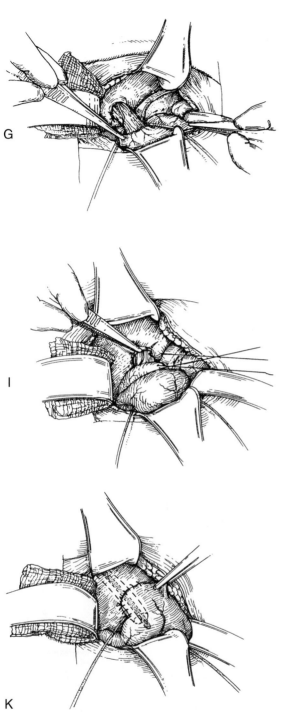

FIGURE 39-4—cont'd ■ The limbs of the Dacron tape are spread so that the fundus of the stomach may be brought up between them and sutured to the anterior half of the esophagus. None of the short gastric vessels needs to be divided to perform this fundoplication. A continuous suture is used, beginning at the greater curve of the gastroesophageal junction where it is tied, progressively approximating the free wall of the stomach to the esophagus along its left side and moving upward toward the hiatus. This continuous suture at the hiatus includes stomach, esophagus, and hiatus. The continuous suture is carried across the anterior wall of the esophagus. The stomach, esophagus, and hiatus are incorporated in each suture. The continuous suture is completed at the lesser curve of the gastroesophageal junction where it is tied. This method creates an inverted U-like suture line. The dashed lines show the position of the esophagus in relation to the hiatus and the fundus. A nasogastric tube is positioned during the construction of the procedure. The tube may be removed immediately afterward or may be left until the following day, when it is removed. Feedings are then begun. (From Ashcraft KA: Gastroesophageal reflux. In Ashcraft KW, Holder TH [eds]: Pediatric Surgery, 3rd ed. Philadelphia, WB Saunders, 2000.)

some surgeons use the continuous suture, whereas others prefer an interrupted suture technique. With the open approach, the liver is replaced and the abdomen closed. The small incisions are approximated if the laparoscopic route is used.

OTHER DISORDERS OF ESOPHAGEAL FUNCTION

Anatomically, the upper one third of the esophagus is composed of striated muscle, and the remaining lower portion is composed of smooth muscle. Functionally, there are three zones to the esophagus: the upper esophageal sphincter (UES), the body, and the LES. The cricopharyngeus muscle forms the UES and requires participation of the inferior pharyngeal constrictors and the circular muscle of the proximal esophagus for proper function. After pharyngeal contraction but before esophageal peristalsis, the UES relaxes, contracting again when swallowing is completed. Each swallow is followed by a monophasic pressure wave that traverses the esophagus aborally crossing the striated and smooth muscle. Approximately 90% of swallows are followed by this "primary peristalsis." "Secondary peristalsis" is not preceded by a swallow but is induced by the failure of a bolus to pass into the stomach or by the reflux of gastric contents into the esophagus. "Tertiary peristalsis" is initiated in the smooth muscle of the esophagus.

Compared with GER, esophageal neuromotor disorders are rare in children. These disorders include achalasia, diffuse esophageal spasm, and scleroderma. The diagnosis of these disorders is based on clinical suspicion, contrast esophagography, manometry, and, occasionally, pH monitoring. Dysphagia is usually a prominent symptom with these esophageal motor disorders.

Achalasia

Achalasia is a motor disorder usually affecting the entire length of the esophagus. Although the cause of achalasia is unclear, approximately 10% of cases occur in children. Even though this disease is relatively uncommon in children, it seems to be increasing in frequency. Two thirds of affected children are boys. Whether the condition is being diagnosed at an earlier age or there is a true increase in its incidence is unclear. This disorder is caused by failure of the LES to relax and failure of the peristaltic wave to propagate. It seems to be similar functionally and pathologically to Hirschsprung's disease in that the distal myenteric ganglion cells are absent in each disorder causing functional obstruction and proximal dilation. There also has been shown to be a paucity of vasoactive intestinal polypeptide–containing nerve fibers in the distal esophagus in these patients. Vasoactive intestinal polypeptide is known to relax smooth muscle in the LES, and its absence may lead to this disorder. Nitric oxide also has been shown to be important in relaxation of the LES muscle.

Most children with achalasia present with symptoms of several months' to several years' duration consisting typically of vomiting of undigested food, severe halitosis, and significant dysphagia. These children also may have prolonged coughing spells after meals. Weight loss becomes a common component of the symptoms because nutritional status is markedly affected. Children often complain of substernal pain or burning secondary to esophageal irritation from retained food. Usually there is a delay in establishing a diagnosis. An upright chest radiograph may show a wide mediastinum and an air-fluid level in the posterior mediastinum (Fig. 39-5A). The diagnosis usually is suspected after an upper GI series that shows significant narrowing at the

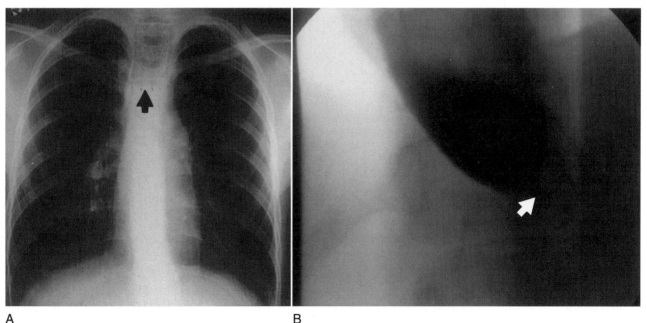

A   B

FIGURE 39-5 ■ **A,** Chest radiograph shows an air-fluid level in the mediastinum (arrow). **B,** Upper GI study shows dilation of the proximal esophagus (arrow) with failure of relaxation of the LES, creating a bird beak deformity.

LES with considerable dilation of the proximal esophagus (bird beak deformity) (Fig. 39-5B). In addition, there is no relaxation of the LES on contrast radiography. The diagnosis is confirmed by manometric evaluation revealing a markedly elevated resting pressure in the esophagus without evidence of relaxation of the LES (Fig. 39-6). There also is absence of coordinated peristaltic contractions in the body of the esophagus. If esophagoscopy is performed, it is usually nondiagnostic. There is often a significant amount of retained undigested food in the esophagus, however.

The ideal treatment of patients with achalasia is controversial. In 1971, Van Trapp introduced the concept of pneumatic dilation for adult patients. Balloon dilation is used in children but seems to be less successful in relieving symptoms than pneumatic dilation in adults. The incidence of postdilation GER may be higher in children, and the procedure is technically more difficult in younger patients. Other approaches for relief of symptoms include injection of botulinum toxin into the LES. Although this technique has gained popularity in more recent years, its effectiveness usually lasts only a few months. Medical management is also not successful. Calcium channel blockade with nifedipine or verapamil has had limited efficacy but may be useful in some patients as a temporizing measure between diagnosis and operative management. Because nonoperative therapy is rarely successful, especially for a prolonged period, most children with achalasia require esophagomyotomy for long-term relief.

In 1913, Heller described extramucosal esophagomyotomy for relief of symptoms referable to achalasia. With advancements in minimally invasive surgery, this myotomy has become an attractive approach for surgical management. Although esophagomyotomy has been reported using either the laparoscopic or the thorascopic route, the laparoscopic route is now favored. There are many reports in the adult literature describing the efficacy of a laparoscopic Heller myotomy for relief of symptoms resulting from achalasia, but the experience in the pediatric literature is not nearly as large.

The most controversial aspect of performing a laparoscopic esophagomyotomy in a child is whether or not an antireflux procedure should be added. This controversy also exists in the adult literature. Most adult surgeons favor the performance of an antireflux operation because it is relatively easy to accomplish and prevents the need for a second procedure if GER develops. The preferred technique is an anterior (Dor) fundoplication performed at the time of the laparoscopic esophageal myotomy, but the posterior (Toupet) fundoplication also has been described. The primary advantage of the anterior fundoplication is that the fundoplication covers the esophagomyotomy.

Esophagomyotomy

For the laparoscopic esophageal myotomy, the patient is positioned at the foot of the operating table in the so-called French position, which is identical to that used by most surgeons for laparoscopic fundoplication. In addition, placement of the incisions is similar to that used for fundoplication (Fig. 39-7). Identical instruments are employed for a laparoscopic esophageal myotomy as for a laparoscopic fundoplication.

With an operative plan of myotomy and anterior fundoplication, the initial step is to divide the most cephalad two or three short gastric vessels to mobilize the fundus of the stomach. This can be accomplished with cautery or with the ultrasonic scalpel. Next, the anesthesiologist is asked to introduce an appropriate-sized bougie through the mouth and into the stomach to stent the lower esophagus. Some surgeons also use esophagoscopy for this reason, but the major disadvantage of concomitant esophagoscopy is distention of the stomach owing to insufflation, which impairs visualization of the esophagus.

The first step in performing the myotomy is careful separation of the esophageal muscle fibers 1 to 2 cm

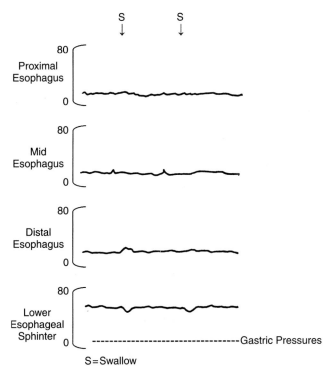

FIGURE 39-6 ■ Manometric study shows a markedly elevated resting pressure in the esophagus without evidence of relaxation at the LES.

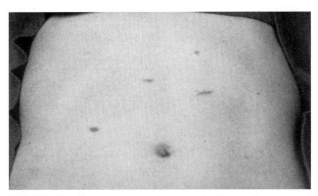

FIGURE 39-7 ■ Postoperative photograph shows placement of the incisions for laparoscopic esophagomyotomy and anterior fundoplication.

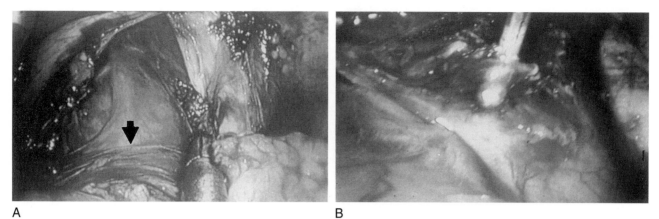

FIGURE 39-8 ■ **A,** The esophagomyotomy was initiated above the LES and progressed caudally. The fibers of the LES (arrow) are seen traversing the inferior margin of the esophagomyotomy. **B,** The technique of hooking the esophageal muscle fibers and pulling these fibers away from the underlying submucosa.

above the LES (Fig. 39-8A). This usually is performed with the hook cautery. When the esophageal submucosa is visualized, the muscle fibers are gently hooked, pulled away from the submucosa, and cauterized (Fig. 39-8B). In this manner, a vertical plane is created from the initial starting point down onto the stomach for approximately 1 cm. Visualization of these muscle fibers is excellent, and it is usually possible to distinguish the esophageal muscle fibers from the submucosa. Great care must be taken, however, during this part of the operation not to cauterize too deeply, creating a perforation. The myotomy usually is extended cephalad a little above the phreno-esophageal ligament. With myotomy to this level, usually the myotomy length is 6 to 8 cm (Fig. 39-9). If a longer esophageal myotomy is desired, further caudal esophageal retraction is required. A Penrose drain or umbilical tape can be placed through the retroesophageal space and the esophagus retracted caudally for this purpose. If there is concern about the completeness of the myotomy, the bougie can be removed and esophagoscopy performed to confirm that an adequate myotomy has been accomplished. If required, the esophagomyotomy can be extended more caudally onto the stomach. An anterior fundoplication is performed by rotating the fundus anteriorly and to the patient's right and sewing it to the phrenoesophageal ligament and the open edges of the esophageal muscle with interrupted silk sutures. A standard Thal fundoplication or a posterior Toupet fundoplication also can be established.

The postoperative management varies from surgeon to surgeon. Some proceed with a liquid diet the evening of the operation with discharge the following morning. Others prefer to decompress the stomach overnight with a nasogastric tube. Some may prefer to perform an esophagogram the following morning to ensure there is no evidence of perforation followed by a liquid diet if no perforation is noted on the contrast study. A mechanical soft diet usually is employed for several days, after which a regular diet may be initiated. There is usually no need for additional radiographic evaluation unless symptoms recur.

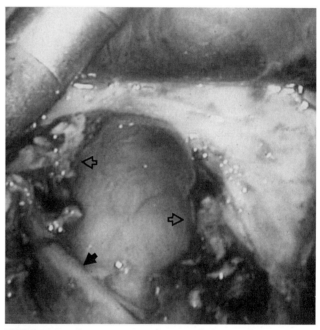

FIGURE 39-9 ■ Intraoperative photograph depicts the completed esophagomyotomy to a length of 8 cm. The muscle fibers are widely separated (open arrows), and the anterior vagus nerve crosses the submucosa (solid arrow).

Diffuse Esophageal Spasm

Diffuse esophageal spasm is even less common than achalasia. Symptoms of this disorder are similar to symptoms seen with achalasia. Patients present with a long-standing history of dysphagia, regurgitation of undigested food, halitosis, and weight loss. Children also may complain of substernal chest pain of a pressure or burning nature. Pulmonary symptoms, such as pneumonia or asthma, also may be present. Cold beverages may exacerbate these symptoms. The diagnosis usually is made with manometry and an upper GI study. On contrast esophagogram, localized segmental contractions of the esophagus are seen, giving the appearance of a distorted corkscrew or rosary bead with to-and-fro stasis of a barium bolus. On manometry, there are repetitive high-amplitude prolonged synchronous pressure peaks in the distal one half to two thirds of the esophagus with relaxation of the LES.

Little is written on the management of children with this disorder. In adults, there have been reports of successful treatment with injection of botulinum toxin in the LES, psychosomatic treatment with antidepressants, and ingestion of peppermint oil along with nitroglycerin. Pneumatic dilation and surgical myotomy also have been employed with intermittent success. Neither of these invasive approaches is totally satisfactory.

Scleroderma

Scleroderma is a connective tissue disorder in which esophageal motor dysfunction is only one part of the syndrome. Although esophageal dysmotility can occur in other connective tissue disorders, it is most common in scleroderma and is found eventually in 80% of patients. In addition, delayed gastric emptying also is seen often in these patients. The development of esophageal dysfunction in patients with scleroderma also has been found to correlate with the development of pulmonary disease.

Pathologically the abnormality is manifested by periarterial inflammation in the distal two thirds of the esophagus associated with collagen deposition and atrophy of the smooth muscle. This results in poor contractions of the esophagus and in decreased LES tone, leading to GER and complications of esophagitis, stricture, aspiration, malnutrition, and growth failure. In children with scleroderma, GI involvement seems more frequent than the clinical symptoms indicate. An active diagnostic evaluation for GI dysmotility and GER is necessary to detect these complications.

There is no effective treatment for this disorder. Oral calcitriol has been studied but has not been found to be any more effective than placebo in adults with scleroderma. An antireflux procedure can be performed if the symptoms of GER cannot be managed medically. If the esophageal length is shortened, Collis gastroplasty may be necessary. A partial fundoplication may be more appropriate than a complete Nissen fundoplication because of the potential for obstruction at the gastroesophageal junction with the latter operation.

SUGGESTED READINGS

Chung DH, Georgeson KW, Winters DC: Laparoscopic gastrostomy as adjunctive procedure to laparoscopic fundoplication in children. Surg Endosc 10:1106-1110, 1999.

The authors describe their technique for laparoscopic fundoplication and the U-stitch technique for laparoscopic gastrostomy.

Dalla Vecchia LK, Grosfeld JL, West KW, et al: Reoperation after Nissen fundoplication in children with gastroesophageal reflux: Experience with 130 patients. Ann Surg 226:315-321, 1997.

In a series of 130 patients, of whom 78% were neurologically impaired, a breakdown of the fundoplication occurred in 42%, and migration of the wrap through a hiatal hernia occurred in 30%. Both problems developed in 21% of the patients.

Danielson PD, Emmens RW: Esophagogastric disconnection for gastroesophageal reflux in children with severe neurological impairment. J Pediatr Surg 34:84-86, 1999.

The authors describe 27 patients who required esophagogastric disconnection. All patients were severely neurologically impaired. This procedure was performed primarily in 26 of the patients.

Fonkalsrud ER, Ashcraft KW, Coran AG, et al: Surgical treatment of gastroesophageal reflux in children: A combined hospital study of 7,467 patients. Pediatrics 101:467-468, 1998.

This is a retrospective review of the authors' combined clinical experience with surgical treatment of symptomatic GER in children over 20 years. This is the largest cohort of patients who have undergone surgical treatment of GER.

Hurwitz M, Bahar RJ, Ament ME, et al: Evaluation of the use of botulinum toxin in children with achalasia. J Pediatr Gastroenterol Nutr 30:509-514, 2000.

Botulinum toxin was used in 23 children. Because many of the children eventually will require an additional procedure (dilation or esophagomyotomy), the authors recommend this technique only in children who are poor candidates for either dilation or surgery.

Patti MG, Albanese CT, Holcomb GW III, et al: Laparoscopic Heller myotomy and Dor fundoplication for esophageal achalasia in children. J Pediatr Surg 36:1248-1251, 2001.

A small series of children underwent laparoscopic esophagomyotomy and anterior fundoplication for achalasia. All patients were discharged within 2 days of the procedure.

Patti MG, Pellegrini CA, Horgan S, et al: Minimally invasive surgery for achalasia: An 8-year experience with 168 patients. Ann Surg 230:587-593, 1999.

In this large series of 168 adults, the authors describe the evolution in their surgical technique and their clinical results.

Poirier NC, Taillefor R, Topart P, et al: Antireflux operations in patients with scleroderma. Ann Thorac Surg 58:66-72, 1994.

Fourteen patients with scleroderma underwent an antireflux procedure. Reflux symptoms were relieved in 10 of the patients through a variety of operations. Antireflux procedures in patients with scleroderma can palliate esophageal injury caused by GER without jeopardizing esophageal function.

Rudolph CD, Mazur LJ, Liptak GS, et al: Guidelines for evaluation and treatment of gastroesophageal reflux in infants and children: Recommendations of the North American Society for Pediatric Gastroenterology and Nutrition. J Pediatr Gastroenterol Nutr 32(Suppl 2):S1-31, 2001.

This article describes clinical practice guidelines for the management of GER in children that were formulated by the GER Guideline Committee of the North American Society for Pediatric Gastroenterology and Nutrition. The guidelines provide recommendations for management by the primary care provider, including evaluation, initial treatment, follow-up management, and indications for consultation by a specialist. It also provides recommendations for management by the pediatric gastroenterologist. These guidelines have been endorsed by the American Academy of Pediatrics.

Snyder CL, Ramachandran V, Kennedy AP, et al: Efficacy of partial wrap fundoplication for gastroesophageal reflux after repair of esophageal atresia. J Pediatr Surg 32:1089-1091, 1997.

The authors review their experience with 59 children who required Thal fundoplication for surgical management of GER after correction of esophageal atresia and tracheoesophageal fistula. In this series, 15% of the children required reoperation compared with a failure rate of 4.3% in the authors' experience of patients without esophageal atresia.

Storr M, Allescher HD, Classen M: Current concepts on pathophysiology, diagnosis and treatment of diffuse esophageal spasm. Drugs 61:579-591, 2001.

This article describes current concepts regarding the physiology, diagnosis, and treatment of patients with diffuse esophageal spasm.

PART VI

Abdominal Wall, Peritoneum, and Diaphragm

40

Abdominal Wall Defects

The first description of an abdominal wall defect is credited to Paré in 1634. Visick was the first to treat an infant with a ruptured omphalocele successfully with a skin closure in 1873. The skin flap method of closure developed by Gross in Boston in 1948 was an important advance in the surgical management of infants with omphalocele and improved the outcome for neonates with gastroschisis. Lack of availability of infant ventilators and inability to maintain adequate nutrition during the prolonged adynamic ileus that accompanies gastroschisis played a role in the poor outlook for these infants before the 1960s.

In 1965, Dudrick and associates described their experience with total parenteral nutrition (TPN) in the laboratory and clinical setting. At the same time, the first infant pressure ventilators and then volume ventilators became available for clinical use in neonates. In 1967, Schuster reported the successful application of a temporary extra-abdominal housing for the bowel in instances of large omphaloceles using an inner lining of polyethylene sheeting and an outer layer of polytetrafluoroethylene (Teflon) mesh. This technique also was applied to infants with gastroschisis and was modified by others, including Allen and Wrenn, using Dacron-reinforced Silastic, an alternative prosthetic material. Their silo method was a simpler technique and promptly was adopted by most pediatric surgeons. These three events in the 1960s significantly changed the outcome for infants with abdominal wall defects. Since then, recognition of abdominal wall defects in utero by prenatal ultrasonography, improved understanding of associated chromosomal abnormalities in infants with omphalocele, continued advances in neonatal intensive care by development of more effective infant ventilators, and significant improvements in monitoring in the neonatal intensive care unit (NICU) and operating room have influenced further the overall management of these patients.

There is some controversy regarding the exact embryologic basis of abdominal wall defects and whether gastroschisis and omphalocele are distinctly separate entities. Based on embryologic and prenatal ultrasound studies, some authors suggest that gastroschisis is the result of an early intrauterine rupture of the umbilical cord or an early intrauterine rupture of an omphalocele with subsequent resorption of the remnants of the sac. The fact that serious associated anomalies are rare—and trisomy syndromes, Beckwith-Wiedemann syndrome, and exstrophy of the bladder and cloaca are never seen with gastroschisis—strongly suggests that these two anomalies are different.

Studies concerning serial sections of human fetuses in the Carnegie Embryologic Collection seem to confirm the impression that gastroschisis and omphalocele are different conditions. A more in-depth examination of the embryology is beyond the scope of this chapter, which reviews some of the similarities and differences between gastroschisis and omphalocele (Table 40-1) and describes the current diagnostic and therapeutic management of infants with these congenital abdominal wall malformations.

TABLE 40-1 ▪ Clinical Findings in Infants with Abdominal Wall Defects		
Factor	Omphalocele	Gastroschisis
Location	Umbilical ring	Lateral to cord
Defect size	Large (2-10 cm)	Small (2-4 cm)
Cord	Inserts in sac	Normal insertion (left of defect)
Sac	Present	None
Contents	Liver, bowel	Bowel, gonads
Bowel	Normal	Matted, inflamed
Malrotation	Present	Present
Small abdomen	Present	Present
Gastrointestinal function	Normal	Prolonged ileus
Associated anomalies	Common (30-70%) (often major)	Unusual (bowel atresia 10-15%)
Syndromes	Common: Beckwith-Wiedemann syndrome, trisomies 13-15, trisomies 16-18, lower midline syndrome, Cantrell's pentalogy	Not observed

GASTROSCHISIS

Gastroschisis (Greek for "belly cleft") is a defect of the anterior abdominal wall just lateral to the umbilicus. The defect is almost always to the right of an intact umbilical cord and in some cases is separated from the cord by an intact skin bridge. This anomaly is probably the result of a defect that occurs at the site where the second umbilical vein involutes. In contrast to instances of omphalocele, there is no peritoneal sac so that antenatal evisceration of the bowel occurs through a relatively small defect during intrauterine life. The irritating effects of amniotic fluid (pH 7.0), which contains fetal urine and various growth factors, on the exposed bowel wall results in a chemical form of peritonitis characterized by a thick edematous membrane that is occasionally exudative. The exposed viscera may be congested, and the bowel appears matted and foreshortened (Fig. 40-1). There is a varying degree of mesenteric venous and lymphatic obstruction resulting from the small abdominal wall defect. Nonrotation always accompanies this condition, and the bowel is not fixed to the abdominal wall. In contrast to infants with omphalocele, the incidence of associated anomalies in patients with gastroschisis is relatively infrequent. The exception is the occurrence of intestinal atresia, which may complicate gastroschisis in 10% to 15% of patients. Atresia of the bowel often is related to intrauterine volvulus, intussusception, or an interruption of the blood supply to a segment of exposed intestine by compression in a tight defect in the abdominal wall (Fig. 40-2). The liver is almost never eviscerated; the stomach, small bowel, and large intestine usually reside outside the defect. The bowel may be perforated in approximately 5% of patients. Occasionally the ovaries and fallopian tubes in girls and an undescended testis in boys are found outside the defect. The abdominal cavity is often small. The sexes are equally affected. Most patients are born to young mothers; 25% are born to teenaged mothers. Of patients,

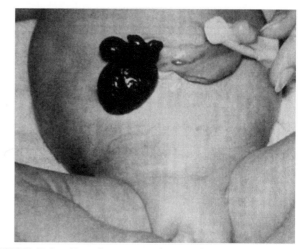

FIGURE 40-2 ■ Bowel compressed in a tight gastroschisis defect, resulting in bowel atresia.

40% are either premature or small for gestational age. Gastroschisis is more common than omphalocele, with a ratio of 1.5:1 to 2:1 at most major pediatric surgical centers. Occasionally there is a maternal history of a previous infant with gastroschisis. Chromosomal syndromes almost never are encountered in infants with a gastroschisis defect.

Gastroschisis frequently can be detected on a prenatal ultrasound study. The sonogram often shows dilated bowel free in amniotic fluid adjacent to the umbilical insertion (Fig. 40-3). When identified prenatally, the pregnant woman should be referred to a high-risk obstetric unit with an NICU and pediatric surgical expertise. Although an elective preterm delivery theoretically may minimize the irritating effect of amniotic fluid exposure, evidence does not suggest that early cesarean section improves the outcome. Spontaneous vaginal delivery is a reasonable choice for most of these infants, unless the eviscerated intestine appears unusually large.

When delivered, infants with gastroschisis may experience various problems as a result of an increase in insensible fluid and heat losses related to exposure of the eviscerated bowel. Hypothermia, hypovolemia, and sepsis are the major problems to avoid. Significant third-space fluid deficits and hypoproteinemia occur as the result of extra-abdominal and intra-abdominal sequestration of interstitial fluid. The lower half of the infant (including the eviscerated bowel) is placed into a sterile bowel bag, feet first, up to the level of the axillae (Fig. 40-4). This plastic bag is available in almost every operating room and helps retain the infant's heat, reduces evaporative insensible losses, reduces the risk of sepsis, and collects sequestered fluids that can be measured and replaced accurately.

Fluid requirements in a neonate with gastroschisis are two to three times that of a normal newborn in the first 24 hours of life. In a large group of infants with gastroschisis, the average fluid requirement was approximately 175 mL/kg/day. As a general rule, the more matted and inflamed the exposed viscera appear, the greater the fluid requirements necessary to resuscitate the infant. The infant is resuscitated with a bolus of 20 mL/kg

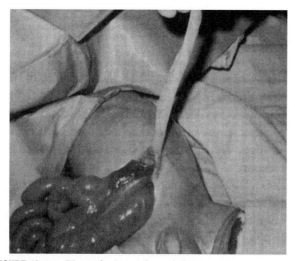

FIGURE 40-1 ■ Typical gastroschisis defect just to the right of an intact umbilical cord. The eviscerated bowel is matted, edematous, and foreshortened. No sac is observed. (From Grosfeld JL, et al: Congenital abdominal wall defects: current management and survival. Surg Clin North Am 61:1037, 1981.)

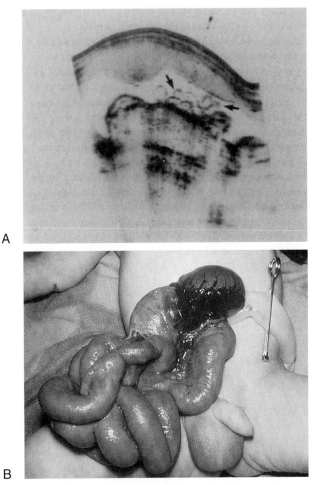

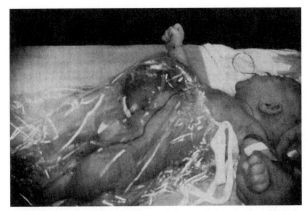

FIGURE 40-4 ■ Newborn infant with an abdominal wall defect placed feet first in a bowel bag.

FIGURE 40-3 ■ Gastroschisis. **A,** Obstetric sonogram at 34 weeks' gestation shows dilated bowel (arrows) free in amniotic fluid adjacent to the umbilical cord insertion site. Previous sonograms at 27 and 31 weeks showed the bowel contained near the base of the cord, suggesting rupture of a small omphalocele (hernia of the cord) late in gestation. **B,** Typical gastroschisis after delivery at 35 weeks. Bowel edema and inflammation are minimal.

has adynamic ileus. The infant is given parenteral antibiotics in divided doses (ampicillin, 50 to 100 mg/kg/day, and gentamicin, 5 to 7 mg/kg/day in 3 doses). When the acidosis is corrected and urine output is established, the infant is taken to the operating room for repair. With the infant under well-monitored general endotracheal anesthesia, the abdominal wall and exposed viscera are cleansed carefully of loose debris with warm sterile saline and prepared with an iodophor solution. Alcohol or alcohol-containing solutions should not be applied directly on the bowel because they have an irritating effect. The bowel is inspected carefully for accompanying atresia or perforation. The umbilical cord is inspected and the number of umbilical arteries noted. The abdominal wall defect is enlarged 1 to 2 cm cephalad and caudad to improve the mechanical advantage for reducing the exposed viscera (Fig. 40-5). The stomach, duodenal, and upper jejunal

of 10% dextrose in lactated Ringer's solution given over 30 minutes. Additional fluids (additional bolus of 10 mL/kg of human plasma protein fraction [Plasmanate] and lactated Ringer's solution at a rate of 150 to 200 mL/kg/day divided into hourly aliquots) are administered until urine output is established, and the pulse rate and tissue perfusion improve. Although most patients require rigorous fluid resuscitation, there are two subsets: a "low group" and a "high group." The low group is usually premature, is physiologically stable, and requires only 90 to 125 mL/kg/ 24 hours for maintenance. The high group is often small for gestational age, has elevated hematocrit levels, and requires 190 mL/kg/24 hours (see Chapter 4). Acid-base balance is monitored closely because metabolic acidosis commonly is observed as a result of poor perfusion related to hypovolemia.

An orogastric tube is placed into the stomach to remove swallowed air and to aspirate gastrointestinal contents because the infant with gastroschisis almost invariably

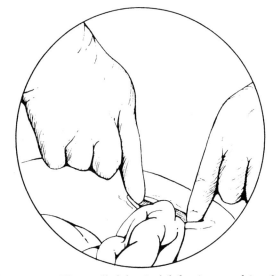

FIGURE 40-5 ■ The small abdominal defect is opened 1 to 2 cm cephalad and caudad to improve the mechanical advantage when attempting reduction of the herniated viscera. The abdominal cavity is stretched manually in an attempt to increase the right of domain for the bowel.

contents are aspirated through the previously placed orogastric tube, and meconium in the transverse, descending, and sigmoid colon and rectum is evacuated manually through the anal orifice by external compression of the viscera. An enterotomy to decompress the bowel is unnecessary and should be avoided because it may result in a leak with subsequent peritonitis or an enterocutaneous fistula. Similarly, if an asymptomatic Meckel's diverticulum is present, it should be left in place and not excised. The abdominal wall is stretched manually to enlarge the relatively small peritoneal cavity (see Fig. 40-5).

Primary reduction of the viscera is attempted using a maximum ventilatory pressure of 35 cm H_2O as a safe reference guide; this is successful in more than 50% of patients. Inferior vena caval and intragastric pressure measurements occasionally have been used to monitor the ability to perform a primary closure of the abdominal wall safely. When there is considerable visceroabdominal disproportion, attempts to close the abdomen primarily under moderate tension increase the risk of bowel perforation or leak. The abdominal wall closure is accomplished using one layer of full-thickness interrupted 3-0 nonabsorbable polypropylene sutures that do not include the skin. Often the umbilicus can be preserved for cosmetic purposes. Several surgeons create an umbilicus with a purse-string suture during skin closure.

After primary closure, most infants are maintained on ventilator support for 24 to 48 hours and are weaned and extubated safely in the NICU. Although previously surgeons often performed an adjunctive gastrostomy in infants with abdominal wall defects, this has been found to be unnecessary in most cases, and it may interfere with abdominal closure and cause a higher complication rate. An orogastric tube is tolerated well by infants and does not interfere with nasal breathing.

Primary abdominal repair may not be possible in 40% to 50% of reported cases of gastroschisis. Too tight a closure may result in cardiorespiratory compromise from diaphragmatic elevation and ventilatory restriction, vena caval compression that reduces venous return to the right side of the heart, and compression of the bowel mesentery, resulting in diminished bowel perfusion and intestinal ischemia and necrosis. Some infants require a staged closure using a Dacron-reinforced Silastic silo as a temporary extra-abdominal housing. The edge of the prosthetic material is sutured to the rim of the fascia or skin at the edge of the defect with continuous or interrupted 3-0 or 2-0 nonabsorbable monofilament sutures. The walls of the prosthetic silo should be constructed parallel to each other as a straight-walled structure so that the base is as wide as the top, preventing a conical narrow entry to the abdominal cavity (Fig. 40-6). The upper end of the silo is ligated with umbilical tape, which is suspended loosely from the top of the infant's Isolette unit. An antibiotic ointment (povidone-iodine [Betadine]) is placed around the base of the silo at the skin-prosthesis interface. A sterile support dressing is applied to prevent the silo from tilting over and kinking the contained viscera. The viscera can be reduced gradually by gentle pressure and placing the ligature on the silo lower starting on the second to third postoperative day using sterile technique at the bedside in the NICU. The silo

usually can be removed and closure of the abdominal wall completed within 1 to 3 weeks in most cases. The infant is returned to the operating room for fascial closure using interrupted full-thickness 3-0 or 2-0 nonabsorbable monofilament sutures. Parenteral antibiotics are discontinued shortly after the silo is removed.

As a result of prolonged adynamic ileus, almost all infants with gastroschisis require TPN for adequate caloric support. A central venous catheter is inserted at the time of abdominal closure. TPN is started when the fluid derangements observed at birth are corrected (24 to 48 hours later) and may be required for 3 to 4 weeks. The solution contains 25% glucose, 2.5% amino acids, and 3 to 4 g/kg/day of fat using 10% or 20% Intralipid, trace minerals, and vitamins. The infants should receive 125 to 130 calories/kg/day. Most infants begin to tolerate oral intake by 2 to 3 weeks of age and usually can take all of their calories enterally by 1 month. Dilute 1/4-strength to 1/2-strength formula is given initially, and the volume is increased slowly, depending on the volume of gastric residuals. In the first few weeks of life, patients with gastroschisis have decreased absorption of carbohydrates, protein, and fat; however, absorptive function returns to normal for all three caloric sources by 6 months of age.

In infants with associated intestinal atresia, a temporary enterostomy occasionally is constructed at the time of the initial abdominal wall repair. Closure can be accomplished within 1 to 3 months. Primary anastomosis can be performed in the neonatal period after abdominal closure in most patients within 1 to 2 weeks as an elective procedure when the intestinal edema and inflammation have largely subsided, and the gastric, biliary, and pancreatic drainage is controlled with an orogastric suction catheter. Anastomosis at birth often is complicated by stricture or leak in many patients. Patients with atresia often have longer delays in recovery of gastrointestinal function and a more complicated and prolonged hospitalization. In some instances, the entire midgut may be involved by ischemia as a result of being trapped in a small defect in utero or by a volvulus resulting in short-bowel syndrome. The only remaining bowel may be atretic and significantly thickened, inflamed, and dilated with abnormal intestinal motility. After a temporary enterostomy is fashioned in the neonatal period to allow time for the thickened and inflamed bowel wall to return to near normal, a tapering enteroplasty and bowel anastomosis subsequently can be performed. Occasionally a Bianchi procedure, which longitudinally divides the dilated intestine into two independent segments and increases its length, may be considered. Intestinal atresia complicating gastroschisis may require long-term TPN support and innovative enteral feeding programs best carried out with small hourly drip feedings maximally to stimulate adaptation and villus hyperplasia. Enteral feedings also maximize gallbladder contraction and reduce the risk of TPN-related cholestasis and the formation of pigment gallstones.

In addition to prolonged adynamic ileus, other postoperative complications after repair of a gastroschisis defect include sepsis, aspiration pneumonia, abdominal wall cellulitis, temporary groin and lower extremity edema,

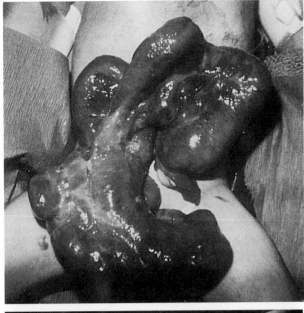

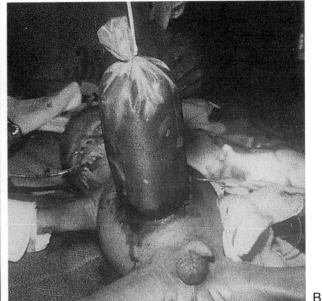

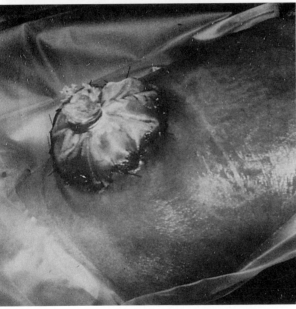

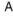

FIGURE 40-6 ■ **A,** An infant with gastroschisis and antenatal evisceration of the bowel. **B,** The intestine could not be completely reduced and was placed in a temporary Dacron-reinforced Silastic "silo." **C,** The viscera is reduced gradually in the NICU with repeated gentle downward pressure on the upper end of the silo. The infant is returned to the operating room, the bowel is completely reduced, and a primary abdominal wall closure is performed.

necrotizing enterocolitis, and TPN-related cholestasis. Symptomatic gastroesophageal reflux and inguinal hernia may occur from increased intra-abdominal pressure as a result of replacement of the herniated viscera in a relatively small abdominal cavity. Few patients require an antireflux procedure, however. Rarely the patient with gastroschisis remains obstructed for more than 4 to 5 weeks as the result of severe visceroabdominal disproportion with intestinal edema and matting, a missed second atresia, or distal intraluminal web that was masked by the inflammatory process present at the initial procedure. Patients with a prolonged obstructive course should undergo radiographic intestinal contrast studies in an attempt to locate a mechanical cause of obstruction.

With appropriate neonatal resuscitation, surgical treatment, and nutritional support, the current survival rate in infants with gastroschisis is greater than 90%.

Most deaths are related to prematurity or sepsis or late complications occurring in infants with atresias and short-bowel syndrome, including progressive liver disease related to TPN. Most surviving patients have normal growth and development, tolerate a full diet, and have normal bowel habits.

OMPHALOCELE

An omphalocele is a covered defect of the umbilical ring into which abdominal contents herniate. The defect is related to a central defect of the umbilical ring and the medial segments of the lateral embryonic abdominal wall folds. This defect is thought to occur in the third week of intrauterine life when the midgut elongates and resides in the yolk sac outside of the embryonic coelom. This is referred to as the *middle celosomia* or a *central omphalocele*.

Omphaloceles are covered by a sac composed of an outer layer of amnion and an inner layer of peritoneum. The umbilical cord inserts into the sac. A separate compartment containing Wharton's jelly also may be observed. The omphalocele defect may reside in an epigastric location as a result of a defective cephalad abdominal wall fold development, usually in association with many other defects involving the diaphragm, sternum, and heart. An omphalocele defect also may reside in the hypogastrium as a result of defective development of the caudal abdominal wall fold and coexist with other defects affecting the genitourinary system, the primitive hindgut, and the caudal neural tube.

The incidence of omphalocele is approximately 1 in 5000 live births. Boys are affected more often than girls. Infants with an omphalocele have a high incidence of associated anomalies. More than 50% of cases have other serious defects involving the alimentary tract and the cardiovascular, genitourinary, musculoskeletal, and central nervous systems. Many infants born with an omphalocele are premature. Others may be affected by many chromosomal syndromes, including Beckwith-Wiedemann syndrome characterized by gigantism, macroglossia, and an umbilical defect in the form of either an umbilical hernia or an omphalocele. Infants with Beckwith-Wiedemann syndrome have visceromegaly and pancreatic islet cell hyperplasia that may result in significant hypoglycemia complicated by seizures in the neonatal period. These infants also have an increased incidence of malignant tumors, including Wilms' tumor, neuroblastoma, and adrenocortical tumors. Omphalocele may occur in infants with other serious chromosomal abnormalities, such as trisomies 13 through 15, trisomies 16 through 18, and trisomy 21.

When the omphalocele is located in the hypogastrium, it often is associated with a lower midline syndrome, which includes exstrophy of the bladder or cloaca, vesicointestinal fissure, colon atresia, imperforate anus, sacral vertebral defects, and a lipomeningocele or meningomyelocele (Fig. 40-7). Duplications of the appendix and atretic colon commonly are observed. The genitalia are often ambiguous, with a highly limited phallus in boys, and sex assignment must be considered carefully at an early stage. An epigastric omphalocele may be part of Cantrell's pentalogy, which includes omphalocele, anterior diaphragmatic hernia, sternal cleft, a downward displaced heart, intracardiac defects (most commonly a ventricular septal defect), and occasionally a diverticulum of the left ventricle that may extend down into the abdominal portion of the sac (Fig. 40-8).

An omphalocele defect may vary from 2 cm to greater than 10 cm in diameter. The smaller the defect, the better the prognosis. Many smaller defects (<4 cm) probably represent herniation of the umbilical cord—a minor form of the defect. These smaller defects probably occur in the 8th to 10th week of gestation as a result of failure of the umbilical ring to close. An umbilical cord hernia usually contains only small bowel. In contrast, although the true omphalocele sac also may contain bowel, frequently the liver (in 35% of patients) (Fig. 40-9), colon, and stomach may be present within the sac. The extraabdominal location of the viscera in utero results in a small

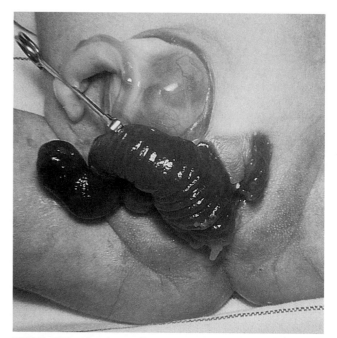

FIGURE 40-7 ■ Lower midline omphalocele with exstrophy of the cloaca and imperforate anus with colon atresia. The halves of the bladder are separated by a vesicointestinal fissure with prolapsing right colon.

abdominal cavity that may make attempts at reducing the sac contents extremely difficult. In addition, anomalies of rotation and fixation almost always are present as a coexisting anomaly. Meckel's diverticulum also is seen with increased frequency in these patients.

The diagnosis of omphalocele can be obtained by prenatal ultrasound examination (Fig. 40-10). The early detection of this defect allows for maternal counseling,

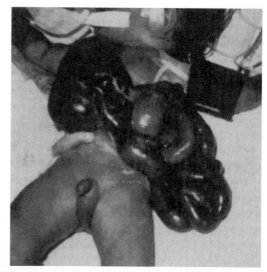

FIGURE 40-8 ■ Example of a ruptured epigastric omphalocele with the liver and the entire gastrointestinal tract eviscerated. A congenital heart defect, sternal cleft, and anterior diaphragmatic defect also were present. (From Grosfeld JL: Congenital abdominal wall defects: Current management and survival. Surg Clin North Am 61:1037, 1981.)

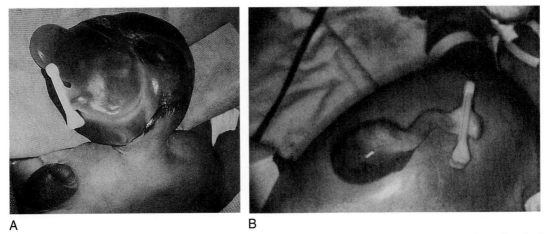

A   B

FIGURE 40-9 ■ **A,** Large omphalocele sac containing the liver and the intestine. **B,** In contrast, this infant had a small hernia of the umbilical cord that contained a few loops of intestine.

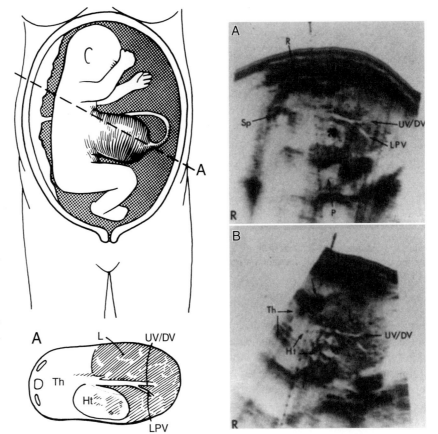

FIGURE 40-10 ■ **A** and **B,** Prenatal diagnosis of omphalocele and ectopia cordis by ultrasound. The drawings on the left illustrate the anatomic relations seen in the sonograms. **A,** Transverse scan in the plane illustrated in the drawing shows a large mass that extends beyond the anterior limit of the thorax. The umbilical vein/ductus venosus (UV/DV) complex joins the left portal vein (LPV). A sonolucent structure (cursor) adjacent to the UV/DV is investigated further in **B.** By slowing the rate of transducer motion, the sonolucent structure seen in **A** can be identified definitely as the fetal heart (Ht) by characteristic wall motion. P, placenta; Sp, spine; R, rib; Th, thorax; L, liver. (From Harrison MR, Golbus MS, Filly RA, et al: Management of the fetus with a correctable congenital defect. JAMA 246:774, 1981.)

optimal delivery planning, and referral of the affected mother to a high-risk delivery center supported by a contemporary NICU and pediatric surgical expertise. Prenatal ultrasound studies can help distinguish between lesions with a good prognosis, such as a small omphalocele or hernia of the umbilical cord, and lesions with a more guarded outcome, including a large omphalocele in fetuses with multiple anomalies and related syndromes that have a high perinatal morbidity and mortality. If the liver is recognized outside the abdomen within the sac, the defect is usually large; the infant's prognosis also depends on the presence or absence of serious associated anomalies. If the defect is large, the mother commonly requires a cesarean section. With the exception of a large omphalocele, cesarean delivery has little advantage over a vaginal delivery in the management of most fetal

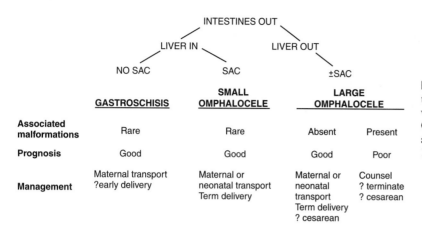

	GASTROSCHISIS	SMALL OMPHALOCELE	LARGE OMPHALOCELE	
Associated malformations	Rare	Rare	Absent	Present
Prognosis	Good	Good	Good	Poor
Management	Maternal transport ?early delivery	Maternal or neonatal transport Term delivery	Maternal or neonatal transport Term delivery ? cesarean	Counsel ? terminate ? cesarean

FIGURE 40-11 ■ Prenatal diagnosis and perinatal management of the fetus with an abdominal wall defect. (From Nakayama DK, Harrison MR, Gross BH, et al: Management of the fetus with an abdominal wall defect. J Pediatr Surg 19:408, 1984.)

abdominal wall defects (Fig. 40-11). Elevated α-fetoprotein levels have been observed in the amniotic fluid from amniocentesis samples in some infants with an omphalocele, even in the absence of associated neural tube defects. Fetoscopy may allow for fetal blood sampling and detection of serious chromosomal abnormalities. This is particularly useful in women with advanced maternal age (35 to 45 years) in whom the age-specific risk of the fetus having a trisomy is two to three times greater than in younger women.

At birth, the emergency care of neonates with omphalocele includes the insertion of an orogastric tube to decompress the stomach and prevent swallowed air from causing bowel distention, which may interfere with attempted reduction of the viscera at the time of repair. The intact omphalocele sac should be kept covered with a plastic sheet, protected from injury, and transported in a thermally neutral environment. Wet dressings may macerate the sac, cause temperature loss by cooling and evaporative loss, and adhere to the sac. If the sac is large and unstable, causing collapse to one side or the other, resulting in kinking of the enclosed viscera and even obstruction of the inferior vena cava, the sac should be supported by a sterile gauze roller dressing (Kerlix) that wraps around the infant's back. Intravenous fluids are administered using 10% dextrose in water and 0.25% normal saline solution if the infant is hemodynamically stable. The fluid losses are usually not excessive because the viscera are covered by an intact sac.

Approximately 10% of patients have a rupture of the omphalocele sac. In these instances, fluid losses are significantly greater and similar to fluid losses of infants with gastroschisis. These patients require more vigorous fluid resuscitation using 20 mL/kg of 10% dextrose in lactated Ringer's solution as a priming bolus given over 30 to 60 minutes followed by an increased maintenance volume. Perioperative parenteral antibiotics are administered (ampicillin, 50 to 100 mg/kg/day, and gentamicin, 5 to 7 mg/kg/day in 3 doses). The infant's general condition should be assessed carefully in regard to cardiorespiratory status and the possible occurrence of additional congenital anomalies.

Because the viscera are covered by a physiologic sac, the pediatric surgeon has many options available regarding omphalocele treatment. Case management depends on the set of clinical circumstances and the anatomy that

presents in each patient. Small defects (2 cm) can be managed by direct primary closure of the abdominal wall. Medium-sized defects are managed by careful removal of the sac at its base with suture ligation of the umbilical vein, the two umbilical arteries, and the urachus. The abdominal wall is stretched manually on both sides to enlarge the size of the relatively small abdominal cavity. The liver and then the bowel are reduced into the abdomen. Reduction of the liver must be done carefully to avoid torsion of the hepatic veins, portal vein inflow, and injury to the hepatic capsule, which may result in significant, potentially life-threatening hemorrhage that is difficult to control. Primary closure of the abdominal wall is not advisable for patients with large omphaloceles and visceroabdominal disproportion. If the abdominal wall fascia cannot be approximated, skin closure with creation of a small ventral hernia may be used in some patients. If the skin flaps are not extensively undermined, the subsequent ventral hernia remains small and is easier to repair at a later date. Some surgeons prefer to bridge the defect by insertion of a prosthetic material, such as Gore-Tex, Marlex, or absorbable patches.

Primary abdominal wall repair is usually not possible for infants with large omphalocele defects. These infants often require a staged abdominal wall closure using a Dacron-reinforced Silastic silo as a temporary extra-abdominal locale for the bowel. This technique first was described by Schuster in 1967 and has had a positive impact on survival in these difficult cases. Similar to infants with gastroschisis, the prosthetic material is sutured to the skin at the edge of the abdominal wall defect with a polypropylene or other nonabsorbable monofilament suture. The vessels in the umbilical cord are ligated, but the covering sac need not be excised before placing the Silastic silo. The silo should be constructed with its walls perpendicular to the abdominal wall and parallel to each other to avoid a conical base and difficulty in attempted reduction of the herniated viscera. Iodophor or antibiotic ointment is placed around the base of the sac on the skin-prosthesis interface. The contents of the sac are supported by umbilical tape suspended from the top of the Isolette and attached to the apex of the prosthesis. The viscera can be reduced gradually over 3 to 10 days under sterile technique in the NICU. The infant is returned to the operating room for removal of the prosthesis and a formal closure of the abdominal wall. When the silo is removed, the major portion of the sac is excised except for the segment that is adherent to the liver. Some surgeons remove the sac at the initial operation to evaluate the intra-abdominal viscera for possible bowel atresias, vitelline duct anomalies, or other intra-abdominal defects.

On rare occasions, when the defect is large (>10 cm) and takes up much of the anterior abdominal wall and the infant has a small abdominal cavity with limited right of domain for the herniated viscera, or in cases of suspected chromosomal syndromes (trisomies 13 through 15 or trisomies 16 through 18), nonoperative management using topical application of an escharotic agent is an alternative choice of treatment. Topical therapy is also useful as a temporizing measure in infants with severe unstable cardiac defects (hypoplastic left heart, hypoplastic aortic arch) and in premature infants with an omphalocele complicated by hyaline membrane disease, persistent pulmonary hypertension, or sepsis. As long as the sac remains intact, definitive repair can be delayed until the infant's cardiac condition is treated or the pulmonary status is improved. Escharotic agents include 0.25% merbromin (Mercurochrome) and 0.5% silver nitrate solution. Twice-daily applications allow the sac to thicken and epithelialize. The initial use of merbromin in Europe employed a 2% solution. This concentration resulted in instances of mercury poisoning, however, and was abandoned. The current concentration of 0.25% has not been associated with any significant complications. Silver nitrate solution is bacteriostatic and encourages epithelialization. Because the 0.5% solution is hypotonic, loss of sodium from the sac into the dressing has been observed and may cause hyponatremia. Silver nitrate solution also stains linens, bed sheets, and the infant's and caretakers' skin gray-black. Large sheets of Op-site as a semipermeable wound cover over the intact sac has been suggested by some investigators. Epithelialization can occur beneath the Op-site, and downward pressure over the sac contents aids in the reduction process. If sac rupture occurs, the remaining sac and its contents may be covered temporarily with a biologic dressing, such as amnion, a homograft of human skin, or pigskin heterografts. The disadvantages of topical therapy include the potential for subsequent sac rupture, local infection, prolonged hospitalization, and a huge residual ventral hernia. The topical therapy should be used for only a few weeks at most because the abdominal muscles should be stretched as early as possible or the resulting massive skin-covered ventral hernia will be difficult to repair and be associated with high mortality. These factors have convinced us to use this technique sparingly.

After operative repair, infants with an omphalocele have a moderate risk of developing complications. Sepsis may occur and may be related to the presence of a prosthetic silo. The infant with an omphalocele can be nourished by enteral feedings much more quickly than neonates with gastroschisis. Because the sac is intact in most patients, the bowel has not been exposed to the irritating effects of amniotic fluid and is relatively normal in appearance and function. Some infants with omphalocele manifest gastroesophageal reflux postoperatively as a result of increased abdominal pressure caused by the repair of the smaller than normal abdominal cavity. In a few patients, an antireflux procedure may be necessary to allow discharge from the hospital. There is also an increased risk of inguinal hernia because of the elevated intra-abdominal pressure.

The overall survival for infants with omphalocele depends on the size of the defect, whether the infant is premature, if the sac ruptures, and how many and of what severity associated anomalies coexist. Mortality is related directly to the severity of coexisting defects and the presence of chromosomal conditions inconsistent with long-term survival. Infants with chromosomal syndromes and infants with Cantrell's pentalogy have a significant mortality (75%). Most infants with Cantrell's pentalogy die as a result of cardiorespiratory failure and sepsis. Infants with lower midline syndrome rarely have congenital heart disease, and even if there is a myelomeningocele, they rarely have problems with hydrocephalus. Repair of infants with lower midline syndrome is often complex, with bladder reconstruction commonly performed with intestinal augmentation and Mitrofanoff drainage, reconstruction of the genitalia, orthopedic repair of the widely separated pubic rami, and cutaneous enterostomy. There is a small group of infants with omphaloceles who have hypoplastic lungs. These infants require long-term ventilator support, often have permanently limited respiratory reserve, and frequently have a high postoperative mortality. Overall mortality ranges from 25% to 60% in reports from various institutions and in our own experience has been 30%.

SUGGESTED READINGS

Allen RG, Wrenn EL Jr: Silon as a sac in the treatment of omphalocele and gastroschisis. J Pediatr Surg 4:3, 1969.

This article describes a simple modification of the Schuster technique currently adopted by most pediatric surgeons for cases of gastroschisis that cannot be repaired primarily.

Fonkalsrud EW, Smith MD, Shaw KS, et al: Selective management of gastroschisis according to degree of visceroabdominal disproportion. Ann Surg 218:742, 1993.

How to determine which patients may have primary repair and which require staged repairs.

Grosfeld JL, Weber TR: Congenital abdominal wall defects: Gastroschisis and omphalocele. Curr Probl Surg 19:157, 1982.

A thorough discussion of all aspects of the major abdominal wall defects.

Pokorny WJ, Harberg FJ, McGill CW: Gastroschisis complicated by intestinal atresia. J Pediatr Surg 16:261, 1981.

This important early report documents the care of infants with gastroschisis complicated by intestinal atresia.

Schuster S: A new method for the staged repair of large omphaloceles. Surg Gynecol Obstet 125:261, 1967.

The classic description of staged repair of giant abdominal wall defects.

Disorders of the Umbilicus

The anterior abdominal wall is believed to develop by a combination of lateral infolding and acute ventral flexion beginning in the fourth fetal week. Between 6 and 10 weeks' gestation, the developing gastrointestinal tract is partially extruded into the extraembryonic coelomic cavity within the body stalk (Fig. 41-1). The viscera return to the abdominal portion of the coelomic cavity by the 10th week. By 12 weeks' gestation, approximation of the two rectus muscles toward the midline is complete except at the site of the umbilical ring, where the muscles are separated by undifferentiated somatopleure.

By the time of birth, the umbilical ring has become entirely closed by the developing abdominal wall except for the space occupied by the cord, which contains the umbilical vein, paired umbilical arteries, and the fibrous remnants of the urachus (allantois), and omphalomesenteric duct (yolk sac). After ligation of the cord, the vessels thrombose, and the cord dries and sloughs, leaving a granulating surface that heals by cicatrization and becomes covered by epithelium. This is followed by scar contraction and retraction of the umbilicus.

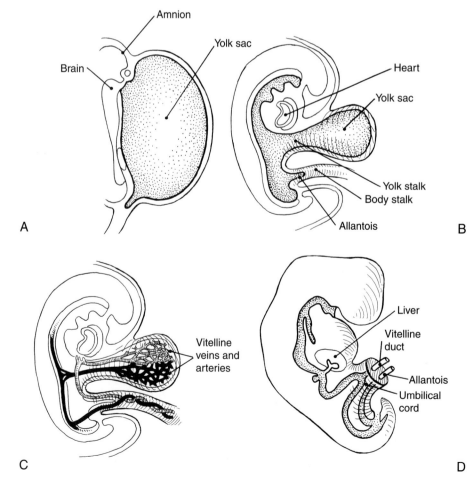

FIGURE 41-1 ■ Development of umbilical cord. **A,** Embryonic disk. Yolk sac in contact with the entire ventral surface of the developing fetus. **B,** Ventral attachment of the yolk sac narrowed and lengthened as a result of folding of the embryo. Intracoelomic portion of the yolk sac forms gut. Allantois buds from the hindgut into the body stalk. **C,** Vitelline and umbilical vessels develop in the yolk and body stalks. **D,** Yolk and body stalks fused into the umbilical cord. Development of the abdominal wall narrows the umbilical ring.

The normal umbilicus consists of a dense cicatrix covered by peritoneum on its undersurface and skin with little subcutaneous tissue superficially. The presence of a fascial layer between the peritoneum and scar tissue, corresponding to the linea alba and the remainder of the midline, is inconstant. Most umbilical hernias may occur through the cephalad portion of the umbilical ring, where the contracted scar around the obliterated umbilical vein is less dense than in the caudal portion of the scar.

UMBILICAL DRAINAGE

Drainage from the umbilicus during the early weeks of life after division of the umbilical cord may be from the presence of vestigial embryonal structures derived from the vitelline duct, urachus, umbilical vessels, umbilical infection (omphalitis), or a combination. The vitelline duct usually disappears by 7 weeks' gestation, although the umbilical portion of the vitelline artery and vein may persist for longer periods. Remnants of duct include omphalomesenteric sinus, fistula, Meckel's diverticulum, cysts, polyps, and vitelline bands.

Although umbilical drainage caused by local sepsis commonly is associated with a vestigial sinus in older children, umbilical sepsis in infants may be associated with retained umbilical cord elements or ectopic tissue. Most commonly, however, it represents poor hygienic practices or nosocomial infection. Omphalitis may progress dramatically from mild erythema of the umbilical area to florid cellulitis and sepsis within hours and must be treated vigorously when its earliest manifestations are recognized. In the past, omphalitis was a common cause of inflammation of the portal vein and portal vein thrombosis. In rare instances, omphalitis is associated with the use of umbilical venous catheters. Culturing of the umbilical area in infants who show any evidence of abnormal umbilical healing may identify pathogenic organisms sufficiently early to prevent major infection. Omphalitis associated with defective neutrophil function has been described in a few newborns with delayed separation of the umbilical cord. These infections may respond poorly to medical measures and may require excision of the cord remnant. Rarely, even in previously healthy infants, omphalitis may be fulminant. Although *Staphylococcus aureus* is the most common organism encountered, *Clostridium* may be the causative agent at times associated with induration erythema and spreading necrosis of subcutaneous fat and fascia. Although clostridial infection is uncommon, the mortality is high. Treatment must be aggressive and include intravenous antibiotics and excision of necrotic skin, subcutaneous tissue, fascia, and muscles. The cord remnants must be removed. Often the excision must extend to the peritoneal cavity.

After normal separation of the cord, a friable pink excrescence of granulation tissue may persist in the umbilical dimple that may enlarge into a large mass called an *umbilical granuloma*. This lesion often is associated with resistant umbilical drainage and swelling with erythema of the surrounding skin. Small granulomas may be eradicated by one or two applications of silver nitrate at an early stage. Larger granulomas may require excision with cauterization of the base. Epithelialization occurs in most patients with complete healing. If cellulitis is present, local measures and antibiotics are helpful.

An umbilical polyp is a glistening, cherry-red nodule that may be seen in the umbilical dimple after separation of the cord. This nodule is a remnant of the vitelline duct, usually consisting of isolated small intestinal mucosa. Rarely the polyp may contain gastric mucosa that may produce slight erosion of the periumbilical skin. Umbilical polyps are often mistaken for granulomas. They do not yield to silver nitrate treatment, however, and must be excised. A central core of the umbilicus should be excised in continuity with the polyp to identify and remove the contiguous intra-abdominal vitelline duct vestiges.

URACHAL SINUS

The urachus usually persists as a cord-like structure extending from the dome of the bladder to the lower border of the umbilical ring, flanked by the two umbilical ligaments (arteries). The mucosa-lined urachal lumen may persist throughout life, although usually it collapses or becomes occluded by desquamated epithelial cells. The urachus may produce symptoms if it communicates widely between the bladder and umbilical skin as a urinary fistula, if cysts develop along its course, or if either its umbilical or bladder ends remain widely patent, resulting in a persistent urachal sinus or bladder diverticulum. Occasionally, infants with a persistently draining urachal sinus may have some type of bladder outlet obstruction (e.g., posterior urethral valves), which may increase intravesical pressure, leading to persistent patency of the urachus. A voiding cystourethrogram is helpful in evaluating these infants. Because the patent urachus provides ready access for bacteria to enter the bladder, recurrent episodes of cystitis may occur. Surgical repair is done most easily through a small curvilinear infraumbilical incision, with excision of the urachal sinus to within a few millimeters of the bladder with ligation using absorbable suture.

Urachal cysts may occur anywhere along the urachal tract from the bladder to the umbilicus and may escape detection in infancy, causing symptoms in older children or adults as an enlarging suprapubic or infraumbilical mass. Infection of urachal cysts with abscess may produce an ovoid, painful, tender midline mass accompanied by systemic signs of acute infection. Urachal abscesses may drain through the umbilicus; rupture into the peritoneal cavity, causing peritonitis; or cause a spreading infection of the anterior abdominal wall or retroperitoneal tissues. Urachal abscesses may occur in infancy but are more common in adolescents and young adults. Urachal cysts should be excised in continuity with the rest of the urachal tract using either an open or a laparoscopic approach. Urachal abscesses should be drained promptly. In some cases, the infection may destroy the secretory cyst lining, preventing recurrence, although persistence is common when abscesses are treated by drainage alone. Usually excision of the cyst is necessary after infection has resolved.

PATENT OMPHALOMESENTERIC SINUS

A persistent vitelline fistula or sinus may permit drainage of small intestinal contents from the umbilicus. The intestinal communication is almost invariably at the site of a Meckel's diverticulum (Fig. 41-2). Frequently the ileum may prolapse through the patent vitelline sinus and project onto the abdominal wall as a bicornuate segment of prolapsed intestine in the newborn period. This type of umbilical prolapse is common when the vitelline duct is large. Prolapse rarely progresses to bowel obstruction or compromise of circulation of the prolapsed intestine. Surgical correction with resection of the communication with the intestine usually may be performed without loss of more than a few centimeters of intestine. Vitelline cysts may develop as mucosa-lined pockets along the course of the vitelline duct and may become large at birth. These cysts should be resected shortly after they are identified.

When the vitelline duct obliterates, it may leave a residual cord extending from the serosal surface of the distal ileum or from the tip of a Meckel's diverticulum to the umbilical ring. These cords provide a point of fixation to the abdominal wall about which a volvulus or internal hernia of small intestine may occur. The patient presents with acute closed-loop intestinal obstruction. Gangrene of the involved bowel is frequent with volvulus. The cords occasionally may extend to the mesentery or retroperitoneum. Intra-abdominal cords may necessitate prompt surgical exploration and, when identified, should be excised along with the Meckel's diverticulum.

An accurate delineation of the site of communication of a draining umbilical sinus may be obtained by a fistulagram after injection of water-soluble contrast material. Omphalomesenteric sinuses and fistulas are excised most easily through a curvilinear infraumbilical incision. The fascia may be opened more widely in a vertical direction to improve exposure of the ileum at the site of attachment of the Meckel's diverticulum. When intestinal obstruction is present, a standard laparotomy incision with wider exposure is needed.

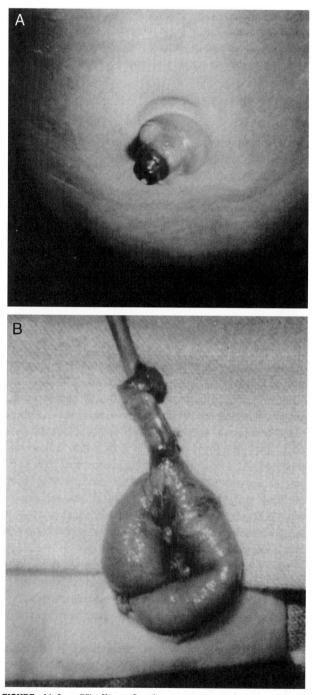

FIGURE 41-2 ■ Vitelline fistula (patent omphalomesenteric sinus). **A,** Ileostomy-like umbilical protrusion draining stool in a 2-week-old girl. **B,** Fistula, including Meckel's diverticulum and ileum, delivered through an infraumbilical incision.

UNUSUAL UMBILICAL MASSES

Although rare, dermoid cysts and vascular malformations may occur in the umbilicus. Ectopic liver has appeared as an umbilical nodule, probably as a result of entrapment of the tip of the right lobe during closure of the umbilical ring. Adenocarcinoma of the urachus may present as a supraumbilical mass and has a poor prognosis. This neoplasm is rare in adolescents, with more than 70% occurring in middle-aged or elderly patients.

UMBILICAL HERNIA

Failure of closure of the fascial ring through which the umbilical cord protrudes at birth causes the development of an umbilical hernia. Because the peritoneum and skin are intact, this is the mildest form of anterior abdominal wall anomaly. When the umbilical vein, vestigial umbilical arteries, and possibly urachal remnants dry up, a small opening is left in the abdominal wall, which usually is closed by extension of the fascia of the rectus muscles on each side of the opening. The defect usually is noticed within a few weeks after separation of the cord. Incomplete development, imperfect attachment, or weak areas in either ligamentous or fascial structures may predispose to herniation at the umbilicus.

Incidence

Umbilical hernia is one of the most commonly encountered abnormalities in the early months of infancy.

There is a distinct racial predilection, with black infants having a greatly increased incidence. In one comparative study, umbilical hernia was present in 32% of black infants younger than 6 weeks of age compared with 4% of white infants of the same age. At 1 year of age, the incidence was 13% in black infants and 2% in white infants. Another predisposing factor is low birth weight. More than 80% of infants weighing less than 1200 g have at least transient umbilical hernias compared with approximately 21% of infants with a birth weight greater than 2500 g.

Age is another important factor in the incidence of umbilical hernia. Most umbilical hernias close spontaneously so that only a few children have a hernia that persists beyond 4 or 5 years of age. Hernias occur with equal frequency in boys and girls.

Although usually an isolated abnormality in an otherwise healthy child, umbilical hernia occurs with Down syndrome (trisomy 21), congenital hypothyroidism (cretinism), mucopolysaccharidoses, and Beckwith-Wiedemann syndrome (omphalocele-macroglossia-gigantism).

Diagnosis

Umbilical hernias usually are recognized in the early weeks of life after the cord sloughs and the umbilicus heals. They are rarely symptomatic and simply are observed as a bulging at the umbilicus (Fig. 41-3). At times, the skin over the defect may become severely stretched and resemble a mushroom or occasionally a large phallus. When the infant strains or cries, the umbilical mass tenses, and with relaxation the sac is readily reduced. Digital examination of the umbilicus reveals a well-defined rim of the defect, the diameter of which varies from a few millimeters to a few centimeters. Most are smaller than 1.5 cm. The skin overlying the umbilicus, although redundant, is usually otherwise normal.

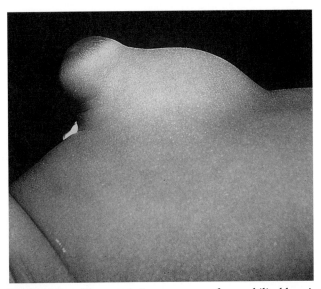

FIGURE 41-3 ■ Characteristic appearance of an umbilical hernia in a 4-month-old boy. The fascial defect measures only 1.5 cm.

Complications

Complications of umbilical hernia are uncommon. Incarceration is infrequent, and strangulation is rare in contrast to inguinal hernia, although the fascial defect may be small, and omentum or bowel often may be present in the sac transiently. The supine position of the infant favors spontaneous reduction. Because fewer than 1% of umbilical hernias ever incarcerate, concern about this possible complication is not considered an indication for surgical repair. Other complications of umbilical hernia include erosion of the overlying skin and, rarely, injury to the protruding hernia or spontaneous rupture with evisceration. Pain rarely occurs with umbilical hernia, and other causes should be sought for this complaint.

In contrast to the benign course of umbilical hernia in infants, the few adult patients who experience the disorder frequently develop incarceration. Adults at high risk for incarceration include obese adults and multiparous women.

Treatment

The rationale for management of umbilical hernia is based on the high incidence of spontaneous closure in the early years of life. During this time, no treatment other than parental reassurance is necessary. Umbilical strapping with a coin or pledget placed over the hernia to maintain it in a reduced position has not been shown to promote early closure of the fascial defect. This technique rarely is recommended because of the discomfort to the child and the likelihood of causing skin irritation.

Surgical repair of umbilical hernia is reserved for three groups: patients whose hernias have incarcerated, patients with persistent hernias, and patients with large protruding hernias. The rare infant who develops incarceration that requires reduction by a physician should have prompt repair. Most of these children undergo surgery because the defect has not closed spontaneously. Repair is considered appropriate for children with a large fascial defect (>1.5 cm) who are older than age 3 years. Children with small defects may be observed 4 to 5 years, although spontaneous closure is unlikely thereafter. Although a few hernias that have not closed by the time the child is 5 years old may do so subsequently, many remain open into adult years, when complications are more frequent and serious. In general, we prefer repair of all umbilical hernias before school age, when children begin to participate in physical activities.

Operative Technique

Surgical repair is performed on an outpatient basis using a light general anesthetic. A transverse curvilinear infraumbilical incision usually is made within a skin fold and extended down to the linea alba at the inferior rim of the umbilical ring. A plane around the hernia sac at the level of the linea alba is defined by blunt and sharp dissection. The sac either is dissected from the skin or is divided, leaving a disk of sac attached to the undersurface of the umbilical skin. The edges of the fascial defect should be mobilized and defined clearly. The fascial defect may be closed in either a transverse or a vertical direction with interrupted absorbable or nonabsorbable sutures. The undersurface of the dome of the umbilical sac is sutured to the fascia near the surgical repair. The skin is closed with fine absorbable subcuticular stitches. Thorough hemostasis is achieved with electrocautery to avoid hematoma. A fluffed sponge is pressed into the umbilical dimple, and a pressure dressing is applied for 72 hours to minimize the risk of wound hematoma, the most common and troublesome complication after repair. Wound infection is a rare complication after umbilical herniorrhaphy. Recurrent hernia is rare. Surgical techniques for repair in which a two-layer or three-layer fascial closure is performed (e.g., vest-over-pants closure) are unnecessary.

SUGGESTED READINGS

Lassaletta L, Fonkalsrud EW, Tovar J, et al: The management of umbilical hernias in infancy and childhood. J Pediatr Surg 10:405, 1975.

This is one of the largest reported clinical studies indicating the role of surgery for umbilical hernias in infancy and childhood.

Luchtman M, Rahav S, Zer M, et al: Management of urachal anomalies in children and adults. Urology 42:426, 1993.

A thorough description is provided of the various problems associated with urachal remnants.

Scherer LR, Grosfeld JG: Inguinal hernia and umbilical anomalies. Pediatr Clin North Am 40:1121, 1993.

This article provides a good review of the diagnosis and management of umbilical hernias and other anomalies.

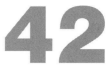

Disorders of the Inguinal Canal

INGUINAL HERNIA AND HYDROCELE

Inguinal hernia is a common condition of infancy and childhood, and repair is the most frequently performed general surgical operation in childhood. This chapter discusses the embryology, incidence, clinical presentation, treatment, and results of surgery in children with various anomalies of the inguinal canal, including inguinal hernia, hydrocele, and cryptorchidism.

Embryology

The occurrence of a congenital inguinal hernia and undescended testis is related to events that result in formational descent of the testis and formation of the processus vaginalis. At approximately 3 months' gestation, the testis descends under androgen influence from a retroperitoneal location following the course of the gubernaculum testis, a fold that is attached to the caudal part of the gonad. The gubernaculum passes distally through the internal ring and the inguinal canal; the testis descends behind it. As the testis comes through the internal inguinal ring, a diverticulum of peritoneum, the processus vaginalis, follows it through the ring into the inguinal canal. In the third trimester, the gubernaculum extends down to the scrotum, leading the testis and processus to their final destination. Although this process is related in part to androgen stimulation and adequate end-organ receptors, evidence indicates that the genitofemoral nerve also has a role in this process. The genitofemoral nerve supplies the cremasteric muscle, and the cremaster develops within the gubernaculum. Experimental division or injury to both genitofemoral nerves in the fetus prevents testicular descent. In approximately 90% of children, the processus vaginalis involutes by spontaneous obliteration, leaving a small remnant attached to the testis, the tunica vaginalis. Persistent patency of all or part of the processus vaginalis may result in various inguinal anomalies, including (1) complete patency associated with scrotal hernia; (2) obliteration of the distal processus and proximal patency (an inguinal hernia); (3) a narrow proximal opening at the internal ring, with a distal sac that changes in size because of fluctuation of fluid content resulting from an exchange of fluid from the peritoneal cavity and the sac (a communicating hydrocele); (4) a hydrocele of the spermatic cord, which presents as a mass in the inguinal canal and frequently has a small connection to the peritoneal cavity at the internal ring; and (5) an isolated hydrocele of the tunica vaginalis (Fig. 42-1). The rate of persistent patency of the processus vaginalis is related to the gestational age of the infant and whether the testis descends or not. In girls, only the round ligament penetrates into the inguinal canal so that hernias are less common than in boys. Inguinal hernia and, more rarely, a hydrocele may occur along the round ligament (canal of Nuck), often presenting as a bulge or mass in the labia majora.

Incidence

Congenital inguinal hernias are indirect hernias. The sac enters the inguinal canal through the internal ring lateral to the epigastric vessels and passes distally through the canal and may descend through the external ring into the scrotum. In contrast, a direct hernia (which is usually acquired) bulges into the canal medial to the epigastric vessels through a defect in the transversalis fascia. Approximately 3% to 5% of term infants may be born with a clinically apparent inguinal hernia. Preterm infants have a considerably higher incidence (9% to 11%). In infants less than 28 weeks' gestation, the incidence is 35%. A cryptorchid testis is found in 1 of 125 boys by age 1 year. Cryptorchidism occurs more frequently in preterm boys (30%) and almost always is associated with an indirect inguinal hernia, although most are not symptomatic. Clinical presentation of inguinal hernia occurs on the right side in 60% of patients and the left in 25%; 15% are bilateral. The higher incidence on the right side most likely is related to a later descent of the right testis compared with the left and delayed obliteration of the processus vaginalis. Inguinal hernia is much more common in boys than girls; however, bilateral presentation may be higher in girls.

In addition to prematurity, several other conditions are associated with an increased risk of inguinal hernia, including hydrops, chylous ascites, abdominal wall defects, meconium peritonitis, a positive family history for inguinal hernias, exstrophy of the bladder or cloaca, hypospadias, epispadias, certain connective tissue disorders (Marfan syndrome, Ehlers-Danlos syndrome), and

437

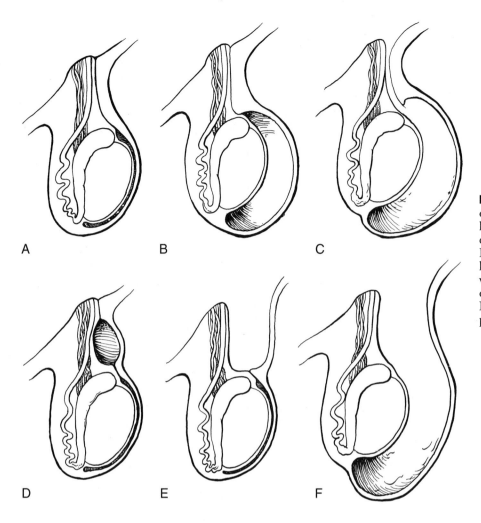

A   B   C

D   E   F

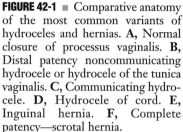

FIGURE 42-1 ■ Comparative anatomy of the most common variants of hydroceles and hernias. **A,** Normal closure of processus vaginalis. **B,** Distal patency noncommunicating hydrocele or hydrocele of the tunica vaginalis. **C,** Communicating hydrocele. **D,** Hydrocele of cord. **E,** Inguinal hernia. **F,** Complete patency—scrotal hernia.

testicular feminization syndrome and other forms of ambiguous genitalia (Fig. 42-2). An increased incidence of inguinal hernia also is observed in patients receiving continuous ambulatory peritoneal dialysis and infants with a ventriculoperitoneal shunt for hydrocephalus. In both of these situations, an increased amount of fluid in the abdominal cavity raises the intra-abdominal pressure, which opens and enlarges the processus.

Physical Examination

The most common presentation of inguinal hernia in male infants is a bulge in the groin or the scrotal sac. The bulge is seen more easily during straining or crying but is sometimes difficult to identify. If infants are relaxed, the mass may reduce spontaneously. Infants should be examined supine and erect. The mass is often reducible. In girls, the bulge presents in the upper portion of the labia majora. If a mass is palpable, it is usually an ovary. If gonads are palpable on both sides in girls, one should suspect testicular feminization syndrome, in which case the vagina is short when probed. When the examination is performed in boys, it should be noted whether the testis is within the scrotal sac to avoid mistaking a retractile testis for a hernia. In some instances, it may be difficult to show the presence of a hernia. It is generally unwise to rely on the physical finding of another physician or parent as an indication for surgery. If the physical examination is unconvincing, it is safer to re-examine the patient another day or ask the parents to photograph the bulge. The surgeon should document the presence of a hernia before an operation is undertaken. Patients with a small patent connection at the internal ring frequently present with a scrotal mass that changes in size according to the infant's activity from morning to evening. As previously noted, this is called a *communicating hydrocele*. One sometimes can observe the changing size on physical examination by gentle compression of the scrotum. A noncommunicating hydrocele of the tunica vaginalis usually presents as a soft, nontender, fluid-filled sac that may transilluminate. This form of hydrocele does not actively fluctuate in size, and it may gradually involute spontaneously in the first 12 months of life. Hydroceles that persist beyond that time probably are associated with an inguinal hernia or patent processus vaginalis and require operative intervention. Occasionally, hydroceles in older children may follow trauma, inflammation, or tumors affecting the testis. Rarely a hydrocele may enlarge significantly and extend through the internal ring into the abdomen (abdominoscrotal hydrocele).

Incarcerated Hernia

The most common complication of inguinal hernia is incarceration. An *incarcerated hernia* is defined as an irreducible mass that carries the risk of vascular compromise

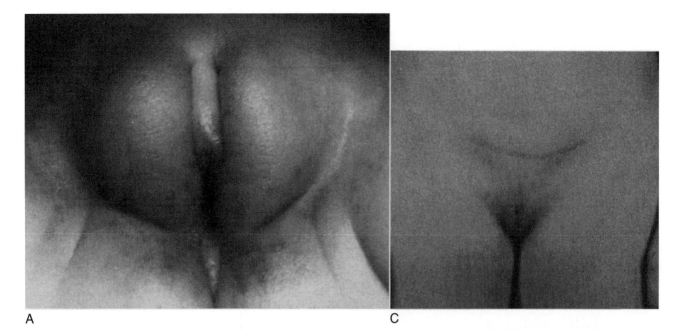

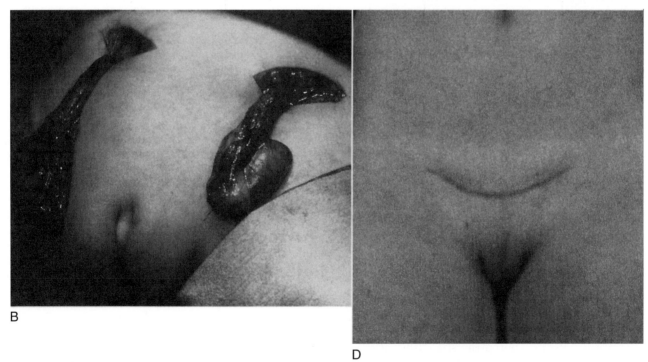

FIGURE 42-2 ■ Complete androgen insensitivity presenting with bilateral inguinal hernias. **A,** Appearance of the external genitalia. **B,** Testes. **C,** Patient presenting with failure to menstruate. The history is of bilateral inguinal hernia repairs as an infant with the 46XY karyotype. The testes were removed through a Pfannenstiel incision. **D,** Sister (46XY karyotype) of the patient in **C** with an identical history.

to the incarcerated omentum or bowel trapped within the sac. Incarceration is more common on the right side than the left, and approximately 12% of all children (<12 years old) with hernia have incarceration. This event is far more common in the first year of life, when the incidence of incarceration may be 30%. Clinical presentation is that of an acute tender mass in the inguinal canal. The mass may extend into the scrotum and be edematous, erythematous, and tender. Failure to reduce the incarcerated viscera may result in hypoxic changes, leading to

strangulation obstruction. Because of the risk of incarceration (especially in the first few months of life), elective hernia repair should be scheduled shortly after the diagnosis is made. While waiting for an early elective repair, parents of infants or children with a documented inguinal hernia should be counseled carefully regarding the need to call immediately if the hernia becomes irreducible or any discoloration occurs. In instances of incarceration, the infant is sedated with a short-acting barbiturate or analgesic and placed in the Trendelenburg position.

When the infant quiets, spontaneous reduction may occur or gentle taxis often manually reduces the hernia and obviates the need for an emergency operation. Because of the risk of recurrent incarceration, in most cases these infants should be admitted to the hospital and undergo elective surgery the next day. Complications of incarceration include late testicular atrophy, gonadal infarction, intestinal obstruction (10% of patients), and gangrenous bowel (3% to 7% of patients). The complication rate after emergency surgical care of infants with incarcerated hernia is greater than 10%, compared with a postoperative complication rate of 1.5% after elective surgery. Postoperative complications include wound infection, recurrent hernia, and injury to the vas deferens and spermatic vessels.

Inguinal Hernia in the Premature Infant

With the advent of neonatal intensive care, many infants, particularly premature infants, now recover from serious conditions such as respiratory insufficiency, sepsis, and necrotizing enterocolitis. Because of prematurity, they also are at risk for developing an inguinal hernia. During hospitalization, premature infants with an inguinal hernia can be kept under close observation in the neonatal intensive care unit. Manual reduction of the incarcerated hernia can allow the infant time to recover from the underlying neonatal illness without being subjected to the additional stress related to undergoing anesthesia and an emergency operation. As a general rule because of the high incarceration in premature infants, the hernia should be repaired just before the infant's discharge from the neonatal intensive care unit. These infants require postoperative monitoring for episodes of apnea and bradycardia. For premature infants who have the hernia diagnosed after discharge from the hospital, repair is done when they are approximately 60 weeks' gestation equivalent. These infants require either an extensive postoperative observation period or 23-hour admission to observe for apnea and bradycardia.

Treatment

In most instances, inguinal hernia repair in infants and children can be done in the ambulatory setting. Ambulatory surgery for infants and children requires skilled pediatric anesthesiologists and nursing staff, a pleasant environment, appropriate-sized pediatric equipment and monitoring equipment, and the ability to admit to a pediatric inpatient facility if necessary. Outpatient surgery for inguinal hernia is safe, effective, and well tolerated. Benefits of ambulatory surgery include minimizing the psychological trauma associated with hospitalization and separation from loved ones, reduced cost of hospitalization, and a lower risk of cross-infection. In selected patients who have other associated abnormalities, such as congenital heart disease or a ventriculoperitoneal shunt, antibiotics can be administered as indicated.

In addition to an obvious inguinal hernia, other lesions requiring operative exploration for inguinal anomalies in infants include a hydrocele of the canal of Nuck or spermatic cord, a communicating hydrocele, a tense hydrocele that may cause gonadal ischemia, and hydroceles of the tunica vaginalis that persist for 1 year or more.

Although occasional surgeons use local anesthetic or spinal anesthesia for small infants during inguinal operation, a well-administered general anesthetic is often preferred. Body temperature is maintained in the normal range. Temperature, electrocardiogram, blood pressure, pulse, oxygen saturation, and end-tidal carbon dioxide are monitored. An intravenous line is started, and endotracheal anesthesia is initiated.

The incision is made in the lowest inguinal crease on the ipsilateral side. Bleeding is usually minimal and can be controlled with a fine-tipped electrocoagulator. Scarpa's fascia is opened, and the external oblique fascia is noted and traced laterally then inferiorly along the inguinal ligament to identify the external inguinal ring. The external oblique fascia is opened extending laterally from the ring following the long axis of its fibers. The external ring does not need to be opened. The ilioinguinal nerve is spared, and the cremasteric muscle is opened on the anteromedial surface, exposing the hernia sac, which usually presents as a white, glistening membrane (Fig. 42-3). At this point, an ilioinguinal and iliohypogastric nerve block using bupivacaine 0.5% may be performed for pain control. The sac is retracted medially, which allows lateral and posterior dissection of the spermatic vessels and vas deferens away from the diverticular-like hernia sac. Dissection is continued to the level of the internal inguinal ring until preperitoneal fat is identified. To avoid injury, the vas deferens should not be grasped with forceps. If the sac extends into the scrotum, it may be divided, leaving the distal sac in place. High ligation of the proximal twisted sac at the level of the internal ring is accomplished using two 4-0 nonabsorbable suture ligatures. The distal end of the sac simply can be opened widely on its anterior surface to avoid injury to the testis and periscrotal tissues. If there is a separate associated hydrocele that does not communicate with the hernia sac, however, this should be excised or opened. If the internal ring is excessively large, it can be narrowed with an interrupted 4-0 suture that approximates the transversalis fascia edges below the cord structures; this is rarely needed. Too tight a closure may result in venous congestion and testicular swelling. Rarely the posterior wall of the inguinal canal is weak, or an associated direct defect in the transversalis fascia is present. One or two interrupted sutures placed from the conjoined tendon to the iliopubic tract suffice to strengthen the floor. Prosthetic mesh or plugs are not needed except perhaps in older teenagers. The testis always should be replaced in an intrascrotal location; the scrotum always should be prepared into the operative field.

Closure of the wound can be accomplished in layers with interrupted fine absorbable suture. The skin is closed with fine subcuticular sutures of absorbable material. The skin edges can be sealed with collodion or in older children who are continent of urine with Steri-strips. In some instances, the parents may request that a circumcision be performed at the same time as the hernia repair. Preparation of the foreskin is best delayed until the completion of the hernia repair because early retraction may lead to significant edema formation by the time the hernia is repaired.

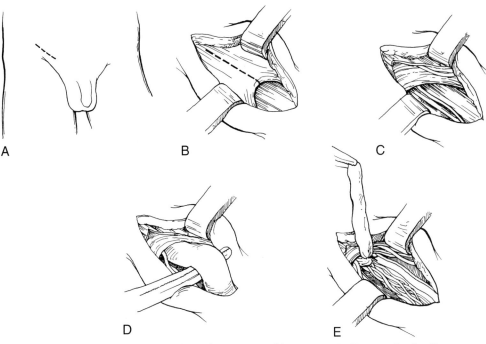

FIGURE 42-3 ■ Technique for indirect inguinal hernia repair. See text for details.

There is considerable controversy as to whether the contralateral side should be explored in childhood. At least 5% of infants and children have a clinically identifiable hernia on both sides before operation. Children younger than age 2 years have a high incidence of contralateral patent processus vaginalis. Because only 12% to 15% of adolescents and adults have bilateral indirect inguinal hernias, most patent processes close spontaneously and are not precursors of a hernia. Several reports indicate an incidence of only 7% of a late occurrence of a hernia on the contralateral side in patients who had one side repaired previously. This low incidence suggests that bilateral exploration is not indicated. It has become popular to pass a peritoneoscope through the sac at the time of repair to view the contralateral internal ring from inside the abdomen, but this technique only verifies the presence of an open processus and not an actual hernia. Some pediatric surgeons still routinely explore both groins in children younger than age 2 years, in older boys with a clinical hernia that presents on the left side, and in girls younger than age 10 years because bilaterality is more common. Contralateral exploration may be undertaken if the surgeon is skilled and experienced, the anesthesia support is at a high level, and there are no major risk factors. The risk of injury to the vas and spermatic vessels during hernia repair is higher in infants than in older patients.

In patients with an incarcerated hernia that requires emergent repair, the infant should be given perioperative antibiotics at least 30 minutes before the incision. The operation is carried out through the standard inguinal incision, and the incarcerated viscera is inspected carefully to ensure viability. A rapid return of pink color to the intestine with visible peristalsis and sheen usually indicates a viable bowel. The Doppler probe is occasionally useful to determine bowel viability. If peritoneal fluid is malodorous or cloudy, it should be cultured for aerobic and anaerobic organisms. If the bowel reduces during the induction of anesthesia, it is rare for a patient to have devascularized bowel. In the rare setting in which purulent or bloody fluid is noted in the hernia sac or there are suggestive clinical findings of bowel infarction, a laparotomy should be done to inspect the reduced segment of bowel. Surgery for incarcerated inguinal hernia occasionally can be difficult because of tissue friability, edema, and the presence of the mass that initially can obscure the anatomy. For this reason, some prefer the transperitoneal Cheatle-Henry approach, especially in infants.

Occasional infants have a sliding hernia in which the medial part of the sac is composed of a viscus such as the cecum, appendix, bladder, sigmoid colon, ovary, or fallopian tube (Fig. 42-4). The ovary and fallopian tubes can be invaginated into the peritoneal cavity through a carefully placed circumferential purse-string suture at

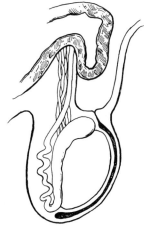

FIGURE 42-4 ■ Sliding inguinal hernia.

the base of the outside of the sac without dissecting the ovary and tube from the wall of the sac. Sliding hernias of the ovaries or fallopian tube are observed in 15% of girls with inguinal hernia. Ovarian torsion can occur within the sac, and although the presence of an incarcerated ovary does not present the same high risk as incarcerated bowel, prompt operation is in order.

In experienced hands, complications, such as injury to the ilioinguinal nerve, vas deferens, and spermatic vessels, are uncommon after an elective hernia repair. If the vas deferens is inadvertently divided, it should be repaired with interrupted 8-0 monofilament sutures using either an operating microscope or a magnifying loupe. Intraoperative bleeding is unusual. The floor of the inguinal canal does not require a formal repair, although many surgeons approximate the internal oblique muscle to the shelving edge of the inguinal ligament over the spermatic cord with one or two nonabsorbable sutures.

Postoperative complications include wound infection, scrotal hematoma, postoperative hydrocele, and recurrent inguinal hernia. The wound infection rate is approximately 1% in most institutions but may be higher with incarceration. Recurrent inguinal hernia occurs in about 2% of uncomplicated cases. Causes of recurrence include infection, missed hernia sac, unrecognized tear in the base of the sac, failure to repair an excessively large internal ring, operative injury to the floor of the inguinal canal resulting in the development of a direct inguinal hernia, and previous surgery for an incarcerated hernia. Patients with cystic fibrosis, ascites, peritoneal dialysis, and connective tissue disorders have a much higher risk of recurrence. Because of scarring, surgery for recurrence in boys can be technically challenging, and it may be helpful in these patients to use the preperitoneal approach. In instances in which direct inguinal hernia is observed, a formal Cooper's ligament repair or use of a prosthetic patch may be necessary.

Femoral hernias are unusual in the pediatric age group and are noted more commonly in girls. Occasional patients may develop a postoperative hydrocele that usually resolves. If it persists, aspiration may be useful because there is no longer a connection to the peritoneal cavity. Rarely a persistent symptomatic postoperative hydrocele requires formal repair and excision.

Although laparoscopic hernia repair has become a popular alternative in adults, there is a limited role for this minimally invasive technique in infants and young children. The multiple incisions required for adequate visualization and tissue manipulation and the increased length of operative time and prolonged anesthesia are of concern. Because conventional inguinal hernia repair during infancy and childhood can be performed through a small incision in 20 to 30 minutes and is associated with little morbidity and almost no mortality, with prompt return to normal activity, laparoscopic repair in infants and young children offers no advantage.

UNDESCENDED TESTIS

Undescended testis is one of the most common surgical disorders in childhood. Cryptorchidism occurs in approximately 0.8% to 1.3% of boys. Surgery is the cornerstone of therapy for the correction of true undescended testis.

Embryology

The testes originate in the mesonephric ridge on each side of the fetal spine and are drawn downward through the retroperitoneal space and out through the abdominal wall during the seventh and eighth months of gestation by the gubernaculum. The gubernaculum is attached superiorly to the proximal tip of the vas deferens and is believed to divide distally into several tails extending to the dartos muscle and fascia in the scrotum, Colles' fascia in the perineum, the pubic tubercle and crest, the inguinal ligament, and the fascia in the femoral triangle. The testicle descends through the external inguinal ring into the scrotum during the eighth and ninth months of gestation. Although the testicle normally follows the course of the scrotal extension, occasionally it may follow one of the other gubernacular tails to an ectopic location in the perineal, suprapubic, or femoral areas. An extension of the peritoneal cavity, the processus vaginalis, is drawn into the scrotum with the testicle and eventually becomes the tunica of the gonad with obliteration of the processus within the inguinal canal. After the gonad reaches the scrotum, the gubernaculum becomes indistinct as an identifiable structure. Many aspects of embryologic and morphologic development of the testicle remain undefined.

Hormonal Influences

Testicular descent into the scrotum is influenced greatly by maternal gonadotropic hormones that stimulate production of androgenic hormones by the fetal testis. Gonadotropic hormones are present in the human maternal circulation until the third trimester, when they begin to decrease. Failure of the testicle to descend through the inguinal canal during the third trimester may be related to inadequacy of the maternal gonadotropic hormones, failure of the testis to respond to them, inadequate gubernacular traction, or various other factors because more than 80% of undescended testes are unilateral. There is no clear evidence that true cryptorchid testes with mechanical obstruction would descend into the scrotum in response to exogenous or endogenous hormones after the first 3 months of life.

Empty Scrotum

An empty scrotum is found in 20% to 30% of premature infants and 1.2% to 4% of mature newborns. The diagnosis of true undescended testis may be difficult to determine before age 6 months, particularly in premature infants. Thereafter the testicle should be able to be placed into the low scrotum with gentle manipulation. The empty scrotum may be caused by a retractile testis or by true testicular pathology: ectopic testes (3%), dysgenetic or atrophic testes (5%), absent testes (3%), or true undescended testes (89%).

Retractile Testes

An empty scrotum in a young child may be the result of a retractile testis caused by an overactive cremaster muscle and inadequate gubernacular attachment of the

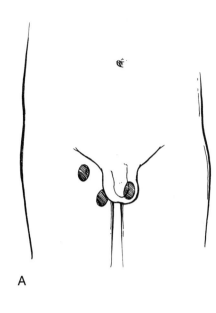

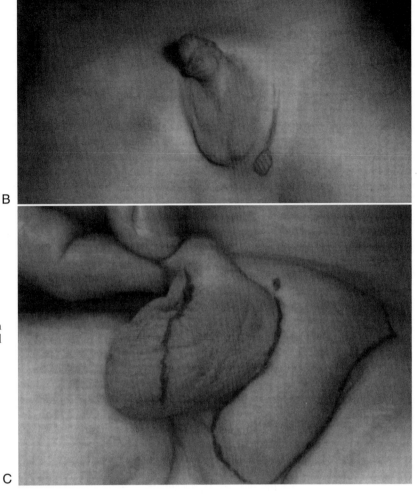

FIGURE 42-5 ■ Ectopic testes. **A,** Common locations. **B,** Perineal location. **C,** Femoral location associated with femoral hernia.

testicle to the scrotum. These testes descend into the scrotum spontaneously when children are asleep or relaxed and can be manipulated into the low scrotum on examination. Retractile testes are usually bilateral and remain in the scrotum after early adolescence when the testicle becomes heavier and larger than the external inguinal ring and the cremaster muscle becomes less active. Testicular volume and function of retractile testicles are believed to be normal in adulthood. No surgical treatment is indicated. The use of luteinizing hormone–releasing hormone and human chorionic gonadotropin to accelerate descent is controversial.

Ectopic Testes

The ectopic testis is drawn into the thigh, groin, or superpubic area by an abnormally positioned gubernaculum and places the gonad at risk for trauma (Fig. 42-5). These testes usually function normally but should be placed into the scrotum surgically by age 2 years.

Hypoplastic or Absent Testes

Approximately 8% of children with an empty scrotum have absence or hypoplasia of the testicle. Although hormonal factors may be influential, torsion or obstruction to testicular blood flow during fetal development is believed to be the major cause. The ipsilateral scrotum is usually underdeveloped, and occasionally ipsilateral renal and ureteral agenesis are present. The vas deferens in these patients is usually hypoplastic and ends blindly at the internal inguinal ring or in the canal. Exploration to identify a nonpalpable high undescended testis is necessary inasmuch as total absence is uncommon. Although abdominal ultrasound studies and computed tomography scans assist in identifying intra-abdominal testes, surgical exploration, usually with laparoscopy, is necessary to establish the diagnosis because dysplastic or intra-abdominal testes have a high predilection for malignant degeneration. A testicular prosthesis can be inserted into the scrotum for psychological benefit.

True Undescended Testes

The undescended testis that does not descend into the scrotum spontaneously, with hormone therapy, or with operation by age 4 years probably will not achieve normal spermatogenic function in adolescence. The higher the testis resides above the scrotum, the more dysgenetic the morphologic features of the gonad are likely to be. Because of maldescent, most cryptorchid testes are prevented from reaching the scrotum because the spermatic artery is shorter than normal.

Inasmuch as more than 80% of true undescended testes are unilateral, a specific hormonal deficiency to account for the cryptorchidism has been difficult to identify. Children with bilateral cryptorchidism are more likely to have an endocrinologic disturbance with hormonal deficiency than children with unilateral descent. They also tend to have anatomic disturbances limiting descent of the testis (e.g., exstrophy of the bladder, gastroschisis, prune-belly syndrome, hypospadias, and intersex anomalies).

Descent within the first 9 months of life occurs in most infants with an empty scrotum. After the first year of life, true undescent is pathologic, occurring in approximately 1.2% at that age. Examination of testicular weight, diameter of seminiferous tubules, and spermatogonia counts shows that the young child's testes have a linear development patterned before puberty. Damaging influences causing morphologic changes in the undescended testis generally are considered to begin by 9 to 18 months of age. Using spermatogonia counts and qualitative examination of the ultrastructure of interstitial tissue, a few authors have shown that the undescended testis has few histomorphologic changes during the first year of life. After the second year, the spermatogonia counts decrease significantly. The spermatogonia counts in low-lying testes are much higher than counts in high-lying testes regardless of the type of treatment.

Testicular degeneration may occur from the higher temperature in the abdomen compared with that of the scrotum. Heat applied to the scrotal testis similarly may cause degeneration. Placing a scrotal testis into the abdomen causes degeneration of germinal epithelium. Normal testicular volume is less than 2 mL up to age 11 years. At age 12, the volume is 2 to 5 mL; at age 13, 5 to 10 mL; and at age 15, 12 to 14 mL.

With increasing age, the true undescended testis develops interstitial fibrosis and poor tubular development. Spermatogenesis decreases because of atrophy of seminiferous tubules with fibrosis caused by decreased vascularization and expansion of the connective tissue.

The unilateral cryptorchid testis is believed possibly to produce autoantibodies that adversely affect development and function of the contralateral descended testis. Similar adverse effects on the descended contralateral testicle have been observed after unilateral testicular torsion with severe vascular insult to the gonad that is not removed. The basement membrane of the seminiferous tubules may act as an immunologic barrier that under normal circumstances keeps antibodies from penetrating into the seminiferous tubules. Under pathologic conditions, the basement membrane may become porous, exposing parts of the seminiferous tubules to antibodies, leading to an antigen-antibody reaction. Azathioprine has improved spermatogonia counts in dystopic and orthotopic testes of experimentally cryptorchid dogs. More recent studies indicate that luteinizing hormone–releasing hormone administration improves the biopsy appearance of undescended testes repaired after age 2. If the cryptorchid testis is not placed into the scrotum at an early age, despite the presence of a descended contralateral testis, fertility decreases.

Kiesewetter and associates showed that young children who undergo orchiopexy subsequently show an increase in the spermatogonia count. Other, more recent studies confirmed this observation and found further that this improvement is mainly seen when orchidopexy is performed by age 2 years.

Treatment

Retractile testes almost always descend after exogenous gonadotropin therapy; however, few reports document reliable benefit for true unilateral undescended testes. Hormone therapy may be beneficial if a mechanical barrier is not present, particularly in cases of bilateral undescended testicles. A trial of luteinizing hormone–releasing hormone and human chorionic gonadotropin combination therapy may cause descent of retractile testes in 60% of cases from European trials, although this has not been confirmed uniformly in U.S. trials. High doses and long-term use of human chorionic gonadotropin may produce tubular degeneration, precocious puberty, and early epiphyseal closure. Combination hormone therapy before orchiopexy enlarges the testis and the spermatic vessels, making the technical repair easier, particularly in children with a small scrotum, and it may promote maturation after repair based on biopsy information.

Orchiopexy

The major indications for performing orchiopexy are to enhance fertility, to reduce the likelihood of torsion, to repair a concomitant hernia, to prevent trauma or pain, to provide easier examination for testicular tumor, and for psychological effect and appearance. Surgically the limiting factor for placement of the testis in the scrotum is the length of the spermatic artery, which is placed under tension when the testis is pulled inferior to the external inguinal ring. Surgical correction consists of mobilizing the spermatic artery and veins medially and the vas deferens in such a manner that the vessels may descend directly into the scrotum rather than passing through the circuitous course through the internal inguinal ring, inguinal canal, and external inguinal ring. Obliteration of the triangle of normal descent usually provides sufficient length for the vessels to extend into the low scrotum. The inferior epigastric vessels are divided, and the posterior wall of the inguinal canal is opened wide to permit sufficient mobilization of the spermatic vessels and to divide the lateral spermatic fascia. High ligation of the hernia sac is performed; however, the peritoneum is not intentionally opened unless it is necessary to bring an intra-abdominal testis down. The testis is secured in the low scrotum using the dartos pouch technique, in which the scrotum is stretched

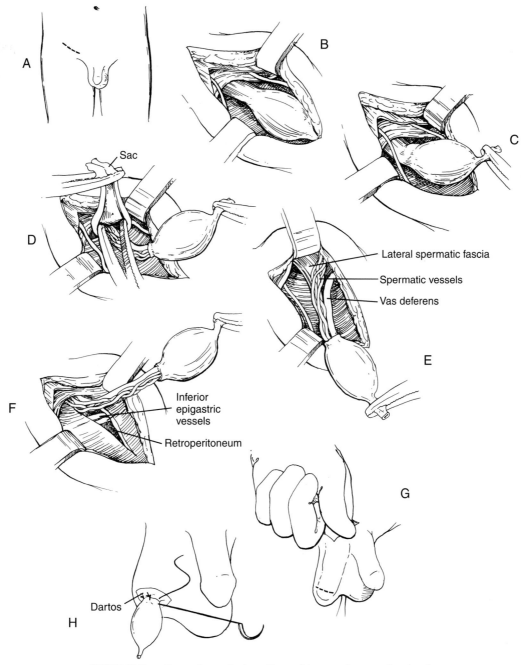

FIGURE 42-6 ■ Operative technique for orchiopexy. See text for details.

forcibly with a finger, and a space is developed between the scrotal skin and the dartos fascia. The procedure is performed through an extended hernia incision with a counterincision in the lowermost point of the ipsilateral scrotum (Fig. 42-6). The operation is performed with the patient under general anesthesia, usually on an outpatient basis.

Epididymal abnormalities are present in approximately 35% to 40% of cryptorchid testes, are more common with high situated gonads, and may affect fertility. Testicular biopsy may be performed selectively as indicated when postoperative hormone treatment is contemplated.

For high cryptorchid testes, a few surgical techniques have been used effectively. The midline transabdominal or the muscle-splitting preperitoneal approaches are especially useful for children with bilateral high undescended testes, making it possible to bring both testes down to the scrotum through a single incision. The Fowler-Stephens "long-loop vas" orchiopexy provides length for the testicle to reach the scrotum by dividing the spermatic artery and veins high in the retroperitoneal space. The testis derives its blood supply entirely from the vessels of the vas deferens, collaterals from the deep epigastric vessels, and branches entering the posterior wall of the processus vaginalis in the area of the gubernaculum. A two-stage repair in which the testicle is placed as low as possible in the first operation, then mobilized further 1 or 2 years later occasionally has been effective. The initial high ligation and division of the spermatic vessels of intra-abdominal testes can be accomplished laparoscopically, and this approach is useful when no testis can be palpated. Microsurgical techniques for anastomosis of the spermatic vessels to vessels of the thigh or branches of the inferior epigastric vessels have been reported with occasional success in the management of the high undescended testis, although this technique has found only limited application.

When the testis cannot be located after laparoscopy or after extensive exploration of the retroperitoneal space, transperitoneal exploration through the same inguinal incision slightly extended (La Roque maneuver) should be performed to exclude completely the presence of a gonad. An intra-abdominal testis may be missed during retroperitoneal dissection because it may be suspended in the peritoneal cavity by the mesorchium, as with the normal ovary. Currently, laparoscopy is probably the best way to identify the site of an intra-abdominal testis or document anorchia in boys with an empty scrotum and nonpalpable testis. Of these children, 10% to 15% have a truly absent testis. To secure the diagnosis, one must identify surgically the blind-ending vas and the blind-ending spermatic vessels. Because of the occurrence of epididymal-gonadal disunion, identification of a blind-ending vas alone is not diagnostic. Occasionally an atrophic testis may be encountered either in the inguinal canal or within the scrotum. Because this likely is a sequela of previous torsion, it may be wise to consider contralateral scrotal orchiopexy. If an atrophic testis is found (confirmed by biopsy), and the contralateral gonad is normal, orchiectomy should be performed. One generally waits until puberty to remove other dysgenetic testes for a possible hormonal advantage. If the testis is absent, a scrotal prosthesis can be placed.

Results

Complications from orchiopexy include injury to the vas (approximately 1%), spermatic vascular injuries leading to testicular atrophy (1% to 8%), and retraction of the testis to the external ring (5% to 10%). Fertility in patients with uncorrected unilateral undescended testis has been reported between 30% and 60%. Fertility in patients with unilateral descended testis repaired before age 9 years is near 85%, indicating the importance of early surgical repair. For children with untreated bilateral undescended testes, 100% are infertile, although testosterone production is often normal. If orchiopexy for bilateral undescended testes is performed in children before age 5 years, 50% are fertile, and 30% are normospermic. In instances of bilateral undescended testes, maturation is at the same stage in both testes for 39%. Follicle-stimulating hormone levels increase inversely with spermatogenesis; elevated luteinizing hormone levels suggest Leydig cell dysfunction and gonadal atrophy. Patients who undergo bilateral orchiopexy before age 2 years are reported to have greater than 65% fertility, whereas patients repaired after age 13 have approximately 12% fertility.

Malignancy

Approximately 12% of testicular tumors arise in cryptorchid testes. Conversely, 5% of cryptorchid testes may become malignant. A tumor in a cryptorchid testis is 30 to 50 times more likely than in a normal testicle. Atrophic and intra-abdominal testes may have a 200-fold increase in the incidence of tumor. Orchiopexy may *not* decrease the likelihood of tumor. The average age when a tumor is found is 26 years. Malignant tumors originating from cryptorchid testes include seminoma, teratocarcinoma, embryonal carcinoma, and adult teratoma. The incidence of tumor has been lower in cryptorchid testes placed into the scrotum before age 5 years compared with cryptorchid testes repaired in adolescence. Current belief is that children 14 years or older with a unilateral high undescended testis should undergo ipsilateral orchiectomy rather than orchiopexy because the risk of developing a neoplasm seems to increase directly with age at the time of orchiopexy. Testes in the low inguinal canal that grossly appear normal should be biopsied to determine if dysplasia is present before performing orchiectomy. A close relationship may exist between the development of neoplasm in the testicle and the degree of dystopia. When the testicle is removed or in the case of anorchia, regardless of the patient's age, a testicular prosthesis should be placed into the scrotum.

The higher the testis resides above the scrotum, the more dysgenetic the morphology. Patients with high testes rarely respond to luteinizing hormone–releasing hormone and human chorionic gonadotropin and should have an orchiopexy by age 2 years. Low testes may descend with hormone treatment at age 2 to 3 years; if not, patients should undergo orchiopexy. Unilateral cryptorchid testes that are dysplastic or located high should be removed before adolescence. The unilateral cryptorchid testis may produce adverse effects on the contralateral descended testis after age 2 years. Fertility in children with unilateral undescent repaired before age 2 years is near normal.

ACUTE CONDITIONS OF THE SCROTUM

The most common causes of acute scrotal disorders are testicular torsion, torsion of the appendage, epididymitis, and orchitis (Fig. 42-7). Trauma, tumor, and hemorrhage also may present as an acute condition. The differential diagnosis is often age dependent. In children younger than 6 years old, testicular torsion predominates. The incidence of torsion of testicular or epididymal appendages increases in early adolescence. Epididymitis and orchitis are the most frequent diagnoses in young adults; however, these conditions may be encountered in a significant number of adolescents and occasionally young children. Often a history of sexual contact may be elicited and may influence antibiotic therapy. Young children with epididymitis should be evaluated for an anatomic anomaly of the urinary tract (e.g., bladder outlet obstruction from posterior urethral valves or urethral stricture, Cowper's duct anomaly, or insertion of an ectopic ureter into the genital tract). More rare entities that may present with acute scrotal conditions include spermatic vein thrombosis, scrotal fat necrosis, idiopathic scrotal edema, and scrotal peritonitis (e.g., ruptured appendix associated with a patent processus vaginalis).

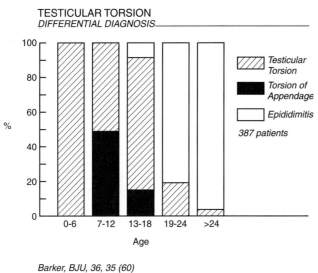

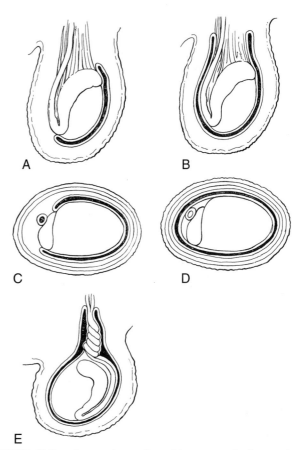

FIGURE 42-7 ■ Relative incidence of the most common causes of acute scrotal conditions in children as a function of age. (From Sheldon CA: The acute scrotum. Surg Clin North Am 65:1321, 1985.)

Testicular Torsion

Testicular torsion (torsion of the spermatic cord) may interrupt blood flow to the testis and epididymis. The degree of torsion may vary from 360 to 720 degrees. The extent and the duration of torsion and the presence or absence of intermittent torsion have prominent influences on the degree of testicular injury. The two most common types of testicular torsion are extravaginal torsion, which occurs predominantly in the perinatal period, and intravaginal torsion, which occurs predominantly in older children (Fig. 42-8).

Intravaginal torsion is related to an anomalous lack of testicular fixation in the tunica vaginalis that has been called the *bell-clapper anomaly* (Fig. 42-9). Normal testicular suspension ensures firm fixation of the epididymal-testicular complex posteriorly and effectively prevents twisting of the spermatic cord. The testis may lie in a plane more transverse than normal so that the epididymis is located more superiorly with respect to the testis.

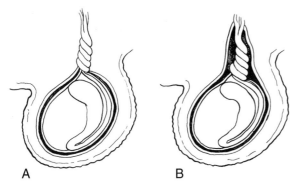

FIGURE 42-8 ■ Classification of testicular torsion. **A,** Extravaginal. **B,** Intravaginal.

FIGURE 42-9 ■ Anatomic predisposition to testicular torsion. **A** and **B,** Normal anatomy. **C** and **D,** Bell-clapper anomaly. **E,** Testicular torsion.

Contraction of the cremasteric muscles shortens the spermatic cord and may initiate testicular torsion. Progression of torsion is promoted by increasing testicular and epididymal congestion. Often, testicular torsion occurs spontaneously. The onset of sudden severe scrotal pain is almost pathognomonic. In some patients, however, a history of scrotal trauma or other scrotal disease (including torsion of appendix testis or epididymitis) may precede the occurrence of subsequent testicular torsion.

On physical examination, the epididymis may be located in a position other than immediately posterior to the testis. The testis itself is enlarged and tender and often is elevated within the scrotum. Often the contralateral testis has a transverse orientation. Urinalysis is generally normal; however, this is not always a reliable finding.

In most cases, the diagnosis is apparent and should be confirmed by prompt scrotal exploration. This is the appropriate course for any patient presenting with a characteristic picture of testicular torsion or in whom a less than characteristic picture is associated with a duration of symptoms approaching or exceeding 6 hours. Two diagnostic tests that may be useful include Doppler testicular flow study and testicular radioisotope imaging, but often clinical findings are sufficient for diagnosis.

Radioisotope testis imaging is the more reliable modality. Characteristically, with torsion, absence of isotope uptake within the testis is shown, surrounded by a

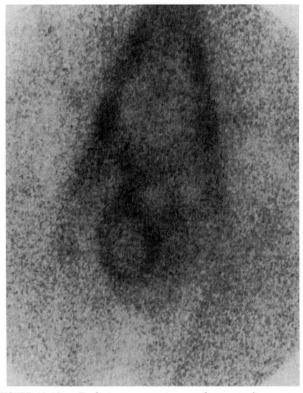

FIGURE 42-10 ■ Radioisotope testis scan for testicular torsion. The central area of decreased isotope uptake (testis) is surrounded by a halo of uptake (scrotum).

halo of scrotal perfusion (Fig. 42-10). The halo is accentuated in delayed torsion as a result of surrounding inflammatory hyperperfusion. Occasionally the testis scan suggests an alternate diagnosis by showing normal blood flow and an area of increased perfusion within the ipsilateral scrotum (e.g., epididymitis and occasionally torsion of an appendix testis). Some limitations of radioisotope imaging exist in obese boys with extremely elevated testes housed in a small scrotal compartment. The testicular scan should be performed promptly to avoid unnecessary delays. Radioisotope testicular imaging is indicated when the diagnosis of testicular torsion is considered unlikely by clinical criteria but when a definitive diagnosis of torsion of an appendix testis or epididymitis cannot be made.

Treatment of testicular torsion varies according to the age of the patient. Testicular torsion encountered in the perinatal period may have its onset either before or after birth. Patients who are born with testicular torsion are managed by early, selective exploration and contralateral orchiopexy. The potential for salvage of such a testis is nil, making the risk of immediate surgery before complete stabilization of the newborn unwarranted. In sharp contrast, the testis found to be normal at birth but that subsequently undergoes torsion demands immediate exploration. Although prenatal testicular torsion is usually extravaginal, postnatal torsion may be intravaginal. Although controversy exists whether the contralateral testis always should undergo orchiopexy for extravaginal torsion, the fact that bilateral synchronous extravaginal torsion, bilateral asynchronous extravaginal torsion, and

extravaginal torsion followed by intravaginal torsion all have been reported indicates that routine contralateral orchiopexy is warranted.

Testicular torsion in older children is managed by immediate surgical exploration. After the induction of anesthesia, repeat examination unhindered by pain and tenderness is suggested and occasionally may show the presence of an incarcerated hernia or testicular tumor, either of which is managed through an inguinal incision rather than the scrotal incision used for testicular torsion. The operation is performed through the midline scrotal raphe (Fig. 42-11). The ipsilateral scrotal compartment is entered and the testis delivered and detorsed. The testis is evaluated for viability based on color and its ability to bleed from an incision in the tunica albuginea after detorsion. Necrotic testes are removed because their retention often results in prolonged debilitating pain and tenderness and may exacerbate the potential for subfertility, presumably because of the development of an autoimmune response, which may affect the contralateral normal testis.

The contralateral scrotal compartment is entered, and the normal contralateral testis is delivered. The presence of a bell-clapper deformity in the contralateral testis is common and mandates routine contralateral four-point fixation. As shown in Figure 42-11C, the tunica albuginea is approximated to the scrotal wall, deeply within the scrotal compartment, employing nonabsorbable suture material, but does not traverse the scrotal wall. Four nonabsorbable sutures are placed on each testis. The testis should not be fixed too superficially within the scrotal compartment because scrotal closure may be difficult.

Patients who require orchiectomy for nonviability of the testis may benefit from the placement of a testicular prosthesis. This placement should be delayed, usually for 6 months, until complete healing and resolution of inflammatory changes have occurred. Prosthetic placement is performed through an inguinal incision.

Prognosis depends on the duration of testicular torsion. The incidence and the extent of testicular atrophy are exacerbated by delayed surgical intervention.

Torsion of Testicular Appendages

Torsion of an appendix testis and appendix epididymis are common causes of torsion. Occasionally, examination of the scrotum reveals a "blue dot sign." Characteristically a firm, tender nodule can be palpated at the junction of the epididymis with the testis. The nodule is mobile within the scrotum, and the testis itself is normal. Patients who present after torsion of the appendix testis may have these characteristic findings obscured by the presence of a reactive hydrocele or edema.

Treatment generally consists of bed rest, analgesia, and reassurance. Because torsion of the appendix testis may precipitate reactive epididymitis, prophylactic antibiotics may be helpful in selected patients. Patients in whom testicular torsion cannot be excluded or who have resistant incapacitating pain require scrotal exploration and excision of the involved appendage. Prognosis is excellent.

Epididymitis and Orchitis

Epididymitis may have an infectious or inflammatory cause. Most commonly, epididymitis occurs from the

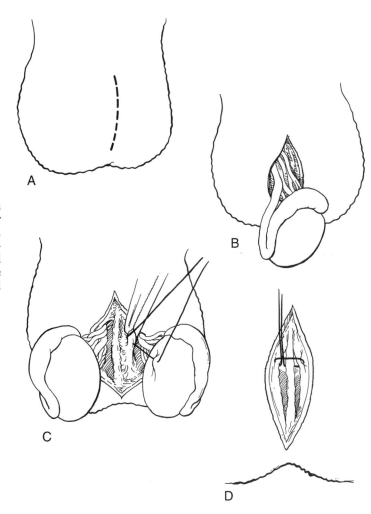

FIGURE 42-11 ■ Technique of scrotal exploration and orchiopexy for testicular torsion. See text for details. **A,** Incision through midline scrotal raphe. **B,** Testis is mobilized into the wound, and spermatic vessels and vas are placed in the normal position. **C,** The gonad is sutured to the wall of the scrotum with quadrant stitches. **D,** The scrotal wound is closed with deep and superficial sutures.

reflux of infected urine or from sexually acquired disease caused by gonococci and *Chlamydia*. This distinction is important because alterations in antibiotic therapy may be necessary. Occasionally, epididymitis develops after excessive straining or lifting and the reflux of urine into the vas deferens, which causes a chemical epididymitis; this usually resolves promptly. Any non–sexually active child, especially a prepubertal child who develops epididymitis, should be evaluated for a urinary tract abnormality.

Evaluation begins with an attempt to elicit a history of sexual activity or urethral discharge. Physical examination characteristically reveals a normal, nontender testis with an epididymis located directly posteriorly and that is large, tender, and firm.

Patients with mild symptoms of epididymitis may be treated with oral antibiotics on an outpatient basis. Because of the potential for progressive, chronic epididymal injury, patients with severe epididymitis and patients who are very young should be treated with intravenous antibiotics. Pain and tenderness commonly resolve within 72 hours; however, induration may persist for weeks.

A renal ultrasound study to exclude the presence of hydronephrosis from ectopic ureter and a voiding cystourethrogram to exclude the presence of bladder outlet obstruction should be obtained in the prepubertal patient and older children who are not sexually active.

Orchitis is uncommon in infants and young children. Most cases are associated with a viral infection, including mumps. The testis is tender, and the scrotal skin is usually erythematous and edematous. Urinalysis is normal, but the white blood cell count may be elevated. Testis isotope scan shows hyperemia. The treatment includes bed rest and observation. In most cases, testicular function is normal. Young adults with mumps orchitis may be at risk for postinfectious subfertility.

Varicocele

Varicoceles occur predominantly in the left hemiscrotum. This occurrence probably is related to the drainage of the spermatic vein into the left renal vein. Varicoceles may be idiopathic, in which case incompetent venous valves are demonstrable, or may occur as a result of venous obstruction secondary to renal vein thrombosis or a retroperitoneal tumor.

The occurrence of a varicocele may be complicated by discomfort or pain, testicular atrophy, traumatic hematoma, and subfertility. The cause of testicular atrophy and subfertility is largely unknown; however, temperature and metabolic etiologies have been implicated.

Most children are prepubertal or pubertal when they present for evaluation after the detection of a varicocele on routine examination. The varicocele is usually an obvious nest of dilated veins in the subcutaneous space along the cord augmented by either a cough or a Valsalva maneuver. Accurate measurement of testicular dimension is important because testicular atrophy is the predominant indication for surgical correction in childhood. Visible varicoceles (grade II or III) should be operated on. Retroperitoneal ultrasound examination should be considered whenever a varicocele is encountered in the right hemiscrotum, has sudden onset, or occurs in a prepubertal child because it may be caused by compression of the spermatic vessels by a hydronephrotic kidney or tumor. Indications for surgery include pain, discomfort from the associated mass, evidence for testicular injury, subfertility, and a measured alteration in the hypothalamic-pituitary-gonadal axis.

At operation, the entire spermatic vascular bundle is isolated carefully above the internal ring. The spermatic artery is identified and preserved; this may be assisted by intraoperative Doppler evaluation. The dilated spermatic veins are doubly ligated and divided. An intraoperative spermatic venogram allows demonstration that all collateral venous tributaries have been divided. Collateral communication with pelvic veins may be shown, and these venous tributaries must be divided to minimize the risk of recurrence. Laparoscopy has an increasing role in the surgical management of varicocele, especially to permit mass ligation of the testicular veins and artery in the retroperitoneal space as recommended by Palomo. Fewer postoperative hydroceles are seen with this approach.

Testicular and Paratesticular Tumors

The occurrence of any solid testicular or paratesticular mass requires immediate evaluation. The most common testis tumors in children are teratomas, yolk sac tumors, rhabdomyosarcoma, and testis infiltration by non-Hodgkin's lymphoma or leukemia. A chest film, β-human chorionic gonadotropin, and serum α-fetoprotein levels are obtained. Surgery is performed through an inguinal incision with isolation of the cord structures first, which are occluded by a vascular clamp at the internal ring. The testis is delivered for evaluation. A high inguinal orchiectomy is undertaken if examination reveals a neoplasm. With the exception of leukemic involvement, testicular tumors should never be approached through a scrotal incision. These entities are discussed in detail elsewhere in this book.

SUGGESTED READINGS

Fowler R, Stephens FD: The role of testicular vascular anatomy in the salvage of high undescended testis. Aust N Z J Surg 29:92, 1959.

This classic article describes the surgical management of the high intra-abdominal testis.

Grosfeld JL: Inguinal hernia in the premature neonate. In Grosfeld JL (ed): Common Problems in Pediatric Surgery. Chicago, Year Book Medical Publishers, 1991.

This article describes the problems associated with inguinal hernia presenting in seriously ill neonates treated in the neonatal intensive care unit and suggests a management program.

Hadziselimovic F, Herzog B: Cryptorchism, its impact on male fertility. Horm Res 55:6, 2001.

This symposium series of 13 papers covers virtually all the important considerations of cryptorchidism, including the place of biopsy, hormone therapy, aspects of fertility and neoplasms, germ cell development over time and with repair, and a variety of surgical considerations.

Puri P, Guiney EJ, O'Donnell B: Inguinal hernia in infants: The fate of the testis after incarceration. J Pediatr Surg 19:44, 1984.

This article documents the high incidence of incarceration (31%) seen in premature infants and young infants with inguinal hernia that persists throughout the first year of life.

Schwobel MG, Schramm H, Gitzelmann CA: The infantile inguinal hernia—a bilateral disease? Pediatr Surg Int 15:115-118, 1999.

This is one of three more recent follow-up studies showing that the incidence of late occurrence of an inguinal hernia on the asymptomatic contralateral side in patients undergoing unilateral repair is only 7%.

Skoag SJ, Roberts KP, Goldstein M, Pryor JL: The adolescent varicocele: What's new with an old problem in young patients? Pediatrics 100:112-122, 1997.

This is an excellent review of varicocele, indications for treatment, pathophysiology, and long-term implications.

Steinau G, Treutner KH, Fecken G, Schumpelick V: Recurrent inguinal hernias in infants and children. World J Surg 19:303-306, 1995.

A good contemporary review of the factors that predispose to failure of hernia repair, timing of recurrence, and approach to secondary repair.

43

Disorders of the Peritoneum and Peritoneal Cavity

MECONIUM PERITONITIS

Meconium peritonitis is an intense chemical and foreign body reaction of the peritoneum caused by spillage of meconium from an antenatal perforation of the intestinal tract. It occurs in 1 of 20,000 to 40,000 live births. The following classification of meconium peritonitis is useful:

1. *Pseudocyst.* The intestinal perforation does not immediately seal, and meconium continues to leak into the peritoneal cavity. The necrotic bowel segment, the adjacent bowel loops, and the omentum contain the perforation by forming a pseudocyst. Calcium deposits line the cyst wall.
2. *Plastic.* Meconium escapes into the peritoneal cavity, causing a marked generalized inflammatory reaction. Dense, fibrous adhesions are formed. Calcium deposits are scattered throughout. Frequently the perforation is sealed by the intense reaction and cannot be identified.
3. *Generalized.* Perforation occurs perinatally. The perforation is open, and the leak continues. Meconium is distributed throughout the peritoneal cavity, essentially producing a meconium ascites. The fluid is thin and bile stained, and the bowel loops adhere by thin, fibrinous, rather than fibrous, adhesion. Flecks of calcium deposits are seen throughout the peritoneum.

Etiology

The causes of intrauterine perforation are listed in Table 43-1. In 53% of the affected patients (from a collected series of 1084 cases), meconium peritonitis was associated with intrauterine intestinal obstruction. The basis of the obstruction was intestinal atresia in 66% and cystic fibrosis with meconium ileus in 34% of these patients. The combination of meconium peritonitis and intestinal atresia may be the result of intestinal vascular compromise leading to necrosis, perforation, and spillage of meconium. The necrotic segment of the bowel may be absorbed, and the proximal and distal ends of the bowel seal to form a classic intestinal atresia. Atresia also may develop without initial meconium spillage, but later the proximal, dilated, atretic segment of bowel may rupture and release meconium. When meconium ileus is present,

intrauterine volvulus of a redundant, meconium-filled segment of bowel may cause vascular necrosis and spillage. Perforation also may occur in meconium ileus as a result of pressure on the bowel wall caused by an intraluminal meconium mass, leading to localized necrosis. Other causes of obstruction in the fetus that have been associated with meconium peritonitis include intussusception, volvulus, and congenital bands. Perforation without obstruction has been reported after Meckel's diverticulitis, fetal appendicitis, and iatrogenic perforation during amniocentesis and in association with mesenteric vascular insufficiency. The progression from intestinal obstruction to meconium peritonitis in a fetus has been studied by serial prenatal ultrasonography. The first finding was polyhydramnios and dilated obstructed loops of fetal intestine. Fetal ascites then developed, and the dilated loops decompressed. Later intraperitoneal calcifications were noted.

Pathology

The site of perforation is found in two thirds of patients, with the most common sites being the ileum and the jejunum equally. Meconium is composed of amniotic fluid, fatty acids, squame cells, bile salts and pigments, and pancreatic and intestinal enzymes and is intensely irritating to the peritoneum. It is formed in the third month of life and moves down to the ileum by 4 months. Meconium spillage results in marked fibrinous exudates,

---

TABLE 43-1 ■ Causes of Intrauterine Intestinal Perforation

Obstruction
 Intestinal atresia
 Volvulus
 Intussusception
 Meconium ileus (cystic fibrosis)
 Vascular accident
 Extrinsic pressure from congenital bands
Perforation without obstruction
 Appendicitis
 Meckel's diverticulum
 Iatrogenic (e.g., from amniocentesis)

---

fibroblastic proliferation, granuloma formation, and giant cell reaction. Calcifications develop within 2 to 6 days as a result of the generation of free fatty acids by pancreatic enzymes and subsequent saponification.

Clinical Presentation

Polyhydramnios is present in the mother in 10% of these patients. One third of the patients are premature. The most common presentations are abdominal distention (70%) and bilious vomiting (60%). Despite the high incidence of intestinal obstruction, 10% will have passed meconium. The flow of meconium from the peritoneal cavity into a patent processus vaginalis can lead to a hydrocele with a calcified scrotal mass at birth. Rarely, meconium peritonitis is found incidentally in an asymptomatic patient as a result of the evaluation of a scrotal mass or identification of calcifications on abdominal film. In these patients, the perforation usually has sealed, and there may be no intestinal obstruction.

Imaging

Ultrasonography

In the past, meconium peritonitis was diagnosed prenatally only when maternal pelvimetry identified fetal calcification. As a result of the widespread use of fetal ultrasonography, meconium peritonitis now is detected frequently. Ultrasound findings include polyhydramnios, acoustic shadowing from calcific foci, fetal ascites, and intestinal dilation. Calcifications are found less frequently by prenatal ultrasound in cystic fibrosis patients with meconium peritonitis. These patients have reduced pancreatic enzymes compared with normal patients, and this may inhibit the precipitation of calcium.

Radiographic Findings

Postnatal abdominal radiographs usually reveal dilated loops of intestine and intra-abdominal calcifications. The calcifications caused by meconium peritonitis must be differentiated from other causes of calcification, such as intraluminal meconium calcification, adrenal hemorrhage, and tumors. Meconium peritonitis calcifications are linear and located on the outer surface of the bowel and intra-abdominal organs. The calcifications also may be speckled or in clumps or line portions of the peritoneum. Calcifications along the course of the patent processus vaginalis and in the scrotum are pathognomonic.

Management

The indications for operation are evidence of intestinal obstruction, free intraperitoneal air, abdominal mass, cellulitis of the abdominal wall, sepsis, or clinical deterioration. Asymptomatic infants with incidental meconium ascites or calcification in the scrotum or peritoneum should be observed carefully.

When operative intervention is required, the procedures may be long and tedious and involve significant blood loss. A balance is sought between excessive dissection and operative trauma with preservation of as much intestinal length as possible. If the perforated necrotic segment of intestine is short, it is resected, and a primary anastomosis is performed. Sometimes much of the intestine is contained within the pseudocysts. Usually, preservation of bowel length requires that the cyst be entered and broken up and as much gut as possible freed and retained. If the proximal bowel can be traced into the cyst and the distal bowel identified leaving the cyst, and their combined length is more than 50% of the entire small intestine, the cyst and its contained bowel can be resected, and the proximal and distal limbs can be anastomosed or exteriorized. Because of the high incidence of cystic fibrosis, sweat tests should be performed postoperatively on all patients with meconium peritonitis, and pancreatic enzyme supplements should be given enterally if indicated.

OMENTAL AND MESENTERIC CYSTS

Omental and mesenteric cysts are rare lesions. Collected series have analyzed light and electron microscopic histology and the clinical and ultrasound findings, and the results indicate that cystic lymphangiomas are the most common form of cyst of the omentum and mesentery in children. These lymphangiomas are large multicystic lesions most frequently found in boys. True mesothelial cysts are less common and are found most often in women. They are relatively small and asymptomatic. Table 43-2 compares the characteristics of the two lesions and their management.

Children with mesenteric and omental cysts most commonly present with abdominal pain, vomiting, and a mass in the abdomen. Mesenteric and omental cysts must be differentiated from nonpancreatic pseudocysts, enteric duplications, and the mesothelial cysts previously mentioned that are more common in adults. Computed tomography (CT) scans and ultrasound frequently are able to identify lymphangiomas, which are usually multiloculated, are located in the mesentery, and show no discernible wall. Most cysts in children are located in the mesentery, usually in the terminal ileum. Less common sites are the mesentery of the jejunum, omentum, mesocolon, and retroperitoneum. Because of the frequent association of the cysts with the small bowel mesentery, complete excision may require bowel resection. Pseudocysts that develop after ventriculoperitoneal shunting are common. Treatment of these lesions requires unroofing the cyst using an open or laparoscopic approach and repositioning the peritoneal portion of the ventriculoperitoneal shunt, usually over the liver.

ASCITES

Excessive fluid accumulation in the peritoneal cavity leading to abdominal distention has a multitude of causes in pediatric patients. Ascites may be secondary to cardiovascular or hepatorenal disease or caused by highly specific lesions. Radiographic signs of ascites consist of haziness, bulging of the flanks, separation of the intestinal loops, and central positioning of the intestinal gas pattern. Ultrasonography is the most reliable method of differentiating a generalized fluid collection from a cystic or solid lesion. A CT scan may delineate existing pathologic conditions. Paracentesis and examination of the

				Pathology and		
TABLE 43-2 ■ Cystic Lymphangiomas versus Mesothelial Cysts						
Cyst	**Mean Age (yr)**	**Location**	**Signs/Symptoms**	**Histology**	**Sex**	**Treatment**
Lymphangioma	10	Commonly mesentery; rarely omentum	88% symptomatic Rarely ascites Large lesion	Endothelial cells, foam cells, lymphoid tissue, smooth muscle; chyle in cyst, commonly multiloculated	Males 75%	Excision—often bowel resection necessary
Mesothelial cyst	44 (66% >40)	Common in omentum and mesentery	35% symptomatic Rarely ascites Small lesion	Cuboidal cell lining, no muscle or lymphoid tissue; rare chyle, uniloculated	Females 60%	Excision—omental lesions can be excised without difficulty

fluid microscopically and chemically is of great value in determining a diagnosis.

Conditions such as pancreatic and ovarian ascites usually are caused by specific pathology. In pancreatic ascites, the etiologic factor is usually pancreatitis, and ascites is an early stage in the development of a pseudocyst. Ovarian ascites frequently is associated with an ovarian cyst or tumor. Fetal, chylous, urinary, and biliary ascites are of particular pediatric surgical significance. The various characteristics are outlined in Table 43-3.

PERITONEAL ADHESIONS

Intra-abdominal surgery is the most common cause of intestinal obstruction. The incidence is not as high in children as in adults. In one series, colectomy for ulcerative colitis was the most common procedure leading to obstruction, followed by surgery for Meckel's diverticulum, Ladd procedure for malrotation, nephrectomy for Wilms' tumors, reduction and resection of intussusception, hepatectomy for tumor, and Nissen fundoplication. In several series, adhesive obstruction was one of the most common complications after fundoplication for gastroesophageal reflux. Formation of adhesions is part of the normal healing process of an injured peritoneum. Bowel loops adhere to each other by fibrinous adhesions that are replaced by fibroblasts and developing capillaries. Initially the adhesions are thick and vascular, but over 3 months the vascularity decreases, and the adhesions are composed mainly of dense fibrous tissue. Trauma to the peritoneal surface by drying, abrasion from sponges, irritation by foreign bodies such as talc, and stripping of the intestinal serosa stimulate an intense fibroblastic reaction in the peritoneum. Obstruction is the result of a loop of intestine that is kinked by an adhesive band, by an internal hernia developing from a pocket formed by adhesions, or by volvulus of a segment of intestine around an adhesive band.

Intestinal obstruction developing immediately after laparotomy frequently is caused by small bowel intussusception rather than adhesion. Early obstruction from inflammatory adhesions sometimes may be seen, however, soon after operation for a ruptured appendix.

In patients who have had previous operations for adhesive small bowel obstruction and who have signs of incomplete intestinal obstruction, a contrast examination of the gastrointestinal tract can be useful. Thin barium gives the best contrast, although occasionally it may cause an impaction above the obstruction. Isotonic radiopaque contrast solutions also are effective and provide good visualization, even in infants, but dilution may limit visualization distally. Failure of the contrast agent to pass into the distal small bowel, along with the presence of dilated proximal bowel, suggests a high-grade intestinal obstruction. For distal obstructions, contrast material may be instilled best from below to confirm the presence of collapsed distal bowel.

All patients with intestinal obstruction should be treated initially with a nasogastric tube, intravenous hydration, and administration of broad-spectrum antibiotics. Correction of hypovolemia is important before considering laparotomy. If there is hypertonic dehydration, care must be taken not to correct the hyperosmolality rapidly because of the fear of seizures. In this case, we correct the hypovolemia by administering adequate isotonic replacement fluids and continue correction of the hypertonicity intraoperatively and postoperatively for 24 to 48 hours.

Surgery for intestinal obstruction can be as simple as dividing a single adhesive band or involved because of dense adhesions obliterating the entire peritoneal space. Because adhesions are usually multiple, it is important to identify the responsible band by finding the proximal dilated loop and the collapsed distal loop (transition zone). Some surgeons believe that it is important to free the entire peritoneal cavity of adhesions. Others believe that only the adhesions that obstruct the intestine should be divided because the other adhesions have fixed the remaining bowel in a nonobstructed position. In most instances, this appears to be the most prudent approach. Adhesions are best divided sharply, aided by countertraction by the assistant. The decision to resect a segment of bowel is based on an estimate of its viability.

Because of the increasingly difficult problems faced by a patient who has had repeated operations for extensive adhesions (often with multiple bowel resections), many mechanical and chemical approaches have been developed

TABLE 43-3 ■ Ascites				
Ascites	**Causes and Pathogenesis**	**Diagnostic Evaluation**	**Treatment**	**Comment**

Fetal immune and nonimmune ascites	Maternal-fetal Rh incompatibility, now less common
	Nonimmune ascites and hydrops most common
	Most common causes due to
	    Cardiac anomalies
	    Chromosomal disorders
	    Congenital anomalies
	    Thalassemia
	    Twin-twin transfusion
	Cause can be established in 84% of cases
		Ultrasound study
		Coombs' titers, blood typing, blood cell count
		Amniocentesis
		Fetoscopy
		Karyotyping
		Fetal ECG
		Glucose-6-phosphate deficiency screen
		Assessment for infections
		Meconium ascites—calcification
		Urinary ascites—hydronephrosis
		Prenatal paracentesis for analysis
			Prenatal paracentesis
			Some cases of unknown cause disappear spontaneously and have an excellent prognosis
				Meconium ascites may show calcifications
				Many causes of postnatal ascites (urine, bile, and chyle) are present in fetus also
				Often associated with generalized fetal edema (hydrops)
				Overall survival of nonimmune ascites as high as 98%

Urinary ascites	Most common cause of neonatal ascites Posterior urethral valves and ureteropelvic junction obstruction most common underlying pathology Other causes include bladder neck obstruction, urethral atresia, spontaneous bladder rupture, ureterovesical obstruction, bladder hematoma Male-to-female ratio 7:1 Perforation identified in 64% Leak often from kidney May first leak into retroperitoneum and cause peritoneal transudate	Clinical presentation—abdominal distention, oliguria, hyponatremia, and hyperkalemia Analyze ascites for creatinine clearance, serum urea nitrogen value, and a potassium level higher than serum Ultrasound study Contrast studies—IVP and CT scan: halo sign (dye around kidney) Voiding cystourethrogram	May require paracentesis to relieve respiratory distress Excision of urethral valve may be curative In most instances obstruction must be relieved by proximal drainage or by immediate correction of lesion	
Chylous	Congenital malformations 39%, inflammation 15%, neoplasm 3% Associated with malrotation, adhesive bands, incarcerated hernia, lymphangiomas, mesenteric cyst, and trauma Operative injury to the cysterna chyli	Can present acutely, resembling peritonitis, or nonacutely and present with distended abdomen Paracentesis fluid clear if infant not fed; chyle appears if fed Paracentesis—fat globules stained by Sudan III; T lymphocytes, high triglyceride levels Most common in infancy Film of abdomen Sonogram Upper GI series to identify malrotation CT scan	56% respond to NPO and TPN, followed by low-fat diet with MCT No response 4–6 wk exploration; feed cream preoperatively If cause such as cyst—remove; if no cause search for leaks and suture If ascites persists ventriculoperitoneal shunt may be successful	If no definite cause found at operation, suture of suspected leak seldom successful

TABLE 43-3 ■ Ascites—cont'd				
Ascites	**Causes and Pathogenesis**	**Diagnostic Evaluation**	**Treatment**	**Comment**
Biliary	No known cause— suggested pathogenesis is mural defect in common duct; because simple drainage of abdomen usually cures condition, structured abnormality such as obstruction is unlikely Perforation is usually at junction of cystic duct and common bile duct Pseudocyst usually forms rather than generalized ascites	Present between 1–12 wk Usually indolent but may present as peritonitis Usual signs: jaundice, acholic stools, and abdominal distention If infection develops, patient becomes acutely ill Paracentesis—high bilirubin level Ultrasound study; collection at porta hepatis HIDA scan often shows leak	Operative cholangiogram through gallbladder to identify leak and rule out obstruction Local drainage and no attempt to repair leak Cholecystostomy for postoperative evaluation; healing takes 1 mo Antibiotics and TPN or feed with fat-free diet	

ECG, Electrocardiogram; IVP, intravenous pyelography; CT, computed tomography; GI, gastrointestinal; NPO, nothing by mouth; TPN, total parenteral nutrition; HIDA, hepatoiminodiacetic acid.

to prevent repeat obstruction from adhesion formation. Some surgeons have used internal stenting with a long intestinal tube (Baker or Leonard tube). At operation, the tube can be passed into the stomach and the balloon inflated and manipulated down the length of the small bowel. It also may be introduced through a gastrostomy or an enterotomy. These stenting techniques have proved useful in patients who have had multiple operations for recurrent adhesions and may be of value in select pediatric patients.

Several chemical methods have been studied experimentally, and a few have been used clinically to prevent adhesions, including heparin, fibrinolytic compounds, nonsteroidal anti-inflammatory drugs, antihistamines, calcium channel blockers, prokinetic agents, and corticosteroids. The most extensively studied agent is low-molecular-weight dextran. This solution prevents adhesions experimentally and has been used in several series of patients. Some evidence suggests that in the presence of bowel injury or anastomosis dextran may inhibit intestinal healing and possibly lead to intestinal leakage and peritonitis. Presently the most practical method for preventing adhesions is gentle surgical technique.

SUGGESTED READINGS

Akgur FM, et al: Adhesive small bowel obstruction in children: The place and predictors of success for conservative treatment. J Pediatr Surg 26:37, 1991.

A review of factors to consider when deciding to operate on a child with adhesive small bowel obstruction.

Athow AC, Wilkinson ML, Saunders AJS, et al: Pancreatic ascites presenting in infancy, with review of the literature. Dig Dis Sci 36:245-250, 1991.

This is one of the most comprehensive reviews of pancreatic ascites in childhood.

Dirbes K, Crombleholme TM, Craigo SD, et al: The natural history of meconium peritonitis diagnosed in utero. J Pediatr Surg 30:979-982, 1995.

This article describes the various presentations of meconium peritonitis based on its pathophysiology and diagnostic appearance.

Hebra A, Brown MF, McGeehin KM, et al: Mesenteric, mental, and retroperitoneal cysts in children: a clinical study of 22 cases. South Med J 86:173-176, 1993.

This is a review of 22 cases of peritoneal and retroperitoneal cysts, specifically in children; all were lymphangiomas.

Machin GA: Diseases causing fetal and neonatal ascites. Pediatr Pathol 4:195-211, 1985.

The causes of fetal ascites based on the literature and three new cases are reviewed.

Wilins BM, Spitz L: Incidence of postoperative adhesions and obstruction following neonatal laparotomy. Br J Surg 73:762-764, 1986.

In this unique study, 649 neonates who were operated on and followed for the complication of adhesions and obstructions; 8.3% of the group developed obstruction. Gastroschisis and malrotation patients had the highest incidence of obstruction requiring operation.

44

Congenital Diaphragmatic Hernia

Although congenital diaphragmatic hernia (CDH) was described by Bochdalek in 1848, the first successful repair in a neonate was not done until 1946 by Gross. The true extent of the physiologic problems involved and the associated mortality were not evident until more recently.

EMBRYOLOGY

The diaphragm forms between 4 and 8 weeks' gestation and divides the coelomic cavity into the pleural and peritoneal cavities. The central tendon derives from the transverse septum, and the peripheral muscular portion of the diaphragm arises from the posterolateral pleuroperitoneal membranes, which eventually fuse with the transverse septum. Failure of this fusion is the cause of posterolateral diaphragmatic hernia (so-called foramen of Bochdalek hernia). Because the left side of the diaphragm closes after the right side, most diaphragmatic hernias occur on the left. The muscular portion of the diaphragm derives from the pleuroperitoneal folds, the innermost layer of thoracic mesoderm, and the migratory myoblasts

from the cervical, infrahyoidal mesoderm. This may explain why the innervation of the diaphragm is from the phrenic nerve, to which C3, C4, and C5 contribute.

Anomalies of the diaphragm are either from fusion defects, as previously described, or from defects in formation of the diaphragmatic muscle. These muscular defects may be focal or may involve the entire hemidiaphragm. Examples of focal defects are posterolateral diaphragmatic defects in the muscle with a hernia sac present or a foramen of Morgagni hernia. Diffuse muscular defects are represented by diaphragmatic eventration. CDH has been produced experimentally by exposing pregnant rats to herbicides; about 50% of the offspring developed right-sided defects.

ANATOMY

The posterolateral hernia is the most common CDH, with an incidence of 1 in 4000 to 5000 live births (Fig. 44-1). If stillbirths are included, the incidence is 1 in 2000 births. The defects can vary significantly in size from 1 to 2 cm

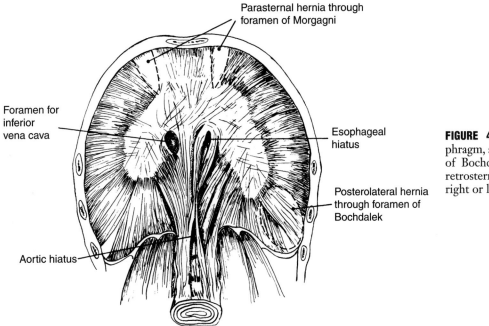

Parasternal hernia through foramen of Morgagni

Foramen for inferior vena cava

Esophageal hiatus

Posterolateral hernia through foramen of Bochdalek

Aortic hiatus

FIGURE 44-1 ■ Anatomy of the diaphragm, showing position of the foramen of Bochdalek. Morgagni hernias occur retrosternally, in the midline or to the right or left of the midline.

to complete absence of the hemidiaphragm. Although prognosis is not always related to the size of the defect, large defects with essentially complete absence of the diaphragm are associated with early symptoms and poor survival. In general, survival is related to the degree of associated pulmonary hypoplasia in the ipsilateral and contralateral lung and the responsiveness of the infant's transitional circulation. A posterolateral rim almost always is found covered by pleura or peritoneum. This finding is important in facilitating the subsequent repair of the defect. A hernia sac is present in 10% to 20% of patients and can be missed easily at surgery. If the hernia sac is not excised, a residual cyst is present on the postoperative radiographs and may compress the lung. Of CDHs, 85% to 90% are on the left side, and most of these contain small bowel, spleen, stomach, and colon; occasionally the left lobe of the liver is found in the defect. Right-sided hernias usually contain the right lobe of the liver and intestine, and they sometimes have a delayed presentation. Nonfixation of the midgut is present in all instances because the intestine has been displaced into the thoracic cavity before its fixation to the posterior abdominal wall. The nonfixation usually is not addressed at operation because of the possible need for extracorporeal membrane oxygenation (ECMO) and anticoagulation, and obstructive duodenal bands are rarely present.

PATHOPHYSIOLOGY

The pathophysiology reflects an interface between pulmonary hypoplasia and pulmonary hypertension. Displacement of the abdominal viscera into the thoracic cavity during gestation prevents normal growth and development of the ipsilateral lung (Fig. 44-2). In addition, the mediastinal shift that occurs during gestation contributes to pulmonary hypoplasia of the contralateral lung, although more recent experimental data question this theory. Histologic evaluation of these fetal lungs shows development only up to the gestational age of 14 to 16 weeks. The numbers of bronchopulmonary generations are permanently reduced in both lungs, resulting in a significant reduction in the number of alveoli. The alveoli themselves have the appearance of fetal alveoli.

Pulmonary hypoplasia is bilateral, but much worse on the ipsilateral side. Pulmonary hypoplasia causes inadequate gas exchange. Compounding pulmonary hypoplasia is the presence of significant pulmonary hypertension because of a hypoplastic pulmonary vascular bed. The pulmonary arteries also have hypertrophied muscle, which contributes further to pulmonary hypertension. Hypertrophy of the media of the pulmonary arterioles results in highly reactive vessels that are sensitive to systemic metabolic change, such as hypoxia, acidosis, hypercarbia, and hypocarbia. Pulmonary hypertension contributes to persistent fetal circulation with shunting of blood from right to left through the patent ductus arteriosus and the patent foramen ovale. Pulmonary hypoplasia is probably the cause of hypercarbia, and pulmonary hypertension probably is the cause of hypoxemia. Because pulmonary vascular tone is extremely sensitive to arterial oxygen tension, hypoxemia creates a vicious cycle that perpetuates pulmonary hypertension and hypoxemia.

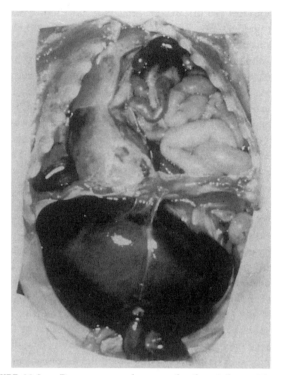

FIGURE 44-2 ■ Postmortem photograph of an infant with congenital diaphragmatic hernia. The infant developed respiratory distress and cyanosis immediately after birth and died before surgery could be performed. Note the hypoplastic left lung. The right lung is also smaller than normal; expansion of intestine in the left side of the chest caused further compression, shifting the mediastinum to the right.

There are several mediators of pulmonary vascular tone; however, the prostaglandins seem to be the most important. Prostaglandin E_1 and E_2 and prostacyclin are pulmonary vasodilators, and thromboxane A_2 and B_2, leukotrienes, and the prostaglandin F series are pulmonary vasoconstrictors. The exact role of these mediators in infants with CDH is not known; however, the prostaglandin E series often is used clinically to reduce pulmonary artery hypertension and to prevent closure of the ductus arteriosus in infants with congenital heart disease. In newborns with CDH, several pharmacologic agents have been used to reduce pulmonary hypertension, such as prostaglandin E, acetylcholine, histamine, bradykinin, nitroprusside, fentanyl sedation, general anesthesia, and tolazoline. Tolazoline has been the most widely used agent; it seems to act directly on vascular smooth muscle. No consistent beneficial effects have been noted with this drug in several series, however. Inhaled nitric oxide has been shown to be a potent pulmonary vasodilator, but it has been disappointing in that few seriously ill infants receive significant benefit. Inotropic agents, such as dopamine and dobutamine, seem to help the pulmonary hypertension by increasing systemic blood pressure, which minimizes right-to-left shunting through the patent ductus arteriosus. Acidosis and hypercarbia increase pulmonary vascular resistance, whereas alkalosis and hypocarbia cause pulmonary vasodilation. Spontaneous low mean airway pressure ventilation and permissive hypercapnia have shown great promise.

CLINICAL FINDINGS

Most CDHs are discovered prenatally on routine maternal ultrasound. If the liver, stomach, or both are in the chest on prenatal ultrasound, the mortality is high. Because most infants with CDH are born with severe respiratory distress and require immediate resuscitation with mechanical ventilation and often ECMO, these mothers should be cared for in a facility that can provide this type of care. At birth, most infants are in severe respiratory distress with severe hypercarbia and hypoxemia. The infrequent infants who are born asymptomatic and remain so for the first 12 to 24 hours of life have an uneventful course after surgery and represent a different group of patients physiologically.

Physical examination reveals a scaphoid abdomen and prominence of the ipsilateral chest. Breath sounds are diminished on the side of the hernia, and heart sounds are deviated into the contralateral chest. The diagnosis can be made with a plain chest film, which shows loops of air-filled intestine within the thoracic cavity and the absence of intestine in the abdominal cavity (Fig. 44-3). If an orogastric tube is in place, the tube is seen coursing down the esophagus and into the stomach, which lies in the chest. A shift of the mediastinum to the contralateral side also is typical of this entity. Occasionally, cystic adenomatoid malformation or intralobar sequestration of the lower lobe may be confused with CDH; however,

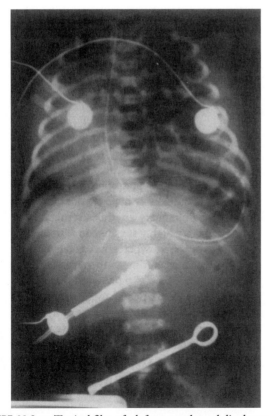

FIGURE 44-3 ▪ Typical film of a left posterolateral diaphragmatic hernia shows several loops of bowel in the left chest with shifting of the mediastinum to the right side and compression of the right lung. There is a paucity of bowel gas in the abdomen.

in both of these malformations the stomach bubble is seen below the diaphragm. If the diagnosis is not certain, an upper gastrointestinal series allows one to differentiate these latter two entities from CDH. Computed tomography also may be used.

Associated anomalies occur in 15% to 25% of infants with CDH, the most common being cardiovascular anomalies. Neonates with persistent pulmonary hypertension almost always have a patent ductus arteriosus. Other associated cardiovascular anomalies include ventricular septal defect, vascular rings, and coarctation of the aorta. Chromosomal abnormalities (trisomy 13), central nervous system malformations (myelomeningocele, anencephaly, and encephalocele), and pulmonary sequestration are other anomalies seen with CDH.

TREATMENT

Preoperative

All newborns with CDH require operative repair; however, the key factor is the timing of the operation. In the past, it was believed that emergency surgery was required to reduce the hernia and allow expansion of the ipsilateral lung. It is now clear that operative reduction of the hernia often has no significant immediate beneficial physiologic effect on pulmonary function. Operative repair may impair pulmonary function by elevating the diaphragm on the contralateral side, reducing contralateral lung compliance. Postoperative results seem to depend on the degree of ipsilateral and contralateral pulmonary hypoplasia and the degree of pulmonary artery hypertension. Intensive preoperative management is crucial in determining the ultimate postoperative result. Preoperative management includes orogastric decompression of the stomach and intestine; mechanical ventilation to reduce the hypercarbia, hypoxemia, and acidosis; and vasodilators to improve pulmonary artery hypertension. If the mechanical ventilation involves high pressures, barotrauma can result fairly quickly. To minimize barotrauma and oxygen toxicity, the evolving standard of respiratory care is a strategy based on spontaneous respiration and permissive hypercarbia.

Treatment decisions are based on preductal oximetry. Inotropic agents, such as dopamine and dobutamine, are helpful in increasing systemic arterial pressure and reducing right-to-left shunting. Monitoring of arterial blood gas levels is essential in evaluating therapy; especially important is measuring preductal and postductal arterial blood gas levels to determine the degree of shunting. Pulse oximetry is also helpful in evaluating oxygenation, and two probes (one on the right arm and one on the lower leg) can detect shunting. One must observe the infant carefully for the development of pneumothorax on the contralateral side. The main goal of preoperative supportive therapy is to stabilize infants so that they can undergo definitive repair of the hernia on an elective basis. If the measures previously mentioned are unsuccessful in adequately resuscitating the infant, additional strategies are required. High-frequency ventilation has been used to reduce barotrauma; high pressures are avoided, and carbon dioxide elimination is effective. The latter technique does not seem to be as effective, however, as spontaneous respiration with permissive hypercapnia or ECMO.

If ventilation is unsuccessful in stabilizing the infant preoperatively, ECMO should be instituted. Although uniform criteria for initiation of ECMO have not been well established, most centers place infants with CDH on ECMO if, after maximum therapy, the preductal oxygen pressure (Po_2) is less than 50 mm Hg and the carbon dioxide pressure (Pco_2) is greater than 50 mm Hg on a fractional inspired oxygen concentration (Fio_2) of 100%. ECMO can be carried out only in major neonatal centers because of its complexity and expense. The purpose of ECMO and permissive hypercapnia in these patients is to provide respiratory support until persistent pulmonary hypertension is resolved, and the sensitivity of the pulmonary vasculature to vasoconstrictor stimuli is reduced. ECMO and permissive hypercapnia ventilation provide this type of respiratory support without creating barotrauma or oxygen toxicity, which is associated with conventional mechanical ventilation. In the 1990s, ECMO was used principally in patients who had undergone repair of CDH and subsequently developed severe respiratory distress during the first 12 to 24 postoperative hours. Using this approach, infants who have undergone CDH repair and have been placed on ECMO postoperatively have been able to achieve an 80% overall survival rate. Now most institutions place neonates with CDH on ECMO preoperatively because of severe respiratory distress that cannot be corrected by any other means. Initially, hernia repair was done while the patient was on ECMO, but currently most institutions do the repair after ECMO is no longer needed. The best results have been obtained with post-ECMO repair, when the infant is more stable, and bleeding complications are avoided.

SURGICAL TECHNIQUE

The CDH is repaired transabdominally through a subcostal incision in most major centers; however, a few institutions recommend transthoracic repair of this anomaly. The disadvantage of the transthoracic approach is the inability of the surgeon to create a ventral hernia, if necessary, to relieve intra-abdominal pressure. Also the ipsilateral lung is exposed to physical injury with this approach.

The first step after opening the abdomen is to reduce all the abdominal viscera into the peritoneal cavity (Fig. 44-4). After this, the posterior diaphragmatic rim,

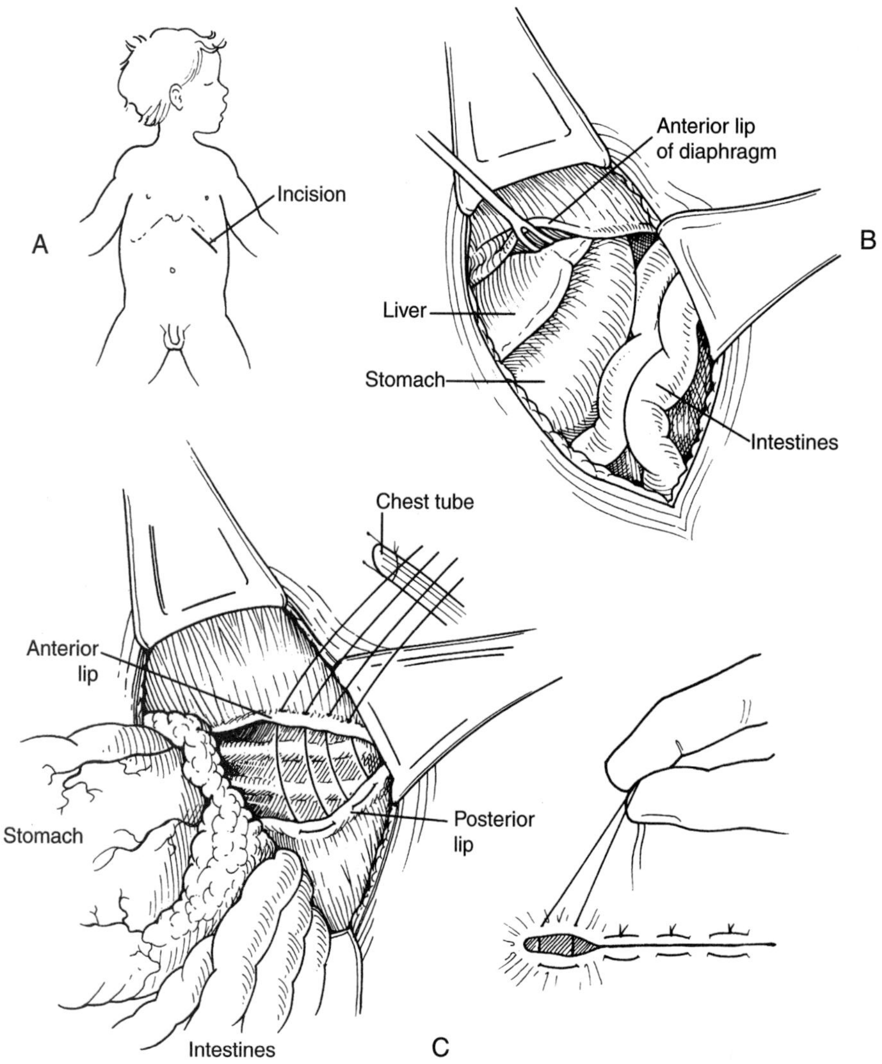

FIGURE 44-4 ■ Technique for congenital diaphragmatic hernia repair. **A,** The diaphragm is approached through a left subcostal incision. Stomach, liver, and multiple loops of intestine enter the chest through the posterolateral defect. Viscera are reduced by gentle traction. It may be necessary to lift the muscular margin of the defect to allow air into the chest to overcome the negative pressure in the thorax. **B,** The posterolateral defect usually is outlined by a definite anterior layer of muscular diaphragm. Posteriorly a rim of diaphragm is seen behind the continuous layers of posterior parietal pleura and peritoneum. This layer is incised, and the rim of diaphragm is unrolled. The left lung is too small to be seen through the defect. **C,** Mattress sutures of 2-0 nonabsorbable material are placed to approximate the two muscle edges and close the defect. An intercostal tube is placed before tying the sutures.

which is covered by peritoneum or pleura, is dissected so that the repair can be done more easily. Standard defects are closed by approximating the upper and lower lips of the defect with interrupted sutures. If the defect is too large to close primarily, transversus abdominis muscle flaps can be used to bridge the gap. If a muscle flap is inadequate to close the defect, a synthetic patch (i.e., Gore-Tex) must be inserted. These patches are associated with complications, such as disruption with recurrence of the hernia and leakage of peritoneal fluid and blood through the suture line, producing a persistent hydrothorax on the affected side. More recently, other synthetic materials have been used because of the high rate of recurrent hernias with Gore-Tex patches. A chest tube is left in the ipsilateral thoracic cavity only if there is an active air leak or bleeding. If, after stretching, the abdomen is too tight for primary closure, skin flap closure may be performed. For infants with a small abdominal cavity, a Silastic/Dacron mesh pouch may be placed temporarily. Stretching the abdominal wall or creation of muscle or skin flaps should be avoided if ECMO is needed because of the potential need for anticoagulation.

The timing of the operation is still debated, but currently most surgeons recommend waiting until the pulmonary hypertension has resolved as evidenced by resolution of preductal and postductal shunting and weaning to minimal supportive care. In the postoperative period, it is essential that the oxygen concentration be weaned slowly because small decreases in the FIO_2 may result in significant pulmonary vasoconstriction and a redevelopment of persistent fetal circulation and pulmonary hypertension.

Although appealing, in utero repair of fetal CDH has been disappointing and currently is not offered as a treatment option. Significant problems remain with patient selection, appropriate surgical techniques, and postoperative maternal management. A direct extension of the fetal repair was the observation that fetal tracheal ligation accelerated fetal lung growth and reversed the alveolar hypoplasia and abnormal pulmonary vascular pattern in a fetal lamb model of CDH. Tracheal occlusion of the fetus resulted in improved oxygenation and ventilation after birth compared with untreated control animals. Limited clinical trials of fetal tracheal occlusion are under way. As survival for isolated CDH improves, the rationale for fetal intervention is questioned. Liquid ventilation techniques have advanced to the point of clinical applicability. Hirschl and associates reported the use of partial liquid ventilation in a few infants with CDH while on ECMO, with good results, but its application is as yet unproved.

Another experimental approach is the use of lung transplantation in infants with CDH who have undergone repair and are on ECMO but are unable to be weaned because of severe bilateral pulmonary hypoplasia. Transplantation has been done in only two infants with one long-term success. The concept is to transplant a downsized lobe of an adult donor into the ipsilateral thoracic cavity of the infant. The lung transplant can be allowed to heal while the patient remains on ECMO. The infant then would be able to be weaned from ECMO and have reasonable pulmonary function from the transplanted lobe. The transplanted lobe could function as a temporary assist until the contralateral lung matures or could have long-term function in the infant.

RESULTS

The overall survival for infants with CDH who are symptomatic within the first few hours of life has remained around 50% for 20 years. In a few centers, this figure has improved to 80% or more with the use of ECMO, lung-sparing respiratory care strategies, and preoperative stabilization. Children who survive the neonatal period usually have normal growth and development. Extensive pulmonary function studies on children who have survived repair of CDH are not available; the few studies available suggest normal pulmonary function in many of these children. More recent survivors of CDH repair performed with ECMO support seem to have significant long-term pulmonary dysfunction, however, which in many cases may largely be iatrogenic.

FORAMEN OF MORGAGNI HERNIA

The foramen of Morgagni hernia (Fig. 44-5) is a defect in the anterior diaphragmatic muscle where it attaches to the sternum. This defect can be in the midline or on either side. This rare defect accounts for less than 2% of all CDHs. It usually presents after several weeks or months and occasionally in older children; the symptoms are usually intestinal obstruction instead of respiratory distress.

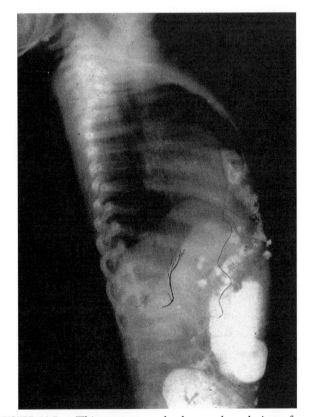

FIGURE 44-5 ■ This contrast study shows a lateral view of an infant with a foramen of Morgagni hernia, which was repaired laparoscopically.

The hernia occasionally is discovered incidentally on a chest film obtained for other reasons. Typically a hernia sac is present and contains either liver or transverse colon; occasionally, stomach and small intestine are seen in the sac. Incarceration of intestine is extremely unusual.

Operative repair is performed easily through an upper abdominal incision by either open or laparoscopic technique. The herniated viscera are reduced, and the diaphragm is sutured to the undersurface of the sternum and the posterior rectus sheath.

EVENTRATION OF THE DIAPHRAGM

Eventration of the diaphragm may be congenital or may be secondary to damage to the phrenic nerve. The abnormality consists of abnormal elevation of the entire diaphragm or a portion of the diaphragm. Congenital eventration usually is caused by a defect in the muscularization of the diaphragm, with most of the diaphragm being principally membranous. In acquired eventration, the diaphragmatic muscle is normal; it merely lacks innervation, often associated with Erb's palsy or after cardiac surgery. Most congenital eventrations are on the left side. The diagnosis is made easily by fluoroscopy or ultrasound. Ultrasound is more accurate in distinguishing a congenital diaphragmatic eventration from a CDH. Also, infants with eventration do not show the extreme

physiologic problems seen in CDH patients. Fluoroscopy usually shows an intact hemidiaphragm that is elevated and has a paradoxical motion on respiration. If the diagnosis cannot be made by fluoroscopy or ultrasound, an upper gastrointestinal series helps make the diagnosis. Many infants with congenital eventration are asymptomatic, whereas most children with acquired eventration develop significant symptoms from the abnormality. Asymptomatic patients should be observed only (Fig. 44-6). Patients with significant respiratory symptoms from the eventration, mainly respiratory distress with poor gas exchange, require operation. If the elevation of the diaphragm in a young infant is so high as to compress severely the ipsilateral lung, repair should be considered even though the patient may be largely asymptomatic.

Most eventrations are repaired best transthoracically, although some surgeons use the transabdominal approach. The diaphragm can be plicated alone, which avoids injury to the phrenic nerve, or occasionally the excess diaphragmatic tissue can be excised and the diaphragm reapproximated with interrupted sutures.

PARAESOPHAGEAL HIATUS HERNIA

Primary paraesophageal hiatus hernia is a rare condition in children; they may or may not be asymptomatic. Vomiting is a common chronic symptom of this condition;

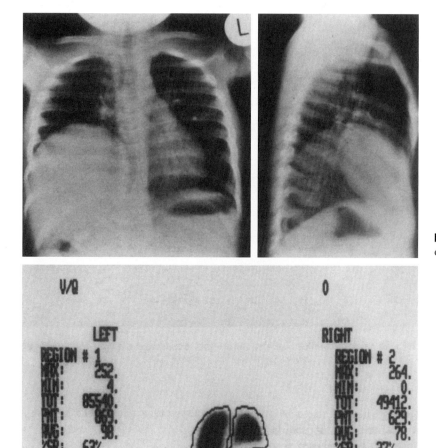

FIGURE 44-6 ■ Eventration of the right diaphragm in an infant.

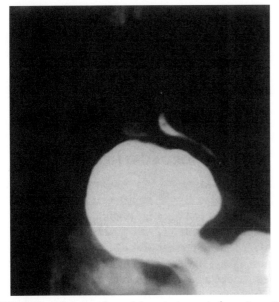

FIGURE 44-7 ■ Paraesophageal hernia in an infant. Associated gastroesophageal reflux was shown on barium swallow and upper gastrointestinal series.

however, this abnormality may present in infants and children as an acute emergency with incarceration and strangulation of the stomach. If not treated immediately, this condition can result in death. The diagnosis is made easily by upper gastrointestinal series; the repair can be performed transabdominally by reducing the incarcerated stomach and closing the diaphragmatic defect (Fig. 44-7). In most cases, because of the significant incidence of gastroesophageal reflux, fundoplication also is done. Paraesophageal hernia after gastroesophageal fundoplication is one of the most common complications, occurring most frequently in patients with neurologic impairment or chronic lung disease. Dysphagia and recurrent reflux are the most frequent symptoms. Secondary repair with reconstruction of the slipped fundoplication is necessary for most patients.

SUGGESTED READINGS

Adzick NS, Harrison MR, Glick PH, et al: Diaphragmatic hernia in the fetus: Prenatal diagnosis and outcome in 94 cases. J Pediatr Surg 20:357, 1985.

This important study shows the high mortality of infants with CDH diagnosed in utero.

Boloker J, Borteman D, Wung JT, Stolar CJA: Congenital diaphragmatic hernia in 120 infants treated consecutively with permissive hypercapnia, spontaneous respiration and elective repair. J Pediatr Surg 37:357, 2002.

This article describes a pioneering study of a series of neonates with CDH. They were treated primarily with slow, gentle ventilation rather than with ECMO for pulmonary support.

Clark RH, Hardin WD, Hirschl RB, et al: Current surgical management of congenital diaphragmatic hernia: A report from the Congenital Diaphragmatic Hernia Study group. J Pediatr Surg 33:1004, 1998.

A comprehensive review is presented of the current management of CDH based on the combined experience from 62 neonatal centers.

Glick PL, Leach CL, Besner GE, et al: Pathophysiology of congenital diaphragmatic hernia: III. Exogenous surfactant therapy for the high-risk neonate with CDH. J Pediatr Surg 27:866, 1992.

Infants with CDH may be surfactant deficient and may benefit from exogenous surfactant therapy.

Hedrick MH, Estes JM, Sullivan KM, et al: Plug the lung until it grows (PLUG): A new method to treat congenital diaphragmatic hernia in utero. J Pediatr Surg 29:5, 1994.

Fetal lung plugging is an experimental method that seems to be more effective than intrauterine repair.

VanderWall KH, Skarsgard ED, Filly RA, et al: Fetendo-Clip: A fetal endoscopic tracheal clip procedure in a human fetus. J Pediatr Surg 32:970, 1997.

This is one of the earliest reports introducing fetal endoscopic tracheal occlusion for management of CDH.

PART VII

Stomach, Duodenum, and Small Intestine

Hypertrophic Pyloric Stenosis

45

Hypertrophic pyloric stenosis is the most common surgical disorder producing emesis in infancy, with an incidence of approximately 1 in every 400 live births in the United States. This incidence varies with ethnic origin, and the disorder is most common in white infants and less frequent in African-American and Asian infants. Male infants are four times more likely to have pyloric stenosis than females; firstborn males are more likely to be affected than their siblings. Approximately 5% of the sons and 2% of the daughters of fathers who have had pyloric stenosis develop the disorder; the frequency increases threefold if the infant's mother had the disorder.

PATHOPHYSIOLOGY

The cause of infantile hypertrophic pyloric stenosis has not been defined clearly. Many investigators have evaluated the morphologic changes in the intrinsic nerves and ganglion cells, including the degree of maturity, distribution, and degeneration of these cells, with no unanimous agreement. No clear relationship has been identified with respect to onset of allergies, variations of infant feedings, or other specific clinical disorders. Increased production of gastrin in either mother or infant does not seem to be a causative factor. An association with blood groups O and B and with maternal stress in the last trimester of pregnancy has been suggested. The etiology is considered multifactorial, with a proven genetic X-linked factor and an uncertain environmental one.

Although the designation as congenital is questioned by some, the presence of a partial obstruction at the pylorus in some ways is analogous to congenital duodenal webs, which may not produce symptoms for several days or a few weeks after birth. It is doubtful that pyloric stenosis would produce such severe symptoms predictably within the first 3 to 5 weeks unless a major component of the disorder were congenital.

The pathogenesis of pyloric stenosis is believed by some to be postnatal work hypertrophy, possibly following a congenital delay in the opening of the pyloric sphincter. Others have suggested a congenital redundancy of the pyloric mucosa. Another theory suggests that milk curds passing through the narrow channel cause additional edema and swelling with eventual complete occlusion, which subsides if nothing is taken by mouth for a few days or if only clear fluids are given. This theory is consistent with the course of the lesion because it disappears after the obstruction is relieved. Vasoactive intestinal peptide decreases the intensity and duration of pyloric contraction in a dose-dependent manner, suggesting vasoactive intestinal peptide could play a role in etiology. Studies implicate unbalanced function of the peptidergic nervous system, but the precise relationship is not yet proven.

The musculature of the pylorus in patients with pyloric stenosis is markedly thickened and edematous. There is hypertrophy of the circular muscle fibers but no increase in their number. The spindle-shaped swelling of the hypertrophied muscles of the pylorus usually measures approximately 2.0 to 2.5 cm long and protrudes into the duodenum, analogous to the cervix into the vagina. The pyloric muscle is usually firm and discrete and likened to a tumor, although it becomes softer in older infants. The proximal portion is less abrupt and fuses with the normal antral musculature. The gastric muscle is usually thickened, and the mucosa is frequently edematous and congested, occasionally leading to bleeding. After pyloromyotomy, the pyloric muscle gradually becomes completely normal, and when visualized at subsequent operations, only a fine scar in the area of the myotomy can be identified. Approximately 7% of infants with pyloric stenosis have associated anomalies, with esophageal hiatal and inguinal hernias being the most frequent.

SYMPTOMS

Classically, projectile nonbilious emesis, the presence of a palpable pyloric tumor, and visible gastric waves on the abdomen in a 3- to 5-week-old infant are the clinical features of hypertrophic pyloric stenosis. Most infants experience emesis of small amounts by 2 weeks of life, then develop nearly complete obstruction with vomiting of almost all feeds by 2 to 4 weeks. The range of presentations is 1 to 12 weeks of age. Shortly after emesis, infants usually crave further feedings. Although withholding feedings for a short period may provide slight resolution of mucosal edema, allowing the infant to retain clear liquid feedings, this apparent improvement is almost invariably short-lived, and emesis recurs when small milk feedings are resumed. The emesis is characteristically projectile or forceful because of the high pressure generated by the hypertrophied gastric muscles. Infants who are allowed to continue with symptoms for more than a few days often lose weight and may become dehydrated with metabolic alkalosis or even malnourished. Repeated emesis that is allowed to persist for several days may produce gastritis with mild bleeding.

DIAGNOSIS

Observation of the abdomen after a feeding in infants with well-established pyloric stenosis often reveals contractions of the stomach that proceed from left to right across the epigastrium. These gastric waves eventually terminate in an episode of emesis. Similar but less prominent waves can be seen in other conditions, such as severe pylorospasm or gastric duplication. Careful palpation of the epigastrium slightly to the right of the midline often discloses a firm, olive-sized mass that can be manipulated slightly upward or downward. The hypertrophied pyloric muscle is identified most easily when the stomach is empty, either after emesis or after tube decompression of the stomach. Elevating and gently moving the lower extremities while allowing the infant to suck on a pacifier or a bottle of sugar water during the examination may relax the abdominal musculature, permitting a more accurate examination. Repeated examinations over a few hours occasionally may be necessary in an active, crying infant, but sedation is rarely necessary. The pyloric mass is pathognomonic, and depending on the experience and patience of the examiner, it can be identified in 70% to 90% of infants with hypertrophic pyloric stenosis.

Hypertrophic pyloric stenosis may be simulated by many other causes of vomiting in infants. Overfeeding is the most common and is a frequent practice in many families. There is a frequent history of formula changes because of a suspected milk allergy or intolerance to the current formula. Improved feeding technique, frequent burping, and time are all that is needed for most of these disorders to resolve. Pylorospasm, gastroesophageal reflux, delayed gastric emptying of undetermined etiology without mechanical obstruction, and several anomalies including malrotation with duodenal bands, duodenal or antral webs, and pyloric duplications rarely may simulate pyloric stenosis. Emesis also may be associated with metabolic disorders, inborn errors of metabolism, central nervous system lesions, and sepsis. A good clinical rule of thumb that aids in the differential diagnosis is that a child with pyloric stenosis will continue to be hungry and active unless severely dehydrated. Infants with metabolic disorders or increased intracranial pressure are likely to be lethargic and feed poorly, and the vomitus is often bilious.

Abdominal ultrasonography is performed on infants in whom a tumor cannot be palpated. This study is highly reliable and is currently the preferred approach when the pyloric mass cannot be felt. The most commonly used criteria are a pyloric muscle thickness of 4 mm or more and a pyloric channel length of 16 mm or more (Fig. 45-1). The barium upper gastrointestinal (UGI) series is used for the occasional infant in whom physical examination and ultrasound are not diagnostic. The UGI series often

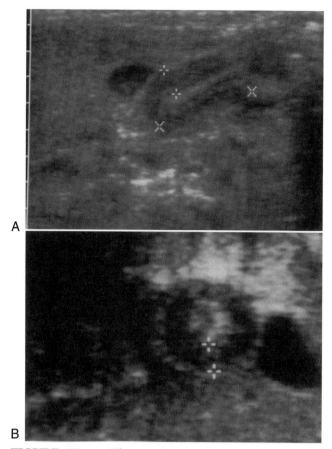

FIGURE 45-1 ■ Ultrasound images of the hypertrophied pylorus in a 5-week-old infant. **A,** A longitudinal view is shown with the pyloric length (X-X) measuring 18 mm and the pyloric muscle thickness (+-+) measuring 5.2 mm. **B,** A transverse view illustrating muscle thickness (+-+). (**A** courtesy of Dorothy Bulas, MD.)

shows a distended stomach with an elongated and narrowed pyloric canal—the "string sign" (Fig. 45-2). Gastroesophageal reflux noted on UGI series usually resolves within 1 month after pyloromyotomy. If a barium UGI series is performed, any excess barium should be lavaged from the infant's stomach before the induction of anesthesia to minimize the risk of aspiration.

Occasionally the diagnosis may be made as early as the fourth or fifth day of life and, in rare instances, as late as 4 months. In our experience, the average onset of symptoms occurs at 3 weeks. Vomiting is the initial sign, and the emesis is always free of bile. Initially the infant may vomit once or twice a day; however, as the obstruction progresses, the emesis becomes more constant and forceful or projectile, extending several inches from the face. The infants characteristically have a ravenous appetite shortly after an episode of emesis. Occasionally the emesis in infants with more protracted vomiting may become brownish or blood-streaked as a result of bleeding from ruptured capillaries in the gastric mucosa induced by the frequent vomiting.

Vomiting with an open pylorus generally results in a loss of an isotonic mixture of duodenal, biliary, and pancreatic secretions. In contrast, vomiting caused by pyloric stenosis

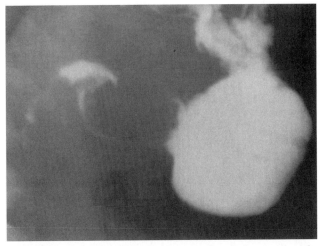

FIGURE 45-2 ■ Upper gastrointestinal study from a 6-week-old boy shows narrowing of the pyloric channel and the characteristic string sign. Note distention of the stomach and minimal contrast distal to the pylorus.

results in the loss of chloride-rich fluid (130 to 150 mEq/L), with lower concentrations of sodium (60 to 100 mEq/L) and potassium (10 to 20 mEq/L). The excess chloride loss depletes extracellular chloride and, along with the loss of luminal hydrogen ions, produces a metabolic alkalosis.

The initial response of the kidney is to maintain blood pH by excreting an alkaline urine. This increase in urinary bicarbonate coupled with potassium and sodium ions results in a net hydrogen resorption by the renal tubular cells. With continued vomiting, the volume deficit progresses, however, and the response of the kidney is to expand the extracellular volume rather than maintain blood pH. There is increased sodium resorption and a marked loss of potassium via an aldosterone-mediated mechanism. The resulting hypokalemia leads to excretion of hydrogen ion, producing a "paradoxic aciduria." The major loss of potassium is from the kidney, and serum hypokalemia occurs only when cellular potassium is severely depleted. Acid urine and hypokalemia are late signs in infants with pyloric stenosis.

Jaundice occurs in approximately 2% of infants with pyloric stenosis. Although the cause is not defined clearly, it is presumed to be related to the combination of acute starvation and an immature liver. Histochemical studies of liver biopsy specimens and the preponderance of indirect serum bilirubinemia in these infants indicate defective hepatic glucuronyl transferase activity. The condition is comparable to Gilbert syndrome. No specific treatment is necessary because the jaundice resolves spontaneously within 5 to 7 days after pyloromyotomy.

NONOPERATIVE TREATMENT

Rare infants with mild vomiting and proven hypertrophic pyloric stenosis have been reported to improve over time (3 to 6 months) with the administration of antispasmodics, such as atropine or scopolamine, and intravenous nutrition. Because this approach, originally reported from Sweden, usually fails, however, it is of historical interest only.

OPERATIVE TREATMENT

Preoperative care is aimed at restoring fluid and electrolyte losses. Because the diagnosis of pyloric stenosis usually is made earlier than in previous years, few infants are seen in an advanced state of severe dehydration, malnutrition, and alkalosis. Most infants with pyloric stenosis can be operated on within 12 hours after admission to the hospital. Although a clear liquid feed may be tolerated preoperatively, most pediatric anesthesiologists prefer that these infants not be fed for 8 to 12 hours preoperatively because of delayed gastric emptying. In some cases, it is necessary to lavage the stomach with normal saline solution to remove obstructing milk curds or barium.

For most infants, intravenous fluids are initiated as the infant is being admitted to the hospital for treatment. A solution containing 5% dextrose in 0.45% saline is administered intravenously at a rate of approximately 150 to 175 mL/kg/24 hours, depending on the amount of hydration necessary. After the infant has voided, 10 to 15 mEq of potassium chloride is added to each 500-mL intravenous bottle. The total amount of potassium chloride in the fluids administered should not exceed 40 mEq/L in 24 hours. Dehydration with more severe electrolyte deficits requires the administration of normal saline solution at a rate of 175 to 185 mL/kg/24 hours until the infant voids. Dehydrated patients occasionally require resuscitation for 24 to 36 hours. When the stomach has been emptied, most infants with pyloric stenosis stop vomiting.

The Ramstedt-Fredet pyloromyotomy, performed with the infant under general anesthesia, is universally accepted as the preferred operation. The stomach should be emptied again just before induction of anesthesia to minimize the risk of aspiration. The procedure can be performed through a variety of approaches, although the one used most frequently is a transverse skin incision followed by a vertical splitting of the right rectus muscle and fascia. The right upper abdominal transverse muscle-splitting gridiron incision (Robertson) is used by many. Because it provides a better cosmetic appearance, a supraumbilical, curvilinear incision has been used by some surgeons; however, there is a higher incidence of wound-related complications. After entering the abdomen, the omentum can be readily retrieved into the wound, which when elevated lifts the transverse colon and leads directly to the gastric antrum. The lower stomach may be elevated with gentle traction using moistened gauze to minimize slipping as the pyloric mass is delivered into the wound. A vertical incision is made on the mid anterior surface through the serosa and superficial muscularis extending from approximately 2 mm proximal to the pyloric vein (an avascular area) to a point 0.5 cm onto the lower antrum (Fig. 45-3). Although most surgeons use a straight, longitudinal incision, a superficial V-shaped extension at the duodenal end of the myotomy incision has been helpful in reducing the risk of duodenal mucosal injury. The circular muscle is opened bluntly using the Benson pyloromyotomy spreader or the back of the knife handle. Gentle upward traction on the exposed lower gastric submucosa with a gauze pledget lowers the risk of duodenal mucosal injury as the muscle separation is continued caudally. With completion of the myotomy, the

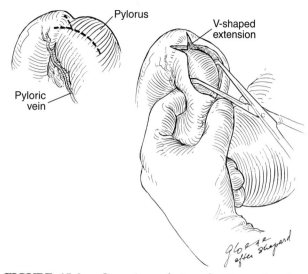

FIGURE 45-3 ■ Operative technique for Ramstedt pyloromyotomy with V-shaped extension of the incision down to the duodenum. The incision is approximately 3 cm long for most infants. Note the Benson spreader used to separate the muscularis.

gastric submucosa protrudes outward, indicating relief of the obstruction. Rarely the duodenal mucosa may be entered, as noted by the appearance of bilious fluid. The disruption is best repaired with interrupted fine monofilament nonabsorbable sutures placed in a transverse direction and covered with omentum. Closure of a mucosal perforation rarely compromises the pyloromyotomy. If this occurs, the pylorus can be rotated 45 to 90 degrees and a fresh pyloromyotomy performed, but this is rarely required. It is helpful to have the anesthesiologist instill air into the stomach at the completion of the pyloromyotomy to check the integrity of the duodenal mucosa. Before the pylorus is returned to the abdomen, any major bleeding sites should be controlled with electrocautery.

Laparoscopic pyloromyotomy has been performed successfully by several authors and has the advantage of using slightly smaller incisions than the open procedure. The endoscopic pyloromyotomy often has a longer operating time, is more expensive, thus far has been associated with more duodenal perforations, and does not result in more rapid recovery or hospital discharge. As more experience is gained with this technique, the results are likely to improve.

After the operation, the gastric tube is removed as soon as the infant awakens from the anesthetic. For infants in whom the duodenal mucosa has been perforated, the gastric tube may be left for an additional 24 hours to ensure gastric decompression. Parenteral fluids are administered to maintain adequate hydration and urine output until oral intake is sufficient. Oral feedings usually are initiated 4 hours after surgery, provided that the infant is alert and has a good sucking reflex. A variety of postoperative feeding regimens have been used, depending on the weight of the infant. An effective regimen begins 4 hours postoperatively with 15 mL of Pedialyte solution every 2 hours for two feeds, then 30 mL of Pedialyte or full-strength formula every 2 hours × 2, then 30 mL full-strength formula every 2 hours × 2, then 60 mL every 3 hours × 2, then 75 mL

every 3 hours × 2, and then 90 mL every 4 hours. If the mother's breast milk is available, it may be substituted for formula (from breast pump), and breast-feeding may be started after 24 hours. Regardless of the feeding schedule, small episodes of regurgitation occur in less than 20% of patients, and most infants may be discharged from the hospital within 36 to 48 hours after surgery. The long-term results after pyloromyotomy have been excellent with no increased frequency of gastrointestinal symptoms compared with the general population.

COMPLICATIONS

Gastritis and gastroesophageal reflux are the most common causes of persistent postoperative vomiting. Incomplete pyloromyotomy as a cause of persistent vomiting is rare but should be considered if vomiting continues for more than 7 to 10 days postoperatively, if it is forceful, and if it follows every feeding. It is usually due to an incomplete separation of the muscles on the antral side of the pylorus. Contrast radiography in this instance may diagnose gastroesophageal reflux or show whether the stomach readily empties, but it is of little help in diagnosing an incomplete myotomy because the radiographic appearance of pyloric stenosis has been relieved. If a second myotomy is deemed necessary, which is rare, the procedure consists of a fresh pyloromyotomy in an area that is well away from the original incision. This is done by turning the pylorus 45 to 90 degrees to either side and performing the standard pyloric incision.

The rare unrecognized duodenal perforation is identified by the postoperative presence of emesis, distention, fever, and peritonitis. In this instance, prompt reoperation is mandatory, consisting of simple duodenal repair and placement of a tongue of omentum over the closure. Wound infections with *Staphylococcus* occasionally occur and may be related to the proximity of the umbilical stump. Postoperative incisional dehiscence and delayed incisional hernias are uncommon. The mortality associated with pyloromyotomy is less than 0.4% in the experience of almost all major children's centers. The rare deaths encountered in most instances have occurred in patients with multiple congenital anomalies.

SUGGESTED READINGS

Lynn H: The mechanism of pyloric stenosis and its relationship to preoperative preparation. Arch Surg 81:453, 1960.

This is a classic review of the clinical manifestations of congenital pyloric stenosis and its surgical management.

Najmaldin A, Tan HL: Early experience with laparoscopic pyloromyotomy for infantile hypertrophic pyloric stenosis. J Pediatr Surg 30:37, 1995.

This article covers a technical approach for relief of pyloric stenosis. Whether it will replace open pyloromyotomy will be determined from outcome studies.

Schwartz MZ: Hypertrophic pyloric stenosis. In O'Neill JA, Rowe MI, Grosfeld JG, et al (eds): Pediatric Surgery, 5th ed. St Louis, Mosby–Year Book, 1998, p 1111.

This thorough review includes etiology, occurrence in premature infants, and various aspects of diagnosis and treatment.

Duodenal Obstruction

Duodenal atresia and stenosis are the most common causes of intrinsic duodenal obstruction in the newborn. The first description of duodenal atresia is credited to Calder, who described two cases of duodenal atresia in newborns in 1733. Scattered reports concerning this defect appeared in the European literature over the next two centuries. The first survivor was not recorded until 1914 by Ernst in Denmark. More than 250 cases of duodenal atresia were reported by 1931, with only 9 survivors documented at that time. During the past 60 years, gradual improvement in the survival of infants with this condition has been achieved.

ETIOLOGY

The etiology of duodenal atresia and stenosis is probably related to a failure of recanalization of the duodenal lumen from its solid cord stage. The duodenum is derived from the distal portion of the foregut and develops at the same time as the extrahepatic ductal system and pancreas. Vacuolization of the solid cord stage begins at 8 to 10 weeks' gestation, resulting in a lumen. Failure of recanalization leads to a variety of intrinsic anomalies, including atresia, stenosis, and formation of a mucosal web. During duodenal development, the pancreas also is developing from dorsal and ventral buds coming from the liver. Duodenal atresia and stenosis frequently are associated with an annular pancreas. The dorsal portion of the fetal pancreas comes from the dorsal wall of the duodenum, whereas the ventral portion arises from an area between the duodenum and hepatic bud. As the process of bowel rotation occurs, the ventral pancreas extends around the right side of the duodenum to merge with the dorsal bud, fusing the ventral duct with the dorsal pancreas to form Wirsung's duct.

Anomalous development of the paired, ladder-shaped embryonic vitelline veins contributes to the myriad of complex anatomic defects in this region. An anterior portal vein (preduodenal portal vein) is related to persistence of a primitive vitelline vein that, rather than passing inferior and behind the pancreas on its cephalad path to the liver, crosses over the top of the duodenum and pancreas. Annular pancreas and preduodenal portal vein may contribute to extrinsic compression of the second part of the duodenum.

Although annular pancreas often is associated with duodenal atresia or stenosis, some cases are not detected until laparotomy is performed when the patient is an adult. Anomalies of bowel rotation and fixation also frequently are noted in association with duodenal anomalies. Various biliary and pancreatic anomalies have been observed in patients with duodenal atresia and stenosis. These include biliary atresia, choledochal cyst, pancreatic lipomatosis, dual pancreatic duct, and bile duct insertion with communication between the proximal and distal atretic segments as a result of persistence of the primitive dual duct stage of development of the bile duct.

CLASSIFICATION

The most useful classification of duodenal atresia divides these anomalies into three major types (Fig. 46-1). A type 1 defect is most common and represents a mucosal diaphragmatic membrane (atresia) with an intact muscle wall. The duodenum proximal to the atresia is dilated, and the distal portion is narrowed. Occasionally a membrane in the shape of a "windsock" web may be noted. The site of the origin of the windsock may be a few centimeters proximal to the obstruction. The web almost always is intimately involved with the entry of the bile ducts at the papilla of Vater. Type 2 duodenal defects have a short fibrous cord connecting the two ends of the atretic duodenum. The rare type 3 defect is one in which there is complete separation of the two ends of the atretic duodenum. Most of the unusual biliary duct anomalies that coexist are seen in infants with a type III defect.

CLINICAL PRESENTATION AND DIAGNOSIS

The diagnosis of neonatal duodenal obstruction may be suspected before birth. The presence of a high intestinal obstruction in the fetus always should be considered in any pregnant woman with polyhydramnios. Although polyhydramnios may be idiopathic, from maternal causes and other fetal conditions and not pathognomonic, its presence raises a high index of suspicion. Prenatal ultrasonography should be performed in all pregnancies associated with amniotic fluid abnormalities, including polyhydramnios. Of infants born with duodenal obstruction,

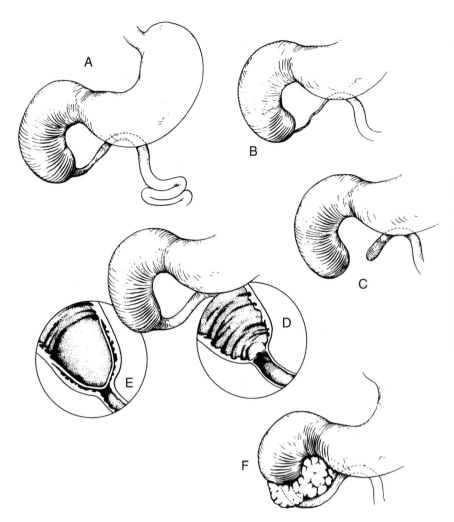

FIGURE 46-1 ■ Classification of anomalies causing duodenal obstruction. **A,** Type 1 atresia with intact membrane producing marked discrepancy in size between proximal and distal segments. **B,** Blind ends (type 2) of duodenum connected by a fibrous cord. **C,** Blind ends (type 3) are separated, and the mesentery is absent at the separation. **D,** Intraluminal membrane with a perforation. **E,** Windsock anomaly. An incision in the distal portion of the dilated segment is still beyond the obstruction. **F,** Annular pancreas.

30% to 59% have a history of maternal polyhydramnios. Prenatal ultrasound documents polyhydramnios and may show the presence of duodenal obstruction with a dilated fluid-filled stomach and duodenum (Fig. 46-2) by the seventh or eighth month of intrauterine life. A normal ultrasound examination in the presence of polyhydramnios does not rule out the diagnosis of duodenal obstruction. Similarly, an initial ultrasound that shows duodenal obstruction and subsequently is followed by a normal scan simply may be an indicator of fetal vomiting changing the appearance of the study. Duodenal stenosis is not usually detectable by prenatal ultrasound.

If prenatal ultrasound was not performed and the infant is born with an unsuspected defect, the clinical presentation of duodenal atresia usually is characterized by the onset of vomiting within a few hours of birth and intolerance of attempted feedings. Because 85% of cases of duodenal obstruction are distal to the entry of the bile duct into the duodenum, vomiting is most often bilious. Because of the high level of obstruction, abdominal distention is not observed. Occasionally the epigastrium appears full as a result of gastric dilation. Meconium may be passed.

In contrast to atresia, the diagnosis of duodenal stenosis may be delayed because these infants are able to tolerate some feedings as a result of the incomplete nature of the obstruction. The presence of bilious vomiting is always a

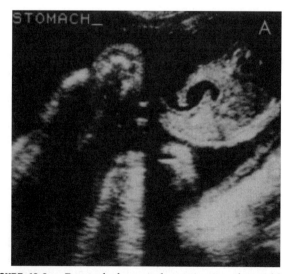

FIGURE 46-2 ■ Prenatal ultrasound examination shows dilated stomach and duodenum filled with fluid consistent with duodenal obstruction. The mother had polyhydramnios, which prompted the study.

warning signal, however, and must be considered a pathologic finding and evidence of intestinal obstruction until ruled otherwise. Of cases of congenital duodenal obstruction, 15% occur proximal to the bile duct entry, and these patients have nonbilious emesis. Approximately one third of infants born with duodenal atresia and stenosis have Down syndrome (trisomy 21).

Untreated infants with duodenal obstruction tend to become dehydrated and lose electrolytes because of vomiting and an inability to tolerate fluid intake. Passage of an orogastric tube usually yields significant amounts (>30 mL) of bile-stained gastric fluid. The tube should be left in place to reduce the risk of vomiting and aspiration. Erect and recumbent radiographs of the abdomen usually document the presence of an air-filled stomach and first portion of the duodenum—the classic double bubble sign diagnostic of duodenal obstruction (Fig. 46-3). If no air is observed beyond the second bubble, the infant has an atresia. Scattered small amounts of air seen distal to the obstruction are consistent with duodenal stenosis. There is little indication for the use of upper gastrointestinal contrast radiographs in most infants with duodenal atresia, but occasionally instillation of air before obtaining plain films may facilitate the diagnosis.

Some patients with duodenal stenosis may go unrecognized for several weeks or months. Partial obstruction usually results, however, in recurrent vomiting, failure to thrive, and aspiration over months to years. Some cases are not recognized until adult life, usually in association with peptic ulceration, reflux esophagitis, or obstruction of the duodenum proximal to the stenosis by a bezoar or foreign body. Patients with symptoms of partial obstruction should undergo an upper gastrointestinal contrast study to help differentiate duodenal stenosis, web, annular pancreas, duodenal duplications, and conditions associated with external pressure on the duodenum, such as preduodenal portal vein or malrotation with Ladd's bands. In more recent years, infants and older children have been evaluated with fiberoptic gastrointestinal endoscopy, although the radiographic approach is usually sufficient. Endoscopic retrograde cholangiopancreatography has been used occasionally to document abnormalities of the bile duct and pancreatic ductal system in older patients, but more recently, magnetic resonance imaging cholangiopancreatography has been preferred.

CLINICAL MANAGEMENT

Although duodenal atresia is a relative emergency, the patient should not be rushed to the operating room until hemodynamic status and fluid and electrolyte status are normalized. It is usually possible to operate on infants with duodenal atresia semielectively while orogastric drainage and intravenous fluids are given. Because of the high incidence of associated anomalies, a prompt system review should be done to rule out other congenital defects, particularly cardiac. The abdomen is entered best through a transverse right upper quadrant supraumbilical incision. The stomach and first portion of the duodenum are usually thickened and dilated. Full exposure of the duodenum on either side of the obstruction is important. There may be an associated annular pancreas or malrotation in at least 36% each of patients and an anterior portal vein in 4% (Table 46-1).

The orogastric tube may be passed distally to locate the point of obstruction without opening the stomach. A type 1 defect is detected easily by this maneuver. The duodenum distal to the site of the obstruction is small, whereas the proximal duodenum is thickened, floppy, and dilated. It is best when feasible to perform a duodenoduodenostomy. A standard side-to-side or, preferably, proximal transverse-to-distal longitudinal (diamond-shaped) anastomosis may be performed using fine interrupted suture (Fig. 46-4). If the proximal duodenum is excessively floppy and distended, an antimesenteric tapering duodenoplasty may be useful. Alternatively the

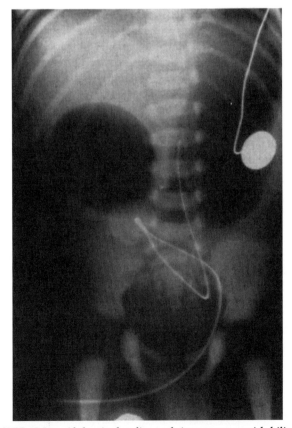

FIGURE 46-3 ■ Abdominal radiograph in a neonate with bilious vomiting shows a double bubble with no distal air, consistent with duodenal atresia.

TABLE 46-1 ■ **Associated Abdominal Conditions at the Time of Operation for Duodenal Atresia or Stenosis***

Condition	Cases (%)
Annular pancreas	36
Malrotation	36
Anterior portal vein	4
Second distal web	3
Biliary atresia	2

*Annular pancreas and anomalies of rotation and fixation were the most common associations in a review of 503 cases of duodenal atresia.

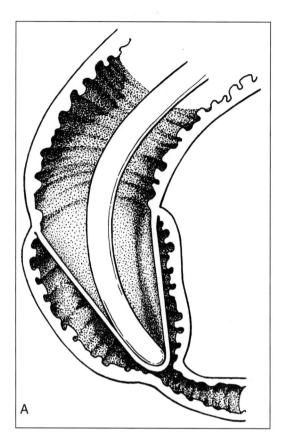

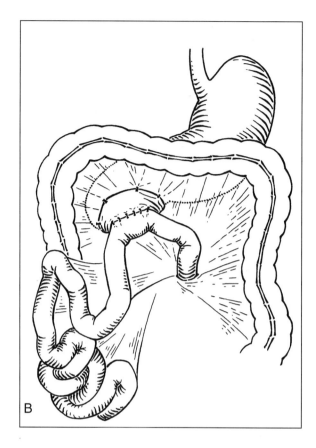

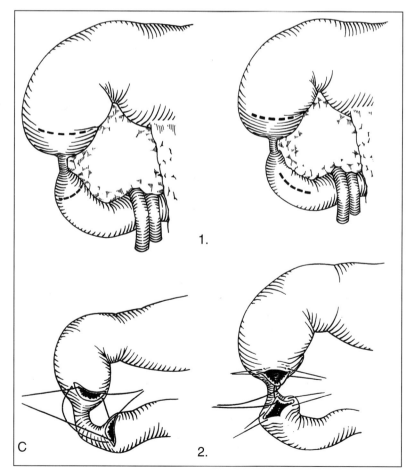

FIGURE 46-4 ■ **A,** Pressure on the tube at the bottom of the web produces an indentation in the duodenal wall, indicating the point apex of the web. The incision should be placed at that point. **B,** Duodenojejunostomy. A loop of proximal jejunum is brought through an opening in the transverse mesocolon and anastomosed to the most dependent portion of the obstructed duodenum. This approach now is used only when direct duodenal anastomosis is not feasible. **C,** Duodenoduodenostomy. 1, Standard side-to-side anastomosis. 2, Diamond-shaped duodenoduodenostomy.

redundant proximal anterior duodenal wall may be plicated (imbricated) with interrupted sutures over a dilator. To identify the location of the papilla of Vater, it is useful to press gently on the gallbladder to see where the bile enters the duodenum. Failure to see any bile in the proximal atretic segment may indicate a postatretic bile duct entry. In some patients with a type 3 defect, dual bile ducts may be present and should be identified to avoid injury to these structures. In patients with an annular pancreas, the pancreatic tissue should not be divided to avoid fistula formation, but duodenoduodenostomy should be performed. At the time of the procedure, a small red rubber catheter can be passed distally through the opening made in the distal segment because a second duodenal mucosal web may exist in 1% to 3% of patients. Failure to recognize the second web may result in postoperative obstruction distal to the anastomosis.

In patients with a windsock web variant, the pancreas is usually normal. By passing the orogastric catheter down to the level of obstruction to detect a site of indentation of the wall of the duodenum proximal to the level of obstruction, the origin of the web can be identified and the duodenum opened at the base of the web so that it simply can be excised. During web excision, the papilla of Vater must be preserved. The web can be opened carefully along the lateral side because in most cases the papilla is located in the medial portion of the web. The web should be excised partially, leaving the medial portion containing the papilla in place. After documenting that there is no distal obstruction, simple closure of the duodenotomy usually is performed in these patients. This can be done either in a longitudinal or in a transverse manner.

In patients with associated malrotation, a Ladd procedure should be performed. An appendectomy is suggested because of the unusual location of the appendix after the Ladd procedure. Some infants with duodenal atresia have a prolonged delay in gastric emptying and duodenal transit after repair, although less so since duodenoduodenostomy replaced duodenojejunostomy. Gastrostomy is employed occasionally, although complications of gastrostomy and the late development of gastroesophageal reflux in these patients has prompted more frequent use of an orogastric tube without gastrostomy in most patients. The patient is kept without oral intake until intestinal function is regained. Although transanastomotic feeding tubes were used in the past, short-term intravenous nutrition is used now for support until gastrointestinal function resumes.

The survival of infants with duodenal anomalies has improved gradually from 68% to greater than 90% over the past 25 years so that now the only deaths are related to associated malformations. Improved survival is most likely the result of advances in neonatal intensive care, such as respiratory management, improved monitoring and surveillance, nutritional support, improvements in pediatric anesthesia, and an early systems work-up to document potentially salvageable anomalies in other systems. Most deaths are related to severe cardiac defects.

COMPLICATIONS

Although the improved early survival data are gratifying, several reports documenting the occurrence of late complications in patients with congenital duodenal anomalies are of concern. Late complications are reported to occur in 12% to 15% of patients. Long-term complications such as blind loop syndrome, megaduodenum with abnormal duodenal motility, duodenogastric reflux and esophagitis, pancreatitis, cholecystitis, and cholelithiasis indicate that a reassessment of treatment must be considered. Most cases of blind loop syndrome have been observed in patients treated by duodenojejunostomy, now rarely done. Blind loop syndrome can be corrected by conversion to a duodenoduodenostomy. Late occurrence of megaduodenum has been treated successfully by reoperation and a tapering duodenoplasty or plication. These findings suggest that instances of duodenal atresia with significant distention of the proximal atretic segment may benefit from a tapering procedure at the time of the initial operation. Endoscopic excision of an obstructing duodenal web also is of questionable efficacy in preventing late complications. Other complications, such as duodenogastric reflux and gastritis, can be ameliorated by medical management because these patients may respond to the administration of parasympathomimetic drugs, such as bethanechol, or a prokinetic agent (metoclopramide) to improve gastric and duodenal emptying. Antacids and H_2-antagonists (cimetidine and ranitidine) may be useful in the management of peptic ulcer and gastroesophageal reflux. Long-term follow-up is essential for infants treated for congenital duodenal anomalies. Further observations regarding outcome as related to changes in surgical management ultimately will determine future recommendations regarding optimal treatment.

SUGGESTED READINGS

Fonkalsrud EW, deLorimier AA, Hays DM: Congenital atresia and stenosis of the duodenum: A review compiled from the members of the Surgical Section of the American Academy of Pediatrics. Pediatrics 43:79, 1969.

This report concerning 503 cases of duodenal atresia is an important early contribution to the understanding of this congenital anomaly.

Grosfeld JL, Rescorla FJ: Duodenal atresia and stenosis: Reassessment of treatment and outcome based on antenatal diagnosis, pathologic variance, and long-term follow-up. World J Surg 17:301-309, 1993.

This article evaluates long-term survival and late morbidity.

Kimura K, Mukahara N, Nishijima E, et al: Diamond shaped anastomosis for duodenal atresia: An experience with 44 patients over 15 years. J Pediatr Surg 25:977, 1990.

This report documents the efficacy of the diamond-shaped anastomosis for cases of duodenal atresia.

Skandalakis JE, Gray SW: Embryology for Surgeons, 2nd ed. Baltimore, Williams & Wilkins, 1994, p 184.

This textbook describes the classification of duodenal anomalies clearly and concisely.

Weaver E, et al: Operative management of duodenal atresia. Pediatr Surg Int 10: 332, 1995.

This article provides an excellent description of all the various approaches useful to the management of the spectrum of duodenal obstruction.

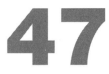

Rotational Anomalies and Volvulus

Midgut volvulus, internal hernias, and certain congenital duodenal and colonic obstructions are the result of abnormalities of intestinal rotation and fixation. Delays in diagnosis and improper management result in significant mortality and lifelong morbidity. Prompt and effective treatment is based on the surgeon's understanding of the embryology of intestinal rotation. Without this knowledge, the surgeon may be confused during laparotomy because of the variability of these cases and incompletely reduce a volvulus, fail to achieve intestinal stabilization, return the intestines to the abdomen improperly, or injure important structures while attempting to reduce an internal hernia.

At about 1 month of gestational age, the midgut, the intestine from the primitive duodenum to the midtransverse colon, is a short, straight, continuous tube suspended from the superior mesenteric artery, which arises posteriorly. Rotation and fixation of the intestine take place during the first 3 months of gestation. The two most important events, rotation of the duodenojejunal and cecocolic loops, occur simultaneously but for the sake of simplicity are best described as separate events.

The duodenojejunal loop originally lies above or anterior to the superior mesenteric artery. It first rotates counterclockwise 90 degrees to the right of the artery, then another 90 degrees under the artery. The loop finally rotates 90 degrees across the spine and upward so that the duodenojejunal junction lies to the left of the spine and superior mesenteric artery and slightly above the duodenum in an area that eventually becomes the ligament of Treitz (Fig. 47-1).

The cecocolic loop originally hangs beneath the superior mesenteric artery. Rotation is also counterclockwise. The loop moves to the left of the artery 90 degrees, then above the artery 90 degrees, and finally to the right and

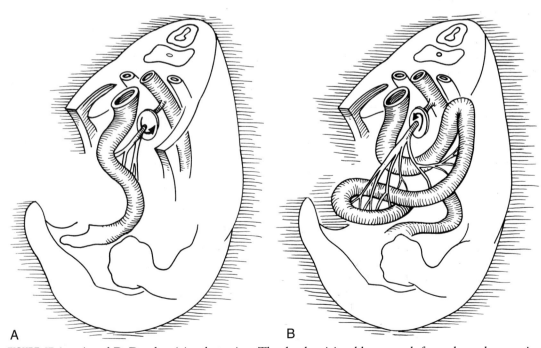

A   B

FIGURE 47-1 ■ **A** and **B,** Duodenojejunal rotation. The duodenojejunal loop travels from above the superior mesenteric artery counterclockwise to the right of the artery, below the artery, and finally across the spine to the left, then above the superior mesenteric artery.

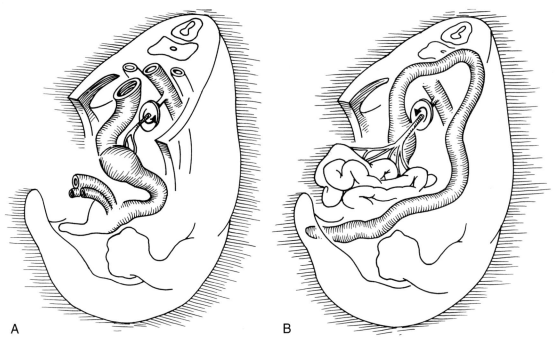

FIGURE 47-2 ■ **A** and **B**, Cecocolic rotation. Cecocolic loop rotation begins with the loop below the superior mesenteric artery. It travels counterclockwise to the left, then above to the right, then below the artery.

downward 90 degrees, forming the typical horseshoe configuration of the colon. The left colon lies to the left of the superior mesenteric artery, the transverse colon is draped across the artery, and the right colon lies to the right with the cecum in the right iliac fossa (Fig. 47-2).

Rotation of the two loops and lengthening of the gut begin at about 1 month of gestational age. Fixation of the intestine to the posterior abdominal wall occurs during the process of rotation and continues after rotation is complete. If fixation does not take place, the intestine remains suspended by the thin stalk of the superior mesenteric vessels and is susceptible to volvulus. As rotation begins, the intestine moves outside the abdomen into the base of the umbilical cord. At about 10 weeks' gestation, the intestine returns to the abdomen, and rotation and fixation continue. Although fixation of the duodenojejunal loop is accomplished early, colonic attachment takes place gradually until term. This accounts for the "mobile right colon" or high cecum of term and premature infants.

ACUTE MIDGUT VOLVULUS

Normal rotation and fixation securely anchor the bowel to the posterior abdominal wall, preventing the bowel from twisting on itself. The major source of stabilization of the small bowel is the broad base of the mesentery, beginning in the right iliac fossa at the ileocecal junction and running obliquely upward across the abdomen to the ligament of Treitz in the left upper abdomen (Fig. 47-3). When rotation and fixation are complete, the duodenum is fixed securely to the retroperitoneum in the pattern of a C-loop. The ascending and descending colon are attached to the retroperitoneum on their respective sides of the abdomen.

If the course of intestinal rotation and fixation is interrupted, two conditions may develop that make the gut vulnerable to volvulus: (1) nonrotation of the midgut and (2) normal or partial rotation of the duodenojejunal loop with nonrotation of the colon. In both of these conditions, the midgut is supported exclusively by a narrow pedicle that contains its entire blood supply. Distention and peristalsis may initiate torsion of the intestine around the superior mesenteric artery and vein and lead to acute volvulus and necrosis of the complete midgut.

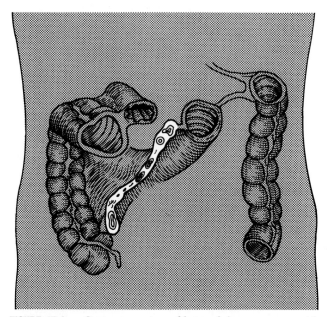

FIGURE 47-3 ■ Cutaway section of base of the mesentery with normal rotation. Broad attachment prevents volvulus.

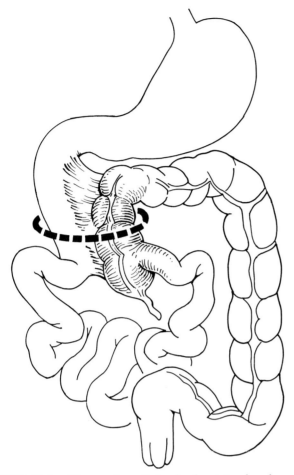

FIGURE 47-4 ■ Nonrotation of the duodenojejunal and cecocolic loops. Duodenojejunal and ileocecal junctions lie close together in the midline; the mesenteric base is narrow.

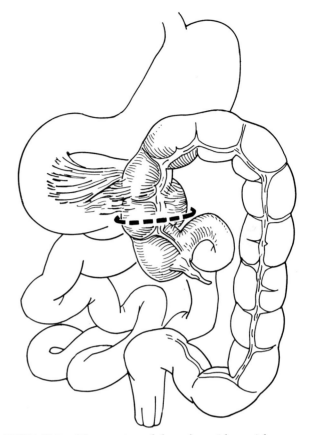

FIGURE 47-5 ■ Nonrotation of the colon with partial or complete rotation of duodenojejunal loop. The mesentery base is narrow, and volvulus can occur.

In nonrotation (Fig. 47-4), there is lengthening of the midgut without rotation of the duodenojejunal or cecocolic loops. The midgut hangs on a thin stalk containing the superior mesenteric vessels. The duodenum lies near the midline, slightly to the right of the spine, and descends downward. The small bowel fans out below on the right until the terminal ileum is reached. The cecum and first part of the colon lie close to the midline on the left, running parallel to the duodenum. Stability of the midgut is poor because of the narrow base of the mesentery.

Similarly with nonrotation of the colon and normal rotation of the duodenum and jejunum, the cecum and first part of the colon lie close to the midline against the third portion of the duodenum over the superior mesenteric vessels (Fig. 47-5). The base of the mesentery is narrow and unstable. Volvulus can occur early or even in utero.

At operation in both anatomic configurations, when the volvulus has been reduced and the small intestine is laid out as a fan on the lower abdominal wall, the narrow mesenteric pedicle can be seen. The base can be encircled by the thumb and index finger and contains the duodenojejunal junction, ascending colon, and superior mesenteric artery and vein (Fig. 47-6). A layer of peritoneum runs across the ascending and descending loops of intestine. Dividing the peritoneum, often called *Ladd's bands*, and moving the colon to the left, away from the duodenum and jejunum, is an essential step in broadening the base of the mesentery.

CLINICAL FINDINGS

Most patients who present with acute midgut volvulus are infants; 30% present within the first week of life, and more than 50% present within the first month. The most common symptom is vomiting (95%). Vomitus initially may contain gastric secretions but soon becomes bilious. When intestinal necrosis develops, vomitus is bloody. Stools are grossly bloody in a third of patients; half have abdominal distention. Pain and tenderness in neonates may be subtle but appear to be universally present and are most obvious with bowel ischemia. Infants commonly appear acutely ill with grunting respirations; as the process advances, the infant appears dehydrated and lethargic and may show frank signs of peritonitis and shock.

DIAGNOSIS

Plain films reveal either a gasless abdomen or dilated intestine, suggesting intestinal obstruction. In about 20% of patients, a double bubble sign signifying duodenal

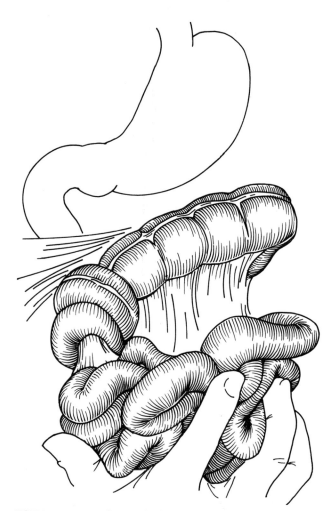

FIGURE 47-6 ■ Midgut volvulus. The colon is tightly coiled around the base of the small bowel mesentery. The bowel must be rotated in a counterclockwise manner to reduce volvulus.

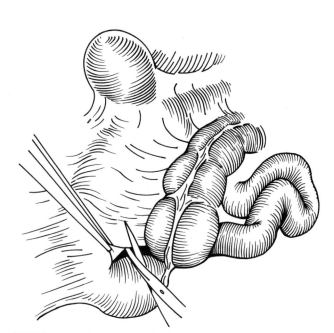

FIGURE 47-7 ■ Incising Ladd's bands so that the cecocolic loop can move to the left across the duodenum.

PREOPERATIVE PREPARATION

When the diagnosis of volvulus is considered, preoperative preparations must be made quickly because bowel necrosis can develop rapidly and involve the entire small bowel and half of the large intestine. Broad-spectrum antibiotics are administered. The GI tract is decompressed by a nasogastric or orogastric tube placed on intermittent suction. Intravenous fluids are administered rapidly to correct hypovolemia and continued in the operating room so that there is no delay in intervention.

OPERATION

A right supraumbilical transverse incision is made so that the entire intestine can be delivered from the peritoneal cavity. Blood-stained fluid indicates vascular compromise. Often chylous ascites is encountered, indicating lymphatic disruption from a volvulus. The colon is not immediately visible but is found tightly encircling the base of the small bowel mesentery (Figs. 47-6 and 47-7). The proximal duodenum is dilated and passes into the encircling coils of the large intestine. The small bowel is often edematous and hemorrhagic and may appear frankly necrotic. All volvulus is clockwise so that the small bowel must be rotated in a *counterclockwise fashion*. One to three complete turns are necessary to reduce the volvulus and bring the transverse colon and the cecum into view. The small bowel is fanned out over the lower abdominal wall, spreading the mesentery out as much as possible. The anatomy of the mesenteric base is then visible. The duodenum and ascending colon lie parallel to each other. The mesenteric vessels lie behind and between these two structures. The space between is called the *duodenocolic isthmus*. Peritoneal folds pass from the ascending colon to the duodenum and into the right lateral gutter. These folds, called *Ladd's bands*, are incised along the medial

obstruction is often present, but the duodenum is less dilated than with duodenal atresia. These plain film findings, along with clinical findings suggesting impending bowel necrosis, such as bloody vomitus and stool and abdominal tenderness, necessitate immediate operation. If the diagnosis is in doubt, and there is no evidence of compromised bowel, an upper gastrointestinal (GI) contrast study may be helpful. Experienced pediatric radiologists often use ultrasound to determine the position of the superior mesenteric artery to confirm the diagnosis.

With malrotation, the upper GI series usually shows an abnormal position of the duodenum. The duodenum and jejunum may lie to the right of the spine, and the entire opacified small bowel is on the right. The duodenum may cross the spine partially, but then travel downward, rather than be positioned upward and to the left at the ligament of Treitz. With volvulus, there is usually duodenal obstruction with a corkscrew appearance of the proximal duodenum at the point of obstruction. Distally the mucosal folds of the jejunum may be thickened because of mucosal edema. In the rare patient in whom obstruction is complete, there is a beak appearance at the site of duodenal obstruction.

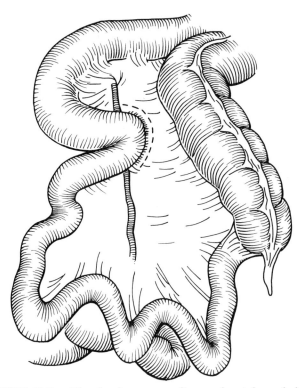

FIGURE 47-8 ■ The duodenum now lies to the right and the cecocolic loop to the left. The anterior layer of the mesenteric peritoneum must be incised to broaden the mesentery.

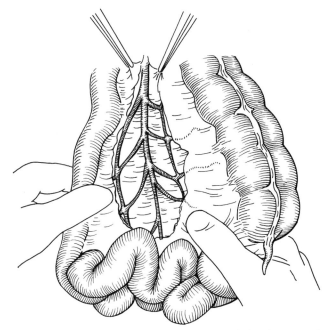

FIGURE 47-9 ■ The peritoneum is incised, and duodenojejunal and cecocolic loops are moved farther apart. Final check of reduction of volvulus and proper orientation of the bowel is now done. The loops of small bowel are fanned out. The left hand encircles the first part of the jejunum, and the right hand encircles the terminal ileum. The remainder of the small bowel is below the hands to form an irregular U.

aspect of the duodenum (see Fig. 47-7). When this incision is made, the course of the duodenum is clarified. The duodenum passes in a sinuous manner to the right of the spine. When the duodenum and ascending colon are exposed clearly by incision of the peritoneal folds, the underlying tissue of the anterior leaf of the mesentery is divided until the superior mesenteric artery is visualized. This allows the ascending colon and cecum to move to the left, away from the duodenum, widening the base of the mesentery (Fig. 47-8). Dissection continues until the cecum and ascending colon lie in the left upper abdomen. Care must be taken to ensure the duodenum is uncoiled completely. At this point, the viability of the involved intestine is checked and proper alignment of the intestine is confirmed by placing the left hand around the proximal jejunum and the right hand around the ileocecal junction. The left hand and right hand should be on opposite sides of the abdomen, on the same level, and the small bowel laid out below in a U shape (Fig. 47-9).

Previously, it was recommended that the intestine be fixed by duodenal sutures to the right lower abdomen and colonic sutures to the left upper abdomen, but this was proved to be ineffective. The incidence of recurrent volvulus was 5% to 8%, whether or not fixation was accomplished. Because of the abnormal position of the appendix in the left upper abdomen after widening of the mesentery, most surgeons perform an appendectomy, often using inversion appendectomy. Exploration and operative management can be carried out laparoscopically and by open approach, but if there is any question about the

completeness of a procedure done laparoscopically, conversion to an open procedure is in order.

The procedure previously described is carried out if there is no question of viability of intestine. The guiding principle when operating on patients with midgut volvulus with compromised bowel is rapid reduction of the volvulus and preservation of maximum length of intestine. One always should lean toward leaving rather than resecting intestine. Three possible situations may be encountered when there is compromised intestine: (1) A short segment of intestine is necrotic, and the remaining bowel appears healthy. The necrotic bowel is resected, and an anastomosis is performed. (2) A relatively short segment of bowel is frankly necrotic, but after resection, variable lengths of proximal and distal bowel are of questionable viability. Both ends should be brought out as stomas. After 24 to 48 hours, if the ends of the stomas appear necrotic, the patient is operated on again, and further necrotic intestine is resected. If the stomas are healthy, elective stoma closure is performed later. (3) A significant portion of the small bowel appears necrotic, or there are several alternating areas of necrotic and viable intestine. The intestine is returned to the peritoneal cavity without resection. If the patient does not improve, a second-look procedure is performed in 24 to 48 hours, and definite necrotic intestine is removed and intestinal stomas formed. If necessary, a third or fourth operation is performed, always resecting the absolute minimum length of intestine. In this way, the maximum length of bowel is retained. Injured but not necrotic bowel is allowed to recover, and frankly dead gut has time to declare itself. This cautious approach reduces the frequency of the serious and often fatal complication of short-gut syndrome. Volvulus ranks equally with necrotizing enterocolitis as the most common cause of this syndrome.

MALROTATION BEYOND THE NEONATAL PERIOD

Although clinical problems associated with malrotation usually are thought of as neonatal conditions, several large series have been published reporting clinically significant malrotation abnormalities beyond the neonatal period and into adulthood. Most patients present with chronic symptoms, but 10% to 15% develop midgut volvulus with necrotic bowel. In infants and children older than age 1 month, 30% present with intermittent vomiting, usually bilious, and 20% present with colicky abdominal pain. The most common symptom complex suggests intermittent partial intestinal obstruction. The nutritional status of almost half of patients is below average. Some have malabsorption syndrome with diarrhea and failure to thrive.

Frequently, in the course of evaluating a patient for recurrent abdominal pain, vomiting, or failure to thrive, an upper GI series reveals malrotation. The bulk of evidence suggests that in these patients surgery is indicated because (1) symptoms usually are relieved with surgical correction, and (2) at any age patients with malrotation are susceptible to volvulus and bowel necrosis.

A more difficult problem is the proper course to follow when malrotation is found incidentally by radiograph in an asymptomatic patient or at operation for a nonrelated disease. Some surgeons advise that the abnormality should be corrected only in patients younger than 2 years old. Others follow a more aggressive approach, stating that the complications associated with intestinal malrotation are based on anatomic reasons that do not change with age. They reason that volvulus can occur at any age so that a rotational abnormality should be corrected when it is discovered. Many surgeons do not operate on patients with asymptomatic malrotation. Death from untreated malrotation with volvulus in older patients associated with cardiac anomalies has been reported, but is rare.

DUODENAL OBSTRUCTION

Congenital duodenal obstruction associated with malrotation in neonates sometimes is associated with intrinsic lesions, such as duodenal web. Acute duodenal obstruction without an intrinsic lesion can occur with volvulus, and malrotation alone is sufficient explanation for neonatal duodenal obstruction. The peritoneal bands appear to be drawn tight by the volvulus and obstruct the lumen. The surgeon must suspect an intrinsic lesion when the combination of malrotation and duodenal obstruction is encountered. A gastrotomy is performed, and a Foley catheter is passed the length of the duodenum into the proximal jejunum after the duodenal bands have been incised. If the catheter cannot be passed, an intrinsic

lesion is probably present, and the duodenum must be opened and the obstruction identified.

If the catheter passes from dilated to collapsed bowel through the area covered by bands, the balloon should be inflated and the catheter slowly withdrawn into the dilated duodenum, then the stomach. If the catheter cannot be pulled back, a web may be present. The duodenum should be opened to identify the lesion.

REVERSE ROTATION

Reverse rotation is a rare anomaly, often first seen in adulthood, in which the duodenum and colon rotate in the wrong plane in relation to the superior mesenteric artery and vein. The transverse colon passes beneath a tunnel formed by these vessels, whereas the duodenum and jejunum pass anteriorly to the superior mesenteric vessels, and the duodenal mesentery surrounds the transverse colon. The superior mesenteric artery and vein then lie across the midtransverse colon and may cause acute or chronic colonic obstruction, which can be relieved by mobilizing the duodenum and underlying mesenteric vessels anteriorly and laterally off the transverse colon.

INTERNAL HERNIA

Lack of fixation of the mesentery of the right and left sides of the colon and the duodenum result in the formation of potential mesenteric defects and hernia pouches. Entrapment of the bowel in these pouches can lead to complete obstruction and gangrene. Two internal hernias, right and left mesocolic, are the most common. The right mesocolic hernia can be identified by GI series because the entire small bowel appears to lie high on the right side of the abdomen. At operation, the intestine is encased in a thin pouch of mesentery that carries the blood supply of the right side of the colon. The embryologic explanation suggests that the prearterial limb of the duodenojejunal loop fails to rotate around the superior mesenteric artery, and the intestine is entrapped by the mesentery of the cecum and colon. To reduce the hernia, the lateral peritoneal margin of the right side of the colon is incised, and the colon is reflected to the left. The edges of the mesenteric sac are closed loosely with sutures.

The left mesocolic hernia has as the anterior surface of its sac the mesentery of the left side of the colon. The inferior mesenteric vein forms the neck. At operation, the cecum appears completely rotated and lies in its normal position in the right lower quadrant. The distal ileum enters the sac, and the entire small intestine is trapped within it. Treatment of left mesocolic hernias can be difficult because of the presence of the inferior mesenteric vein in the neck. Sometimes it is possible to reduce the intestine without widening the neck of the sac. If this is not possible, an incision is made in the peritoneum that encases the mesenteric vein so that the vein can be mobilized and raised off the neck of the sac. In this way, enough slack is produced to allow the intestine to be extracted. The peritoneum posterior to the vein is sutured to the posterior abdominal wall peritoneum, obliterating the opening in the sac.

MALROTATION AND OTHER ASSOCIATED CONDITIONS

Malrotation has been called a ubiquitous anomaly because it is found frequently in association with other congenital anomalies and clinical syndromes. It also has been implicated in the pathogenesis of some common GI conditions. Nonrotation almost always accompanies congenital diaphragmatic hernia, gastroschisis, and omphalocele. The incidence is similarly high with prune-belly syndrome. Most surgeons do not perform a Ladd operation when dealing with these patients, unless there is evidence of duodenal obstruction. Malrotation also has been reported in association with Hirschsprung's disease. Some have suggested that there is an association between intussusception and malrotation. In one study of 49 cases of intussusception, 98% of the patients had a mobile cecum, and it was concluded that lack of normal rotation and fixation is an important etiologic factor in idiopathic intussusception. Other studies have found an increased incidence of malrotation in patients who require operation for gastroesophageal reflux. The combination of congenital short gut, malrotation, and functional intestinal obstruction is rare. These patients often have pyloric stenosis. Prognosis is poor, and only a few patients have survived. Malrotation also is associated with congenital heart disease, particularly heterotaxia and asplenia syndromes.

SUGGESTED READINGS

Dott NM: Anomalies of intestinal rotation: Their embryology and surgical aspects with report of five cases. Br J Surg 11:251, 1923.

This is the classic article on this subject with beautiful color diagrams of the various forms of malformations and how they occur.

Gross E, Chen MK, Lobe TE: Laparoscopic evaluation and treatment of intestinal malrotation in infants. Surg Endosc 10:936, 1996.

This article describes a minimally invasive approach to correction of malrotation, verifying its utility.

Powell DM, Otherson HB, Smith CD: Malrotation of the intestine in children: The effect of age in presentation and therapy. J Pediatr Surg 24:777, 1989.

Of 70 children presenting with malrotation, 50% were older than age 2 months. The authors concluded that it was impossible to predict which patients would have serious complications of malrotation based on age or presentation. They recommended that all patients with malrotation, even if incidentally discovered, should be operated on.

Rescorla FJ, Shedd FJ, Grosfeld JL, et al: Anomalies of intestinal rotation in childhood: Analysis of 447 cases. Surgery 108:710, 1990.

A large series of different presentations of malrotation is reported. There were 18 cases of volvulus and 54 patients with chronic symptoms of intermittent volvulus or duodenal obstruction. Most patients (n = 331) had malrotation associated with abdominal wall defects or diaphragmatic hernia.

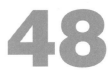

Other Conditions of the Upper Gastrointestinal Tract

Hypertrophic pyloric stenosis is the most common abnormality affecting the stomach in early infancy. This topic is discussed in depth in Chapter 45. Other less well-known but important conditions that affect the stomach of infants and children include pyloric atresia, prepyloric and antral web, pyloric duplication, spontaneous gastric perforation, congenital microgastria, gastric volvulus, and peptic ulcer.

PYLORIC ATRESIA

The first successful repair of pyloric atresia was reported in 1940 by Touroff and Sussman. Pyloric atresia is a relatively uncommon form of intestinal obstruction in newborns and accounts for 17% of all cases of atresia of the alimentary tract. Familial occurrences have been observed in siblings with a probable autosomal recessive inheritance that in some cases can be associated with epidermolysis bullosa. Pyloric atresia occasionally is associated with other intestinal atresias, including esophageal atresia, duodenal atresia, and jejunoileal atresia. Pyloric atresia can be detected on prenatal ultrasonography. Maternal polyhydramnios is observed in more than 60% of these patients, and the α-fetoprotein level in amniotic fluid may be elevated.

Clinical Presentation

At birth, the upper abdomen may become slightly distended with air entering the obstructed stomach. These infants characteristically have nonbilious emesis. A plain abdominal radiograph shows a single upper abdominal gas bubble with no air beyond the stomach or a large gastric air-fluid level (Fig. 48-1). Abdominal ultrasonography may show a dilated pyloric canal. If the diagnosis is delayed, the infant may become dehydrated and develop hypochloremic alkalosis as a result of emesis and loss of potassium and hydrochloric acid. Gastric perforation also may occur with diagnostic delay. An orogastric or nasogastric tube should be inserted for decompression to reduce the risk of aspiration. Intravenous fluids are administered to replace electrolytes and fluid losses from emesis. When adequately hydrated and stable, the infant may be taken to the operating room for relief of the obstruction.

Classification

Pyloric atresias are classified according to the pathologic findings observed at laparotomy (Fig. 48-2). The most common lesion is type I pyloric atresia (58%), in which the stomach and duodenum are intact. Type II atresias (34%) are separated by a fibrous band. In type III pyloric atresia (8%), there is a complete separation of the two ends with a gap between the distal end of the stomach and the duodenum. Patients with a double pyloric membrane also have been described.

Treatment

The procedure of choice for type I pyloric atresia is to perform a gastrotomy and identify the location of the web by passing a firm catheter distally. Through a longitudinal incision across the pylorus, the web can be excised. A catheter should be passed distally to ascertain that a

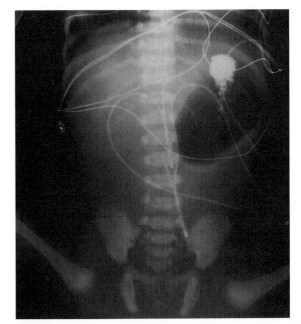

FIGURE 48-1 ■ Plain radiograph of the abdomen in an infant with pyloric atresia shows a single gastric bubble with no distal air beyond the pylorus. No further diagnostic studies are necessary.

485

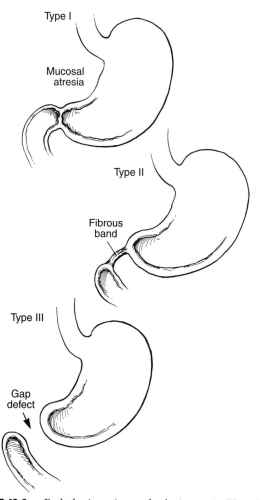

FIGURE 48-2 ■ Pathologic variants of pyloric atresia. Type I is a mucosal atresia. In type II, atretic ends are separated by a fibrous band. In type III pyloric atresia, the two ends of the stomach and duodenum are separated by a short gap.

second web or atresia is not present before the pylorotomy is closed. The incision is closed in a transverse fashion by performing a pyloroplasty. A gastrostomy or a nasogastric or orogastric tube provides safe gastric decompression. In types II and III pyloric atresia, the distal stomach and duodenum are separated, and the operative repair requires performance of a gastroduodenal anastomosis. Postoperatively an orogastric tube is left in place for gastric drainage until normal motility and appropriate gastric emptying are shown. Although overall postoperative survival in a literature review of 114 cases collected over the past 50 years was only 53%, in more recent years survival has been routine, unless there have been serious associated anomalies. Most deaths now are in patients with multiple anomalies and in inherited cases associated with epidermolysis bullosa.

ANTRAL AND PREPYLORIC WEB

Partial gastric outlet obstruction caused by the presence of an antral or prepyloric web is either uncommon in infants and children or not recognized until late. Nonbilious vomiting is the usual presenting symptom.

The diagnosis of antral web is suggested by upper gastrointestinal (UGI) contrast study, which shows indirect evidence of a web and a peristaltic wave with contrast jetting through a ring-like area in the distal antrum. Occasionally a gastric fold can appear similar to a web, and an upper endoscopy should be performed to confirm the diagnosis. The operative description of the web varies from a true diaphragm to a "large fold" of mucosa. In more recent years, all patients with an antral web diagnosed by barium swallow have had endoscopy before attempted surgical correction. This approach has proved to be important because the radiographic appearance of an antral web often cannot be confirmed on endoscopy. If a true antral web is present, it can be excised through a gastrotomy on the anterior wall of the stomach. More recently, webs that are thin have been incised endoscopically, avoiding the need for laparotomy. The prognosis should be favorable in all cases.

SPONTANEOUS GASTRIC PERFORATION IN THE NEWBORN

Etiology

Spontaneous gastric perforation often occurs in infants who require resuscitation or have an episode of hypoxia shortly after delivery. Males are more commonly affected than females, and the incidence is 1:2900 live births. There are two common theories regarding the events leading to gastric perforation. The first postulates that an ischemic insult associated with perinatal stress results in an hypoxic mucosal injury that progresses to perforation a few days later. The second theory is related to gastric overinflation. Gastric overdistention may be the result of aggressive mask resuscitation, accidental esophageal intubation and vigorous insufflation, or proximal distention and perforation related to distal outlet obstruction as in infants with pyloric atresia. Perforation also can occur from passage of a gastric tube or be the result of congenital defects in the muscular wall of the stomach. The incidence seems to be decreasing.

Clinical Findings

Neonatal gastric perforation is observed most commonly between the third and fifth days of life. The most dramatic clinical manifestation is abrupt onset of massive abdominal distention. Tachycardia, lethargy, and evidence of poor perfusion as a result of hypovolemia occur rapidly. Peritonitis, diaphragmatic elevation, and increased respiratory effort occur. If the perforation is not recognized and treated early, shock and cardiovascular collapse result. The diagnosis is usually apparent on a chest or abdominal radiograph that shows significant pneumoperitoneum. An upright or lateral decubitus abdominal film is helpful (Fig. 48-3). The differential diagnosis includes perforated peptic ulcer, necrotizing enterocolitis (see Chapter 52), and massive pneumoperitoneum from air dissecting down from the mediastinum in an infant on mechanical ventilation for respiratory distress. The presence of pulmonary interstitial emphysema and pneumomediastinum in these patients usually indicates that the pneumoperitoneum is from an intrathoracic source, and laparotomy is unnecessary.

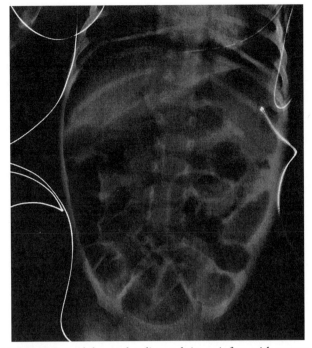

FIGURE 48-3 ■ Abdominal radiograph in an infant with spontaneous gastric perforation shows free air in the peritoneal cavity.

Paracentesis can be used, when necessary, to differentiate these entities. Occasionally infants with Hirschsprung's disease or more rarely colon atresia may present with perforation and pneumoperitoneum.

Treatment

Patients require prompt administration of intravenous fluid; administration should continue at an hourly rate needed to deliver 150 to 200 mL/kg/day. Broad-spectrum intravenous antibiotics (ampicillin and gentamicin) should be administered. An orogastric tube should be inserted and placed on low continuous suction. Endotracheal intubation and respiratory support may be required, and in a dire situation, paracentesis may be necessary to decompress the abdomen.

The operation is performed through an upper abdominal transverse incision. On entering the peritoneal cavity, escape of air and fluid is noted. The contents should be cultured for aerobic and anaerobic bacteria. Clear gastric contents or mildly bile-tinged material usually indicates a perforation of the stomach or duodenum. Dark-stained bilious fluid or feculent drainage suggests small intestine or colonic perforation. Most spontaneous gastric perforations occur along the greater curvature of the stomach just distal to the esophagus. Perforation in infants with peptic ulcer is usually at the pyloroduodenal junction but may be found along the lesser curvature of the stomach at the junction of the antrum and fundus. If the area surrounding the perforation appears viable, the edges at the site of the perforation can be excised and the stomach wall closed in two layers. If the greater curvature of the stomach is involved more extensively, it can be débrided and the stomach closed. If the distal stomach is necrotic, a distal gastrectomy may be necessary. A Billroth I gastroduodenostomy is the preferred anastomosis.

The postoperative course may be stormy, especially if there was a significant delay in diagnosis. Persistent acidosis may be a sign of further tissue necrosis. Repeat abdominal radiographs and direct visualization of the mucosa by careful UGI endoscopy may be necessary to rule out further gastric necrosis. Survival of infants with gastric perforation has improved from 30% in the 1960s to greater than 80% in the present era.

CONGENITAL MICROGASTRIA

The first description of congenital microgastria in the pediatric age group is credited to Caffey, who in 1956 described the radiographic appearance of microgastria associated with incomplete gastric rotation in a 6-month-old infant.

Etiology

Congenital microgastria, a relatively unusual anomaly of the distal primitive foregut, is characterized by a small tubular stomach, megaesophagus, and incomplete gastric rotation. Other associated anomalies have been reported, including nonrotation of the midgut, duodenal web, ileal duplication, absent gallbladder, situs inversus, asplenia, cardiac defects, thoracic hemivertebrae, and various other skeletal abnormalities including micrognathia and radial and ulnar hypoplasia.

Clinical Presentation

The most common presenting findings are failure to thrive, a greatly reduced gastric capacity, and an abnormally enlarged and malfunctioning lower esophagus resulting in gastroesophageal reflux. One or more of the sequelae of gastroesophageal reflux may be present (e.g., aspiration pneumonia, esophagitis, or malnutrition). Rapid gastric emptying also may produce a dumping-like phenomenon. Infants with asplenia are at risk for infection from encapsulated bacterial organisms (e.g., *Haemophilus influenzae* and *Streptococcus pneumoniae*).

Diagnosis and Treatment

A barium contrast UGI study is the most effective diagnostic test. An abnormally dilated esophagus with impaired motility, gastroesophageal reflux, and a small stomach is usually seen. Hourly small feedings through an infant feeding tube should be attempted to provide adequate calories and fluid and to allow stomach growth. This approach is frequently unsuccessful, however.

Surgical management presents a challenge. The stomach is often too small to insert a gastrostomy tube and attach the gastric wall to the undersurface of the anterior abdominal wall. Fundoplication is difficult or impossible to perform because of the small size of the stomach. Creation of a jejunal reservoir (Hunt-Lawrence pouch) is probably the best option. The timing of the procedure also may be important. A temporary catheter jejunostomy can be placed for feedings in the first few months of life. This has been effective in providing enteral calories and avoiding the need for total parenteral nutrition. Patients with asplenia are given a pneumococcal vaccine at 2 months of age and treated with prophylactic antibiotics to avoid overwhelming infection. The size of the stomach is evaluated at 6 months of age, and if increased growth is observed, the same course should be continued. If no growth is detected, a Hunt-Lawrence jejunal pouch should be constructed.

GASTRIC VOLVULUS

Acute gastric volvulus is uncommon in children. A review stated that only 77 childhood cases have been reported. Gastric volvulus has occurred in children from 1 day old to 15 years old (mean age 2.4 years). Of cases, 44% occur in the first year of life, with almost half occurring in the first month; 80% occur within the first 5 years of life. Gastric volvulus occurs more frequently in males than females.

Etiology

The stomach usually is held securely in place by the esophageal hiatus, gastrophrenic ligaments, short gastric vessels, and the gastrocolic ligament. Retroperitoneal duodenal fixation also plays a role in securing the distal stomach. Disorders of gastric rotation play a central role in the development of a gastric volvulus in association with disturbances of attachment. Other contributing causes include gastric displacement in association with diaphragmatic hernia or eventration of the diaphragm, elongation or absence of gastric ligaments (as a result of abnormal fusion of the fetal mesenteries), or congenital bands or adhesions. Mental retardation and congenital asplenia also have been associated with gastric volvulus.

Classification

Gastric volvulus is classified according to the plane of gastric rotation. Three types of gastric volvulus have been described: (1) mesenteroaxial, (2) organoaxial, and rarely (3) a combination of both. Mesenteroaxial volvulus is the most common type seen in children. This type of volvulus occurs in a sagittal plane from greater to lesser curvature with rotation around the long axis of the gastrohepatic omentum, with the pylorus or cardia commonly rotating anteriorly and upward. The opposite rotation also may occur. Torsion may be total (the entire stomach) or partial (limited to the pyloric end). Organoaxial volvulus is more common in adults but also may occur in children. This type of gastric volvulus occurs when the stomach rotates on its long axis in a coronal plane. The greater curvature usually passes anteriorly but in some cases may be displaced posteriorly.

Clinical Presentation and Diagnosis

Symptoms of gastric volvulus depend on the degree of rotation and obstruction of the stomach. The acute onset of epigastric pain usually is followed by gastric distention and retching, often without vomiting. Occasionally, epigastric fullness or a mass may be noted. Borchardt's triad of acute gastric distention, difficulty attempting to pass a nasogastric tube, and nonproductive retching is present in approximately 70% of pediatric patients with this disorder. Dyspnea, dysphagia, chest pain, and dyspepsia also have been described.

Abdominal radiographs are usually diagnostic. Localized distention of the stomach is seen with a paucity of distal gas. Often a hairpin loop with the incisura pointing toward the right upper quadrant is noted. The loop remains fixed despite changing the patient's position. Barium swallow shows a "bird-beak" appearance at the esophagogastric junction. There may be evidence of a hiatal hernia, diaphragmatic hernia, or eventration, and the position of the spleen may be deviated (Fig. 48-4). Early diagnosis is essential to avoid gastric rupture.

Treatment

Acute gastric volvulus requires emergent surgical intervention. At laparotomy, a purse-string suture is placed in the wall of the presenting portion of the stomach, and a trocar or tube is inserted to decompress the dilated viscus promptly to relieve distention, prevent ischemia, and facilitate reduction of the volvulus. This is an important first step because it may not be possible to insert a nasogastric tube preoperatively. When the volvulus is reduced, the associated anatomic defects, especially those affecting the diaphragm (eventration, paraesophageal hernia, or congenital diaphragmatic hernia) can be assessed. The stomach should be inspected carefully to ascertain that there are no areas of ischemia requiring resection. Major gastric resection is usually not necessary; however, a local excision of an ischemic area may be indicated. Gastric fixation must be performed to prevent recurrent volvulus. This is accomplished best by performing a Stamm gastrostomy with fixation of the stomach to the anterior abdominal wall. More extensive anterior gastropexy is advocated by some surgeons. Currently, prompt diagnosis and surgical intervention with decompression, reduction, and fixation are associated with a greater than 90% survival.

OTHER CAUSES OF GASTRIC OUTLET OBSTRUCTION

Aberrant Pancreatic Tissue

Aberrant pancreatic tissue in the stomach usually is located in the pyloric muscle and is an uncommon cause of partial pyloric obstruction in infancy. Most infants present with nonbilious vomiting in the first few days after birth. The symptoms are similar to hypertrophic pyloric stenosis and may be mistaken for this entity. Also, pyloric duplication can have a similar clinical presentation. A UGI study shows asymmetric thickening of the pylorus, which can be differentiated from hypertrophic pyloric stenosis. Ultrasonography may be able to differentiate the two entities. The therapy of choice is surgical intervention. At laparotomy, the mass appears as a yellow-brown nodule located in the pylorus. Excision of the nodule or pyloromyotomy often does not relieve the obstruction. Complete excision of the aberrant nodule with a pyloroplasty is the most effective method of relieving the obstruction. If this procedure is not feasible, a gastroduodenostomy can be performed.

Bezoars

Bezoars (trichobezoar, phytobezoar, and, in neonates, lactobezoar) can cause gastric outlet or intestinal obstruction. Trichobezoars often are noted in children with behavioral

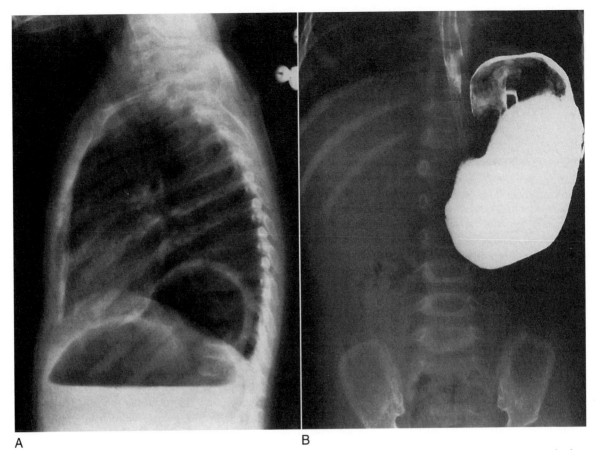

A   B

FIGURE 48-4 ■ **A,** Lateral radiograph of the chest in an infant with eventration of the diaphragm and gastric volvulus. **B,** Contrast study shows the volvulus with the pylorus rotated superiorly.

disorders or mental retardation. These children frequently swallow their own hair and whatever they can get their hands on. Vomiting and failure to thrive are the presenting clinical findings. An epigastric mass, often in the shape of the stomach, may be palpable on physical examination. The diagnosis is recognized easily on a UGI contrast study or by endoscopy. Occasionally, loose bezoars may be broken up and extracted endoscopically. In most patients with complete obstruction, gastrostomy and surgical removal of the intact bezoar is necessary (Fig. 48-5). Attempts at dissolving the bezoar with enzymes (papain) or meat tenderizers have not been efficacious. Phytobezoars are composed mainly of undigested vegetable fibers.

Lactobezoars have been observed in premature infants receiving early feedings of undiluted breast milk. More often lactobezoars are caused by powdered formulas mixed inappropriately and the early premature formulas that were concentrated and had an inappropriate whey-to-casein ratio. The clinical presentation is usually nonbilious emesis and dehydration. The diagnosis usually is suggested by a plain abdominal radiograph and confirmed by UGI study. If the bezoar is not complicated by gastric perforation, conservative nonoperative treatment is the therapy of choice. Cessation of feedings, intravenous hydration, and saline irrigation of the stomach relieve the obstruction. Currently, lactobezoar is an uncommon occurrence.

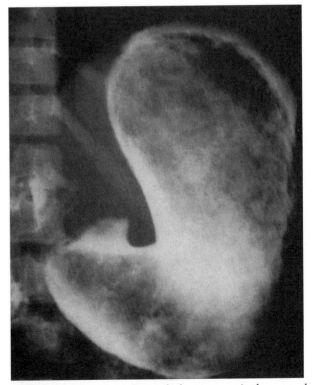

FIGURE 48-5 ■ Contrast radiograph shows a mass in the stomach that proved to be a gastric bezoar.

Pyloric Duplication

Duplications of the stomach and pylorus are uncommon and represent approximately 3% of all duplications in the alimentary tract. Duplications are covered extensively in Chapter 51. The management of only the duplications involving the stomach is described.

Nonbilious vomiting and weight loss are the most common presenting symptoms. A palpable epigastric or right upper quadrant mass may be present. The patient may present in the neonatal period or during the first year of life based on the location in the stomach. Duplication cysts at the pylorus present earlier than cysts attached to the body of the stomach because they produce outlet obstruction. The main differential diagnosis is hypertrophic pyloric stenosis.

Pyloric duplications are slightly more common in females. Gastric and pyloric duplications rarely communicate with the lumen of the stomach and commonly are located in an extramucosal position sharing a common wall. The diagnosis is suggested by an ultrasound examination and contrast studies. In most cases, an extramucosal excision of the mass is possible. If this is not possible, cyst gastrostomy can be performed. If the duplication is extensive, resection of the pyloric area may be necessary.

ACUTE PEPTIC ULCER IN INFANTS AND CHILDREN

Acute peptic ulcers in infancy and childhood are frequently solitary gastric or duodenal lesions. The cause in infants and children is thought to be similar to adults, including *Helicobacter pylori* infection. An ulcer can occur in patients receiving "ulcerogenic" medications, such as steroids, aspirin, or nonsteroidal anti-inflammatory drugs. Stress-related ulcers also have been noted in children suffering from child abuse and children with major systemic disorders, including brain tumors, peritonitis, malnutrition, extensive burns, intestinal pseudo-obstruction, psoriasis, and Reye's syndrome, and medication can be implicated. Acute peptic ulcer can occur in newborns, and approximately 25% of cases are encountered in the first year of life. Hemorrhage is two to three times more common than perforation, and obstruction is a relatively rare occurrence in infancy.

Patients with perforation present in the same manner as infants with spontaneous gastric perforation. There is sudden acute epigastric pain followed by evidence of peritonitis and severe upper abdominal tenderness and muscle guarding on physical examination. Most cases of perforation can be detected by the appearance of free air on an abdominal radiograph.

The therapy of choice for most infants and young children with perforation from an acute peptic ulcer is a simple plication of the site of perforation. In rare situations with multiple perforations affecting the anterior and lateral duodenal wall, a resection may be necessary. Recurrence of a stress ulcer in children is unusual. Prevention of stress-related or medication-related ulcers is the major goal of therapy, and high-risk patients should be treated with acid-suppressing medication. The detailed management of bleeding peptic ulcers and chronic ulcer disease in children is beyond the scope of this chapter.

SUGGESTED READINGS

Acra SA, Nakagawa N, Ghishas FK: Peptic ulcer diseases in children. Compr Ther 17:22, 1991.

This article provides an excellent overview of acute and chronic peptic ulcer disease in childhood.

Grosfeld JL, et al: Gastrointestinal perforation and peritonitis in infants and children: Experience with 179 cases over 10 years. Surgery 120:650, 1996.

This review includes information on spontaneous and iatrogenic gastric perforation in the perspective of other types of gastrointestinal perforation.

Miller DL, Pasquale MD, Seneca RP, et al: Gastric volvulus in the pediatric population. Arch Surg 126:1146, 1991.

A detailed review of the literature concerning gastric volvulus in children is presented. It contains the best data for reference purposes currently available.

Mogilner JG, Vinograd I, Presman A, et al: Pyloric duplication in children. Pediatr Surg Int 5:61, 1990.

This report describes two cases of pyloric duplication and updates the reader on the ultrasound findings in these cases and current surgical trends.

Muller M, Morger R, Engert J: Pyloric atresia: Report of four cases and review of the literature. Pediatr Surg Int 5:276, 1990.

This report from Germany presents the classification of pyloric atresia and updates the subject information available in a literature review.

Neifeld JP, Berman WF, Lawrence W, et al: Management of congenital microgastria with a jejunal reservoir pouch. J Pediatr Surg 15:882, 1980.

This article, one of whose authors (Lawrence) originally described the pouch for patients with a total gastrectomy, was the first to describe this technique in an infant with microgastria.

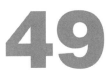

Intestinal Atresia and Stenosis

INTESTINAL ATRESIA AND STENOSIS

Etiology

Goeller is credited with the first description of an ileal atresia in 1684. In 1889, Bland-Sutton proposed a classification of the types of atresia and suggested that they occurred at the site of obliterative embryonic events. In 1900, Tandler proposed the theory that atresia was caused by a lack of recanalization of the solid cord stage of the bowel. Although this theory seemed valid for atresia of the duodenum, most jejunoileal atresias could not be explained by epithelial plugging. In 1912, Spriggs suggested that mechanical accidents, including vascular occlusions, might be responsible for intestinal atresia. The classic experiments reported by Louw and Barnard in 1955 confirmed the role of late prepartum mesenteric vascular accidents as the cause of most intestinal atresias in puppies. These findings were confirmed by several subsequent investigators. Clinical instances of intestinal atresia as a result of intrauterine vascular insults, such as volvulus, internal hernia, intussusception, or constriction of the bowel in a tight gastroschisis defect or omphalocele, supported these experimental studies. In a large series of atresias, 40% to 50% of patients had evidence of either intrauterine bowel necrosis or peritonitis.

Incidence

The incidence of intestinal atresia has been reported to be 1 in 4000 to 5000 live births. Boys and girls are affected equally. Although the mean birth weight in most reports is about 2.7 kg, at least 33% of patients with jejunal atresia, 25% with ileal atresias, and 50% of patients with multiple atresias are of low birth weight. In contrast to infants with duodenal atresia, Down syndrome is uncommon in infants with jejunoileal atresia. Similarly, there is a much lower incidence of associated congenital anomalies. There is a familial pattern of multiple atresias affecting the stomach, duodenum, small bowel, and colon occurring in individuals of French-Canadian background that probably represents a rare autosomal recessive gene inheritance. Other reports of familial atresias involve only the jejunum.

Clinical Presentation

Neonatal intestinal obstruction often manifests with many cardinal signs, including maternal polyhydramnios, bilious vomiting, abdominal distention, and failure to pass normal amounts of meconium in the first 24 to 48 hours of life. Although none of these signs are pathognomonic of a specific obstruction, all are consistent with an obstructive phenomenon and indicate the performance of diagnostic studies. *Polyhydramnios* refers to the presence of excess amniotic fluid in the amniotic sac (>2000 mL). Of amniotic fluid, 25% to 40% is swallowed by the fetus (usually in the fourth or fifth fetal month) and is reabsorbed in the first 25 to 35 cm of jejunum. Jejunal atresia is associated with maternal polyhydramnios in 24% of cases. Although there are other fetal causes of polyhydramnios, any pregnant woman with abnormalities of amniotic fluid should have a prenatal ultrasound examination. Presently, most pregnant women have routine ultrasound screening. The prenatal ultrasound can identify small bowel obstruction associated with atresia, volvulus, and meconium peritonitis. The lesions can be anticipated and an organized management plan developed for delivery and treatment of the infant.

Bilious vomiting is another cardinal sign of intestinal obstruction and is always pathologic. The presence of bile in a gastric aspirate at birth should be investigated carefully. The newborn's stomach usually contains less than 15 mL of clear gastric juice at birth. Greater than 20 to 25 mL of clear gastric juice or any bile may signify the presence of intestinal obstruction. Bilious vomiting also may be seen in instances of neonatal sepsis with adynamic ileus. When mechanical obstruction is present, bile indicates that the level of obstruction is distal to the ampulla of Vater. Bilious vomiting occurs in 85% of infants with jejunal atresia and a lesser number of infants with ileal atresia.

Jaundice occurs in more than 30% of infants with jejunal atresia and 20% with ileal atresia and usually is associated with elevation of the unconjugated fraction of bilirubin. Abdominal distention is a sign of a more distal intestinal obstruction. The normal contour of the newborn abdomen is round, in contrast to the usual scaphoid appearance of the adult. Physical findings associated with distention include visible veins from attenuation of the abdominal wall, visible loops of intestine (intestinal patterning) with or without noticeable peristalsis, and occasionally respiratory distress caused by elevation of the diaphragm.

When obstruction is suspected, recumbent and erect abdominal radiographs must be obtained to evaluate the

TABLE 49-1 ■ Causes of Failure to Pass Meconium After Birth

Distal small intestine or colon atresia
Meconium ileus
Hirschsprung's disease
Meconium plug syndrome
Small left colon syndrome
Infantile neuronal dysplasia
Infant of a diabetic mother
Maternal medications given during
 labor/delivery (e.g., magnesium sulfate)
Sepsis
Hypothyroidism

nature of the distention. Some surgeons use a left lateral decubitus view of the abdomen, particularly in sick, weak infants. Distention may be a result of free air from a perforated viscus, fluid (hemoperitoneum from birth injury to liver, chyloperitoneum), or distended bowel from intestinal obstruction or adynamic ileus. Although distention usually develops 12 to 24 hours after birth, abdominal distention noted immediately at birth suggests the presence of giant cystic meconium peritonitis.

An additional sign of alimentary tract obstruction is failure to pass meconium spontaneously in the first 24 to 48 hours of life. Normal meconium is composed of amniotic fluid and debris (squames, lanugo hairs), succus entericus, and intestinal mucus. Meconium is dark green or black and sticky, and 250 g may be passed rectally. Failure to pass this material the first day of life is often pathologic (Table 49-1). In addition to infants with distal small bowel obstruction, patients with imperforate anus, Hirschsprung's disease, meconium plug syndrome, small left colon syndrome, and colonic neuronal dysplasia may present with failure to pass meconium. Other causes include sepsis with adynamic ileus, hypothyroidism, and narcotic addiction in the mother.

Diagnosis

The diagnosis of jejunoileal atresia usually is confirmed by abdominal x-ray. High jejunal atresia may present with a few air-fluid levels and no further gas beyond that point (Fig. 49-1). The more distal the atresia, the more apparent the clinical abdominal distention and the greater the number of distended intestinal loops and air-fluid levels observed. The atretic loop may be much larger than the other loops of bowel. Occasionally, areas of calcification are seen on plain abdominal radiographs and signify the presence of meconium peritonitis, a sign of intrauterine bowel perforation (12% of patients). The sterile fetal meconium causes a local inflammatory reaction, which includes saponification eventually becoming calcified. In addition, instances of intraluminal calcification ("mummification") may be observed, indicating an antenatal volvulus. In patients with giant cystic meconium peritonitis, plain abdominal radiographs may show an excessively large air-fluid level in a meconium pseudocyst. This type of occurrence is related to a late intrauterine perforation, resulting in an encapsulated mass of perforated bowel and meconium. Because haustral markings rarely are shown on

the abdominal radiograph of a neonate, a contrast enema study must be performed in each case of distal intestinal obstruction. The first enema a newborn should receive is a contrast x-ray enema administered through a soft catheter. Preparation of the colon for this study is unnecessary. The barium or soluble contrast enema study can be used to differentiate small intestine from colonic distention, to determine if the colon is used or unused ("microcolon"), to identify the level of obstruction (e.g., small bowel or colon), and to evaluate the position of the cecum in regard to possible anomalies of intestinal rotation and fixation (Fig. 49-2). Most infants with jejunoileal atresia have a microcolon (unused) on contrast enema study, limiting the obstruction to the small bowel. Microcolon is the result of a lack of distention of the colon because succus entericus does not pass beyond the area of obstruction in the fetal bowel. Malrotation may be observed in 10% of patients with intestinal atresia. There is usually no indication to perform an upper gastrointestinal contrast study in patients with radiographic evidence of complete obstruction; however, in patients with intestinal stenosis who have an incomplete obstruction, this study may be useful.

Differential Diagnosis

Neonates with intestinal obstruction from other causes may present with a clinical picture similar to infants with jejunoileal atresia. These cases include instances of malrotation with or without volvulus, bowel duplication, internal hernia, adynamic ileus with sepsis, meconium ileus, colonic atresia, and total colonic aganglionosis. The two most common causes of distal small bowel obstruction in the newborn are ileal atresia and meconium ileus. The contrast barium enema often yields valuable information that rules out certain causes of obstruction, particularly colon atresia and small bowel aganglionosis. Jejunoileal atresia may coexist with malrotation (10%), meconium peritonitis (12%), meconium ileus (9%), and rarely aganglionosis so that a precise diagnosis beyond obstruction is not always possible. Certain abdominal radiographic findings may help distinguish between instances of ileal atresia and meconium ileus. Infants with uncomplicated meconium ileus often show significant dilation of similar-sized bowel loops with few if any air-fluid levels. A ground-glass appearance in the right lower quadrant (Neuhauser's or "soap bubble" sign) may be observed and represents viscid meconium mixed with air. Although this is not pathognomonic of meconium ileus (e.g., seen in some cases of colon atresia), it is a frequent finding. An enema study commonly shows an unused microcolon similar to cases of ileal atresia; however, reflux of contrast material into the distal ileum may identify the small obstructive concretions of meconium characteristic of this hereditary disorder.

Careful evaluation may avoid unnecessary surgery because at least 50% of these patients with uncomplicated meconium ileus may respond to nonoperative therapy using a hypertonic contrast washout with meglumine diatrizoate (Gastrografin) or other soluble contrast material. Meconium ileus may be complicated by jejunoileal atresia, volvulus, perforation, or giant cystic meconium peritonitis and require operative intervention; the appropriate diagnosis is confirmed at the time of laparotomy. Because 10% of cases of jejunoileal atresia

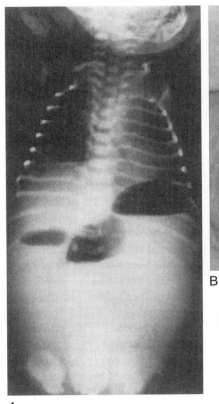

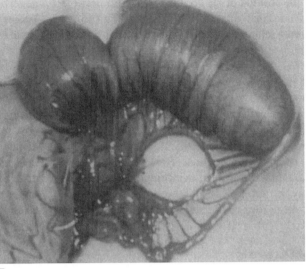

A

FIGURE 49-1 ▪ **A,** Abdominal radiograph in a neonate with bilious vomiting shows a few loops of dilated intestine with air-fluid levels. **B,** At laparotomy, a type I (mucosal) jejunal atresia was observed.

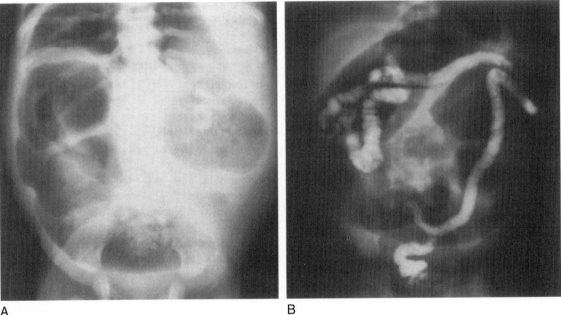

A   B

FIGURE 49-2 ▪ **A,** Abdominal radiograph in a newborn infant with bilious vomiting and abdominal distention shows multiple dilated bowel loops with air-fluid levels. **B,** Barium enema study shows a microcolon, indicating the obstruction is in the distal small bowel. The infant had ileal atresia.

occur in infants with cystic fibrosis, a sweat chloride determination should be obtained in each instance of atresia before hospital discharge.

Pathologic Findings and Classification

Atresias occur slightly more often in the jejunum than in the ileum. Most instances are single (>90%); however, in 10% to 15% of these patients, multiple atresias are observed. The pathologic findings are classified by type (Fig. 49-3). Type I atresias have a mucosal web or diaphragm (possibly from epithelial plugging) with an intact bowel wall and mesentery. Type II atresias have a fibrous cord between two blind ends of the atretic bowel but have an intact mesentery. In type IIIa atresias, there is a complete separation of the blind ends of the atretic bowel by a V-shaped mesenteric gap defect. Type IIIb atresias have an "apple peel" or "Christmas tree" deformity in which fetal occlusion of the proximal superior mesenteric artery occurred with the distal bowel receiving a retrograde blood supply from the ileocolic or right colic artery. Finally, infants with type IV atresias have multiple atresias that often are characterized by a "string-of-sausage" or "string-of-beads" appearance.

Treatment

During the initial evaluation, an orogastric tube is inserted into the stomach, and fluid and electrolyte repletion is accomplished. The umbilical vein should be avoided as a site for fluid administration. Fluid resuscitation is accomplished using 10% dextrose in lactated Ringer's solution given at a rate of 10 mL/kg over 30 minutes while laboratory data are being acquired. Additional fluids may be required to maintain the infant's mean arterial pressure greater than 50 mm Hg and to establish urine flow. A solution of 10% dextrose in 0.25% normal saline is employed for maintenance with potassium chloride added as needed. In most cases, resuscitation and stabilization can be accomplished within a short time, and exploratory laparotomy can be carried out in an expeditious fashion. Perioperative antibiotics, usually ampicillin and gentamicin, are initiated 30 minutes before the procedure.

The infant is taken to the operating room in a thermally neutral environment in an isolette. The operation is done with the patient under well-monitored and controlled general endotracheal anesthesia supplemented with infrared heating lamps and other heating measures. A right upper quadrant transverse supraumbilical incision is ideal in most cases. The abdomen is explored, and the level of obstruction and the type of atresia are determined. In patients with high jejunal atresia, the obstructed proximal dilated atretic segment is often atonic and should be resected back to the ligament of Treitz, provided that there is near-normal bowel length, and an end-to-oblique anastomosis is performed (Fig. 49-4). The distal bowel should be evaluated for additional atresias or stenosis by passage of a soft red rubber catheter or by injection of saline solution. In patients with short-bowel syndrome caused by volvulus, the proximal atretic segment is the only remaining proximal intestine and must be preserved. This can be accomplished by performing an antimesenteric tapering

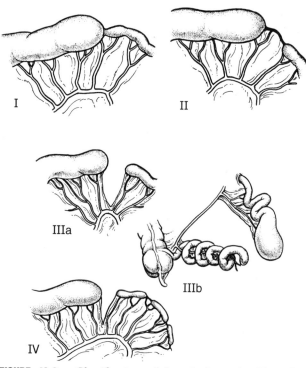

FIGURE 49-3 ■ Classification of intestinal atresia. Type I—mucosal atresia with intact muscularis. Type II—the atretic ends are separated by a fibrous band. Type IIIa—atretic ends are separated by a V-shaped gap defect. Type IIIb—apple peel deformity of the distal atretic segment with retrograde blood supply from the ileocolic or right colic artery. Type IV—multiple atresias (string-of-sausage effect).

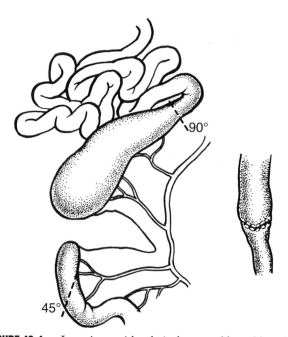

FIGURE 49-4 ■ In patients with relatively normal bowel lengths, the dilated proximal atresia is resected, and an end-to-oblique anastomosis is performed.

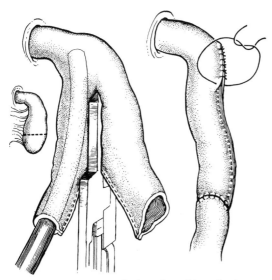

FIGURE 49-5 ■ In infants with short bowel length, the proximal bowel may be preserved by performing a tapering enteroplasty by resection of the antimesenteric border of the bowel using a stapling device.

enteroplasty (Fig. 49-5). An alternative procedure is intestinal imbrication, which also effectively reduces the caliber of distended bowel and allows effective intestinal transit to resume. For the rare infant with very short bowel syndrome and a dilated proximal jejunum, the bowel lengthening procedure described by Bianchi occasionally has been used. Disparity in the size of the dilated proximal bowel and the smaller distal end may be alleviated by an end-to-oblique anastomosis with interrupted 5-0 nonabsorbable sutures.

Most infants with ileal atresia usually have type IIIa pathology, and when reasonably normal bowel length is preserved, operative management includes resection of the dilated atretic loop and an end-to-oblique anastomosis. At the time of the procedure, the distal bowel should be checked for additional areas of atresia or stenosis. In patients with short-bowel syndrome, a tapering ileostomy is performed to preserve an intestinal length compatible with survival. In the presence of severe peritonitis, or when bowel viability is in question, a temporary enterostomy may be required. Infants with ileal atresia who have an intact ileocecal valve have better absorptive capability and survival than infants in whom the ileocecal valve is resected, so if possible, the ileocecal valve should be preserved. This is probably related to prevention of colonization with colonic flora or to improved fat and vitamin B_{12} absorption and an improved enterohepatic circulation of bile from the distal ileum rather than the valve itself (see Chapter 53). In instances of meconium ileus complicated by atresia, bowel resection and anastomosis or temporary enterostomy is required. Anastomotic function may take 7 to 10 days, so the stomach is kept decompressed by an orogastric tube.

Nutritional support is accomplished with postoperative parenteral nutrition until bowel function is restored. When stooling occurs and the gastric volume decreases and clears, the orogastric tube can be removed and feedings instituted. In infants with a temporary enterostomy, feedings can be initiated when stomal function is observed. A low-osmolar, small-curd, easily absorbed formula, such as Pregestimil, or a soybean-based formula can be used. Feedings may be initiated as dilute formulas, then increased in density and volume as tolerated. Most infant formulas contain adequate vitamin and iron supplements. In some formulas that do not contain supplements, iron must be administered on a daily basis for the first year of life: 0.6 mL of ferrous sulfate daily. In instances of short-bowel syndrome, special formulas may be required in addition to long-term total parenteral nutrition to ensure adequate caloric intake for growth. After correction of the obstruction in infants with meconium ileus complicated by atresia, careful family counseling and parental instruction regarding diet, enzyme replacement, and pulmonary toilet using percussion and postural drainage must be done. The parents also must be made aware that these children are at risk of developing meconium ileus equivalent even after several years.

Another less common cause of small bowel obstruction in newborns is intrinsic small bowel stenosis. This condition probably is related to an ischemic injury. These patients present with abdominal distention and bilious vomiting but have a normal contrast enema study and pass meconium within the first 24 hours of life (Fig. 49-6). The indication for operation is continued evidence of partial intestinal obstruction and failure to thrive.

Morbidity and Mortality

The most common cause of death in patients with jejunoileal atresia is infection related to pneumonia, peritonitis, or sepsis. The most significant postoperative complications include functional intestinal obstruction at the site of the anastomosis and anastomotic leak. Other factors that affect morbidity and mortality include respiratory distress, prematurity, short-bowel syndrome, and postoperative volvulus with infarction. In the past, the survival of patients with jejunal atresia was lower than patients with ileal atresia. An increased mortality also was seen in patients with multiple atresias (57%); apple peel atresias (71%); and when atresia was associated with meconium ileus, meconium peritonitis, and gastroschisis. In more recent years, because of improved neonatal intensive care, pediatric anesthesia, total parenteral nutrition, and a better understanding of the overall management of these patients, the survival rate has increased dramatically to 85% to 90% for infants with jejunal and ileal atresia treated at major pediatric surgical centers.

COLON ATRESIA AND STENOSIS

Colon atresia and stenosis as an isolated entity (unassociated with imperforate anus or cloacal exstrophy) is a relatively infrequent cause of neonatal intestinal obstruction. Bininger described the first case in 1673. In 1922, Gaub reported survival of an infant with atresia of the colon after performing a colostomy. The first successful anastomosis for an infant with colon atresia was reported by Potts in 1947.

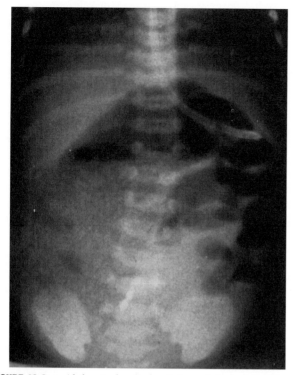

FIGURE 49-6 ■ Abdominal radiograph in an infant with abdominal distention and bilious vomiting. A meconium-filled mass fills the right lower quadrant.

Incidence

The incidence of colon atresia in reported series ranges from 1 in 15,000 to 20,000 live births. The latter figure is probably more correct because most major children's surgical centers see approximately one case per year. In regard to other alimentary tract atresias, only pyloric atresia occurs with less regularity. Some reports suggest that associated anomalies are common. If cases of colon atresia in association with cloacal exstrophy with vesicointestinal fissure and abdominal wall defects (gastroschisis and omphalocele) are excluded, however, the incidence of associated anomalies in infants with colon atresia as an isolated event is low. Colon atresia has been noted in infants with Hirschsprung's disease, jejunal atresia, and some skeletal anomalies including syndactyly and polydactyly on rare occasions.

Etiology

Similar to instances of jejunoileal atresia and stenosis, most cases of colonic atresia and stenosis are the result of in utero vascular compromise of the mesentery to the large bowel. The areas that are most affected are the transverse and sigmoid colon, which have a floppy mesentery and may be prone to volvulus in utero. Atresia also may occur in the right colon.

Classification

The classification of colon atresia is the same as the classification given atresias of the small bowel, but apple peel deformity does not occur in the colon.

Clinical Presentation and Diagnosis

Most infants with isolated colon atresia are usually term and rarely have associated anomalies. Failure to pass meconium in the first 24 hours of life, abdominal distention, and bilious vomiting are the usual clinical manifestations. Erect and recumbent abdominal radiographs show dilated intestine with air-fluid levels and a particularly dilated segment at the point of obstruction. The atretic loop may have a soap bubble appearance from the admixture of meconium and air. Some cases are complicated by perforation and have massive pneumoperitoneum. The diagnosis is confirmed by a contrast enema study that shows a blind distal end of a microcolon. Most instances of colon atresia are type IIIa with a V-shaped gap between the atretic ends (see Fig. 49-6). The sigmoid colon is the second most common site of colon atresia. Rare type I mucosal atresia and type II atresia are more common in the distal colon.

Treatment

The initial resuscitation and management of infants with colon atresia is essentially the same as infants with jejunoileal atresia. At the time of laparotomy, the atretic segment is delivered and inspected. The presence of proximal intestinal (jejunal) and other colon atresias should be ruled out. We, as most, have treated all infants with colon atresia with a preliminary colostomy and subsequent closure with an end-to-oblique ileocolic or colocolic anastomosis at age 3 to 6 months. Some surgeons recommend performing a primary anastomosis for atresia occurring in the right-sided or transverse colon and a temporary colostomy for instances of atresia affecting the sigmoid colon. Surgeons in favor of primary anastomosis in the neonatal period for right-sided atresias recommend resecting the entire atretic segment including the ileocecal valve and performing an ileocolic anastomosis. Complicated cases, such as colon atresia in association with proximal jejunal atresia, are managed best by jejunojejunostomy and distal colostomy. Initial colostomy also is recommended for instances of colon atresia occurring in a patient with gastroschisis.

Results

The current survival for infants with isolated colon atresia is 90% to 100%. Mortality usually is limited to the occasional infant with associated anomalies or when there is a long delay in diagnosis complicated by perforation and peritonitis.

SUGGESTED READINGS

Louw JH, Barnard CN: Congenital intestinal atresia: Observations on its origin. Lancet 2:1065, 1955.

This classic report describes the experiments that documented intrauterine vascular compromise as the cause of most intestinal atresias.

Newman K: Jejunoileal atresia. In Oldham KT, et al (eds): Surgery of Infants and Children: Scientific Principles and Practice. Philadelphia, Lippincott-Raven, 1997, p 1193.

This chapter provides an excellent up-to-date review of intestinal atresia and postoperative care considerations.

Rescorla FJ, Grosfeld JL: Intestinal atresia and stenosis: Analysis of survival in 120 cases. Surgery 98:668, 1985.

This report concerning a large group of infants with intestinal atresia, including colon atresia, documents the currently improved survival data.

50

Meckel's Diverticulum

Although first described 2 centuries earlier, the anatomist Meckel in 1809 identified the origin of the omphalomesenteric duct and called attention to the anatomic abnormality that bears his name as a cause of disease. *Meckel's diverticulum* is caused by a failure of regression of the vitelline duct, a process that normally occurs between 5 and 7 weeks' gestation. Meckel's diverticula are true diverticula with all normal intestinal layers being present. The blood supply is a remnant from the primitive right vitelline artery and arises directly from the mesentery. Obliteration of the vitelline duct at the level of the intestine and persistent patency of the subumbilical area leads to the formation of a vitelline duct sinus. In some instances, proximal and distal obliteration occurs, with the central portion of the duct remaining patent, forming a vitelline duct cyst. In other instances, the entire vitelline duct lumen may obliterate, but the attachment from the undersurface of the umbilicus to the bowel persists as a fibrous cord; volvulus around the band may occur, resulting in intestinal obstruction (Fig. 50-1).

Meckel's diverticulum is the most common congenital anomaly of the gastrointestinal tract and is present in approximately 2% of the population. There is a frequent association with other congenital anomalies, such as cardiac defects, omphalocele, esophageal atresia, malrotation, Hirschsprung's disease, duodenal atresia, and Down syndrome. More than 70% of symptomatic patients with Meckel's diverticulum have heterotopic gastric mucosa in the tip; another 5% have heterotopic pancreatic tissue (Fig. 50-2). For the 95% of patients who are asymptomatic, the occurrence of heterotopic tissue in the diverticulum is less than 15%.

SYMPTOMS

The "rule of 2" often is cited in association with Meckel's diverticulum: 2% incidence, two types of heterotopic mucosa, located within 2 feet of the ileocecal valve, approximately 2 inches in length, and usually symptomatic by 2 years of age. Symptoms result primarily from hemorrhage (40%), obstruction (35%), or inflammation (17%) (Table 50-1). Symptoms related to vitelline duct anomalies vary indirectly with patient age (Table 50-2). In newborns, intestinal obstruction is the most common presentation, whereas bleeding is noted more frequently in slightly older infants and young children. More than 95% of Meckel's diverticula are clinically silent. Surgical removal is indicated if symptoms occur. Whether an asymptomatic, incidentally discovered diverticulum should be removed is controversial.

The most common presentation of Meckel's diverticulum is painless and occasionally massive lower gastrointestinal bleeding, usually in children younger than age 5 years. The stools are characteristically maroon in color and unassociated with vomiting or hematemesis. In many cases, bleeding subsides for a period but recurs intermittently. Bleeding is occasionally excessive and may require blood transfusion. Occasional patients may have melena or hematochezia; however, occult bleeding with anemia is uncommon. Although spontaneous cessation of bleeding is the general rule, occasionally life-threatening hemorrhage may occur. Bleeding is a result of peptic ulceration, commonly located at the base of the diverticulum at the junction of ectopic gastric mucosa and normal ileal mucosa. Occasionally the bleeding may occur in the diverticulum itself.

The second most common presenting symptom with Meckel's diverticula or other vitelline duct anomalies is intestinal obstruction. Obstruction usually occurs in the first few months of life and may be caused by (1) prolapse through a patent vitelline duct, (2) volvulus around a fibrous band originating at the diverticulum and attached to the underside of the umbilicus, or (3) an internal hernia beneath the aberrant right vitelline artery or fibrous band arising from the mesentery and ileocolic intussusception with an inverted Meckel's diverticulum acting as a lead point. Attempted reduction of intussusception caused by Meckel's diverticulum by either a hydrostatic barium enema or air enema is usually unsuccessful, and resection is indicated in any case. Volvulus around a vitelline duct cyst or band may be associated with vascular compromise of the intestine. Rarely, patients with intestinal obstruction from incarcerated inguinal or umbilical hernias have Meckel's diverticulum trapped in the hernia defect (Littre's hernia).

The third most common presentation of Meckel's diverticulum is inflammation, which usually gives a clinical picture similar to that of appendicitis. If the appendix is normal during laparotomy for suspected appendicitis, a careful search for a Meckel's diverticulum should be made.

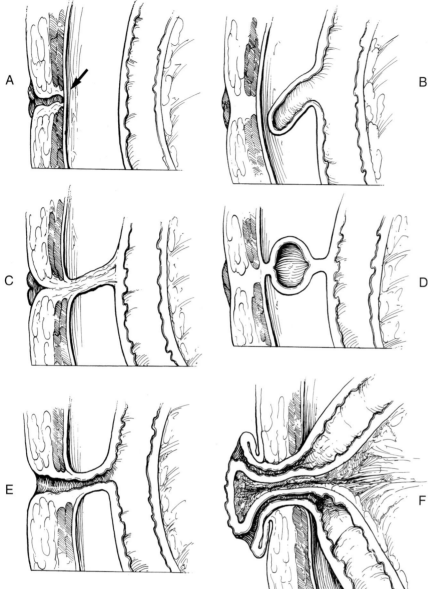

FIGURE 50-1 ■ Various vitelline duct anomalies. **A,** Vitelline duct sinus. The portion of the vitelline duct attached to the bowel has involuted or obliterated; however, a sinus tract remains patent in the umbilicus. **B,** Meckel's diverticulum. The umbilical portion of the primitive vitelline duct has obliterated, leaving an antimesenteric diverticulum communicating with the normal ileum. The diverticulum can bleed, become inflamed, perforate, and act as a lead point for an intussusception. **C,** Persistent fibrous cord. The vitelline duct can be completely obliterated by fibrous tissue; however, volvulus around this band can result in intestinal obstruction. **D,** Vitelline duct cyst. A cystic structure may occur when the umbilical and the bowel margins of the duct obliterate but the central portion remains patent. **E,** Patent vitelline duct. Complete patency of the duct may occur and is characterized by passage of gas or bilious drainage from the umbilicus. **F,** Prolapse. Occasionally a T-shaped prolapse of the proximal and the distal bowel may occur through a patent vitelline duct.

The inflammation often is related to the heterotopic gastric mucosa or pancreatic tissue in the diverticulum. Perforation with diffuse peritonitis or localized abscess occasionally occurs. These patients require aggressive fluid resuscitation and preoperative antibiotic therapy, such as cefoxitin or a combination of ampicillin, gentamicin, and clindamycin or metronidazole. Meckel's diverticulitis is treated by resection, either of the diverticulum alone or together with the involved adjacent ileum. Primary reanastomosis is usually possible; however, on rare occasions, if the child is very ill, exteriorization may be advisable.

Occasional reports have described foreign bodies (e.g., fish or chicken bone) impacted in a Meckel's diverticulum. Stones also have been reported, and even parasitic infections (e.g., ascariasis and schistosomiasis) have been observed in diverticula on rare occasions.

Primary gastrointestinal cancer has been reported sporadically in patients with Meckel's diverticula. Carcinoids, sarcoma, lymphoma, adenocarcinoma, and leiomyoma all have been reported. These lesions are observed rarely in children and are more often a complication in adults. Carcinoids are the most common tumors occurring in Meckel's diverticula and resemble carcinoids found in the appendix in that they are usually small, are asymptomatic, and occur singly. Carcinoids arising from Meckel's diverticula are immunophenotypically and biologically more similar to jejunoileal carcinoids, however, which have a greater metastatic potential than appendiceal carcinoids. Secondary primary cancer occasionally occurs in patients with carcinoids of a Meckel's diverticulum. Resection of the ileal segment that contains the Meckel's diverticulum and its associated mesentery is the treatment of choice.

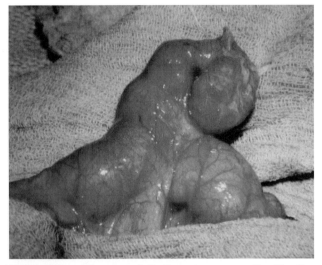

FIGURE 50-2 ■ The typical findings in a case of a bleeding Meckel's diverticulum. The distal part of the diverticulum is thickened where ectopic gastric mucosa is present, and the tip is attached to the site of a bleeding ulcer. Resection with end-to-end anastomosis was done.

TABLE 50-1 ■ Meckel's Diverticulum: Incidence of Complications		
Condition	All Patients (%)	Symptomatic Patients (%)
Bleeding	22	38-56
Obstruction	13	33-42
Inflammation	2	6-14
Umbilical pathology	2	5-6

DIAGNOSIS

Diagnosis of a persistent vitelline duct remnant may be established by performing a lateral contrast x-ray or an umbilical sonogram. Injection of the contrast solution into the external opening usually shows the dye extending into the bowel lumen. The differential diagnosis of draining umbilical lesions includes umbilical granuloma, the most common umbilical abnormality in the newborn, which usually resolves after topical application of silver nitrate. Persistent drainage also may result from an urachal sinus, patent urachus, vitelline duct sinus, or patent vitelline duct. The lateral contrast study or sonogram often shows

TABLE 50-2 ■ Meckel's Diverticulm: Age at Presentation (n = 217)	
	Mean Age (yr)
Symptomatic patients	2.4
Obstruction	0.6
Bleeding	2.8
Inflammation	8.2
Asymptomatic patients	7.1

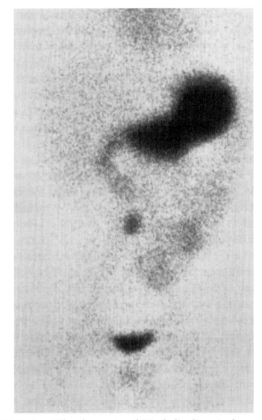

FIGURE 50-3 ■ The diagnosis of Meckel's diverticulum can be obtained by a technetium-99m scintiscan. The isotope can be seen in the stomach and bladder, and the diverticulum is seen in the midabdomen.

extraperitoneal passage of the contrast material inferiorly toward the bladder or even directly into the bladder.

The diagnosis of bleeding Meckel's diverticulum may be made by a technetium-99m pertechnetate isotope scan, which images the gastric mucosa (Fig. 50-3). Administration of pentagastrin enhances technetium scintigraphy. Pentagastrin, 6 μg/kg, is administered 20 minutes before injecting the technetium-99m isotope. Cimetidine causes retention of the radioactive tracer in the gastric secretions of cells and enhances scanning. This scan should be the initial test performed when Meckel's diverticulum is suspected. Barium enema or small bowel radiographic contrast studies are not only futile and unreliable in showing the presence of a Meckel's diverticulum, but also the contrast may interfere with the scintiscans. Although some reports suggest that the isotope is picked up by parietal cells, the isotope is actually taken up by mucus-secreting gastric mucosal cells in the stomach and the ectopic gastric mucosa. Multiple scan views should be obtained to avoid false-negative studies. Changing the patient's position moves the Meckel's diverticulum away from the bladder, where the isotope also may be concentrated. A Foley catheter may be required to eliminate isotope collected in a full bladder, which may obscure uptake from the Meckel's diverticulum. The accuracy of the technetium scan for Meckel's diverticulum is approximately 90%.

Ectopic gastric mucosa also may occur in patients with intestinal duplications, which should be included in the differential diagnosis of rectal bleeding. Other causes of rectal bleeding in children, such as hemangioma, Peutz-Jeghers polyps, nonspecific ileal ulcer, juvenile polyps of the colon, and ulcerative colitis, are ruled out by a positive scintiscan for ectopic gastric mucosa. If the patient is actively bleeding, a visceral angiogram occasionally may be diagnostic when the rate of blood loss is greater than 0.5 to 1.0 mL/min. Tagged red blood cell studies have less sensitivity and less specificity and are rarely necessary. If the Meckel's scan is negative, gastroduodenal endoscopy and colonoscopy should be carried out to look for other sources of bleeding. *Helicobacter pylori* has been isolated only rarely from the ectopic gastric mucosa in Meckel's diverticula and is not believed to be a factor in the inflammation or bleeding complications associated with the lesion.

SURGICAL THERAPY

When the diagnosis of a symptomatic Meckel's diverticulum or other vitelline duct anomaly has been established, surgical resection of the lesion should be performed. Simple diverticulectomy with transverse closure of the ileum is satisfactory treatment for most patients. If there is ulceration or involvement of the ileum at the base of the diverticulum, resection of the involved small bowel and a primary end-to-end anastomosis is recommended. Care should be taken to ligate the separate blood supply to the Meckel's diverticulum, which usually enters the diverticulum directly from the small bowel mesentery. Long-term follow-up of patients comparing simple diverticulectomy versus bowel resection and anastomosis shows no significant difference with respect to late complications between the two groups. Operative reduction of intussusception caused by Meckel's diverticulum as a lead point is rarely feasible and usually requires resection of the obstructed bowel with end-to-end anastomosis. For Meckel's diverticulum with perforation, resection and end-to-end anastomosis commonly is performed if the patient is stable and extensive contamination of the peritoneal cavity has not occurred. For patients who are hemodynamically unstable and who have significant peritoneal soiling, an expeditious temporary enterostomy can be performed. In neonates with a persistent vitelline duct, an infraumbilical curvilinear incision is useful to enter the peritoneal cavity. The duct is identified and traced down to the area of ileum, where it is attached. The portion of the duct attached to bowel can be excised either with resection and primary suture closure of the antimesenteric wall of the small bowel or with a stapling device. Laparoscopic resection of Meckel's diverticulum has been reported with increased frequency with good results.

Although no one questions the need to resect a symptomatic vitelline duct anomaly, controversy persists regarding resection of asymptomatic lesions observed as incidental findings during a laparotomy for other intra-abdominal conditions. The high incidence of symptomatic lesions noted in infants and young children suggests that elective resection of incidental Meckel's diverticulum

probably is indicated. As the patient grows older, the risk of symptomatic complications from a diverticulum seems to decrease. There is no evidence to indicate that resection of a Meckel's diverticulum in older children or adults is necessary because the lifetime risk of a complication occurring from the lesion is only 6%. Resection should be performed, however, if ectopic mucosa is suspected or if the diverticulum is attached to the mesentery or the undersurface of the umbilicus by persistent fibrous bands. Although complications of Meckel's diverticulum rarely may be life-threatening, studies of large numbers of patients with these lesions have been associated with low morbidity and mortality (<2%), related largely to the management of the diverticulum itself. The most common complication after removal of a Meckel's diverticulum is adhesive bowel obstruction, occurring in 5% to 9% of patients. The mortality rate of elective resection for asymptomatic patients should approach zero. The reported mortality rate for the complications of Meckel's diverticula ranges from 1% to 10%.

SUGGESTED READINGS

Soltero MJ, Bill AH: The natural history of Meckel's diverticulum and its relation to incidental removal: A study of 202 cases of diseased Meckel's diverticulum found in King County, Washington over a 15 year period. Am J Surg 132:168-173, 1976.

This is a classic review of the lifetime risk of complications associated with Meckel's diverticulum (4.2% in this series of 202 patients). The risk of complications decreased with the age of the patients.

St. Vil D, Brandt ML, Panic S, et al: Meckel's diverticulum in children: A 20 year review. J Pediatr Surg 26:1289, 1991.

This report reviews a large series of cases of Meckel's diverticulum (n = 164) with a mean age of 5.2 years. The authors document 8.4% morbidity and zero mortality in 117 patients with complications and 6% mortality and 4% complication rate in 25 asymptomatic patients who had an incidental diverticulum resected. The overall morbidity and mortality was 7.3% and 1.8%.

Vane DW, West KW, Grosfeld JL: Vitelline duct anomalies: Experience with 217 childhood cases. Arch Surg 122:542, 1987.

This large retrospective review of 217 infants and children with vitelline duct anomalies documents a relationship of young age and presence of ectopic mucosa with symptomatic lesions. The incidence of symptomatic lesions in infants less than 2 years old was 45%. The overall mortality was 1%. There was no morbidity or mortality observed when resection was performed for an incidental diverticulum.

Yahchouchy EK, Marano AF, Etienne JCF, et al: Meckel's diverticulum. J Am Coll Surg 192:658-662, 2001.

This review summarizes data from several previous reports; the cumulative incidence for operation for complications of Meckel's diverticulum during a lifetime was 6.4%. The overall rate of morbidity of incidental removal of Meckel's diverticulum was 2%. The risk of complications was not found to decrease with age. The authors note that the benefit of incidental diverticulectomy outweighed its attending morbidity and mortality.

Duplications of the Gastrointestinal Tract

51

The term *duplication* is probably a misnomer because most cases are really enteric cysts and not true duplications. The word *duplication* first was used by Fitz, but Ladd used the term to simplify the classification of many forms of the anomaly, including enteric cysts, various forms of diverticula, and truly duplicated small and large intestine. Ladd's classification is used today.

Duplications may occur as a result of abnormal events that take place during the embryologic development of the gastrointestinal (GI) tract. This explanation is based on the occasional association of one or more duplications with GI anomalies, such as atresia or malrotation. Abnormal splitting of the notochord has been suggested to be responsible for the occurrence of neurenteric cysts associated with hemivertebra. Other theories include abnormal fetal luminal canalization or formation of abnormal diverticula and sequestration of portions of endoderm during development. Because duplications take many different forms, a single embryologic theory to explain the cause is probably not valid.

PATHOLOGY

Approximately 75% of duplications are located within the abdomen; 20% are in the thorax; 5% are thoracoabdominal; and the remainder occur at unusual sites, such as the base of the tongue (Fig. 51-1). Of these malformations, 75% are enteric cysts that do not communicate with the lumen of the bowel, and the remaining 25% are true tubular duplications or doubling anomalies that usually communicate with the visceral lumen (Fig. 51-2 and Table 51-1).

All duplications possess at least one coat of smooth muscle, and they are attached intimately to the adjacent portion of the GI tract, sharing a common wall. The relatively thick substance of the wall of a duplication makes it easy to differentiate from the typical thin-walled mesenteric cyst. Duplication cysts typically share a common mesenteric wall with the intestine, as opposed to Meckel's diverticulum, which arises on the antimesenteric border. The lining of the duplication always is composed of some type of GI mucosa. Approximately 25% of duplications have ectopic tissue present, and most of the time it is gastric. In the case of tubular duplications communicating with the normal intestinal lumen, severe peptic

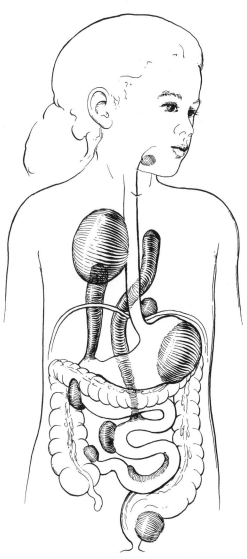

FIGURE 51-1 ■ The many locations where duplications of the alimentary tract may occur (shaded areas). Most are noncommunicating cystic duplications of the terminal ileum, but all parts of the GI tract may be involved. Some are thoracoabdominal.

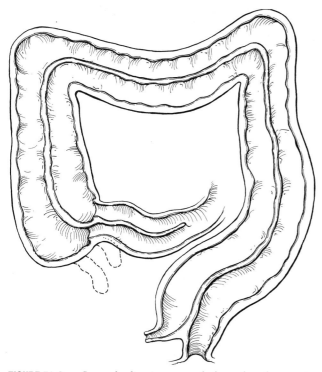

FIGURE 51-2 ■ Some duplications are tubular rather than cystic. Typically the type of duplication depicted here involves the distal intestine or colon. Bleeding is a frequent complication because of the presence of gastric mucosa in many tubular duplications.

ulceration and exsanguinating bleeding may be a significant problem. The mucosal lining of an individual duplication, although enteric, does not always correspond to the typical mucosa of that level of the GI tract where the duplication is found. Occasionally two or three types of visceral lining are found.

In instances in which duplications do not communicate with the adjacent normal lumen, the fluid content is ordinarily clear, colorless, and thinly mucoid. The pH is usually alkaline, but it may be acid in the presence of gastric mucosa. With either high internal pressure or peptic ulceration, blood may be present in the fluid within the duplication. If the duplication communicates with the adjacent lumen, intestinal content is seen. Pancreatic enzymes may be present within the fluid in the occasional

TABLE 51-1 ■ Incidence of Duplications	
Duplications	**%**
Abdominal	75
Thoracic	20
Thoracoabdominal	4
Other	1
Ectopic lining	25
Gastric	20
Other GI	2
Pancreatic	3
Multiple	10

instances in which ectopic pancreatic tissue is present, although these enzymes are usually not activated.

Duplications vary greatly in size and shape. Most are 2 to 4 cm in diameter, round, and cystic, as often seen in the ileocecal area, and can reach huge sizes that may fill the entire thorax. Only in rare cases do the cystic duplications communicate with the adjacent normal bowel. Some duplications resemble giant diverticula extending from one side of the intestine and running adjacent to it for several centimeters, within the mesentery, or extending to distant sites including the mediastinum. Other tubular duplications are attached intimately to a long length of intestine or colon and communicate at one end or the other with the normal bowel. These duplications are generally long and frequently contain large amounts of ectopic gastric lining. When tubular duplications involve the colon and rectum, there may be associated anomalies, such as partial duplication of the external and internal genitalia, rectourethral or rectovaginal fistulas, and duplications of the urinary tract.

CLINICAL PRESENTATION

Approximately one third of patients with duplications present as newborns, another third in the first 2 years of life, and the remainder after that time. Antenatal diagnosis is increasingly frequent. The fact that more than two thirds of patients are recognized before 2 years of age indicates that symptoms become evident early in life, although many still are discovered incidentally. The most common presentation is that of partial intestinal obstruction because an enterogenous cyst or tubular duplication limits the lumen of the adjacent normal intestine. Additionally, accumulation of a large amount of fluid within an enteric cyst may produce abdominal pain. If a duplication becomes excessively large, it may compress adjacent mesenteric vasculature, compromising the adjacent intestine and causing pain, bleeding, or intestinal necrosis. Finally, if a large amount of gastric mucosa is present, peptic ulceration or erosion into adjacent structures may occur. If duplications are located within the thorax, they occasionally may encroach sufficiently on the trachea or lung to produce respiratory embarrassment, or if located strategically within the wall of the esophagus, they may produce dysphagia.

DIAGNOSIS

Plain abdominal films are rarely of diagnostic help. Ultrasound is particularly helpful in screening the abdomen for cystic forms of the anomaly or for large distended tubular duplications. Upper GI radiographic studies and barium enema studies generally are not useful unless it is determined beforehand that there may be a communication between the duplication and the adjacent normal intestinal lumen. Computed tomography (CT) of the abdomen is also useful for diagnostic purposes, but ultrasound is generally sufficient to make a diagnosis sufficient to justify laparotomy. For thoracic duplications, CT with oral contrast material is the preferred approach to diagnostic imaging, and it has virtually replaced the routine barium esophagogram because it provides more

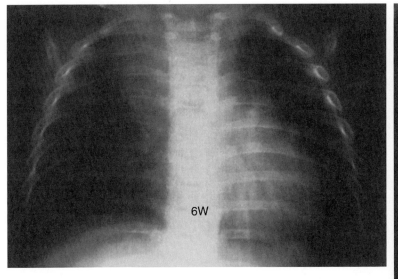

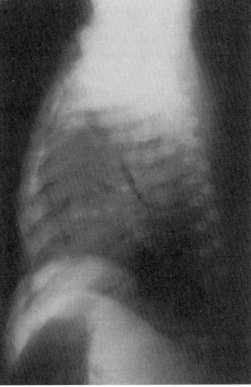

FIGURE 51-3 ■ This 6-week-old infant presented with respiratory stridor. The anteroposterior and lateral films show a large right posterior mediastinal mass, which was shown to be an esophageal duplication cyst by MRI (see Fig. 51-4).

precise information about a thoracic cyst and its relationship to adjacent structures (Fig. 51-3). Endoscopy may be an important diagnostic tool for occasional patients with complicated duplications of the colon and rectum associated with doubling anomalies of the lower genitourinary tract. On CT with intravenous contrast material or magnetic resonance imaging (MRI), an enterogenous cyst usually has contrast enhancement of the outer wall of the cyst but none within it (Fig. 51-4). This pattern helps to differentiate the cyst from a neurogenic tumor such as a neuroblastoma. CT of the chest is also helpful in terms of evaluating a possible communication with the neural canal. MRI, particularly when combined with MRI cholangiopancreatography, is an increasingly useful method for defining the anatomy of pancreaticoduodenal area lesions or if the patient has pancreatitis. In instances in which GI mucosa is believed to be present within a long tubular duplication cyst of the intestine or thorax, a technetium-99m scintiscan using pentagastrin stimulation for enhancement may be diagnostic. If a duplication is found in either the abdomen or the chest, the other body cavity should be screened with ultrasound because 10% of patients have more than one duplication.

ABDOMINAL DUPLICATIONS

Stomach

Almost all gastric duplications are cystic and may occur anywhere within the stomach. A barium upper GI series usually shows a smooth-outlined filling defect impinging on the gastric lumen along the greater curvature (Fig. 51-5). Ultrasound confirms the cystic nature of the lesion. Frequently, when gastric duplications become

evident in neonates, they produce abdominal distention, a large mass, and vomiting. If gastric bleeding occurs, it is usually the result of compromise of mucosal blood supply related to increasing tension within the duplication cyst. Complete excision with primary closure of the stomach is usually possible, but in the case of large duplications, it is sometimes necessary to excise the cyst partially and strip

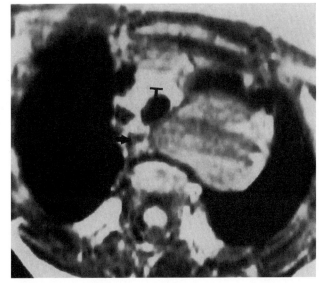

FIGURE 51-4 ■ MRI of patient in Figure 51-3 shows a large right posterior esophageal duplication cyst impinging on the trachea (T) and attached to the esophagus (arrow). MRI is useful for the evaluation of the spinal canal in patients with thoracic duplications with an intradural component.

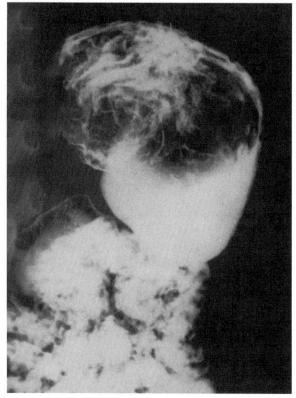

FIGURE 51-5 ■ Barium contrast study shows a large fundic filling defect caused by a cystic duplication of the stomach. The patient presented with vomiting and mild hematemesis.

the mucosa from the common wall or to drain the lesion internally into the stomach.

Duodenum

Duodenal duplications may be either cystic or diverticular. They tend to cause compression of the first or second portions of the duodenum, producing partial obstruction. Whenever possible, they should be excised completely, but frequently the location on the mesenteric border of the duodenal duplication makes this approach unfeasible because of potential danger to the common bile and pancreatic ducts. These lesions are managed best by duodenotomy, partial excision and mucosal stripping, or a re-entry procedure. If internal drainage into the duodenum is not possible, Roux-en-Y drainage into the jejunum may be necessary. Cholangiography should be performed when indicated.

Small Intestine

Duplications are found most commonly in the ileum or jejunum. Ultrasound may be a helpful adjunct, but most imaging modalities are unrevealing. The most common presentation is partial intestinal obstruction or abdominal pain, but occasionally the mode of presentation is severe GI bleeding (Fig. 51-6). Sometimes small intestinal duplications are found incidentally at the time of correction of intestinal atresia or other newborn anomalies associated with intestinal obstruction. Some duplications produce small bowel intussusception or intestinal volvulus in association with signs and symptoms of

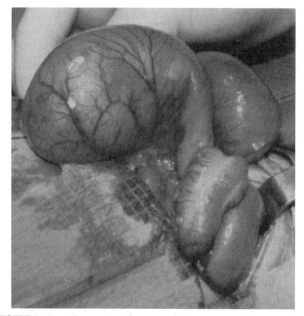

FIGURE 51-6 ■ Operative photograph shows a typical cystic ileal duplication that caused partial intestinal obstruction.

intestinal obstruction. Approximately 10% of patients with small bowel duplications have associated thoracic duplications.

Most small bowel duplications are cystic, and they can be managed by primary resection and end-to-end anastomosis. With long tubular diverticular duplications of the small intestine, complete resection is usually possible. In the case of complete duplication of the small bowel, patients may be managed by partial resection with internal drainage at the distal end. If gastric mucosa is present, mucosal stripping facilitated by sequential transverse incisions and eversion of the lining should be performed to avoid subsequent GI hemorrhage. The most common site for ectopic gastric mucosa is in the ileum.

Colon and Rectum

Patients with colonic and rectal duplications frequently have associated anomalies, including exstrophy of the cloaca, double urethra and vagina, spina bifida, and omphalocele. Other genitourinary anomalies frequently are seen. Partial intestinal obstruction associated with abdominal pain is the primary presenting symptom, but many patients with hindgut duplications are asymptomatic. Hemorrhage rarely occurs with colonic duplications because they rarely contain gastric mucosa, as opposed to ileal and esophageal duplications, in which ectopic gastric lining frequently is found.

Similar to small intestinal duplications, those found in the colon and rectum are treated best by resection and primary anastomosis. In most instances, rectal duplications can be excised with preservation of the anal canal either through the abdomen or via a posterior sagittal approach. Protective colostomy occasionally may be required.

For the long tubular double colon, it is usually sufficient to provide internal drainage at the distal end because both walls seem to have propulsive capability. Thorough imaging is required for appropriate planning

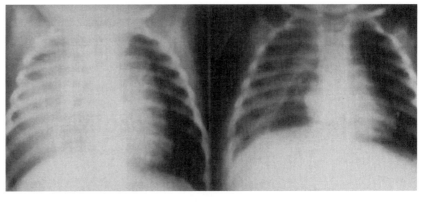

FIGURE 51-7 ■ Composite of two chest films shows a large right-sided thoracoabdominal gastric duplication that looked opaque when full (left) and air filled when it emptied into the native stomach (right). Thoracoabdominal duplications frequently have different appearances on radiography, making evaluation difficult on plain film alone, so CT or MRI is usually necessary.

of operative management of complicated colorectal duplications associated with genitourinary anomalies.

THORACIC DUPLICATIONS

Almost all thoracic duplications are cystic and are located within the posterior mediastinum. Occasionally, these lesions may be present at the base of the tongue or anywhere along the esophagus, but most commonly they are in the lower half of the esophagus. When the lesions are large, there may be respiratory embarrassment and associated shift of the mediastinum to the contralateral side. Approximately 30% of esophageal duplications have ectopic gastric mucosa, and frequently bleeding and erosion into adjacent structures are problematic. Esophageal duplications are seen occasionally in association with posterolateral diaphragmatic hernia and esophageal atresia.

Esophageal duplications virtually always can be excised completely, although at times the procedure may be complicated because of severe inflammation related to peptic ulceration within the cyst. Care should be taken to avoid injury to the esophagus, but if it occurs, primary repair and protective gastrostomy usually takes care of the problem. Because 10% of patients with thoracic duplications have associated abdominal duplications, abdominal ultrasound should be performed for screening purposes in any patient found to have a thoracic duplication. In patients with thoracic duplications associated with vertebral anomalies, CT, CT myelography, or MRI of the spine and mediastinum should be performed to determine whether an intraspinal component exists because, when present, it should be excised as well.

THORACOABDOMINAL DUPLICATIONS

Duplications involving the abdomen and the chest are unusual and usually represent long diverticula originating from the stomach or intestine extending into the chest (Fig. 51-7). Symptoms may be related simply to distention of the intrathoracic portion of the cyst, or if gastric lining is present, there may be hemorrhage or diarrhea related to passage of excessive acid secretions into the intestinal tract. Similar to thoracic duplications, thoracoabdominal duplications are more than twice as common on the right than on the left. Complete resection of thoracoabdominal duplications is required, and this usually entails separate thoracic and abdominal incisions. The procedure may be performed in one or two stages, depending on the condition of the patient.

SUGGESTED READINGS

Alrabeeah A, Gillis DA, Giacomantonio M, et al: Neurenteric cysts—a spectrum. J Pediatr Surg 23:752, 1988.

This article from a large Canadian center describes the essential features of duplication cysts that involve the spinal canal and their appropriate management.

Holcomb GW III, Gheissari A, O'Neill JA: Surgical management of alimentary tract duplications. Ann Surg 209:167, 1989.

In this review, all forms of enteric duplications are classified, and each type is described in terms of clinical presentation, diagnosis, and treatment.

LaQuaglia MP, Feins N, Craklis A, et al: Rectal duplications. J Pediatr Surg 20:980-984, 1990.

This article describes the various presentations of rectal duplications and the approach to diagnosis and treatment.

Pokorny WJ, Goldstein IR: Enteric thoraco-abdominal duplications in children. J Thorac Cardiovasc Surg 87:821, 1984.

This article describes approaches to diagnosis and treatment of the most challenging forms of duplications.

52

Necrotizing Enterocolitis

HISTORY

In 1888, Paltauf may have described the first cases of necrotizing enterocolitis (NEC) by reporting three infants with full-thickness necrosis and multiple perforations. In 1943, Agerty was the first to close successfully an ileal perforation that may have resulted from NEC. The real evolution of NEC began in the 1960s as a result of the development of neonatal intensive care units, which were capable of supporting premature infants. One of the first reports was published in 1964 from Babies' Hospital in New York, which described the clinical and radiographic characteristics of NEC. Since the 1960s, NEC has remained a major cause of morbidity and mortality in premature infants.

INCIDENCE

The approximate incidence of NEC is 25,000 cases per year, and the mortality averages 20% to 30%. NEC is the most serious and frequent gastrointestinal (GI) disorder of low-birth-weight infants. For infants weighing less than 1500 g, the incidence is 6% and accounts for 15% of deaths occurring after 1 week of life. NEC was responsible for 4% of low-birth-weight, infection-associated, late deaths in 1968, but by 1980, it was 37%. The result of dramatic improvements in the management of the pulmonary and nutritional needs of premature infants has exposed premature infants now living longer to a higher risk of NEC.

PATHOGENESIS

Despite extensive study, the cause of NEC is uncertain. The cause is likely to be multifactorial, but intestinal ischemia and infection are central to the process. Perinatal events causing hypotension, hypovolemia, or hypoxia, such as birth asphyxia, cannulation of the umbilical artery, patent ductus arteriosus, hyaline membrane disease, and exchange transfusions, have been implicated as additive factors. It is apparent, however, that other factors also may play a role.

More recent clinical and experimental studies indicate that there are two important factors in the pathogenesis of NEC: (1) circulatory insufficiency with an inciting agent, probably bacteria, and (2) a vulnerable host, which most often is a premature infant. The role of bacteria in NEC is supported by the following observations: (1) NEC occurs in episodic epidemic waves; (2) initiation of infection control measures usually prevents further spread of these epidemics; and (3) when cases occur in clusters, specific microorganisms frequently are identified in affected patients and nursery personnel.

The following is a unifying hypothesis for the pathogenesis of NEC. Newborn premature infants are vulnerable to developing NEC because of an immature gut barrier defense. Lack of breast-feeding results in the absence of secretory IgA and other important breast milk components, such as oligosaccharides, lactoferrin, growth factors such as epidermal growth factor, and immune cells. The immature goblet cells secrete only scant quantities of mucus. The mucosal cells themselves are poorly developed and may receive inadequate nutrients to maintain optimal cell function. Gastric, pancreatic, and intestinal secretions are diminished. In addition, premature infants are born with an immature immune system, with moderate-to-severe hypogammaglobulinemia, absence of immunoglobulin A and immunoglobulin M, deficient complement levels, and poor phagocyte function. The infant is admitted to a neonatal intensive care unit usually for treatment of respiratory distress and is exposed to pathogenic "intensive care" bacteria. Antibiotics frequently are administered, which alter the patient's intestinal flora, and formula feeding provides substrate for bacterial growth. Secondary ileus permits overgrowth and colonization by pathogenic bacteria.

Depending on the quantity and virulence of the microorganisms and the presence or absence of mucosal damage, bacteria breach the mucosal layer. Because of the reduction of the components of specific and nonspecific immune defense systems, bacterial killing is not effective when the microorganisms enter body tissues. The inflammatory reaction involving macrophages, bacteria, and bacterial byproducts results in release of various cytokines, including platelet-activating factor and tumor necrosis factor, which damage the mucosa and bowel wall. More bacteria can invade through the mucosal breaks, and progressive bowel damage results in full-thickness necrosis and intestinal perforation.

PATHOLOGY

The most common site of involvement of NEC is the terminal ileum followed by the colon. Together the large and small intestine are involved in 44% of these patients. The disease can involve single (50%) or multiple segments of intestine. A fulminating form of NEC, pan-necrosis, is characterized by necrosis of at least 75% of the intestine. Pan-necrosis occurs in 19% of all patients with NEC, and the mortality approaches 100%.

The gross findings in NEC include patchy areas of hemorrhage, often with intramural gas. Some areas have a normal appearance, whereas other areas of the bowel may be necrotic. Fibrinous exudate can be present on the serosal surface. The mucosa is ulcerated with wide areas of slough.

The most common microscopic lesion is bland or coagulation necrosis of the superficial mucosa (89%). There is loss of cellular detail but ghost-like preservation of cellular and tissue structure. Edema and hemorrhage in the submucosa precede mucosal necrosis and ulceration. Pneumatosis intestinalis occurs as a result of a breach in the mucosal barrier by gas-forming bacteria and appears first in the submucosa and later may extend to the muscularis and subserosa. Despite the presence of bacteria in the bowel wall, inflammation is minimal early and becomes prominent later during healing. Epithelial regeneration, granulation, and early fibrosis suggesting suppurative processes of at least a few days' duration is common. Exuberant granulation and fibrosis leading to stricture formation is a late finding in 5% to 10% of patients who recover from the initial episode.

CLINICAL SYMPTOMS

Abdominal distention is almost universal and is the most common physical finding. The abdomen is usually soft, but as the disease progresses, it may become firm and tender. Dilated bowel loops and crepitus may be palpable. Edema and erythema of the abdominal wall are encountered in approximately 5% of patients, suggesting underlying peritonitis. A mobile or fixed mass occasionally can be palpated. Bilious emesis occurs in three fourths of these infants. Diarrhea occurs in 20% of patients early before ileus is established. Guaiac-positive stools or gross blood in the stool is common, although massive bleeding is rare. Nonspecific clinical findings represent physiologic instability and include lethargy, temperature instability, apnea, and bradycardia; shock may be the outcome.

LABORATORY FINDINGS

The total white blood cell count is highly variable and can be elevated or low. There is usually a predominance of polymorphonuclear leukocytes and an increase in band forms. A depressed white blood cell count indicates a more severe sepsis and a poorer prognosis.

Thrombocytopenia is the result of platelet binding to gram-negative endotoxin. Greater than 80% of patients have platelet counts less than 100,000/mm^3, sometimes associated with disseminated intravascular coagulation. Metabolic acidosis (70% to 90%) is the result of physiologic instability and decreased tissue perfusion. Examination of the stool for occult and gross blood is helpful because of the high frequency of rectal bleeding. Breath hydrogen excretion is elevated when fermentation is increased. Although highly accurate, it rarely is used because of the difficulty performing the test. None of the laboratory tests are specific for NEC despite extensive research since the 1960s. Serial decreases in the platelet count are probably the most helpful indication of progressive NEC.

IMAGING

Abdominal Radiography

Because the clinical and laboratory features of NEC are nonspecific, radiographic findings have served as the cornerstone of diagnosis. Radiographs of the abdomen and chest are taken in the anteroposterior and left lateral decubitus projections. Occasionally, cross-table lateral projections are helpful. The findings most commonly associated with NEC are pneumatosis intestinalis, portal vein gas, pneumoperitoneum, intraperitoneal fluid, and persistently dilated intestinal loops.

Pneumatosis Intestinalis

Intramural gas is the pathognomonic sign of NEC, occurring in 98% of patients. Pneumatosis is fleeting and commonly is an early rather than a late finding. Intramural air is seen more frequently in infants who have been fed compared with unfed infants but eventually is seen in all. In patients with fulminating NEC and pan-necrosis, extensive pneumatosis involving large portions of the small and large intestine is seen.

Two forms of pneumatosis intestinalis are recognized: cystic and linear (Fig. 52-1). The cystic form, which is more common, has a granular or foamy appearance and represents gas in the submucosa. Frequently, it is confused with fecal material in the large intestine. Linear pneumatosis either coexists with the cystic form or can develop later and represents subserosal air, which often outlines a segment of intestine.

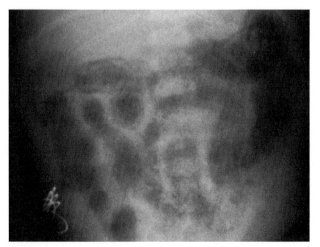

FIGURE 52-1 ■ Cystic and linear pneumatosis. The patient had multiple segments of necrotic bowel.

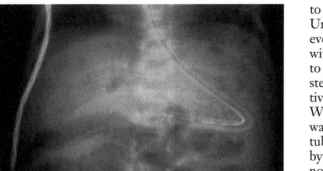

FIGURE 52-2 ■ Portal vein gas in a patient with paninvolvement.

Portal Vein Gas

Portal vein gas is recognized as an arborizing pattern in the right upper quadrant (Fig. 52-2). The gas in the bowel wall is absorbed into the mesenteric venous system and is trapped in the intrahepatic branches of the portal vein. The presence of gas in the portal venous system is fleeting and accounts for the low incidence (10%). In many patient series, the presence of portal vein gas is associated with a poor prognosis. In cases of pan-necrosis, portal vein air is present in 60% of patients.

Pneumoperitoneum

Free air in the peritoneal cavity, as a result of perforation of the intestine, can be shown in 10% to 20% of patients with NEC. It is seen best on a lateral decubitus radiograph. Intestinal perforation proven at laparotomy is associated with radiographic evidence of free air in only two thirds of the patients, indicating that perforation can occur without evidence of free air in the abdomen.

Ascites

The radiographic findings of free fluid in the peritoneal cavity, seen in 10% of patients, consist of a grossly distended abdomen with gas-filled loops of bowel in the center of the abdomen surrounded by opacity in the flanks and increased haziness within the abdomen. The combination of ascites and portal venous gas has been associated with high mortality. A fourth of patients with surgically proven intestinal perforation have ascites, but 15% of patients with proven intestinal perforation have neither ascites nor free air on abdominal radiographs.

Fixed Loop Sign

The finding of a single loop or several loops of dilated small bowel that remain unchanged in position and configuration for 24 to 36 hours is referred to as the *persistent loop sign* and suggests lack of peristalsis secondary to full-thickness bowel necrosis.

Contrast Studies

Contrast studies of the GI tract for NEC are performed infrequently, and contrast enemas have been considered to be contraindicated because of risk of perforation. Under certain circumstances, they may be of value, however, to improve diagnostic accuracy in premature infants with ambiguous clinical and radiographic signs of NEC, to differentiate NEC from volvulus, or to verify late stenosis. Early diagnosis of NEC and prompt nonoperative treatment may decrease the morbidity and mortality. When upper GI contrast studies are done, an iso-osmolar, water-soluble agent is injected through a small orogastric tube, and the progress of the contrast material is followed by serial portable radiographs. Soluble contrast agents do not damage the bowel mucosa, are slowly absorbed systemically, and if they leak into the peritoneal cavity are rapidly reabsorbed. Findings strongly suggestive of NEC during contrast imaging include mucosal ulceration or speculation, spasm and bowel wall thickening, luminal narrowing, subtle pneumatosis intestinalis (noted because of enhanced bowel opacification), and intramural extravasation of contrast material. These findings may identify questionable patients with NEC, while allowing early resumption of feedings in patients with negative studies. Contrast studies are rarely indicated.

Ultrasonography

Although plain radiographs are usually all that is required for diagnosis, ultrasound has been used by some as well. The principal ultrasound sign is echogenic portal venous gas. Occasionally, pneumatosis can be identified by ultrasound. The most helpful information from ultrasonography is identifying free fluid in the peritoneal cavity, however. These findings may be important in deciding whether to use paracentesis as a diagnostic maneuver or to consider abdominal exploration.

CLASSIFICATION

Previously, considerable emphasis was placed on a classification introduced by Bell and colleagues as follows: stage I, infants who show features suggestive of NEC; stage II, infants who are designated as definite cases; and stage III, infants who are in the advanced stages of NEC with evidence of necrosis of the bowel. The value of staging is related more to outcome reporting, and it does not determine management.

NONOPERATIVE SUPPORTIVE TREATMENT

Unless there is evidence of intestinal necrosis or perforation, the initial treatment of NEC is nonoperative. It is essential to decompress the GI tract with an orogastric tube maintained on low continuous suction. Hypovolemia must be corrected to diminish the risk of further intestinal ischemia. In addition to appropriate and continuous fluid resuscitation and monitoring, serum electrolytes and pH should be maintained in the normal range. Intravenous nutrition should be initiated as soon as it is practical to do so. The remaining cornerstone of care is broad-spectrum antibiotics. The choice of antibiotic regimens has been based principally on bacteriologic studies of the stool, peritoneal cavity, and blood. The most common organisms grown in the stool are

Escherichia coli, *Klebsiella pneumoniae*, *Enterobacter cloacae*, *Pseudomonas*, coagulase-negative staphylococci (*Staphylococcus epidermidis*), and *Clostridium perfringens*. In the blood, the organisms are *E. coli*, *K. pneumoniae*, *Staphylococcus aureus*, coagulase-negative staphylococci, enterococci, *C. perfringens*, and *Pseudomonas*. Infants maintained in newborn intensive care units frequently become colonized with *Klebsiella*. Anaerobes are sparse in premature newborns compared with adults.

Antibiotic regimens vary according to local infection surveillance profiles, but ampicillin, gentamicin, and vancomycin have been the most common combination because of the organisms involved. In some units, cefotaxime is used with vancomycin. Depending on culture results, other antibiotic combinations may be needed, especially when fungal organisms are found.

The course of NEC is monitored by serial physical examination, radiographs of the abdomen every 6 to 8 hours, serial platelet and white blood cell counts, and blood gas and pH determinations. Antibiotics are continued for a minimum of 10 days. Tube decompression of the intestinal tract is continued until there is evidence of complete recovery of peristalsis, or a minimum of 7 to 10 days. The patient is monitored carefully for abdominal distention, emesis, or nonspecific signs and symptoms of NEC. If there are no signs of recurrence, small quantities of dilute formula are administered. Feedings are advanced progressively to the infant's caloric goal.

INDICATIONS FOR OPERATION

The optimal time for operative intervention is just before bowel necrosis or perforation. There is no specific marker for these impending events. Numerous studies in the past revealed that abdominal exploration in the absence of specific evidence of dead or perforated bowel led to a higher mortality. We rely on specific indications for surgical exploration. The clearly recognized indication for surgical exploration is pneumoperitoneum indicative of bowel perforation or necrosis. "Relative" indications include clinical deterioration despite aggressive resuscitation, persistent acidosis, progressive thrombocytopenia, erythema of the abdominal wall, abdominal mass, a fixed dilated loop of intestine, positive paracentesis, and portal vein gas. None of these signs, symptoms, or laboratory findings by themselves indicate dead or perforated bowel. Probably the best available sign of established gangrene is progressive thrombocytopenia in the absence of any other cause. Profound septicemia also can lead to many of these findings.

Pneumoperitoneum

Infants who present with pneumoperitoneum or develop it during the course of medical treatment and infants with progressive physiologic deterioration require operative intervention. Not all patients who have intestinal perforation have free air. The decision to proceed with abdominal exploration is often one of clinical judgment integrating multiple findings.

Paracentesis

Kosloske and colleagues recommended abdominal paracentesis for infants with extensive pneumatosis intestinalis or who have failed to improve on medical management. These authors recommended paracenteses within 48 hours, whereas others use this procedure selectively. If peritoneal fluid is not encountered, peritoneal lavage is performed by instilling normal saline solution into the abdominal cavity. If bacteria are seen on Gram stain or if bile-stained fluid is found, operation is indicated because several studies have confirmed the accuracy of this finding. Some have suggested that paracentesis should be viewed only as another tool for diagnosis of intestinal gangrene; that the results of paracentesis must be considered in the context of all other clinical and laboratory findings; and that laparotomy should be performed if the infant continues to deteriorate, even when paracentesis is negative.

Fixed Intestinal Loop

The finding of a fixed loop of dilated featureless intestine for more than 24 hours is uncommon but indicates no peristalsis and strongly suggests full-thickness necrosis. It is not universally accurate, however, as shown in one patient series in which necrosis was found in 57% of patients, but 43% never developed gangrene and recovered without operation.

Ascites

The radiographic finding of ascites must be interpreted with care. After nasogastric suction, an infant with NEC may have a gasless abdomen. If there are other radiographic signs of ascites (see earlier) or ascites is confirmed by ultrasonography, 20% to 40% of patients have bowel necrosis. If ascites is present, paracentesis may be performed. If organisms are noted on smear, the incidence of necrosis is close to 100%.

Portal Vein Gas

Several reports have indicated that the finding of portal venous gas is a relative indication for operation. We have studied our patients and reviewed reported series to determine the significance of portal vein gas in relationship to bowel necrosis, pan-necrosis, and mortality. An additional goal of the review was to determine the outcome of patients with portal vein gas who did not receive surgical treatment. A total of 616 patients were collected; 118, or 19%, had portal vein gas on an abdominal radiograph. Of these 118 patients, 102, or 85%, eventually underwent operative exploration. All of them had full-thickness bowel necrosis; 52% had pan-necrosis.

The overall operative mortality for patients with portal vein gas was 55%. Fifteen patients who had portal vein gas did not undergo abdominal exploration initially. Six patients eventually were found to have full-thickness necrosis, and five died of bowel perforation and peritonitis. One patient developed an abscess and stricture but survived. These data strongly indicate that in patients with portal vein gas, most (>90%) have full-thickness necrosis, and a relatively large percentage (52%) have pan-necrosis.

OPERATIVE MANAGEMENT

Under optimal circumstances, the premature infant's condition should be stabilized with agressive resuscitation to establish normal vital signs and good urine output (1 to 2 mL/kg/hr). In reality, this may not be possible. Packed red blood cells, fresh-frozen plasma, and platelets should be administered as appropriate to correct coagulation abnormalities. A mild-to-moderate coagulopathy may be tolerated, but if a significant coagulopathy is present, it must be corrected. In the operating room, heat loss and evaporative water loss must be minimized. All preparation and irrigating solutions should be kept at 38°C. During surgery, the bowel is kept within the peritoneal cavity as much as possible.

Figures 52-3 and 52-4 outline treatment options when there is segmental involvement and paninvolvement of the bowel with necrosis. The abdomen is approached best by a right transverse supraumbilical incision using electrocautery to reduce blood loss and operating time. Samples of peritoneal fluid are taken for aerobic and anaerobic culture. The entire GI tract is examined systematically for perforations and necrosis. Pale white areas signify full-thickness ischemic necrosis. A thinned area of the intestine that balloons out and is covered by a thinned, discolored, semitransparent serosa has undergone necrosis of the mucosa, submucosa, and muscularis and will rupture shortly. Often there are long segments of purple or dull greenish black intestine. It is difficult to determine whether these color changes are caused by subserosal hemorrhage and edema or are the result of full-thickness necrosis. Palpation is sometimes helpful. Relatively firm, resilient bowel is usually viable, and lax bowel that dents on compression is often necrotic. The guiding principle is to resect only perforated or unquestionably necrotic tissue and preserve as much bowel as possible. Every effort is made to preserve the ileocecal valve. When a single necrotic segment of bowel is encountered, it should be resected and a proximal stoma and mucosa fistula created. If multiple segments of intestine are necrotic, and there are intervening segments of viable small intestine that together provide enough length to maintain nutrition, it is appropriate to excise each individual necrotic segment rather than perform a massive resection. If the individual segments are of adequate length, multiple stomas can be created. Often the bowel segments are too short to create two stomas (proximal and distal), or the mesentery is contracted and edematous, making it impossible to bring the ends to the abdominal wall. In this situation, a stoma may be created in the most proximal bowel, allowing for diversion of the intestinal stream.

The individual segments can be closed proximally and the distal ends brought out as stomas or anastomosed together with four to six full-thickness noninverting stitches. The proximal end of the most distal bowel segment is closed as a Hartmann's closure, and the distal end of the anastomosed segments is brought to the abdominal wall as a single stoma or left in continuity with the remaining intestine.

Approximately 20% of patients have pan-necrosis. Often only a small portion of proximal bowel close to the

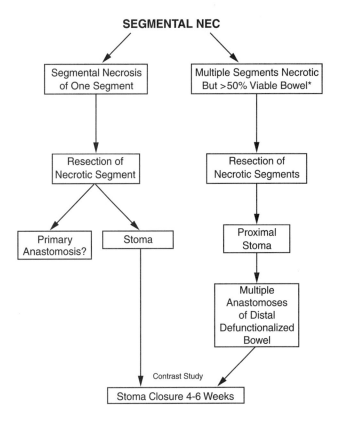

FIGURE 52-3 ■ Management plan for patients with necrotizing enterocolitis and segmental necrosis. *(1)* Segmental necrosis can involve a single bowel segment or multiple bowel segments, but less than 50% of the small intestine is involved. Perforation may or may not be present. *(2)* Single segment: *(a)* The single segment of necrotic bowel is resected. *(b)* In selected cases, a primary anastomosis may be performed. *(c)* The safest approach is to perform a stoma at the proximal end of the divided bowel and bring out the distal end as a mucosal fistula. The distal end also may be closed and returned to the peritoneal cavity (Hartmann's pouch). *(d)* In 4 to 6 weeks, a contrast enema is performed, and if there are no strictures, the stoma is closed, and intestinal continuity is restored. *(3)* Multiple segments: *(a)* The necrotic, perforated segments are resected. *(b)* A proximal stoma is created: *(I)* If the necrotic bowel segments are close to each other and sufficient uninvolved bowel would remain, a single resection is performed. The proximal end is brought out as a stoma and the distal end as a mucosal fistula. *(II)* If there are multiple segments resected with intervening viable bowel, multiple anastomoses are done in the distal defunctionalized bowel. *(c)* After a normal contrast study, the stoma is closed in 4 to 6 weeks, and continuity of the bowel is re-established.

ligament of Treitz is viable, and the distal bowel appears completely necrotic. At this point, some surgeons elect to close the abdomen and forego further treatment. In rare instances, diverting the intestinal stream with a proximal stoma has led to survival of some bowel segments, however. If the patient does not improve in 48 hours after creation of the proximal stoma, a decision must be made whether to discontinue further surgical treatment or re-explore the patient. If the patient's physiologic

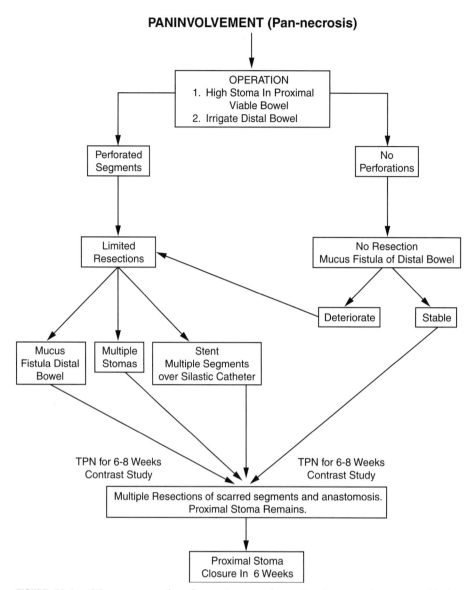

FIGURE 52-4 ■ Management plan for patients with paninvolvement (pan-necrosis) (an attempt to avoid short-bowel syndrome). In some instances, it is possible to determine that all the intestine is necrotic, and the situation is hopeless under these circumstances; the abdomen may be closed and care terminated. If the degree of necrosis and its extent are uncertain, however, the following steps may be taken: (1) All patients with paninvolvement are managed operatively by (*a*) a high stoma in the most proximal viable bowel, usually the upper jejunum, or (*b*) suctioning of distal bowel. (2) If the distal bowel has a *single* or *multiple* perforations: (*a*) The perforated segment or segments are resected; these are limited, not wide, resections. (*b*) If only one resection is done, the distal bowel end is brought out as a mucosal fistula. (*c*) If several resections are required for multiple perforations, several proximal and distal stomas may be created in the defunctionalized bowel. (*d*) If creation of multiple stomas would reduce significantly the amount of remaining intestine, a Silastic catheter is threaded through the individual segments of the distal bowel; the bowel segments are held loosely together with a few absorbable sutures, and these joined segments are left in the abdomen. (*e*) The patient receives TPN for 6 weeks, then the proximal stoma is closed, restoring intestinal continuity. (3) Paninvolvement without perforation: (*a*) No resection is done; the bowel is divided through the junction of clearly viable and severely involved bowel, and a high proximal stoma is done. The distal end is brought out as a mucosal fistula. (*b*) If there is progressive clinical deterioration, the patient is re-explored, and frankly necrotic or perforated bowel is resected (second-look procedure). (*c*) If the patient is clinically stable, the patient receives TPN. A contrast study is done in 6 weeks. (*d*) Multiple resections of the scarred segments of defunctionalized bowel are done, and the segments are anastomosed together. (*e*) Six weeks later, the proximal stoma is closed, and bowel continuity is restored.

condition remains stable and it is believed that there is a sufficient amount of viable small intestine ultimately to support adequate enteral nutrition, a central venous line is placed, and the patient is maintained on total parenteral nutrition (TPN). At 6 to 10 weeks, the patient can be re-explored, and segments of viable bowel can be anastomosed to restore continuity.

No matter what length of intestine is necrotic during laparotomy, the length of viable intestine should be measured along the mesenteric border. The proximal stoma and mucosa fistula are brought out through separate ostomy sites or occasionally through the wound. There seems to be no increase in wound complications by using the laparotomy incision to place the stomas, although it is more difficult to place an ostomy appliance over the proximal stoma.

To perform the enterostomy, the intestine is attached to the peritoneum or only to the skin by several interrupted sutures. Approximately 1 to 1.5 cm of bowel is left protruding from the abdominal wall and no attempt need be made to mature the end. If the viability of the stoma is in doubt in the postoperative period, a small portion of full-thickness bowel can be excised and the cut surface observed for bleeding.

There is no universal agreement on when to close a stoma and restore intestinal continuity. If there is sufficient intestinal length, the enteral feedings are tolerated, and satisfactory weight gain is taking place, most surgeons delay closure for a minimum of 2 months. The patient frequently is sent home for a time to reach an arbitrary body weight (often >3 kg). Some patients tolerate enteral feedings poorly, although they have sufficient intestinal length. Because of failure to thrive or continued salt and water loss, these patients may require earlier stoma closure. Stomal dysfunction from stenosis is common because of the tenuous nature of the exteriorized intestine. If the infant is more than 4 weeks postoperative, many surgeons close the stoma rather than revise it. Infants with insufficient functional bowel to maintain adequate nutrition by enteral means must be maintained on TPN while adaptation takes place, often for 1 year. These patients should have stomal closure as soon as possible if they develop recurrent central line infections or TPN-associated liver disease. Kosloske and colleagues compared the complications between patients closed less than 3 months postoperatively, 3 to 5 months postoperatively, and more than 5 months postoperatively. They found no difference in the complication rate. They also found that there was no difference in complications between patients closed at a body weight less than 2.5 kg, 2.5 to 5.0 kg, or greater than 5.0 kg.

When a segment of the intestinal necrosis is localized and the remaining intestine appears undamaged, success with resection and primary anastomosis has been reported. This approach avoids the morbidity associated with enterostomy and a second operation. To obtain the optimal outcome, the necrotic area of bowel should be localized to a short segment; the surrounding intestine should be healthy; and the patient's general condition should be good.

Ein and associates described the use of peritoneal drainage under local anesthesia to treat 15 extremely ill infants with perforated bowel. The overall mortality was 54%, and the mortality directly caused by NEC was 27%. In 1990, Ein and associates updated their series to 37 patients. The overall survival was 56%. Of these patients, 88% weighed less than 1500 g and 65% weighed less than 1000 g. These authors' current feeling is that peritoneal drainage is used best as a temporizing measure until the infant can be stabilized for operation even though recovery with drainage alone has been reported. The Pittsburgh group reported 92 surgically treated patients, of whom 51 (55%) underwent peritoneal drainage. Patients with a primary laparotomy had an 83.7% survival, whereas patients with peritoneal drainage had a 57% survival. The patients who underwent drainage weighed significantly less, however, and were more premature (average weight of 1.158 kg and gestational age of 28.8 weeks). These patients also had lower preoperative platelet counts and a higher incidence of patent ductus arteriosus and intraventricular hemorrhage.

The ideal management of complicated NEC is primary laparotomy when the patient's condition is acceptable. Peritoneal drainage may be a helpful adjunct to therapy, however, in the high-risk infant with peritonitis, respiratory failure, and shock. The drainage of infected peritoneal fluid may reduce bacterial invasion and further reduce peritoneal contamination. The patients most likely to benefit from peritoneal drainage are infants weighing less than 1000 g with free air shown radiographically and who are physiologically unstable. The procedure is done at the bedside. A small (1 cm) incision is made in the right lower quadrant and a Penrose drain is placed, or a clamp is passed across the abdomen along the underside of the anterior abdominal wall to the left lower quadrant. A stab wound is made over the tip of the clamp in the left lower quadrant. A Penrose drain is grasped by the clamp and passed from left to right across the abdomen, allowing drainage from both wounds. After drainage, the infant is monitored closely. There is controversy regarding the subsequent management after Penrose drainage is established. Some reports suggest that if there is no improvement over 24 hours the infant should be explored. Of infants who do respond, there is controversy regarding the need for exploration. Several reports have suggested that some infants recover without the need for further surgical intervention.

INTESTINAL STRICTURES

The first report of the development of an intestinal stricture after recovery from acute NEC was in 1968. Stricture results from healing of an area of severe intestinal injury. The reported overall incidence varies between 11% and 35%. Whether the stricture follows operative or nonoperative therapy, the most common site of involvement has been the colon (70%), followed by the terminal ileum (15%). Of colonic strictures, 60% involve the left side of the colon, and the most common colonic site is the splenic flexure (21%). Most patients have a single stricture, but multiple strictures are common after operative management. Colonic strictures are typically asymptomatic in patients who have had operative treatment because the stricture usually forms distal to an intestinal stoma. Of the patients treated nonoperatively, slightly more than half with colonic strictures are symptomatic and present with signs and symptoms of high-grade, partial intestinal obstruction. Strictures become established 3 to 4 weeks after the initial injury, so stomal closure should be done before that time. Because of the danger of closing a proximal intestinal stoma in the presence of a distal obstruction, it is appropriate to perform a contrast study of the distal bowel before stoma closure. If a stricture is found, it can be resected during the procedure to close the intestinal stoma. Current consensus is that patients treated nonoperatively who develop delayed signs of partial intestinal obstruction should have distal contrast studies. If a stricture is found, resection and primary anastomosis is in order.

Schwartz and colleagues conducted a prospective evaluation of premature infants with medically managed NEC. A contrast enema was performed 6 weeks after recovery. They noted an overall incidence of 35% of intestinal stenosis. Asymptomatic patients were followed, and approximately one third of these patients had resolution of stenosis. This finding suggested that the areas of narrowing seen radiographically likely were not true strictures but stenotic areas from mucosal granulation tissue. The most important finding from this study was the high incidence (>50%) of asymptomatic lesions. Although all the infants did not require initial surgery, approximately one third became symptomatic after hospital discharge. Because the stenosis was known, there was no delay in proceeding with prompt resection before the infant became seriously ill.

If the contrast enema study shows a stricture in a symptomatic patient, surgery is indicated. Management of an asymptomatic patient with only radiographic evidence of a postoperative colonic stricture is less clear, however. Some of these patients have been treated successfully with balloon dilation. Other infants have been observed, and on follow-up contrast studies the stenotic area had resolved. Patients who develop GI symptoms or fail to thrive are readmitted, the contrast radiographs are repeated, and operative intervention is performed when indicated.

SURVIVAL

There has been a steady improvement in the operative and nonoperative survival of patients with NEC. The increased survival has been most noticeable in infants weighing less than 1000 g with gestational age less than 28 weeks. The improved survival has been attributed to earlier diagnosis and selective and more effective treatment. The progress made in the physiologic management of low-birth-weight, critically ill infants also has contributed to this reduced mortality. Overall survival in the 1970s averaged 35% to 40%. In the 1980s, survival improved to 65% in surgical series, and presently the survival averages 65% to 70% in large series reported by Grosfeld, O'Neill, and Snyder and their respective groups.

LATE OUTCOME

Long-term follow-up of patients by Stevens and colleagues and Welsh and colleagues and large series indicate that long-term neurologic and other developmental impairment is related primarily to the degree of immaturity of the patient. GI-related malabsorption, short-bowel syndrome, and associated delayed development are still significant considerations despite all of the advances in nutritional and other forms of support. The more advanced the degree of NEC, the more impairment of growth and development, although recovery usually eventually occurs. In most large series, 25% to 30% of survivors have some form of impairment.

NEC in premature infants is one of the greatest challenges to neonatologists and pediatric surgeons. Despite remarkable and steady advances in overall care of markedly premature infants, diagnosis and timing of management remain difficult to determine. Decisions must be made on indirect or cumulative information because definitive indications frequently are lacking. All premature infants with NEC have varying degrees of systemic sepsis. This can result in multiple organ failure in the absence of perforated or necrotic bowel. We still are forced to make judgments when definitive data are lacking.

SUGGESTED READINGS

Ahmed T, Ein S, Moore A: The role of peritoneal drains in treatment of perforated necrotizing enterocolitis: Recommendations from recent experience. J Pediatr Surg 33:1468-1470, 1995.

An excellent review of the indications and techniques for peritoneal drainage for NEC.

Cooper A, Ross AJ, O'Neill JA, Schnaufer L: Resection with primary anastomosis for necrotizing enterocolitis: A contrasting view. J Pediatr Surg 16:743-746, 1983.

This analysis of a series of 27 patients who had resection and primary anastomosis from a total series of 198 surgical cases indicated that the role of primary anastomosis is limited and risky in a population of critically ill, low-birth-weight, premature infants with multiple comorbidities.

Ehrlich PF, Sato TT, Short BL, Hartman GE: Outcome of perforated necrotizing enterocolitis in the very low-birth weight neonate may be independent of the type of surgical treatment. Am Surg 67:752-756, 2001.

These authors did a multivariate analysis of 70 surviving infants weighing less than 1000 g in terms of GI-related and non–GI-related morbidity and mortality and found that it is best to tailor the therapeutic approach according to the individual patient situation.

Grosfeld JL, Cheu H, Schlatter M, et al: Changing trends in necrotizing enterocolitis. Ann Surg 214:300, 1991.

This large series shows reduced mortality for surgical NEC. The authors point out that even "micropremies" have satisfactory survival similar to more mature infants. The poor prognostic implications of pan-necrosis and portal vein air are emphasized.

Musemeche CA, Kosloske AM, Ricketts RR: Enterostomy in necrotizing enterocolitis: An analysis of techniques and timing of closure. J Pediatr Surg 22:479, 1987.

This is the only study that examines time of closure and weight of patient in determining when the stoma should be closed. Closure less than 3 months after creation of the stoma did not increase the complication rate.

Moss RL, Dimmitt RA, Henry MCW, et al: A meta-analysis of peritoneal drainage versus laparotomy for perforated necrotizing enterocolitis. J Pediatr Surg 36:1210, 2001.

A summary is provided of the indications for peritoneal drainage versus laparotomy for the management of NEC with perforation.

O'Neill JA: Necrotizing enterocolitis. In Puri P (ed): Surgery and Support of the Premature Infant. Basel, Karger 1985, pp 40-49.

This chapter reviews the cause of NEC, supportive care, indications for operation, and the various approaches available for contemporary management.

Schwartz MZ, Hayden CK, Richardson CJ, et al: A prospective evaluation of intestinal stenosis following necrotizing enterocolitis. J Pediatr Surg 17:764, 1983.

This study analyzes the time course and incidence of intestinal stenosis resulting from NEC, including many cases that were asymptomatic and resolved spontaneously.

53

Short-Bowel Syndrome

There are numerous definitions for short-bowel syndrome (SBS). The simplest definition is that there is inadequate length of functional intestine to maintain normal enteral nutrition. Because infants and children require increased caloric needs to maintain normal growth and development, SBS can have a more devastating effect in these patients.

Before the availability of total parenteral nutrition (TPN), most infants and children with SBS died from malnutrition. The true incidence of SBS is unknown because of the variation in definition used in different reports. A Canadian study suggested that the incidence was 4.8 per 1 million population using the criteria that the patient required TPN for more than 6 weeks or had residual small intestine of less than 25%. SBS typically is the result of a catastrophic event involving the small intestine and possibly the colon. Necrotizing enterocolitis and midgut volvulus from malrotation are the two most common causes of SBS. Other causes are listed in Table 53-1.

NORMAL PHYSIOLOGY

The small intestine is derived from the midgut and is anatomically complete by 20 weeks' gestation. Most of its intrauterine growth occurs in the third trimester. Before 27 weeks' gestation, the average length of the small intestine is 115 cm. This length increases to approximately 250 cm with a diameter of 1.5 cm after 35 weeks' gestation. In contrast, the adult intestine is 600 to 800 cm in length and 4 cm in diameter. The mucosal surface area changes markedly with age. Infants have 950 cm^2; adults have 7500 cm^2.

The intestine has an enormous capacity to absorb secretions and ingested fluids (Fig. 53-1). There is considerable redundancy in the absorptive capability of normal intestine, which is why a major loss of the intestine may not result in SBS. Absorption occurs through the interface of luminal contents and the mucosal lining of the small intestine. The mucosa comprises villi, crypts, lamina propria, and muscularis mucosa. The luminal surface of the mucosa consists of a single layer of columnar epithelial cells that line the crypts and villi. Undifferentiated mucosal cells arise in the crypts at the bottom of the villi. As these cells migrate toward the villus tip, they mature

TABLE 53-1 ■ Etiology of Short-Bowel Syndrome in Infants and Children
Necrotizing enterocolitis
Midgut volvulus from malrotation
Multiple intestinal atresias
Gastroschisis
Trauma
Inflammatory bowel disease

and acquire absorptive properties. They are cast off when they reach the tip and are replaced by new cells. Receptor sites for nutrients, vitamin B_{12}, calcium, iron, and bile acids are located on the epithelial cells. Mucus covers the surface of the enterocyte and acts as a trap to hold nutrients in contact with the cell surface. Mucus also acts as a bacterial barrier.

Dietary fats, principally triglycerides, are hydrolyzed by pancreatic lipases into fatty acids, mainly monoglycerides and diglycerides. Fatty acids combine with bile acid to form micelles that are absorbed through the intestinal lymphatics. The micelles are transferred via the thoracic duct to the venous system. Carbohydrates as polysaccharides and glycogen are hydrolyzed to simple sugars in the intestinal lumen by amylases from the saliva and pancreas and by disaccharidases produced at the brush border of jejunal mucosa cells. Then they are absorbed through the mucosal cell into the portal circulation to be processed by the liver. Proteins are broken down by peptidases, trypsin, chymotrypsin, and elastinase. These enzymes are principally pancreatic, and only a few are from the brush border. Dipeptides and tripeptides are the end point of protein digestion rather than amino acids. The peptides are absorbed through the mucosa and enter the portal circulation to the liver.

PATHOPHYSIOLOGY

In patients with SBS, intestinal function depends on multiple factors (Table 53-2). The most crucial factor is the length of the remaining intestine. Excision of the stomach, jejunum, or colon is better tolerated than ileal resection. The stomach digests nutrients by the action of acid and

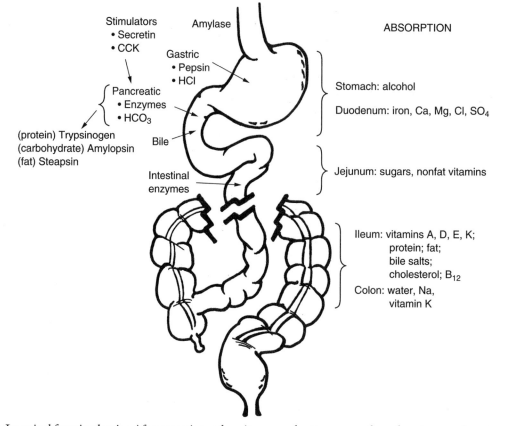

FIGURE 53-1 ■ Intestinal function by site. After resection, other sites may adapt to assume those functions, as there is overlap of some absorptive function between sites.

pepsin and produces intrinsic factor essential for vitamin B_{12} absorption. The stomach reacts to massive intestinal resection by secreting large volumes of high acid–containing gastric juices at least for a time. The jejunum is the site of absorption of most macronutrients and minerals, such as calcium, magnesium, and iron. Cholecystokinin and secretin, stimulants of pancreaticobiliary secretions, are produced in the jejunum. With removal of the jejunum, there is loss of the jejunal brush border carbohydrate enzymes and decreased carbohydrate digestion and absorption, then higher concentration of luminal sugars provides substrate for bacterial growth. The interaction of bacteria and carbohydrates (fermentation) produces lactic acid. The colonic absorption of increased concentrations of lactic acid can lead to lactic acidosis. After jejunal resection, cholecystokinin and secretin production are decreased, and pancreaticobiliary secretions are altered. Fat and

protein digestion may be reduced significantly. Calcium and magnesium losses are increased. If there is adequate ileum remaining after jejunal resection, however, the loss of the jejunum is better tolerated.

Carbohydrate, protein, fluid, and electrolytes are absorbed in the ileum. The ileum is the principal source of absorption of bile acids; vitamin B_{12}; and the fat-soluble vitamins A, D, E, and K. Removal of most of the ileum results in vitamin B_{12} and fat-soluble vitamin deficiencies and diarrhea. The diarrhea is from three factors: (1) Large volumes of fluid are passed because of decreased transit time and loss of absorptive surface. (2) Bile salt absorption is markedly reduced, and excess bile salts pass into the colon, resulting in impaired electrolyte absorption and increased colonic mucosal secretory activity. (3) A paradoxical relative bile salt deficiency occurs. Because the enterohepatic cycle of bile is interrupted, the liver cannot synthesize enough bile to replace the loss. Micelle formation is reduced, and fat cannot be absorbed, resulting in steatorrhea.

The ileocecal valve's major function is to increase the pressure gradient between the ileum and the colon to prevent reflux of colonic fluids with high concentrations of bacteria. Nutrient transit time across the small bowel is increased in the absence of the valve, and nutrient contact time against the gut absorptive surface is prolonged when the valve is present.

Removal of the colon has a minimal effect on digestion and absorption. The colon is the site of absorption

TABLE 53-2 ■ Factors Influencing Intestinal Function in Short-Bowel Syndrome
Total remaining small intestinal length
Etiology of intestinal loss
In utero versus postnatal intestinal loss
Residual intestine (jejunum or ileum)
Presence of the ileocecal valve
Length of time from intestinal resection

of fluid and sodium and the excretion of potassium and bicarbonate. In SBS, the presence of the colon is of value because it increases the absorptive surface area for fluids and electrolytes and decreases diarrhea. The colon can induce certain adverse effects, however. Exposure to higher concentrations of bile salts can lead to a form of colitis. There is an increase in absorption of oxalates by the colon, which are excreted in the urine and can lead to renal calculi. Also the colon can serve as an absorptive site for abnormally produced lactic acid with the subsequent development of lactic acidosis. Finally, in the absence of the ileocecal value, reflux of bacteria into the ileum can lead to small intestine bacterial overgrowth.

ADAPTATION

Loss of a significant percentage of the small intestine produces physiologic and anatomic changes in the bowel called *intestinal adaptation*. The result is an increase in intestinal surface area and a compensatory increase in absorption and digestion. The first and most significant adaptive change is villus hyperplasia. Elongation of the villi, thickening of the muscularis, and increasing luminal diameter are the end points of adaptation. There is an upper limit to this phenomenon. The mechanism or signal that turns the adaptive process off is unknown, as is the mechanism that induces it. Adaptation begins almost immediately after resection and can take 2 years to complete. The most important site of hyperplasia after bowel resection is the small intestine; however, mucosal hyperplasia also occurs in the large intestine, resulting in a modest increase in water and electrolyte absorption.

Although the specific mechanisms that initiate and control adaptation are not known, there is a large body of information on factors that influence the adaptive process (Table 53-3). Providing intravenous calories is sufficient to support growth and development, but it does not support the adaptive process. Patients on TPN exclusively develop mucosal atrophy. This condition can be reversed with a small amount of enteral nutrition, typically referred to as *trophic feeds*. The composition of the trophic feeds influences the adaptive process with complex nutrients being more effective. Unsaturated fats seem to induce the greatest stimulus.

Normal endogenous secretions in the gastrointestinal (GI) tract promote the adaptive process. Biliary and pancreatic secretions are trophic to the small intestine mucosa with pancreatic secretions having the greatest effect. Experiments in which the ampulla of Vater was transplanted to the ileum, bypassing the jejunum, resulted in jejunal mucosal hypoplasia, whereas the ileal mucosa in the area where the ampulla was implanted (and exposed to pancreaticobiliary secretions) resulted in marked mucosal hyperplasia.

Perhaps the most important influence on intestinal adaptation is humoral factors. These substances may be hormones, growth factors, or cytokines. The relationship between growth factors and intestinal adaptation has been known since the 1960s. In the 1980s and 1990s, specific hormones or peptides were identified that on an experimental basis induce mucosal hyperplasia or increase mucosal cell function. At present, the only substance that

TABLE 53-3 ■ Factors Influencing Intestinal Adaptation
Humoral factors
Hormones (gastrin, cholecystokinin, glucagon)
Candidate hormones or intestinal peptides (e.g., epidermal growth factor, hepatocyte growth factor, glucagon-like peptide-2, interleukin-11)
Gastrointestinal secretions
Pancreatic secretions
Intestinal secretions
Bile
Luminal nutrients
Exogenous (food)
Endogenous

has reached clinical trials is glucagon-like peptide-2 (GLP-2). Data are insufficient to determine its benefit, however. The source of these humoral factors includes saliva, enteroendocrine cells lining the GI tract, and peptides secreted into the blood from distant sites.

The mechanism of cellular adaptation has not been delineated. There is general agreement, however, that it is multifactorial. There is increasing evidence that the naturally occurring polyamines (putrescine, spermidine, and spermine) may play a crucial role. Experimentally, massive small bowel resection results in a marked increase in polyamines and the enzyme that controls polyamine synthesis, ornithine decarboxylase (ODC). If ODC is blocked after small bowel resection, polyamine concentrations are markedly reduced, and mucosal hypertrophy does not occur.

MANAGEMENT

In the early recovery period after significant intestinal loss, attention is directed toward maintenance of fluid and electrolyte balance. Central TPN is begun. Excess secretions that are lost through stomas or diarrhea must be monitored, and fluid volume and electrolytes must be replaced. Blood levels of calcium, magnesium, trace elements, and vitamins and blood pH must be monitored. Intravenous fat emulsion (40% of calories) is given daily or at least three times per week.

As soon as GI function has resumed, enteral feeds are introduced gradually. This is usually accomplished through a gastrostomy or orogastric or indwelling nasogastric tube. Infants and young children must be fed at least in part orally, however, to establish firmly their sucking and eating patterns. Because adaptation begins early after bowel resection, the initial object of limited early enteral feeding is not to provide nutrition but to stimulate adaptive mechanisms. Small volumes of isotonic liquid feedings are introduced first. Several variables must be controlled during feedings: (1) osmolality, (2) volume, (3) composition, and (4) method (continuous versus bolus). A trial-and-error method maximizes the results.

In the past, there was considerable interest in the use of elemental diets to feed patients with SBS. These diets have the theoretical advantage of being better absorbed because they are already in elemental form. Because they do not require intraluminal digestion, they do not stimulate digestive secretions. In addition, the simple sugars and amino acids that compose an elemental diet result in a high osmolality that may initiate diarrhea. Experimental evidence and some clinical evidence suggest that complex diets are more trophic to the GI tract and accelerate adaptation. Because elemental diets contain amino acids rather than peptides, they offer no advantage regarding protein digestion, as peptides are absorbed through the mucosa. From a practical vantage point, elemental diets have the disadvantage of being more expensive than complex diets.

Well-tolerated diets contain peptides as the major protein source and glucose polymers as the carbohydrate source. Glucose polymers have a lower osmolality and are readily hydrolyzed by pancreatic secretions. Long-chain triglycerides and short-chain fatty acids are important and should be added gradually to the diet because they stimulate mucosal hyperplasia. In the past, patients were not fed complex fats because of the fear of increasing steatorrhea. Several clinical studies have shown that this is incorrect. Medium-chain triglycerides are absorbed readily through the mucosa without lipase digestion or bile acids. They have a theoretical advantage in SBS, but they do not stimulate intestinal adaptation.

The volume and complexity of feedings are increased gradually. Consideration should be given to adding fiber to the diet, particularly pectin. Vitamins B_{12}, A, D, E, and K may be required. As more nutrients are absorbed, the volume of parenteral nutrition is decreased. At this point, cycling of TPN should begin. This prepares the patient for discharge and maintenance by home TPN. During hospitalization and at home, stools should be monitored periodically for reducing substances, water content, frequency, volume, and the presence of undigested fat.

PHARMACOTHERAPY

Reducing Gastric Acid Output

There is evidence that gastric hypersecretion complicates the first phase of adaptation to the SBS. In addition to aggressive monitoring and replacement of fluid and electrolyte deficits, early medical treatment should address hypergastrinemia and subsequent increase in gastric fluid secretion, which characterize the first several months after massive small bowel loss. In the early postoperative period, antacids or sucralfate may be administered via a nasogastric tube (and later by mouth) to reduce the elevated risk of peptic ulcer disease in these patients. Histamine-2 receptor blockers can be especially useful in decreasing water and sodium losses related to the secretory diarrhea that results from gastric hypersecretion; studies have shown that this can be accomplished in SBS patients with cimetidine or ranitidine. Clinically, we typically have used cimetidine in doses of 10 to 20 mg/kg/day orally or intravenously divided every 6 hours. If a more potent agent is required to reduce gastric output, proton-pump inhibitors can be used. Oral and intravenous forms of omeprazole have been shown experimentally to decrease stool weight and fecal sodium losses in SBS patients. In children, omeprazole can be administered, 0.6 to 0.7 mg/kg once or twice daily.

Antimotility and Antisecretory Agents

Medications that slow peristalsis and increase intestinal transit time have been used for several decades to treat SBS. By prolonging transit, there is a longer contact time between ingested nutrients and enterocytes, allowing for better absorption and less diarrhea.

Loperamide hydrochloride is a synthetic, peripherally acting opioid analogue, which inhibits motility in the small bowel and colon. In children, this agent is safely administered enterally as 1- to 1.5-mg doses three times a day. Loperamide has few side effects and essentially no risk of physiologic tolerance or abuse. Numerous controlled trials have shown the efficacy of loperamide in chronic diarrhea.

Diphenoxylate (Lomotil) is another opioid antidiarrheal agent that is well absorbed and metabolized to the active compound, defenoxin hydrochloride. Its oral form contains atropine to discourage drug abuse by producing anticholinergic side effects at higher doses. Because diphenoxylate in children has been linked to at least 36 cases of serious central nervous system, respiratory, and cardiac side effects related either to its opioid or to its atropine component, it is important to use this medication cautiously. As enteral feeds are gradually increased, if a second-line agent is required in addition to loperamide, it is possible to add another opiate drug, such as codeine (0.5 to 1.0 mg/kg per dose orally every 6 hours) to retard small intestinal motility further. Deodorized tincture of opium (Paregoric) also may be effective and has the benefit of slow titration by a few drops at a time to achieve desirable results, while minimizing the risk of side effects. The treatment plan should be individualized for each patient based on the length of the remaining intestine, the presence of the ileocecal valve, and the length of colon in continuity. Treating SBS patients, especially patients lacking an ileocecal valve, with antimotility agents most likely increases the risk of bacterial overgrowth in dysmotile, dilated portions of intestine. Diagnosis of significant bacterial overgrowth in patients experiencing increased pain and diarrhea mandates cessation of antimotility agents, a course of appropriate antibiotics (usually oral metronidazole), and occasionally saline enemas.

The absence of the terminal ileum increases diarrhea as a result of the high concentration of bile acids and bile salts entering the colon instead of being absorbed as part of the enterohepatic circulation. Colonic bacteria deconjugate bile salts to increase the free bile acid concentration, which stimulates the secretion of water and electrolytes into the colonic lumen. Bile acid sequestrants, such as cholestyramine, decrease stool losses by exchanging chloride ions for bile acids to form nonabsorbable complexes for excretion in the feces. Treatment of pediatric patients with SBS is usually with 100 to 250 mg/kg/day of cholestyramine divided into three doses.

Although binding bile acids in the small intestine may alleviate choleretic diarrhea, it may exacerbate malabsorption and steatorrhea when enteral fats are introduced into the diet as the bile acid pool diminishes to a level below the concentration necessary for creating micelles. The efficacy of cholestyramine must be determined empirically on an individual basis.

Somatostatin is a peptide hormone with a wide distribution throughout the GI tract. It has potent inhibitory effects on a wide range of GI peptides and hormones. Somatostatin and its synthetic analogue, octreotide, can reduce gastric acid secretion, gastric emptying, gallbladder contraction, exocrine pancreas function, bowel motility, and small intestinal secretions. Increasing intestinal transit time and reducing intestinal secretions can result in improved fluid, electrolyte, and substrate absorption and is thought to be the mechanism by which somatostatin is beneficial. Somatostatin and octreotide have been shown to decrease intestinal fluid losses in SBS patients. Because octreotide has a long duration of action and may be given via subcutaneous injections, it has been proposed as a potential long-term treatment to improve the lifestyles of SBS patients. Its use in this population has not been studied extensively, however, and the mechanism by which somatostatin analogues benefit patients with SBS is unclear. An increase in transit time results in improved absorption. It also increases contact time between the mucosa and luminal trophic factors, which could facilitate adaptation. Treatment with octreotide has been shown in humans, however, not only to reduce levels of numerous GI hormones, such as insulin, gastrin, glucagon, peptide YY, and growth hormone (GH), but also to lower the uptake of amino acids destined for pancreatic or mucosal protein synthesis. The net effect of octreotide on intestinal adaptation and function is not clear. These studies also help to illustrate the concept that intestinal adaptation is likely the result of multiple peptides and mechanisms.

Other issues regarding octreotide include the possible side effects of abdominal pain, nausea, increased incidence of gallstones, facial flushing, and headache. At this time, the role of octreotide in managing SBS patients seems limited. Although it is unlikely that patients whose intestinal output is greater than their oral intake would wean completely from parenteral support with the administration of octreotide, certain patients can enjoy an improved lifestyle with reduced intravenous fluid requirements. Therapeutic doses of octreotide in the pediatric age group usually range from 1 to 10 mcg/kg/24 hours subcutaneously or intravenously.

Glutamine and Growth Hormone

Glutamine and GH, as individual agents and as parts of the same regimen, have been the factors most extensively studied in humans with SBS. Glutamine is an essential amino acid, which serves as an energy source for enterocytes and colonocytes. In vitro experiments have shown that glutamine stimulates intestinal cell proliferation. In animal studies, adding glutamine supplements to parenteral nutrition prevents mucosal atrophy and encourages mucosal hyperplasia after massive small bowel resection. Glutamine has been shown to induce levels of ODC by enterocytes in vitro. ODC is important in the pathway for the synthesis of polyamines, which are abundant in enterocytes undergoing proliferation.

Human GH is a single-chain peptide synthesized as a prehormone in the anterior pituitary gland. Studies have focused on the role of the anabolic effects of recombinant human GH on intestinal adaptation. Exogenous administration of GH in animals has been shown to enhance bowel growth and to increase ion transport. GH also has been shown to induce small bowel lengthening in newborn piglets.

Wilmore and associates have studied extensively patients with SBS undergoing treatment with a combination of GH, enteral and parenteral glutamine, and a high-carbohydrate diet. Of patients, 43 had a colonic remnant and an average of 50 cm of small intestine, whereas the remaining 4 patients had no colon and approximately 100 cm of combined jejunoileal length. At the end of a 4-week treatment period, these authors reported that 27 patients (57%) were completely weaned from TPN, 14 patients (30%) had reduced TPN requirements, and only 6 patients (13%) were receiving the same amount of TPN. Patients were discharged and maintained on the modified diet and enteral glutamine. In follow-up at 1 year, these values were still impressive at 40%, 40%, and 20%. Several criticisms of these results have been cited. The patients in Wilmore's initial absorption study were not randomized among the groups receiving modified diet alone, glutamine, GH, or the combination. Findings of a randomized, prospective study were in contrast to Wilmore's results. Because the end point of their study was the discontinuation of TPN (and not measurements of increased nutrient absorption), it is possible that the same reductions in TPN might have been attainable with their strict inpatient dietary regulation alone. It is also possible that some of the subjects in their heterogeneous, nonrandomized group were less "TPN-dependent" than others. The role of glutamine and GH in the treatment of SBS is unclear. More controlled studies in greater numbers of patients with and without colons are necessary to justify the widespread use of glutamine and GH.

Other Growth Factors

The concept that endogenous or exogenous circulating factors could produce alterations in small intestinal morphology and function is not new. The specific factors that induce this phenomenon are unclear, however. Over 20 years, Schwartz and associates have studied numerous peptides that have been discovered and subsequently shown in animal studies to enhance intestinal adaptation. Most of these peptides have not yet been studied in humans, however.

Numerous animal studies of epidermal growth factor (EGF) and insulin-like growth factor (IGF-1) suggest that these factors stimulate intestinal adaptation in patients with SBS. EGF is an endogenous peptide hormone secreted by the salivary glands and the endocrine cells of the small intestine. Using a rat short-bowel model, luminal EGF and IGF-1 were each capable of enhancing substrate absorption beyond the normal adaptive response, an effect that was sustained 2 weeks after cessation of treatment. Parenteral EGF significantly reduces mucosal atrophy in rats receiving TPN. It has been shown that systemic administration of interleukin-11 to rats after massive small bowel resection significantly increases mucosal mass and absorptive function beyond normal adaptation. Future clinical trials are necessary to define the roles of these and other growth factors as potential treatments for SBS.

Two peptides probably have the greatest clinical potential as growth factors for the small intestine. GLP-2 is a

33-amino acid peptide that is liberated from the carboxy-terminus of proglucagon in small and large intestine L cells by the action of tissue-specific proteases. It belongs to a specific class of compounds called *proglucagon-derived peptides*. Studies have shown that GLP-2 and GLP-2α enhance mucosal mass and absorptive function in rat models of SBS, ischemia-reperfusion injury, and normal intestine. Preliminary studies in humans also support its possible role in the treatment of SBS. It is believed that GLP-2 is one of the most promising trophic peptides for the small intestine. Phase II clinical trials are now under way to evaluate the role of exogenous GLP-2 in patients with SBS, using a protease-resistant GLP-2 analogue called *ALX-0600*.

Numerous studies have shown that hepatocyte growth factor (HGF) is also a potent trophic factor for the small intestine. Originally discovered in the serum of partially hepatectomized rats, HGF stimulates hepatocyte DNA synthesis, but it also has been shown in numerous other organs, including the small intestine. In vitro studies have implicated roles for HGF in intestinal epithelial cell repair and in stimulating the migration of human fetal intestinal cells.

HGF has been evaluated in several studies regarding its enhancement of small intestinal growth and absorptive function. In rats after massive small bowel resection, it initially was shown that HGF increases mucosal mass and enhances absorption of carbohydrate (galactose) and amino acid (glycine) beyond the normal adaptive response. It also has been shown that 3 weeks after cessation of the peptide exposure the enhanced absorption persists. Luminal delivery of HGF produces a greater trophic response than when given systemically. The HGF receptor has been identified in the brush border membranes of enterocytes, suggesting a mechanism for the trophic effect of luminal HGF. It has been shown that luminal administration of HGF significantly increases the expression of genes encoding the sodium/glucose cotransporter SGLT1 and the facilitative glucose transporter GLUT5 in the rat model of SBS.

Continued research aimed at further elucidating the process of intestinal adaptation may allow clinicians to employ therapeutically the various peptides and hormones that act as growth factors for the bowel mucosa. Exogenous administration of these growth factors ultimately will lead to the future success of definitively treating SBS. Knowledge gained from these studies combined with gene therapy techniques will result in the permanent enhancement of intestinal function beyond the normal adaptation process, eliminating the dependence on TPN, and avoid the need for intestinal transplantation.

SURGERY

Most operations developed to treat SBS are designed to slow transit time or to increase the mucosal surface area for improved absorption.

Reversed Intestinal Segment

To slow transit time and increase mucosal contact time, a 2- to 3-cm segment of small intestine is isolated with its blood supply, reversed and anastomosed in situ, re-establishing intestinal continuity. Reversed segments longer than 3 cm lead to intestinal obstruction and bacterial stasis and overgrowth. There have been only anecdotal reports of improved enteral nutrition after this procedure.

Recirculating Loop

A loop is constructed to allow nutrients and secretions to pass by the mucosa for several transits, increasing the opportunity for absorption. This procedure seldom has been clinically successful and has been abandoned.

Artificial Ileocecal Valves

Because of the importance of the ileocecal valve, attempts have been made to construct valves after ileal resection. Procedures have included the prolapse of a segment of small bowel into the large intestine and tunneling of a segment of ileum into the muscularis of the colon. Experimentally, these valves have reduced reflux of colon contents into the small intestine and increased transit time. Severe small bowel stasis and bacterial overgrowth still can occur, however. There have been few successful clinical reports using this technique.

Colon Interposition

Segments of colon (8 to 24 cm) have been interposed in the small bowel to slow transit time. Although this procedure has been successful in experimental animals, only a few encouraging clinical reports exist.

Small Intestine Tapering

Tapering of the dilated small intestine reduces stasis and bacterial overgrowth and the resulting malabsorption. By reducing small bowel bacterial overgrowth, bacterial translocation also may be decreased. This procedure has been used frequently. It has allowed some patients fully to adapt enterally and discontinue parenteral nutrition, but the results reported have not been uniformly good.

Intestinal Lengthening

Bianchi originally described intestinal lengthening in pigs. Because the terminal mesenteric vessels within the leaves of the mesentery separate and course to either side of the intestine, the mesenteric vasculature can be converted into two systems. The dilated small intestine can be split into two parallel segments, each with its own blood supply. This reduces the diameter of the dilated intestine by half and doubles its length. An intestinal stapling device expedites the procedure. A few successful cases have been reported in which the patients have been converted totally to enteral feedings and bouts of recurrent sepsis reduced. Patient selection is important. The intestinal diameter must be increased, resulting in poor peristalsis and increased risk of bacterial growth.

Neomucosal Patching

To grow neomucosa in the small bowel and increase the intestinal absorptive surface, a portion of the small bowel is opened. A patch of abdominal wall or colonic serosa is sutured over the resulting defect. Small intestinal mucosa grows over the inner aspect of the patch, increasing the total absorptive surface. Although this procedure has been effective in experimental animals, it has not been used clinically.

Intestinal Pacing

Retrograde pacing of the small intestine by electrodes implanted in the gut slows intestinal transit time and increases mucosal nutrient contact. This procedure has been effective in the treatment of experimental SBS, but there are no reported clinical cases.

Small Intestine Transplantation

Small intestine failure or inadequate intestinal length leads to the indications for small intestine transplantation in (1) patients with SBS who have failed to adapt, (2) patients unable to be maintained on enteral feedings and who are developing liver disease as a result of TPN, or (3) patients who have lost central venous access and TPN is no longer possible. Before the introduction of cyclosporine as an immunosuppressive agent, there were no long-term successful small bowel transplants. Cyclosporine with supplementary azathioprine and corticosteroids has resulted in improved but still less than optimal long-term survival. Improved immunosuppressive regimens, which include tacrolimus and better means of identifying rejection, have improved survival further. To date, more than 200 adults and children have undergone small intestine transplantation either as an isolated graft or in combination with the liver. The complications of small intestine failure are numerous and unique. Recurrent sepsis (in large part from bacterial translocation), lymphoproliferative disease from the adverse effects of aggressive immunosuppression, and bouts of rejection are common and life-threatening.

Rejection is a major issue in small intestine failure. Differentiating between infection and rejection can be difficult. No specific marker or test for rejection exists. Endoscopic small intestine transplant biopsy remains the standard, but this is subject to sampling errors. Also, interpretation of what constitutes histologic evidence of rejection has changed.

A report from the University of Pittsburgh indicated a 1-year graft and patient survival of 65% and 70%. This decreased to 50% and 55% at 3 years. Patients surviving small intestine failure were free of TPN in 92% of cases. In the pediatric age group, isolated small intestine transplant was more successful. This was not true for infants younger than age 2 years, however. The incidence of rejection was 92%. Because the incidence of death occurring while on the waiting list is still 50%, in some patients isolated liver transplants have been done when patients showed 50% enteral tolerance.

PROGNOSIS

Numerous series of SBS patients have been reported with survivals ranging from 25% to 80%. Although few of these series are comparable, adaptation did not seem to be related to the presence or absence of the ileocecal valve or even to a particular length unless it was 20 cm of small intestine or less. The overall incidence of adaptation and successful weaning to enteral diets for the 146 surviving patients in the combined series was 63%.

The management of SBS has changed considerably since the 1970s. Although before TPN there was little hope for survival, the current modalities offer an acceptable-to-good quality and quantity of life. TPN provides appropriate caloric needs. Improved enteral formulas can facilitate the absorptive capacity of the small intestine, and surgical manipulation, especially intestinal lengthening, may maximize the absorptive surface area. The results of small intestine transplant are improving, and when indicated, this procedure offers an acceptable option. The most promising modality for the future is the use of growth factors to stimulate growth of enterocytes and to improve their absorptive efficiency. Because most SBS patients adapt within 2 years after resection, ample time should be allowed for adaptation to occur before small intestine transplant is considered.

SUGGESTED READINGS

Abu-Elmagd K, Reyes J, Bond G, et al: Clinical intestinal transplantation: A decade of experience at a single center. Am Surg 234:404-417, 2001.

This report of 155 patients from Pittsburgh provides a thorough description of all aspects of small bowel transplantation and serves as an excellent summary of this undertaking.

Byrne T, Morrissey TB, Wattkom TV, et al: Growth hormone, glutamine, and a modified diet enhance nutrient absorption with severe short bowel syndrome. J Parenter Enteral Nutr 19:296-302, 1995.

This article from Wilmore's group describes a supportive approach to the management of SBS in a preliminary clinical trial that has proved to be useful.

Reyes J: Intestinal transplantation for children with short bowel syndrome. Semin Pediatr Surg 10:99-104, 2001.

This author from the Pittsburgh transplant center presents results with intestinal transplantation in childhood, which are representative of what currently can be expected as the outcome of this procedure.

Schwartz MZ, Kuenzler K: Pharmacotherapy and growth factors in the treatment of short bowel syndrome. Semin Pediatr Surg 10:81-90, 2001.

The authors summarize current clinical and experimental information on drug treatment of intestinal insufficiency.

Thompson JS: Surgical treatment of the short bowel syndrome. Pediatr Surg Int 3:303-311, 1988.

This is one of the best available descriptions of the various surgical procedures that have been used to treat SBS.

Vanderhoof JA, Young RJ: Enteral nutrition in short bowel syndrome. Semin Pediatr Surg 10:65-70, 2001.

An up-to-date review is provided of the various dietary compounds available for patients with SBS.

54

Intussusception

Although intussusception was described by Hunter in 1793, it was not until 1876 that the first series of hydrostatic reductions of intussusception in children was reported by Hirschprung. In 1913, Ladd published the first radiograph of a contrast enema in intussusception. Ravitch published his first article on a large series of successful barium enema reductions of intussusception in 1948 with standard guidelines.

INCIDENCE

The incidence of intussusception in the United States is 1.9 to 4 per 1000 live births. This also seems to be the incidence in other parts of the Western world. There is a male preponderance with a 3:2 ratio. Although there seems to be a higher incidence in whites than in blacks, many series do not substantiate this perceived difference. Idiopathic intussusception of infancy is seen most commonly between 6 and 10 months of age, with 65% of the children being less than 1 year of age. There seems to be a seasonal incidence, with two peaks occurring (1) in spring and summer and (2) in the middle of winter, corresponding to times of the year with an increased incidence of viral gastroenteritis and upper respiratory tract infections.

PATHOLOGY

Most cases of idiopathic intussusception of infancy have no distinct lead point; however, 2% to 8% of intussusceptions in this age group are secondary to a recognizable lesion of the bowel, such as polyp, Meckel's diverticulum, segment of ectopic pancreas, enterogenous cyst, or lymphosarcoma, which usually is found in slightly older children. With idiopathic intussusception, many viruses have been cultured from the stools of affected children, including rotaviruses, reoviruses, and echoviruses. It generally is believed that viral gastroenteritis leads to hypertrophy of Peyer's patches in the terminal ileum, which act as a lead point for the intussusception. Intussusception can occur with Henoch-Schönlein purpura, secondary to hematomas in the intestinal wall acting as lead points. Finally, children with cystic fibrosis have a significant incidence of intussusception. The etiology probably is related to the markedly thickened inspissated stool.

Another common cause in children is postoperative small bowel intussusception seen after abdominal or thoracic operations. Intussusception secondary to a long intestinal decompression tube also is seen occasionally.

The pathophysiology of intussusception starts with venous compression from the invagination of the bowel and its mesentery, which progresses to venous stasis and edema (Fig. 54-1). As the edema increases, arterial blood flow ceases, and bowel necrosis occurs. The goal of therapy is to relieve the intussusception before arterial compromise occurs.

CLINICAL FINDINGS

The characteristic clinical picture is that of a well-nourished male infant about 9 months old who suddenly awakens from sleep with colicky abdominal pain. The pain may pass, and the infant may go back to sleep, only to be awakened shortly with a similar clinical picture that does not remit. Pain is followed by repeated bouts of vomiting that may become bilious, then the passage of bloody mucus rectally, which may have the appearance of currant jelly. If this condition continues untreated, complete intestinal obstruction ensues, which if uncorrected may be fatal in 2 to 4 days. Pain is seen in 100% of children with intussusception and vomiting in about 80%. Blood in the stool is present in 95% of infants with idiopathic intussusception. Occasionally, infants present with signs of toxicity and are lethargic or stuporous. In these cases, the diagnosis may be confused with meningitis.

Physical examination reveals a sausage-shaped mass, usually in the right upper abdomen, in about 85% of patients. If the mass cannot be palpated abdominally, it rarely may be palpated on rectal examination. Associated with the mass is a sense of emptiness in the right lower quadrant (Dance's sign) because the intussusception has moved up to the hepatic flexure of the colon. Fever is common with intussusception in infants.

The thin barium enema study has been the traditional diagnostic test for evaluation and treatment of intussusception, but hydrostatic reduction with air is used in most cases now. Currently, abdominal ultrasound is the most widely used diagnostic study.

Hydrostatic reduction of an intussusception with air or barium can be successful if the principles outlined by

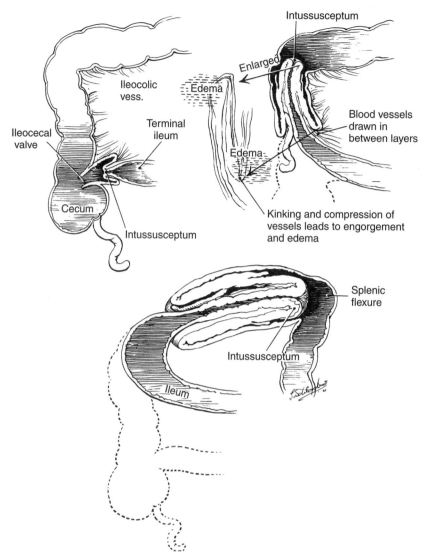

FIGURE 54-1 ■ Most cases of intussusception in infants and children are of the kind shown here. The intussusception begins at or near the ileocecal valve without an obvious precipitating anatomic lesion. Simultaneous interference of the patency of the alimentary canal and the vascular supply of the intussusceptum occurs. The mesenteric vessels are compressed between the layers of the intussusception. Interference with lymphatic and venous drainage results in edema and an increase in tissue pressure. This further increases resistance to the return of venous blood. Venules and capillaries become engorged, and bloody, edematous fluid drips into the lumen. The mucosal cells swell, and goblet cells discharge mucus, which mixes with the bloody transudate in the lumen and forms the currant jelly–like stool. Edema increases until venous inflow is completely obstructed. As arterial blood continues to enter the area of intussusception, tissue pressure rises until it is higher than arterial pressure, and gangrene ensues. The outer coat of the intussusceptum (middle layer of the intussusception) is isolated between two sharp bends and is the first to become gangrenous.

Ravitch are followed. The patient is admitted to the hospital when the diagnosis is confirmed. In the emergency department, a broad-spectrum antibiotic is administered intravenously. The patient is taken to the radiology suite for diagnosis and reduction of the intussusception (Fig. 54-2). A nasogastric tube usually is inserted. Anesthesia is not used, but sedation may be helpful during the study and reduction. In the radiology suite, the patient is restrained, and a Foley catheter is inserted into the rectum and strapped in place. The balloon is inflated and pulled down against the levator muscles to create a seal. Some radiologists prefer to use a straight catheter and tightly strap the buttocks rather than use a balloon catheter. If barium is used, it is allowed to run into the rectum from a height of 3 feet above the table, and fluoroscopy is used intermittently to observe the flow of the barium column. If air is used, instillation pressure should not exceed 120 cm H_2O (usually 60 to 80 cm H_2O). If reduction does not occur immediately, a few more attempts should be made before abandoning the procedure, and at times it may be worthwhile to administer glucagon intravenously as a last resort and attempt the reduction again. Complete reduction of the intussusception is marked by free flow of contrast material into

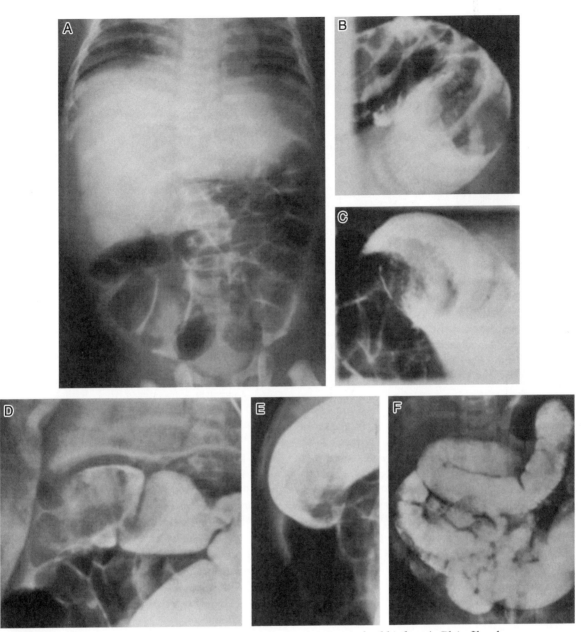

FIGURE 54-2 ■ Barium enema reduction of an intussusception in a 3-month-old infant. **A,** Plain film shows numerous distended loops with a picture of intestinal obstruction. **B,** Intussusception is at the splenic flexure, where a filling defect is seen with the seepage of barium around the intussusceptum, giving the appearance of a coiled spring. **C,** Intussusceptum is being displaced proximally. **D,** Intussusceptum is in the midtransverse colon. **E,** Filling defect is seen now in the hepatic flexure. **F,** Intussusception rapidly gives way, and the filling of numerous loops of small bowel gives evidence of complete reduction.

several loops of small bowel with simultaneous expulsion of feces. This usually is accompanied by disappearance of the abdominal mass and marked clinical improvement in the child. After successful reduction, the child is admitted for observation overnight. The next morning the antibiotics are stopped, feedings are started, and the child is discharged shortly thereafter.

If the reduction is not successful, the child is taken to the operating room for manual reduction of the intussusception (Fig. 54-3). The operation usually is performed through a right lower quadrant incision. The intussusception is palpated and reduced intra-abdominally by pushing the lead point rather than pulling it. Pulling of the intussuscepted bowel can result in serosal tears and perforation. After successful reduction, an appendectomy is carried out, and a search is made for lead points. The ileocecal valve often is markedly edematous after the reduction and can look like a large polyp. It is best not to perform a cecotomy to visualize this because it is extremely rare to find a polyp in the cecum of an infant acting as a lead point. If the intussusception cannot be reduced, bowel resection, usually involving the terminal ileum and proximal right colon, is required. Likewise, if necrotic bowel is found at laparotomy, resection of the involved

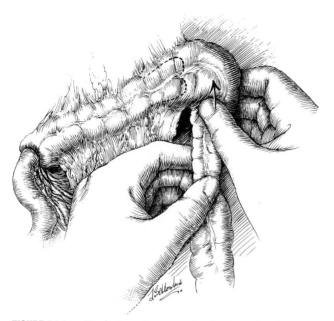

FIGURE 54-3 ■ Technique for manual reduction of an intussusception. The intussusception is being pushed rather than pulled. If reduction cannot be achieved without creating significant serosal tears, resection is required.

area is required. Primary anastomosis usually is performed, unless there is severe fecal contamination of the peritoneal cavity or unless the patient is highly toxic. In these latter two situations, temporary ileostomy is needed. After operative reduction, feedings usually are started the day following surgery, and the child often can be discharged the following day. As is the case with hydrostatic reduction, antibiotics are continued for 24 hours postoperatively.

Ultrasonography also has been used as a means of reducing the intussusception. Under ultrasound, saline solution appears as a contrast agent; the intussusception can be reduced successfully with saline solution enemas under ultrasound control. This technique is being evaluated further in a few centers.

The incidence of recurrence with intussusception is the same whether hydrostatic or surgical reduction is carried out; it varies between 5% and 7%. The current mortality rate in children with intussusception in developed countries is less than 1%. Mortality usually is related to delay in diagnosis, inadequate intravenous fluid and antibiotic therapy, delay in recognizing residual intussusception after nonsurgical reduction, and surgical complications.

SUGGESTED READINGS

Daneman A: Intussusception: Issues and controversies related to diagnosis and treatment. Radiol Clin North Am 34:743, 1999.

Controversies in the diagnosis and management of intussusception are reviewed.

Meyer JS, Dangman BC, Buonomo C, et al: Air and liquid contrast agents in the management of intussusception: A controlled, randomized trial. Radiology 188:507-511, 1993.

This controlled study showed that air is as effective as liquid contrast material for diagnosis and treatment.

Ravitch MM, McCune RM Jr: Reduction of intussusception by barium enema: A clinical and experimental study. Ann Surg 128:904, 1948.

This is an excellent review of the diagnosis and management of intussusception by one of the pioneers in the field.

55

Crohn's Disease

Regional enteritis was described and recognized as being different from other inflammatory conditions of the small intestine by Crohn and colleagues in 1932. Although originally believed to occur only in the ileum, it became evident that the colon is often involved and, less frequently, other segments of the intestinal tract. The colonic form of the disease was not differentiated from ulcerative colitis until 30 years later.

Crohn's disease (CD) occurs with equal frequency in men and women and is five times more prevalent in whites than in blacks, with a marked increase among Jews. Epidemiologic studies from England and Norway indicate a progressive increase in incidence. The peak onset is in the mid to late teens to early 20s; however, approximately 5% of patients are younger than 5 years of age. Children of parents with CD and siblings of affected children have a higher (35-fold to 70-fold) risk.

ETIOLOGY

The cause of CD is unknown, although the same causative factors suggested for ulcerative colitis may be implicated. No dietary habits or specific dietary ingredients have been implicated consistently with development of CD. A genetic factor and transmissible infection are considered as likely possibilities, inasmuch as both are observed in many patients with CD. The *HLA B27* gene is known to predispose to the development of inflammatory bowel disease and is the basis of a unique animal model of inflammatory bowel disease. Some investigators have indicated that nonsteroidal anti-inflammatory drugs, toxins, and infections may reduce the ability of the intestine to regulate the mucosal diffusion of luminal bacterial products. Because lymphangiectasia and prominent mesenteric lymphadenopathy are frequent pathologic features in CD, obstructive lymphangitis also has been suggested as a possible etiologic factor. Smoking has been recognized as one of the strongest exogenous risk factors for the development of CD.

PATHOLOGY

In CD, the intestinal wall is thickened by submucosal edema, fibrosis, and lymphatic dilation. Small slit-like ulcers may appear in the mucosa, which enlarge into serpiginous ulcers, producing a cobblestone appearance (Fig. 55-1). Except for the mucosa adjacent to these ulcers, the gland tubules and goblet cells are generally normal. Fissures often occur parallel to the long axis of the intestine, particularly notable on the mesenteric side. These ulcerations may penetrate deeply or into the muscularis and can produce sinus tracts, fistulas, adhesions, and chronic abscesses. Characteristic epithelioid cell granulomas containing multinucleated giant cells are present in approximately 60% of patients (Fig. 55-2). Granulomas chiefly occur in the submucosa but may be found in the muscularis, subserosally, or in regional lymph nodes. Although noncaseating granulomas are a valuable diagnostic feature of CD, their presence is not specific for the diagnosis and does not imply activity. The bowel wall is usually thickened where transmural inflammation is present.

Frequently the surgeon can estimate the extent of gross involvement with CD at the time of operation based on

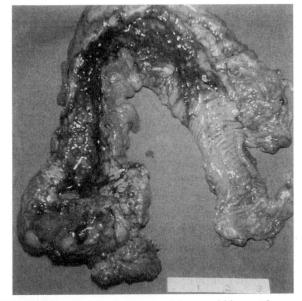

FIGURE 55-1 ■ Right colon from a 16-year-old boy with severe granulomatous colitis. Note the severe thickening of the intestinal wall and linear ulcerations through the mucosa. An abrupt line of demarcation is noted between normal and diseased intestine.

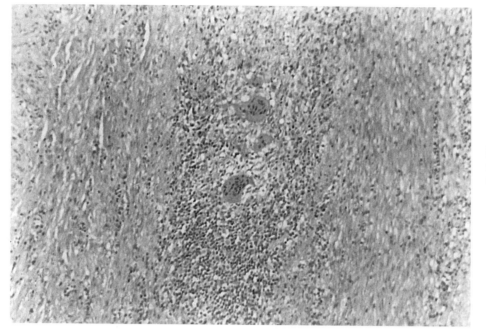

FIGURE 55-2 ■ Histologic section from distal ileum shows non-caseating granulomas.

the degree of intestinal thickening, the extent of fat surrounding the intestine, an increase in subserosal vascularity, or the presence of a firm stricture. It is not unusual to observe skip areas of involved intestine with intervening normal segments.

NATURAL HISTORY

Although CD typically affects young adults, it has been recognized increasingly in children. In a review of more than 600 cases at the Mayo Clinic, 14% of patients had symptoms before age 15 years. Similarly, Rogers and associates found that in 21% of 489 patients with CD, the onset occurred before age 15. Although CD has been reported more often at an earlier age and with more severe symptoms than noted previously, medical treatment, while rarely curative, often helps to alleviate acute symptoms. Early dominant complaints include weight loss (90%), abdominal pain (70%), diarrhea (67%), and fever (25%). Extraintestinal manifestations including arthritis also may become apparent early in the course of the disease.

Bloody diarrhea is common with CD of the colon, although rectal bleeding occurs less frequently than in patients with ulcerative colitis. Diagnosis delayed more than 1 year after onset of symptoms has occurred in more than two thirds of affected children. More than one third initially were believed to have nongastrointestinal disorders.

Children with CD have a more chronic, continuous course in contrast to patients with ulcerative colitis, who tend to have alternating remissions and relapses. Perianal ulcers, abscesses, and fistulas are frequent in children with CD of the colon in contrast to patients with ulcerative colitis. Perianal lesions are often the first manifestation of CD. Ileocolitis is the most common form of CD in children requiring surgery (55%). In approximately 34%,

the colon was the only site of involvement, and disease confined to the small intestine was present in 10%.

Many of the extraintestinal manifestations reported for ulcerative colitis also occur with CD, including growth retardation, weight loss, lack of sexual maturation, arthralgias, skin lesions (erythema nodosum, pyoderma gangrenosum), sclerosing cholangitis, cholelithiasis, nephrolithiasis, uveitis, anemia, and stomatitis (Table 55-1). Biopsy of the oral lesions may show granulomas typical of CD. Some children with severe CD manifest digital clubbing.

PHYSICAL FEATURES

Children with CD often have growth retardation and are underweight for age. A tender mass in the right lower abdomen is a common finding in patients with ileocecal disease. Perianal ulcers or sinuses are typical in children with colorectal disease. The ulcers are often painful, extending widely in the perineum with sinuses and undermining the bowel wall with indolent granulation tissue at the base (Fig. 55-3). With extensive ulceration, the perineal muscles may become damaged. Sigmoidoscopic examination is often normal in children with CD of the small intestine and in children who have localized colonic involvement, but with rectal sparing. In patients with rectal disease, the mucosa may resemble that seen in ulcerative colitis but is usually less friable and often contains linear mucosal ulcerations.

Laboratory findings in children with CD usually indicate anemia, elevation of the erythrocyte sedimentation rate, hypoalbuminemia, increase of immunoglobulin A, and prolonged prothrombin time. Vitamin B_{12} absorption may be abnormal if there is extensive distal ileal involvement. Stool cultures are consistently negative for pathogenic bacteria and parasites.

The radiographic appearance in CD can reveal abnormalities of any site from the esophagus to the rectum,

TABLE 55-1 ■ Crohn's Disease: Extraintestinal Manifestations

Eyes
    Anterior uveitis
    Iritis
    Episcleritis
Mouth
    Aphthous ulcers
    Liver
    Pericholangitis
    Sclerosing cholangitis
    Chronic hepatitis
    Cholelithiasis
Kidneys
    Oxalate stones
    Hydronephrosis
    Pyelonephritis
    Urinary tract infection
Joints
    Migratory arthritis
    Ankylosing spondylitis
    Clubbing
Skin
    Erythema nodosum
    Pyoderma gangrenosun
    Hyperkeratosis
Miscellaneous
    Amyloidosis
    Thromboembolic phenomena

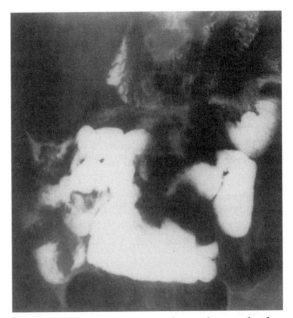

FIGURE 55-4 ■ Small intestine radiographic study from a 13-year-old girl with ileocolonic Crohn's disease with ileoileal and ileocutaneous fistulas.

but they chiefly occur in the distal ileum and colon. The small bowel mucosa may appear flattened, thickened, or distorted, and thickening of the bowel wall may show separation of contrast-filled bowel loops. Mucosal ulcerations, luminal narrowing, intestinal fistulas, sinus tracts, or intra-abdominal abscesses may be present (Fig. 55-4). Benign strictures and skip lesions are frequent.

COMPLICATIONS

Sinuses and internal fistulas are characteristic of CD and should be suspected when a flare-up of symptoms is associated with the development of persistent abdominal pain, localized abdominal tenderness, and the presence of a mass. The fistula often is located between the terminal ileum and right colon or sigmoid colon. Development of a draining sinus after an appendectomy may indicate CD, although a sinogram occasionally shows that the internal opening leads into the distal ileum and not the base of the appendix. Fistulas from the intestine to the bladder or urethra occasionally occur. Urinary tract infection in a patient with CD suggests enterovesicle fistula; pneumaturia or fecaluria confirms this complication.

In contrast to ulcerative colitis, toxic megacolon rarely occurs with CD. Free perforation into the peritoneal cavity is uncommon but can happen during an acute exacerbation of chronic disease, particularly in the presence of distal obstruction. Rarely is steroid therapy implicated as a major factor in the development of a perforation.

Adenocarcinoma of the intestine is an uncommon complication of CD, is less frequent than with chronic ulcerative colitis, and is rare in children. Nonetheless, the incidence of colorectal carcinoma is approximately 20 times greater in patients with CD than in the general population. Carcinoma usually is found to be contiguous with areas of high-grade dysplasia.

MEDICAL MANAGEMENT

Because CD is a chronic relapsing inflammatory condition, therapy is directed at reducing the inflammation and providing symptomatic relief. Most children with CD can be managed on an ambulatory basis for long periods with dietary modifications, including high-calorie,

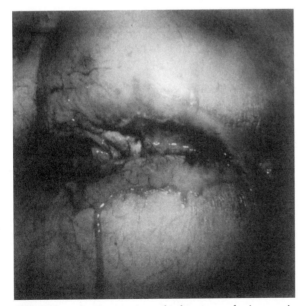

FIGURE 55-3 ■ Severe perirectal abscess and sinuses in a 17-year-old boy with colorectal Crohn's disease of 6 years' duration.

TABLE 55-2 ■ **Pharmacologic Options in the Management of Crohn's Disease**

Acetylsalicylic acid–based substances
  Sulfasalazine
  5-Aminosalicylic acid
  Mesalamine (Rowasa suppositories, enemas)
Corticosteroids
  Prednisone
  Budesonide
Antibiotics
  Metronidazole
  Ciprofloxacin
Immunosuppressants
  Azathioprine
  6-Mercaptopurine
  Cyclosporine
  Tacrolimus (Prograf)
Anticytokine and anti–tumor necrosis factor agents
  Infliximab (Remicade)
  Etanercept
Growth factors (experimental)
  Hepatocyte growth factor
  Interleukin-11
Angiogenesis antagonist
  Thalidomide

high-protein, low-roughage foods. Milk is eliminated for children with milk intolerance. In patients with steatorrhea, a low-fat diet with added medium-chain triglycerides is recommended. Between-meal nutritious snacks are encouraged.

Sulfasalazine (Azulfidine) or mesalamine is the initial treatment for CD, although they tend to be less effective than for ulcerative colitis (Table 55-2). Certain antibiotics, such as metronidazole and ciprofloxacin, in low dosage have helped to relieve symptoms with minimum side effects in several patients. Steroids (prednisone) are administered when other medical measures have failed to achieve improvement and indications for operation are not yet present. Some studies have indicated that budesonide, a glucocorticosteroid almost as effective as prednisone, but without the steroid-associated side effects, may be equally effective. Steroids also are given to acutely ill hospitalized children in toxic condition to treat uncomfortable extraintestinal manifestations, such as arthralgias and skin lesions unresponsive to other measures, and to children with extensive enteritis considered to be inoperable. Topical mesalamine (Rowasa) as an enema or suppository may be helpful in patients with distal rectal or anorectal CD.

Immunosuppressant medications, such as azathioprine (Imuran) and 6-mercaptopurine, have been used as secondary drugs to treat children with chronic CD, with occasional success. Patients receiving long-term azathioprine and prednisone therapy have a 5% incidence of de novo tumors, estimated to be 80 times greater than that of the general population. Cyclosporine suppresses cell-mediated immunity by interfering with interleukin-2 synthesis and release and has been administered to patients unresponsive to other therapy with better results than reported for azathioprine. Long-term use of this medication may produce serious side effects, such as nephrotoxicity and increased susceptibility to infections. Tacrolimus (Prograf), another immunosuppressive drug, has been shown to have a beneficial effect in the management of chronic CD.

The observation of increased mucosal levels of tumor necrosis factor-α in inflamed CD intestine has prompted the experimental use of certain anti–tumor necrosis factor medications, such as infliximab (Remicade) and etanercept, in the treatment of patients with chronic CD unresponsive to other medications. The high cost of these agents has been a limiting factor. Thalidomide, an angiogenesis antagonist, also has been reported to be of some benefit in the treatment of persistent CD. In experimental models of inflammatory bowel disease, hepatocyte growth factor, interleukin-11, and blocking agents have shown promise in clinical trials.

Cholestyramine resin may be beneficial in treating diarrhea after ileal resection. Antispasmodics on a continuous basis may be helpful in alleviating diarrhea and abdominal cramps. Long-term analgesic medications should be avoided because of the addictive potential. Similarly, nonsteroidal anti-inflammatory drugs should be used rarely because of the potential for exacerbating intestinal inflammation.

Hospitalization for children with CD is advised when symptoms become severe and there is progressive nutritional deficiency despite therapy on an ambulatory basis. Parenteral alimentation; bowel rest; and electrolyte, vitamin, and trace element repletion may produce improvement in many patients. The ready accessibility of a sympathetic and interested family and physician on whom the patient can rely does much to reduce the severity of the disease.

OPERATIVE THERAPY

Surgery for selected patients with CD may produce marked clinical improvement and make it feasible to reduce the dose or discontinue medications. Surgical treatment is rarely curative, however, and is associated with a high incidence of recurrent disease. Surgery is indicated for the complications of CD, including intestinal obstruction, growth retardation, medical intractability, enterocutaneous or enteric fistulas, perirectal fistulas or abscess, intestinal bleeding, abdominal pain, or abdominal abscess. A judicious combination of complete bowel rest with total parenteral nutrition before and after operation has helped to reduce the complications of surgery and restore most of these patients to an improved quality of life.

During the 24 years from 1967 through 1991, 72 patients, 18 years old or younger, underwent operations for CD and its complications at UCLA Hospital. The 49 male and 23 female patients had a median duration of symptoms before operation of 3.2 years. Inflammatory bowel disease was present in immediate family members in 12 of the 72 patients (16%). During the same 24 years, at least 60 other children with CD were treated by medical therapy without operation.

Although CD generally is recognized as a diffuse condition involving primarily the small intestine and cecum, three general patterns of the condition were identified

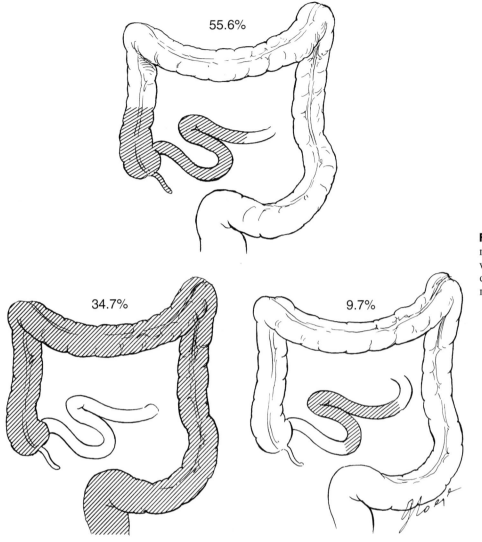

FIGURE 55-5 ■ Location of primary involvement in the intestine with Crohn's disease from 72 children who underwent operative management.

in the 72 children who had been operated on (Fig. 55-5). Of patients, 40 had disease in the terminal ileum and cecum or ascending colon, whereas 25 had involvement of the colon and rectum. Seven children had disease limited to a portion of the small intestine.

Intestinal obstruction was the condition requiring initial operation in children with ileocecal disease (90%), whereas only three of the patients with colorectal disease (12%) had obstruction (Table 55-3). Protracted diarrhea was a prominent symptom in only 8 of the 40 children with ileocecal disease, whereas almost all children with colorectal inflammation had severe diarrhea. Rectal bleeding occurred in only five from the latter group. Growth retardation and delayed development of secondary sex characteristics were present in 33% of children with ileocecal disease and 48% of children with colorectal inflammation.

Primary or secondary enterocutaneous fistulas were present in 8 of the 40 patients with ileocecal disease and in 3 of the 25 patients with colorectal inflammation. In two children, the fistulas developed 2 years after appendectomy. Six children with ileocecal disease had

TABLE 55-3 ■ Symptoms of Crohn's Disease Related to Location*				
	Terminal Ileum and Cecum (40 Patients)		Colon and Rectum (25 Patients)	
Symptoms	**No.**	**(%)**	**No.**	**(%)**
Intestinal obstruction	36	90	3	12
Diarrhea	8	20	24	96
Growth failure	13	33	12	48
Internal or external fistulas	14	35	4	16
Anal fistula or abscess	2	5	19	76
Arthralgias	12	30	10	40
Mean age at first operation	17.3 yr		15.2 yr	

*UCLA data.

TABLE 55-4 ■ Major Indications for Operation	
Indication	No. Operations (72 Children)
Intestinal obstruction	39
Perianal fistula, ulcer, abscess	36
Growth failure, persistent diarrhea, pain, fever	27
Recurrent small intestinal disease after previous resection	18
Enteroenteric fistula	11
Enterocutaneous fistula	5
Cholelithiasis	5
Abdominal pain of undetermined cause	4
Total	145

TABLE 55-5 ■ Operations for Crohn's Disease	
Operation	No. Operations (72 Children)
Resection of distal ileum and right side of the colon with anastomosis	39
Drainage, débridement of perianal sinus, fistula, abscess	36
Total proctocolectomy and ileostomy	24
Small bowel resection with anastomosis or ileostomy	14
Resection of distal ileum and >50% of colon with anastomosis	7
Resection of distal ileum and segment of colon with ileostomy and colostomy	6
Exploratory laparotomy and appendectomy	5
Cholecystectomy	5
Ileostomy without intestinal resection	3
Exploratory laparotomy with resection	3
Colon resection with anastomosis	1
Diverting colostomy	1
Gastroenterostomy	1
Total	145

enteroenteric fistulas, including one that communicated with the bladder.

Anal fistulas, abscesses, or indolent fissures are often the earliest manifestation of CD and are more than 15 times as common in colorectal disease as in ileocecal disease. Palder and associates observed that 62% of 325 children with CD had perianal disease. Four required intestinal resection or enterostomy for progressive perianal disease. Others were treated medically with local surgical measures. There is a limited role for extensive surgery, but there is a great need for meticulous perianal care. Nitroglycerin 0.2% has been used locally with some success. Perianal disease may be simple, as with a fissure or ulcer, or more complex, with an abscess or a fistula that may be simple or more extensive and occasionally lead to a rectovaginal fistula.

Resection of a short segment of the ileum for obstruction was performed on three of the seven children who had localized disease of the small intestine. Strictureplasty has been reserved for patients with localized obstruction associated with extensive small bowel disease. Three other children with CD of the ileum experienced sudden onset of abdominal pain, which was diagnosed as appendicitis. Each of these patients underwent exploratory laparotomy during which an uninflamed appendix was found, but a diseased distal ileum in the absence of obstruction was noted; each underwent an uneventful appendectomy. The inflammatory disease in each was managed successfully by nonoperative therapy.

Primary indications for surgery in the 72 children are listed in Table 55-4, although many had more than one indication. Intestinal obstruction with resultant pain, malnutrition, and fever was the most common reason and was present before 39 of the 145 operations. Growth failure, frequently accompanied by persistent diarrhea, pain, and fever, was the indication for operation on 27 occasions. Operation for treatment of perianal fistulas, sinuses, or abscesses that caused severe discomfort was performed on 21 patients, all but 2 of whom had persistent colorectal inflammation. Either diverting ileostomy or proctocolectomy eventually was performed on all but two of these patients. Laparotomy and intestinal resection

for enteroenteric fistulas with or without localized abscess and obstruction were performed on 11 children.

Parenteral nutrition was administered to 61 of the 72 patients and has been used routinely in the perioperative period in almost all children undergoing operation during the past 25 years. Corticosteroids, sulfasalazine, mesalamine, or a combination was used during the course of medical management at some time in the preoperative period in 70 of the 72 children; most were receiving steroids at the time of operation.

During the 24 years of this study, 145 operations were performed on the 72 children (Table 55-5). Resection of the distal ileum and ascending colon with reanastomosis was the dominant intra-abdominal operation, performed on 39 patients. Drainage or débridement of perianal sinuses, fistulas, or abscesses was performed on 36 occasions. Total proctocolectomy with cutaneous ileostomy was performed on 24 patients; however, in only 11 patients was this procedure carried out as the initial operation (Fig. 55-6). The other 12 patients with colorectal disease previously underwent a diverting ileostomy or colostomy or ileocolonic resection with or without anastomosis. In nine patients, additional distal ileum was resected within 8 years after ileostomy and proctocolectomy for localized recurrence.

Appendectomy had been performed on 11 children, 6 in other hospitals during the 6 years before resection; only 2 of the patients had acute appendicitis (18%). In three of these patients, enteric fistulas developed later, which appeared to originate in the cecum. Five patients in whom cholelithiasis and cholecystitis developed after ileal or colonic resection later required cholecystectomy.

RESULTS

With a follow-up period of 5 months to 29 years, all 72 patients who underwent surgery survived for more than

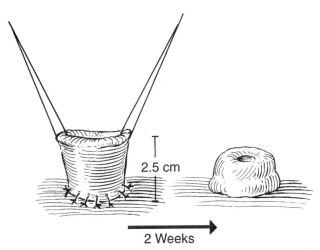

FIGURE 55-6 ■ For construction of an end ileostomy in children, the mesentery is mobilized from the distal 2.5 cm of ileum. The side of the ileum is sutured to dermis circumferentially with interrupted absorbable suture. No fascial sutures are used. The stoma will mature spontaneously without sutured eversion.

10 years. Inflammatory disease of the small intestine recurred in 10 of the 40 patients with ileocecal disease (25%). Recurrence occurred in each of the 15 children with colorectal disease (100%) who had a lesser operation than proctocolectomy; 62% had recurrence after proctocolectomy, and 9 of the 25 patients required further operation. Two of the three with primary ileal disease who underwent resection subsequently developed recurrent disease.

In most patients, recurrent disease was managed successfully with mesalamine or sulfasalazine, steroid therapy, bowel rest with partial or total parenteral nutrition, or metronidazole therapy for varying periods. Recurrent disease in the small intestine in patients who had primary colorectal involvement was occasionally severe, extending to the duodenum in two patients and involving internal fistulas in three. In contrast, recurrent disease was more localized and milder in patients with primary ileocecal involvement. Five required reoperation owing to persistent perineal sinus after proctocolectomy. Nine others required resection of a short segment of terminal ileum with revision of the ileostomy stoma.

COMPARISON OF METHODS

Removal of the diseased intestine with reanastomosis is the optimal operative procedure for treatment of CD. Although it was previously common practice to resect several centimeters of normal intestine proximal and distal to the involved area, studies by Hamilton and associates showed that reanastomosis of intestine with mild disease rarely interferes with healing and is less likely to lead to short-intestine syndrome. Skip areas of involved small intestine are usually not resected, unless they cause obstruction or other symptoms. Although strictureplasty has been reported to benefit patients with multiple small intestinal segments of stricture to avoid multiple resections and possible subsequent short-bowel syndrome, minimal experience has been reported with this technique in children.

Colectomy with ileosigmoid anastomosis may be performed in children with mild rectal involvement who do not have perianal sinuses or fistulas. Even in this small group, recurrent inflammation in the ileum requiring subsequent operation is common. The endorectal ileal pull-through procedure with reservoir and the continent ileostomy (Kock pouch) generally are contraindicated because of the high frequency of recurrent disease in the distal ileum. Resection of an inflammatory mass involving the distal ileum and cecum may endanger the right ureter, mandating cautious dissection. Identification of the ureter before extensive dissection into the retroperitoneal tissues is highly advisable. Enterovesicle fistulas are treated by resection of the diseased intestine with simultaneous closure of the bladder.

Ileostomy without colon resection or bypass operations is followed by a higher incidence of complications and far lower degree of clinical improvement than are limited resections or strictureplasty. End rather than loop ileostomies are preferred in the surgical management of CD. Internal fistulas involving intestine near the site of resection are removed along with the specimen. Fistulas to intestine at a distance from the site of resection are divided. If the distal intestine appears healthy, simple closure of the fistula is done. If the distal intestinal segment evidences active disease, a second resection is performed.

Appendectomy is indicated when laparotomy is performed for abdominal pain and there is no active disease in the cecum or distal ileum. Laparoscopic appendectomy permits more thorough evaluation of the abdomen than open appendectomy. The incidence of subsequent fistula formation is more than sixfold higher in children with ileocecal inflammation than in patients without CD. Acute appendicitis is less common in children with CD than in the normal population. Crohn's disease of the duodenum causing obstruction is treated best by gastrojejunostomy and vagotomy to prevent jejunal ulceration, although recurrent symptoms are likely to occur.

The reported recurrence rate of 50% within 3 years after operation for CD, which gradually increases to 90%, indicates that surgical therapy rarely cures this condition. Recurrent CD often develops proximal to an ileostomy stoma.

Operation for recurrent CD is necessary in approximately 30% of patients who have had a previous primary resection. The success rate of the second operation is more than 50%. In a review by Greenstein of 100 postoperative patients with CD of the ileum or colon, 58 patients required reoperation; there was a cumulative reoperation rate of 89% and clinical recurrence rate of 94% by the 15th postoperative year; the reoperation rate diminished with each succeeding operation; and the annual rate of operation from the time of onset was 15% per year.

For patients who retain diseased intestine, perianal wounds heal poorly or not at all. Simple débridement or adequate drainage is sufficient for treatment of perianal wounds and chronic infection in many patients. Satisfactory healing usually follows complete extirpation of the diseased bowel if the perianal lesions are well débrided and the patient's nutritional state is good.

SUMMARY

Despite the high incidence of recurrent disease after operation in children with CD, there is a gratifying response with relief of major symptoms in many patients. Most gain weight and are free of pain and extraintestinal symptoms for extended periods. When necessary, additional resections are performed, and the patient's condition is likely to improve again. The goal of a one-time curative operation for CD is rarely achievable, however. For most children with CD, treatment includes many years of intermittent medical therapy with occasional operations for the treatment of specific complications, with the goal of preserving as much length of intestine as feasible. Most of these patients experience fewer, milder symptoms and require less vigorous therapy as they progress into adulthood.

SUGGESTED READINGS

Block GE, Michelassi F: Crohn's disease. Curr Probl Surg 30:177, 1993.

This is an authoritative extensive review of the management of Crohn's disease.

Fazio VW, Galandiuk S, Jagelman BG, et al: Stricturoplasty in Crohn's disease. Ann Surg 210:621, 1989.

An evaluation by the authority in the field of the role of stricturoplasty in the surgical management of Crohn's disease with obstruction.

Fazio VW, Wu JS: Surgical therapy for Crohn's disease of the colon and rectum. Surg Clin North Am 77:197, 1997.

This is a review of the surgical management of Crohn's disease of the colon and rectum by a leading authority.

Fonkalsrud EW, Ament ME, Fleisher D, et al: Surgical management of Crohn's disease in children. Am J Surg 138:15, 1979.

This is one of the largest published reviews of clinical experience in the surgical management of Crohn's disease in childhood.

Greenstein AJ, Sachar DB, Pastemack BS, et al: Reoperation and recurrence in Crohn's colitis and ileocolitis. N Engl J Med 293:685, 1975.

A thorough review of factors leading to recurrence and reoperation after resection for Crohn's disease based on the clinical experience at one of the largest centers in the United States. There has been no change in the incidence of recurrence since this report.

Palder SB, Shandling B, Billick R, et al: Perianal complications of pediatric Crohn's disease. J Pediatr Surg 26:513, 1991.

An extensive review of perianal disease based on clinical experience with a large number of patients is presented.

Podolsky DK: Inflammatory bowel disease. N Engl J Med 347:417-429, 2002.

An in-depth review is given of the entire subject of inflammatory bowel disease, describing not only modern management but also discussing the issue of differentiating the various forms of inflammatory bowel disease.

Telander RL: Surgical management of Crohn's disease in children. Curr Opin Pediatr 7:328, 1995.

This article reviews the surgical management of children with Crohn's disease.

PART VIII

Colon, Rectum, and Anus

56

Gastrointestinal Bleeding

Bleeding from the gastrointestinal (GI) tract may present with hematemesis, hematochezia, melena, or occult blood in the stool. Although peptic ulcer disease, diverticular disease of the colon, and angiodysplasia are the most common causes of GI bleeding in adults, these conditions are seen rarely in children. The causes of GI bleeding in infants and children can be categorized into diagnostic age groups in which the age of the patient, the amount of bleeding, the presence of blood on passage of a nasogastric (NG) tube, and the color of the blood passed rectally often provide some guidance to the probable source of bleeding. Pediatric patients can be divided conveniently into four main age groups: (1) neonates, (2) infants, (3) toddlers and preschool children, and (4) older children and teenagers (Tables 56-1 and 56-2).

NEONATES (BIRTH TO 1 MONTH OLD)

A common cause of hematemesis or return of blood on NG tube placement and passage of blood rectally in neonates is related to swallowing maternal blood at the time of birth. The newborn in this instance is hemodynamically stable and has a steady hematocrit value. The Apt test for maternal blood usually resolves the issue regarding the source of blood. This test is accomplished by mixing the bloody stool or emesis with 1% sodium hydroxide. Fetal hemoglobin resists oxidation and remains pinkish red, whereas maternal hemoglobin changes to a dark brown color. Swallowed maternal blood is to be distinguished from stress gastritis, which may be seen occasionally with neonatal distress. NG tube lavage followed by administration of H_2-blocking agents usually suffices for treatment of stress gastritis.

An anal fissure is the most common cause of rectal bleeding in neonates. This condition often presents with coating of the stool with streaks of *bright* red blood. Direct inspection of the anal canal, if necessary with a nasal speculum, often allows visualization of the fissure. Rectal examination may reveal anal stenosis. Treatment with stool softeners, sitz baths, and rectal dilation, if a stenosis is present, resolves the problem in most patients.

Passage of occult or gross *dark* blood per rectum, especially when associated with the passage of mucus or mucosa, suggests necrotizing enterocolitis, particularly in low-birth-weight neonates. Increased gastric residuals and abdominal distention also may be observed in infants with this process. Although not typical, *bright* red rectal bleeding may indicate colonic involvement with necrotizing enterocolitis. A plain abdominal radiograph may show pneumatosis intestinalis, free air from a bowel perforation, or the presence of portal venous air. This condition is discussed in Chapter 52.

Another relatively common cause of rectal bleeding in neonates is malrotation with midgut volvulus (Fig. 56-1). The infant usually passes *dark* blood mixed with the stool. Occasionally, sloughed mucosa also is passed. Most of these patients have a clinical presentation with sudden onset of bilious vomiting. Although immediate operation rarely is required in newborns, malrotation with volvulus is one diagnosis that represents a surgical emergency. Later the vomitus may become bloody. Although often associated with necrotic bowel, bleeding may be associated with venous congestion. Plain abdominal radiographs and, especially, an upper GI (UGI) contrast study usually document the problem (see Chapter 47 for a more thorough discussion of this condition).

Rectal bleeding in newborns may be caused by more unusual medical conditions that affect neonates, including hemorrhagic disease of the newborn, hypoprothrombinemia, and thrombocytopenia. These conditions are associated with either a prolonged prothrombin time or a history of maternal intake of medications that interfere with vitamin K metabolism (e.g., sulfa drugs). In most instances, bleeding responds to the administration of parenteral vitamin K. Thrombocytopenia may be related to maternal or neonatal idiopathic thrombocytopenic purpura or sepsis or may be a sign of necrotizing enterocolitis.

In the evaluation of patients in all age groups, including neonates, an orogastric or NG tube should be passed to rule out the possibility of bleeding from a source in the UGI tract. Although colonoscopy often is done early in the work-up of adults with rectal bleeding, this procedure is rarely necessary in newborns. Despite careful assessment, the cause of GI bleeding in 50% of neonates may remain unexplained.

INFANTS (3 TO 12 MONTHS OLD)

Beyond 1 month of age, the most common causes of GI bleeding include anal fissure; esophagitis, usually associated with gastroesophageal reflux; gastritis;

TABLE 56-1 ■ Common Causes of Gastrointestinal Bleeding in Children by Age

Age Group	Cause of Bleeding	Diagnostic Studies
Neonates (birth to 1 mo)	Swallowed maternal blood Hemorrhagic disease of newborn NEC Malrotation and volvulus	Apt test, platelet count, PT, PTT, orogastric tube, anorectal examination, plain abdominal radiographs (NEC), UGI contrast study (malrotation)
Infants (3-12 mo)	Anal fissure Intussusception Intestinal volvulus Duplication Gastroenteritis Esophagitis Peptic ulcer disease	Platelet count, PT, PTT, bleeding time, orogastric tube, anorectal examination, fecal cultures, plain abdominal radiographs, barium or air contrast enema, UGI ± small bowel contrast study, upper endoscopy ± test for *H. pylori*, colonoscopy and isotope scan for duplication if enema study does not show intussusception
Toddlers and preschoolers (1-5 yr)	Juvenile polyp Anal fissure Rectal prolapse Gastroenteritis Meckel's diverticulum Peptic ulcer disease Intussusception Gastroenteritis Inflammatory bowel disease Hemolytic uremic syndrome Henoch-Schönlein disease Duplication Telangectasias Bowel ulcers Hemangiomas	Platelet count, PT, PTT, bleeding time, urinalysis, orogastric tube, fecal culture, plain abdominal radiographs, barium or air contrast enema, UGI ± small bowel contrast study, anorectal examination, upper endoscopy ± test for *H. pylori*, colonoscopy; if negative, isotope scan for Meckel's diverticulum; if negative, labeled red blood cell isotope scan, or if rapid bleeding is present, selective arteriography; if negative, laparoscopy or laparotomy
Older children and teenagers (6-18 yr)	Polypoid diseases Inflammatory bowel disease Hemorrhoids Meckel's diverticulum Gastroesophageal varices Hemangiomas Peptic ulcer disease Duplication Gastritis Telangectasias Bowel ulcers Hemolytic uremic syndrome Henoch-Schönlein disease	Similar to above

NEC, necrotizing enterocolitis; PT, prothrombin time; PTT, partial thromboplastin time.

intussusception; and intestinal volvulus. Although unusual, bleeding in the UGI tract may be due to esophagitis, usually secondary to reflux, and rarely to peptic ulcer disease. Both problems are assessed by UGI endoscopy and usually respond to H₂-blocking and prokinetic agents. Work-up for reflux with a UGI radiographic or pH probe evaluation (or both) may be required. Patients with reflux who are unresponsive to medical treatment may require fundoplication.

Anal fissure continues to be the most common cause of rectal bleeding in the first year of life. Diagnosis and treatment are similar to that alluded to in the preceding section. When the infant changes from formula to table foods, a high-fiber diet may be an effective method of maintaining a soft stool. If the fissure appears large and is surrounded by bruising, child abuse must be suspected.

From age 3 months to 3 years, a common cause of rectal bleeding is idiopathic ileocolic intussusception (Fig. 56-2). Of cases, 75% to 80% occur by the time children are 2 years old. This subject is discussed in Chapter 54. Bleeding ranges from occult to large "currant jelly" stools mixed with blood and mucus.

Intestinal volvulus is a relatively common cause of rectal bleeding in infants. Malrotation and volvulus present in the first year of life in 90% of cases. A segmental volvulus or intestinal volvulus around a persistent omphalomesenteric duct also may present with symptoms of bowel obstruction and GI bleeding, which indicates impending, if not already present, bowel necrosis.

Rectal bleeding also may be a manifestation of an intestinal duplication with ectopic gastric mucosa. This bleeding more commonly originates in the small bowel

TABLE 56-2 ■ Incidence of Causes of Gastrointestinal Bleeding Ranked in Descending Order in Patients Younger and Older than 1 Year of Age

% Patients <1 Year Old (n = 263)	Disorder	% Patients >1 Year Old (n = 169)	Disorder
30	Anal fissure	56	Colonic polyp
19	Intussusception	12	Intussusception
18	Unexplained bleeding	7	Esophageal varices
7	Hemorrhagic disease	6	Anal fissure
5	Prolapse	5	Gastric ulcer
5	Gangrenous bowel	5	Duodenal ulcer
5	Swallowed maternal blood	5	Ulcerative colitis
4	Duodenal ulcer	2	Meckel's diverticulum
3	Gastric ulcer	1	Regional enteritis
2	Meckel's diverticulum	1	Hemorrhoids
1	Ileal hematoma		
1	Duplication-colon		

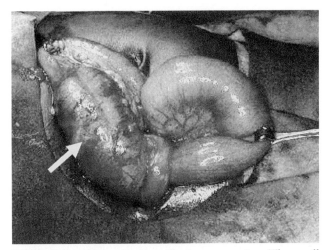

FIGURE 56-2 ■ Idiopathic ileocolic intussusception. The small bowel (the intussusceptum) is inside of the right colon (the intussuscipiens, arrow). In this case, the bowel involved in the intussusception was necrotic and had to be resected. Venous congestion commonly occurs in the intussusceptum resulting in gastrointestinal bleeding even before necrosis develops.

because the incidence of ectopic gastric mucosa is low in colonic duplications. The bleeding may be in the form of melena or hematochezia. The diagnosis is suspected when a technetium-99m pertechnetate scan shows uptake of the isotope in the lower abdomen extrinsic to the stomach. The differential diagnosis includes Meckel's diverticulum, which also contains ectopic gastric mucosa. A duplication should be suspected because bleeding from a Meckel's diverticulum is uncommon in young infants. Pyloric stenosis is an uncommon cause of hematemesis in infants. Rectal bleeding also may be due to bacterial or viral gastroenteritis (see later).

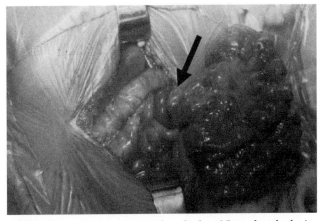

FIGURE 56-1 ■ Malrotation with volvulus. Note the clockwise twist at the base of the small bowel (arrow) and the ischemic, dark small bowel. Bleeding from the bowel typically indicates venous congestion, if not necrosis.

TODDLERS AND PRESCHOOL CHILDREN (1 TO 5 YEARS OLD)

Bleeding from various types of polyps is the most common cause of GI hemorrhage in toddlers and preschool children and includes juvenile polyps of the colon (most common), Peutz-Jeghers polyps, polypoid lymphoid hyperplasia, and rarely adenomatous polyps. Polypoid diseases of the GI tract are discussed in Chapter 57. Colonoscopy is the most efficient diagnostic test and should be performed before obtaining any contrast studies. Most juvenile polyps are single (50%) and usually are located in the colon, only occasionally being present in the small intestine, with 49% in the rectosigmoid area. Juvenile polyps comprise 80% of the polyps found in children (Fig. 56-3). They are seen most commonly in 3- to 5-year-olds. They are hamartomas, which often have an ulcerated surface that leads to the GI hemorrhage. In most cases, the polyp spontaneously passes without treatment. In instances in which bleeding has occurred, the polyp can be snared and excised endoscopically without the need for laparotomy. Occasionally a rectal polyp prolapses from the anus, where it can be excised. Children also can develop hyperplastic submucosal lymphoid aggregates, which form lymphoid polyps that can ulcerate and bleed. These lesions have a peak incidence at age 4 years and usually regress by age 5.

Anal fissures may occur from the passage of hard feces in patients with constipation and are treated as indicated previously. Rectal prolapse may be the cause of blood on the diaper or underwear because the exposed mucosa bleeds easily from external contact or passage of stool. The prolapse may be visualized and reduced manually. Rectal prolapse often follows severe straining as a result of constipation or tenesmus associated with a severe bout of diarrhea. Rectal prolapse is more common in children

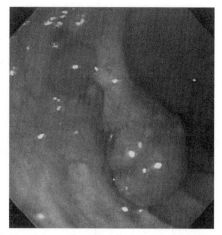

FIGURE 56-3 ■ A juvenile polyp present in the colon. Note the nonsessile nature of the polyp. These juvenile polyps typically are found in the colon and are excised easily using colonoscopy and a snare. In most cases, however, the polyp undergoes autoamputation.

with cystic fibrosis and may be associated with pinworm infestation. A sweat chloride determination and examination of a stool specimen for the presence of ova and parasites are suggested. Most patients with simple rectal mucosal prolapse respond to conservative measures, including the use of stool softeners and enemas. Instances of persistent prolapse despite application of these conservative measures may require rectal cautery or placement of a Thiersch wire or suture circumferentially around the anus.

Bleeding from a Meckel's diverticulum is a relatively common cause of painless rectal bleeding in this age group. The stool is often maroon and usually is accompanied by a significant decrease in hemoglobin. If this condition is suspected, most physicians perform a technetium-99m scintiscan because the tracer is secreted by the gastric mucosa, which is universally present in Meckel's diverticula that are associated with bleeding. This subject is discussed in Chapter 50.

Peptic ulcer disease is the most common cause of UGI bleeding in this age group. Although observed in patients with associated diseases (burns, head trauma, malignancy, and sepsis) and in patients taking salicylates, nonsteroidal anti-inflammatory drugs (NSAIDs), and cyclooxygenase type 2 inhibitors, gastric and duodenal inflammation and ulcers are associated most commonly with *Helicobacter pylori* infestation. The diagnosis of *H. pylori* infection may be made by assay for serum IgG antibody to *H. pylori*, assay for fecal *H. pylori* antigen, hematoxylin-eosin or silver stain pathologic assessment of endoscopic gastric biopsy specimen, and presence of *H. pylori*–produced urease on placement of a gastric biopsy specimen into urea-rich medium. The urease results in hydrolysis of the urea into ammonium, which leads to an increase in pH and change in color of the medium. Assay for exhaled labeled carbon dioxide in patients after consumption of carbon 13–labeled or carbon 14–labeled urea also can be used to make the diagnosis. Treatment with antibiotics (metronidazole, amoxicillin, clarithromycin) plus an acid

suppressor (ranitidine, omeprazole) for 14 days is usually effective. Some practitioners choose to add an antimicrobial agent, such as bismuth subsalicylate, to the regimen.

Rectal bleeding may be a manifestation of idiopathic intussusception as discussed previously or of severe intestinal infection caused by bacterial or viral gastroenteritis. *Campylobacter, Shigella, Clostridium difficile,* toxigenic *Escherichia coli,* rotavirus, *Entamoeba,* cytomegalovirus (in immunosuppressed patients or transplant recipients), or other species may be the offending organisms. Appropriate stool cultures and specific titers usually identify the organism and allow initiation of selective treatment.

Although uncommon, instances of inflammatory bowel disease (ulcerative colitis and Crohn's disease) occasionally may be encountered in 2- to 5-year-olds. Early fiberoptic colonoscopy and biopsy and a contrast barium enema study and small bowel series clarify the diagnosis.

Children with hemolytic uremic syndrome or Henoch-Schönlein purpura also can present with rectal bleeding. The presence of abdominal pain, thrombocytopenia, and elevated blood urea nitrogen levels suggests the former condition, which may be associated with left colon ischemia and gangrene. The presence of a rash (palpable purpura), thrombocytosis, proteinuria, and abdominal pain and GI bleeding should make one suspect Henoch-Schönlein disease, which may be complicated by small bowel intussusception.

SCHOOL-AGE CHILDREN AND TEENAGERS

Some of the causes of GI bleeding observed in the toddler and preschool child are more common in school-age children and teenagers. These include polypoid diseases of the lower GI tract (familial polyposis, Gardner's disease, and Peutz-Jeghers syndrome) and especially instances of inflammatory bowel disease as a result of ulcerative colitis or Crohn's disease, which are much more prevalent in preadolescents and teenage children. Other conditions seen in the previous age group also can be observed in older children, including gastritis or peptic ulcer disease with or without *H. pylori* infection, Meckel's diverticulum, duplication, Henoch-Schönlein disease, and hemolytic uremic syndrome. Bleeding from internal hemorrhoids is encountered occasionally in older children as well.

Polypoid disease of the GI tract continues to be a common source of hemorrhage in patients older than age 5 years. Juvenile polyps, as described previously, continue to be the most common presenting polyps. Diffuse juvenile polyposis or juvenile polyposis coli, with greater than five juvenile polyps throughout the GI tract in the former and limited to the distal sigmoid and rectum in the latter, frequently presents with rectal bleeding. Other polypoid syndromes begin to appear in older children: occult blood loss secondary to ulceration of the hamartomas in Peutz-Jeghers syndrome and rectal bleeding or anemia or both in familial polyposis syndrome.

Inflammatory bowel disease may be associated with GI bleeding and anemia. This is especially true of ulcerative colitis, in which profuse, bloody diarrhea almost always is associated with the disease (Fig. 56-4).

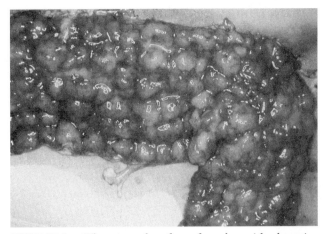

FIGURE 56-4 ■ The mucosal surface of a colon with ulcerative colitis. Note the pseudopolyps. This is a relatively frequent cause of gastrointestinal hemorrhage in older children and adolescents.

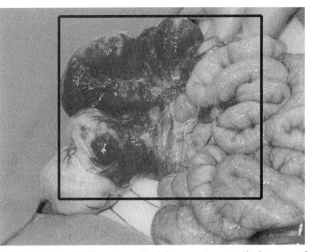

FIGURE 56-6 ■ Diffuse intestinal hemangiomas (dark area of bowel enclosed in the box) of the terminal ileum and right colon, which may lead to gastrointestinal bleeding.

Approximately two thirds of patients with ulcerative colitis have anemia from GI blood loss. UGI and contrast enema radiography, colonoscopy, and biopsy are diagnostic and delineate the extent of inflammatory bowel disease. Management with immunosuppressive medications, tumor necrosis factor-α in Crohn's disease, and resection when indicated leads to resolution of the hemorrhage.

Gastric and esophageal varices secondary to portal vein thrombosis, cirrhosis, and resulting portal hypertension may become apparent beyond age 2 to 3 years and are more common by age 5 (Fig. 56-5). Massive hematemesis is often the first symptom. Esophagoscopy usually confirms the diagnosis and when combined with sclerotherapy may control the bleeding and treat the varices. Only rarely is a portosystemic venous shunt required, unless hypersplenism and symptomatic thrombocytopenia occur as a result of the portal hypertension.

Hemangiomas of the bowel can be localized or diffuse (Fig. 56-6). Most hemangiomas are small, but some can become large (>2 cm). The larger lesions tend to occur in

the rectum and can be capillary or cavernous. They present with slow rectal bleeding often associated with iron deficiency anemia and usually can be diagnosed by colonoscopy. Diffuse intestinal hemangiomatosis usually involves the small intestine and the stomach and colon. Occasionally a hemangioma can act as a lead point for an intussusception. The lesions should be excised locally. If this is not possible, a limited bowel resection must be performed.

Telangiectasias are small, spider-like vascular lesions found on cutaneous, mucocutaneous, and mucosal surfaces and are usually part of the Osler-Weber-Rendu disease (hereditary hemorrhagic telangiectasia). Similar vascular lesions may be seen in children with von Willebrand's disease and in patients with chronic renal failure. Most children have had recurrent bleeding from the GI tract and nosebleeds by the time they are 10 years old. Telangiectasias are common in the small bowel and stomach and may be seen on gastroscopy.

Rectal bleeding also may be caused by a stercoral ulcer of the rectum as a result of severe obstipation in institutionalized older children and teenagers with neurologic impairment. This can be managed by disimpaction and endoscopic local control of the ulcerated area with a heat probe. Dietary change and stool softeners usually resolve the problem.

Another unusual cause of rectal bleeding in children is a nonspecific small bowel ulcer. Small bowel ulcers most commonly occur in the ileum, are of unknown etiology, and result in slow chronic blood loss and iron deficiency anemia. The bleeding may be in the form of melena, or the stool may test positive for occult blood. The treatment of choice is resection of the segment of bowel containing the ulcer. Occasionally an intestinal anastomosis bleeds chronically many years after the initial operation and requires resection.

MANAGEMENT

The clinical management of GI bleeding in children depends in part on the age group in question. In all

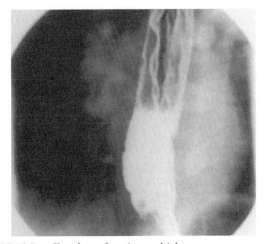

FIGURE 56-5 ■ Esophageal varices, which are a common cause of upper gastrointestinal bleeding in children with portal hypertension, are seen in this barium swallow.

patients who are actively bleeding, the physician must formulate a careful plan of action that includes resuscitation to stabilize the infant or child's hemodynamic status, prompt investigation of the cause of bleeding, and treatment of the problem. Vital signs are monitored closely. The patient's hemoglobin and hematocrit values and clotting studies (prothrombin time, partial thromboplastin time, bleeding time, and platelet count) are evaluated routinely. The patient's blood is typed and blood made available for type-specific crossmatch. Passage of an NG tube usually rules out bleeding originating from the proximal GI tract. In older children and teenagers, in whom bleeding from reflux esophagitis, peptic ulcer disease, or esophageal varices is more common, esophagogastroduodenoscopy is advisable. Digital rectal examination and colonoscopy can identify a colorectal cause of bleeding promptly.

In neonates, plain abdominal radiographs are obtained to rule out necrotizing enterocolitis, and a GI contrast study may be performed to evaluate for midgut volvulus. In infants in whom an intussusception is suspected, an ultrasound or diagnostic air or barium enema study is performed. In older patients with acute rectal bleeding, contrast studies have little to offer because they are usually uninformative and may preclude the use of other techniques, causing delays in the work-up. Colonoscopy may be performed instead and frequently identifies the cause of bleeding in children with hemangioma, polyps, and ulcerative colitis. If colonoscopy is negative, the source of bleeding is probably in the small bowel, and precise localization of the site may be difficult. If bleeding from a Meckel's diverticulum is the suspected source of bleeding, a technetium-99m pertechnetate scan is obtained. If the scintiscan is negative, judgment must be used to determine whether laparoscopy should be performed to examine the small intestine for the presence of a Meckel's diverticulum, especially when colonoscopy and UGI endoscopy are normal. Isotopic scanning with labeled autologous red blood cells using either chromium 51 or technetium-99m may be useful in children with continued blood loss that is not rapid or in children experiencing intermittent bleeding. The labeled red blood cell scan can detect bleeding at a rate of 0.5 mL/min. This is not a highly sensitive test in patients who have a single instance of bleeding or multiple hemorrhages with long periods between events. The resolution is sometimes poor, and accurate localization may be difficult. The test usually can differentiate the site of bleeding, however, between the small bowel and colon. Angiographic identification and embolization may be useful in patients with active bleeding that exceeds 1 mL/min, but too-extensive vascular occlusion may threaten bowel viability.

If continued blood loss is apparent and the site of bleeding cannot be identified by radiographic, isotopic, or endoscopic studies, laparoscopy or a laparotomy should be performed. The cause of bleeding often may be observed directly (hemangioma, small bowel polyp, nonspecific ileal ulcer). If no obvious source of bleeding is noted, the bowel must be carefully palpated and transilluminated, looking for an intraluminal abnormality. Intraoperative enteroscopy or simultaneous on-table colonoscopy with the surgeon guiding the colonoscope into the distal small bowel also may prove useful.

SUGGESTED READINGS

Arensman RM: Gastrointestinal bleeding. In O'Neill JA Jr, Rowe MI, Grosfeld JL, et al (eds): Pediatric Surgery, vol 2, 5th ed. St Louis, Mosby, 1998, pp 1253-1256.

Bass B, Alvarez C: Acute gastrointestinal hemorrhage. In Townsend CM Jr, Beauchamp RD, Evers BM, Mattox KL (eds): Sabiston's Textbook of Surgery, 16th ed. Philadelphia, WB Saunders, 2000, pp 816-834.

Chamberlain SA, Soybel DI: Occult and obscure sources of gastrointestinal bleeding. Curr Probl Surg 37:861-916, 2000.

These references deal with the various childhood disorders associated with GI bleeding as well as modern approaches to diagnostic localization and treatment.

Polypoid Diseases of the Gastrointestinal Tract

Polypoid disorders of the gastrointestinal (GI) tract include epithelial tumors that are adenomatous polyps (neoplasias) and tumor-like lesions, such as hamartomas (juvenile polyps, Peutz-Jeghers polyps), hyperplastic (metaplastic) polyps, and many miscellaneous diseases that may present polypoid masses in the lumen of the intestine (Table 57-1). Some patients with intestinal polyps have associated disorders in other areas of the body and are classified in specific polyp syndromes. With the advancement of genetic analysis of many of these patients and their families, better understanding and classification of these conditions have occurred. This chapter discusses these genetic conditions and lays out specific guidelines for following these patients and screening for intestinal and extraintestinal malignancies. Table 57-2 summarizes common polyposis syndromes.

INFLAMMATORY POLYPS

Juvenile Polyps

The concept of juvenile polypoid disease was established more than 50 years ago, when it was recognized that this condition represents a distinct pathologic entity distinguishable from other benign polypoid lesions of the colon. Before that time, juvenile polyps usually were classified as adenomas. Although juvenile polyps are regarded as benign lesions, the practice of equating intestinal polyp with adenoma was ingrained so deeply in the past that treatment of juvenile polyps often has been unnecessarily radical. Single or multiple juvenile polyps currently are regarded as benign with no relation to adenomatous polyps.

Pathology

Juvenile polyps, which also are called *retention, inflammatory,* or *cystic polyps,* are the most common type of polypoid lesion found in the GI tract in children and account for more than 80% of polyps in children. They are generally pedunculated but occasionally sessile, particularly when small, and are composed of dilated glands filled with mucus and inspissated inflammatory debris, giving a cystic appearance (Fig. 57-1). Ultrastructural and tissue culture studies support the hamartomatous nature of these lesions. The polyps are uniformly smooth, glistening, and reddish and range from a few millimeters to several centimeters in size. The average juvenile polyp is approximately 1 cm long and has a thin stalk covered by normal colonic mucosa, which is ulcerated on the surface. The eroded surface often is replaced by proliferating granulation tissue. In areas adjacent to the erosions, the regenerating epithelium may show some cytologic atypism.

These lesions are typically solitary and usually occur in the rectum or sigmoid colon. When there are multiple colonic polyps, the patient may have juvenile polyposis syndrome (see later). Before the era of aggressive colonoscopy, it was believed that approximately 70% of juvenile polyps occurred in the rectum, 15% occurred in the sigmoid colon, and the remainder were scattered

---

TABLE 57-1 ■ **Classification of Polypoid Tumors of the Large Intestine***

Epithelial tumors
  Adenoma: familial adenomatous polyposis (Gardner's and two thirds of Turcot's syndrome families), attenuated adematous polyposis coli
  Endocrine tumors
  Carcinoid tumors
  Nonepithelial tumors
    Leiomyoma, leiomyomatosis
    Lipoma, lipomatosis
    Vascular tumors: hemangioma, lymphangioma
    Neurogenic tumors: neurolemoma, neurofibroma (neurofibromatosis type 1), granular cell tumor, ganglioneuroma
Tumor-like lesions
  Harmartoma: Peutz-Jeghers polyps, Cronkhite-Canada and Cowden's syndromes, juvenile polyposis, hereditary mixed polyposis syndrome, Gorlin's syndrome
  Hyperplastic (metaplastic) polyps
  Lymphoid polyps
  Inflammatory polyps (pseudopolyps), ulcerative colitis
  Heterotopic tissue (gastric, pancreatic)
  Lesions secondary to mucosal prolapse, colitis cystica profunda

*Modification of the World Health Organization (WHO) Classification of Benign Tumors of the Large Intestine.
Modified from Jass JR, Sobin LH: WHO International Classification of Tumors: Histological Typing of Intestinal Tumors, 2nd ed. Berlin, Springer-Verlag, 1989.

TABLE 57-2 ■ Summary of Key Polyposis Syndromes

	Familial Adenomatous Polyposis	Peutz-Jegher Syndrome	Multiple Juvenile Polyposis
Colon	100s to 1000s adenomatous polyps	Entire colon	Juvenile polyps throughout colon
Rest of bowel	None	Throughout GI tract	Rest of GI tract, although minimally
Mutations	*APC* gene	*STK11*	*SMAD4, BMPR1A, PTEN*
Colon screening starts	10-12 yr	Late teens, or sooner with symptoms	Early teens
Prophylactic colectomy	Mid to late teens	With neoplastic or dysplastic changes	With neoplastic or dysplastic changes
Extraintestinal manifestations Includes	Desmoid tumors, osteomas Gardner's, Turcot's, and attenuated syndromes	Associated malignancies Melanin pigmentation	Few None

throughout the more proximal colon to the cecum. More recent studies have shown that 60% of polyps are proximal to the rectosigmoid. Additionally, more than one polyp is identified in greater than 50% of children.

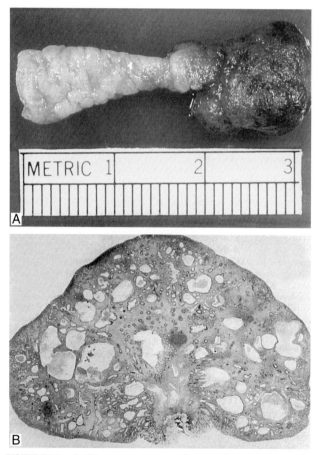

FIGURE 57-1 ■ A, Gross appearance of a juvenile polyp. Note the typical polyp has a long stalk attached to it. **B,** Low-power microscopic appearance of a juvenile polyp. Note the epithelial surface is flat with tubular cystic spaces within the polyp. (From Lelli JL, Coran AG: Polypoid disease of the gastrointestinal tract. In O'Neill Jr JA, Rowe MI, Grosfeld JL, et al [eds]: Pediatric Surgery, 5th ed. St. Louis, Mosby, 1998.)

Juvenile polyps do not seem to occur in the small intestine. Studies of patients at St. Mark's Hospital in London showed that the relative risk of developing a future colon cancer is not increased in children who have had a juvenile polyp removed.

The cause of juvenile polyps is undetermined and has been attributed to hereditary, congenital, inflammatory, allergic, and neoplastic causes. The initial stage is ulceration and inflammation of the mucosa, which cause obstruction of one or more small colonic glands. The blocked gland then proliferates, branches, and dilates to give the appearance of a mucous cyst, exposing a larger surface of the mucosa that becomes ulcerated and inflamed. Granulation tissue develops on the ulcerated surface, and the cycle continues until the entire lesion is sufficiently large to extend into the intestinal lumen. Mucosal ulceration on the polyp may produce hemorrhage. The flow of the fecal stream usually causes the stalk to elongate. The polyps often spontaneously twist on their pedicle, infarct, and slough.

Clinical Features

The incidence of juvenile polyps is undetermined, although various reports suggest that they occur in 1% of children. The polyps are slightly more common in boys than in girls. Juvenile polyps are seen most frequently in children between the ages of 2 and 8 years with peak incidence of 4 to 5 years, although occasional polyps have been identified during the first year of life. Juvenile polyps rarely are seen after early adolescence, and there have been only rare reports in adults.

The most common presentation of juvenile polyps is bleeding caused by inflammation and mucosal ulceration. Blood loss is usually minimal, appearing as streaks of fresh blood on the outside of the stool. Bleeding from polyps in the proximal colon may be darker and mixed with the stool. Hemorrhage is usually intermittent and is rarely of great magnitude. Rarely, autoamputation may expose a feeding vessel at the base, which may produce brisk bleeding, sometimes requiring transfusion. An occasional polyp located low in the rectum may prolapse or protrude from the anus and cause prolapse of the anal and rectal mucosa. Children occasionally experience abdominal cramps believed to be caused by traction on a polyp during peristaltic activity, and in rare instances, the lesion may initiate an intussusception. Most juvenile polyps are believed to slough eventually.

Rectal examination occasionally discloses the presence of a palpable rectal polyp. Colonoscopy under anesthesia is the preferred way of identifying and evaluating juvenile polyps. A barium enema radiographic study with air contrast helps to identify pedunculated polyps of the colon in patients of all ages, but colonoscopy is the standard.

The differential diagnosis of juvenile polyposis includes the common causes of rectal bleeding in young children, such as anal fissures, which generally can be visualized; acute and chronic inflammatory bowel disease, which usually is accompanied by diarrhea; and blood dyscrasias, such as Henoch-Schönlein purpura. Bleeding from Meckel's diverticulum or duplication of the intestine is usually of greater magnitude and mixed with stool. Bleeding from intussusception is usually darker and accompanied by severe cramping abdominal pain. The diagnosis of juvenile polyps is made from the history, rectal examination, air contrast studies, barium enema, and colonoscopy. Laboratory studies should include a hemogram to evaluate for anemia and blood dyscrasias and stool culture and examination for ova and parasites.

Therapy

Many polyps are located in the rectum and lower sigmoid colon and can be removed through a flexible sigmoidoscope. Some of these lesions can be prolapsed through the anus and removed by suture ligation of the pedicle. For higher lesions, a snare and cautery through a colonoscope may be performed. Increasingly, polyps have been identified at more proximal locations in the colon, so if one removes a polyp via a sigmoidoscope, colonoscopy should follow. If fewer than five additional total polyps are identified, the proximal polyps are observed. Excision is indicated only with symptoms (i.e., bleeding). It is rarely necessary to perform a laparotomy with colotomy for removal of a juvenile polyp. If 5 to 10 polyps or more are identified, a colonoscopic excision of the polyps should be performed. This latter clinical scenario (≥5 to 10 polyps) or a single polyp with a family history of juvenile polypsis is consistent with the diagnosis of juvenile polyposis syndrome and would place the child at risk for future malignancies (see later).

Complications after endoscopic removal of juvenile polyps have been rare. Subsequent bleeding from additional or recurrent juvenile polyps is believed to be approximately 5%. The natural history of juvenile polyps is that they are self-limited and seem to disappear, presumably by autoamputation. Older patients with juvenile polyps containing dysplasia or adenomatous transformation should be in a clinical follow-up program to facilitate the detection of early malignancy.

Juvenile Polyposis Syndromes: Juvenile Polyposis Coli and Generalized Juvenile Polyposis

Juvenile polyposis coli and generalized juvenile polyposis are rare but distinct conditions that have a propensity for future development of colon cancer. The polyps are similar to solitary juvenile polyps in that they are inflammatory by histology. In contrast to children with single or multiple juvenile colonic polyps, the diagnosis of juvenile polyposis coli is made with the presence of multiple polyps. Although numbers vary, the diagnosis should be entertained with 5 to 10 or more juvenile polyps. In juvenile polyposis coli, polyps are found in the entire colon. In generalized juvenile polyposis, polyps (inflammatory type) are seen in the entire GI tract. Patients with these conditions have different clinical and genetic implications. Approximately one third of cases of juvenile polyposis are found to have familial inheritance with an autosomal dominant pattern. Patients with a family history present with polyps at an older age (9.5 years) compared with patients without a family history (4.5 years). The incidence of juvenile polyposis is 1 in 100,000 individuals. In patients with the familial form, congenital defects, including cardiac anomalies, cranial anomalies, cleft palate, polydactyly, and intestinal malrotation, have been described. Genetic mutations in the familial forms have been described in several genes, including *SMAD4* (on chromosome 18), bone morphogenetic receptor 1A (*BMPR1A*), and *PTEN*.

The condition is characterized by anemia caused by GI bleeding, diarrhea, occasional rectal prolapse or intussusception, and, less commonly, protein-losing enteropathy producing malnutrition and anasarca. Almost all patients have gastric polyps that may cover most of the gastric mucosa, cause bleeding, and occasionally require gastric resection. The prognosis is related to the extent of intestinal involvement with juvenile polyps. Beyond infancy, accurate histologic interpretation of the polyps is essential to distinguish the syndrome from familial polyposis coli, familial juvenile adenomatous polyposis, and Peutz-Jeghers syndrome. Although polyps in this disorder are usually benign, patients with this condition may have a 10% risk of developing cancer (significantly less than patients with a family history of familial polyposis coli; see later). The average age for the diagnosis of cancer is 34 years. Additionally, gastric, duodenal, and pancreatic cancers have been reported. In contrast to sporadic juvenile polyps, new polyps almost always form after a polyp is removed, and polyps continue into adulthood. The occasional rapidly debilitating course in this life-threatening disease in young children seems to justify aggressive operative therapy. Genetic testing should be done in familial cases because mutations can be used to diagnose other family members who will manifest the disease. Colonoscopy should begin in the early teens even without symptoms and should be repeated every 3 years. Total colectomy with mucosal proctectomy and the endorectal ileal pouch pull-through constitute the recommended operative technique, although colectomy and ileal-rectal anastomosis are options chosen by some surgeons. Because of the risk of gastric and duodenal malignancies and potential complications of benign polyps, an upper GI endoscopy should be performed every 3 years starting in the early teens.

HAMARTOMATOUS POLYPS

Peutz-Jeghers Syndrome

The association of intestinal polyps with abnormal mucocutaneous pigmentation first was described by

Peutz in 1921, when he called attention to the hereditary aspects of the condition. In 1949, Jeghers and associates defined the syndrome and analyzed 22 cases, 10 of their own. In subsequent years, additional information has accumulated regarding the increased incidence of malignancy in the GI tract and elsewhere in patients with intestinal polyposis associated with mucocutaneous pigmentation.

Pathology

Peutz-Jeghers syndrome is characterized by GI polyps and circumoral buccal or lingual pigmentation. Similar pigmentation may be found on the palms and soles. The pigmented lesions resemble freckles but do not show seasonal change and are present in areas where freckles are normally absent. Freckles are sparse near the mouth and rarely involve the palms or buccal mucosa. The mucocutaneous lesions vary from light brown to black and may be linear, oval, or irregular. They are usually small (<5 mm), flat, and hairless and do not coalesce. Microscopically the pigment is present in vertical bands in the basal layer of the epidermis; however, the pigmented cells are not melanoblasts. The relationship of mucocutaneous pigmentation to polyposis is unknown; intestinal polyps are not pigmented. The pigmented lesions may be seen in infancy. The lesions of the lips and skin begin to fade at puberty, whereas those of the buccal mucosa remain.

Polypoid lesions occur most frequently in the small intestine but also may occur in the nasal cavity, esophagus, stomach, colon, rectum, urinary bladder, and bronchus. GI polyps associated with Peutz-Jeghers syndrome are usually multiple and widely scattered, although greater than 90% are located in the small intestine. In more than one third of patients, polyps are found in the rectum (28%), colon (42%), and stomach (38%). Only rarely have patients with an isolated polyp been reported. The size may vary from a few millimeters to several centimeters. The polyps are hamartomas, not adenomas. Despite this benign appearance, 38% of patients have a lifetime risk of developing colon carcinoma. Whether the carcinoma develops in the hamartomatous polyp or elsewhere in the mucosa is unknown. Table 57-3 shows the relative lifetime risk of other intestinal and extraintestinal malignancies. Almost 10% of female patients with Peutz-Jeghers syndrome develop ovarian neoplasms, half of which are sex cord tumors with a high percentage being hormonally active. Other malignancies include pancreatic, stomach, and breast.

Genetics

Peutz-Jeghers syndrome arises from mutations in the *STK11* gene. This gene is a kinase that is involved with intracellular growth signals. Only half of the involved families have this mutation. It appears another yet unidentified gene is involved in the remaining families. If a mutation in the *STK11* gene is present, other family members should be screened with a near 100% accuracy.

Clinical Features

Peutz-Jeghers syndrome is rare (1 in 200,000), the sex distribution is approximately equal, and the condition has been described in all racial groups. A family history is present in half of patients. The syndrome is an autosomal dominant genetic abnormality. Approximately half of the descendants of patients with the syndrome are affected. Although Peutz-Jeghers syndrome is diagnosed most often in childhood, the ages in reported cases extend from 2 to 82 years with a mean of 29 years. The condition rarely is detected in infants younger than 1 year of age. The primary features of the syndrome are a frequent occurrence in family members; mucocutaneous pigmentation; GI polyposis; repeated episodes of abdominal pain caused by intussusception, melena, or occult blood loss from the intestine; and anemia. The pigmented spots are distinctive and, when present, should lead to investigation for intestinal polyps. Pigmentation is often the initial manifestation, with abdominal symptoms rarely becoming apparent before age 6 to 8 years.

TABLE 57-3 ■ Cancer Risk and Screening Recommendations for Patients with Peutz-Jeghers Syndrome

Cancer	Frequency (Lifetime Risk, %)	Screening Recommendations
Colon	38	Colonoscopy starting in late teens without symptoms; interval determined by number and type of polyps (at least every 3 yr)
Pancreatic	35	Endoscopy or ultrasound every 1-2 yr starting at 30 yr
Stomach	27	Upper GI endoscopy every 2 yr starting at age 10 yr
Small bowel	13	Annual hemoglobin, small bowel x-ray every 2 yr, both starting at age 10 yr
Esophagus	2	None
Breast	53	Annual breast examination and mammography every 2-3 yr starting at age 25 yr
Ovarian	20	Annual pelvic examination with Pap smear; annual pelvic or vaginal ultrasound or uterine washings. Both start at age 20 yr
Uterine/cervix	9-10	See Ovarian
Sex cord tumor with annular tubules, in almost all women		See Ovarian
Sertoli cell tumor (men), unusual	8	Annual testicular examination, start at 10 yr. Testicular ultrasound with feminizing features
Lung	12	None

Adapted from Burt RW: Polyposis syndromes. Clin Perspect Gastroenterol January/February, 2002.

Partial intestinal obstruction characterized by recurrent attacks of crampy abdominal discomfort caused by transient intussusception is characteristic. Plain radiographs often show dilated small bowel with air-fluid levels. Complete obstruction is uncommon, with most episodes of small bowel intussusception resolving spontaneously. The episodes of obstruction occur periodically with intervals of quiescence lasting months to years. Occult GI bleeding with secondary anemia occurs in approximately one third of patients. Occasional patients manifest growth failure.

Barium enema radiographs with air contrast and sigmoidoscopy or colonoscopic examination identify the 30% to 35% of patients who have rectal and colonic involvement. Transient ileal intussusception is shown occasionally. Gastroscopy is helpful in identifying the relatively uncommon gastric polyp. Upper GI series with small bowel follow-through sometimes allow visualization of small bowel polyps.

Therapy

Surgery is often unnecessary for the treatment of Peutz-Jeghers syndrome. The patient and family should be advised regarding the rare necessity to operate for the brief transitory episodes of intussusception. Surgery is necessary for persistent intussusception or for prolonged or extensive intestinal bleeding. Resection is necessary only for the rare unreducible intussusception. Enterotomies to remove large bleeding polyps in either small or large intestine are occasionally necessary, and some patients require multiple operations. Intestinal resection should be avoided whenever feasible. The prognosis for patients with Peutz-Jeghers syndrome is good, with most patients living into advanced adult life. Although rare, death may result from the complications of intussusception, blood loss, and the necessary operations for treatment.

Patients with Peutz-Jeghers syndrome have a lifetime risk of greater than 30% to develop colon carcinoma. Colonoscopy should be performed at least every 3 years starting in the late teens. Resection is indicated with neoplastic or dysplastic changes. The high frequency of extraintestinal cancer in patients with Peutz-Jeghers syndrome, including carcinoma of the pancreas, breast, lung, uterus, and ovary and multiple myeloma, must be emphasized. Routine screening for these lesions is shown in Table 57-3.

Cowden's Syndrome

Cowden's syndrome is an uncommon autosomal dominant genodermatosis first described in 1963 and subsequently called *multiple hamartoma syndrome*. The incidence of the disorder is 1 in 200,000 individuals. The syndrome is due to mutations of the *PTEN* gene on chromosome 10. The associated ectodermal, mesodermal, and entodermal anomalies present a clinical picture of facial trichilemmomas, acral keratosis, and oral mucosal papillomas. Associated breast, thyroid, and GI tract lesions have a propensity for malignant degeneration. Two thirds of patients have a goiter, with a 10% lifetime risk of carcinoma. Screening should start in the patient's teens. Three fourths of women have breast lesions, with a 50% incidence of breast carcinoma at a mean age of 41 years. Screening for breast malignancies should start by 25 years.

In Cowden's syndrome, GI polyps are frequently present and are hamartomatous. Colorectal lesions may include hamartomatous colonic polyps, juvenile and lipomatous polyps, multiple small inflammatory rectal polyps, ganglioneuromatous polyps, epithelioid leiomyomas of the rectum, nodular lymphoid hyperplasia of the rectum, and adenocarcinoma of the cecum. The actual risk of colorectal malignancies has not been well described but is probably minimal. Nonintestinal abnormalities that occasionally have occurred in association with Cowden's syndrome include adenoid facies, hyperkeratotic verrucous papular lesions, keratoderma of the palms and soles, thyroglossal cysts, malignant melanoma, vitiligo, pseudoacanthosis nigricans, facial hypertrichosis, dermal fibroma, trichilemmoma, scoliosis, pectus excavatum, bone cysts, supernumerary digits, high arched palate, clubfoot anomalies, lipomas, hemangiomas, papules of the larynx and oral mucosa, enlarged tongue, and various other lesions.

SYNDROMES OF ADENOMATOUS POLYPOSIS

Adenomatous Polyps

Adenomatous polyps are rare in children except in familial polyposis coli. The adenomatous polyp, often referred to as the *adult* or *neoplastic* polyp, consists of a proliferation of glandular elements with much branching and little stroma and connective tissue. There is usually little evidence of the inflammation frequently seen in juvenile polyps. The epithelium is often multilayered with atypism, mitotic figures, and hyperchromatic nuclei. When a solitary adenoma is identified in a child, extensive investigation should be undertaken to determine if familial polyposis is present. Careful follow-up of the patient and investigation of family members are recommended.

Familial Adenomatous Polyposis (Famial Polyposis Coli)

Although multiple polyposis of the colon had been recognized previously, the hereditary nature of the disease was described in 1882. A few years later, the familial occurrence was noted, and the early malignant changes of the polyps were documented. Lockhart-Mummery established the genetic background of colonic polyposis, noting it to be an autosomal dominant trait. It subsequently was determined that the disorder was inherited as a mendelian autosomal non–sex-linked dominant trait. In families in which polyposis develops early in life, cancer frequently occurs within 10 to 15 years, whereas in families in which polyposis is recognized later, the precancerous latency period is longer. Since the 1990s, a tremendous advancement in the understanding of the pathophysiology and genetics of this disorder has occurred. Categorization of familial adenomatous polyposis (FAP) now includes Gardner's syndrome, attenuated FAP (also called *attenuated adenomatous polyposis*), and approximately two thirds of cases of Turcot's syndrome. The incidence of FAP is 1 in 8000 births.

Pathology

Characteristic features of FAP include innumerable polyps carpeting the entire colon from anus to cecum,

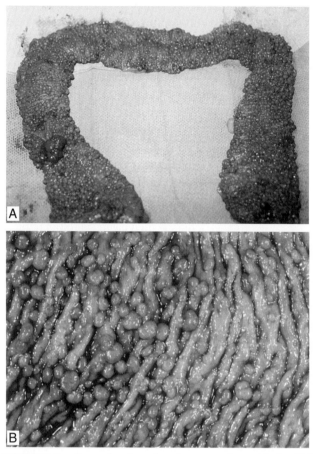

FIGURE 57-2 ■ Example of a colon from a patient with familial adenomatous polyposis. **A,** Gross specimen shows thousands of adenomatous polyps throughout the colon. **B,** Close-up view of the mucosa shows a diffuse carpet of small adenomatous polyps from same patient. (From Lelli JL, Coran AG: Polypoid disease of the gastrointestinal tract. In O'Neill Jr JA, Rowe MI, Grosfeld JL, et al [eds]: Pediatric Surgery, 5th ed. St. Louis, Mosby, 1998.)

including the appendix (Fig. 57-2). The polyps are the adult adenomatous type and may vary in size from 2 mm to 2 cm. Although polyps less than 3 mm occasionally may be hyperplastic, they must be distinguished clearly from adenomatous polyps, which also may be small. Adenomatous polyps are benign, gland-forming neoplasms that can contain cytologically malignant cells within the basement membrane of the crypts; these areas are designated *intraepithelial carcinoma*. Extension beyond the basement membrane into the lamina propria is termed *intramucosal carcinoma*. Neither intraepithelial nor intramucosal carcinoma has a great potential for metastasis, provided that all the neoplastic tissue is removed, because there are no lymphatics in the lamina propria of the colon. When neoplastic cells are contained within the basement membrane of the colonic epithelium, the term *in situ carcinoma* is used. When malignant cells extend beyond the basement membrane, the tumor is microscopically invasive. In the colon, where there are no mucosal lymphatics, lymphatic invasion and nodal metastases are unlikely until the tumor invades through

the muscularis mucosae into the submucosa, where lymphatics are present. Carcinoma in an adenomatous polyp of the colon is not considered invasive until it extends through the mucosa into the submucosa. In some polyps with foci of cancer, it is difficult to determine whether malignant cells have extended into the submucosa.

Clinical Features

Although familial polyposis coli syndrome has been observed in infancy and early childhood, it is recognized much more frequently in early adolescence. Although most patients are asymptomatic, some may experience increased stool frequency and occasionally rectal bleeding, anemia, and tenesmus; rarely abdominal pain may occur. Most children are asymptomatic and are identified by investigation on the basis of another member of the family having FAP. The diagnosis is established most frequently by family history, colonoscopic examination, and sometimes rectal examination. Colonoscopy may show a carpet of polyps covering the entire surface of the colon and rectum. Biopsy of one of the polyps establishes the diagnosis when adenomatous features are shown. Although barium enema with air contrast radiographs may show many filling defects with extensive involvement of the colon, many patients with small polyps have a normal-appearing radiographic contrast enema study. When the diagnosis is established, careful investigation of all family members should be initiated (see Genetic Mutations and Recommendations for Testing). Members of the family are at high risk of developing carcinoma of the colon because there is an inherited predisposition of the colonic mucosa to undergo malignant change at an early age.

Many associated malignancies may occur in patients with FAP (Table 57-4). More than 50% of patients with FAP are likely to develop gastric polyps, although this is infrequent before age 18 years. Most gastric polyps are hamartomas and not precancerous. Less than 15% of gastric polyps are believed to be adenomas. Duodenal polyps occur with much lower frequency than polyps in the stomach, although they are more likely to be adenomatous. Gastric and duodenal (periampullary) polyps initially were believed to occur primarily in patients with Gardner's syndrome; however, they are a frequent occurrence in all patients with FAP. Most patients with gastric and duodenal polyps are asymptomatic, although occasional patients may experience bleeding or gastritis. Endoscopic biopsy usually reveals inflammation and hyperplasia. The patient's symptoms are often improved with antacids and H$_2$-blocking agents, yet the polyps may persist for varying periods. Desmoid tumors of the small intestinal mesentery or abdominal wall occur in at least 10% of patients, but less frequently than in patients with Gardner's syndrome. Malignancy usually does not appear until late adolescence or early adult life, although the syndrome may have been recognized early in life. In patients recognized to have the disorder before age 13 years, carcinoma has been identified in only 6%. At least 50% of patients with FAP develop carcinoma of the colon or rectum by age 42 years. When it occurs, carcinoma is frequently multicentric. Hepatoblastoma may be seen in approximately 1.5% of patients with FAP.

TABLE 57-4 ■ Cancer Risk and Screening Recommendations in Familial Adenomatous Polyposis

Cancer	Frequency (Lifetime Risk, %)	Screening Recommendations
Colon	100	Sigmoidoscopy annually beginning at age 10-12 yr
Duodenal or periampullary	5	Upper GI endoscopy (with side viewing) every 1-3 yr starting at age 20 yr
Pancreatic	2	Possibly periodic ultrasound after age 20 yr
Thyroid	2	Annual thyroid examination starting at age 10-12 yr
Gastric	0.5	Same as for duodenal
Central nervous system (Turcot's syndrome)	0.5	Annual physical examination, possibly periodic CT scans in affected families
Hepatic (hepatoblastoma)	1.5	Hepatic ultrasound and α-fetoprotein annually during first decade of life

CT, computed tomography.
Adapted from Burt RW: Polyposis syndromes. Clin Perspect Gastroenterol January/February, 2002.

Therapy

Colectomy for familial polyposis coli is recommended at any age if the child is symptomatic; however, it is usually deferred until age 10 to 14 years when children are more capable of managing their own care after surgery. Because the major cause of death is colorectal cancer, prophylactic proctocolectomy soon after diagnosis is the recommended management. In general, the most favorable option has become the rectal mucosectomy and the endorectal ileal pouch pull-through procedure. Although each of the operations has its advocates, if any rectal mucosa remains, the patient must be followed closely with at least annual sigmoidoscopic examination until the rectum is removed because of the risk of carcinoma developing in the remaining rectal stump. Of patients who have the rectum preserved, 60% develop carcinoma within 20 to 30 years. In contrast to ulcerative colitis, a much more extensive mucosectomy must be performed with this disorder.

Several reports of clinical experience with the endorectal ileal pull-through procedure indicate that stool frequency, urgency, and continence are equally good or better than with ulcerative colitis. A temporary diverting ileostomy typically is performed postoperatively; however, some have reported good experience with a one-stage procedure.

Use of nonsteroidal anti-inflammatory drugs (e.g., sulindac) and inhibitors of cyclooxygenase-2 (e.g., celecoxib) has been shown to lead to a regression of FAP-associated adenomas in several studies. The use of sulindac in a prospective study to prevent the development of adenomas failed to show efficacy, however.

Genetic Mutations and Recommendations for Testing

It has been well appreciated that FAP is inherited by an autosomal dominant pattern. With the linkage of several *APC* kindreds to the *APC* locus, a true genetic etiology and pathophysiology of the disease could be appreciated. At least 95% of affected families have a mutation in the adenomatous polyposis coli (*APC*) gene, which is located on chromosome 5q21. To date, there are at least 34 mutations in this gene. Of newly diagnosed cases, 30% arise from new mutations and are without a family history. The *APC* gene is a tumor suppressor gene by maintaining normal levels of cell growth and apoptosis. The *APC* gene guides growth through the normal growth cycle (WNT pathway). Normally the APC protein associates with β-catenin, which (after phosphorylation) finds regulatory transcriptional factors preventing cell growth. With normal growth signals, or with *APC* mutations, APC is uncoupled from β-catenin, and cell growth occurs. Both alleles of the *APC* gene must be mutated for the gene function to be lost. In FAP, one allele is inherited in a mutated form; when the second allele is mutated, the tumor suppressor function is lost. Genetic analysis of colorectal adenocarcinomas from non-FAP patients also shows mutations in the *APC* gene.

Genetic testing is now a crucial part of managing families with FAP. The proper way to manage a family is to begin with the person known to have the adenomatous polyposis. This allows one to determine which genetic mutation is present in the particular family and allows guidance as to how to screen additional family members. In children at risk for disease, testing should begin by age 10 years. Genetic testing should be done in a person who has greater than 100 colorectal adenomatous polyps. Testing also should be done in a person with more than 20 cumulative adenomas (this also may detect patients with attenuated FAP). Finally, first-degree relatives of a patient confirmed to have FAP who are 10 years old or older should be screened, based on the specific mutation of the known FAP individual.

Gardner's Syndrome

In 1953, Gardner and Richards described a familial form of colonic polyposis that occurred in association with osteomas of the skull and facial bones and in some instances with multiple soft tissue tumors, such as lipomas, desmoid tumors, leiomyomas, sebaceous cysts, and dental abnormalities, including multiple unerupted and supernumerary teeth and multiple dental caries (Fig. 57-3). The polyps, which are adenomatous, often involve the small intestine and duodenum. Genetic analysis has shown that virtually all patients with Gardner's syndrome have a mutation of the *APC* gene and are essentially FAP patients. Mutations in these patients tend to occur in the most distal third of the gene. Inheritance (dominant) is the same as other FAP patients, and cancer and genetic screening should be followed similarly.

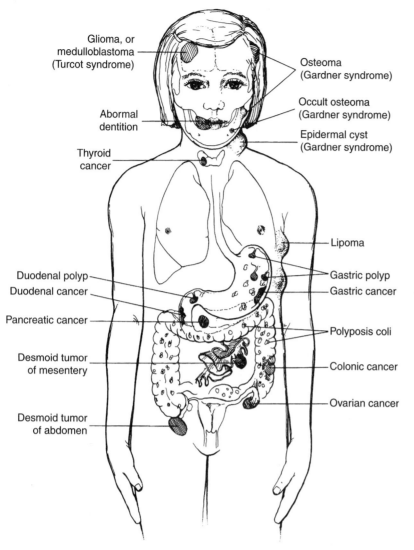

Glioma, or
medulloblastoma
(Turcot syndrome)

Osteoma
(Gardner syndrome)

Abormal
dentition

Occult osteoma
(Gardner syndrome)

Epidermal cyst
(Gardner syndrome)

Thyroid
cancer

Lipoma

Duodenal polyp
Duodenal cancer

Gastric polyp
Gastric cancer

Pancreatic cancer

Polyposis coli

Desmoid tumor
of mesentery

Colonic cancer

Ovarian cancer

Desmoid tumor
of abdomen

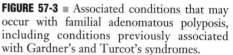

FIGURE 57-3 ■ Associated conditions that may occur with familial adenomatous polyposis, including conditions previously associated with Gardner's and Turcot's syndromes.

Desmoid tumors of the abdominal wall or mesentery of the small intestine occur in approximately 20% of patients with Gardner's syndrome, which is a much higher rate than most patients with FAP. Desmoid tumors are a leading cause of death with FAP. This lesion is a dense fibroplastic proliferation that may be localized or extend widely, as is common when the mesentery is involved. In approximately 20% of patients, the desmoplastic tumor may be recognized before the diagnosis of polyposis coli is established. The fibrous desmoplastic lesions occasionally have a family predisposition. All stages of fibrous dysplasia, desmoid tumor, and, rarely, fibrosarcoma have been reported. When present, desmoid tumors of the mesentery may limit the surgical options because of shortening caused by fibrous contraction around the mesenteric vessels. Because desmoid tumors are not malignant, local excision without bowel resection is recommended whenever feasible; however, excision of desmoid tumors of the mesentery is rarely possible. Radiation therapy has been minimally effective. Clinical improvement was observed in several patients with desmoid tumors of the mesentery after an extended course of therapy with tamoxifen and sulindac (Clinoril).

Clinical trials with many nonsteroidal anti-inflammatory drugs have been conducted with moderate success. When untreated, desmoid tumors may cause progressive contracture and eventually intestinal obstruction that may be surgically uncorrectable, resulting in death.

Turcot's Syndrome

Turcot's syndrome is characterized by adenomatous polyposis occurring in conjunction with a malignant tumor of the central nervous system, most often cerebellar medulloblastoma or glioblastoma (see Fig. 57-3). Other associated lesions include ependymoma and carcinoma of the thyroid. In contrast to familial polyposis coli or Gardner's syndrome, Turcot's syndrome is transmitted by an autosomal recessive gene, although some workers suggest that the syndrome may be a variant of Gardner's syndrome. There is a high risk for colon cancer, which develops at a relatively young age. Careful follow-up of the patients and their relatives is recommended.

Attenuated Adenomatous Polyposis

This disease is also due to mutations of the *APC* gene and inherited in an autosomal dominant pattern. These patients

58

Ulcerative Colitis

Ulcerative colitis first was described almost 150 years ago. Despite significant advancements in the knowledge of inflammatory bowel disease (IBD), this disorder's cause and definitive treatment remain unresolved. Although classically thought of as a disorder of adults, many children are affected. The pediatric surgeon is often instrumental in caring for patients with this disabling disease.

ETIOLOGY

No etiology has been determined, although several theories have been suggested. A clear association with many factors suggests that all IBD is due to a combination of genetic predisposition and environmental exposure to either enteric organisms or dietary factors. The identification of an *IBD1* gene locus in Crohn's disease supports the genetic association with IBD. Although such a gene has not been identified in ulcerative colitis, linkages with genes on chromosomes 3, 5, 7, and 12 have been found in some studies. Genetics clearly play a role; however, the fact that only 45% of identical twins develop IBD suggests that other processes are also important. Environmental factors, including enteric organisms, may influence whether IBD actually develops. An immunologic response to luminal bacteria is supported by clinical responsiveness to antimicrobials. This finding also is supported by the fact that murine models of IBD fail to develop colitis without the addition of enteric organisms. Others believe that bacteria or viruses are secondary invaders rather than primary agents and that dietary factors have a more important role.

Approximately 15% of patients with ulcerative colitis are from families with members who have IBD. Studies of HLA antigens, particularly the W27 isoform, in patients with idiopathic ankylosing spondylitis, uveitis, and ulcerative colitis suggest a genetic predisposition, although no definite predictable relationship has been determined. Although many workers suggest that psychological factors may play a causative role, there seems to be no "premorbid personality." Psychological factors and stress may provoke relapses, contributing to the chronicity of the disease, yet not causing the condition.

PATHOLOGY

Ulcerative colitis is primarily a disease of the rectal and colonic mucosa and submucosa. The rectum is involved in more than 95% of patients, and inflammation extends proximally in a contiguous manner. When the entire colon is involved (pancolitis), the most severe pathologic changes are present in the rectum and sigmoid colon. Crypt abscesses are the most characteristic microscopic feature, leading to mucosal ulceration with undermining of the adjacent mucosa. Mucosal bridging and pseudopolyp formation often result. As the disease progresses, in the acute phase, the colon distends, peristalsis decreases, and the muscularis becomes thin and diffusely hemorrhagic; this may progress to toxic megacolon (Fig. 58-1). Conversely, with chronic ulcerative colitis, the colon becomes stiff, thickened, and foreshortened with atrophic mucosa and loss of haustral folds. This often gives the appearance of a "lead pipe" in the descending and sigmoid colon (Fig. 58-2). In remission, the mucosa may revert to a near-normal microscopic appearance. Mucosal biopsy helps to confirm the diagnosis and assess the activity of the disease.

From an immune perspective, the mucosa in ulcerative colitis consists of a dominant CD4+ population of T lymphocytes. These T cells have an atypical phenotype with an increased production of transforming growth factor-β and interleukin (IL)-5. These cells seem to be activated by antigen presentation from adjacent epithelial cells. Additional mediators of inflammation are derived from activated macrophages, which express many inflammatory cytokines, including tumor necrosis factor, IL-1, and IL-6. These latter inflammatory factors form the basis for much of the newer medical management of this disease.

CLINICAL FEATURES

Ulcerative colitis chiefly affects persons after the second decade of life, but at least 22% of all patients manifest initial symptoms before age 18. Males and females are equally affected; however, the condition is four times more prevalent in whites than in blacks, Hispanics, or Asians. Ulcerative colitis is at least three times more common in Jews than in non-Jews. The disease seems to be increasing in the United States and in Europe, although it remains uncommon in Asia.

In approximately 4% of patients with ulcerative colitis, the onset of disease occurs before age 10 years.

557

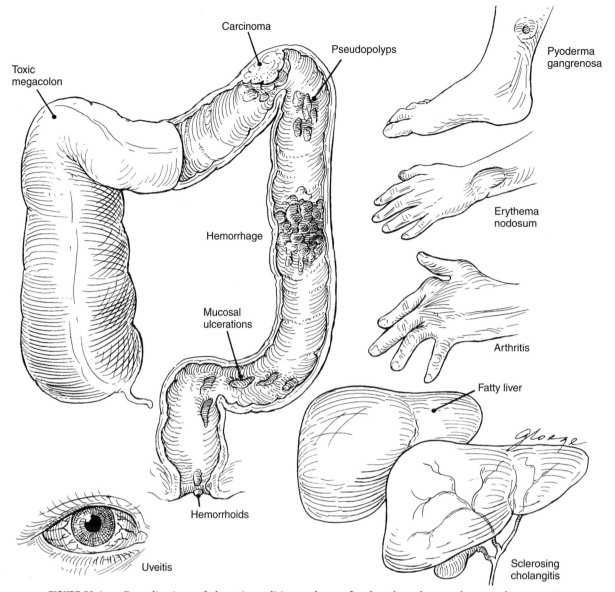

FIGURE 58-1 ■ Complications of ulcerative colitis may be confined to the colon, or they may be systemic.

In 18%, symptoms appear between 10 and 20 years, but the onset is most frequent during the mid-20s. Symptoms typically begin insidiously with persistent diarrhea followed by the appearance of blood, mucus, and pus in the stool. Cramping lower abdominal pain and tenesmus are common. Anorexia, weight loss, and growth retardation from chronic inflammation, poor appetite, and prolonged use of corticosteroids tend to occur when the disease is chronic. As a result, many children experience feelings of inferiority and lack a desire to participate in social and physical activities. Most develop unremitting colitis with periodic relapses precipitated by emotional stress or intercurrent infection. After a few years, some patients may achieve permanent remission, although most experience chronic colitis with shorter and less frequent remissions. A single attack with complete remission occurs in less than 10% of children.

In approximately 15% of children, the onset of ulcerative colitis is acute and fulminating with profuse bloody diarrhea, severe abdominal cramps, fever, and occasionally sepsis, requiring prompt treatment. Although most improve for varying periods with medical therapy, approximately 5% of patients develop toxic megacolon, requiring urgent operation. At least 60% of children with colitis eventually require surgical resection.

Cancer of the colon or rectum has been reported in 3% of patients during the first 10 years of disease, increasing by 20% in each subsequent decade. Cancer may develop even in patients with apparent remission. Cancer is more common in patients who have pancolitis, in patients whose symptoms began in childhood, and in patients who have frequent flare-ups of symptoms. Evidence of dysplasia of the colonic mucosa on the biopsy specimen indicates a high risk for development of carcinoma.

Extracolonic manifestations include growth retardation, arthralgias, skin lesions, failure of sexual maturation, anemia, liver disease, osteoporosis, nephrolithiasis,

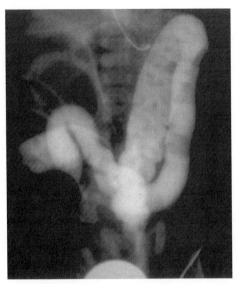

FIGURE 58-2 ■ Barium enema radiograph shows a shortened and narrow left-sided colon with absence of haustral folds, giving a "lead pipe" appearance. Also note the presence of pseudopolyps in the transverse colon.

uveitis, and stomatitis (see Fig. 58-1). Growth retardation with delay in bone age frequently accompanies chronic ulcerative colitis in adolescents. Delayed sexual maturation may be in part because of abnormally low levels of 24-hour urinary gonadotropins. Growth hormone levels are usually normal for the patient's age.

Arthralgias occur in approximately 20% of patients with ulcerative colitis, usually involving the knees, ankles, and wrists. Joint symptoms occasionally precede the onset of intestinal symptoms, sometimes being confused with juvenile rheumatoid arthritis. Ankylosing spondylitis may be seen in 1% to 6%, and sacroiliitis may be seen in 4% to 18% of patients. Both of these conditions may be permanently disabling. Aphthous stomatitis, gingivitis, and erythema nodosum are seen occasionally in patients with ulcerative colitis, but more frequently in Crohn's disease. A more common skin lesion in ulcerative colitis is pyoderma gangrenosum.

Abnormal liver function tests are found in approximately 15% of patients and may stem from a variety of hepatic disorders. Of patients with ulcerative colitis, 80% have some abnormality of the liver on biopsy specimen. The predominant lesions are a pericholangitis. Approximately 50% to 90% of patients have a fatty infiltration of the liver. Of greater long-term concern is the development of sclerosing cholangitis, which may be seen in 1% to 4% of patients with ulcerative colitis. Patients may have pruritus and right upper quadrant pain with this condition. Although adults manifest this condition with an elevation of alkaline phosphatase, evaluation of this parameter must be done with caution in adolescents and children, who normally have higher alkaline phosphatase levels. Diagnosis is made by endoscopic retrograde cholangiopancreatography. Sclerosing cholangitis may persist after proctocolectomy but typically does not occur if it has not developed before the patient's proctocolectomy. Anemia is common, usually the result of overt or occult

blood loss in the stool. Osteoporosis and osteomalacia may occur from decreased calcium absorption associated with diminished uptake of fat-soluble vitamins and by increased urinary losses of calcium resulting from steroid therapy. Nephrolithiasis occurs in about 8% of patients, largely because of inadequate fluid intake to compensate for diarrheal losses and increased oxalate absorption in the terminal ileum. Uveitis is an inflammation of the iris found in less than 2% of patients.

Children with mild ulcerative colitis or children who experience a period of remission may manifest few if any positive findings on examination, although sigmoidoscopy may show friable and edematous mucosa with a thin purulent exudate. These children often show evidence of delayed growth, lack of sexual maturation, anemia, pallor, and cushingoid features from long-term corticosteroid therapy. With more severe acute disease, children may develop fever, dehydration, and symptoms of systemic toxicity. Pain during palpation over the sigmoid colon is common. Although external hemorrhoids frequently develop from stool frequency, anal sinuses, fissures, and abscesses are much more indicative of Crohn's disease. On sigmoidoscopy, the mucosa is often edematous and hemorrhagic and contains superficial ulcers. The mucosa is covered with a purulent, bloody exudate.

Anemia resulting from blood loss occurs in approximately two thirds of patients. The erythrocyte sedimentation rate is typically elevated, and the prothrombin time is prolonged. Serum albumin level is usually low. Hyponatremia and hypokalemia may occur with protracted diarrhea. Stool cultures are consistently negative for pathogenic bacteria and parasites.

Although barium enema radiographs have been used for many years to establish the extent and severity of ulcerative colitis, most physicians recognize that better information can be obtained from flexible colonoscopy. A contrast enema can precipitate the acute manifestations of colitis. When performed, the radiographic enema study may reveal a shortened, narrow, and rigid colon with loss of haustral folds and extensive pseudopolyp formation with chronic ulcerative colitis (Fig. 58-3). In acute colitis, the bowel contour may have an irregular serrated border from mucosal ulcerations. The edematous mucosa between areas of ulceration appear as pseudopolyps. Swollen, inflamed mucosa can form symmetric defects along the borders, known as *thumbprinting*.

Differentiation of ulcerative colitis from other pathologic states is essential. An upper gastrointestinal series with small bowel follow-through is crucial because Crohn's disease often may be confused with ulcerative colitis. Culturing of stool to rule out an infectious cause is essential because several organisms may mimic the symptoms of ulcerative colitis. Additionally an accurate pathologic review of multiple biopsy specimens from colonoscopy and, if indicated, upper endoscopy is essential for the diagnosis. Nevertheless, 10% of patients may not be assigned accurately to either Crohn's disease or ulcerative colitis and have a diagnosis of indeterminate colitis. To address more accurately the differentiation between these two disorders, a panel of serologic tests has been developed. These include antineutrophil cytoplasmic antibody (ANCA), with a perinuclear staining

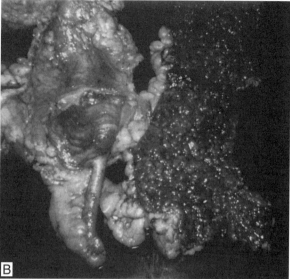

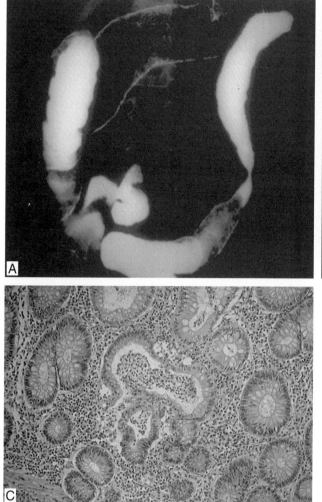

FIGURE 58-3 ■ **A,** Barium enema radiograph shows mucosal details of the transverse colon. Note the irregular mucosa with thumbprinting. **B,** Gross specimen of colon shows mucosal details. Note the extensive pseudopolyps over the entire surface. **C,** Histologic appearance of the mucosa. The crypts are filled with neutrophils (crypt abscesses).

pattern being observed in ulcerative colitis patients (pANCA). Conversely, antibody to *Saccharomyces cerevisiae* (ASCA) had been identified in nearly 50% of patients with Crohn's disease. An additional antibody, anti–cathepsin G, has been identified in 63% of ulcerative colitis patients and is particularly prevalent in patients with active disease. Use of these antibodies has prompted numerous studies. Because of the relatively low predictive value, application of these studies is restricted to confirming a clinical and pathologic diagnosis at present. A potential use of these antibodies for the surgeon is in the 10% of patients who have the diagnosis of an indeterminate colitis, for whom surgery is contemplated. In these cases, although a fair amount of overlap exists, the use of these antibodies may help direct the surgical approach. Table 58-1 shows the relative frequency of these serologic markers in indeterminate colitis.

NONOPERATIVE TREATMENT

Medical therapy for ulcerative colitis is nonspecific and is based on measures to provide symptomatic relief. At present, it is unlikely, however, that the ultimate

course of the disease can be altered or a cure achieved by nonoperative treatment. Medical management may be stratified based on the clinical severity of the disease process (Table 58-2). Patients with stable disease or who are in remission may benefit from the use of 5-aminosalicylate-based compounds, such as sulfasalazine (Azulfidine; Procter & Gamble, Cincinnati, OH). These drugs are a mainstay for the treatment of patients with mild or moderate forms of the disease. The function of these drugs seems to be in the 5-aminosalicylate portion of the compound, which blocks the production of prostaglandins and leukotrienes. Additional actions include the blocking of bacterial peptide–induced neutrophil chemotaxis, adenosine-induced secretion, and scavenging of reactive oxygen metabolites. Use of different derivatives of these compounds may direct therapy to a targeted site. This includes the use of a suppository or enema for proctitis and oral compounds that are not broken down in the small bowel for targeting colonic tissue (mesalamine [Rowasa enema or oral Pentasa]).

For patients who have an acute exacerbation of symptoms, corticosteroid therapy is much more effective. Topical corticosteroids, such as hydrocortisone

TABLE 58-1 ■ Ability to Predict the Correct Diagnosis of Disease in a Group of Patients with an Initial Diagnosis of Indeterminate Colitis

	Diagnosis	Sensitivity (%)	Specificity (%)	PPV (%)	NPV (%)
ASCA+/pANCA–	CD	67	78	80	64
ASCA–/pANCA+	UC	78	67	64	80

PPV, positive predictive value; NPV, negative predictive value; CD, Crohn's disease; UC, ulcerative colitis.
From Joossens S, Reinisch W, Vermeire S, et al: The value of serologic markers in indeterminate colitis: A prospective follow-up study. Gastroenterology 122:1240-1447, 2002.

(Cortenema), can be used for a severe, distal inflammatory process. Oral prednisone is used for severe ulcerative colitis, and intravenous dosing is given for patients who are hospitalized. In general, patients respond to steroids within 7 to 10 days. Steroid therapy should be given only as long as there is an acute inflammatory process. Tapering should be instituted, with a transition to other medications. While on corticosteroids, patients should receive an H_2-blocking agent. Additionally, side effects of corticosteroids should be anticipated, including growth failure, osteoporosis, hypertension, hyperglycemia, and cushingoid features. Patients also should be placed on calcium, vitamin D, and bisphosphonates.

Immunosuppressive therapy (azathioprine, 6-mercaptopurine, cyclosporine) has been advocated for patients with chronic or refractory ulcerative colitis. Azathioprine and mercaptopurine work on long-lived subgroups of T cells, which require a prolonged length of administration before their action takes effect. These drugs should be started while the child is tapering off of corticosteroids. These drugs are toxic, and monitoring of the white blood cell count is essential. Additionally, both drugs may cause pancreatitis and drug-induced hepatitis. The drugs are not only helpful in allowing steroid therapy to be tapered, but also are useful in maintaining remission. Cyclosporine works by preventing T-cell activation and by inhibition of IL-2 and IL-2 receptor expression. Its onset of action is much faster than azathioprine. It has been shown to have equal efficacy to corticosteroids in treating patients with severe ulcerative colitis. It is useful in severe steroid-refractory disease.

Cyclosporine does have shortcomings, however, in that it is highly immunosuppressive. Additionally the success of the drug may not preclude future surgery. Approximately 30% to 70% of patients who have been treated with cyclosporine for an acute exacerbation of ulcerative colitis undergo a proctocolectomy within 6 months to 1 year.

Still controversial is the use of anti–tumor necrosis factor therapy (infliximab; Centorcor, Malvern, PA). Although conventionally used in patients with Crohn's disease, a limited study of 17 adults showed that 16 responded within 6 days, with a sustained response in 2 to 10 months. Colectomy was required in only one patient.

Psychotherapy may help a patient with chronic ulcerative colitis adjust to the disease, its complications, and its side effects. Even more important than psychotherapy is the ready availability of a sympathetic and interested physician and an understanding family on whom the patient can rely.

During acute flare-ups of ulcerative colitis, most patients require hospitalization with intravenous fluid administration, bowel rest, increased doses of steroids, and parenteral nutrition. These measures correct the patient's metabolic deficit and often reduce the clinical symptoms, yet do not alter the course of the colitis. The primary benefit of intravenous nutrition is to reduce surgical risk by improving the patient's nitrogen balance. Progression of the colitis or failure to respond to therapy is an indication for urgent operation. When the acute attack subsides, the patient may begin consuming a bland high-calorie diet.

TABLE 58-2 ■ Therapeutic Options for Medical Management of Patients with Ulcerative Colitis

Clinical Condition	Distal Ulcerative Colitis	Extensive Ulcerative Colitis
Mild disease	Oral or rectal aminosalicylates, rectal corticosteroids	Oral aminosalicylates
Moderate disease	Oral or rectal aminosalicylates, rectal corticosteroids	Oral aminosalicylates
Severe disease	Oral or rectal aminosalicylates, rectal corticosteroids	Oral or parenteral corticosteroids, intravenous cyclosporine
Refractory disease	Oral or rectal aminosalicylates, rectal corticosteroids	Oral or intravenous corticosteroids, in addition to azathioprine or mercaptopurine; consider anti-TNF
Remission	Oral or rectal aminosalicylates, rectal corticosteroids	Oral aminosalicylates, oral azathioprine or mecaptopurine

anti-TNF, antibody to tumor necrosis factor.
Adapted from Podolsky DK: Inflammatory bowel disease. N Engl J Med 347:417-429, 2002.

Antidiarrheal medications, such as diphenoxylate hydrochloride with atropine sulfate (Lomotil) or loperamide hydrochloride (Imodium), may reduce the number of bowel movements and decrease rectal spasm, but they should be used with care because these drugs as well as opiates occasionally may induce toxic megacolon. Dietary modification may be useful to minimize intestinal stimulants (e.g., elimination of chocolate, vinegar, spicy foods, fresh vegetables, and nuts). Marked anemia and hypoalbuminemia may necessitate blood or albumin infusion.

OPERATIVE THERAPY

Ulcerative colitis can be cured by surgically removing the diseased colon and rectum. When this treatment implied a permanent ileostomy, operation often was delayed until the patient was severely ill, the operative risk was high, and the complication rate was excessive. Since the development of the mucosal proctectomy and endorectal ileal pull-through procedure, serious consideration should be given to operation for any patient with chronic ulcerative colitis before severe disability and major complications develop.

Surgery in children with ulcerative colitis can be elective or emergent. Elective operation is performed on patients with chronic disease who experience continued symptoms despite medical therapy, growth retardation, severe limitation of activities, and an unacceptable quality of life. Emergency indications for operation include fulminant disease refractory to medical therapy, extensive rectal bleeding, and toxic megacolon. Careful monitoring and the use of steroids have reduced the number of operations in an emergency setting. If the indication for surgery is growth failure, the diseased colon should be removed while the epiphyses are still open to allow for growth and development. Evaluation of the child's condition should be done periodically during the course of therapy by the surgeon and the gastroenterologist to consider alternatives to long-term medical therapy.

Surgical options are discussed in detail beforehand with the patient and the parents. It is helpful if the patient speaks to another child of the same sex and similar age who has undergone surgery to alleviate fears and concerns about an ileostomy and to support the decision for surgery. Preoperative discussion with an enterostomal therapist also helps to prepare the child and parents for an ileostomy. A short course of parenteral hyperalimentation is used if the patient is severely malnourished. Anemia, hypoalbuminemia, and electrolyte abnormalities are corrected preoperatively. Corticosteroid therapy is maintained to avoid an acute flare-up preoperatively. Oral intake is restricted to clear liquids for 48 hours before surgery. Cleansing enemas are avoided because they may precipitate an acute flare-up of colitis. Oral antibiotics are given on the day before the operation, and intravenous antibiotics are given preoperatively.

Complete proctocolectomy with permanent ileostomy is curative for ulcerative colitis and is done as a one-stage operation. It has been used with low morbidity and mortality for more than 50 years. A major concern of patients, particularly children, is the required lifetime ileostomy appliance. Although the care of an ileostomy usually is mastered easily by a child, the presence of a stoma often creates embarrassment during physical and social activities. Although postoperative impotence or bladder dysfunction after proctocolectomy in children are uncommon, these major concerns have caused many children, parents, and physicians to defer operation until severe debilitation by the colitis or steroid therapy causes irreversible systemic complications. Other operations less commonly employed include a subtotal colectomy with preservation of the rectum and an ileorectal anastomosis. Active disease in the rectum in most of these patients requires continued medical therapy and eventual surgical removal because of the risk of cancer. The Kock continent ileal reservoir with nipple valve construction obviates the need to wear an ileostomy drainage bag for most patients. Drainage is provided by inserting a Silastic catheter into the reservoir several times daily. Complications related to stasis and distention from incomplete emptying, with chronic reservoir inflammation and incompetence of the nipple valve, leads to multiple reoperations and eventual removal in many patients. The procedure currently is used primarily for patients who already have a permanent ileostomy and who are severely handicapped by it.

Inasmuch as ulcerative colitis is primarily a disease of the mucosa, a modification of the rectal mucosal stripping procedure described by Soave in 1963 for treatment of Hirschsprung's disease has become the treatment of choice for children and adults. Removal of the entire rectal mucosa down to the dentate line does not interfere appreciably with anorectal sphincter function or the ability to discriminate between gas and liquid or solid contents. Clinical use of the endorectal ileal pull-through procedure in children was not adopted until a successful outcome was reported in 15 of 17 children with a straight ileal pull-through operation. Pouch procedures had been reported previously in adults.

Although numerous modifications of the endorectal pull-through were made during the ensuing years, it now is generally accepted as a highly desirable option for surgical treatment of ulcerative colitis and familial polyposis. Appealing features of this operation include absence of a permanent stoma, lack of repeated catheterization (as needed with a Kock pouch), and development of a near-normal pattern of defecation. Despite these advantages, patient expectations need to be addressed preoperatively. Stooling frequency is typically high initially regardless of whether a pouch is used or not. Another problem is nocturnal incontinence. This latter problem is particularly prevalent in younger children, with the process resolving as the child matures. Finally, it is common for children to be on multiple medications to control stooling frequency; however, most of these patients eventually wean off most of these medications.

The approach to the operation involves either a straight pull-through or the creation of a pouch. Choice of either depends on weighing the risks and benefits of each procedure. The pouch is associated with fewer bowel movements, particularly in the first year after the procedure. A pouch has the attendant risk of pouchitis, however, which may occur in 50% of patients after 10 years following pull-through. The straight pull-through avoids the risk of pouchitis; however, it is associated with more frequent bowel movements in the first postoperative year. Regardless of the type of procedure performed, as long as the lower 4 cm of the rectal muscle is not damaged, the anal sphincter resting pressure and the anal sphincter squeeze pressure approach normal values within 6 weeks.

Early surgical experience with pull-through operations indicated that a completely diverting, protecting ileostomy for approximately 2 months is advisable to minimize the risk of pelvic infection. Children with chronic ulcerative colitis who receive long-term steroids are often malnourished and frequently have a suppressed immune response, which increases the risk of anastomotic leak. Anastomotic leak has been found in approximately 10% to 15% of patients and has the attendant risk of leading to anal stricture. Nonetheless, some adult series have been reported in which protective ileostomy has not been used.

Four basic reservoir types have been used clinically: the S-shaped reservoir, the J-shaped reservoir, the lateral isoperistaltic reservoir, and the W-shaped reservoir (Fig. 58-4). In general, the W-pouch and lateral isoperistaltic reservoirs have been abandoned. The S-shaped and the W-shaped reservoirs must be hand-sutured, requiring longer operating time than that needed for other pouches. The blood supply to the lower ileum of these two pouches may be obstructed partially by bending the mesentery, particularly if it is thick. Pouch stasis is common with these two reservoirs, and an irrigating catheter often is required for adequate emptying. After several months, the reservoir tends to enlarge, and the spout elongates. When using the S-pouch, it is crucial to make the distal spout extremely short (1 to 1.5 cm in length).

The J-shaped reservoir, the most common pouch currently used (see Fig. 58-4), is usually constructed with a stapling instrument. A major advantage is the placement of the lower end of the reservoir close to the anus without a spout. The drawback is that it is sometimes difficult to bring the side of the ileum down to the anus without tension, particularly in heavy or tall patients. The S-pouch has the same overall mesenteric length as a straight pull-through. It is a useful technique in patients who desire a reservoir, but in whom adequate length cannot be achieved with a J-pouch.

Intravenous steroids are tapered rapidly after surgery, and oral prednisone usually can be discontinued within 3 weeks. Most children are discharged from the hospital by the seventh postoperative day. A water-soluble contrast enema is performed within the first 2 months to ensure that the ileal reservoir has healed securely, and there are no leaks or sinus tracts. Most children resume full physical activities within 3 weeks.

Approximately 2 months after the first operation, the child is rehospitalized for ileostomy closure and sigmoidoscopy; the ileoanal anastomosis is dilated at this time. Management of patients when the stoma has closed may be challenging. When oral feedings are begun, it is important initially to withhold some foods that may cause excess stooling, including chocolate, vinegar salad dressings, and spicy foods. Medical management starts with a combination of pectins in the form of Kaopectate and low doses of Imodium. Imodium dosing increases as needed. Small amounts of fiber (Metamucil or Fibercon) may be given to increase fecal bulk for the first few weeks, if necessary. Occasional rectal examinations are performed to maintain the patency of the rectal anastomosis. Use of oral metronidazole may be helpful in controlling episodes of frequent stooling because it leads to considerable bulking of the stool.

RESULTS

Regardless of the type of pull-through, stool frequency and continence are similar in large series of patients followed for many years. Complications are multiple, and children need long-term follow-up and care to attend to these problems.

Leakage from the anastomosis may occur in 20% of patients if there is no protective stoma. Although many of these leaks resolve with subsequent formation of a protective stoma, patients are left at increased risk for anastomotic stricture and potential problems with future continence. Although inconvenient to the patient, it has been our practice to perform a diverting stoma in most patients.

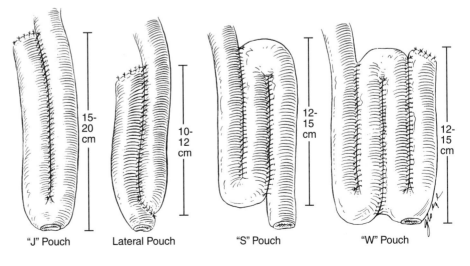

FIGURE 58-4 ■ Ileal reservoir configurations in current clinical use for patients undergoing an endorectal ileal pull-through procedure. The length of the reservoir for the J-pouch is often much shorter in children (10 to 12 cm).

"J" Pouch   15-20 cm

Lateral Pouch   10-12 cm

"S" Pouch   12-15 cm

"W" Pouch   12-15 cm

Despite the advantages of a stoma, several problems are associated with its use, including retraction, parastomal hernias, dehydration, and most commonly obstruction owing to fecal material or excessive fascial tightness. Patients who present with signs of a bowel obstruction often may be relieved of the blockage with the passage of a large red rubber catheter through the proximal limb of the stoma.

Small bowel obstruction is a common problem with reported frequencies of 15% to 25%. Adhesions are the major cause of the obstruction; however, internal hernias and outlet obstruction from the ileostomy are other common causes.

Pouchitis first was described by Kock as an inflammatory state resulting from stasis within the reservoir. Incidence may be 50% in patients followed for more than 10 years. Patients with a positive pANCA serologic marker are most at risk to develop pouchitis. The process may relate to the original disease because pouchitis is seen infrequently in patients with familial polyposis. Symptoms include low-grade fever, pelvic pain, bloody stools, diarrhea, and malaise. Treatment with antibiotics (metronidazole or ciprofloxacin) is usually successful. Occasionally, patients may benefit from steroid enemas. The use of probiotics may be beneficial in preventing recurrence of pouchitis when the patient is in remission. Recurrent pouchitis may be a manifestation of Crohn's disease, and biopsy specimens should be obtained. It has become apparent that pouchitis is more common in larger reservoirs, which empty only partially with each defecation. Although stenosis at the ileoanal anastomosis or lower end of the reservoir may seem to be a mild, annoying problem, it can cause reservoir distention, stasis, and pouchitis if not corrected early.

Fistulas from the pouch to the perianal skin or vagina seem related to technical problems at the time of the pull-through. Fistula formation may be seen in 4% to 7% of patients. Pouch loss resulting from multiple, often failed procedures may be 30%. Although technical problems may be a major causative factor, the possibility that the patient has Crohn's disease must be excluded by extensive biopsy specimens of the pouch and more proximal bowel.

Other complications include the rare occurrence of pouch perforation, erectile dysfunction, reduced fertility, and incorrect diagnosis. Temporary ileostomy may be needed in certain patients, particularly if growth and development during adolescent years are not progressing at optimal rates. After the reservoir reconstruction has been completed, and the child has resumed normal growth, the ileostomy may be closed safely. Long-term follow-up must include proctoscopies every 2 to 3 years with biopsy specimens of the retained 1 to 2 cm of rectal cuff to rule out malignancy.

SUGGESTED READINGS

Coran AG: A personal experience with 100 consecutive total colectomies and straight ileoanal endorectal pull-throughs for benign disease of the colon and rectum in children and adults. Ann Surg 212:242-248, 2002.

This is the largest review of patients undergoing a straight pull-through for ulcerative colitis and familial polyposis. The frequency of stooling was no higher in these patients compared with patients with a reservoir by 1 year after the closure of the ileostomy.

Devroede GJ, Taylor WF, Sauer WG, et al: Cancer risk and life expectancy of children with ulcerative colitis. N Engl J Med 185:17, 1971.

This is one of the most authoritative and extensive reviews of the relationship between the length and severity of ulcerative colitis and the development of cancer.

Ekbom A, Helmick C, Zack M, Adami HO: Ulcerative colitis and colorectal cancer: A population-based study. N Engl J Med 323:1228-1233, 1990.

A well-controlled, population-based analysis of the risk of colorectal carcinoma in patients (including children) with ulcerative colitis is reported.

Fonkalsrud EW, Loar N: Long-term results after colectomy and experience with endorectal ileal pull-through procedure in children. Ann Surg 215:57, 1992.

This article contains the largest reported clinical experience with the endorectal ileal pull-through procedure for ulcerative colitis in childhood.

Joossens S, Reinisch W, Vermeire S, et al: The value of serologic markers in indeterminate colitis: A prospective follow-up study. Gastroenterology 122:1240-1447, 2002.

An excellent review is provided of the value of serologic markers to help clinicians determine if a patient has Crohn's disease or ulcerative colitis.

Kock NG, Darle N, Kewenter J, et al: The quality of life after proctocolectomy and ileostomy: A study of patients with conventional ileostomies converted to continent ileostomies. Dis Colon Rectum 17:287, 1974.

This is one of the most extensive and authoritative reviews of the role of the continent ileostomy in the surgical treatment of ulcerative colitis.

Pemberton JH, Kelly KA, Beart RW Jr, et al: Ileal pouch-anal anastomosis for chronic ulcerative colitis. Ann Surg 206:504, 1987.

This article contains an extensive discussion and review of the current restorative proctocolectomy in the surgical treatment of ulcerative colitis by leading authorities in the field.

Podolsky DK: Inflammatory bowel disease. N Engl J Med 347:417-429, 2002.

This article is a good review of the medical treatments and etiology of IBD.

59

Appendicitis

Acute appendicitis is one of the most common causes of abdominal pain in childhood. This diagnosis must be considered in all age groups but is more common between the ages of 4 and 15 years. The function of the appendix is unknown. However, in rabbits and other animals the cecum is similar in shape to the appendix and plays a role in digestion of food: the cecum of rabbits is associated with a disease known as typhlitis, which is similar to appendicitis. This blind-ending diverticular structure arising from the cecum at the confluence of the three taenia coli has a lumen that may be irregular and somewhat narrow because of the presence of abundant lymphoid follicles in the submucosa. The blood supply comes from the appendicular branch of the ileocolic artery. In most patients the appendix is located in the right lower quadrant, but its site may be variable because of malrotation, situs inversus, or a mobile cecum.

The pathophysiology of acute appendicitis is most likely the result of a "closed-loop" obstruction of its lumen related to a fecalith or, less commonly, resulting from hyperplasia of submucosal lymphoid follicles caused by a viral infection or, rarely, from obstruction from pinworm or other helminthic infestation. Occasionally, obstruction is caused by a carcinoid tumor that if less than 1 cm requires no further therapy after appendectomy with reasonable margins. In the presence of obstruction, the mucosa continues to secrete, resulting in an accumulation of mucoid material and increasing intraluminal pressure. Bacteria located within the lumen of the appendix proliferate in the presence of stasis and obstruction. The flora of the appendix includes both aerobic and anaerobic organisms typical of those found in the large intestine. Continued mucus production and proliferation of gas-forming bacteria cause a further rise of intraluminal pressure, resulting in the development of acute appendicitis with edema, lymphatic obstruction, and necrotizing ulceration of the mucosa. Translocation of bacteria across the wall of the appendix may occur. If the diagnosis of appendicitis is not made early, the process will continue and obstruction of venous and lymphatic drainage and arterial thrombosis will ensue, causing gangrenous changes in the appendiceal wall and subsequent perforation (Fig. 59-1).

CLINICAL PRESENTATION

A careful clinical history and thorough physical examination are the hallmarks of arriving at an early and accurate diagnosis of appendicitis. The classic presentation of acute appendicitis usually begins with abdominal pain, frequently localized to the periumbilical area and epigastrium. This is commonly followed by development of anorexia, and most children with appendicitis show no interest in their favorite foods. Anorexia is followed by the onset of nausea and vomiting. The patient with abdominal pain is less likely to have appendicitis in the absence of anorexia and nausea/vomiting. In time, the abdominal pain eventually shifts to the right lower quadrant. The pain in appendicitis is continuous and generally does not get better during the course of the disease process. The pain is also present even when the patient is lying still. Localized pain is related to inflammation of the parietal peritoneum. Because the appendix is a finger-like projection, it may be in various locations and

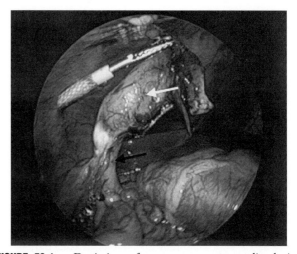

FIGURE 59-1 ■ Depiction of a gangrenous appendix during laparoscopic appendectomy. Note the enlarged, edematous appendix (*white arrow*) with a relatively normal appendiceal base (*black arrow*).

produce localized pain in the right upper quadrant under the gallbladder, in the pelvis, across the top of the bladder, and in a retrocecal site (Fig. 59-2.) In approximately 15% of patients, the appendix lies in a retrocecal, extraperitoneal location. When the appendix lies behind the cecum or in the pelvis, irritation of the parietal peritoneum often does not occur and the classic shift of pain to the right lower quadrant may be absent. Many patients have a history of constipation, which is a common cause of abdominal pain in and of itself; however, in some patients diarrhea will be present and may be related to pelvic inflammation and irritation of the rectum, although a viral cause is most common. The physician should search for a history of upper respiratory tract infection symptoms, such as cough and runny nose, and for recent gastroenteritis in the patient or the remainder of the family. Symptoms of urinary tract infection should be elicited. Occasionally, a child complains of right lower abdominal pain while walking or refuses to stand up or walk. Obtaining an accurate history from an infant or a very young child (<3 years old) may be problematic because communication is difficult in this younger age group, contributing to

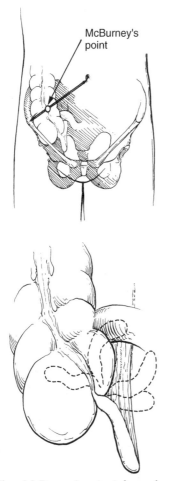

FIGURE 59-2 ■ Top, McBurney's point is located one third of the distance along a line from the anterior iliac spine and umbilicus. **Bottom,** The appendix is a finger-like projection that can extend inferiorly in the pelvis, medially toward the midline, superiorly, or into the retrocecal area.

a high rate of perforated appendicitis in this population. Most children with appendicitis have a low-grade fever of 38°C to 39°C [100.4°F to 102.2°F]; however, some patients have no elevation of temperature. It is unusual for patients with appendicitis to present with a temperature above 39°C (102.2°F). When the temperature is this high, viral gastroenteritis should be considered.

PHYSICAL EXAMINATION

The physical examination is the most important diagnostic determinant in children with acute abdominal conditions. The physical examination must include a careful and meaningful abdominal and rectal examination with the patient cooperative enough to make the evaluation valid. Examination of a small child with appendicitis may be a challenge. A youngster who is ill and in pain is often frightened by an unfamiliar environment such as a hospital emergency department. Examination under these circumstances can be extremely difficult and may require great skill, patience, and experience. Time spent taking the history from the child's parents serves an additional purpose of indicating to the child that the "stranger" physician is nonthreatening. Observation of the child before the actual physical examination will often detect signs suggestive of appendicitis: the patient usually lies quietly with the knees flexed or on the side with the knees drawn up. How the patient turns on the examining room table is informative; the patient with appendicitis moves slowly and carefully, avoiding any sudden movements. These are some of the many signs and symptoms of peritonitis for which the physician is searching. These peritoneal signs are due to irritation of the parietal peritoneum from the inflamed appendix and consist of pain or tenderness associated with movement of the abdominal wall. Such peritoneal signs are the hallmark of appendicitis. The abdominal examination should be initiated anywhere but the right lower quadrant, with that area left for last. Potentially unpleasant parts of the examination such as evaluation of the throat with the use of a tongue blade or looking at the tympanic membranes with an otoscope or performing a rectal examination also should be left for last. Careful examination of the neck and auscultation of the chest are important, because occasionally streptococcal pharyngitis with lymphadenopathy or pneumonia may mimic appendicitis, particularly if right middle lobe or lower lobe inflammation exists.

With the patient supine, the knees are flexed during the examination to reduce any tension on the rectus muscles and to make the abdomen somewhat softer and easier to palpate. The child can be asked to "point with one finger at the spot where it hurts the most," which is usually found in the right lower quadrant at McBurney's point, which is one third of the distance from the right anterior superior iliac spine toward the umbilicus (see Fig. 59-2). The examiner should begin with percussion of all four quadrants of the abdomen to elicit peritoneal signs. This should be followed by gentle and shallow palpation to identify subtle signs of peritoneal irritation. Such gentle palpation may elicit significant, localized tenderness in the right lower quadrant and suggest the diagnosis of appendicitis. Peritoneal signs can also be elicited by moving the palpating fingers in a short, rapid, up-and-down motion, thus shaking the abdominal quadrant. The typical description of rebound tenderness by pressing deeply and then releasing to elicit signs of peritonitis is unnecessary in the child with abdominal pain. Rather, gentle palpation and shaking of the parietal peritoneum can elicit similar symptoms and signs. Rovsing's sign, which consists of the production of pain in the right lower quadrant on palpation of the left lower quadrant, should be elicited in a similar fashion. Once the examination using percussion and gentle palpation has been completed, deep palpation in all quadrants of the abdomen should be performed unless the diagnosis is already clear. Having a patient raise the hips and buttocks off of and then drop them onto the examining table may elicit pain consistent with peritonitis. It is critical to have the child in whom the diagnosis is in question get off of the examining room table and jump up and down. Jumping elicits peritoneal signs. A patient with appendicitis will rarely jump up and down more than once and will have pain with doing so. Holding a hand above a child's head and challenging him or her to jump and touch it is irresistible to most children, except those in whom pain is produced.

The classic psoas sign is elicited by placing the child on the left side and extending the leg and hip posteriorly. The presence of a psoas sign can also be determined by having patients push the knee anteriorly against the resistance of the examiner's hands. Particularly in young children, it is difficult to differentiate discomfort due to palpation from true tenderness. Children will often answer yes if asked whether an area is tender. The child should be distracted by being engaged in a conversation about pets, siblings, or school while the examination is being done. Auscultation of the abdomen is of little diagnostic importance in diagnosing appendicitis. However, the stethoscope may serve as a tool to palpate the abdomen to search for tenderness in young patients who believe that the device is being used for auscultation. Tenderness can usually be detected by watching changes in the patient's facial expression.

A rectal examination should be performed in most patients with acute abdominal pain unless the diagnosis is clear. The rectal examination may detect a fecal impaction caused by severe constipation, which may be a cause of abdominal pain. Localized right rectal vault tenderness is common with appendicitis and may allow detection of an inflamed pelvic appendix. In some patients one can palpate a mass consistent with an abscess. In teenage girls with a nonvirginal introitus, a routine pelvic examination is indicated. However, in most cases a routine pelvic examination is not necessary unless indicated by the information obtained in the history. Instead, an adequate pelvic examination, including evaluation of cervical motion tenderness, can be performed during rectal examination and can include bimanual abdominal palpation. A positive obturator sign is also indicative of pelvic appendicitis. This sign is elicited by placing the child supine and abducting and adducting the flexed right leg to rotate the obturator internus muscle.

LABORATORY TESTS

Laboratory tests are not especially helpful in the diagnosis of early acute appendicitis. Approximately 90% of the patients with appendicitis have a white blood cell count elevated between 10,000 to 15,000/mm^3; however, under certain circumstances a normal white blood cell count can be observed, and in some patients with perforated appendicitis leukopenia may be noted. The differential blood smear may be of more importance and usually shows some shift to the left, with excessive numbers of polymorphonuclear leukocytes and band forms. Urinalysis may be of importance if gross or microscopic hematuria or excessive numbers of white blood cells are present in the urine, consistent with a diagnosis of renal stone or urinary tract infection. An abnormal urinalysis may also be observed in patients with appendicitis when the inflamed appendix rests on or near the ureter or bladder. Elevated urine-specific gravity is consistent with hypovolemia and dehydration. In teenage female patients a urine human chorionic gonadotropin level should be obtained to rule out pregnancy. Other laboratory tests are usually unnecessary unless the patient is severely dehydrated and hypovolemic. In these patients serum electrolyte levels are obtained.

DIAGNOSTIC TESTS

Chest and erect and recumbent abdominal radiographs are rarely obtained. The chest radiograph should only be performed if there is a concern for pneumonia. Abdominal radiographic findings are rarely helpful but in 15% of patients demonstrate the presence of a calcified fecalith in the right lower quadrant that is diagnostic of appendicitis. Ultrasound examination is especially useful in teenage girls in whom pelvic inflammatory disease and/or some other gynecologic condition such as torsion of a right ovarian cyst is being considered. Ultrasonography suggests appendicitis when the diameter of the appendix is greater than 6 mm and fluid is noted in its vicinity. The typical finding is an oval, tender, noncompressible, blind-ending tubular structure consisting of an anechoic lumen centered by an echogenic mucosa and a zone of decreased echoes adjacent to the cecum. Recently, computed tomographic (CT) scans have played a role in the diagnosis of appendicitis. Dedicated CT for appendicitis may be performed either without contrast material or with administration of rectal contrast material such that it fills the cecum and, it is hoped, the appendix in a retrograde fashion. Some radiologists use an oral contrast agent instead. CT images of the right lower quadrant are then evaluated for an enlarged, edematous appendix, which often presents as a "target sign" (Fig. 59-3). Fat stranding in the right lower quadrant is also indicative of adjacent inflammation, which may be secondary to appendicitis. Studies in children have demonstrated a sensitivity and specificity of 97% for CT evaluation for appendicitis. In fact, CT evaluation appears to reduce the number of negative exploratory procedures and to achieve cost savings when compared with clinical evaluation of pediatric patients with a *questionable* presentation of appendicitis. However, in patients with a *clear clinical picture* of appendicitis a CT scan may be

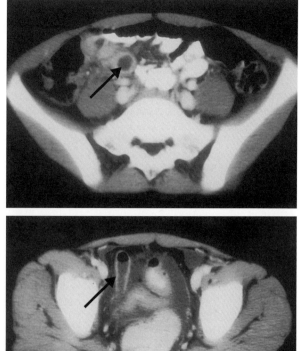

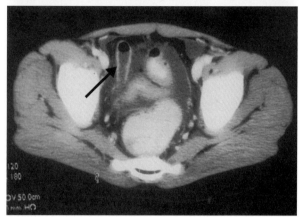

FIGURE 59-3 ■ CT images of acute appendicitis. **A,** The typical target sign of the appendix with evidence of surrounding inflammation and fat stranding in the right lower abdomen is demonstrated by the arrow. **B,** A different cut through an inflamed appendix.

TABLE 59-1 ■ Differential Diagnosis of Appendicitis
Gastrointestinal Tract
Gastroenteritis (viral, bacterial)
Inflammatory bowel disease
Intestinal obstruction
Intussusception
Mesenteric adenitis (bacterial, viral)
Meckel's diverticulum
Peptic ulcer
Severe constipation
Typhlitis
Gynecologic
Mittelschmerz
Pelvic inflammatory disease
Ruptured ovarian cyst
Ruptured tubal pregnancy
Torsion of normal ovary or ovarian cyst or tumor
Hepatobiliary/Pancreatic
Cholecystitis/cholelithiasis
Pancreatitis
Trauma
Rectus hematoma
Solid/hollow organ injury
Trauma to a previously unsuspected mass (e.g., Wilms' tumor, lymphoma)
Urinary Tract
Cystitis
Hydronephrosis
Pyelonephritis
Renal stone
Other Causes
Diabetic ketoacidosis
Helminthic infestation
Hemolytic-uremic syndrome
Hemophilia A
Henoch-Schönlein purpura
Lupus erythematosus
Porphyria
Primary peritonitis
Right-sided pneumonia
Sickle cell crisis
Streptococcal infection
Torsion of appendix epiploica
Torsion of omentum

wasteful from a cost point of view and unnecessary from a radiation exposure point of view. As such, CT scan should be used in the diagnostic armamentarium to augment the clinical findings and is most useful in patients in whom the diagnosis of appendicitis is unclear.

Diagnostic laparoscopy with appendectomy is the final diagnostic test in the patient with unrelenting pain and continued concern for appendicitis. Although costly, the minimally invasive nature of this technique makes it reasonable in the presence of a persisting diagnostic dilemma.

DIFFERENTIAL DIAGNOSIS

Although appendicitis is a common childhood condition, the typical history may be absent in 50% of patients, and arriving at the diagnosis may be difficult. One third to one half of patients with perforated appendicitis have already been seen in a physician's office or an emergency department and are sent home with an incorrect diagnosis. The differential diagnosis of acute appendicitis is extensive, and errors in diagnosis may be common in infants, very young children, mentally retarded children, patients initially hospitalized for other conditions, and teen-age girls (30% to 40%), in whom various gynecologic problems

may also present as lower abdominal pain (Table 59-1). A careful menstrual history often yields important diagnostic clues. In addition, observation of a vaginal discharge, cervical tenderness, and bilateral lower pelvic abdominal pain on physical examination is often indicative of pelvic inflammatory disease. Torsion of either a normal ovary, an ovarian cyst, or a tumor-bearing ovary and a ruptured tubal pregnancy are also diagnostic considerations. In addition, mid-monthly cycle ovulation characterized by rupture of a follicular cyst may cause significant peritoneal irritation ("mittelschmerz") and be a cause of concern because of its associated pain. Gastroenteritis is a frequent cause of abdominal pain in young children. Vomiting, watery diarrhea, and high fever may accompany the abdominal pain.

Other conditions that may be misdiagnosed as appendicitis in childhood include Crohn's disease, mesenteric adenitis (*Campylobacter, Yersinia*, viruses), and, less commonly, pancreatitis, perforated peptic ulcer (with material draining downward along the right gutter causing lower abdominal pain), and cholecystitis and cholelithiasis. Abdominal pain may also be caused by constipation, urinary tract infection (pyelonephritis and cystitis), renal calculus, and various other conditions, including lupus erythematosus (associated with serositis), Henoch-Schönlein purpura (abdominal cramps, rash, hematuria, albuminuria, elevated platelet count), hemolytic-uremic syndrome (thrombocytopenia, hematuria, rectal bleeding, elevated blood urea nitrogen value), sickle cell crisis, diabetic ketoacidosis, hemorrhage into the mesentery (in a boy with hemophilia A), streptococcal septicemia, right lower lobe pneumonia, torsion of the omentum, inflamed Meckel's diverticulum, traumatic hematoma of the rectus sheath, and hemorrhage caused by trauma of a previously unsuspected mass (Wilms' tumor, lymphoma).

In children younger than 3 years of age, gastroenteritis and idiopathic ileocolic intussusception are two of the more common conditions included in the differential diagnosis. Appendicitis has been described in neonates in whom a perforation of the appendix is observed, and sometimes Hirschsprung's disease is the cause. Primary peritonitis, in which the peritonitis has no intra-abdominal cause, should also be included in the differential diagnosis, especially in children with ascites as a result of the nephrotic syndrome or cirrhosis of the liver. In immunosuppressed children (often patients with leukemia) inflammation of the cecum and right colon as a result of bacterial invasion of the intestinal wall (typhlitis) may be the cause of severe localized right lower quadrant pain and may be difficult to distinguish from appendicitis. The CT scan in patients with typhlitis may demonstrate thickening of the wall of the cecum and right side of the colon with edema and pericecal fluid collection.

In the clinical setting, children with appendicitis usually fit into one of three groups (Fig. 59-4). The first are patients who present with an obvious case of acute appendicitis with point tenderness in the right lower quadrant, leaving no doubt as to the diagnosis. The second group of patients are those who clearly do not have appendicitis. Finally, the third and most perplexing group of patients are those children with abdominal pain in whom the diagnosis is unclear. Here, adjunctive tests including ultrasonography or CT may be required. In most patients the combination of history, physical examination, and imaging will allow a determination of whether appendicitis is likely or unlikely. With the former, operation is indicated, whereas with the latter, patients are observed closely from home. It is rare that admission for observation and serial examination is required.

TREATMENT

Persistent localized right lower quadrant pain and tenderness indicates that the patient may have appendicitis; and, in the absence of findings to suggest otherwise, operation should be performed. The time interval between onset of symptoms and perforation is quite variable but appears to be on the order of 36 to 48 hours. Gangrenous or perforated appendicitis occurs in approximately one third of patients admitted to most children's hospitals.

The advent of treatment of perforated appendicitis with antibiotics followed by interval appendectomy created the need to distinguish between perforated and nonperforated appendicitis. Patients with perforated appendicitis tend to appear more ill, more often have fevers, and have a higher white blood cell count, diffuse versus localized tenderness, and a longer period of symptoms. However, any one of these individual symptoms or even a combination does not distinguish between perforated and nonperforated appendicitis with sufficient accuracy. CT evaluation may distinguish between perforated versus nonperforated appendicitis by identification of the presence of one or more abscesses or a phlegmon, but not with a high degree of accuracy (Fig. 59-5). The physician, in effect, must make a judgment and is usually not sure whether the patient has "perforated" versus "nonperforated" appendicitis based on the overall clinical and radiologic picture. As such, most physicians choose to use the term "advanced" versus "early" appendicitis instead of perforated versus nonperforated appendicitis, respectively.

In instances of early acute appendicitis, the child should receive administration of intravenous fluids; cefotetan or triple antibiotics (ampicillin, gentamicin, and clindamycin or metronidazole); and narcotics for pain relief. Once antibiotics are administered, the process leading toward perforation appears to be halted and is accompanied by a reduction in pain and tenderness in many children. As such, in most instances, antibiotics and narcotics should not be administered until the diagnosis of appendicitis has been made by the surgeon. The need for emergent operation is also removed, and most appendectomy cases can await the daylight hours. A nasogastric tube may be inserted after endotracheal intubation and rapid-sequence induction of general anesthesia. Appendectomy is accomplished at many centers through a laparoscopic approach. The operating costs with laparoscopy are greater than with an open approach, but the hospital stay is shorter in some instances. A laparoscopic approach can be performed in the same time that it takes to perform an open procedure. One benefit, other than the cosmetic advantage, is the ability to perform a complete evaluation of the adnexae and other intra-abdominal structures should the appendix appear normal. Visualization during appendectomy is also excellent. The laparoscopic approach can be performed through either a 3- or 2-port approach. With a three-port technique, a 12F port is placed either through the umbilicus or the left lower quadrant, with the former being of advantage from a cosmetic point of view. Two other 5-mm ports are placed so that a total of three ports are placed, respectively, in the umbilicus, the left lower quadrant, and the right mid abdomen. A window is created in the mesoappendix adjacent to the base of the appendix (Fig. 59-6). A stapler is first fired across the mesoappendix and then across the base of the appendix. The appendix can be removed through the 12-mm port or an endoscopic bag if required. The pelvis and right pericolic gutter can be inspected for the presence of an abscess and irrigated. With the two-port technique a 5-mm port is placed through the umbilicus, through

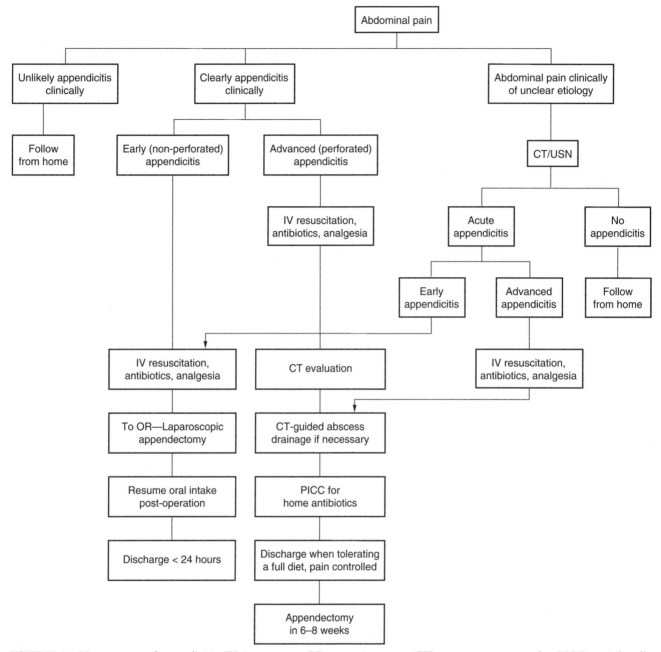

FIGURE 59-4 ■ Management of appendicitis. IV, intravenous; OR, operating room; CT, computer tomography; PICC, peripherally inserted central catheter; USN, ultrasound.

which the laparoscope is introduced. A 10-mm port is placed in the right lower quadrant, and the appendix is grasped under direct vision and brought up through the 10-mm port site as the port is removed. An extracorporeal appendectomy is then performed with ligation of the mesoappendix. The base of the appendix is ligated, after which it is returned into the peritoneal cavity. The 10-mm port is then replaced, the abdomen insufflated, the base of the appendix inspected for hemostasis, and the pelvis and right pericolic gutter inspected for abscesses and irrigated. The latter technique is applicable to situations in which either an early acute appendicitis is present or a normal appendix is encountered.

Open appendectomy is performed through a right lower quadrant (Rockey-Davis) transverse incision. The technique consists of mobilization of the cecum, division and ligation of the appendiceal vessels within the mesoappendix, ligation of the base of the appendix, and appendectomy (with or without inversion of the stump, Figure 59-7). Primary wound closure is accomplished because the incidence of postoperative wound infection is exceedingly low even in the setting of perforation. Peritoneal cultures have been shown to be of low utility and rarely are helpful because of the spectrum of standard antibiotic regimens. Antibiotics are continued postoperatively only in patients with perforated appendicitis.

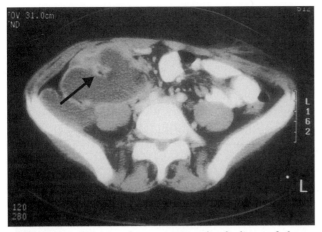

FIGURE 59-5 ■ CT scan demonstrating the findings of abscess (*arrow*) and inflammation in the right lower abdomen of a child with perforated appendicitis.

In the setting of advanced or perforated appendicitis, children may or may not have signs and symptoms of systemic sepsis. If so, the patient may be dehydrated and have diminished urine output, high body temperature (greater than 39°C [102.2°F]), rapid pulse, and adynamic ileus related to peritonitis. Tenderness may be localized or diffuse. The patient should be resuscitated with intravenous fluids and triple antibiotics or cefotetan administered to treat infection from aerobic and anaerobic organisms. Pain medication is administered. When stable, the patient may be taken to the operating room

Patients can usually resume oral intake after operation and, in most cases of nonperforated appendicitis, are discharged within 24 to 48 hours regardless of whether a laparoscopic or open technique is used.

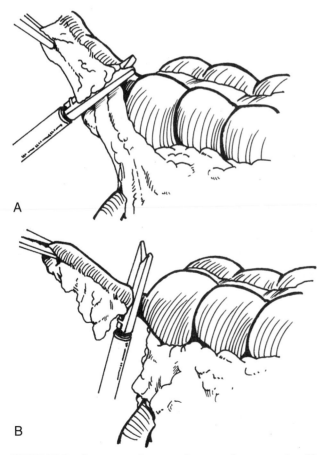

FIGURE 59-6 ■ Laparoscopic appendectomy demonstrating (**A**) creation of a window in the mesoappendix adjacent to the base of the appendix and division of the mesoappendix using a stapler, followed by (**B**) excision of the appendix using a stapler.

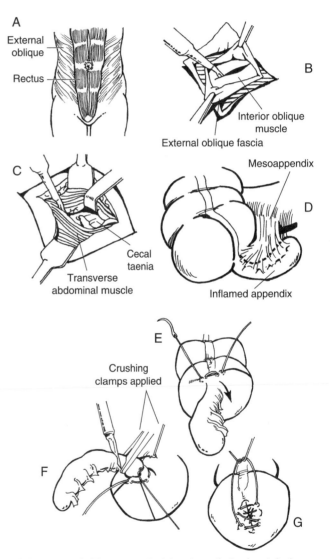

FIGURE 59-7 ■ **A,** Transverse incision is made in the right lower quadrant over the lateral musculature. **B,** The external oblique fascia is incised, exposing the internal oblique fascia and muscle. **C,** The transverse abdominal muscle and peritoneum is opened and the cecum identified. **D,** An inflamed appendix is identified and the mesoappendix is isolated, clamped, divided, and tied. **E,** A purse-string suture is placed in the cecal wall. **F,** The base of the appendix is crushed and tied. The appendix is excised, and **G,** the appendiceal stump is inverted into the cecal wall and the purse-string suture tied.

for appendectomy. In some cases of advanced appendicitis, an approach applying interval appendectomy is used: patients are first treated with intravenous antibiotics to allow resolution of the acute infectious and inflammatory process. Abscess formation is managed with CT-guided percutaneous aspiration and/or drain placement. Appendectomy is performed after a 6- to 8-week interval. This approach is effective in many patients and may be associated with a reduction in the complication rate associated with an acute operation. Intravenous antibiotics are continued until the patient's temperature returns to normal, the white blood cell count diminishes, and diet is tolerated. A peripherally inserted central catheter may be placed and the patient discharged home on intravenous antibiotics once a diet is tolerated and pain is controlled on oral medication. Parenteral nutrition may be necessary until adequate nutrition can be acquired orally. Once intravenous antibiotics are discontinued, some practitioners continue to treat potential infection with 1 to 2 weeks of oral antibiotics.

MORTALITY AND COMPLICATIONS

The mortality of appendicitis in children has gradually decreased over the past three decades to the point where it is now almost never the primary cause of death. The availability of broad-spectrum antibiotics along with CT imaging and interventional radiologic drainage of abscesses have made deaths from appendicitis almost unheard of and the incidence certainly less than 1%. Wound infection is an infrequent postoperative complication after appendectomy for acute appendicitis even after perforation (3%). Pelvic abscesses are also fairly uncommon (less than 5%) and can usually be managed by CT-guided percutaneous drain placement, transrectal drainage, or continued antibiotic administration in the case of multiple, small abscesses. There is a 3% to 5% risk of postoperative adhesive small bowel obstruction. Previous negative laparotomy rates were approximately 20% and were thought to be appropriate to avoid ruptured appendicitis. Currently, over 90% of children operated on for appendicitis indeed have the disease. The incidence of ruptured appendicitis has not increased even though the negative laparotomy rate has decreased.

CHRONIC APPENDICITIS

Although the existence of chronic appendicitis is controversial, most surgeons have managed patients with recurrent abdominal pain that resolved with appendectomy. In some cases, the history consists of intermittent right lower quadrant abdominal pain and, in fact, the appendiceal pathology demonstrates chronic changes consistent with recurrent inflammation and fibrosis. Some surgeons have suggested that identification of a nonfilling or partially filling appendix on contrast enema or CT, as well as the failure of contrast to drain from the appendix after a few days after contrast medium administration, is suggestive of chronic or recurrent appendicitis in the patient with chronic abdominal pain. Although one should perform a thorough evaluation of the patient with chronic abdominal pain before operative intervention, laparoscopy with appendectomy is a minimally invasive means for intraperitoneal evaluation and appendectomy in the child with unrelenting lower abdominal pain.

SUGGESTED READINGS

These three references outline current practice issues related to the diagnosis and treatment of acute appendicitis.

Anderson KD, Parry RL: Appendicitis. In O'Neill JA Jr, Rowe MI, Grosfeld JL, et al (eds): Pediatric Surgery, 5th ed. St. Louis, CV Mosby, 1998, vol 2, pp 1369-1377.
Blakely ML, Spurbeck WW, Laksman S, et al: Laparoscopic appendectomy in children. Semin Laparosc Surg 5:14-18, 1998.
Irish MS, Pearl RH, Caty MG, Glick PL: The approach to common abdominal diagnoses in infants and children. Pediatr Clin North Am 45:729–772, 1998.

Hirschsprung's Disease

60

HISTORICAL BACKGROUND

Descriptions of children with megacolon date back to the 17th century, when Ruysch (1691), a Dutch anatomist, described a 5-year-old girl who died of intestinal obstruction. The first clinical description of congenital megacolon was presented at the Berlin Society of Pediatrics in 1886 by Hirschsprung. He thought that the disease was caused by distention of the colon, as evidenced by the title of his presentation: "Constipation in Newborns Due to Dilation and Hypertrophy of the Colon." As a result of Hirschsprung's presentation, however, attention was focused on the consequences of the abnormality rather than the pathophysiology of the disease.

An understanding of the pathogenesis of Hirschsprung's disease took several more decades. An appreciation that the distal colon was the actual abnormality initially was advanced by Tittel (1901), who identified an absence of ganglion cells in the distal colon of a child with Hirschsprung's disease. Because some children with primary constipation were included in the diagnosis of Hirschsprung's disease, confusion about the etiology continued until the late 1940s. Ehrenpreis in 1946 was the first to appreciate that the colon became secondarily dilated owing to distal obstruction. Although several other workers presented series of cases that resembled those described by Hirschsprung, it was Ehrenpreis who observed the motility disturbance present from birth in 10 infants with Hirschsprung's disease in 1940. In 1946, Ehrenpreis also identified the colonic dilation as an acquired abnormality that occurred secondary to the more distal colonic motility disturbance rather than the primary problem. Finally, between 1946 and 1948, three groups published data that established the absence of ganglion cells in the myenteric and submucosal plexus as the primary abnormality. Although Whitehouse and Kernohan described the neurologic abnormality in a review of many previous reports and 11 of their own cases in which the ganglion cells of the myenteric plexus were absent, Bodian and colleagues identified the narrowed colonic segment as lacking ganglion cells. Swenson and Bill in 1948 were the first to advocate full-thickness rectal biopsy to make the definitive diagnosis and to recommend a treatment plan. This plan involved resection of the aganglionic bowel and its replacement with normally innervated proximal intestine. Since then, many refinements have been introduced in the evaluation of the constipated child and the newborn with intestinal obstruction that have improved the outcome.

Over the past 50 years, with increasing awareness of the presentation, the diagnosis of Hirschsprung's disease has been identified increasingly as a form of neonatal bowel obstruction. In more recent reviews, more than 45% of all patients with Hirschsprung's disease were diagnosed in the neonatal period. Data obtained by Kleinhaus and colleagues in their 1979 review of 1196 patients supported this trend. Until 1955, the mean age at diagnosis was 45 months compared with a mean age of 6 months reported between 1971 and 1975. The percentage of patients diagnosed by age 3 months increased from 20% before 1955 to 64% between 1971 and 1975. The percentage diagnosed by age 1 month simultaneously increased from 5% to 50% during the same periods. Missing the diagnosis in this time period places a child at increased risk for the development of complications of the disease, including enterocolitis and perforation of the intestine. The trend is evident in the striking decline in mortality associated with this disease. Klein and Scarborough in 1954 reported a 70% mortality rate, Hoffman and Rehbein in 1966 reported a 28% mortality, and Shimm and Swenson in 1966 reported a mortality of 33%. More recent series, also such as that from Rescorla and colleagues in 1992 (6%) and Teitelbaum in 2000 (1%), have shown a marked decline in mortality. Additional improvements in the perioperative care of surgical patients have contributed to these excellent results.

EMBRYOLOGY

Congenital intestinal aganglionosis (Hirschsprung's disease) is the result of arrested fetal development of the myenteric nervous system, but the precise pathogenic mechanisms involved are unknown. Normally, neuroblasts derived from neural crest precursors become discernible in the foregut by 5 weeks' gestation. Cranial to caudal migration subsequently occurs with vagal nerve fibers to complete the myenteric nervous system. Normal ganglion cells are recognized in the esophagus at 6 weeks, the transverse colon by 8 weeks, and the rectum by

12 weeks. The initial caudal migration of intermuscular neuroblasts is followed by intramural dispersal of neuroblasts to the superficial and deep submucosal nerve plexus. Concurrent and subsequent maturation of neuroblasts into ganglion cells occurs and normally seems to continue well into infancy.

GENETIC INHERITANCE

It has long been appreciated that Hirschsprung's disease may affect more than one family member in 3.6% to 7.8% of cases, and some kindreds of Hirschsprung's disease have a 50% inheritance rate. According to Passarge, siblings of female patients with Hirschsprung's disease have a 7.5% risk of being born with the disease (360 times that of the general population), and siblings of male patients with Hirschsprung's disease have a 2.5% to 6% higher incidence (130-fold higher incidence) of the disease. The studies also indicate that the longer the segment of aganglionosis, the higher the rate of familial incidence. It is important to educate families about these risks because future children and relatives of the parents are at risk of having children with Hirschsprung's disease.

GENETIC MUTATIONS

The first association of a specific genetic defect in Hirschsprung's disease was reported in 1992 by Martucciello and colleagues. This group found a deletion in the long arm of chromosome 10. This child had total colonic Hirschsprung's disease and no family history. Further investigation by this group and others narrowed the location of this mutation between 10q11.2 and q21.2. This allowed the investigators to narrow the search for a "Hirschsprung's gene" to a 250-kb region that overlapped the region of the *RET* proto-oncogene. Investigations have

transpired over the past several years that have shown that Hirschsprung's disease is one of the first identified polymorphic, multifactorial human diseases with a defined multigenetic etiology (Table 60-1).

RET Proto-oncogene

RET is a transmembrane receptor with tyrosine kinase activity. This receptor contains a cadherin-related sequence (used for cell-to-cell interactions) in the extracellular domain, which is important in control of normal cell growth and differentiation. In particular, the *RET* proto-oncogene seems to play a major role in the development of the enteric nervous system. Genetic errors in *RET* also are found in patients with multiple endocrine neoplasia types 2A and 2B; this may explain why a few patients with Hirschsprung's disease also have multiple endocrine neoplasia 2A. Many groups have shown actual point mutations affecting the *RET* proto-oncogene. The *RET* proto-oncogene consists of 20 exons (exons are the codable portion of the gene that produces RNA and eventually the *RET* product). Of these, mutations have been found in exons 2, 3, 5, 6, 11, 13, 15, and 17. The mutations have been noted in patients with sporadic Hirschsprung's disease and in patients with a family history. The genetic defect in any group with a family history seems to be the same mutation; however, the phenotypic expression (i.e., length of aganglionosis) may vary. The *RET* proto-oncogene also has been identified as the genetic defect in a rat model of aganglionosis.

GDNF

After the realization that *RET* mutations could lead to the development of Hirschsprung's disease, investigators began to examine the ligand for *RET*, the glial cell line–derived neurotrophic factor (*GDNF*). *GDNF* is a distant member of the transforming growth factor-β

	TABLE 60-1 ■ Listing of the Known Genetic Mutations Associated with Hirschsprung's Disease			
Predominant Name	**Model or Human**	**Chromosome**	**Strain if Present or Percent of Humans**	**Phenotype**
Endothelin receptor B gene	Mouse and rat	13q22	Piebald—lethal, spotting lethal	Distal colon aganglionosis
	Humans		Mennonites and sporadic types	
Endothelin-3 gene	Mouse and rat 2 human cases	20q13.2-q13.3	Lethal spotted	Variable length of aganglionosis
SOX10/sox10 gene	Mouse	22q12-q13	Dominant megacolon	Absent melanocytes and aganglionosis
	Human			Waardenburg-Shah syndrome
Ret proto-oncogene	Mouse	10q11.2	20-25% of humans	Aganglionosis, trend to long segment disease
	Humans			
GDNF gene	Mouse	5p12-p13.1	Knock-out	Small and large bowel aganglionosis
	Humans			
Neuturin	Humans			
Not identified	Human	2q22-q23		Hirschsprung's with microcephaly, mental retardation, and facial features
Not identified	Human	20p11.22-p11.23		Hirschsprung's with autism
L1CAM gene	Humans	Exon 18 of *L1CAM* gene		Hydrocephalus, cleft palate, micrognathia and Hirschsprung's

superfamily and has a potent action in maintaining the dopaminergic neuronal cells of the substantia nigra and central cholinergic neurons. It is now known that *GDNF* is the ligand for *RET*, and mutations of *GDNF* can be seen in patients with Hirschsprung's disease. Subsequently, it has been shown that GFRα1 is the primary receptor for *GDNF* and *RET* a secondary, although important receptor. Additionally, neuturin and persephin are homologues that can bind and signal the GFRα1 receptor. A mutation in neuturin has been found in a patient with Hirschsprung's disease.

Endothelin-B Receptor and Endothelin-3 Genes

As with *RET* signaling via *GDNF*, endothelin receptor-B (*ENDRB*) is a receptor that transduces an intracellular signal after binding to three closely related isoforms (*ET-1, ET-2,* and *ET-3*). Although originally found only in the brain, kidney, lung, and heart, *ENDRB* also has been identified in the human colon in the myenteric plexus, mucosal layer, and ganglion cells. The endothelins initially were shown to support long-lasting vasopressor activity; however, Puffenberger and colleagues identified a mutation of this gene (mostly W276C) in an inbred group of Mennonites who had a high rate of Hirschsprung's disease. This mutation also was observed in mice with a targeted disruption of the *ENDRB* gene (piebald lethal) and *ET-3* gene (lethal spotted). It appears that signaling between these two molecules (*ENDRB* and *ET-3*) is crucial to the normal development of ganglion cells.

Other Genetic Mutations

Many other mutations have been described (see Table 60-1).

SOX10 and *sox10:* The *SOX10* mRNA is expressed in humans, and *sox10* mRNA is expressed in mice. It is found in adult brain, heart, small intestine, and colon, and strong expression of *sox10* occurs throughout the peripheral nervous system during mouse embryonic development. Mutations in *SOX10* have been identified in patients with the Waardenburg-Shah syndrome (lateral displacement of the medial canthi, partial albinism, and deafness).

Chr 20p: Michaelis and colleagues described an interstitial deletion of 20p in a patient with Hirschsprung's disease and autism. The location was between 20p11.22 and p11.23. The deleted region was close to the region characterized for Alagille syndrome, although the precise gene has not yet been identified.

Chr 2q22-q23: Mowat and colleagues identified six children with distinctive facial features (cleft palate, iris coloboma), microcephaly, mental retardation, and Hirschsprung's disease. These children were found to have interstitial deletions of chromosome 2q.

Neuturin: Mutations in neuturin, a related protein to *GDNF*, have been identified in some patients with Hirschsprung's disease. Doray and colleagues reported the association of a neuturin (19p13.3) mutation (missense) in family with four children

with Hirschsprung's disease. Each of these family members also were identified as having a *RET* mutation, suggesting that a missense in neuturin was insufficient alone to cause Hirschsprung's disease.

Interaction of Genetic Mutations and the Development of Hirschsprung's Disease

A common theme among many of the mutations listed previously is the fact that these mutations are incompletely penetrant so that some family members with the mutation are completely asymptomatic. Although the loss of both copies of the gene generally leads to a much more severe variant of the disease in mice, the loss of one copy of the *RET* proto-oncogene in humans often results in the development of Hirschsprung's disease (dominant effect). How this interplay of these multiple ligands and receptors works is still not fully understood, but it seems to be a major factor in the development of Hirschsprung's disease. Figure 60-1 summarizes a potential schema of how mutations may play a role in the development of Hirschsprung's disease. Signaling from multiple sites is required to lead to normal ganglion development. Mutations in these signaling proteins may lead to a lack of development. Because of the redundancy of the system, however, one single mutation may not be sufficient to form Hirschsprung's disease.

Trisomy 21

About 15% of patients with Hirschsprung's disease have trisomy 21. The precise relationship of this genetic abnormality to the development of Hirschsprung's disease has yet to be defined.

Loss of Nitric Oxide

The finding that nitric oxide is the mediator for nonadrenergic, noncholinergic smooth muscle relaxation led to investigations of its role in Hirschsprung's disease. Several investigators have shown a loss of staining for

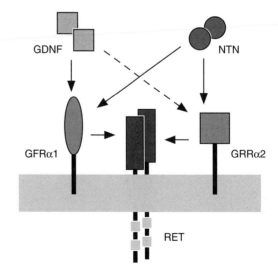

FIGURE 60-1 ■ Potential schema of how mutations may play a role in the development of Hirschsprung's disease. Signaling from multiple sites is required to lead to normal ganglion development.

nitric oxide synthetase in much of the aganglionic segments of intestine in patients with Hirschsprung's disease. From a genetic point of view, it is tempting to associate this loss to known genetic mutations. There is a close association between the signaling of endothelin to endothelin receptors 1 and 3 with the subsequent formation of nitric oxide. Although this relationship has been studied primarily in relation to its effects on vascular smooth muscle, it is possible that the loss of signaling in the embryo may lead to a loss of nitric oxide formation.

Alterations in the Extracellular Matrix

Another way in which migration may be inhibited is by an alteration in the extracellular matrix, including fibronectin and laminin. Fibronectin and laminin are two of several vital glycoproteins that facilitate nerve migration and neural cell growth. Abnormally large amounts of laminin accumulate in the extracellular spaces of aganglionic bowel and may prevent migration of ganglion cells into their new environment. The interrelationship between genetic mutations and the development of laminin accumulation has been addressed. There is evidence that the absence of endothelin-B activation by *ET-3* leads to increased expression of laminin that may result in the premature differentiation of neural crest–derived cells. This premature differentiation may contribute to their incomplete colonization of the gut.

Alteration in Neural Cell Adhesion Molecules

Kobayashi and colleagues studied neural cell adhesion molecule (NCAM) reactivity in colonic specimens of Hirschsprung's disease patients and compared them with age-matched and sex-matched controls. Bowel containing ganglion cells had strong NCAM reactivity, whereas there was an absence of NCAM-positive nerve fibers in the myenteric plexus of aganglionic segments. NCAM is believed to be important in neurocyte migration and localization of neurocytes to specific sites during embryogenesis. These findings are in conflict with an earlier report that found increased NCAM activity in aganglionic tissue. Ikawa and colleagues identified a loss of L1CAM, another associated neural cell adhesion molecule, in the aganglionic segments of the colon. If NCAM or L1CAM is absent in aganglionic tissue, it is possible that this loss may lead to an inability of migrating ganglion cells to adhere to the involved areas of the colon.

THERAPEUTIC IMPLICATIONS OF GENETIC FINDINGS

Rats with a targeted disruption of the *ENDRB* gene or with the sl mutation (spotting lethal), have been "treated" by the embryonic transfection of rats with the *ENDRB* gene. This procedure has resulted in the complete expression of *ENDRB* and presence of colonic ganglion cells in these rats, with the prevention of a megacolon. This exciting new area of investigation opens the question as to whether these therapeutic maneuvers could ever be applied to humans with such disorders. A better understanding of the mutations associated with Hirschsprung's disease and the detection of these disorders in a prenatal setting may be essential. Another challenge would be the timing of such an approach. The embryonic stage seems to be the time in which this therapy would be required to effect the adequate expression of ganglion cells. Detecting a genetic disorder this early and being able to transfect genetic material to an embryo would be extremely difficult challenges to undertake.

PATHOLOGIC ANATOMY

Aganglionosis is confined to the sigmoid colon or rectum in 75% to 80% of affected infants. The transition between normal and abnormal bowel may be found anywhere between the esophagus and anus and occurs in the small bowel in only 5% of affected infants. The remaining 15% of patients have progressively longer lengths of colonic aganglionosis. Classically the proximal bowel is distended with histologic evidence of muscular hypertrophy, although this is age dependent, and these findings may be subtle in newborns with obstruction of short duration. The proximal bowel has a normal myenteric nervous system. The characteristic lesion in the distal bowel is the absence of ganglion cells in the intermuscular and the submucosal plexus. In addition, many large, thickened, nonmyelinated nerve fibers are found within the muscularis mucosa, lamina propria, submucosa, and Auerbach's intermuscular plexus. These represent postganglionic fibers from proximal normal ganglion cells and disordered preganglionic parasympathetic fibers without discernible distal synaptic connections. Although adrenergic and cholinergic nerve fibers are increased by histochemical analysis, most of these fibers are cholinergic. An important diagnostic test involves histochemical staining for acetylcholinesterase (AChE). Adrenergic fibers appear diminished in aganglionic segments of bowel.

Interposed between normal ganglionated proximal bowel and the abnormal distal bowel is a transition zone characterized by hypoganglionosis and a progressive increase in the number of thickened nonmyelinated neurons as one moves distally. Externally the transition is usually a short funnel or a cone-shaped segment of the colon. Correlation between the gross and microscopic anatomy is not precise, so histologic confirmation is always necessary for intraoperative decision making. The transition zone is often obvious grossly or radiographically by a few weeks of age as the obstruction leads to progressive proximal dilation and to "congenital megacolon." Neonates with classic rectosigmoid aganglionosis and older children with transition zones in the small intestine may have subtle or undetectable bowel lumen discrepancies. The identification of the transition zone is problematic for the surgeon or radiologist with these particular patients. A normal barium enema study can never rule out the diagnosis of Hirschsprung's disease. Although a few reports of discontinuous aganglionosis have appeared, most evidence supports the concept that Hirschsprung's disease is a continuous disorder starting in the distal rectum and moving proximally. Although the rectal segment involved may be short, a correctly obtained rectal biopsy specimen showing ganglion cells precludes the existence of Hirschsprung's disease.

PATHOPHYSIOLOGY

Normal intestinal motility depends on a coordinated segmental contraction wave immediately preceded by smooth muscle relaxation as it propagates caudally. Patients with Hirschsprung's disease lack a functional myenteric nervous system in the affected distal intestine and have ineffective distal peristalsis. This situation seems to be the result of a cholinergic (propulsive) neuronal disorder and the absence of adrenergic and nonadrenergic inhibitory input. The clinical outcome is an incomplete distal small bowel obstruction in neonates or chronic constipation in older children. Reliable diagnostic manometric studies are feasible. Typically, patients with Hirschsprung's disease lack the normal reflex internal sphincteric relaxation induced by rectal dilation.

CLINICAL PRESENTATION

Hirschsprung's disease often presents in newborns as distal intestinal obstruction with or without sepsis. Although the incidence of enterocolitis is variable, this complication makes the diagnosis and early treatment of Hirschsprung's disease urgent. In the mildest case, delayed passage of meconium may be the only abnormality. In several large series, most patients failed to pass meconium within the first 48 hours of life. At the other end of the spectrum is the acutely ill newborn whose presentation is consistent with low intestinal obstruction. In these patients, abdominal distention, bilious or feculent vomiting, and failure to pass meconium are the presenting signs. Plain abdominal films commonly show multiple dilated loops of bowel with air-fluid levels consistent with low intestinal obstruction (Fig. 60-2A).

In the most fulminant presentation, infants may present with a picture of overwhelming sepsis. This picture may create confusion in making the diagnosis because intestinal dysfunction often accompanies neonatal sepsis. This clinical presentation demands the most urgent medical attention. The clinical presentation in this case is altered by other findings of sepsis in newborns, including progressive respiratory failure, hypovolemia, shock, coagulopathy with decreased platelet count, decreased urine output, and temperature instability. Finally a few infants present with peritonitis from intestinal perforation.

These variations in the clinical presentation are substantiated by several large series. Swenson, in his review of 501 patients, verified that 94% of patients had delayed passage of meconium beyond 24 hours. This well-quoted finding is not always seen. In a series of 35 newborns managed at the University of Michigan Medical Center, 54% showed abdominal distention, 46% failed to pass meconium after 48 hours, 34% presented with constipation, 26% presented with vomiting, and 6% had intestinal perforation. Enterocolitis occurred in 12% of patients. A similar rate of delayed passage of meconium (37% failed to pass meconium in 48 hours) was seen in the series by Rescorla. Each child has a unique presentation. The passage of meconium within 48 hours does not exclude the diagnosis of Hirschsprung's disease in a child with other gastrointestinal abnormalities. The pediatric surgeon must maintain a high index of suspicion for the disease

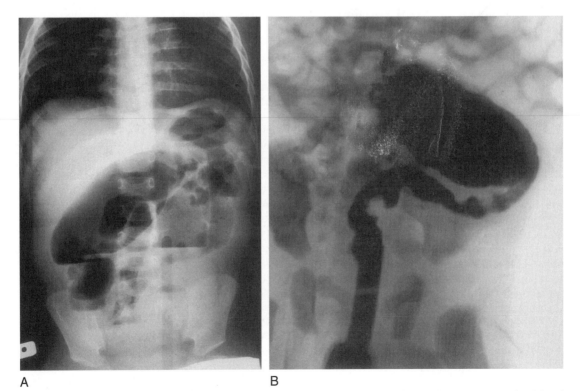

A   B

FIGURE 60-2 ■ **A,** Plain abdominal radiograph of an infant with rectosigmoid aganglionosis. Note the dilated bowel without a clear distinction between large and small bowel loops. **B,** Characteristic contrast enema in an infant with rectosigmoid aganglionosis. Note the typical saw-toothed pattern of the rectosigmoid.

and have a low threshold for performing a suction rectal biopsy.

The age at diagnosis varies widely, but approximately half of patients in the United States are diagnosed in the neonatal period, and most of the remainder are diagnosed before the age of 2. In older children or occasionally adults, Hirschsprung's disease is discovered during evaluation for chronic constipation. Symptoms range from minimal to severe, but chronic abdominal distention is characteristic. Malnutrition and failure to thrive may be seen in these patients, but this has become relatively uncommon in more recent years in the developed world.

DIFFERENTIAL DIAGNOSIS

The differential diagnosis of Hirschsprung's disease must include all the entities responsible for low mechanical intestinal obstruction of the distal small bowel or colon (Table 60-2). These entities are discussed in detail in their respective chapters.

DIAGNOSIS

When the clinical suspicion of Hirschsprung's disease has been raised, plain abdominal radiographs in the anteroposterior projection, as a cross-table lateral, or in left lateral decubitus position are obtained to look for evidence of intestinal obstruction or free intraperitoneal air or both. These studies can be followed by an unprepared barium enema or anorectal manometry and full-thickness or suction rectal biopsy. In Ehrenpreis' original work, he based the diagnosis on barium enema findings. Some workers have questioned the usefulness of the barium enema study in the newborn period because of the absence of a transition zone in many cases, but we find it useful. The diagnostic accuracy of a barium enema in the

first month of life as variously reported ranges from 21% to 96%. This study is essentially diagnostic if there is demonstration of a spasmodic distal intestinal segment with dilated proximal bowel. A suggestive finding is failure to evacuate barium from the colon within 24 hours of the performance of the study. Avoidance of passing anything into the anal opening increases the diagnostic accuracy of the procedure. Figure 60-2B shows a characteristic series of radiographs with the typical saw-toothed pattern of the rectosigmoid in a patient with standard Hirschsprung's disease.

Many investigators have continued to use anorectal manometry in establishing the definitive diagnosis of Hirschsprung's disease. This technique has the advantage of bedside performance and the immediate availability of results. The study is fairly noninvasive and can be performed in an outpatient setting. There have been no reported complications from this procedure. Hito and colleagues suggested that the test is unreliable only in cases in which the gestational age plus the age after birth is less than 39 weeks and the weight is less than 2.7 kg. Loening-Baucke reported that anorectal manometry is more difficult in newborns because of the sensitivity of the equipment and the ease of malposition of the balloons. In her study, there was only one false-negative diagnosis out of 21 studies performed, however, suggesting that manometry is useful in excluding the diagnosis of Hirschsprung's disease. Tamate studied 65 neonates, including several premature newborns, 60 of whom had normal manometric findings and subsequently were shown not to have Hirschsprung's disease by rectal biopsy. In the remaining five of these newborns, the diagnosis was confirmed by biopsy. There were no false-negative or false-positive results in this series, which was attributed to sophisticated equipment and the experience of the personnel. There have been several reports of the use of radiography and manometry.

Based on the observations by Robertson and Kernohan and Tiffen and colleagues of abnormalities in ganglion cell populations, Swenson established the full-thickness rectal biopsy as the standard for diagnosis in 1955, reporting a 98% accuracy rate in follow-up studies. This technique has several disadvantages, however, including the need for general anesthesia and the occasional report of postbiopsy rectal bleeding. Subsequently, detailed pathologic studies reported by Aldridge and Campbell led to the use of the suction rectal biopsy, which has several advantages, including simplicity, absence of need for anesthesia, performance at the bedside or outpatient setting, and absence of complications. Its widespread use has been supported by several studies that report an accuracy rate of 99.7% with no complications. An experienced pathologist can interpret the biopsy specimen easily and provide a report within 24 hours. Frozen section interpretation is possible, although it is much more difficult to read and is not recommended. Finally, in contrast to full-thickness rectal biopsy, the suction rectal biopsy does not interfere with the subsequent pull-through procedure. Histochemical techniques are helpful in making the diagnosis. The presence of increased AChE content in the nerve fibers of the lamina propria and muscularis mucosae in patients with Hirschsprung's

---

TABLE 60-2 ■ Differential Diagnosis of Hirschsprung's Disease

Mechanical Obstruction
Meconium ileus
  Simple
  Complicated (with meconium cyst or peritonitis)
Meconium plug syndrome
Neonatal small left colon syndrome
Malrotation with volvulus
Incarcerated hernia
Jejunoileal atresia
Colonic atresia
Intestinal duplication
Intussusception
NEC
Funtional Obstruction
Sepsis
Intracranial hemorrhage
Hypothyroidism
Maternal drug ingestion or addiction
Adrenal hemorrhage
Hypermagnesemia
Hypokalemia

disease is the basis of this test. Wakely and McAdams reported a 95% accuracy rate with this technique versus 85% with hematoxylin-eosin staining, but stressed that the diagnosis is not made on the presence or absence of AChE but on the pattern of nerve distribution. Barr and colleagues in 1985 reported on 101 suction rectal biopsy specimens stained for AChE with only 3 false-negative results. They also stressed the use of AChE only in biopsy specimens of the rectum and left side of the colon because there is no AChE activity proximal to the splenic flexure. Monoclonal antineurofilament antibodies and neuron-specific enolase also have been used to increase the accuracy of diagnosis, especially in newborns in whom ganglion cells may be sparse and immature. Occasionally the diagnosis of Hirschsprung's disease is made at exploratory laparotomy for intestinal obstruction, especially in patients with total colonic aganglionosis. If no clear-cut gross transition zone is seen, many surgeons perform an appendectomy with frozen section evaluation for ganglion cells. Further biopsy specimens are obtained either more proximally or more distally to establish the point of histologic transition. Anderson and Chandra reported on a single patient, however, who had aganglionosis of the appendix but ganglion cells in the ascending and right transverse colon, a rare happening. There were no ganglion cells in the distal colon. They also reviewed 46 appendices from patients with Hirschsprung's disease; all patients with total colonic aganglionosis had no ganglion cells in the appendix. All patients without Hirschsprung's disease and patients with sigmoid Hirschsprung's disease had ganglion cells in the appendix.

TREATMENT

The successful treatment of infants and children with Hirschsprung's disease depends on prompt diagnosis and early treatment. The decision to perform a primary pull-through when the diagnosis is established depends on the condition of the child and the response to initial treatment. A prompt decompression of the colon with a large-caliber soft tube should be performed, followed by serial washouts, leaving the catheter within the rectal vault. Broad-spectrum antibiotics are given, and hemodynamics are corrected with intravenous fluids and, on occasion, pressors. The safest approach to an unstable child is the performance of a leveling colostomy. A stable child with a milder enterocolitic episode can be decompressed over several days and subsequently undergo a definitive, primary pull-through. Infants with longer lengths of aganglionosis may not respond to washouts and require a colostomy on a more urgent basis.

In the past, a blind right transverse colostomy was the procedure of choice; presently a leveling colostomy at the transition zone is standard. The blind right transverse loop colostomy has the advantage of being faster to perform in that intraoperative frozen sections may not be required. Surgeons who favor the transverse colostomy leave it in place after the definitive procedure and close it at a third operation after recovery from the pull-through. The disadvantage of this approach is the need for three rather than two procedures.

We favor the use of a leveling colostomy or enterostomy. The colostomy is pulled through at the time of the definitive operation, and no back-up colostomy is performed. Operative mortality is almost nonexistent, aside from an infant with enterocolitis. The most common complications of colostomy are prolapse, occasional leaks when the colostomy is sutured to the fascia, and rare strictures.

Definitive Pull-Throughs

Historical Background

The first definitive operation was described by Swenson and Bill in 1948. This procedure involves resection of the aganglionic bowel and anastomosis of the distal rectum to ganglionated colon by a combined abdominoperineal approach. Essential to this operation is maintenance of the dissection immediately adjacent to the rectal wall to avoid injury to the pelvic nerves responsible for rectal and bladder innervation and sexual function. The results presented by Swenson in a 25-year follow-up are excellent. In this series, there were no cases of impotence or urinary incontinence, a 1.4% incidence of permanent colostomy or ileostomy, and a 3.2% incidence of permanent soiling. Of these patients, 90% experienced normal bowel habits. These results have not been consistently reproduced by surgeons with less experience, however.

Duhamel introduced the retrorectal pull-through technique in 1956. In this procedure, the pelvic dissection is limited to the retrorectal space, where dissection is carried down to the pectinate line entirely behind the rectum, avoiding potential injury to the pelvic nerves. Normally the innervated bowel is brought down posteriorly and anastomosed end-to-side to the remaining rectal stump. To minimize the pelvic dissection, however, a relatively long rectal stump is left, predisposing to formation of a retained septum. Grob and Martin and Altmeier introduced modifications to attempt to decrease the relatively high incontinence rate and to deal with the retained septum. The advantage of this procedure is that it is technically easy to perform and can be used in the case of a failed Swenson procedure.

The Soave or endorectal pull-through was introduced by Soave in 1960. Conceptually, this procedure consists of removing the mucosa and submucosa of the rectum and pulling ganglionic bowel through a short aganglionic muscular cuff. The initial procedure was done without a formal anastomosis, but the procedure was modified by Boley by performing a primary anastomosis at the anus, then further modified by Coran with the eversion of the submucosal/mucosal tube onto the perineum to facilitate the performance of the anastomosis. The procedure now is performed commonly as a primary pull-through in neonates without the need for an initial leveling colostomy. By remaining within the muscular cuff of the aganglionic segment, important sensory fibers and the integrity of the internal sphincter are preserved. Although leaving behind aganglionic muscle surrounding normal bowel conceptually might lead to a high incidence of constipation, this has not been the experience clinically. A schematic of the various types of pull-through procedures for Hirschsprung's disease is shown in Figure 60-3.

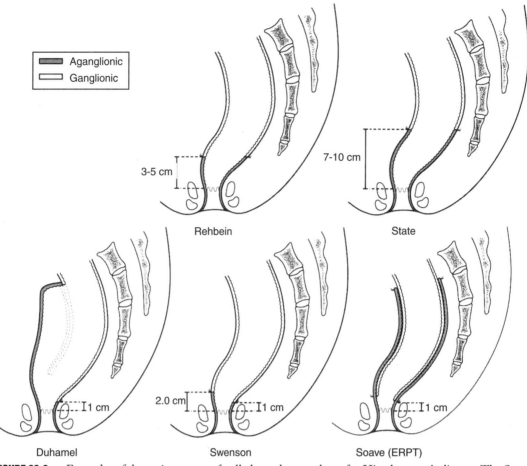

Aganglionic
Ganglionic

3-5 cm

Rehbein

7-10 cm

State

1 cm

Duhamel

2.0 cm   1 cm

Swenson

1 cm

Soave (ERPT)

FIGURE 60-3 ■ Examples of the various types of pull-through procedures for Hirschsprung's disease. The State procedure is shown only for historical purposes because it is no longer performed. The 1-cm length of bowel above the dentate line is shown only for reference because in young infants this distance may be 0.5 cm.

Primary Pull-Through for Hirschsprung's Disease

In 1980, So presented a 10-year experience with primary endorectal pull-through in neonates without the use of a preliminary colostomy. In two thirds of his patients, the definitive pull-through was performed by the fourth week of life with no deaths or major complications. A subsequent multi-institutional analysis of the primary pull-through showed it to be equally effective and safe compared with a two-stage approach in patients with a mean age of 7 days.

Preoperative Preparation

Surgical Preparation for Elective Two-Staged Repair

The patient is placed on a clear liquid diet at home 24 hours before the operation and is admitted to the hospital the day of surgery. Saline is used as an irrigant via the rectum and via the proximal and distal limbs of the colostomy to cleanse the colon. Some use 1% neomycin solution for the last irrigation. Intravenous broad-spectrum antibiotics are administered in the immediate perioperative period. Commonly the distal, aganglionic rectum has retained stool that never passed. This stool should be aggressively removed before surgery.

Surgical Preparation for a One-Stage Approach

In the newborn period, serial saline rectal washouts (10 mL/kg) and digital dilations of the rectum are performed before beginning the pull-through. The last of the rectal irrigations has 1% neomycin added to it. Intravenous antibiotics are given before the beginning of surgery and continued for 1 to 2 days after surgery.

Endorectal Pull-Through

Transabdominal Approach

The child is placed in a supine position, with the buttocks brought to the end of the operating table, and propped slightly up with a folded towel. The legs are padded carefully and placed on wooden skis extending off the end of the table. A Foley catheter is placed, and the entire field is prepared and draped. The operating table is placed in a slightly Trendelenburg position. A left lower quadrant oblique incision is made incorporating the leveling colostomy, if present. The level of aganglionosis is established with frozen section if a leveling colostomy is not present. Ganglionic bowel is mobilized proximally and is transected at the transition level with a stapling device. The distal colon is mobilized fully and resected to about 4 cm above the peritoneal reflection. Traction sutures are placed on either end of the distal bowel. The endorectal

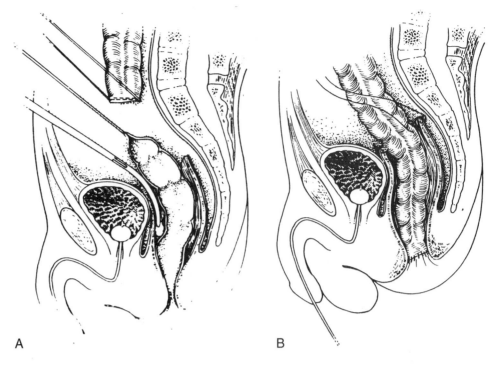

FIGURE 60-4 ■ Endorectal pull-through. **A,** The dissection is progressed distally using blunt dissection with a hemostat or a Kitner dissector. **B,** Anastomosis of endorectal pull-through.

A   B

dissection is started about 2 cm below the peritoneal reflection.

The endorectal dissection usually begins by completely clearing the serosa of mesentery and fat over a 2-cm length of bowel. The seromuscular layer is incised with either sharp dissection or cautery. When the submucosal layer is reached, the seromuscular layer is divided circumferentially. Dissection is progressed distally using blunt dissection with a hemostat or a Kitner dissector (Fig. 60-4A). In the newborn period, a cotton-tipped applicator is the most effective tool for this dissection.

After the dissection plane is established, it is continued distally and facilitated by an assistant pulling upward on the already dissected mucosal-submucosal tube for countertraction. As the muscular cuff begins to develop, traction sutures also are placed in the muscle, one in each quadrant. Larger communicating vessels are coagulated; however, most of these vessels are not cauterized during the dissection without incurring significant blood loss, particularly in the newborn period. Dissection is carried down to within 1.5 cm of the anal opening in older children and less than 1 cm in a newborn, all from the abdominal approach.

One of the operating surgeons then moves to the foot of the table. Narrow retractors (phrenic or Army-Navy) are placed at the anal-mucocutaneous junction, a ring or Kelly clamp is inserted into the rectum, and the mucosal/submucosal tube is everted. The mucosal/submucosal tube is incised on the anterior half, 1 cm above the dentate line (or 0.5 cm above the dentate line in the neonate). A Kelly clamp is inserted into this opening, and the ganglionic bowel is brought down to this point by grasping the two previously placed traction sutures. Great care is taken not to twist the bowel as it is brought through the muscular cuff.

The anterior half of the ganglionic colon is incised and is anastomosed to the anterior half of the anus

with 4-0 Vicryl suture. Following this, the posterior two quarters are sequentially anastomosed. Gloves are changed, and attention is directed to the abdominal field. The pulled-through colon is attached with seromuscular bites to the muscular cuff (Fig. 60-4B). This prevents the colon from prolapsing in the early postoperative period.

Duhamel Operation

Preoperative Preparation

The child usually has a leveling colostomy, which was placed several months previously. This colostomy decompresses the bowel and returns it to normal caliber. The operation generally is performed when the child is 6 to 12 months old with a weight of 10 kg (see Laparoscopic Approach later). More recently a primary Duhamel pull-through has been performed with good results.

Operative Technique

A hockey-stick or oblique incision is made incorporating the colostomy. The bowel is mobilized proximally to the former colostomy, and the proximal bowel is mobilized to ensure adequate length for the pull-through. In general, the colon must reach to the level of the perineum when drawn over the child's pubis with only modest tension. Occasionally the mesentery is foreshortened, and it is necessary to ligate the inferior mesenteric artery near the aortic root. By preserving the remainder of the arcades, the bowel should maintain its viability. The ureters are identified carefully, and the peritoneal reflection between the rectum and bladder is incised. The distal rectum is mobilized for approximately 4 cm below the reflection. The colostomy site is then removed. A retrorectal space is created, with dissection carried out directly in the posterior midline. This dissection is carried down to the pelvic floor so that an assistant's finger can be felt when inserted no further than 1 to 1.5 cm into the anus.

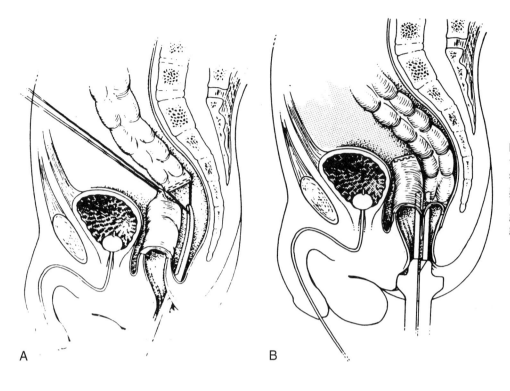

FIGURE 60-5 ■ Duhamel pull-through. **A,** Retrorectal dissection clears a space for the ganglionated bowel. **B,** Stapling between the anterior aganglionic segment and the ganglionic bowel posteriorly.

When the retrorectal dissection is done, redundant aganglionic bowel is resected to just above the peritoneal reflection with an automatic stapling device. Tacking sutures are placed on left and right sides of this bowel so that it can be retracted anteriorly during the pull-through. The ganglionic bowel is labeled mesenteric and antimesenteric to allow the surgeon working on the pulled-through segment to maintain correct orientation of the bowel. At this point, the surgeon's attention is directed to the perineum. Both legs are drawn upward allowing a clear view of the anus. Narrow anal retractors are placed and held in position by two assistants. Using cautery, a full-thickness incision is made 1 cm (less in a younger patient) proximal to the dentate line for 180 degrees posteriorly. Care is taken to maintain this distance by curving the incision as one moves laterally in each direction. One then enters the retrorectal space. Three 4-0 silk sutures are placed on the inferior aspect of this incision, one in the midline and one each on the left and right sides; needles are left on the sutures for eventual creation of an anastomosis. Sutures are directed from the mucosal side to the retrorectal space. This is done so that the suture needle can be directed later from the serosal surface of the ganglionic bowel, once it is pulled through. Three additional absorbable sutures are placed on the upper portion of this incision in similar positions. Each suture is held in position with hemostats. The different suture types prevent confusion of orientation when the ganglionic bowel is pulled through.

The surgeon operating on the anus inserts a long ring clamp into the retrorectal space and carefully pulls down the ganglionated bowel (Fig. 60-5A). The surgeon remaining in the abdominal field makes sure that the bowel does not rotate as it is brought down. When the bowel is pulled through, a single-layered anastomosis is created, starting with the previously placed sutures. An extra long automatic stapling device (80 to 90 mm, with 4.8-mm staples) is placed with one arm in the native anal canal and the other in the neorectum. The stapler is fired directly in the midline. Hemostasis along the suture line is checked. The operation from below is completed at this point (Fig. 60-5B).

Typically a complete anastomosis between the ganglionic and aganglionic bowel requires a second firing from the abdomen via a colotomy. The surgeon must palpate to ensure no remaining spur is left between the two bowel segments. The anastomosis is completed by suturing the proximal end of the rectum to the enterostomy in the ganglionic colon in two layers. The neorectum is reperitonealized to prevent internal herniation of the bowel, and the abdomen is closed.

Laparoscopic Approach to Hirschsprung's Disease

The use of advanced laparoscopic techniques for Hirschsprung's disease has been advanced by Georgeson and others. This approach and the pure perineal method have gained wide use in the pediatric surgical community.

Laparoscopic Endorectal Pull-Through

After bowel preparation, smaller children and infants are positioned transversely at the end of the operating table, and older children are positioned in stirrups in the lithotomy position. The first trocar is placed in the right upper quadrant. Two more trocars are placed in the right and left lower quadrants, and a fourth trocar is placed in the suprapubic position for placing traction on the colon (Fig. 60-6A). The level of the transition zone is determined first by obtaining seromuscular biopsy specimens with a fine grasper and scissors.

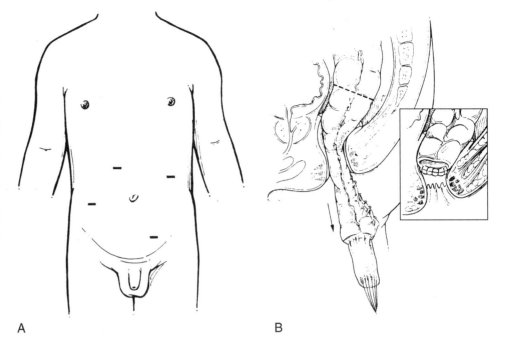

FIGURE 60-6 ■ Laparoscopic endorectal pull-through. **A,** Shows placement of trocars if a laparoscopic portion is used. **B,** Transanal approach for an endorectal dissection. (From Georgeson KE, Cohen RD, Hebra A, et al: Primary laparoscopic-assisted endorectal colon pull-through for Hirschsprung's disease: A new gold standard. Ann Surg 229:678-682, 1999.)

A

B

Dissection is begun by establishing a plane at the rectosigmoid junction 5 to 10 cm above the peritoneal reflection adjacent to the colon. Mesenteric vessels are divided proximal to the level of the transition zone using an ultrasonic scalpel, electrocautery, or clips. The inferior mesenteric artery also can be divided below the level of the vascular arcades to gain length for the pull-through. Adequate mobility of the colon pedicle can be determined by grasping the colon 10 to 20 cm above the transition zone and pushing this portion of colon deep into the pelvis. After the proximal dissection is complete, attention is directed to the rectum, which is circumferentially dissected to the level of the prostate or cervix anteriorly and the coccyx posteriorly.

A mucosal incision is made 0.5 cm above the dentate line transanally with electrocautery. When the plane between the submucosa and muscularis is identified, multiple fine sutures are placed in the proximal mucosal sleeve for traction. The proctectomy is continued in the submucosal plane using fine scissors, cautery, and blunt dissection. When the level of the intracorporeal dissection is reached, the rectum begins to prolapse through the anus. A marked decrease in bleeding in the submucosal plane also is noted. These features identify the level of the intracorporeal dissection. The muscular wall is divided circumferentially at this level, and the colon is pulled through the rectal cuff. The cuff is split posteriorly to provide room for a neorectal reservoir. The rectum is amputated approximately several centimeters above the transition zone, and an anastomosis is performed with absorbable sutures (Fig. 60-6B).

Laparoscopic Duhamel Pull-Through

A Duhamel pull-through is performed on patients with a right colon transition zone or total colonic aganglionosis. The trocars are placed as for the endorectal pull-through. Attention first is directed to determining the transition zone. Biopsy specimens are obtained as previously

described just above the suspected transition zone. If necessary, the appendix may be removed to establish the diagnosis of total colonic aganglionosis. The gastrocolic ligament is divided using electrocautery or an ultrasonic scalpel. The mesentery is divided to the transition zone.

The presacral space is dissected using a hook cautery and blunt dissection. The bowel is divided with an endoscopic stapler, leaving a rectal stump length of 5 to 10 cm. One or two graspers are wedged deep in the pelvis, and a transanal incision is made in the posterior rectum 1 cm above the dentate line onto the wedged graspers. The bowel is brought down through the presacral space, through the defect in the posterior rectal wall and through the anus. The bowel is amputated 10 to 20 cm above the transition zone. An anastomosis of the neorectum to the anorectal mucosa is performed transanally with interrupted, absorbable sutures. The endoscopic stapler is inserted from below to obliterate the septum between the rectum and ganglionated bowel.

Transanal One-Stage Endorectal Pull-Through

Transanal one-stage endorectal pull-through originally was described by Mondragon and has been advanced by Langer. Essentially the approach is similar to the laparoscopic endorectal pull-through except that it relies on the mobilization of the rectum via the perineum. Because of the relative limitation on the length of bowel that can be mobilized, this approach is best reserved for rectosigmoid disease.

Exposure can be facilitated by either many retraction sutures or the placement of an anal retractor (Lone Star Medical Products, Houston, TX). The rectal mucosa is circumferentially incised using cautery, approximately 0.5 cm from the dentate line, and a submucosal plane is developed. The proximal cut edge of the mucosal cuff is tagged with multiple fine sutures, which are used for traction. The endorectal dissection is carried proximally, staying in the submucosal plane until the free peritoneal cavity is reached (similar to Fig. 60-5B). The posterior muscular wall is incised in a linear fashion down to the internal sphincter, and the full thickness of the bowel is pulled down. At this point, the mesenteric vessels are ligated under direct vision. The repair is completed in a similar fashion to the above-described laparoscopic approach.

INTESTINAL NEURONAL DYSPLASIA

Intestinal neuronal dysplasia (IND) initially was described by Meier-Ruge in 1971. This disorder was classified as a colonic dysplasia, although the disease can involve any portion of the gastrointestinal tract. IND has a varied histologic appearance with hyperplasia of the enteric ganglia, and increased AChE staining is characteristic (Fig. 60-7). Two basic forms of the disease have been described. Type A IND is characterized by (1) absent or hypoplastic sympathetic innervation of the myenteric and submucosal plexuses; (2) moderately increased parasympathetic nerve fibers in the lamina propria, muscularis mucosae, and circular muscle; (3) hyperplasia of the myenteric plexus; and sometimes (4) inflammatory changes in the colonic mucosa. In type B IND, the following histologic features are noted: (1) dysplasia of the submucosal plexus with giant ganglia and thickened nerve fibers, (2) increased AChE staining, and occasionally (3) isolated ganglion cells in the lamina propria. Type B IND is seen much more commonly than type A, and symptoms in type B are milder. The typical presentation of IND is variable. Children with type A present at a younger age than children with type B. Most children have complaints of abdominal distention. Some have constipation and develop enterocolitis. The extent of IND may range from a short colonic segment to the entire length of the gastrointestinal tract. In contrast to Hirschsprung's disease, the internal sphincter relaxation reflex is absent or atypical in only 75% of patients

with IND. The association of IND and Hirschsprung's disease also has been noted by some authors. The incidence ranges from 0 to 75% in reported series. Because the symptoms of Hirschsprung's disease may mask those of IND, the diagnosis often is not made until the patient develops stooling problems after a definitive pull-through.

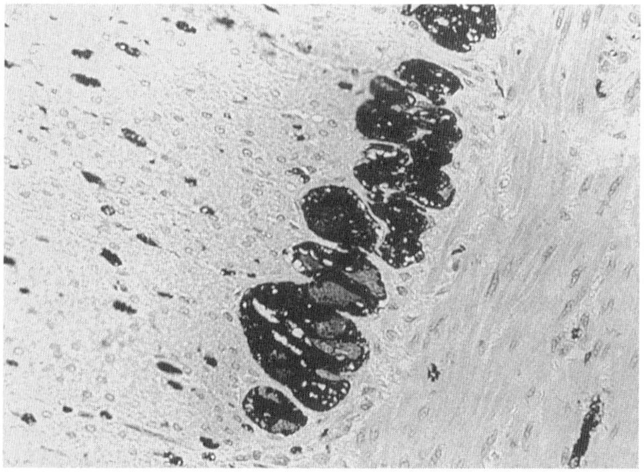

The significance of IND, as seen on pathologic examination, was evaluated by Koletzko and colleagues, who examined the pathology and manometric findings of 57 children with constipation. In this study, the finding of IND histologically correlated poorly with the severity of the constipation, colonic transit time, and manometric studies. Based on these findings, the authors advised placing little emphasis on the histologic findings of IND and suggested that one should rely predominately on the clinical presentation of constipation for planning any subsequent surgical intervention. This underscores an important point about IND; the precise criteria for the diagnosis are lacking. This lack of rigid criteria most likely explains the variability in the incidence of this disorder. This problem also was shown by Schofield's review of 498 suction rectal biopsy specimens from 456 children. IND was found in 38 biopsy specimens from 38 patients who showed mild-to-moderate increases in AChE staining and abundant submucosal ganglia (≥5 per high-power field). Despite the histologic diagnosis, these 38 patients represented a heterogeneous population, including those with prematurity, small left colon syndrome, and meconium plug syndrome. Several other causes, including gastroschisis and protein-sensitive enteropathy, were identified. Virtually all of these children had a benign clinical course with few residual gastrointestinal complaints. Caution should be observed when making the diagnosis of IND, and a conservative approach to surgery for this disorder should be used.

VARIANTS OF HIRSCHSPRUNG'S DISEASE

Enterocolitis

Enterocolitis of Hirschsprung's disease remains the major cause of significant morbidity and mortality today. The entity is manifested clinically by explosive diarrhea, abdominal distention, and fever. Pathologically, enterocolitis is defined as an acute inflammatory infiltrate into the crypts and mucosa of either the colonic or the small intestinal epithelium. As the disease progresses, the mucosal epithelium becomes ulcerated, and the lumen of the intestine becomes filled with fibrinopurulent debris. If the process is left to proceed unabated, perforation of the intestine may occur.

The pathophysiology of the enterocolitis of Hirschsprung's disease has not been elucidated fully; however, based on experimental and clinical studies, several contributory factors have been identified: intestinal stasis with bacterial invasion of the luminal wall, decrease in intestinal defense mechanisms, and abnormal mucins. Patients with trisomy 21 are known to have an increased risk for developing enterocolitis. The diagnosis of enterocolitis is made on the basis of a clinical history

FIGURE 60-7 ■ Enteric ganglia showing increased acetylcholinesterase staining consistent with intestinal neuronal dysplasia.

of diarrhea with distention (69%), vomiting (51%), fever (34%), and often lethargy (27%). Along with the history and physical examination, the finding of an "intestinal cutoff sign" on abdominal x-rays has a high degree of sensitivity (74%) and specificity (86%) for enterocolitis. Most commonly, enterocolitis presents in the post-pull-through period. This form of enterocolitis may be due to an excessively tight pull-through or may be related to spasm of the internal anal sphincter.

The treatment of Hirschsprung's disease–associated enterocolitis begins with a series of aggressive washouts using a large-caliber rectal tube to decompress the colon above the anal sphincter. Enemas alone are ineffective because they do not allow for adequate decompression of the colon. These serial washouts should be accompanied by either intravenous antibiotics or oral metronidazole. Recurrences of enterocolitis are common and may be due to mucosal changes that occurred early in the life of the child. Mild cases of enterocolitis may be treated with oral metronidazole.

Hirschsprung's Disease in the Older or Adult Patient

Rarely, Hirschsprung's disease may present in the adolescent or adult. Over a 10-year period, two adolescents and one adult were found at our institution with a diagnosis of Hirschsprung's disease (3% of all patients). In general, these patients have adapted to their disease by a compensatory dilation of their proximal bowel and through the regular use of cathartics and enemas. In general, complication rates with most procedures on adults and adolescents seem to be higher than in children. Often a primary pull-through without colostomy cannot be performed because of the markedly dilated nature of the colon. Although some have advocated the performance of a posterior anorectal myectomy, we would advocate a standard pull-through, unless the patient has an ultra-short segment. The Duhamel procedure is usually the easiest to perform in this sort of patient, although some prefer the Swenson procedure.

Ultra-Short Hirschsprung's Disease

The term *ultra-short Hirschsprung's disease* has prompted a great deal of confusion among clinicians. This confusion relates to the diagnosis, treatment, and even the occurrence of this entity. The major problem with ultra-short Hirschsprung's disease is the fact that the gold standard for making the diagnosis of standard Hirschsprung's disease—the rectal biopsy—may show ganglion cells. Many of these children not only have chronic constipation, often for many years, but also fecal soiling, which makes its differentiation from encopresis difficult. In general, ultra-short Hirschsprung's disease consists of a 2- to 4-cm distal segment of aganglionosis. A contrast enema may not show a transition zone. Finally, despite these negative findings, manometry shows a failure of anorectal reflex relaxation with rectal distention. It is possible that several children with this entity may be overlooked because many centers do not perform anorectal manometry routinely. The preferred treatment of a definitive case of ultra-short segment Hirschsprung's disease is an anorectal myectomy, provided that one has

confirmed ganglion cells from a prior biopsy specimen at 4 cm or more above the dentate line.

Long Segment and Total Colonic Hirschsprung's Disease

Long segment disease represents a significant proportion of cases of Hirschsprung's disease diagnosed in newborns, representing 22% of neonates in a series reported by Fraser and Wilkinson, 26% by Bowring and Kern, and 37% by Polley and colleagues. The mortality in this group of infants is also generally higher and probably is related to the increased incidence of enterocolitis present at the time of diagnosis. The enterocolitis rate in the entire series reported by Kleinhaus was 14% in patients with standard rectosigmoid disease versus 25% in patients with long segment disease. Delay in diagnosis, which is more common in long segment disease, leads to an increased incidence of enterocolitis and a resultant increased mortality.

Total colonic aganglionosis accounts for approximately 3% to 12% of infants with Hirschsprung's disease. These patients comprise a unique subset of patients because of the associated increased morbidity and mortality. The diagnosis of total colonic aganglionosis can be difficult. Radiographic studies may show dilated loops of bowel, and a contrast enema may show a question mark–shaped colon owing to rounded edges of the splenic and hepatic flexures (Fig. 60-8). Radiographic studies are diagnostic, however, in only 20% to 30% of all patients with total colonic aganglionosis. The diagnosis generally is made at the time of an exploratory laparotomy for a suspected bowel obstruction or for a leveling colostomy for Hirschsprung's disease. A frozen section of the appendix is almost always diagnostic and significantly reduces

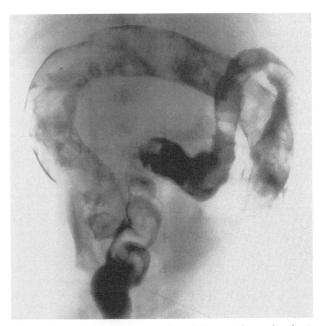

FIGURE 60-8 ■ Barium enema of an infant with total colonic aganglionosis. Note the characteristic rounding of the hepatic and splenic flexures, creating what is often termed the "question mark" sign.

operative time. A family history of Hirschsprung's disease can be found in many of these children (12.4% to 33%). The male-to-female ratio also is decreased and approximates almost an equal proportion of males and females. In one series, the proximal extent of aganglionosis was the terminal ileum in 76%, mid ileum in 19%, and jejunum in 5%. Complications associated with total colonic aganglionosis are numerous and considerably higher than for standard length Hirschsprung's disease. Many infants with total colonic Hirschsprung's disease require parenteral nutrition, making catheter sepsis, failure to thrive, stomal dysfunction, electrolyte imbalance, and dehydration commonly encountered complications. Mortality ranges from 0 to 44% depending on the series of patients, which emphasizes the severity of this variant of Hirschsprung's disease. Conventional treatment for total colonic aganglionosis begins with the creation of a properly formed enterostomy. More recently, we have been successful in managing a few of these patients with a primary pull-through. Fluids and electrolytes are monitored closely. In general, the performance of a pull-through procedure should be withheld until the child is toilet trained because excoriation of the perineum can be severe in this disease. Although this approach is the most commonly used, we have performed endorectal pull-throughs on three newborns with comparable continence and stooling frequency to those seen in older children with total colonic Hirschsprung's disease undergoing a pull-through. Several operative approaches can be considered. In general, however, as Hoehner and colleagues have shown, a standard-length Duhamel or endorectal pull-through yields the best results compared with other methods, including the Martin (extended) Duhamel technique.

CONCLUSION

Hirschsprung's disease is an important part of the differential diagnosis of intestinal obstruction in newborns. The increased rate of diagnosis in the newborn period is the result of improvements in diagnostic techniques, including suction rectal biopsy, expertise in pathologic interpretation, increased experience with barium enema study interpretation, addition of histochemical and immunohistochemical analyses, and increased physician awareness. This increasing awareness has led to a shift in the average age of diagnosis from childhood to the newborn and infant age group. Most importantly, this increased awareness has led to prompt institution of appropriate resuscitation and treatment, resulting in a decrease in mortality. Finally, refinements in surgical technique and preoperative and postoperative care have reduced mortality and morbidity greatly and have improved significantly the long-term outcome for these patients.

SUGGESTED READINGS

Georgeson KE, Cohen RD, Hebra A, et al: Primary laparoscopic-assisted endorectal colon pull-through for Hirschsprung's disease: A new gold standard. Ann Surg 229:678-682, 1999.

This article is a definitive review of laparoscopic-assisted pull-through from several institutions.

Kleinhaus S, Boley SJ, Sheran M, et al: Hirschsprung's disease: A survey of the members of the Surgical Section of the American Academy of Pediatrics. J Pediatr Surg 14:588, 1979.

This is an important review of various operations for Hirschsprung's disease.

Langer JC, Minkes RK, Mazziotti MV, et al: Transanal one-stage Soave procedure for infants with Hirschsprung's disease. J Pediatr Surg 34:148-151, 1999.

This is an excellent review of the one-stage transanal approach for Hirschsprung's disease.

Polley TZ Jr, Coran AG: Hirschsprung's disease in the newborn: An eleven year experience. Pediatr Surg Int 1:80, 1986.

This represents a large experience with the surgical management of newborns with Hirschsprung's disease.

Swenson O: Hirschsprung's disease: A review. Pediatrics 109:914-918, 2002.

Swenson O, Sherman JO, Fisher JH, et al: The treatment and postoperative complications of congenital megacolon: A twenty-five year follow-up. Ann Surg 182:266, 1985.

Classic reviews of Swenson's lifetime experience with Hirschsprung's disease are presented.

Teitelbaum DH, Cilley R, Sherman NJ, et al: A decade experience with the primary pull-through for Hirschsprung's disease in the newborn period: A multi-center analysis of outcomes. Ann Surg 232:372-380, 2000.

This is a review of the outcome of primary pull-throughs for Hirschsprung's disease from several institutions compared with a staged repair.

Wartiovaara K, Salo M, Sariola H: Hirschsprung's disease genes and the development of the enteric nervous system. Ann Med 30:66-74, 1998.

This article presents a good review of some of the genetic aberrations in Hirschsprung's disease and a conceptual picture of how each of these genes may interact with each other.

61

Anorectal Disorders and Imperforate Anus

EMBRYOLOGY OF THE ANUS AND RECTUM

A series of developmental steps are involved in the formation of the normal anatomy of the lower end of the anus, rectum, and genitourinary (GU) tract. By the fourth week of embryologic development, the cloaca and the cloacal membrane are present (Figs. 61-1 and 61-2A). This membrane separates the internal from the external portions of the cloaca. At this stage, the internal portion of the cloaca receives the allantois, the wolffian ducts, and the portion of the hindgut that becomes the rectum. Between the fourth and sixth weeks of development, the upper part of the cloaca begins to be divided by the urorectal septum, growing caudally from above. The descent of the urorectal septum is associated with simultaneous

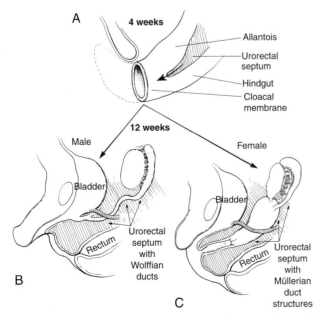

FIGURE 61-1 ■ **A,** Early anorectal development from the cloacal stage; **B,** at approximately 4 weeks' gestation to full separation of the hindgut and the genitourinary tract in the male; **C,** at 12 weeks' gestation in the female.

lateral ingrowths that result in an anterior chamber receiving the allantois and the wolffian ducts and a posterior chamber receiving the rectum. Failure of the cloacal membrane to develop posteriorly results in the development of an anteriorly placed hindgut opening (Fig. 61-2B). The extent of the failure of development of the posterior aspect of the cloacal membrane determines the degree of misplacement of the fistula: A mild failure results in a perineal fistula, whereas a severe developmental failure results in a rectourethral or even a rectovesical fistula in boys and a rectovaginal fistula in girls. Failure of development of the anterior and posterior cloacal membranes may result in the formation of a cloaca with a common hindgut and urogenital opening (Fig. 61-2C).

During the time that the previously mentioned events are occurring, at the level of the perineum, mesodermal tissue develops on the surface, resulting in the formation of a genital tubercle, genital folds, and an anal tubercle in the region of the external cloaca. By the sixth week of development, the cloacal membrane gradually atrophies, permitting the future GU tract and rectum to empty into the external cloaca. Between 6 and 10 weeks' gestation, the urorectal septum, now representing a uroanal septum, gradually grows caudally into the external cloaca, and at the same time, there is inward migration of the genital folds on either side, gradually fusing to form the perineum, separating the genitourinary and anal canals. The anal orifice develops as a separate structure by the ringlike fusion of the right and left anal tubercles around the anal orifice. Patency of the anal canal usually is established by 7 or 8 weeks' gestation followed by a secondary occlusion resulting from adhesion of the anorectal walls followed later by recanalization secondary to apoptotic cell death. Failure of recanalization of the secondarily occluded anal canal results in a normally located imperforate anal membrane, such as that observed with a membranous covering, or a bucket-handle deformity. Between this point and 10 to 12 weeks' gestation, there is continued elongation of the urethra and anal canals, but the external genitalia are not yet developed. By 14 to 16 weeks' gestation, male and female differentiation becomes evident.

The various anorectal anomalies appear to depend on the degree of failure of development of the cloacal

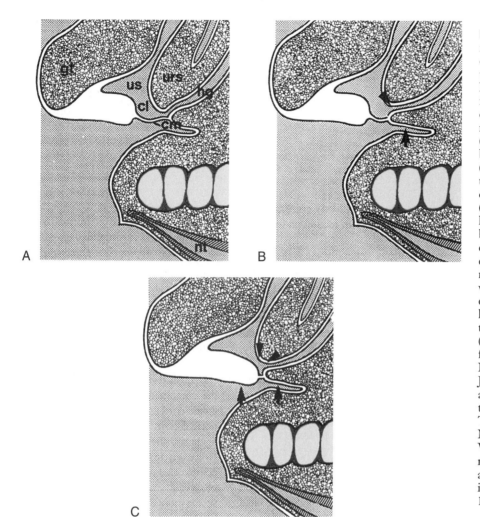

FIGURE 61-2 ▪ Sagittal schematic representations of the caudal region of the human embryo just before rupture of the cloacal membrane. **A,** Normal situation. **B,** Anorectal malformation with anterior ectopic anal orifice. The dorsal part of the cloacal membrane and cloaca are absent (arrow), and the hindgut opening becomes more anteriorly located (arrowhead). **C,** Cloacal malformation. The dorsal and the ventral part of the cloacal membrane are absent (arrows), and as a consequence, the hindgut and urogenital opening become more anteriorly and posteriorly located (arrowheads). Only the central part of the cloaca and cloacal membrane persists, which coincides with the common cavity and channel. cl, cloaca; gt, genital tubercle; hg, hindgut; nt, neural tube; urs, urorectal septum; us, urogenital sinus. (Reprinted, in part, with permission from John Wiley Sons. From Nievelstein RAJ, Van Der Werff JFA, Verbeek FJ, et al: Normal and abnormal embryonic development of the anorectum in human embryos. Teratology 57:70-78, 1998; in Nievelstein RAJ, Vos A, Valk J, Verjeig-Keers Chr. Magnetic resonance imaging in children with anorectal malformations: Embryologic implications. J Pediatr Surg 37:1138-1145, 2002.)

membrane or of recanalization of the secondarily closed anal canal.

NORMAL ANORECTAL ANATOMY AND FUNCTION

Continence is related to normal function of the sphincters surrounding the anus and rectum and the degree to which they are present and appropriately innervated. Development of the sacrum occurs at around the same time as development of the anus, rectum, and sphincters. This is an important consideration because the S2 to S4 nerve roots supply the muscle sphincters. Figure 61-3 shows normal sphincter anatomy. Each of the major components of the anal canal is considered subsequently.

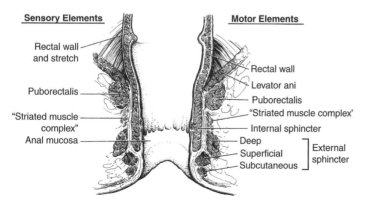

FIGURE 61-3 ▪ Demonstration of the many crucial components of the anatomy of the anorectal canal and their contributions to sensory and motor function. The function of these structures is highly coordinated.

Lining of the Anorectal Canal

The epithelial lining of the anal canal stops at the pectinate or dentate line, which separates the skin of the anus from the mucosa of the rectum. Distal or external to the pectinate line, the epithelium changes from stratified columnar epithelium to stratified squamous epithelium, below which sebaceous glands and hair follicles appear. The stratified columnar epithelium lining the zone of the anal columns contains sensory receptors important for continence. At the pectinate line, anal crypts and papillae are present within the columns of Morgagni, which secrete mucus and appear to be responsible for the development of perirectal abscesses and fistula-in-ano. Internal hemorrhoids exist above the pectinate line, whereas external hemorrhoids present below the area of the pectinate line. Procedures internal to the pectinate line are not painful because there is only visceral sensation, whereas procedures external to the pectinate line are accompanied by the pain typically associated with skin sensation.

Muscle Sphincters

The specialized sphincters that surround the anus and the rectum have voluntary and involuntary components. Three levels of muscles exist: the external sphincter, internal sphincter, and levator complex.

External Sphincter

The external sphincter consists of voluntary striated muscle that completely surrounds the anus from the anal orifice to the anal papillae. The external sphincter is attached anteriorly to the perineal body and posteriorly

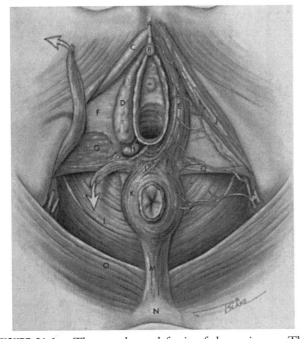

FIGURE 61-4 ■ The muscles and fascia of the perineum. The following are related to anorectal physiology: I, perineal body; K, external anal sphincter; L, levator ani muscle; M, anococcygeal body; N, coccyx. (From Hamond CB: Gynecology: The female reproductive organs. In Townsend E [ed]: Sabiston Textbook of Surgery, 16th ed. Philadelphia, WB Saunders, 2001.)

to the anococcygeal body (Fig. 61-4). The subcutaneous portion of the external sphincter is attached to the skin of the anus. The external sphincter is differentiated further into superficial and deep portions moving inward. The deep portion, which ends at about the level of the pectinate line, blends in with the so-called striated muscle complex, which fuses with the lowermost portion of the levator ani, often referred to as the *puborectalis sling*. The external sphincter muscles also contain sensory receptors and are innervated via the inferior rectal nerve and a perineal branch of the fourth sacral nerve. The mucosa of the anal canal is sensitive to differentiating solids, gas, and liquids, and in response, the external sphincter is responsible for preventing the passage of solid and liquid stool and gas. One of the major functions of the external sphincter is to maintain continence by increasing tone in response to rectal distention and internal sphincter relaxation. The external sphincter also prevents incontinence when increased intrarectal pressure results in what otherwise would be imminent defecation.

Internal Sphincter

The circular smooth muscle intrinsic to the rectum becomes thicker just below the dentate line, forming the internal sphincter. The internal sphincter is joined by the fibers of the levator ani to form the conjoined longitudinal muscle, which extends down to and joins the external sphincter muscle. The internal sphincter is bound closely to the external sphincter and attached to the skin by muscular strands, ensuring that the activity of the internal and external sphincters relative to opening and closing of the anal canal is coordinated. Sensory receptors also exist in the internal sphincter muscle to enable this coordination.

Levator Ani

Although arbitrary, the striated muscle of the levator ani is divided into the ileococcygeus, pubococcygeus, and puborectalis portions. The puborectalis is the portion most closely associated with the rectum, and it contains the largest number of sensory receptors of the levator ani complex. The fibers of the levator ani blend into the internal and external sphincters so that its activity is coordinated closely with their function. The various portions of the levator ani muscle are shaped like a cone surrounding the anus and rectum and tend to pull the rectum forward, increasing the angle between the longitudinal axis of the rectum and the anal canal. This rectoanal angle helps to maintain continence by preventing formed stool from entering the anal canal. Anteriorly the levator ani is firmly fixed and blends into the sphincters of the urethra and vagina, the puborectalis, and the pubovaginalis muscles. The levator ani muscles are supplied by the fourth sacral nerve and the inferior rectal or perineal branches of the pudendal nerves.

Innervation of the Anus, Rectum, and Their Sphincters

Sacral segments S2 to S4 constitute the sensory receptor–motor effector arc for the anus and rectum, urethra, bladder, and vagina, including the various components of the levator ani complex. As a general rule, if a sacral segment is missing, its corresponding nerve root is likely absent also. Although the external sphincter is innervated primarily through S4, its function can be coordinated appropriately with the other sphincters only if S2 to S4 are functional. Different degrees of sacral agenesis result in varying levels of defective innervation of the anus and rectum. The S2 to S4 segments also serve as the cutaneous sensory receptors of the anus and perianal areas. The anoderm and perianal skin are extremely sensitive to pain, touch, cold, pressure, tension, and friction distal to the dentate line and to a point 0.5 to 1.5 cm cephalad to this level. Evidence suggests that similar sensory receptors are located in the puborectalis and surrounding pelvic musculature. These receptors are able to distinguish between contents that are solid, liquid, and gas.

The sympathetic and parasympathetic nerves of the anus and rectum pass through Auerbach's and Meissner's plexus and ganglia and coordinate peristalsis and tone in the internal sphincter. The sympathetic nerve supply is inhibitory to the musculature of the rectum and stimulatory to the internal sphincter and tends to promote continence. In contrast, the parasympathetic nerve supply stimulates the musculature of the rectum and inhibits the internal sphincter, enhancing defecation. The sympathetic nerves pass through the L2 to L4 ganglia, whereas the parasympathetic nerves arise from S2 to S4. The anal canal and the rectum above the dentate line are mostly insensitive to pain but are sensitive to distention.

Fecal continence is possible only when the sensory afferent impulses from the anal mucosa, the rectal wall, and the coordinated sphincter muscles are received and integrated within the brain and enabled by motor efferent fibers to the various sphincter muscles. The receptors in the rectum primarily appreciate distention and can sense a balloon in the rectum as small as 10 mL. As the

rectum fills, the rectoanal inhibitory reflex results in relaxation of the internal sphincter. The degree of relaxation is proportional to the volume in the rectum. As the rectum distends, however, pressure in the distal and canal is increased via simultaneous external anal sphincter contraction, maintaining continence. As the internal sphincter relaxes, rectal contents are allowed to come into contact with the anal canal, where the sensory nerve endings are capable of distinguishing between solids, liquids, and gas. The contents of the rectum can be recognized and a conscious determination made of whether to let those contents through. Gas may be passed, relieving the rectal distention. The rectoanal inhibitory reflex is followed by an accommodation response, which consists of relaxation of the rectum to accommodate the fecal mass.

Under normal circumstances, the anal canal is closed by the resting tone of the internal and external sphincters and the lower portion of the levator ani. The puborectalis muscle provides a sling-like effect around the anal canal, drawing it forward and creating an 80-degree to 90-degree angle between the rectum and anal canal, preventing solid feces from entering the anal canal (Fig. 61-5). Under these circumstances, increased abdominal pressure accentuates this angle, further preventing defecation. Between the sphincters and the levator ani, a high-pressure zone is created in the anal canal at rest (average 25 to 120 mm Hg) compared with the pressure in the rectum (average 5 to 20 mm Hg). When defecation is to occur, the individual squats, which decreases the rectoanal angle, and a reflex ensues in which the Valsalva maneuver increases abdominal pressure and causes the pelvic floor to descend as the puborectalis, external sphincter, and internal sphincter relax. The feces are evacuated followed by return of the levator and sphincter muscles to baseline tone.

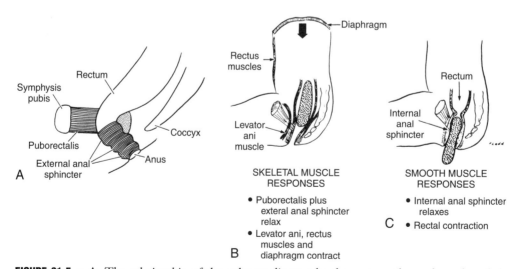

FIGURE 61-5 ■ **A,** The relationship of the puborectalis muscle, the rectum, the anal canal, and the external sphincter. Note the approximately 90 degree orientation between the rectum and the anal canal, which contributes to fecal continence. **B and C,** During defecation, squatting along with relaxation of the puborectalis straightens out the anorectal angle, which, along with performance of the Valsalva maneuver and relaxation of the sphincter muscles, allows evacuation of the fecal bolus from the rectum. (From Schiller LR: Fecal incontinence. In Feldman M [ed]: Sleisenger and Fordtran's Gastrointestinal and Liver Disease, 6th ed. Philadelphia, WB Saunders, 1998, pp 160-171.)

FECAL INCONTINENCE

Fecal incontinence is associated with three major causes: congenital anomalies, mental retardation, and childhood encopresis with constipation. The most common congenital anomaly resulting in fecal incontinence is myelomeningocele. Other disorders of the spinal cord resulting in neural deficiency, such as tethered cord and lipomeningocele, also may result in fecal incontinence. In the same fashion, deficiencies of pelvic musculature and innervation related to high forms of anorectal atresia may result in incontinence. Varying degrees of incontinence result, depending on the number of sacral segments missing or deformed. In general terms, absence or deficiencies of S4 and S5 usually are associated with normal innervation of the bladder and anorectal muscles. Patients missing three sacral segments have variable innervation and muscle development, but most are incontinent. Patients with deficiencies of four or all five sacral segments are all incontinent because of inadequate development of the levator and sphincters and absence of crucial innervation.

Fecal incontinence also may be acquired after trauma to the sacrum and spinal cord or destruction of the anal sphincters by a systemic disease, such as Crohn's disease, severe proctitis, or extensive anorectal infection. Incontinence also may result from inappropriate anorectal reconstruction for imperforate anus, Hirschsprung's disease, and ulcerative colitis.

Children who are neurologically handicapped have varying degrees of incontinence, mostly dependent on the degree of impairment. The most common form of acquired fecal incontinence is associated with chronic constipation, however, whereby liquid feces are evacuated around a large obstructing stool plug in the rectum. This is called *encopresis* and generally occurs in patients older than age 2 years. For a variety of reasons, most commonly associated with problematic toilet training or painful defecation, such children contract the anal canal during defecation. The result is retention of feces, which induces rectal distention, reflex anal relaxation, and soiling.

Diagnosis

History and physical findings often are all that are needed to make a diagnosis. If a child previously had normal bowel movements and now presents with intermittent incontinence, it is usually psychologically based. A history of congenital anomalies, perirectal disease and operations, neurologic impairment, and trauma should be elicited. The physical examination should begin with abdominal palpation for evidence of a mass or feces. Stroking of the perianal skin should elicit an anal wink. Absence of this reflex suggests a problem with the peripheral sensory or motor nerves or the reflex arc. Rectal examination can be used to evaluate for the presence of large amounts of stool, which suggests the presence of encopresis. The strength of the anal sphincter should be assessed at baseline and with the patient voluntarily squeezing. One should palpate all areas of the sphincter during this maneuver to identify focal areas of weakness. The puborectalis muscle can be palpated posteriorly and laterally. The examiner should push posteriorly against the puborectalis to assess for laxity. The examining finger should be pushed forward by the puborectalis muscle when the patient is asked to prevent fecal passage.

Patients who have a lax anus, decreased perianal sensation, absence of the external sphincter reflex (anal wink), and urinary incontinence likely have either a congenital or an acquired neural deficiency. These findings may be associated with anorectal malformations. Sacral spine films should be obtained to evaluate for anomalies and ultrasound or magnetic resonance imaging (MRI) to evaluate for a tethered cord. MRI also allows evaluation of the levator and sphincter complex, especially the position of the anus relative to these structures after an anorectal operation. Anorectal manometry may allow evaluation of anorectal sphincter reflexes, sensation, and coordination. Typically a three-balloon probe is inserted into the rectum (Fig. 61-6). Rectal sensation can be assessed by inflating the rectal balloon with air or water and identifying the volume at which the balloon is first

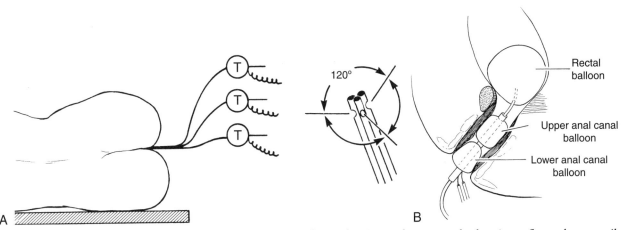

FIGURE 61-6 ■ Anorectal manometry. Balloon manometry can be used to assess the rectoanal relaxation reflex and contractile response, rectal sensation, and rectal compliance. (From Schiller LR: Fecal incontinence. In Feldman M [ed]: Sleisenger and Fordtran's Gastrointestinal and Liver Disease, 6th ed. Philadelphia, WB Saunders, 1998, pp 160-171.)

sensed (typically 10 mL). Delayed sensation may prevent an adequate cortical response to prevent incontinence. During rectal balloon inflation, the rectum can be assessed for adequate compliance, which may be compromised by ischemia or fibrosis. Appropriate internal sphincter relaxation in response to rectal distention (rectoanal inhibitory reflex) can be shown with inflation of the rectal balloon to 20 mL. The rectoanal inhibitory reflex is absent in patients with Hirschsprung's disease. The lower balloon allows assessment of external sphincter contraction under conditions of rectal distention (rectoanal contraction). This is a response that may be absent in patients with a variety of causes of incontinence.

Electrophysiologic assessment via a pudendal nerve terminal motor latency study may complement anorectal manometry. A glove with a stimulating and recording electrode on the tip and base of the finger is inserted into the rectum until the pudendal nerve is stimulated. The time for the nerve impulse to travel down the pudendal nerve is recorded. A prolonged latency indicates the presence of a pudendal neuropathy.

Occasionally, defecography may provide useful information. Barium is instilled into the rectum, and a marker is placed on the anal verge. The patient sits on a radiopaque toilet and first coughs; then bears down while attempting to maintain continence; and finally defecates while videofluoroscopy is used to assess the rectoanal angle, completeness of emptying during defecation, and descent of the pelvic floor, which should remain within 1 cm of a line drawn between the middle point of the pubic bone and the coccyx (pubococcygeal line).

Treatment

Three approaches to treatment of fecal incontinence are available: (1) control of stool consistency, (2) conditioning or biofeedback therapy, and (3) operations to strengthen the sphincter muscles. Incontinence related to neurologic deficiency, associated myelomeningocele, and other spinal malformations and variants of high imperforate anus is usually manageable by dietary or pharmacologic manipulation to thicken the stool and regular emptying of the rectum each morning with glycerin suppositories, saline enemas, or bisacodyl (Dulcolax) suppositories. The suppository or enema should be administered optimally within 30 minutes of a meal to take advantage of the gastrocolic reflex. Biofeedback therapy may play a role in patients with decreased sphincter function: A rectal balloon manometry device is placed into the rectum, and the rectal and sphincter pressures are shown to the patient. The rectal balloon is inflated, and the patient is encouraged to contract the external sphincter in response. The sensation of rectal distention and external sphincter contraction is learned, which may enhance continence.

In patients with encopresis associated with chronic constipation, incontinence is relieved when constipation is alleviated. These patients are managed best with initial evacuation of stool via an aggressive enema program along with administration of stool softeners, such as mineral oil or MiraLax (polyethylene glycol). Occasionally, disimpaction is required and may be performed in the operating room or via rectal water-soluble contrast agent administration under fluoroscopic guidance. Because many patients with constipation and encopresis contract, rather than relax, the external sphincter during defecation, biofeedback therapy may be important in resolving the dysfunction in patients with psychogenic incontinence. As described earlier, a balloon manometer is placed into the rectum, and the anal pressures are shown to the patient. The patient is taught to contract the abdominal wall muscles and to relax the external sphincter during an attempt to defecate. Some studies have suggested, however, that biofeedback therapy provides no contribution over laxative therapy in the constipated child. Other options to maintain continence and to treat constipation include a Malone appendicocecostomy or a sigmoidostomy tube for antegrade colonic enema administration.

If patients are incontinent after repair of imperforate anus with a normal sacrum and appropriately positioned and functioning sphincter muscles, control can be enhanced by dietary manipulation and regular evacuation of the rectum with saline solution washouts. If the rectum is positioned inappropriately outside the levator or external sphincter muscles on physical examination, MRI, or electromyographic localization, remedial operative correction via the posterior sagittal approach is indicated. Some success has been reported after surgical transplantation of one or both gracilis muscles around the external sphincter, especially with stimulation of the muscle with an implanted device during times when continence is desired. In preliminary studies, perianal autologous fat injection may enhance continence in patients with partial incontinence. Finally, reports of use of an artificial anal sphincter device have been encouraging, but this approach probably should be a last resort because of the severity of potential complications.

CHRONIC CONSTIPATION

Individuals with chronic constipation defecate infrequently, often less than once a week, which results in retention of bulky, firm stool that is increasingly difficult to evacuate. Any child who has a hard stool less frequently than once every third day should be considered to have constipation. As with incontinence, constipation may result from congenital or acquired causes.

Congenital causes of chronic constipation include neurologic disorders in which colonic dysmotility is present; Hirschsprung's disease, in which there is a deficiency of the intrinsic neural plexus; hypothyroidism; and intestinal pseudo-obstruction. In all of these conditions, the difficulty is not with rectal emptying, but rather filling of the rectum. Newborns who are breast-fed may have infrequent stools but often have minimal stool present on rectal examination and are not "constipated." It is likely that the breast milk is so well absorbed that production of feces is reduced. Other congenital causes of constipation include variants of low imperforate anus, such as anal stenosis and rectoperineal fistula, which are determined easily on physical examination.

The most common cause of significant chronic constipation in childhood is characterized by a history of a normal stooling pattern abruptly changing to severe constipation, sometimes associated with a stressful environmental factor, such as toilet training or family difficulties.

As mentioned previously, this functional constipation is most commonly due to problematic toilet training or painful defecation resulting in contraction of the anal canal during defecation. Stool retention occurs, and as hard, large stools develop, defecation becomes more painful, increasing stool retention. The rectum becomes more distended, and the encircling sling of the levator ani and lower sphincter muscles gradually become stretched as impacted feces accumulate, eventually shortening the anal canal. The result is constant leakage of feces or encopresis. Children frequently would prefer to endure this overflow incontinence rather than the pain associated with the anal stretching necessary to permit the evacuation of a large constipated stool. As the retention of feces increases, the continuing stretch of the sphincters results in sensory loss and a diminution in the defecation reflex. Rectal peristalsis becomes less effective. Although constipation in general does not affect the child's health directly, the family often is emotionally affected by the disorder. Other acquired causes of chronic constipation include chronic dehydration; use of drugs, such as opiates and anticholinergics; and metabolic disorders, such as hypothyroidism, disorders of calcium metabolism, lead poisoning, and cystic fibrosis.

Diagnosis

As with incontinence, history and physical examination are the mainstays of diagnosis. Age is an important factor. In newborns, an anatomic or mechanical abnormality, such as anal stenosis, rectoperineal fistula, or Hirschsprung's disease, is often the cause. With Hirschsprung's disease, constipation has a typical onset in the newborn period with passage of meconium at greater than 48 hours after birth. Patients with Hirschsprung's disease rarely give a history of encopresis. Patients with onset of constipation at an older age usually have functional constipation, which most commonly develops between 2 and 4 years of age. Many patients report nonspecific abdominal pain. On physical examination, the underwear should be examined for soiling. The position of the anus should be ascertained to be directly on a line between the ischial tuberosities. An anteriorly displaced anus with a posterior shelf is an occasional cause of constipation. The rectal examination typically shows a large amount of hard stool with an anal canal that is shorter than the typical 4 cm of a 5-year-old to 10-year-old child. Hard feces may be palpable on abdominal examination. An unprepared barium enema is helpful if Hirschsprung's disease is a consideration. The contrast enema in a patient with functional constipation typically shows a large amount of feces with a markedly dilated colon down to the anal verge (Fig. 61-7). Other tests, such as anorectal manometry, can help to distinguish functional constipation and Hirschsprung's disease; functional constipation is associated with external sphincter contraction during defecation, whereas the internal sphincter fails to relax during rectal distention (rectoanal inhibitory reflex) in patients with Hirschsprung's disease. The definitive study for evaluation of Hirschsprung's disease is a rectal biopsy. Patients with metabolic disorders or drug-related causes of constipation are identified by specific studies directed at the underlying cause.

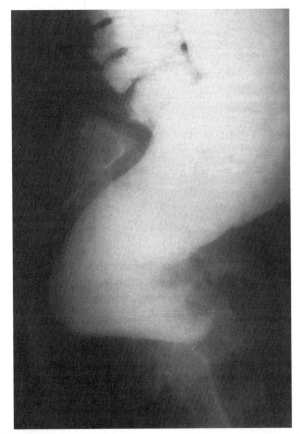

FIGURE 61-7 ■ Typical barium enema findings in a patient with severe chronic constipation. Rectal dilation extends to the anus and balloons posteriorly, which differentiates this disorder from Hirschsprung's disease.

Treatment

Patients with anal stenosis, anterior anus, or rectoperineal fistula have symptoms alleviated for the most part by appropriate anatomic repair. The management of patients with functional constipation is approached best in a fashion similar to the patient with encopresis, which includes dietary manipulation to soften the stool, use of stool softeners such as mineral oil or polyethylene glycol, saline enemas, glycerin or bisacodyl suppositories, and biofeedback therapy. The key goals of treatment include initial evacuation of retained feces, effective stool softening, and establishment of a normal, regular pattern of evacuation. This program is continued for many months with gradual weaning first of enemas and suppositories, then stool softeners. Multivitamins should be administered if mineral oil is used for more than a few months.

An occasional patient with severe constipation fails to respond to the aforementioned regimen. Alternatives include creation of an appendicocecostomy (the Malone procedure), which can be cannulated and through which antegrade colonic enemas can be performed. The Malone procedure can be performed laparoscopically and has been effective in controlling incontinence and constipation in numerous patients. The major complication is stenosis of the appendicocecostomy. An alternative in patients with isolated rectosigmoid constipation is the percutaneous placement of a sigmoidostomy tube using a technique analogous to placement of a percutaneous gastrostomy tube. Direct sigmoid enemas may be performed, which are effective at washing out the fecal material from the rectum.

RECTAL PROLAPSE

Prolapse of the rectum through the anus may involve only a small ring of mucosa or more commonly all layers of the rectum (Fig. 61-8). With mucosal prolapse, one observes radial folds adjacent to the anal skin, whereas with full-thickness prolapse, circular folds are seen in the prolapsed mucosa. The most common form of rectal prolapse is idiopathic. The average child with idiopathic rectal prolapse is 1 to 3 years old. At this age, the child's muscle mass is not well developed, the rectum is loosely adherent to the underlying muscles, intra-abdominal pressure is directed toward the anus instead of the hollow of the sacrum as in the infant, and the child is working to develop continence. Frequently, these children spend long periods straining to evacuate their rectum as they concentrate to develop voluntary control of defecation. Under these circumstances, the rectum herniates through the anus. In many cases, this is a self-limited problem that alleviates itself within 1 to 2 years. In all cases, the prolapse is mucosal.

Children with conditions that tend to promote tenesmus, such as rectal polyps, worms, proctitis, ulcerative colitis, and cystic fibrosis, also may have mild rectal prolapse. Rectal prolapse is common in patients with myelomeningocele and exstrophy of the bladder and similar conditions associated with deficiencies in either the pelvic musculature or its innervation.

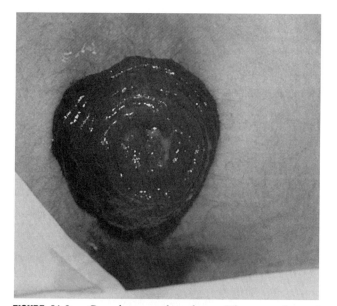

FIGURE 61-8 ■ Complete rectal prolapse. The everted rectal wall appears as a tubular mass composed of several concentric mucosal folds. (Reprinted permission of Mayo Foundation. From Nelson H, Dozois RR: Anus. In Townsend C [ed]: Sabiston Textbook of Surgery, 16th ed. Philadelphia, WB Saunders, 2001, pp 974-996.)

History and physical examination usually provide enough information to indicate the cause of the prolapse. Rectal prolapse often occurs with defecation or crying and reduces spontaneously or with minimal manipulation. It may be difficult to reproduce the prolapse in the clinic, but a picture or videotape taken by the parents can document the prolapse. When prolapse is present, it is not possible to insert an examining finger in the space between the prolapsed bowel and the anus. If intussusception is present, the finger can be inserted into the rectum, however, between the prolapsed bowel and the anal opening. In similar fashion, a prolapsed colonic or rectal polyp can be differentiated from a prolapsed rectum. In the initial work-up of patients with idiopathic prolapse, appropriate studies should be performed to rule out cystic fibrosis and parasites, especially because one fifth of patients with cystic fibrosis have rectal prolapse. If a polyp is suspected, colonoscopy should be performed.

Treatment

Most patients with rectal prolapse do not require any specific form of treatment other than measures to prevent excessive straining. A program consisting of administration of mineral oil or polyethylene glycol with occasional use of enemas is usually effective. Within a few months, the condition is alleviated in most patients. If the prolapse persists, many surgical approaches have been developed. One of the most effective is injection of saline or a sclerosing solution, such as 5% phenol in glycerin, 30% saline, or 50% glucose. Another approach is linear electrocauterization of the rectum down to the level of the submucosa from just short of the dentate line up and over the dome of the prolapse in each of four quadrants. These techniques are designed to produce a perirectal inflammatory reaction to induce scarring and prevent prolapse. Injection of a sclerosant or linear electrocauterization may be combined with placement of a temporary Thiersch suture to prevent prolapse. The Thiersch technique consists of a small incision in the perianal skin at 6 and 12 o'clock, which facilitates placement of a circumferential no. 2 PDS or polyglactin (Vicryl) suture in the perianal subcutaneous tissues. This suture is tied over a 12 (infant) to 20 (adolescent) Hegar dilator or the surgeon's index and middle fingers placed into the rectum, allowing for defecation with temporary resolution of the prolapse.

In severe cases of prolapse, especially in adolescents, operation with resection or rectopexy is performed. A full-thickness rectal resection is performed in the Altemeier procedure starting 1 or 2 cm above the pectinate line. The redundant rectum is resected, and a full-thickness anastomosis is performed. Rectopexy may be performed with or without resection via a transabdominal approach. The rectum is secured, often with mesh, to the presacral tissues. This procedure can be performed by a laparoscopic approach.

ANAL FISSURE

One of the most common causes of rectal bleeding in newborns and infants is an anal fissure, which results from a superficial tear of the anal mucosa. In most instances, the anal fissure is produced by excessive stretching during the evacuation of a large, constipated stool. The stool may be streaked with blood. This is a painful process and may result in the infant retaining stool, further complicating the problem. In some instances, an anal fissure occurs in patients who have normal or soft stool. Fissures are observed most frequently in the posterior midline. If fissures become chronic and fail to heal, they often are associated with hypertrophy of the anal papilla at the dentate line and a skin tag at the anal verge. Anal fissures also may be seen in anorectal Crohn's disease and as a complication of immunodeficiency states.

The diagnosis of a fissure is made by retracting the skin at the anus and having the patient bear down, which allows visualization of the anal canal. Occasionally, examination under anesthesia is warranted, along with sigmoidoscopy or colonoscopy and biopsy, when the diagnosis of Crohn's disease is suspected. Gentle anal dilation and administration of mineral oil or polyethylene glycol to soften the stools are usually all that is needed to treat acute anal fissures, which often heal within 1 to 2 weeks. Chronic fissures may be treated effectively with topical application of nitroglycerin. Lateral subcutaneous internal anal sphincterotomy, in which the internal sphincter is divided, may be necessary in patients with chronic fissures. Fissures associated with Crohn's disease and leukemia are treated best with metronidazole.

PERIANAL AND PERIRECTAL ABSCESS

Perianal abscesses and fistulas are seen commonly in male infants younger than 1 year of age with a peak incidence at 4 months of age. Histologic examination of excised fistula specimens shows an epithelial lining of the tract mixed with stratified squamous, transitional, and columnar epithelium, suggesting a congenital source for the problem. The process is limited to the perianal region, in contrast to the perirectal abscesses seen in older children. Drainage of the abscess can be performed in the clinic and often relieves pain and accompanying fever. Antibiotic treatment is usually not necessary. Approximately one third of abscesses recur, and approximately one third develop into a fistula-in-ano. A recurrent abscess or fistula can be treated effectively and simply by placing a probe through the fistula to the anal papilla, where the probe passes through or creates an opening. The overlying skin down to the probe is opened, and the base of the fistula is cauterized. Recurrence is observed in 15% of cases.

In older children, a perianal or perirectal abscess almost always is related to a crypt abscess descending through the intersphincteric plane, presenting either subcutaneously around the anus or in the ischiorectal fossa. Superficial abscesses ordinarily contain staphylococci or occasionally gram-negative organisms, but perirectal infections generally contain anaerobes. Perianal and perirectal abscesses in older children frequently are the first signs of Crohn's disease, leukemia, or immunodeficiency disorders. Perianal and perirectal abscesses are associated with fever and pain. Although perianal abscesses

are evident on physical inspection, perirectal infections may be evident only on rectal examination. These abscesses should be incised and drained as soon as they are identified. Systemic antibiotics ordinarily are not required for localized perianal abscesses, but they are indicated in patients with perirectal disease. Recurrence is common, and 25% to 50% of patients with crypt abscesses develop fistulas-in-ano.

FISTULA-IN-ANO

Fistula-in-ano is the end result of a perianal abscess that extends from a crypt to the perianal skin. Its presence should be suspected whenever there are multiple recurrences of an abscess. The fistula usually extends through the external sphincter, exiting laterally. In contrast to older patients, in infants fistulas do not follow Goodsall's rule, which predicts that all fistulas anterior to the midportion of the anus will track radially, whereas all fistulas posterior to this point will track to the posterior midline. All fistulas in infants extend radially from the involved crypt. Figure 61-9 shows the typical appearance of a fistula-in-ano. Some surgeons suggest that nonoperative therapy of a fistula in an infant is followed by spontaneous resolution over the next 6 to 12 months. Others suggest that the treatment of fistula-in-ano should be operative. With the patient under general anesthesia, a lacrimal duct probe is passed through the fistulous tract. It ordinarily can be seen exiting at or close to an anal papilla. It is then possible to cut down on the probe to perform the fistulotomy. The base of the tract is cauterized extensively to prevent recurrence.

In older patients, primary fistulotomy is the definitive treatment for superficial fistulas. Complex and high transphincteric fistulas, in which greater than one fourth to one half of the sphincter muscle would be divided, are treated best by drainage of ongoing infection and placement of a seton, which consists of a suture placed through the fistula and tied to itself. The fistula often heals as the seton is tightened and works its way through the

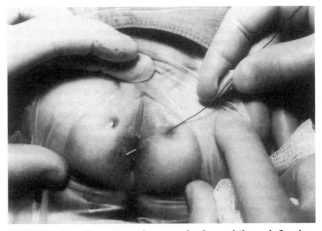

FIGURE 61-9 ■ Operative photograph shows bilateral fistulas-in-ano. The small probe passes from the cutaneous opening to one of the anal columns. In most children, the fistulous tracts are straight as shown.

tissues or is removed. Injection of fibrin glue into these fistulas may result in healing in approximately 60% of patients, although late recurrences are common. Crohn's disease should be ruled out in all older children with chronic fistulas.

IMPERFORATE ANUS

Classification

In both sexes, anorectal deformities are divided into high, intermediate, and low anomalies as related to the level of the puborectalis portion of the levator ani muscle and whether there is a fistula to the urinary tract in males or the vagina in females. Cloacal anomalies, in which the urethra, vagina, and rectum all empty into a single conduit, are considered as a separate category because of the critical associated GU malformations. The most common of these anomalies are depicted in Figure 61-10. The incidence of anorectal malformations is approximately 1 in 5000 live births. They occur slightly more commonly in boys, and boys are twice as likely as girls to have high or intermediate anomalies. In boys with an intermediate or high anomaly, 85% have a rectourinary fistula (Fig. 61-11). Most high anomalies in girls are variants of cloaca; a high anomaly with a rectovaginal fistula is rare. In terms of low-lying anomalies, 35% of boys have a thin membrane covering the anal fistula, whereas 93% of girls have an external fistula. Although imperforate anus may occur as an isolated malformation, it coexists with duodenal atresia, esophageal atresia, vertebral and renal anomalies, Down syndrome, and congenital heart disease in 50% to 60% of patients. The VATER or VACTERL syndrome (*v*ertebral, *a*nal, *c*ardiac, *t*racheo*e*sophageal, *r*enal, and radial *l*imb anomalies) occurs in approximately

15% of patients. A tethered cord and other types of spinal cord abnormalities are observed in half of patients with imperforate anus. Approximately 60% of patients with high or intermediate forms of imperforate anus have some form of associated GU malformation or vesicoureteral reflux. The incidence of GU malformation with low anomalies is only 15% to 20%; however, associated anomalies of the GU tract are particularly important to recognize early if deterioration of renal function is to be avoided.

Initial Management of the Newborn with Imperforate Anus

The first decision in the assessment of the newborn with an anorectal anomaly is whether a colostomy is required. Although it is always better to err on the side of performing a colostomy, there are many anomalies in which one is unnecessary. Examination of the perineum is paramount because it may provide evidence of a low-lying fistula or meconium beneath a membranous covering typical of a low lesion. In contrast, a flat or "rocker-bottom" perineum may be observed, which indicates the poor sphincter or levator muscle development typical of a high anomaly (Fig. 61-12). It is best to wait 24 hours to allow progression of gas or meconium down close to or onto the perineum before finalizing the assessment. Of female malformations, 95% are of the low variety, whereas most male anomalies are high.

Imperforate Anus in Boys

Figure 61-13 is an efficient algorithm for the initial management of anorectal malformations in boys. As mentioned previously, the distinction between a low or intermediate/ high anomaly can be assessed by clinical examination,

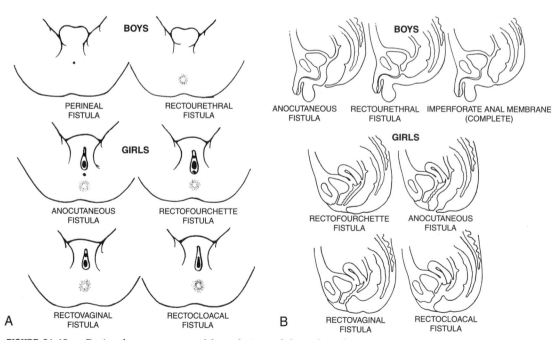

FIGURE 61-10 ■ Perineal appearance and lateral view of the pelvis showing anorectal anomalies in males and females. (From Grosfeld JL: Anorectal malformations. In Zuidema G, Condon RE [eds]: Surgery of the Alimentary Tract, vol 4, 3rd ed. Philadelphia, WB Saunders, 1990.)

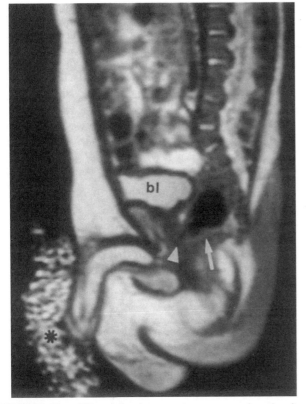

FIGURE 61-11 ■ T2-weighted magnetic resonance imaging in a boy with a high anorectal malformation and rectourethral fistula. The rectal pouch ends above the levator ani muscle (arrow), and the fistula (arrowhead) extends anteriorly to the urethra. Feces have been passed through the urethra (asterisk). bl, bladder. (From Nievelstein RAJ, Vos A, Valk J, Verjeig-Keers Chr: Magnetic Resonance Imaging in Children with Anorectal Malformations: Embryologic Implications. J Pediatr Surg 37:1138-1145, 2002.)

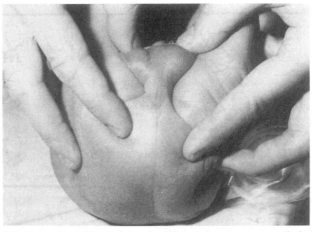

FIGURE 61-12 ■ Typical "rocker-bottom" appearance of the perineum in a newborn boy with anorectal atresia and rectourethreal fistula, a high anomaly. Note the poorly formed gluteal folds characteristic of absent innervation from sacral agenesis.

the presence of gas in the bladder or meconium in the urine, and a prone cross-table lateral film of the abdomen. If an external opening is visible in the perineum, one can predict the presence of a low anomaly with an anocutaneous fistula or anal stenosis. At times, the meconium may be seen extending up the raphe as a continuation of the fistula. This is often white meconium, which consists of the first and most distal meconium that has not been colored by the more proximal bile. Hypertrophied folds over the expected site of the anus, often referred to as a "bucket handle," or a well-formed anus and gluteal crease suggest the presence of a low anomaly with a membranous covering, which may be observed in one third of boys.

FIGURE 61-13 ■ Algorithm for treatment of newborn boy with anorectal malformation. (From Kiely EM, Pena A: Anorectal malformations. In O'Neill J (ed): Pediatric Surgery, volume 2, 5th ed. St Louis, Mosby, 1998.)

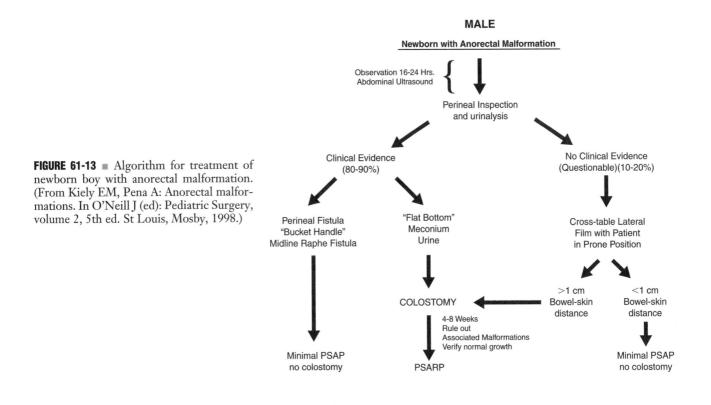

MALE

Newborn with Anorectal Malformation

Observation 16-24 Hrs.
Abdominal Ultrasound

Perineal Inspection
and urinalysis

Clinical Evidence
(80-90%)

No Clinical Evidence
(Questionable)(10-20%)

Perineal Fistula
"Bucket Handle"
Midline Raphe Fistula

"Flat Bottom"
Meconium
Urine

Cross-table Lateral
Film with Patient
in Prone Position

COLOSTOMY

>1 cm
Bowel-skin
distance

<1 cm
Bowel-skin
distance

4-8 Weeks
Rule out
Associated Malformations
Verify normal growth

Minimal PSAP
no colostomy

PSARP

Minimal PSAP
no colostomy

At times, a tiny amount of meconium staining can be seen through the membrane. After 24 hours of life, a speck of meconium may indicate the location of a tiny fistulous orifice. When no anal orifice or fistula is seen at the level of the perineum, gentle massage of the urethra may produce meconium at the meatus or in the urine, which would indicate a high or intermediate anomaly with a fistula. If air is seen in the bladder, the anomaly may be presumed to be high with either a proximal urethral or rectovesicular fistula. In patients in whom the anal opening appears to be normal, but there is intestinal obstruction or passage of small-caliber stools, gentle probing of the anus shows an anal membrane, anorectal stenosis, or rectal atresia.

If a boy has an associated cleft scrotum or proximal hypospadias, one should suspect a high or intermediate anomaly. If there is complete absence of the gluteal fold, the so-called rocker bottom; if no anal wink can be elicited; and if sacral anomalies are able to be determined on palpation or by radiograph, a high anomaly is usually present.

Other approaches to evaluation of the level of the rectal pouch include ultrasound and prone cross-table lateral abdominal radiography. If the rectum is noted on radiograph or ultrasound to be less than 1 cm from the perineum at the site of the expected anus, a low anomaly may be presumed and an anoplasty performed. One problem with ultrasound is that compression with the probe on the perineum may decrease the natural distance between the anal skin and the rectum, and diagnosis of a low anomaly may be made inappropriately.

In addition to the preceding studies, the patient should be assessed for components of the VACTERL syndrome. Ultrasound evaluation of the kidneys and ureters should be performed to diagnose a potential obstructive uropathy. In boys, this is treated best at the time of surgery for imperforate anus. A voiding cystourethrogram may be performed at the time of birth or later but should be performed before initial discharge to rule out vesicoureteral reflux so that appropriate therapy can be instituted. Ultrasound evaluation for a tethered cord also should be performed.

Patients with clinical features suggestive of diminished innervation of the pelvis, such as myelomeningocele, sacral agenesis, and features of a rocker bottom, should be evaluated for neurogenic bladder. Generally, these patients have a compressible bladder, and on voiding cystourethrography the bladder is large and empties poorly. Determining whether a patient has a neurogenic bladder is important because it would be necessary to perform intermittent catheterization and to provide antibacterial prophylaxis.

Imperforate Anus in Girls

Figure 61-14 shows the diagnostic approach to girls with an anorectal anomaly. The internal anatomy of girls with imperforate anus usually can be predicted from a careful study of the visible orifices in the perineum. At times, the vulva is closed, and the labial folds must be opened so that all orifices can be inspected. Three orifices typically are seen. Usually the urethral and vaginal openings are normal, and the third orifice represents a fistula either at the level of the normal anus or more commonly as an opening at an abnormal site anteriorly. The common anomalies are anovestibular fistula, anocutaneous fistula, and anal stenosis. If a small hemostat is placed in the posterior opening, it is frequently possible to tell by pushing posteriorly and inferiorly that the rectal pouch forms a low anomaly as the end of the hemostat is palpated in the site where the anus normally is located (Fig. 61-15). Figure 61-15 depicts a typical low anomaly in a girl that would be managed effectively with an anoplasty. If the

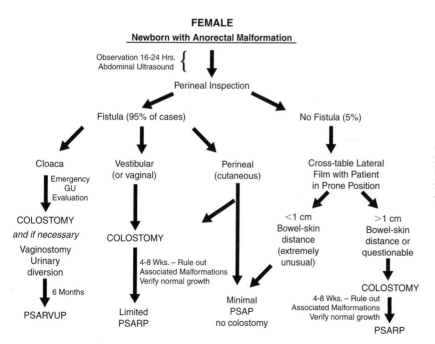

FIGURE 61-14 ■ Algorithm for treatment of newborn girl with anorectal malformation. (From Kiely EM, Pena A: Anorectal malformations. In O'Neill J (ed): Pediatric Surgery, volume 2, 5th ed. St. Louis, Mosby, 1998.)

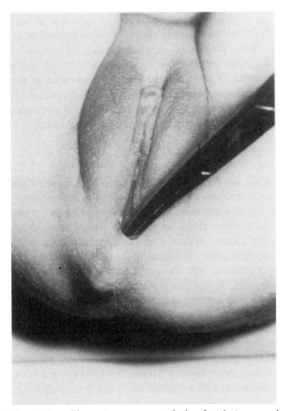

FIGURE 61-15 ■ Clamp in an anovestibular fistula in a newborn girl. The clamp shows that the rectal pouch is low adjacent to the skin. Repair of anomalies of this type usually can be done in the newborn period.

hemostat tends to go upward, a catheter should be passed, and a contrast study should be performed to rule out a rectovestibular fistula, which is an intermediate anomaly.

If only two orifices are seen in the perineum, including the urethra and vagina, and meconium is seen coming from the vagina, a rectovaginal fistula or cloacal variant is present. It is not possible to determine under these circumstances whether the rectovaginal fistula is high or low in the vagina. At times, it is possible to pass a catheter into the fistula and to do a contrast injection study or to perform endoscopy to obtain further information. In either case, an intermediate/high anomaly can be presumed, and a colostomy can be performed.

If neither a fistula nor meconium is noted on or just beneath the perineum, ultrasound or a prone cross-table lateral abdominal radiograph may be performed to assess for proximity of the rectum to the anal skin (<1 cm). In the circumstance in which the rectum is within 1 cm of the presumed anus, an anoplasty may be performed. In most cases, however, an intermediate or high anomaly should be presumed, and a colostomy should be performed.

If only one orifice is seen in the vulva, it must be assumed that there is a cloaca constituting a common opening for the urethra, vagina, and rectum. Usually urine and meconium exit from a common orifice. These are generally complicated anomalies that require colostomy and, at times, vaginostomy or urinary diversion or both.

Panendoscopy of patients with cloacal malformations is helpful in terms of determining the exact internal anatomy, and selective injection studies are performed to delineate the anatomy precisely. All girls with imperforate anus should be screened for vesicoureteral reflux and other severe associated GU and VACTERL malformations.

Surgical Management

Initial Treatment in the Neonate

Male and female newborns who have low anomalies in the form of an anocutaneous fistula, an anovestibular fistula, or anal stenosis usually can be treated initially with dilation. In the past, anocutaneous fistulas regularly were dilated and repair performed several months later, but in more recent years, most pediatric centers have been performing anoplasty shortly after birth unless contraindicated by some other condition. Male and female infants suspected of having intermediate or high-lying deformities and infants whose internal anatomy cannot be determined with certainty should have a colostomy performed. The most satisfactory approach is to perform a colostomy at the junction between the descending colon and the sigmoid colon, leaving a sufficient length to permit a subsequent pull-through procedure without having to take down the colostomy. In essence, the colostomy should be performed as proximally as possible on the sigmoid colon. Although some surgeons prefer to bring the two ends of the colostomy out as separate openings, many surgeons believe that it is possible to do a loop colostomy performed in such a fashion that it later can be divided to make it totally diverting. At the time the colostomy is performed, all distal meconium should be washed out to avoid contamination of the urinary tract. A definitive pull-through operation can be performed when the infant is believed to be thriving and of appropriate size. Timing is based on medical judgment rather than on an arbitrary interval, but typically is performed at any point beyond 8 to 10 weeks of age. Most boys require a colostomy, but most newborn girls with imperforate anus are able to have an anoplasty performed because most have low-lying lesions.

Repair of Low-Lying Lesions

In the setting of a membranous covering over a low anomaly, some surgeons prefer to puncture the membrane followed by enlargement of the tract with Hegar dilators, whereas others do a formal anoplasty. In the case of other low-lying anomalies, either an anoplasty or an anal transposition procedure is required. Figure 61-16 shows two methods of cutback anoplasty. The first (Fig. 61-16A) is the so-called classic cutback procedure whereby a hemostat is placed in the anus and the tissue is cut back with cautery exactly in the midline to the posterior border of the external sphincter. The latter is identified by stimulation and observation of the extent of the external sphincter. The mucosa and anoderm at the cut edges are approximated with absorbable suture. A more desirable approach is shown in Figure 61-16B, 1-3. The external sphincter fibers are identified precisely using a nerve stimulator on the skin. The skin is incised in a Y fashion, the sphincter muscles retracted posteriorly,

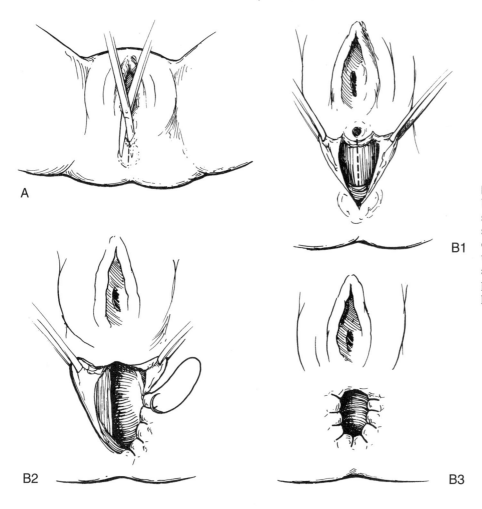

A

B1

B2

B3

FIGURE 61-16 ■ **A,** The classic "cutback" procedure still used by many surgeons. **B1, B2, B3,** The various steps used for Y-V anoplasty repair of anal atresia with rectoperineal fistula. The latter procedure is not appropriate for more anteriorly placed fistulas, which require transposition posteriorly.

and a long posterior midline incision performed in the rectal pouch to convert the Y incision to a V, widening the opening extensively. The external sphincter is reconstructed around the newly opened rectum in the process.

In many girls and rarely in boys, the anterior margin of the anus would lie too far anteriorly using the Y-V anoplasty technique. Anal transposition is recommended under these circumstances, creating an anterior perineal skin bridge and a satisfactory perineal body in the process. This can be accomplished by one of two techniques. In the first, a "tennis racket" incision is performed around the fistula extending back in the midline to the posterior extent of the external sphincter. The fistula is dissected completely from the vagina in the girl and the rectum transposed to a position within the external sphincter as a neoanus is created. The perineal body is reconstructed. In the second technique, Potts' anoplasty, the perineal body is maintained intact, and the mobilized fistula and rectum are transposed beneath to a separate anoplasty incision posteriorly. If the newborn is ill or too small to permit the anal transposition procedure, the anus can be dilated and the transposition procedure performed several weeks or months later. Typically an anorectal transposition is performed at 3 to 4 weeks of age.

Approximately 3 weeks after anoplasty, anal dilations should be initiated and performed once daily by the parents for several weeks to prevent stenosis. Dilations are weaned slowly over the next few months as long as stricture formation is not observed.

Repair of Intermediate and High Anomalies

Most patients with intermediate and high forms of imperforate anus are recognized shortly after birth. As previously mentioned, all of these infants should have a sigmoid colostomy performed as a staging procedure. Some centers do have laparoscopic anorectal reconstructions in newborns.

At the point that infants are believed to be of sufficient size and condition, a distal colostogram should be performed with soluble contrast material using a Foley balloon catheter in the distal loop of the colostomy (Fig. 61-17). It is usually possible to show the exact site of a rectourethral, retrovesicular, or rectovaginal fistula. If the patient previously had been determined to have vesicoureteral reflux, a repeat voiding cystourethrogram should be performed to verify that no renal effects have been observed. Panendoscopy and contrast injection of all cavities are crucial in girls with cloacal anomalies to plan the operation. Cystoscopy is not usually necessary in boys, unless urethral valves are suspected. A thorough bowel preparation should be performed, and preoperative antibiotics should be administered.

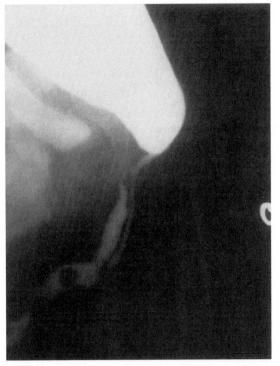

FIGURE 61-17 ■ Before performing definitive pull-through repair in a patient with a high or intermediate imperforate anus, the anatomy should be defined with a distal colostomy injection study using soluble contrast material. This colostogram shows the level and size of the rectal pouch, as well as the rectourethral fistula and its relation to the urethral and bladder neck.

Although numerous surgical approaches have been proposed for the repair of intermediate and high-lying anomalies in boys and girls, currently the posterior sagittal anorectoplasty (PSARP) procedure described by de Vries and Pena is the preferred technique (Fig. 61-18). This approach is also useful for repair of complicated cloacal malformations and for remedial procedures for previously operated patients who are incontinent. At times, an abdominal approach is required in addition to the posterior sagittal approach.

Figure 61-18 shows the major components of the PSARP. The primary principles of the procedure are precise division of all structures in the midline, demonstration of all sphincter muscle components with electrical stimulation, and incision into the rectal pouch with endorectal division of the rectourethral or rectovaginal fistula, if present. Prior placement of a lit endoscope in the pouch via the mucous fistula may aid in identification of the pouch itself and prevent incidental mobilization of or incision into adjacent structures. When the fistula is ligated, a submucosal plane is developed superiorly in the rectal pouch to avoid injury to the closely approximated urethra, prostate, vas deferens, and seminal vesicles. The full-thickness rectal plane is reestablished at a point more superior, and the levator and sphincters are reconstructed about the rectum as the neoanus is formed. In most patients, the entire procedure can be done from a transsacral approach, but occasionally an abdominal component of the operation is necessary, especially when a rectovesical fistula is present. In general, the rectum does not need to be tapered. An attempt is made to save the mucosa close to the point of the fistula because it is believed to have specialized sensory capabilities. Three weeks later, the new anus is dilated gently with a Hegar dilator, and after 6 weeks or so, another colostogram is performed to verify that complete healing has occurred. At that point, the colostomy may be closed.

A laparoscopic approach to repair of high or intermediate imperforate anus in the newborn period or at a later date after colostomy may have distinct advantages over the posterior sagittal approach. The fistula is identified and ligated with a clip. The rectum is mobilized, and the levator ani muscles are viewed through the laparoscope. The perineum is stimulated to identify the location of the external sphincter. A midline incision the length of the external sphincter is performed, and laparoscopy is used to guide development of a tract through the center of the external sphincter and the puborectalis. The tract is dilated followed by delivery of the rectum through the tract with formation of a neoanus on the perineum.

Cloacal anomalies in girls are complicated and vary greatly. The posterior sagittal approach is extremely helpful under these circumstances because it is frequently possible to reconstruct the urethra, vagina, and rectum in a single stage. However, with cloacal malformations, the crucial consideration in the long term is usually the serious associated GU malformations.

Complications

Current mortality rates are low after repair of imperforate anus, and most of these deaths are attributable to anomalies of other organ systems, particularly the cardiovascular system and central nervous system. Sepsis is occasionally a problem in patients with complicated high anomalies involving the GU system. Mortality in patients is in the range of 5% for low anomalies and 15% for high anomalies. After PSARP, the main complications have been prolapse of anal mucosa, anal stenosis, and incontinence. Rare patients have been found to have associated Hirschsprung's disease, a point that should be kept in mind in patients who have unexplained constipation after pull-through for imperforate anus.

Patients who have had repair of imperforate anus must be followed carefully for most of their lives. Greater than 90% of patients who have had a simple anoplasty performed for low-lying lesions are continent, but constipation is a frequent problem, and appropriate management must be provided to avoid the development of megarectum. In patients who have had a PSARP performed, the results in terms of continence are related directly to the level of the anomaly. Patients with intermediate-level imperforate anus anomalies have a higher incidence of continence than patients with high-lying anomalies. Similarly, patients with deficiencies in muscle or innervation and patients with sacral agenesis have a poor prognosis for continence. Satisfactory continence (which may include the need for a bowel

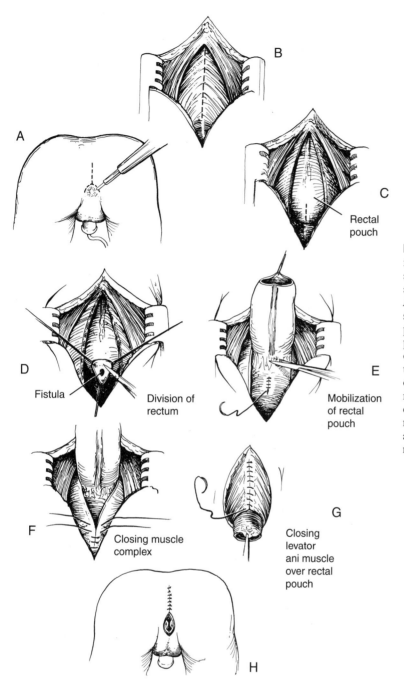

Rectal
pouch

Fistula

Division of
rectum

Mobilization
of rectal
pouch

Closing muscle
complex

Closing
levator
ani muscle
over rectal
pouch

FIGURE 61-18 ■ The essential features of the posterior sagittal anorectoplasty used for intermediate and high malformations, which usually are associated with rectourinary or rectovaginal fistulas. **A,** Electrical stimulation to identify the external sphincter location. **B,** Midline incision through all posterior musculature. **C,** Identification of the rectal pouch and incision into the posterior, inferior wall of the rectum. **D,** Identification and dissection of the rectourethral fistula from the rectum. **E,** Closure of the rectourethral fistula and mobilization of the rectal pouch. **F,** Closure of the striated muscle complex anteriorly. **G,** Closure of the posterior musculature over the rectal pouch. **H,** Skin closure and "double diamond" method of anoplasty to promote sensation and to avoid stricture.

management program) is reported in approximately 75% of patients with intermediate forms of imperforate anus, 65% in boys and girls with high-lying lesions, and 20% or less in girls with cloacal anomalies.

SUGGESTED READINGS

Hassink EA, Rieu PN, Severijnen RS, et al: Are adults content or continent after repair for high anal atresia? Ann Surg 218:196-200, 1993.

This follow-up study of 58 adults with an average age of 26 years, operated on before introduction of the posterior sagittal procedure, had reasonable control of defecation, although none were normal, and 84% were satisfied with their level of cleanliness.

This study indicates that most patients find ways to adapt to their situation.

Hendren WH: Cloaca, the most severe degree of imperforate anus. Ann Surg 228:331-346, 1998.

This review of 195 cases shows the widely variable presentations of cloacal malformations, their diagnosis, treatment, and outcomes. It is the authoritative reference on this subject.

Michof F, Constaglioli B, Leroi A-M, Denis P: Artificial anal sphincter in severe fecal incontinence. Ann Surg 237:52-56, 2003.

This is an encouraging but preliminary report detailing use, complications, and results in patients not amenable to conventional approaches to incontinence.

Rintala RJ, Lindahl H: Is normal bowel function possible after repair of intermediate and high anorectal malformations? J Pediatr Surg 30:491-494, 1995.

A total of 46 patients who had posterior sagittal anorectoplasty and colostomy closure were assessed 3 to 5 years later. Of patients, 70% had satisfactory results, but 30% had poor results. Poor results correlated with absence of a functional internal sphincter, severe sacral anomalies, and constipation.

Schell SR, Toogood GJ, Dudley NE: Control of fecal incontinence: Continued success with the Malone procedure. Surgery 122:626-631, 1997.

The authors describe the use of appendix or tapered ileum for a catheterizable stoma for administration of antegrade enemas. In their hands, the procedure was safe and highly satisfactory in a group of 23 patients followed over 6 years. Results were excellent in 85% of patients.

62

Obturation Obstruction of the Intestine

Obstruction of the intestine and colon related to obturation by meconium or foreign material generally occurs in normal intestine. The most common disorders of this nature in the newborn are meconium ileus, meconium plug syndrome, and neonatal small left colon syndrome. In older children, obturation obstruction generally is associated with foreign bodies, bezoars, or parasites. In each instance, complete or high-grade partial intestinal obstruction is the primary mode of presentation.

APPROACH TO THE INFANT WITH A BOWEL OBSTRUCTION

Evaluation of the newborn or infant with a small or large bowel obstruction is one of the great challenges of pediatric surgery. Figure 62-1 is an algorithm the surgeon may use when evaluating such a patient. The most clinically significant abnormalities should be ruled out first, followed by those that are not immediately life-threatening. If malrotation and volvulus is suspected, an immediate upper gastrointestinal series should be performed. Most proximal (duodenal) and distal (imperforate anus) obstructions are obvious. The surgeon always should inquire if the neonate was delivered with marked abdominal distention. This finding should prompt consideration of four potential disorders: (1) complicated meconium ileus, (2) cystic meconium peritonitis, (3) bilateral ureteral obstruction (posterior urethral valves), and (4) hydrocolpos. Other causes are also possible, including ascites, but can be addressed adequately with plain films looking for calcifications and an abdominal ultrasound. Then a barium enema should be performed. Although not always diagnostic, it often is instructive. A microcolon is found with intestinal atresia, meconium ileus, or, in a rare case, megalocystis and microcolon syndrome. A small left colon may be seen with Hirschsprung's disease, small left colon syndrome, or meconium plug syndrome. A normal barium enema with normal-appearing abdominal radiographs, although suggestive of no pathology, still may be seen with Hirschsprung's disease or with more proximal small bowel atresias.

MECONIUM ILEUS

Meconium ileus is the intestinal obstructive variant of cystic fibrosis (CF) or mucoviscidosis. Approximately 15%

to 20% of infants with CF also present with intestinal obstruction related to meconium ileus. Although it originally was thought that CF primarily affected the pancreas, it now is known that all exocrine and mucus-secreting glands in the body are affected.

Cystic Fibrosis

CF is the most common life-shortening inherited disease in North America. The disease first was described clinically by Andersen in 1938. CF is a complex disorder of the respiratory and digestive systems. The genetics of CF are well understood to be inherited by an autosomal recessive pattern, with families with the disease carrying a one in four chance of having another child with the disorder. The incidence of heterozygous carriers in whites is approximately 1 in 20. People of European extraction have a 1 in 3200 incidence of having a child with CF, whereas the incidence decreases to 1 in 15,000 in African-Americans and is much less in Asians. Collins first identified the genetic mutations responsible for the disorder in 1989. Since this first genetic mutation was isolated, more than 800 mutations have been identified. The loss of a single phenylalanine at position 508 of the gene (ΔF508) represents 70% to 80% of mutations in patients with CF and 50% of those seen in North America.

The CF transmembrane conductance regulator gene (*CFTR*) is a cyclic adenosine monophosphate–regulated chloride channel and is located on chromosome 7q. Functionally the gene encodes a protein that is primarily responsible for regulating the opening and closing of chloride channels. The defect affects all epithelial-lined structures. Although the precise manner in which the deficient chloride transport leads to the numerous manifestations of the disease has not been resolved completely, it seems that the *CFTR* gene also may influence sodium transport and may lead to an overly activated sodium pump. These changes are believed to result in abnormally viscid mucus secretions in the lungs, pancreas, intestine, biliary tree, and elsewhere. This is also why approximately 90% of patients with CF have failure of secretion of pancreatic enzymes into the duodenum, which results in malabsorption of fat and other nutritional substances. Multiple nutritional abnormalities may result in theses cases.

In the intestine, CF leads to the migration of water out of the intestinal lumen with inspissation of meconium

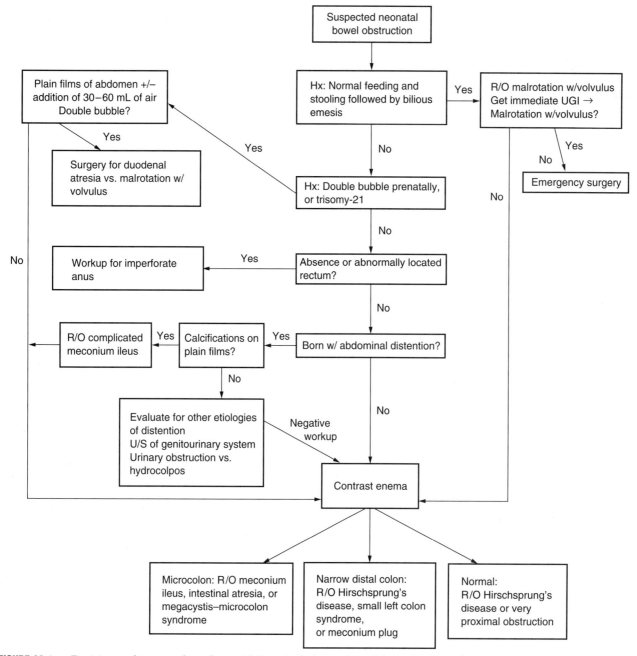

FIGURE 62-1 ■ Decision-making tree for infants with intestinal obstruction with emphasis on obstruction. See text for explanation.

and subsequent obturation obstruction. Diagnosis of CF should be pursued in all children who present with meconium ileus, meconium plug syndrome, rectal prolapse, jejunal/ileal atresias, nasal polyps, neonatal jaundice, portal hypertension, failure to thrive, and pancreatitis.

The diagnosis of CF may be made using a variety of tests. Because it is not possible to test for all of the hundreds of genetic mutations, many approaches are used. Newborns may be tested with a dried blood spot for immunoreactive trypsinogen. This test has a high sensitivity, but a high false-positive rate, which demands that additional testing be performed. Sweat chloride testing (positive if >60 mEq/L) is accurate, and most patients should undergo this test. Only 1% to 4% of CF patients

have a normal test, but the test depends on the ability to collect sufficient quantities of sweat (at least 100 mg obtained after maximal stimulation by pilocarpine iontophoresis), which may be difficult in neonates. Genetic testing is used increasingly. Commercial tests typically examine DNA for 25 to 100 of the most common mutations (95% of all CF patients). Genetic analysis for identifying heterozygotes or for detecting CF in utero has been described, which, although helpful, has ethical considerations.

Pathophysiology of Meconium Ileus

Because the small intestinal mucus glands produce overly thick secretions even in utero, the meconium formed by

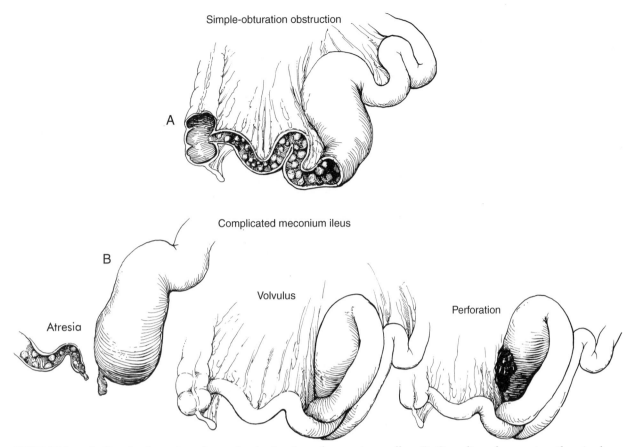

Simple-obturation obstruction

Complicated meconium ileus

FIGURE 62-2 ■ **A,** Simple obturation obstruction by inspissated meconium pellets. **B,** Complicated meconium ileus in three forms: atresia, volvulus, and perforation.

these infants is abnormally viscid, sticky, and adherent. Characteristically in meconium ileus, the proximal ileum is greatly dilated and contains thick, sticky meconium, whereas the distal ileum and colon are collapsed and obstructed by thickly packed, round, mucus plugs that resemble rabbit pellets (Fig. 62-2A). Infants born with this form of the disease have so-called simple meconium ileus or simple obturation obstruction of the intestine. In utero, this may progress, however, to complicated meconium ileus. In such a process, the massively dilated proximal intestine volvulizes or perforates (Fig. 62-2B). If this occurs early in gestation, one or more atresias may be produced. If volvulus of the redundant ileum occurs late in gestation, infants may present with perforation with either free or encysted meconium peritonitis. Each of these presentations has different clinical, radiographic, and therapeutic considerations. Rarely the proximal and distal portions of the volvulized limbs may reanastomose and manifest themselves as ileal stenosis.

Diagnosis

Intestinal obstruction in infants with meconium ileus is generally evident within 24 to 48 hours after birth. Although a family history of CF is helpful, it is present only in 20% of patients. In approximately 20% of patients, particularly patients with complicated meconium ileus, there is a history of maternal polyhydramnios. Although meconium ileus is uncommon in premature infants,

many are dysmature or small for gestational age. Associated congenital malformations are uncommon.

With meconium ileus, three cardinal signs of intestinal obstruction are generally evident: (1) generalized abdominal distention, (2) bilious vomiting, and (3) failure to pass meconium within 48 hours. At times, it is possible to feel a dilated intestinal loop filled with meconium. With complicated meconium ileus, patients generally present either at or shortly after birth because of severe abdominal distention that often is associated with respiratory distress. At times, the abdominal wall is red and inflamed. Progressive hypovolemia may lead to cardiovascular instability, and these infants appear extremely ill. Plain radiographs of the abdomen may be diagnostic. In patients with simple obturation obstruction, the characteristic radiographic features include varying-sized loops of distended intestine, a relative absence of air-fluid levels, and a "soap bubble" appearance of portions of the abdomen (Neuhauser's sign), particularly the right lower quadrant (Fig. 62-3A). Other disorders that may share some of these radiographic findings include Hirschsprung's disease, ileal atresia, and meconium plug syndrome.

Complicated meconium ileus is suggested on plain film of the abdomen when areas of calcification are seen or when there is a large dense mass with a rim of calcification evident, suggesting cystic meconium peritonitis. The development of intraperitoneal calcification may occur within 4 days after perforation of the intestine.

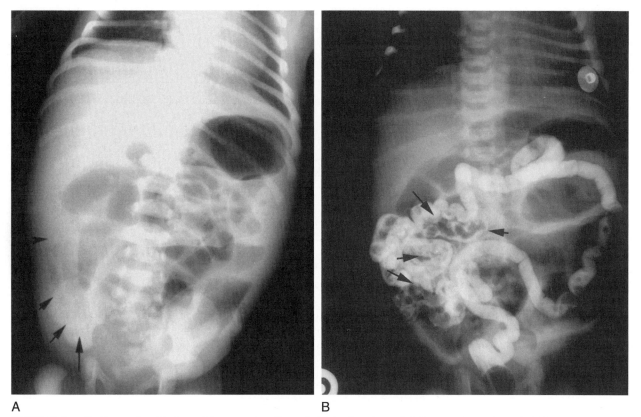

A   B

FIGURE 62-3 ■ Radiographs of infant with meconium ileus. **A,** Plain flat plate of abdomen. Note "soap bubble" appearance in right lower quadrant (arrows) and poorly defined air-fluid pattern. **B,** Contrast enema with microcolon and inspissated meconium in the terminal ileum (arrows).

Liberated lipases and bile salts cause an intense chemical peritonitis and production of soaps, which lead to the deposition of calcium in the peritoneal cavity and within the wall of the intestine. This process may leave the child with a massive pseudocyst formation with diffuse meconium peritonitis. When simple meconium ileus is suspected, a contrast enema study should be performed. The classic finding is a microcolon filled with pellet-like meconium when contrast material is refluxed into the terminal ileum (Fig. 62-3B). In general, it is best to use a nearly iso-osmolar water-soluble contrast material; if the appearance suggests meconium ileus, this material is evacuated and replaced with a water-soluble contrast material of higher osmolarity because efforts then may be used to wash out the obstructing plugs and inspissated meconium. In patients with complicated meconium ileus, a contrast enema study is used primarily to confirm the diagnosis and to determine the position of the colon. In patients with complicated meconium ileus, a contrast enema study is not required before laparotomy because the plain films are often diagnostic. After relief of intestinal obstruction, the diagnosis of CF should be verified.

Treatment

Simple Meconium Ileus

Noblett described a method for washing out obstructing plugs in patients with meconium ileus of an uncomplicated nature. With this method, soluble contrast material, such as diatrizoate meglumine (Gastrografin), is used. Regardless of the contrast material used, it must be water soluble to help loosen the inspissated pellets of meconium. Additionally, water-soluble agents are much safer than barium in case a perforation occurs during the study, which always should be done with fluoroscopic control. Undiluted diatrizoate meglumine has a strikingly high osmolarity (2150 mOsm); this may result in serious fluid derangements. Dilute diatrizoate meglumine, Hypaque (1450 mOsm), and iothalamate meglumine (Cysto-Conray II) (404 mOsm) are being used increasingly. The following criteria must be met before attempting contrast enema management of uncomplicated meconium ileus. The preliminary diagnostic study should have excluded other causes of distal intestinal obstruction, and there should not be any clinical or radiographic signs of complicated meconium ileus. The patient first must have correction of fluid and electrolyte abnormalities. Patients should be given 10 mL/kg boluses of isotonic saline and continued at 1.5 times maintenance fluid rates for at least 8 to 12 hours after the study monitoring urine output. Broad-spectrum antibiotics should be administered, and a nasogastric tube should be passed. Undue pressure must not be used during the procedure, but it may be repeated two or three times over 24 hours, provided that the patient does not show any signs of physiologic deterioration. Otherwise, surgery should be undertaken. Continuing attention to fluid and electrolyte and acid-base balance is mandatory in patients who are being managed in this fashion. Approximately 30% of patients with simple meconium ileus may be managed this way, but the success rate varies widely in reported series. The remainder require operative management.

In simple meconium ileus, the goal of surgery is to evacuate completely the obstructing plugs and meconium from the ileum proximal and distal to the point of obstruction. One method that may be used is to irrigate the intestine and colon clear of plugs of obstructing meconium via an enterotomy in the dilated segment of ileum, which may be closed or brought out as a tube enterostomy. Many surgeons use this approach today. At times, intestinal resection and primary anastomosis may be needed, provided that all of the plugs can be washed out of the distal ileum and colon. An alternative method in patients in whom the distal bowel cannot be cleared or whose condition is precarious is the formation of an ostomy, with a secondary closure when respiratory and nutritional factors are stabilized. Historically a Mikulicz or Bishop-Koop procedure has been advocated. This consists of a Roux-en-Y anastomosis between the end of the dilated proximal segment and the side of the collapsed distal segment approximately 4 cm from the distal open end, which is brought out as an ileostomy (Fig. 62-4). Some surgeons use double-barreled stomas. The distal ostomy provides an opportunity for catheter placement and irrigation of distal obstructing plugs. Although cumbersome, one can place a tube into the distal stoma and introduce gastrointestinal effluent from the proximal stoma.

The Santulli procedure (Fig. 62-4, opposite configuration to a Bishop-Koop) is another approach to the formation of a decompressing stoma but is rarely used. All of the exteriorization procedures may require early closure of the ostomy because of excessive fluid loss except for the Bishop-Koop procedure, which closes on its own 20% of the time.

Complicated Meconium Ileus

By definition, complicated meconium ileus indicates that the infant has intestinal atresia or perforation with varying degrees of meconium peritonitis. Under these circumstances, the findings at operation dictate what should be done. Adhesions are lysed, and inflammatory membranes are decorticated sufficiently to permit identification of enough of the intestine to manage the pathology. These patients require careful preoperative and intraoperative management to replace fluid and blood loss. Necrotic and atretic intestine should be resected, then it is generally best to perform an exteriorization using double-barreled enterostomies. In rare instances, the adhesions are so dense that anatomy cannot be discerned enough to perform a stoma. In these cases, peritoneal drainage tubes can be placed to allow passage of meconium, until the inflammatory process subsides after a couple of months.

Postoperatively, careful attention must be given to fluid and electrolyte and acid-base balance initially and management of pulmonary complications, such as atelectasis and infection. These patients also require careful nutritional management, balancing intravenous and

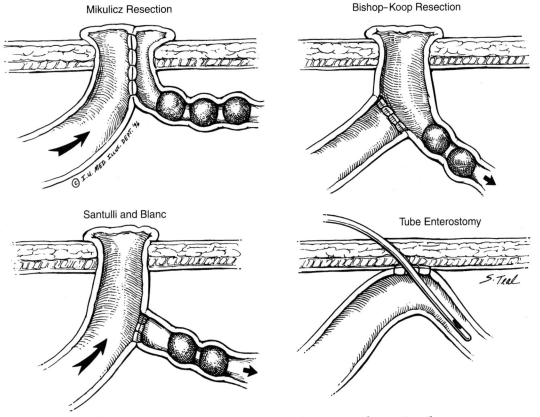

FIGURE 62-4 ■ Operative options for surgical treatment of meconium ileus.

enteral nutrition. Because of pancreatic insufficiency, supplemental pancreatic enzymes and lipid-soluble vitamins are required. Because of varying degrees of protein, fat, and carbohydrate malabsorption, special formulas such as Pregestimil that contain hydrolyzed casein and medium-chain triglyceride oil are generally best. Finally, patients with small bowel stomas may lose large amounts of zinc, magnesium, bicarbonate, and sodium. Monitoring and replacement of these deficiencies are essential. Spot urine sodium checks should be performed because the finding of a urine sodium less than 10 mEq indicates total body sodium depletion. Failure to thrive occurs unless these patients receive sodium supplementation.

Complications

In addition to periodic atelectasis and pulmonary infection, many patients have gastrointestinal complications, including malabsorption, biliary obstruction from inspissated bile, and adhesive intestinal obstruction. In older children who do not comply with enzyme supplementation, a meconium ileus–like picture that has been termed *meconium ileus equivalent* may occur that affects approximately 10% of CF patients. The clinical picture is identical to that of simple meconium ileus in newborns, and meglumine diatriazoate enemas are usually sufficient for relief. Additional pancreatic enzyme supplementation then is provided. These patients also benefit from polyethylene glycol–based oral agents. In the mid-1990s, the use of high concentrations of pancreatic enzymes (mean dose 19,000 U/kg/day) resulted in the development of colonic stricturing in many CF patients that required resection so that appropriate caution is in order.

Results and Outlook

In more recent years, survival has improved, with current operative mortality being 10% to 20%. The long-term outlook is the same as for all patients with CF, in whom the average life expectancy is now in the range of 32 years (based on 1998 statistics). Lung transplantation has become a promising option for selected patients with end-stage pulmonary disease related to CF.

MECONIUM PLUG AND NEONATAL SMALL LEFT COLON SYNDROMES

Although meconium plug and neonatal small left colon syndromes are considered clinically distinct entities, they share sufficient similarities to be discussed together (Fig. 62-5). The basic pathophysiology is that of transient neonatal colonic obstruction most likely due to hypomotility. The principles of diagnosis and management are similar. The important distinction in the recognition of these syndromes is that they are associated with colonic obstruction, as differentiated from the picture seen with meconium ileus, in which the small bowel is involved. Although emphasis previously has been placed on the theory that meconium plug and small left colon syndromes result from obturation obstruction of the colon by abnormal meconium, it is more likely that these disorders result from transient motility disorders of the distal colon related to immaturity.

Diagnosis

These infants present with significant degrees of abdominal distention, bile-stained vomitus, and failure to pass any stool during the first 1 to 2 days of life. In more than 50% of patients with small left colon syndrome, there is a maternal history of diabetes. Plain films of the abdomen show massive intestinal distention with air-fluid levels. Contrast enemas characteristically show a dilated colon proximal to a tapered transition zone at varying levels with meconium plug syndrome and characteristically at the splenic flexure in neonatal small left colon syndrome. Contrast enema suggests Hirschsprung's disease, but characteristically these patients typically improve after the contrast enema, particularly if water-soluble contrast material is used. Occasionally the enema may need to be repeated.

Treatment

Ordinarily, soluble contrast enemas relieve patients with either of these disorders. Surgery rarely is required except in unusual instances in which perforation may have occurred. In infants of diabetic mothers, appropriate perinatal management of hypoglycemia may be necessary. Because the clinical and radiographic picture is similar to that of Hirschsprung's disease, suction biopsy of the rectum may be required to rule it out. Provided that the infant does not have Hirschsprung's disease, there are no long-term complications. CF initially may manifest itself with a meconium plug, so work-up for CF should be performed in infants with this condition.

FOREIGN BODIES AND BEZOARS

A form of obturation obstruction related to foreign material occasionally seen in the perinatal period is that caused by milk curds. The cause of this particular disorder is not known but is presumed to be some sort of malabsorptive state. The clinical picture is similar to meconium plug syndrome or meconium ileus.

Ingestion of foreign bodies is a problem because of the tendency for small children to put everything into their mouths. There may or may not be history of ingestion of a foreign body. If a foreign body does not become impacted in the C-loop of the duodenum or at the ligament of Treitz, it ordinarily passes through the intestinal tract but occasionally may become impacted in a Meckel's diverticulum, the ileocecal valve, or the appendix. A foreign body that perforates the intestine may produce secondary obstruction, and sometimes bleeding occurs.

Bezoars are of many types. Trichobezoars usually are seen in mentally retarded or emotionally disturbed patients. Most patients with bezoars of their own hair are teenage girls. The presentation is one of intestinal obstruction. Plain films of the abdomen, sometimes supplemented by upper gastrointestinal contrast studies with small bowel follow-through, are usually diagnostic. Trichobezoars ordinarily obstruct the stomach, duodenum, and upper jejunum. Phytobezoars of vegetable matter usually obstruct the distal ileum, but also may obstruct the stomach, particularly after vagotomy. Phytobezoars in the

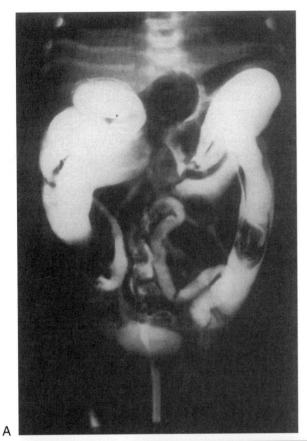

A

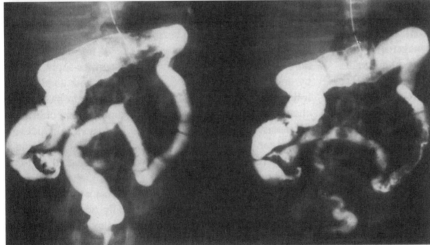

B

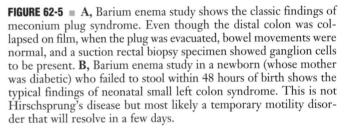

FIGURE 62-5 ■ **A,** Barium enema study shows the classic findings of meconium plug syndrome. Even though the distal colon was collapsed on film, when the plug was evacuated, bowel movements were normal, and a suction rectal biopsy specimen showed ganglion cells to be present. **B,** Barium enema study in a newborn (whose mother was diabetic) who failed to stool within 48 hours of birth shows the typical findings of neonatal small left colon syndrome. This is not Hirschsprung's disease but most likely a temporary motility disorder that will resolve in a few days.

stomach may be broken apart endoscopically. This process may be facilitated by introduction of pancreatic enzymes. Concretions related to use of sodium polystyrene sulfonate (Kayexalate), cholestyramine, or calcium-containing antacids in patients with head trauma being treated with hypothermia usually obstruct the distal intestine and colon. At times a distinct mass can be felt on abdominal examination of the patients even though there is distention.

Trichobezoars that become obstructive must be treated operatively by gastrotomy or enterotomy and removal of the hair. Care must be taken to remove the entire bezoar because this can fragment on removal and be lodged more distally in the small bowel. In instances of obstructing plugs from other causes, if they cannot be dislodged by enema lavage, operative removal by enterotomy generally is required. Colostomy may be needed in patients with colonic obstruction.

Another form of obstruction is caused by parasites, which generally obstruct the mid and distal small bowel. Ascaris lumbricoides is the most common parasite involved. If the obstruction cannot be relieved by the administration of antihelminthic agents, operative enterotomy may be required.

The long-term outlook is generally good, provided that the underlying disorder that resulted in formation of the bezoar is managed appropriately. Psychosocial issues often need to be addressed in children with trichobezoars to prevent reoccurrence.

SUGGESTED READINGS

Berdon WE, Slovis TL, Campbell JB: Neonatal small left colon syndrome: Its relationship to aganglionosis and meconium plug syndrome. Radiology 125:457-462, 1977.

This article emphasizes the occasional association of small left colon syndrome and Hirschsprung's disease.

DelPin CA, Czyrko C, Ziegler MM, et al: Management and survival of meconium ileus, a 30 year review. Ann Surg 215:179, 1992.

This 30-year review provides a valuable follow-up of the extensive experience of Bishop and Koop.

FitzSimmons SC, Burkhart GA, Borowitz Grand RJ, et al: High-dose pancreatic-enzyme supplements and fibrosing colonopathy in children with cystic fibrosis. N Engl J Med 336:1283–1289, 1997.

This is an excellent review of the development of fibrotic stricturing of the colon in CF patients receiving high-dose pancreatic enzymes.

Noblett HR: Treatment of uncomplicated meconium ileus by Gastrografin enema: A preliminary report. J Pediatr Surg 4:190, 1969.

This article contains the original description of the nonoperative approach to uncomplicated meconium ileus that is also applicable to other forms of obturation obstruction of the intestine.

Rescorla FJ, Grosfeld JL: Contemporary management of meconium ileus. World J Surg 17:318-323, 1993.

This is an excellent contemporary view of overall management of infants with CF complicated by meconium ileus.

Rosenstein BJ, Zeitlin PL: Cystic fibrosis (seminar). Lancet 851:277-282, 1998.

An excellent review of CF is provided, including pathophysiology.

PART IX

Liver, Biliary Tract, Pancreas, and Spleen

Benign Liver Tumors and Other Hepatocellular Disorders

Benign hepatic cysts and tumors account for approximately one third of all hepatic neoplasms in childhood. In 1975, members of the Surgical Section of the American Academy of Pediatrics reported the largest compiled series of benign liver tumors in childhood (Table 63-1). The three main categories of benign liver tumors are (1) congenital cysts; (2) solid tumors, including adenomas, hamartomas, and pseudotumors such as focal nodular hyperplasia; and (3) vascular lesions, including hemangiomas, hemangioendotheliomas, and lymphangiomas.

Abdominal enlargement and an abdominal mass, often poorly defined, signal the presence of a benign liver tumor. The appearance of other symptoms, including a sense of fullness, satiety, and abdominal pain, depends on the degree and rapidity of enlargement. An acute abdominal crisis, with severe pain and hypotension, suggests rupture of the tumor with intraperitoneal hemorrhage. A vascular malformation may cause hepatic enlargement and congestive heart failure and produce a bruit audible on auscultation. Discovery of a liver tumor requires expeditious evaluation because of the risk of malignancy. Abdominal radiographs, ultrasound, computed tomography (CT), magnetic resonance imaging, and angiography provide information regarding the size of the lesion, its anatomic position within the segmental anatomy of the liver, whether the lesion is cystic or solid, and the arterial anatomy of the liver.

CONGENITAL CYSTS

Congenital cysts of the liver in infancy and childhood may be classified into cystic mesenchymal hamartomas and nonparasitic cysts. Although mesenchymomas and teratomas may have cystic components, they are basically solid tumors. Table 63-2 lists a complete classification of cysts of the liver.

Nonparasitic cysts tend to be solitary and may vary in diameter from a few centimeters to the size of a grapefruit. Approximately 10% of cysts are unilocular. Liver cysts are three to four times more prevalent in females and are more frequent in white children. The location may vary considerably, but most occur on the inferior aspect of the right lobe. Occasionally a cyst may lie completely within the hepatic parenchyma. Most grow slowly and remain asymptomatic until discovered incidentally during a radiographic evaluation for another condition or during surgery.

Often congenital cysts of the liver are large enough to be detected on physical examination. Ultrasound distinguishes cysts from solid tumors (Fig. 63-1). Usually asymptomatic, cysts may cause symptoms by compressing adjacent viscera. Hemorrhage, perforation, and torsion occur rarely. Cuboidal epithelium, probably of biliary origin, lines the cyst. Cysts may be simple or loculated. Cysts contain clear serous fluid and only rarely communicate with the biliary tree. Current theory asserts that accessory foregut buds are the source of epidermoid cysts.

TABLE 63-1 ▪ Benign Liver Tumors in Childhood	
Tumors	**No. of Patients**
Hemangioma	54
Cavernous	38
Hemangioendothelioma	16
Hamartoma	37
Cysts	16
Simple	10
Hydatid	6
Adenoma	7
Focal nodular hyperplasia	5
Lymphangioma	2
Eosinophilic granuloma	1

From Exelby PR, Filler RM, Grosfeld JL: Liver tumors in children. American Academy of Pediatrics Surgical Section Survey, 1974. J Pediatr Surg 10:329, 1975.

TABLE 63-2 ▪ Cysts of the Liver
Congenital
Solitary unilocular cysts
Polycystic disease
Cystic dilation of common bile duct
Parasitic
Traumatic
Inflammatory

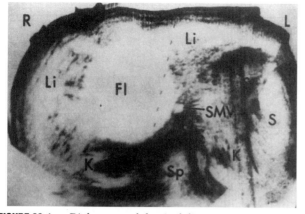

FIGURE 63-1 ■ Right upper abdominal discrete mass in a 3-year-old girl with a congenital cyst of the right lobe of the liver.

The size and location of a solitary cyst dictate treatment options. Operative cholangiography determines where the cyst lies relative to the bile ducts and whether a biliary communication exists. Adjacent major bile ducts and vascular structures may make complete excision of the cyst difficult. Wedge resection or lobectomy may be appropriate options. Internal drainage to a Roux-en-Y limb of jejunum may be the most appropriate option for a large cyst that involves both hepatic lobes. Cysts exposed on the surface of the liver may be completely unroofed and the edges secured with a running absorbable suture. Without a biliary communication, the peritoneum absorbs the small amount of serous drainage. The latter procedure lends itself to video-assisted laparoscopic techniques.

Polycystic disease of the liver is an inherited defect of unknown etiology. Of affected patients, 50% also have polycystic kidneys. Replacement of hepatic parenchyma by cysts generally does not affect liver function until late in the course of disease. No treatment is necessary, unless a large dominant cyst produces symptoms. The dominant cyst undergoes treatment as described for a solitary cyst. When extensive cystic replacement results in hepatic failure (Fig. 63-2), hepatic transplantation may be the sole option.

HEPATIC ADENOMA

Hepatic adenoma is a rare tumor that most commonly affects teenage girls. Glycogen storage disease type I (von Gierke's disease) often accompanies the lesion. The tumor, benign, encapsulated, but highly vascular, usually lies in the right lobe. Imaging studies may reveal large feeding vessels. Infarction and rupture of the tumor cause intraperitoneal hemorrhage and an acute abdominal crisis in one fourth of cases. The tumor has a homogeneous brown parenchyma but no discernible portal structures. Nearly all tumors comprise well-differentiated hepatocytes, but some series report finding areas of dysplasia and hepatocellular carcinoma. Whether the lesion is premalignant is a matter of debate.

Wedge resection or lobectomy with complete resection is appropriate therapy for symptomatic tumors, tumors in which malignancy cannot be ruled out, and large asymptomatic tumors (>5 cm in diameter) to reduce the risk of rupture and malignant degeneration. Recurrence after resection is uncommon. Some authors advocate a nonoperative strategy for small biopsy-proven adenomas that do not cause symptoms.

MESENCHYMAL HAMARTOMA

Mesenchymal hamartoma is a large benign mass composed of multiple cysts of varying size filled with clear liquid or mucoid material and occasional old hemorrhage. Connective tissue stroma combined with bile ducts, liver cells, and angiomatous components characterize this lesion. Approximately 80% are detected in the first year of life. Abdominal radiographs show a soft tissue mass. Ultrasound or CT confirms its cystic architecture. The degree of vascularity varies. When prominent, blood flow through the lesion may precipitate congestive heart failure from arteriovenous shunting. Histopathologic distinction from hemangiomas of the liver may be difficult. Resection is the treatment of choice.

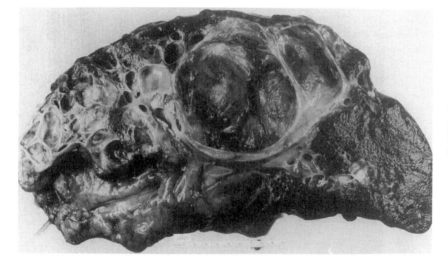

FIGURE 63-2 ■ Transected liver from a patient with severe polycystic disease of the liver. This child also had polycystic renal disease and died as a result of renal failure.

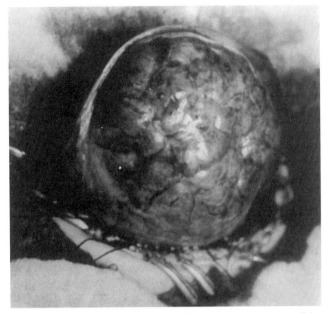

FIGURE 63-3 ■ Focal nodular hyperplasia in the right lobe of the liver in a 1-year-old boy. The large veins coursing over the surface are characteristic of focal nodular hyperplasia. The mass was excised with a wedge resection.

Internal drainage by Roux-en-Y cyst-jejunostomy is a possible approach for large, predominantly cystic lesions that are unresectable. Marsupialization of a cyst into the free peritoneal cavity is another alternative.

FOCAL NODULAR HYPERPLASIA

The cause of focal nodular hyperplasia is obscure. Some believe the lesion arises as a response to a localized injury or infarction or to arterialization by an anomalous artery. The tumor occurs in all age groups, with children younger than age 6 years having been reported. At the time of presentation, most of these lesions are palpable. Torsion of a pedunculated mass may cause pain. Focal nodular hyperplasia is another mass that can rupture and cause intraperitoneal bleeding. Ultrasound or CT shows a solid vascular hepatic mass. With large veins coursing over its surface, focal nodular hyperplasia may resemble a hepatoblastoma, but the tumor is always benign (Fig. 63-3). The cut surface has nodules with central areas of fibrosis. Microscopic examination shows micronodular cirrhosis and hyperplastic regenerative nodules. A preliminary biopsy and frozen section examination avoids an unnecessarily major resection when a more localized resection would be curative.

HEPATIC VASCULAR ANOMALIES

Vascular anomalies of the liver fall into two groups: hemangiomas (90% of all hepatic vascular anomalies) and arteriovenous malformations (10%). The liver is the most common visceral site for hemangiomas. Hemangiomas may be solitary or multiple. Solitary lesions tend to be large when discovered and localized to one lobe, generally the right. Of patients, 20% have lesions in both lobes.

When multiple, cutaneous lesions are present in more than 80%. Large solitary lesions and multiple lesions may have sufficient arteriovenous shunting to cause congestive heart failure. The lesions usually are detected in infancy and generally no later than the third year of life (Fig. 63-4). Hepatic hemangiomas occur at all ages, however, including the fetus. Arteriovenous malformations of the liver are less common and may be indistinguishable from a solitary hemangioma on radiographic evaluation. Arteriovenous shunting also may be sufficient to cause congestive heart failure.

Solitary tumors have a tan, spongy, and smooth outer surface with well-demarcated borders. One to several layers of endothelium line vascular channels separated by pale, myxoid-appearing connective tissue containing fibroblasts and a few smooth muscle cells. Areas may show inflammation, thrombosis, hemorrhage, fibrosis, necrosis, and interstitial calcification. Multiple hemangiomas produce nodules over the entire liver surface. The nodules are red to violet centrally and whitish gray over their surfaces. Arteriovenous connections may cause the nodules to pulsate.

Hepatic hemangiomas have the same natural history of proliferation followed by involution seen in cutaneous hemangiomas. Severely affected infants develop hepatomegaly, anemia, and high-output cardiac failure. In extreme cases, the liver may enlarge to the point of causing respiratory failure and abdominal compartment syndrome.

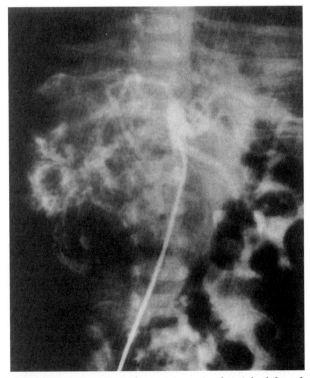

FIGURE 63-4 ■ Cavernous hemangioma in the right lobe of a 4-month-old infant with a bruit over the liver. Selective angiogram shows the right hepatic artery arising from the superior mesenteric artery supplying a large circumscribed mass. Diffuse vascular blushes indicate the presence of extensive arteriovenous communications. Gradual involution of the tumor was monitored by ultrasound over 3 years.

High flow through the lesion may cause a systolic bruit in the epigastrium. Jaundice is rare. Platelets may become trapped within the vascular channels, resulting in thrombocytopenia. Some tumors express type 3 iodothyronine deiodinase, which inactivates circulating thyroid hormone and causes clinical hypothyroidism in some patients. Achieving a euthyroid state may require extremely large doses of hormone replacement. Hepatic hemangiomas have a typical appearance on CT with intravenous contrast material, with an initial arterial blush that evolves into a pattern of multiple areas of pooling during the venous phase. A definitive CT diagnosis obviates biopsy, a hazardous procedure because of the risk of uncontrollable hemorrhage. When detected on fetal ultrasound, the fetus may have hepatomegaly, cardiomegaly, and hydrops.

The clinical spectrum ranges from asymptomatic to rapidly progressive lesions that cause congestive heart failure, respiratory failure, abdominal compartment syndrome, and death. Some no doubt remain asymptomatic and involute without therapy. Small asymptomatic lesions found in the course of work-up for other conditions may be followed with sequential examinations and ultrasound. Treatment addresses larger lesions or lesions causing heart failure. Symptomatic patients require aggressive therapy because mortality approaches 50% in the 2 weeks after onset of sustained heart failure. Digitalis and diuretics may improve a few patients with heart failure. Systemic corticosteroids provide initial therapy for severely affected infants. Patients who do not respond to steroids should receive cyclophosphamide or interferon alfa-2a, a cytokine that directly counteracts the abnormal level of angiogenesis present in the lesions. Lesions that are refractory to pharmacologic intervention may regress with hepatic artery ligation, but hepatic angiography helps guide therapeutic embolization of all feeding vessels, an intervention that has the best chance of success if direct macrovascular shunts can be shown. Irradiation has not been helpful and currently is rarely used. Solitary lesions and arteriovenous malformations confined to a single hepatic lobe undergo resection if all pharmacologic options become exhausted. Transplantation is the sole option for patients in whom partial hepatectomy is not technically feasible.

CHRONIC GRANULOMATOUS HEPATIC DISEASE

Before the discovery and introduction of antibiotics in modern medical practice, hepatic abscess sometimes formed after perforated appendicitis. Today these complications are extremely rare. Currently, chronic granulomatous disease (CGD) of childhood is the principal condition associated with the development of hepatic abscess. Genetically deficient, circulating neutrophils lack bacteria-killing mechanisms that predispose the patient to chronic, recurrent bacterial infections. Recurrent episodes of lymphadenitis, eczema, pneumonia, and perirectal abscesses occur in affected patients in the first months of infancy. Patients develop hepatosplenomegaly. Failure of normal bactericidal function leads to granulomatous reaction and suppuration. Host tissues become infiltrated with large numbers of neutrophils, mononuclear cells, and histiocytes. Abscesses may form in regional nodes (frequently in the neck and axilla), soft tissues, lung, and liver. Of all pyogenic liver abscesses, 40% occur in children with CGD, whereas 30% have a defect of host defense, most commonly acute leukemia. Other causes are umbilical vein catheterization, omphalitis, sickle cell disease, and biliary tract operations. Hepatic abscesses in uncompromised children are uncommon, so occurrence in an otherwise normal child should prompt an immune work-up.

Culture specimens from hepatic abscesses most often grow *Staphylococcus aureus*, *Streptococcus pyogenes*, and *Escherichia coli*. Anaerobic organisms are more likely to arise from cryptogenic abscesses. Culture and sensitivity analyses from abscess specimens should guide the selection of appropriate antibiotics. Interferon-γ has been used to reduce the incidence and severity of infections in children with CGD and may be effective as adjunctive therapy in liver abscess. Prompt abscess drainage is essential for controlling infection. CT-guided or ultrasound-guided catheter drainage is satisfactory in most cases, although some patients need open surgical drainage. With effective drainage and modern antibiotic therapy, mortality for children with pyogenic hepatic abscesses has been reduced to less than 25%.

AMEBIC HEPATIC INFECTION

Entamoeba histolytica causes ulcerative lesions in the colon. Trophozoites from colonic lesions reach the liver through the portal circulation. Most authorities believe that most amebic infections of the liver resolve completely without treatment. The infection may cause thrombosis and liver cell injury, forming a locus from which an abscess may arise. Abscesses arise when large numbers of organisms overwhelm local defenses or host resistance is deficient, such as in immunocompromised patients or patients on long-term steroid therapy. Most pediatric cases occur during infancy. Uncommon in the United States, this condition is endemic in Latin America, much of Asia, and South Africa.

Low-grade fever, malaise, and right upper quadrant tenderness characterize the course of amebic abscess. Pleural effusion is common. Serology or immunoelectrophoresis tests are available to detect an amebic infection. The abscess usually lies in the right lobe. Ultrasonography, CT, and magnetic resonance imaging all can identify the lesion. There is a 10% risk of rupture, so there is some urgency in work-up and drainage. Before drainage, investigations must exclude hydatid disease because the approach to therapy differs.

Metronidazole is the most effective antibiotic against amebic infection, with a dramatic therapeutic response often occurring within a few days of institution. Small cysts (<7 cm in diameter) nearly always resolve on metronidazole without drainage. Closed aspiration of cyst contents under radiographic guidance is the preferred method of treating large lesions and lesions that do not respond to antibiotic therapy. Aspiration yields thick sterile fluid and may collapse the cyst entirely. Repeated percutaneous aspiration may be required.

Alternatively, radiographically guided catheter drainage may be required to treat abscesses that resist antibiotics and cyst aspiration. Open surgical drainage is unnecessary. Prevention of secondary infection by pyogenic organisms is an important aim.

HYDATID DISEASE

The larval stage of *Echinococcus multilocularis*, a microscopic tapeworm found in foxes, coyotes, dogs, and cats, causes hydatid disease in humans. Parasitic tumors form in the liver, lung, and brain. Untreated, it is uniformly fatal. Hydatid disease has a worldwide distribution, but mid-Northern latitudes are the source of most cases: central Europe, Russia, China, Central Asia, Japan, and North America. Human cases in North America, distinctly uncommon, have been reported in Alaska, Manitoba, and Minnesota. Infection may cause fever and toxicity. Imaging studies reveal calcified cysts and "daughter" cysts within and along the margin of dominant cysts. A positive Casoni's skin test confirms the presence of hydatid infection.

Cyst fluid is generally under tension. Daughter cysts may escape into the peritoneal cavity from cyst rupture or during attempts at cyst drainage or aspiration. The risk of intra-abdominal recurrence is high. To minimize this possibility the cyst first is aspirated under radiographic guidance of about one half of its estimated volume. The injection of 20% saline, 96% alcohol, or aqueous iodine into the cyst kills embryos within the cyst. After 5 to 15 minutes, reaspiration completely drains cyst fluid. Most cysts shrink to 22% to 64% of the initial volume, facilitating later resection. Patients receive the antihelminthic antibiotic albendazole for 1 week before percutaneous treatment and for 3 to 6 months thereafter.

SUGGESTED READINGS

Boon LM, Burrows PE, Paltiel HJ, et al: Hepatic vascular anomalies in infancy: A twenty-seven-year experience. J Pediatr 129:346-354, 1996.

This report from the Children's Hospital in Boston, leaders in this field, describes the diagnosis and treatment of infantile hemangiomas and arteriovenous malformations of the liver and early results using interferon alfa-2a in the treatment of refractory hemangiomas.

Daller JA, Bueno J, Gutierrez J, et al: Hepatic hemangioendothelioma: Clinical experience and management strategy. J Pediatr Surg 34:95-105, 1999.

The authors, from the Children's Hospital of Pittsburgh transplantation service, discuss their experience with surgical resection and transplantation for patients who do not respond to pharmacologic treatment of symptomatic hemangiomas.

Kabaalioglu A, Karaali K, Apaydin A, et al: Ultrasound-guided percutaneous sclerotherapy of hydatid liver cysts in children. Pediatr Surg Int 16:346-350, 2000.

In this report from Turkey, the authors describe their protocol for sclerotherapy in the treatment of hydatid liver cysts.

Kumar A, Srinivasan S, Sharma AK: Pyogenic abscesses in children—South Indian experiences. J Pediatr Surg 33:417-421, 1998.

Although their clinical population reflects community-acquired pyogenic liver abscesses and is unique, the authors document resolution of most (10 of 18) cases of pyogenic liver abscesses with antibiotic therapy alone, without aspiration or drainage, over 10 to 40 days.

Meyers RL, Scaife ER: Benign liver and biliary tract masses in infants and children. Semin Pediatr Surg 9:146-155, 2000.

This article discusses the work-up and radiographic findings of benign tumors and cysts of the liver.

Moazam F, Nazir Z: Amebic liver abscess: Spare the knife but save the child. J Pediatr Surg 33:119-122, 1998.

The senior author, one of the leading pediatric surgeons in Pakistan, describes her colleagues' and her approach to amebic abscess in children. Parenteral metronidazole combined with timely aspiration of the abscess in selected cases obviates the need for open surgical intervention.

Terkivatan T, de Wilt JH, de Man RA, et al: Indications and long-term outcome of treatment for benign hepatic tumors: A critical reappraisal. Arch Surg 136:1033-1038, 2001.

From their large series of 208 children and adults with adenoma, focal nodular hyperplasia, and hemangioma, the authors conclude that surgery is necessary only to exclude malignancy, if the lesion causes severe symptoms, or in adenomas measuring more than 5 cm in diameter to reduce the risk of rupture and malignant degeneration.

64

Biliary Atresia and Liver Transplantation

BILIARY ATRESIA

Biliary atresia is a disorder of infants in which an obliteration or discontinuity of the biliary ducts obstructs bile flow. Formerly, it was believed that intrahepatic ductal atresia could be identified as an anomaly separate from extrahepatic ductal atresia and that the two occasionally occurred in combination. The current belief is that these infants have the same basic pathophysiologic process involving the entire biliary ductal system to varying degrees.

The incidence is approximately 1 in 15,000 live births. Biliary atresia is slightly more common in girls (female-to-male ratio of 1.7). Approximately 10% of infants have an associated congenital heart defect.

Embryology

The biliary ductal system originates from the hepatic diverticulum of the foregut at 4 weeks' gestation and differentiates into caudal and cranial components.

The gallbladder, cystic duct, and common bile duct derive from the caudal component, and the proximal extrahepatic ducts derive from the cranial component. Although considerable variation may occur, the three most common anatomic manifestations of biliary atresia tend to follow this embryonic pattern (Fig. 64-1). First, the distal ducts (from caudal component) may obliterate, leaving patent proximal extrahepatic ducts above the level of the cystic duct–common duct junction (6% of cases). Second, the proximal ducts (from the cranial component) may obliterate and leave a patent gallbladder, cystic duct, and common duct below the junction (11%). In the third variation, which is the most common (83%), the entire ductal system is obstructed. Cystic malformations also may occur.

Other important events in organogenesis occur during this time, including formation of the inferior vena cava and portal vein, the beginning of intestinal rotation, and formation of the spleen. Approximately 13% of infants with biliary atresia have associated anomalies in these structures

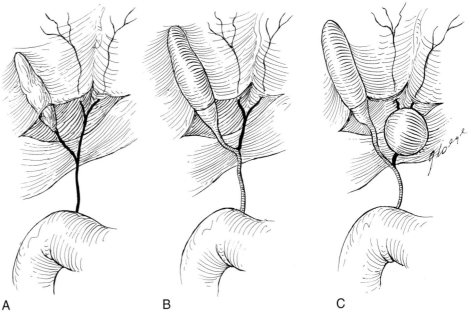

FIGURE 64-1 ■ Appearance of the biliary ductal system in infants with biliary atresia. **A,** Complete fibrous obliteration of the gallbladder and extrahepatic and intrahepatic bile ducts. **B,** Patent gallbladder and common bile duct with atresia of the common hepatic and intrahepatic bile ducts. **C,** The gallbladder is empty and atretic.

A   B   C

(absent inferior vena cava, preduodenal portal vein, intestinal malrotation, and polysplenia), suggesting a common developmental insult early in embryonic development.

Etiology

The cause of biliary atresia has not been defined. Evidence exists for a viral cause (including reovirus, human papillomavirus, rotavirus, and cytomegalovirus), but a definite causal relationship has not been established. Other authors have proposed other mechanisms, including a fetal vascular accident or malunion of the pancreatic and biliary ductal systems. The fact that some infants with definite bile-stained stool at birth progress to biliary obstruction has suggested that biliary atresia is not a single embryologic event, but rather an ongoing inflammatory process that has its onset in the prenatal period or shortly after birth.

The weight of evidence supports the concept that biliary atresia is an inflammatory process analogous to sclerosing cholangitis. Inflammation compresses and may obliterate the lumen of intrahepatic and eventually extrahepatic biliary ducts. Inflammatory cells surround the bile ducts of nearly all infants with biliary atresia. Identifiable at birth, inflammatory cells presumably begin to accumulate in fetal life. In the weeks and months after birth, periductal inflammation progresses. Intrahepatic fibrosis begins to appear first around the bile ducts, then bridges form triad-to-triad characteristic of biliary cirrhosis.

Microscopic studies by Tan and Moscoso of early biliary development in human embryos provide added insight into the pathogenesis of biliary atresia. In normal development, the primitive extrahepatic bile duct maintains continuity with the intrahepatic biliary ductal plate, from which hilar bile ducts are derived. Ductal plate–derived ducts are enveloped by mesenchyme; ducts that are not are deleted. Developing intrahepatic ducts maintain luminal continuity with the common duct from the start of organogenesis. Contrary to previous studies, a "solid cord" stage of ductal development with subsequent vacuolization does not seem to occur. Tan and Moscoso postulated that biliary atresia may be caused by failure of the remodeling process at the hepatic hilum, with persistence of fetal bile ducts poorly supported by mesenchyme. As bile flow increases during the perinatal period, bile leakage from these abnormal ducts may trigger an inflammatory reaction, with subsequent obliteration of the biliary tree.

Regardless of the cause, biliary ductal obstruction leads to progressive periportal fibrosis and cirrhosis, obstruction of the intrahepatic portal veins, and development of portal hypertension and ascites. Esophageal varices cause recurrent episodes of upper gastrointestinal hemorrhage. Hepatosplenomegaly and ascites may cause abdominal distention sufficient to cause respiratory disease and to contribute to atelectasis and pneumonia. Most unoperated infants with uncorrected biliary atresia die before age 20 months, frequently from pneumonia, sepsis, and complications of portal hypertension.

Diagnosis

Neonatal jaundice is common. Immaturity of the enzyme glucuronyl transferase is the cause in most cases. As enzymatic activity increases in response to adequate caloric

TABLE 64-1 ■ Differential Diagnosis of Neonatal Jaundice

Physiologic
Rh, ABO incompatibility
Breast milk feedings
Hemolytic disease (spherocytosis)
Systemic infections (bacterial sepsis; infections caused by togavirus, coxsackievirus, echovirus, cytomegalovirus, herpesvirus, hepatitis B virus, varicella-zoster virus, HIV, *Toxoplasma gondii, Treponema pallidum*
Genetic-metabolic disorders (α_1-antitrypsin deficiency, galactosemia, tyrosinemia, cystic fibrosis, hypothyroidism, Gaucher's disease, Niemann-Pick disease, iron storage disease, fructosemia, excessive copper administration)
Gilbert's disease
Crigler-Najjar syndrome
Neonatal hepatitis
Biliary atresia (intrahepatic, extrahepatic, hypoplasia)
Choledochal cyst
Inspissated bile plug syndrome
Bile duct compression
Parenteral alimentation cholestasis
Bile duct stenosis or stricture
Spontaneous perforation of the bile duct
Intrahepatic cholestasis from arteriohepatic dysplasia (Alagille syndrome), Byler's disease

intake during the first days after birth, jaundice resolves within 7 to 10 days and is considered physiologic. Increased levels of unconjugated bilirubin (indirect fraction) account for almost the entire amount of bilirubin. Jaundice that persists more than 2 weeks after birth is considered pathologic. Elevations of the conjugated (direct) bilirubin fraction often accompany persistent jaundice and may reflect biliary obstruction. Infants with liver dysfunction risk developing sequelae from cholestasis regardless of its etiology. Prompt evaluation of the cause of obstructive jaundice should be done during the first month.

A wide spectrum of disorders may cause persistent jaundice (Table 64-1). Examples include jaundice associated with breast milk feedings, Rh and ABO incompatibility, hemolytic disease, Gilbert's disease, and Crigler-Najjar syndrome. Infants in whom more than 20% of the bilirubin level is direct have either cholestasis or obstruction. Various disorders, some of which require early surgical management, fall into this category, as follows: (1) viral, bacterial, and parasitic systemic infections (toxoplasmosis, rubella, coxsackievirus, echovirus, cytomegalovirus, herpesvirus, hepatitis B, varicella, syphilis, and human immunodeficiency virus [HIV]); (2) genetic-metabolic disorders (α_1-antitrypsin deficiency, galactosemia, tyrosinemia, cystic fibrosis, hypothyroidism, Gaucher's disease, iron storage disease, fructosemia, excessive copper administration); (3) neonatal hepatitis; (4) biliary atresia; (5) choledochal cyst; (6) inspissated bile plug syndrome; (7) bile duct compression; (8) parenteral alimentation cholestasis; (9) bile duct stenosis or stricture; (10) spontaneous perforation of the bile ducts; and (11) cholestasis from arteriohepatic dysplasia (Alagille syndrome) and Byler's disease.

Biliary atresia and choledochal cyst require urgent surgical drainage in infancy and must be separated from other conditions causing cholestatic jaundice but with patent extrahepatic ducts. A series of examinations and measurements identifies most causes of cholestasis that do not require surgical intervention, including the presence of bile in duodenal aspirate, green or brown stool, sweat chloride determination, thyroxine and thyroid-stimulating hormone levels, blood and urine culture, TORCH (toxoplasmosis, other [congenital syphilis and viruses], rubella, cytomegalovirus, herpes simplex virus) screen titers, serologic tests for syphilis, metabolic screen for aminoaciduria, evaluation of urine for reducing substances, and α_1-antitrypsin levels. The nonsurgical causes of neonatal jaundice can be excluded before the age of 4 weeks. If these studies are negative, the diagnostic choice lies between biliary atresia and neonatal hepatitis.

Infants with biliary atresia have persistent, progressive jaundice, with total and direct bilirubin levels that are elevated within 1 week of birth. The direct bilirubin-to-total bilirubin levels may exceed 25% by the end of the first week after birth. Serum alkaline phosphatase levels become characteristically elevated. At 4 weeks, γ-glutamyl transferase levels are significantly elevated in infants with biliary atresia and exceed levels of patients with neonatal hepatitis by 6 weeks.

The stools of infants with biliary atresia are acholic. The urine may appear dark, containing bile but no urobilinogen. The liver becomes large and firm by 4 weeks. Splenomegaly may develop by 6 weeks. Ascites with prominent abdominal veins is evidence of advanced liver disease with portal hypertension but usually does not occur until after 6 months.

None of the clinical features or diagnostic studies are specifically diagnostic of biliary atresia. Abdominal ultrasound may show the absence of a gallbladder, a finding that suggests biliary atresia or, rarely, choledochal cyst. The finding is not absolute, however. In one study, 71% of patients in whom the gallbladder was not seen on ultrasound had biliary atresia, whereas 18% of patients in whom the gallbladder was visualized still had the disorder. The fibrotic remnant of the extrahepatic biliary tree appears as a triangular or tubular-shaped density immediately cranial to the portal vein bifurcation. Finding the triangular cord sign, combined with an abnormally short gallbladder, if present, may have added predictive value for biliary atresia. The intrahepatic bile ducts rarely become dilated or even identified in infants with biliary atresia except late in the disease when cysts known as *bile lakes* may be present.

Technetium-99m diisopropyl iminodiacetic acid (DISIDA) scintiscans are helpful tests because if the administered radioisotope appears in the intestine, complete biliary obstruction can be excluded. Failure of hepatic clearance of the isotope indicates obstruction. Approximately 80% of infants with obstruction on DISIDA scan have biliary atresia.

Magnetic resonance cholangiography clearly depicts the biliary tree in infants, even in the presence of neonatal hepatitis and paucity of bile ducts. The technique holds promise as a means of excluding biliary atresia as a cause of neonatal cholestasis by allowing visualization of the biliary tract.

Percutaneous needle biopsy helps to distinguish between biliary atresia and idiopathic neonatal hepatitis. Pathologic features used to make the distinction are proliferating bile ducts, associated with biliary atresia, and giant cells and focal areas of necrosis, associated with neonatal hepatitis. Patients with biliary atresia may have occasional giant cells in biopsy specimens, however, reflecting a considerable overlap in the pathologic appearances of the two entities. Also, bile duct proliferation may not be evident on needle biopsy until after 3 or 4 weeks of age.

The nonoperative diagnostic work-up should be completed by 6 weeks of age, and no later than 8 weeks, to minimize the deleterious effects of uncorrected obstructive jaundice should the infant have biliary atresia. The final step of the work-up is diagnostic laparotomy for operative cholangiography, wedge biopsy of the liver, and, if biliary atresia is found, a Kasai operation (portoenterostomy). In most infants with biliary atresia, the gallbladder is absent or fibrotic, which makes cholangiography impossible. If the gallbladder is present, injection of dilute water-soluble radiographic contrast material shows whether bile ducts are patent from liver to duodenum, with some hepatofugal flow into the small intrahepatic branches. If the liver is soft, the gallbladder contains bile, and the contrast study shows bile ducts open from liver to duodenum; a wedge biopsy completes the exploration without further surgical interventions. Finding biliary atresia requires extension of the incision, however, and exploration of the porta hepatis for possible portoenterostomy.

Some surgeons have advocated laparoscopic diagnostic cholangiography and direct examination of the liver and gallbladder with needle biopsy. These surgeons note that the liver in biliary atresia appears coarse, irregular in texture, green-brown in color, with angiomas over its surface. In contrast, the liver in neonatal hepatitis is smooth, sharp-edged, and chocolate brown in color.

Surgical Management

Early laparotomy for infants with suspected biliary atresia should be performed before 6 to 8 weeks of age. The prognosis of portoenterostomy for biliary atresia worsens after this time. Because hepatic fibrosis progresses rapidly and becomes irreversible, several authorities question the justification of operative reconstruction after age 3 months. Other surgeons argue that a patient without advanced liver disease who is older than 3 months may benefit from the Kasai operation, with a lower but still acceptable chance of long-term survival with his or her native liver (age at Kasai operation >90 days, 5-year survival with native liver 25%; age <90 days, 5-year survival 35%). Primary liver transplantation best serves patients already in advanced liver failure at the time of diagnosis.

The operation recommended for correction of intrahepatic biliary atresia is a modification of the Kasai hepatic portoenterostomy. Operative cholangiography and dissection of the porta define which pathologic variant exists (see Fig. 64-1). The fibrotic remnants of the extrahepatic ducts in most patients exist as small cords of tissue just anterior to the portal vein and hepatic artery. All tissue lying anterior to the vessels, including the atretic

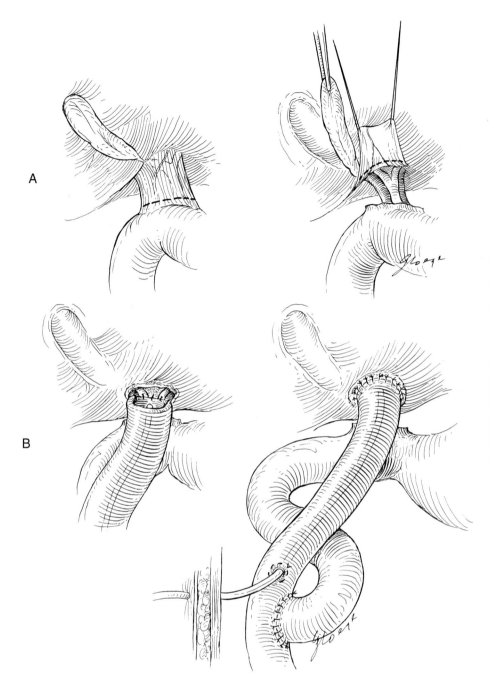

A

B

FIGURE 64-2 ■ **A,** Technique of dissection of hepatoduodenal ligament in an infant with suspected biliary atresia. The fibrous cord and tissue anterior to the portal vein and hepatic artery are mobilized to the liver capsule, exposing the bifurcation of the portal vein. **B,** Roux-en-Y jejunal segment anastomosed to adventitia overlying the portal vein and hepatic artery and to Glisson's capsule on the liver. The drainage catheter, shown here, is used occasionally by some surgeons, but more often the limb is attached to the abdominal wall and marked with a clip so that it can be accessed percutaneously.

gallbladder, common bile duct, and the right and left hepatic ducts, is elevated as an intact flap from the duodenum to the hilum of the liver (Fig. 64-2).

Dissection of the hilum is the crucial phase of the operation. Retraction of the bifurcation of the right and left portal veins and division of short branches that enter the liver directly from the saddle of the bifurcation provide the necessary exposure of the porta. Microscopic biliary ductules lie within the bifurcation of the portal vein at the hilum of the liver. These microscopic ducts seem to be of sufficient size to allow biliary drainage, although some believe these ductules represent lymphatic channels. Microdissection studies reveal that the greatest concentration of ductules lay in the lateral margins of the fibrous plate in proximity to the vascular structures of

the hilum. Transection of the fibrous plate is at the level where the portal veins enter the hepatic parenchyma, although some surgeons extend the dissection upward to include the area adjacent to the segmental portal branches. The liver capsule is not incised intentionally. Pressure and topical thrombin control bleeding from the transected remnant, avoiding cautery, which might injure the ductules.

Fine sutures connect a proximal Roux-en-Y jejunal loop in an anastomosis to the margin of the cut surface of the fibrous plate. Careful placement of sutures avoids damage to the all-important lateral margins of the fibrous plate, using minimal amounts of capsule to secure sutures to the undersurface of the liver, making certain to include the lateral portions of the fibrous plate in immediate relation to the vascular structures of the porta. Placement of the Roux-en-Y loop is usually through the transverse colon mesentery in a retrocolic position. The jejunojejunostomy that completes the Roux-en-Y is placed 40 to 45 cm distal to the portoenterostomy to separate the area from intestinal flora in an effort to decrease the risk of ascending cholangitis. Some surgeons recommend that the side of the Roux-en-Y limb be brought to the abdominal wall as a temporary stoma to assess the volume of bile flow and to decrease the incidence of cholangitis. Most surgeons currently do not use a cutaneous stoma, however, because the site is prone to bleeding if the patient develops portal hypertension. Some surgeons suture the Roux limb to the abdominal wall and mark the site with a clip so that it can be accessed percutaneously. Others have constructed intussuscepted segments and valves using flaps of demuscularized mucosa in efforts to prevent reflux of intestinal bacteria and cholangitis. Cholangitis is a frequent postoperative complication, however, regardless of the type of intestinal anastomosis or venting technique used.

When the gallbladder and distal duct are patent, it is possible in theory to perform an anastomosis between the fundus of the gallbladder and the transected porta (gallbladder Kasai). This modification fails to perform as well as portoenterostomy, however.

Postoperatively, trimethoprim-sulfamethoxazole provides prophylactic bacterial suppression. Patients receive supplemental vitamins, in particular, fat-soluble vitamins. Low-dose phenobarbital stimulates bile flow. Because periportal inflammation progresses despite a technically successful Kasai operation and may contribute to progression of the disease, some advocate corticosteroid therapy sufficient to cause immunosuppression for a minimum of 6 weeks, although statistical proof of benefit is lacking.

Complications

Postoperative complications include cholangitis, progressive cirrhosis with portal hypertension, and eventually liver failure. Cholangitis presumably results from ascending infections from intestinal flora invading the bile ductules and hepatic parenchyma. Recurrent attacks significantly worsen prognosis and decrease liver function. Cholangitis causes a decrease in bile flow, fever, recurrence of jaundice, and leukocytosis. It is often a clinical diagnosis and difficult to document definitively without positive blood cultures and direct samples taken from the Roux loop. Empirical therapy begins with a third-generation cephalosporin antibiotic and choleretics such as phenobarbital, glucagon, and steroids. Patients who do not respond to this regimen receive an intravenous aminoglycoside in addition.

A few surgeons recommend reoperation for recurrent cholangitis. These procedures, although reasonable in theory, are difficult in practice and seldom stem repeated episodes. The only situation that occasionally has led to successful reoperation is when excellent postoperative bile flow ceases abruptly. Several surgeons in this scenario first give a "pulse" of corticosteroids before deciding on reoperation. Most surgeons agree, however, that if bile flow is not present after a technically correct portoenterostomy, reoperation is not successful and should be avoided.

Portal hypertension reflects persistent or worsening intrahepatic disease. The patient has splenomegaly (occasionally with hypersplenism), esophageal variceal hemorrhage, and if a stoma is present, stomal hemorrhage. Advanced liver disease also results in the development of ascites; hypoalbuminemia; hypoprothrombinemia; and deficiencies of fat-soluble vitamins, micronutrients, and long-chain triglycerides. These manifestations usually do not appear until after 2 years of age. Portal pressure in some patients decreases with the development of intrahepatic portosystemic shunts. Most patients have bleeding complications, however. Endosclerosis is generally successful in controlling bleeding esophageal varices. Surgical creation of portosystemic shunts, esophageal devascularization, splenectomy, or LeVeen shunts for ascites are seldom recommended because transplantation is the best therapeutic option for patients who develop advanced liver failure.

Results of Treatment

A successful outcome after hepatic portoenterostomy depends on many clinical factors, including precise performance of the procedure, age of the patient, severity of hepatic fibrosis at the time of operation, presence of microscopic ductules in the hilum, whether the bile flow adequate to clear jaundice is achieved after operation, and occurrence of postoperative cholangitis. Placement of patients into prognostic groups is possible within 4 to 6 weeks postoperatively. Infants who produce bile and clear their jaundice have a good chance of long-term survival and maintenance of near-normal liver function with their native liver. In infants who remain jaundiced but with stabilization of the progression of liver disease, extended survival can be expected. Such patients are likely to require a liver transplant within a few years, however. The Kasai operation has failed if bile does not flow and the liver disease continues to progress. Patients in this category become candidates for transplantation during the first 12 to 16 months of life. Patients who come to medical attention late in the course and show signs of impending or established liver failure require urgent transplantation.

The age of the patient at the time of portoenterostomy is a crucial variable. The younger the patient at the time of operation, the better the overall prognosis. Eight weeks is the important threshold; the likelihood for survival with a functioning native liver begins to fall in patients older than 8 weeks of age. Some surgeons question whether portoenterostomy should be attempted at all in patients older than 3 months of age, reasoning that the liver disease has progressed beyond the point where a Kasai operation would be of benefit and that early transplantation is the best option. Series of patients older than 3 months who have undergone a successful Kasai operation and the scarcity of infant donor livers have led many centers to re-evaluate this attitude.

About one third of patients operated on by 8 weeks of age have a successful outcome and may never require transplantation. An additional third of infants are improved and have an extended survival. Transplantation may not be required until the child is much older and of an age and size when the donor pool is larger, and reduced-size grafts become more of an option. Transplantation is a life-saving procedure for the remaining third of infants who present late in the course of disease or fail to improve after portoenterostomy. The 5-year survival for infants with biliary atresia undergoing liver transplantation is 82%. The current overall 5-year survival for infants born with biliary atresia is 86%.

BILIARY HYPOPLASIA

Biliary hypoplasia is characterized by small but grossly visible and radiographically patent extrahepatic bile ducts. The diagnosis almost invariably is made at exploration for jaundice in infancy with a cholangiogram. The condition is not a specific disease entity but a manifestation of various hepatobiliary disorders that result in decreased bile flow and eventual narrowing of the ductal system. It is unclear whether the primary disorder originates in the bile ducts or is the result of a type of disuse atrophy because of diminished bile flow. It seems that an element of actual structural damage to the ducts is present in most of these cases. Some have suggested that biliary hypoplasia may be an early stage of biliary atresia because the condition seems to be an intermediate between normal patency and complete occlusion. Biliary hypoplasia often is associated with some degree of intrahepatic disease, usually cirrhosis.

It is unclear whether any form of surgical reconstruction can improve biliary hypoplasia. For more severe obstruction, hepatic portoenterostomy, as performed for biliary atresia, is recommended by some, although its effectiveness is unproved. Others have recommended that a cholecystostomy catheter be left in place for extended periods to decompress the biliary system. The prognosis is highly variable, depending on the primary hepatic disease. Some infants recover and may live for many years, often with jaundice and enlarged livers.

INSPISSATED BILE PLUG SYNDROME

In neonates, mechanical obstruction from thick bile sludge in the bile ducts may result from massive hemolysis (e.g., Rh and ABO blood group incompatibility) or thick tenacious bile in patients with cystic fibrosis or patients on parenteral nutrition. Occasionally, inspissation may proceed to the point of precipitation of biliary calculi. Most patients experience gradual resolution of the obstruction. Choleretic agents, such as phenobarbital, ursodeoxycholic acid, and glucagon, may help clear the biliary tract. Operation is rarely necessary and consists of simple irrigation of the biliary tract through a catheter placed in the fundus of the gallbladder. In exceptional patients with bile pigment stones, manual removal of the calculi may be required. Common duct stones in small ducts may be treated expectantly, with irrigation and with temporary diversion through a cholecystostomy catheter, or removed via sphincterotomy. Because of early diagnosis and exchange transfusion for the precipitating disease, inspissated bile syndrome now is seen rarely.

LIVER TRANSPLANTATION

The dramatic increase in the frequency and success of orthotopic liver transplantation is the direct result of advances in immunosuppression; surgical technique; organ procurement methods; new prophylactic and therapeutic antimicrobial agents against pathogenic viruses, bacteria, and fungi; and the development of organ procurement and distribution networks. Reduced-size liver transplantation, split-liver transplantation, and living-related techniques specifically have benefited pediatric liver transplantation.

Indications

Biliary atresia is the most common indication (50% to 75%) for orthotopic liver transplantation in children. Other clinical entities for which transplantation is a therapeutic option include other cholestatic diseases, metabolic diseases, and acute hepatic failure. A group of complex diseases characterized by cholestasis may lead to progressive liver disease and require transplantation. Included are neonatal hepatitis, familial cholestasis, Byler's disease, and arteriohepatic dysplasia (Alagille syndrome). Transplantation may cure liver-based inborn errors of metabolism that result in deficiencies of specific enzymes or the production of abnormal products of hepatic synthesis. Transplantation is needed for some conditions that damage the liver and cause progressive cirrhosis (Wilson's disease and cystic fibrosis) and others that create conditions that injure the liver or increase the risk of malignancy (α_1-antitrypsin deficiency and tyrosinemia). The liver itself may be normal, but its metabolic products may cause neurologic disease (Crigler-Najjar syndrome and ornithine transcarbamylase deficiency) or cardiovascular injury (familial hypercholesterolemia). Complete replacement of the liver may not be necessary in these diseases because correction of the metabolic defect may be possible with auxiliary liver transplantation and, in the future, hepatocyte transplantation. Patients with normal liver structure and function may have fulminant liver failure from virus, hepatotoxins, and drug toxicity. The most common infectious cause in children is hepatitis C. Acetaminophen is the most frequent drug-related cause.

Although hepatic resection is the treatment of choice for hepatobiliary and metastatic malignancies whenever possible, not all liver cancers are resectable. Chemotherapy and radiotherapy do not achieve long-term control. Total hepatectomy, orthotopic liver transplantation, and chemotherapy may cure some patients and provide long-term palliation for others. This approach has a significant recurrence rate, however. Some argue that scarce donor livers should not be devoted to this purpose because of the generally poor survival rate in this group.

Clinical end points that require transplantation include intractable cholestasis, variceal bleeding, ascites, pruritus, failed synthetic function, encephalopathy, unacceptable quality of life, and failure to thrive. Absolute contraindications are becoming less numerous with increased experience; a more recent summary includes HIV seropositivity, systemic sepsis of nonhepatic origin, a life-threatening disorder of extrahepatic origin that is not correctable by transplantation, and extrahepatic malignancy. Relative contraindications include extrahepatic organ system dysfunction that may affect the outcome of transplantation. Children with poor neurologic function with no expected improvement with restoration of hepatic function should not be transplant candidates. In the same category are children with pulmonary complications such as severe pulmonary hypertension, patients with recurrent pulmonary infections (e.g., infections associated with cystic fibrosis), and children with chronic ventilator dependence. Liver failure may cause pulmonary arteriovenous shunting and hypoxemia (hepatopulmonary syndrome), however, which is corrected by liver transplantation. Complex congenital heart disease, especially if accompanied by cyanosis and pulmonary hypertension, imposes an extremely high risk for liver transplantation. Renal insufficiency seldom is a contraindication, however, for transplantation. Renal failure resulting from hepatorenal syndrome resolves with a functioning liver graft.

Donor Organ Options

A shortage of whole-organ livers of appropriate size hampered the development of pediatric liver transplantation. Many pediatric recipient candidates died waiting for a suitable graft. New procedures to divide cadaver donor livers into two functioning grafts (split-liver transplantation) and to harvest a portion of liver from a living donor (living-related transplantation) have maximized donor use and expanded the pool of potential grafts. A functioning component of liver with a suitable vascular pedicle, bile duct, and venous drainage can provide hepatic function for a patient.

Reduced-size liver transplantation first used this principle in children and small adults with an acute need for a graft but when a full-sized cadaver graft was all that was available. The segmental anatomy of the liver allowed reduction in size of the graft to one appropriate for the recipient. Infants and small children usually received the left lateral segments (segments two and three) or the left lobe (segments two, three, and four). The remainder of the liver was discarded, however. Although reduced-size transplantation increased the number of pediatric donor grafts, it did not expand the overall donor pool.

Split-liver transplantation was the next logical step. A whole graft produces two functioning grafts: the left lateral segment for children and the right trisegment (segments four through eight) for adults. *Ex vivo* describes splitting the donor liver on the bench after harvest, whereas *in vivo* is the term for division of the liver before its removal from the donor with its native circulation intact. An in vivo graft may have better hemostasis and control of bile leaks than its ex vivo counterpart.

Living-related transplantation removes the left lateral segment from a living donor, using techniques developed for reduced-size transplantation. Ready availability of the donor allows the optimal preparation of the recipient and potentially eliminates the risk of pretransplant mortality. The graft functions immediately, and, in theory, increased histocompatibility between parent donor and child recipient favors a lower incidence of rejection. Published survival rates in pediatric patients are 88% after living-related transplantation and 82% after cadaver graft transplantation.

SUGGESTED READINGS

Bezerra JA, Balistreri WF: Cholestatic syndromes of infancy and childhood. Semin Gastrointest Dis 12:54-65, 2001.

This is an excellent review of the clinical evaluation of cholestasis in infancy that emphasizes the priority of making an early diagnosis of biliary atresia.

Dillon PW, Owings E, Cilley R, et al: Immunosuppression as adjuvant therapy for biliary atresia. J Pediatr Surg 36:80-85, 2001.

In this nonrandomized study, postoperative corticosteroid therapy is associated with an 88% survival rate (mean follow-up 50 months), with 76% of patients becoming jaundice-free with native liver function. Only 16% failed treatment and required transplantation.

Ghobrial RM, Farmer DG, Amersi F, et al: Advances in pediatric liver and intestinal transplantation. Am J Surg 180:328-334, 2000.

The current status of pediatric liver transplantation is discussed, with a summary of the impact of split-liver and living-related donor organ options.

Jaw TS, Kuo YT, Liu GC, et al: MR cholangiography in the evaluation of neonatal cholestasis. Radiology 212:249-256, 1999.

Magnetic resonance cholangiography clearly depicts the major biliary structures of neonates and small infants and has potential utility as a means of excluding biliary atresia as a cause of neonatal jaundice.

Nio M, Ohi R: Biliary atresia. Semin Pediatr Surg 9:177-186, 2000.

The details of surgical management of biliary atresia are reviewed, from Kasai's home institution.

Ryckman FC, Alonzo MH, Bucuvalas JC, et al: Biliary atresia—surgical management and treatment options as they relate to outcome. Liver Transplant Surg 4(5 Suppl 1):S24-33, 1998.

Results of sequential treatment for biliary atresia are reviewed, with initial portoenterostomy followed by selective transplantation for children with progressive hepatic deterioration or established cirrhosis.

Tan CE, Driver M, Howard ER, et al: Extrahepatic biliary atresia: A first trimester event? Clues from light microscopy and immunohistochemistry. J Pediatr Surg 29:808-814, 1994.

Detailed observations from microscopic examinations of developing human embryos suggest that lack of connection between fetal intrahepatic biliary ducts and the extrahepatic biliary tree allows leakage of bile and inflammatory obliteration of the biliary tract later in fetal life.

65

Choledochal Cyst

The classic clinical classification of the three primary forms of choledochal cyst was described by Alonzo-Lej and colleagues in 1959 based on an analysis of 94 cases from the literature and 2 additional cases of their own. This classification was refined in the 1970s when more data became available from the introduction of accurate cholangiography by Japanese surgeons who published additional forms of choledochal cyst. The Japanese surgeons also pointed out that the incidence of choledochal cyst is severalfold higher in Asian than in non-Asian populations and similarly more common in females.

ANATOMIC CLASSIFICATION

Figure 65-1 shows the five common anatomic forms of choledochal cysts, but variations and combinations of these five types of cysts also occasionally are encountered. Type I, which is cystic dilation of the common duct, represents 85% to 95% of cases in all reported series. In this form of the anomaly, the gallbladder generally enters the choledochal cyst itself; the right and left hepatic ducts and the intrahepatic ducts are normal in size; and the configuration is either saccular or fusiform, depending on the degree of antenatal obstruction at the ampulla of Vater. Type II choledochal cyst is a diverticular malformation of the common bile duct, and the entire intrahepatic and extrahepatic biliary tree is usually normal. Diverticular cysts may be either small or large. Type III choledochal cyst usually is referred to as *choledochocele*, which is usually intraduodenal but occasionally is intrapancreatic. In type III patients, the intrahepatic and extrahepatic biliary tree is normal, and the common bile

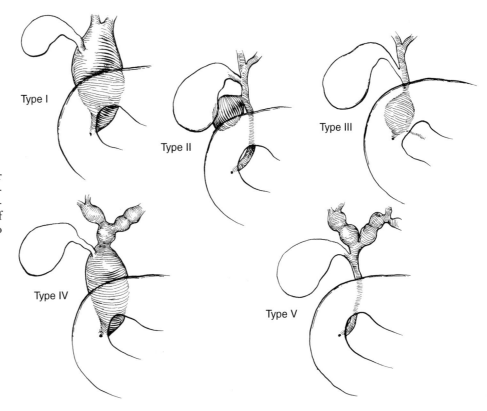

FIGURE 65-1 ■ The five major forms of choledochal cyst malformations as shown by cholangiography. Careful delineation of anatomy dictates the approach to treatment.

duct generally enters the choledochocele within the wall of the duodenum. This entity also has been considered to be a form of duodenal duplication, but this would not explain cases that are intrapancreatic. In most type III malformations, the common bile duct and the main pancreatic duct enter the choledochocele separately, and at times these openings are stenotic because of chronic inflammation. The choledochocele then empties into the main duodenal lumen through a narrow opening. Type IV cysts are multiple and resemble type I cysts except that the intrahepatic biliary tree also is dilated. Type IV choledochal cyst might be considered to be a variation of type I. Type V forms of the anomaly are single or multiple intrahepatic cysts with a normal extrahepatic biliary tree. When these intrahepatic cysts are associated with hepatic fibrosis, they have been referred to as *Caroli's disease*. The difference between Caroli's disease and fibrocystic or polycystic disease of the liver is that in Caroli's disease, the cysts within the liver communicate with the biliary system, whereas in fibrocystic disease, the cysts are filled with bile, but they do not communicate with the biliary tree. Other variants of these five forms of choledochal cysts, such as cystic dilation of the cystic duct or combinations of type I and III malformations, have been described but are uncommon.

PATHOLOGY

Histologic examination of the wall of extrahepatic choledochal cysts shows a thick-walled structure of dense connective tissue interlaced with strands of smooth muscle and with little or no mucosal lining. Although some inflammatory reaction usually is noted within the wall of the cyst and in the tissues surrounding it, in infants it is generally mild, whereas in older children it tends to be more severe, and it is even more severe in adults. Inflammatory reaction has been noted to be particularly severe in patients who have intrahepatic cysts, undoubtedly because of associated cholangitis. Stones have been seen in teenage and older patients within the choledochal cysts and intrahepatic ducts as well, but usually only sludge has been found in younger patients. Occasionally, intrahepatic biliary stones develop after excision of choledochal cysts, primarily when anastomotic stenosis occurs. With regard to the distal common bile duct, two findings have been noted. Most infants have had complete obstruction at the level of the duodenum, but older patients usually have had a patent distal common duct. In most instances, liver biopsy specimens in newborns have been interpreted as being normal or show bile duct proliferation consistent with chronic biliary obstruction. Occasionally, in older patients, mild periportal fibrosis has been seen, and in rare instances progressive biliary cirrhosis has been encountered. Numerous reports of malignant change within the wall of a retained choledochal cyst have been published. It seems that this occurs only in patients who experienced long-standing inflammation of the wall of retained choledochal cysts. In the long-term, 10% to 15% of patients who have retained choledochal cysts may develop carcinomas, which typically have been described as adenosquamous carcinoma with occasional small cell carcinomas occurring.

In one large follow-up series of 1003 patients undergoing biliary enteric drainage, 5.5% of the patients developed primary bile duct cancer with a mean follow-up of 129.6 months, and the incidence in choledochoduodenostomy patients was 7.6%. Malignancy was not observed in patients who had no demonstrated evidence of long-standing postoperative cholangitis. The gallbladder in patients with choledochal cysts is generally normal on histologic examination, but in older patients who have had recurrent bouts of cholangitis, the wall of the gallbladder may show findings consistent with chronic cholecystitis. Portal hypertension has not been a significant accompanying feature in patients with choledochal cyst except for patients who later developed biliary cirrhosis associated with long-standing recurrent cholangitis.

In patients who have had a choledochocele, the cyst usually is lined with duodenal mucosa internally. Inflammation is usually not a prominent feature of this process except in occasional cases in which there is the development of stenosis of the common bile and pancreatic ducts. Normal biliary lining generally is seen on the internal surface of a choledochocele, particularly those in the head of the pancreas, whereas at other times the lining is mixed biliary and duodenal.

ETIOLOGY

A variety of theories have been offered to explain the pathogenesis of choledochal cysts. In more recent years, the development of accurate diagnostic imaging techniques has permitted additional thoughts regarding etiology. Analysis of detailed endoscopic retrograde cholangiopancreatography (ERCP), magnetic resonance cholangiopancreatography (MRCP), and other forms of cholangiographic imaging has shown that most patients with the common form of choledochal cyst have an anomalous arrangement of the pancreaticobiliary ductal system in which the pancreatic duct enters the common duct at an abnormal angle proximal to the circular muscle of the ampulla of Vater. Also, cases of this abnormal pancreaticobiliary junction have been reported in children in whom clinical symptoms suggesting choledochal cyst are present but in whom the extrahepatic biliary tree was found to have only mild dilation. In either case, from an analysis of dynamic injection studies of the biliary tree, this anomalous arrangement of the biliary and pancreatic ducts may permit reflux of pancreatic enzymes containing trypsin and lipase proximally into the common duct with resulting damage to the ductal wall during intrauterine development. Numerous cases now have been documented in which the union of the pancreatic duct and the distal common duct is located at a higher than normal level along the common duct so that it is associated with a long common channel, and no effective sphincter of Oddi around the union of the common duct and pancreatic ducts is present as in normal individuals (Fig. 65-2). Presumably, reflux of pancreatic enzymes into the common duct during fetal development may produce damage resulting in dilation of the common duct, with the saccular form being associated with complete or near-complete obstruction and the fusiform type being associated with lesser degrees of obstruction. This theory

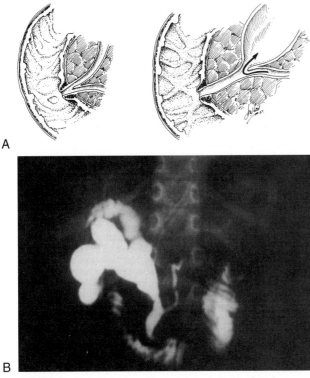

FIGURE 65-2 ■ A, The normal anatomic relationship between the common bile and pancreatic ducts as they pass through the ampullary sphincter (left) and the anomalous relationship (right) constituting a common channel that permits pancreaticobiliary reflux, which is seen in most patients with choledochal cyst. **B,** Operative cholangiogram shows the anomalous pancreaticobiliary relationship in a girl with a fusiform choledochal cyst. (From O'Neill JA: Choledochal cyst. Curr Prob Surg 24:6, 1992.)

does not explain, however, the cause of the diverticular choledochal cyst, choledochocele, or intrahepatic cyst formation. The etiologic significance of the preponderance of females and Asians with this anomaly has yet to be explained fully despite the suggested genetic link.

In recent years, prenatal maternal ultrasound has become a commonplace study. Numerous patients have had serial ultrasound observation in utero, and these studies suggest that choledochal cyst has its origin in midgestation, which might correspond to the prolonged period necessary for pancreatic enzymes to induce lytic damage of the extrahepatic biliary tree. Analysis of the contents of bile of newborn infants with choledochal cysts indicates that newborns secrete trypsin and some lipase but little amylase. The proportion of these enzymes normalizes within a few months of birth.

With regard to type II diverticular forms of choledochal cyst, it has been suggested that the diverticulum is a remnant of an earlier stage of bile duct development, when it represents more of a network of cells than tubular ducts. Others suggest that it is more likely that the large diverticular forms of choledochal cyst represent end-stage healing of prenatal rupture of the common bile duct. Newborn infants who develop spontaneous perforation of the common bile duct do not develop such diverticula, however.

Choledochocele may be the result of primary ectasia of the bile duct or possibly long-standing obstruction at its point of entry into the duodenum. Types IV and V choledochal cysts might be explained on the basis of the common channel theory or primary ductal ectasia or a combination of the two.

CLINICAL PRESENTATION

In all reported series, the preponderance of patients with types I and IV choledochal cysts have been female (female-to-male ratio 4:1), but the sex incidence in types II, III, and V has been noted to be equal. With regard to age and time of presentation, there are two clinically distinct groups of patients. The first group is younger than 6 months of age, with most of these infants presenting with a clinical picture indistinguishable from that of biliary atresia because they have complete biliary obstruction and jaundice. At other times, newborns have evidence of bile flow that ceases after 3 to 6 weeks of age, indicating that the dilated duct may angulate and obstruct or possibly obstruct from inflammation or sludge during this short interval of a few weeks. Infants usually present with jaundice, but the older the patient the more likely there is to be a triad of pain, mass, and jaundice. Jaundice seems to take 1 to 3 weeks to become evident in infants noted to have choledochal cysts on prenatal ultrasound.

The so-called adult form of clinical presentation occurs in patients older than 6 months and usually older than 2 years. In this group of patients, the most common form of presentation has been abdominal pain and jaundice, and occasionally a mass can be felt. The cause of abdominal pain in patients with choledochal cysts may be related to distention of the dilated duct or to cholangitis. Rare patients have presented with signs of pancreatitis, but it is likely that patients who present with mild manifestations of pancreatitis have this on the basis of cholangitis, which is usually present at the same time. The clinical presentation in older patients usually is more confusing and difficult to interpret when the symptoms associated with choledochal cyst are similar to those ordinarily associated with biliary stone disease. This has become evident since the advent of laparoscopic cholecystectomy in adults in whom incidental choledochal cysts have been discovered on routine cholangiography in these patients.

DIAGNOSIS
Laboratory Studies

There are no specific laboratory studies diagnostic of choledochal cyst, but rather studies indicate the patient's condition and possible complications. Because the most common presenting sign of choledochal cyst is jaundice, the primary finding is conjugated hyperbilirubinemia and other serum indicators of obstructive jaundice, such as an elevated level of alkaline phosphatase. Mild increases in serum amylase levels are noted occasionally. In older patients, jaundice may be intermittent and mild, whereas in infants, significant conjugated hyperbilirubinemia is usually present. If biliary obstruction is present for a significant length of time, some patients also have a mildly deranged coagulation profile.

Imaging Studies

Upper gastrointestinal contrast radiographs and oral or intravenous cholangiography are not helpful. Occasionally, computed tomography combined with cholangiography may be helpful in selected older patients. The most helpful initial screening study is probably abdominal ultrasound. Patients with obstructive jaundice, regardless of age,

may benefit from an initial screening with ultrasound because this study is capable of showing the entire intrahepatic and extrahepatic biliary tree, the gallbladder, and the pancreas and its ductal system. In newborns with obstructive jaundice and a dilated extrahepatic biliary tree shown on ultrasound, no further imaging studies may be required preoperatively. Ultrasound and technetium-99m

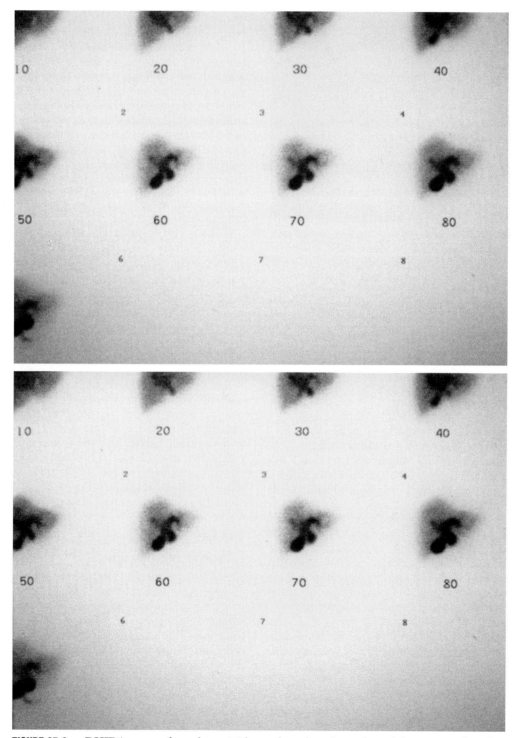

FIGURE 65-3 ■ DISIDA scan performed over 1.5 hours shows hepatic uptake and the pattern of extrahepatic and intestinal excretion in an infant with choledochal cyst. The cyst is seen medial to the gallbladder.

disopropyliminodiacetic acid (DISIDA) scintigraphy are usually sufficient to justify surgery in infants with choledochal cysts (Fig. 65-3). Older patients may require additional studies, however, because of the intermittent nature of the obstructive jaundice. In older patients, percutaneous transhepatic cholangiography, ERCP, or MRCP is probably preferable. These studies have shown the commonly seen anomalous junction of the pancreatic and common bile ducts constituting a common channel. The latter studies also are most useful for defining anatomic detail necessary for planning an appropriate operation. When these studies are combined with operative cholangiography, the appropriate operative approach to all forms of choledochal cyst can be planned safely; this is highlighted by occasional reports of patients with choledochal cyst that is accompanied by aberrant hepatic ducts, which require incorporation into enteric drainage procedures after cyst excision. As mentioned earlier, more patients are presenting in early adulthood as a result of routine cholangiography performed concomitantly with laparoscopic cholecystectomy for cholelithiasis.

Radioscintigraphic studies with DISIDA characteristically show delayed excretion and retarded drainage into the intestine (see Fig. 65-3). When there is complete distal obstruction, no drainage into the intestine is seen. Ordinarily the radionuclide image localizes in the hepatic hilus within 2 to 3 hours, and the pattern is diagnostic. An additional advantage of DISIDA scanning is that it not only provides some idea of the anatomy involved, but also it provides physiologic information related to hepatic uptake and parenchymal function. This information is valuable in older patients who are being evaluated for the possibility of associated cirrhosis.

SURGICAL MANAGEMENT

Simple drainage without excision of types I, II, and IV choledochal cysts no longer is performed (Fig. 65-4). This is because with cyst duodenostomy, most patients develop cholangitis and biliary cirrhosis over time. Although fewer patients who have had Roux-en-Y cyst jejunostomy have had recurrent cholangitis, the incidence has been high enough because of stasis within the cyst that this method also has been abandoned. As mentioned previously, the other consideration with simple drainage of choledochal cyst is that whenever chronic inflammation occurs within a retained cyst, there is an ongoing potential for malignant generation.

The most effective method of avoiding recurrent cholangitis and the late possibility of malignant degeneration in the wall of the cyst is to excise it completely (see Fig. 65-4). In most patients, total cyst excision is possible, and enteric drainage is provided by Roux-en-Y hepaticojejunostomy. Total excision of a choledochal cyst is possible in virtually all infants and young children. Older patients with severe pericystic inflammation are managed best by intramural resection of the cyst, leaving the back wall adjacent to the portal vascular structures in place (Fig. 65-5). In patients who previously have had cyst-enteric anastomosis followed by recurrent bouts of cholangitis, reoperation and cyst excision is needed; the intramural resection technique is preferred. Other forms of enteric drainage that have been described after excision of choledochal cysts include hepaticoduodenostomy, hepatico-valved jejunal interposition hepaticoduodenostomy, and others, but the standard Roux-en-Y hepaticojejunostomy, the simplest procedure, seems to provide superior results to these

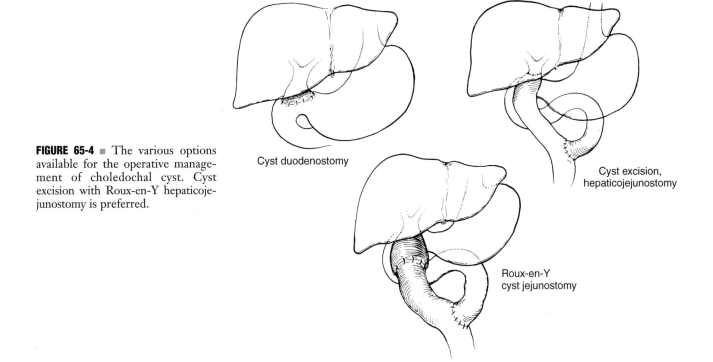

FIGURE 65-4 ■ The various options available for the operative management of choledochal cyst. Cyst excision with Roux-en-Y hepaticojejunostomy is preferred.

Cyst duodenostomy

Cyst excision, hepaticojejunostomy

Roux-en-Y cyst jejunostomy

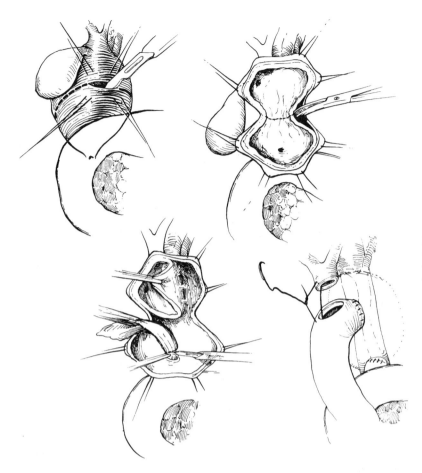

FIGURE 65-5 ■ The steps involved in excision of a choledochal cyst and establishment of enteric drainage. Total resection is performed in patients with no inflammatory reaction surrounding the cyst, whereas intramural excision is performed as shown in patients who have the inflammatory tissue reaction.

more complicated operations. Although there are a few reports of management of type II diverticular forms of choledochal cyst managed by excision of the diverticulum and ductoplasty, the most practical and effective approach is excision of the extrahepatic ductal system with Roux-en-Y hepaticojejunostomy.

Patients with type III choledochoceles are managed best as the anatomy dictates. The general approach is one of lateral duodenotomy with unroofing of the choledochocele to drain the common bile and pancreatic ducts directly into the duodenum with or without associated sphincteroplasty if the ductal openings are stenotic.

Regarding choledochal cysts with intrahepatic involvement, either with or without an extrahepatic component, management is individualized with the primary principle being one of adequate drainage. At times, segmental resection of the liver is necessary, and long-term follow-up is particularly important in patients with intrahepatic cystic disease because progressive cyst formation may occur over time, associated with recurring cholangitis. Drainage may be performed either percutaneously or operatively by open or laparoscopic technique.

RESULTS OF TREATMENT

Most patients treated for types I, II, III, and IV choledochal cysts who do not have preexisting cirrhosis or portal hypertension remain well, provided that their hepatoenteric drainage site remains patent and that any postoperative episode of cholangitis is investigated thoroughly and treated appropriately. Under these circumstances, ultrasound may be helpful to determine the presence of stones. Patients with intrahepatic ductal ectasia may present periodically over many years with recurrent cholangitis related to biliary stasis within the intrahepatic ductal cysts, even after a prolonged period of freedom from symptoms.

SUGGESTED READINGS

Alonzo-Lej F, Revor WB, Pessagno DJ: Congenital choledochal cyst, with a report of 2, and an analysis of 94 cases. Surg Gynecol Obstet Int Abstr Surg 108:1, 1959.

This article is the classic reference on this subject and provides a fundamental understanding of this bile duct anomaly.

Komuro H, Makino S, Momoya T, Niski A: Biliary atresia with extrahepatic biliary cysts—cholangiography patterns influencing prognosis. J Pediatr Surg 35:1771-1774, 2000.

Prognostic information is provided about neonates who present with various types of cystic dilation of the biliary tree associated with complete obstruction.

Ohi R, Yaoita S, Kainiyama T, et al: Surgical treatment of congenital dilatation of the bile duct with special reference to late complications after total excisional operation. J Pediatr Surg 25:613, 1990.

This article provides long-term follow-up information on patients with choledochal cysts treated surgically. The problem of late occurrence of carcinoma is discussed.

O'Neill JA: Choledochal cyst. Curr Probl Surg 29:363, 1992.

This monograph summarizes all currently available information on this subject.

Suita S, Shono K, Kinugasa Y, et al: Influence of age on the presentation and outcome of choledochal cyst. J Pediatr Surg 34:1765-1768, 1999.

This article provides a clear clinical description of how patients with choledochal cysts present and the expected outcome.

66

Portal Hypertension

The profile of portal hypertension in childhood has changed with fewer patients with portal vein thrombosis (PVT) than previously. The etiology and the management of hypertension of the portal venous circulation in infants and children differ in many ways from those in adults (Table 66-1). Portal hypertension continues to be one of the most frequent serious causes of upper gastrointestinal hemorrhage in addition to being a common cause of splenomegaly in childhood. The relatively small size of the mesenteric venous channels and the inferior vena cava in young children makes operative treatment of portal hypertension technically difficult because shunt procedures frequently fail. Temporizing measures, such as sclerotherapy and variceal banding, have become the initial approach to treatment for almost all children with bleeding secondary to portal hypertension.

The approach to management and the long-term outlook for these patients vary considerably, depending on the nature of the underlying pathology. Accurate diagnostic studies are crucial in determining the level of portal obstruction so that appropriate treatment can be undertaken. Basically, portal venous occlusion in children may be caused by obstruction to portal venous flow at one of three levels (Fig. 66-1): (1) the extrahepatic portal veins, (2) intrahepatic obstruction from cirrhosis, and (3) rarely suprahepatic obstruction of the hepatic veins. An individual child with portal hypertension may have few symptoms and readily compensate, or there may be impressive, life-threatening bleeding or severe hypersplenism.

EXTRAHEPATIC (PREHEPATIC) OBSTRUCTION

Pathophysiology

Portal venous obstruction at the extrahepatic, prehepatic level almost always is caused by thrombosis of the main portal vein and various of its tributaries, and there is usually some extension cephalad to involve the proximal intrahepatic branches but not the sinusoids. Thrombotic occlusion may extend into the superior mesenteric and splenic veins to varying degrees, sometimes making shunt procedures not possible. In most cases, the cause of the thrombosis is not obvious. In the past, neonatal omphalitis, intra-abdominal infections, dehydration, and umbilical vein catheterization with fluid infusion were recognized as causative mechanisms, but now most of these entities have responded to either preventive measures or aggressive treatment, so the incidence of extrahepatic portal hypertension has fallen. With PVT, there is always some degree of phlebitis so that the wall of the portal vein and, to a lesser degree, its tributaries are usually thickened and chronically inflamed in some areas. Congenital valves, webs, or stenoses of the portal vein are rare causes of extrahepatic obstruction. The cause of extrahepatic portal hypertension in adults is different and usually results from tumors of the liver or bile ducts, pancreatitis, thrombotic disorders, and use of oral contraceptives.

Clinical Presentation

Extrahepatic portal venous obstruction is the cause of portal hypertension in approximately 30% of cases. That is approximately three times the rate in adults. In children, the diagnosis of PVT usually is made before 6 years of age. The primary feature of PVT is variceal hemorrhage, and more than 90% of patients experience serious bleeding during the course of their disease, most having

TABLE 66-1 ■ Major Causes of Extrahepatic Portal Hypertension		
Children	**Children and Adults**	**Adults**
Congenital venous anomalies/biliary atresia	Hepatic cirrhosis	Neoplasia of liver, bile ducts, and pancreas
Omphalitis	External trauma and operative trauma	Polycythemia
Umbilical vein infusions or exchange transfusions	Intraperitoneal sepsis	Thrombocytosis
Enterocolitis (severe)	Pyelophlebitis	Pancreatitis
Dehydration (severe)	Systemic sepsis and dehydration	Use of oral contraceptives

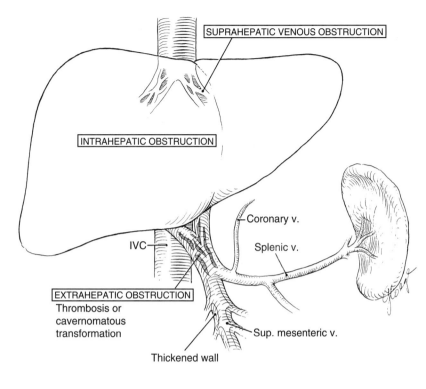

FIGURE 66-1 ■ Various types of portal hypertension in childhood. Extrahepatic portal venous block usually is caused by thrombosis with later cavernomatous transformation of the portal vein, which extends as a phlebitic process into the splenic and superior mesenteric veins. Intrahepatic venous block is caused most often by posthepatic or toxic cirrhosis, biliary atresia, cystic fibrosis, and other hepatocellular disorders. Suprahepatic venous obstruction is usually idiopathic but may result from anomalies of the hepatic veins.

more than one hemorrhage a year. Bleeding from esophageal varices in children frequently follows the onset of an upper respiratory tract infection, although the reason for this relationship is not known.

Portal venography has shown that collateral circulation between the portal and systemic venous systems is extensive, but the flow through these channels is usually insufficient to lower portal pressure appreciably. In the long-term, one fourth of patients eventually may develop collateral portosystemic connections that lower portal pressure sufficiently to prevent recurrent bleeding. The primary route of clinical importance is collateralization from the coronary vein and short gastric veins into the submucosal plexus of the fundus of the stomach and lower esophagus, eventually reaching the azygos system. Direct endoscopic observations have shown that variceal bleeding often comes from a single varix located in the lower portion of the esophagus, but significant varices usually also are present in the fundus of the stomach. In normal patients, portal venous flow is toward and through the liver (hepatopetal), whereas in portal hypertension a major portion of the flow is away from the liver (hepatofugal) and through collateral channels. Normal portal venous pressure is between 5 and 15 cm H_2O.

Varices, which can be shown on esophagogram or endoscopy, extend onto the upper gastric wall in more than half of patients with extrahepatic portal hypertension, whereas in children with intrahepatic disease, gastric varices are less common. It is extremely rare for a child with PVT to die during the first episode of hemorrhage from varices because exsanguinating hemorrhage from PVT is uncommon, even with repeated episodes. Transfusions are required for only approximately one fourth of bleeding episodes. It has not been possible in a variety of reviews to make direct correlation between the frequency and severity of bleeding and the level of portal venous pressure. Generally, bleeding is more severe when it occurs in a patient who has undergone unsuccessful operations for portal hypertension than in a patient who has not been operated on, probably because collaterals have been interrupted.

The second most common initial manifestation of PVT is splenomegaly, which eventually is present in all patients with portal hypertension. Hypersplenism, manifested by mild neutropenia and thrombocytopenia, occurs in 50% of children with extrahepatic portal venous obstruction, but this almost never results in recurrent infection or systemic bleeding, so splenectomy is rarely required.

In infants, portal venous occlusion is accompanied by high portal pressure at a time when minimal collateral circulation has developed, so that transient ascites may be one of the first clinical signs. Malnutrition and pulmonary infection, as a result of diaphragmatic elevation, occasionally may result, but peptic ulceration rarely is seen in association with extrahepatic PVT. It is well known that children with PVT who develop viral infections should never receive medications containing aspirin or other platelet antagonists because bleeding would result.

A characteristic feature of extrahepatic PVT, particularly in older patients, is the large number of hepatopetal collaterals that permit continuing perfusion of the liver by a significant volume of portal blood. Most commonly, this phenomenon occurs through recanalization of the thrombosed portal vein, resulting in a "cavernous transformation" of this structure. Even with cavernous transformation, portal pressures are in the same range as those occurring with intrahepatic portal venous obstruction, ranging from 25 to 50 cm H_2O, which indicates that there is still high resistance in these recanalized veins. The usual finding of normal hepatic wedge pressure further confirms the presinusoidal location of the obstruction in cases of extrahepatic portal hypertension. Cavernous transformation of the portal vein is believed to result from not only recanalization of an old thrombus, but also the development of small intraluminal and extraluminal venous collaterals. The latter vessels may be so small that a portal decompression procedure may not be feasible.

Treatment

Infants with transient ascites caused by acute PVT usually can be treated effectively by repeated infusions of salt-poor albumin to increase intravascular osmotic pressure. Hydrochlorothiazide and spironolactone diuretics are particularly helpful in managing ascites. Paracentesis generally is not needed unless the ascites is so severe that elevation of the diaphragms causes respiratory distress, because the fluid reaccumulates rapidly after removal, and there is increased risk of developing peritonitis. Placement of an indwelling peritoneal catheter, such as that used for long-term peritoneal dialysis, has been helpful in a few patients with rapidly accumulating ascites, but protein depletion is usually so profound that parenteral fluid replacement is often necessary.

Because the liver is almost always normal functionally and histologically in young children with PVT, and massive hemorrhage is rare, nonoperative treatment is preferable until the patient has grown sufficiently for a shunt procedure to have a high likelihood of remaining patent. If variceal hemorrhage occurs, hospitalization with sedation and bed rest, vitamin K administration, intravenous H_2-blockers, oral antacids, and withholding oral feedings are usually successful in stopping the bleeding within 48 hours. If bleeding is persistent, intravenous vasopressin may help to control hemorrhage by decreasing splenic arterial flow and lowering portal venous pressure. When using intravenous vasopressin for active bleeding varices, it may be started at a dose of 0.2 to 0.3 U/min combined with nitroglycerin either as a patch or intravenously at a dose beginning around 40 μg/min. When feasible, esophagoscopy should be performed with injection of a sclerosing solution, such as sodium morrhuate or sodium tetradecyl sulfate. Another useful technique for stopping major recurrent hemorrhage is variceal banding.

When bleeding has been controlled, it is useful to consider long-term pharmacologic treatment to lower portal pressure, including nonselective β-blockers (propranolol and nadolol) and a long-acting nitrate, such as isosorbide mononitrate or dinitrate. Pharmacologic treatment probably should be considered a temporizing measure for children with PVT because long-term compliance is difficult.

Emergency shunt procedures or direct operations on esophageal varices are rarely necessary in children during the first bleeding episode. In a few patients older than 15 years, bleeding may be so persistent and severe, however, as to require balloon tamponade and urgent operation to stop the bleeding. Although the liver tolerates a portosystemic shunt better in patients with PVT than in patients with cirrhosis, encephalopathy still may result, so this has prompted the development of limited and selective shunts over time.

When planning therapy for a patient with PVT, it is essential to appreciate the highly variable bleeding patterns encountered. Some patients may bleed during their first year of life, whereas others may not bleed until a few years later or not at all. Most experience fewer bleeding episodes after age 15 years, but occasional patients bleed repeatedly beyond that time. Patients with PVT who are treated nonoperatively through multiple bleeding episodes have approximately a 2% incidence of transfusion-related hepatitis, and rare cases of human immunodeficiency virus infection have occurred. Rarely, patients die from exsanguination. Approximately 2% of patients die along the way related to operative complications. Of patients, 20% to 25% may develop sufficient portosystemic collaterals so that bleeding does not occur again; if possible, shunt procedures should be reserved for patients with severe, intractable bleeding. It is now evident that patients with PVT who undergo shunt procedures without venographic evidence of adequate-sized vessels for anastomosis and patients who undergo various direct operations on varices may have a higher risk of morbidity and mortality than children managed nonoperatively. Shunt procedures should be undertaken only when absolutely necessary and only when adequate-sized vessels are available for anastomosis. Nonetheless, operation occasionally is needed.

Surgical Management

If, despite repeated sclerotherapy and drug treatment, PVT-based variceal bleeding continues to occur more than two to three times a year, direct surgical intervention eventually may become necessary. As mentioned, shunt procedures rarely are indicated for acute hemorrhage caused by PVT. Direct operations, particularly gastroesophageal devascularization procedures, have been used successfully in many children and adults with PVT. Resection of the varix-bearing portions of the esophagus and upper stomach with subsequent colonic replacement also has been successful in providing long-term relief from bleeding varices in more than half of children who have this procedure. Direct variceal ligation alone rarely is indicated because rebleeding is the rule.

Long-term experience indicates that splenectomy alone for bleeding or for hypersplenism has no place in the management of PVT, particularly in young children, because bleeding almost always recurs, the risk of severe infection is increased, and splenectomy limits the choice of operations available for shunt procedures. Selective distal splenorenal shunt is now one of the operations of choice in children with PVT when the splenic vein is patent. Splenomegaly itself is rarely a serious problem, and splenic rupture rarely occurs even with unrestricted physical activity. In the past, the spleen was useful for splenoportography, but that approach to imaging rarely is used today. Finally the well-documented increase in risk for fatal sepsis and infection in children and adolescents who have undergone splenectomy strongly mitigates against routine removal of the organ for portal hypertension.

When definitive surgical management is considered for patients with variceal bleeding secondary to PVT, it is essential to map portal venous anatomy accurately

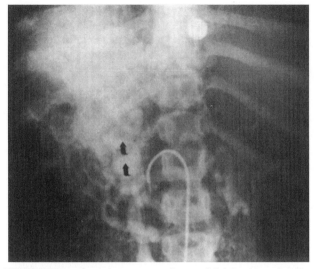

FIGURE 66-2 ■ Superior mesenteric arterial injection of radiographic contrast material shows venous phase in a child with extrahepatic PVT. The recanalized portal vein is shown with multiple collateral channels. Despite PVT, portal flow is hepatopetal (arrows).

using selective superior mesenteric and celiac artery injection with visualization of the mesenteric venous phase (Fig. 66-2). We have preferred to defer all invasive vascular contrast studies until such time as operation is contemplated. Before that time, vascular ultrasound of the portal venous tree and computed tomography scans with contrast injection are usually sufficient. In addition, technetium liver-spleen scans are useful for evaluating hepatic perfusion and function.

Hepatic vein thrombosis or suprahepatic caval obstruction is studied best by transjugular hepatic venography. Liver biopsy is always performed to determine liver histology, particularly when cirrhosis and intrahepatic portal hypertension are present.

At times, operative portography performed through a branch of the superior mesenteric vein is useful. The extent of the thrombosis within the portal system is a vital consideration in planning a shunt operation. If the occlusion extends down the superior mesenteric vein below its junction with the splenic and coronary veins, esophageal and gastric varices are not decompressed by shunting the portion of the superior mesenteric bed that drains the small intestine, and the rate of thrombosis is high. It is only by careful evaluation of the portal system veins that are still widely patent, their size, and their relation to the coronary-esophageal variceal complexes that it is possible to decide if and which type of decompressive surgery would be possible. In several large series of patients with PVT, the results of the various surgical procedures used to control bleeding have been compared. One clear-cut finding is that patients do best if they can have a single successful operation because patients who required a series of operative procedures in an attempt to control bleeding had increasing complications with each succeeding operation. The operations typically became more difficult technically, and postoperative complications of intestinal obstruction, fistula, infection, and wound separation became more common. Accurate and complete angiographic imaging has proved to be crucial.

In a few instances, isolated splenic vein thrombosis may occur with a patent portal vein, usually the result of pancreatitis or pancreatic resection for trauma or tumor. Although there may be sufficient collaterals through gastroepiploic pathways to the patent portal vein to avoid variceal hemorrhage, major bleeding from gastric varices may occur. Under these unusual circumstances, splenectomy may be curative.

Shunt Procedures

The following factors are considered to be essential to achieve a successful portosystemic shunt (Fig. 66-3) in a child:

1. The veins to be used for the anastomosis must be free of phlebitis.
2. The shunt must be of sufficient size to decompress the portal system and to remain patent. Most consider this size to be at least 1 cm in diameter.
3. The shunt anastomosis must be capable of growth with the child, so a modified interrupted suture technique is indicated.
4. The shunt must drain the entire portal venous tree effectively.

For patients with intractable bleeding, a patent portosystemic shunt provides the best protection against future bleeding. The ideal choice of procedure is debatable, with the balancing factors being effective decreasing of portal pressure and avoidance of postshunt encephalopathy. In general, most surgeons now prefer either the classic cavomesenteric shunt or, more recently, the interposition H-graft mesocaval shunt with autogenous jugular vein. In our studies and those of others, cavomesenteric shunts provide an 80% chance of permanent relief from variceal bleeding related to PVT in children who have suitable mesenteric veins for construction of a shunt. Ligation of the inferior vena cava is well tolerated in children, allowing normal growth, but approximately 10% of adults who have had this procedure require temporary elastic supports for the lower extremities to prevent swelling. Interposition H-graft procedures, particularly using autologous veins, have been followed by a low incidence of thrombosis and good control of bleeding over the long-term, although rebleeding sometimes occurs early postoperatively. The classic central splenorenal shunt procedure has a 50% incidence of rebleeding in children, so it is not considered to be a desirable first-choice operation. Distal splenorenal shunts as described by Warren have been used almost with the same level of success as cavomesenteric or H-graft shunts.

Despite some reports to the contrary, shunt procedures in children younger than 8 to 10 years are followed by a high incidence of thrombosis (at least 30%). In addition, nontraditional or makeshift shunts to the mesenteric venous tributaries are associated with a greater than 80% to 90% incidence of rebleeding, making these procedures less desirable than direct devascularization procedures.

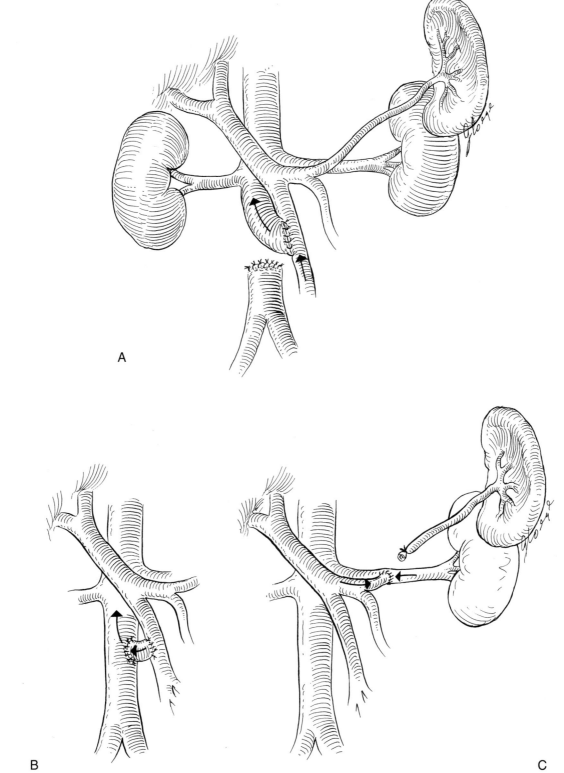

A

B   C

FIGURE 66-3 ■ The most common portal-to-systemic shunts used in children with portal hypertension. **A,** Cavomesenteric shunt with transection of lower vena cava and anastomosis to the side of the superior mesenteric vein. The major direction of the visceral venous flow is toward the vena cava. Hepatopetal flow and potential for hepatofugal flow is depicted. **B,** Interposition mesocaval shunt is hemodynamically similar to the mesocaval shunt but does not interrupt the vena cava. Autogenous vein graft is preferred for creation of this shunt in infants and young children. A prosthetic graft may be used in older children and adults but has a higher incidence of failure in the long term. **C,** In the central splenorenal shunt, there is opportunity for hepatopetal and hepatofugal flow. The spleen is necessarily removed.

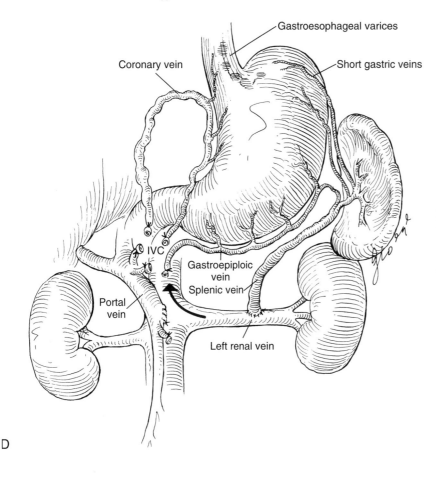

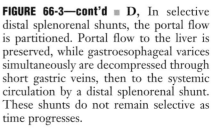

FIGURE 66-3—cont'd ■ **D,** In selective distal splenorenal shunts, the portal flow is partitioned. Portal flow to the liver is preserved, while gastroesophageal varices simultaneously are decompressed through short gastric veins, then to the systemic circulation by a distal splenorenal shunt. These shunts do not remain selective as time progresses.

The incidence of postshunt encephalopathy in patients with extrahepatic portal hypertension has decreased over time with the use of either the distal splenorenal shunt or the H-graft procedure. Even when it occurs in mild form, it usually can be treated successfully by identifying then eliminating the precipitating cause, such as gastrointestinal hemorrhage, excessive diuresis, azotemia, sedatives, infection, and excess protein intake. Mild encephalopathic symptoms have been reported in an occasional older child with PVT who has developed spontaneous portosystemic shunts without operation.

Treatment of the Unshuntable Patient

A portosystemic shunt is not possible in one third to one half of children with PVT because the thrombosis and phlebitis of the portal vein extend into the superior mesenteric and splenic veins. This results in continued bleeding through the years, although some children eventually develop spontaneous shunts. For the three fourths of unshuntable patients who continue to bleed, many other therapeutic options have been devised, including sclerotherapy, pharmacotherapy, and a variety of alternative direct operative approaches to management of the varices. Although none of these direct operative approaches are as successful as a large patent portosystemic shunt, the most successful approach has been the Sigiura gastroesophageal devascularization operation (Fig. 66-4). Rebleeding rates of 37% have been reported, and mortality is low in patients with PVT.

In children who are unshuntable and have repeated bleeding despite nonoperative treatment or a devascularization procedure, esophagogastrectomy, pyloroplasty, and colonic replacement of the esophagus may be a reasonable last resort, with only about one fourth of patients experiencing early rebleeding and none experiencing later rebleeding. Over time, many of the latter patients may form varices in the esophagus above the level of the interposed colon segment or in the stomach. Total esophagectomy usually is reserved for the rare patient shown on portography to have varices extending to the middle and upper third of the esophagus. When necessary, we prefer to use a Sigiura type of gastroesophageal devascularization procedure without an esophageal transection when possible. With the latter modification, we usually have oversewn the bleeding varices through a small gastrotomy, and this has proved to be effective. Pyloroplasty has been used routinely because gastric stasis is common after extensive devascularization procedures. Most of these patients also continue to require periodic endoscopy and endosclerosis. In children, we have preferred not to perform esophageal transection with reanastomosis because of the risk of anastomotic leak, fistula formation, and infection. The Tanner procedure (portoazygous disconnection and gastric division) has a high rebleeding rate and has been replaced by the Sigiura procedure for unshuntable patients. Splenectomy has not been added to devascularization procedures in children because of its inherent long-term risk.

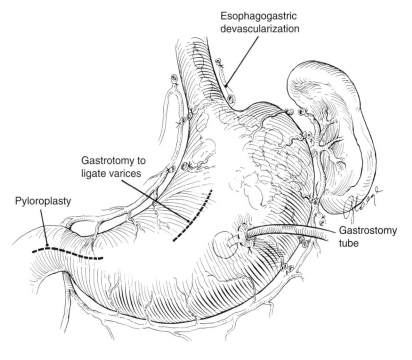

Esophagogastric
devascularization

Gastrotomy to
ligate varices

Pyloroplasty

Gastrostomy
tube

FIGURE 66-4 ▪ Gastroesophageal devascularization operation (modified Sigiura procedure) used in many children with severe variceal hemorrhage as a result of PVT refractory to medical therapy and in whom the portal mesenteric veins are not suitable for shunt procedures. Gastrotomy provides access for oversewing bleeding gastric varices. Because the vagus nerves often are injured during the procedure, pyloroplasty is performed routinely. Temporary gastrostomy is a helpful adjunct in these patients. Esophageal transection is not usually done in children.

Repeated endoscopic variceal sclerotherapy is useful in patients who are unshuntable because it reduces the chance of recurrent bleeding, particularly when combined with pharmacotherapy. Over time, bleeding seems to abate in most patients. The latter methods are used first before considering any patient for a devascularization procedure. Bleeding episodes generally occur less frequently as the child grows older and becomes less susceptible to respiratory infections.

INTRAHEPATIC OBSTRUCTION

The outlook for children with portal hypertension caused by cirrhosis is much less favorable than that with PVT because of the usually progressive nature of the primary liver disease. Intrahepatic obstruction is suggested by a history of jaundice, hepatomegaly with splenic enlargement, ascites, or evidence of impaired liver function. Intrahepatic portal venous hypertension is the result of cirrhosis of the liver, which may follow neonatal hepatitis or exposure to toxic agents or may be associated with congenital hepatic fibrosis, fibrocystic disease, congenital biliary atresia, or, less commonly, a variety of metabolic disorders (Table 66-2). The degree of portal venous hypertension relates to the degree of periportal fibrosis.

Surgical management of intrahepatic portal hypertension in children is determined primarily by the prognosis of the underlying hepatic disease. Although hepatic function is moderately to severely abnormal in most such patients, many conditions in childhood initially produce moderate-to-severe hepatic scarring that causes portal venous obstruction but is not associated with serious injury to the hepatic cell, even though the liver disease is usually progressive. This is the case for children with cystic fibrosis who have experienced variceal hemorrhage but who have only moderately abnormal liver function tests. When variceal bleeding is effectively controlled, long-term survival is possible.

For most patients with intrahepatic portal hypertension associated with severe cirrhosis, such as patients with biliary atresia, treatment plans are best based on their candidacy for liver transplantation. In general, portosystemic shunt procedures are not indicated in patients who are candidates for liver transplantation because this intervention is likely to interfere with the transplantation procedure. Shunt procedures in patients with mild nonprogressive, hepatic fibrosis, such as patients with congenital hepatic fibrosis, may provide long-term relief from bleeding.

Patients with intrahepatic portal hypertension and acute variceal bleeding are best treated initially with bed rest and supportive care and either vasopressin intravenously or intravenous octreotide with a 25-μg bolus followed by 25 to 50 μg/hr for 2 to 5 days. When the

---

TABLE 66-2 ▪ Causes of Cirrhosis Producing Intrahepatic Portal Venous Hypertension in Children

Biliary atresia
Congenital hepatic fibrosis
Cystic fibrosis, focal biliary cirrhosis
α_1-Antitrypsin deficiency
Radiation, chemotherapy
Posthepatitic cirrhosis
Sclerosing cholangitis
Histiocytosis X
Galactosemia
Congenital biliary cirrhosis
Hepatic hemangioendotheliomatosis
Glycogen storage disease

patient's condition has been stabilized, sclerotherapy or banding can be performed. After this, pharmacotherapy as mentioned earlier with nonselective β-blockers is appropriate. If patients continue to bleed repeatedly and excessively despite these measures, placement of a transjugular intrahepatic portosystemic shunt (TIPS) is in order using a percutaneous approach. A TIPS functions effectively as a side-to-side portocaval shunt. Although a TIPS procedure is only a temporizing measure because of subsequent occlusion, it is an excellent bridge to transplantation. Biliary atresia is the most common indication for liver transplantation in children today. Transplantation also is indicated for children with intrahepatic portal hypertension from posthepatitic cirrhosis and occasional patients with diffuse hepatic hemangioendotheliomatosis. Some of the latter patients also are candidates for portosystemic venous shunts. Patients who develop mild hepatic fibrosis from prolonged chemotherapy or radiation therapy for malignant neoplasms also occasionally may require shunt procedures for portal hypertension. Glycogen storage disease may produce portal venous hypertension, but the condition is often reversible with the initiation of night feedings. Shunts are rarely required for this now.

In contradistinction to the lack of mortality with bleeding in patients with extrahepatic portal hypertension, children with intrahepatic portal hypertension who bleed have considerable mortality even with the first major bleeding episode. This is because poor liver function causes malnutrition and coagulopathy, which complicate the treatment of acute hemorrhage. Hyperammonemia, owing to absorption of blood from the colon, also complicates care during an episode of bleeding in these patients.

As mentioned, the treatment of children with cirrhosis and intrahepatic portal hypertension has changed remarkably with the improvements that have been seen in supportive care and liver transplantation. In general, shunt procedures should be considered a last resort except perhaps in patients with conditions involving only mild hepatic fibrosis that is not progressive.

Suprahepatic Obstruction (Budd-Chiari Syndrome)

On rare occasions, children with suprahepatic venous obstruction associated with portal hypertension and ascites are encountered. The presenting signs are variceal hemorrhage, ascites, hypersplenism, and hepatomegaly with only mildly abnormal liver function tests. Hepatic vein obstruction by granulomatosis is common in South America but is extremely rare in North America.

The association between hepatic vein thrombosis and oral contraceptive use is well established. In addition, occasional cases of congenital webs and diaphragms at the junction of the hepatic veins and the suprahepatic vena cava are seen. In most cases, the cause is never clearly identified, however. Symptoms are generally mild at first and not recognized for months to years. There is no specific medical treatment for suprahepatic venous obstruction syndrome other than general supportive care. An acute form of Budd-Chiari syndrome has been recognized, although most patients have a progressively deteriorating course with death eventually resulting from hepatic failure or variceal hemorrhage. Attempts to relieve thrombosis in the hepatic veins by systemic anticoagulation or the administration of fibrinolytic agents have not had much success.

Partially diverting portosystemic shunts have been used with improvement of symptoms and extended survival in 60% of patients with this form of obstruction. Also, mesoatrial shunts have relieved the condition successfully for varying periods in occasional patients, but the best opportunity for complete cure of suprahepatic portal venous obstruction is liver transplantation, which is discussed in detail in Chapter 64.

SUGGESTED READINGS

Orozco H, Takahashi T, Mercado MA, et al: Surgical management of extrahepatic portal hypertension and variceal bleeding. World J Surg 18:246-250, 1994.

The authors describe excellent long-term results with the Sigiura-Futagawa procedure in 38 patients with extrahepatic portal obstruction and normal livers.

Rikkers LF: The changing spectrum of treatment for variceal bleeding. Ann Surg 228:536-543, 1998.

An excellent discussion is presented of sclerotherapy versus shunt procedures versus TIPS in patients with esophageal varices and the place of liver transplantation.

Sharara AI, Rockey DC: Gastroesophageal variceal hemorrhage. N Engl J Med 345:669-681, 2001.

This is an excellent review of approaches to work-up and treatment of patients who have cirrhosis as the cause of variceal bleeding. A thorough discussion of pharmacologic treatment, TIPS, and surgical shunt procedures is presented.

Sigalet DL, Mayer S, Blanchard H: Portal venous decompression with H-type mesocaval shunt using autologous vein graft: A North American experience. J Pediatr Surg 36:91-96, 2001.

This article presents a good option for patients with extrahepatic portal hypertension with good control of bleeding and minimal encephalopathy.

67

Gallbladder Disease

Gallbladder disease, including acute hydrops, acute acalculous cholecystitis, and chronic cholecystitis and cholelithiasis, is common, occurring with increased frequency. This chapter discusses new diagnostic and therapeutic approaches.

CONGENITAL ANOMALIES

Congenital anomalies of the gallbladder are relatively infrequent occurrences. Agenesis, duplication, bilobed gallbladder, and ectopic location are the conditions most commonly observed. More recently, congenital stenosis of the cystic duct has been documented as a cause of gallbladder stasis and obstruction, leading to pain associated with fever and the subsequent development of inflammation and gallstone formation. Most of these conditions are detected incidentally during the work-up of a patient for abdominal pain or during laparotomy for other intra-abdominal conditions.

ACUTE HYDROPS OF THE GALLBLADDER

Acute noncalculous distention of the gallbladder is a well-recognized entity. Hydrops may occur in the neonatal period and in older children. This condition is characterized by the development of severe edema around the gallbladder and common bile duct. Older infants and children may manifest fever, a right upper quadrant mass, and abdominal tenderness on palpation, whereas a mass may be the only finding in neonates. In newborns, acute hydrops has been observed in infants who are septic and has occurred in a patient with cystic duct agenesis. In older infants and children, hydrops may accompany scarlet fever, leptospirosis, and Kawasaki disease. In the last-mentioned condition, the cystic duct and common bile duct are surrounded by enlarged lymph nodes. The diagnosis usually is obtained by abdominal ultrasound. Treatment is expectant with antibiotics, when appropriate for septic patients, and early enteral feedings, when possible, to stimulate gallbladder contraction and emptying. Hydrops should be followed by serial ultrasound examinations, and if distention and pain persist or increase, a cholecystostomy may be performed for temporary decompression. If the gallbladder wall appears gangrenous or if cystic duct obstruction is detected, a cholecystectomy should be performed.

ACALCULOUS CHOLECYSTITIS

Acalculous cholecystitis may occur as a complication during treatment of various disease states. This condition may occur in newborns but is more common in older children. Genders are affected equally. Patients are often severely ill as a result of prior surgery; a severe burn; multisystem trauma; massive blood transfusion; and various infections, including pneumonia, generalized sepsis, typhoid, salmonella, otitis media with meningitis, giardiasis, and Kawasaki disease. Although the cause is unknown, the underlying features involved in the pathogenesis include dehydration, adynamic ileus, gallbladder stasis, treatment with total parenteral nutrition (TPN), and hemolysis from multiple transfusions.

Symptoms include fever, right upper quadrant pain, nausea, vomiting, and occasionally diarrhea when the underlying infection is caused by a pathogenic intestinal organism. Tenderness to palpation and muscle guarding are noted on physical examination. A right upper quadrant mass is sometimes palpable and must be distinguished from acute hydrops. Leukocytosis and jaundice are observed often, and an elevated serum amylase level signifying associated pancreatitis has been noted often. The diagnosis is confirmed on ultrasound that shows gallbladder distention and echogenic debris or sludge. The treatment for mild cases includes nasogastric suction, intravenous fluids, and parenteral antibiotics administered according to blood culture results. The patient's course is followed by serial ultrasound examinations. Persistence of the mass or increased distention and clinical deterioration are indications for operation. Cholecystostomy is a reasonable form of therapy for isolated massive distention; however, cholecystectomy should be done for inflammation, the presence of purulent exudate, or gangrenous changes in the gallbladder wall. Gallbladder infarction also has been observed as a result of arteritis in patients with Kawasaki disease.

CHOLELITHIASIS

Gallstones are relatively uncommon in blacks (except in sickle cell disease), exceptionally common in select groups of Native Americans (especially the Pima Indians) and Hispanics, and a frequent occurrence in whites. Gallstones currently are being recognized in children with increased frequency. Whether this increase in diagnosis is related to an increase in frequency of the disease or an increase in recognition because of the widespread use of ultrasound for abdominal complaints is unclear. The incidence currently is reported to be 0.15% to 0.22% in children. In comparison, cholelithiasis is recognized in approximately 10% of adults.

NONHEMOLYTIC CHOLELITHIASIS

The gallstones in patients with nonhemolytic disease are usually cholesterol in nature. The solubility of cholesterol depends on the concentration of lecithin, bile salts, and cholesterol within bile. Any disturbance in the concentration of these three substances may leave the bile lithogenic and predisposed to the formation of cholesterol stones. These stones result when the bile cannot solubilize all of the cholesterol. Although they often typically are seen in adults with advancing age, in obese patients, and in patients using estrogens or who are pregnant, these stones also can be seen in older children and adolescents without hematologic conditions. Nonhemolytic gallstones often are seen in obese children, in pregnant adolescents, in patients with a family history for cholelithiasis, in women using oral contraceptives, and in children with other chronic illnesses such as cystic fibrosis. In patients with chronic disease, the cause of gallstones may be related more to stasis than any other factor. In some patients requiring chemotherapy for Wilms' tumor, neuroblastoma, Hodgkin's disease, or non-Hodgkin's lymphoma, there also has been noted to be an increased risk for the development of cholelithiasis.

Despite the above-described factors, in most patients with nonhemolytic disease, no predisposing cause can be identified. Although boys and girls usually are affected equally by gallstones in infancy and early childhood, cholelithiasis is more common in girls in adolescents with a female-to-male ratio of 11:1 to 22:1. This increased predominance in girls probably is related to the strong hormonal influences of estrogen and progesterone.

HEMOLYTIC DISEASE

Pigmented stones can be black or earthy brown (calcium bilirubinate). Black pigmented stones usually are associated with a hemolytic process, such as sickle cell disease, hereditary spherocytosis, thalassemia major, pyruvate kinase deficiency, autoimmune hemolytic anemia, and other hemolytic processes. Calcium bilirubinate stones are found in patients with infected bile or biliary strictures. Although the exact cause of the development of pigment stones is unclear, the bile in these patients contains an excess amount of unconjugated bilirubin and β-glucuronidase, an enzyme produced by bacteria that may hydrolyze soluble bilirubin glucuronide to insoluble unconjugated bilirubin and glucuronic acid. Unconjugated bilirubin may form calcium bilirubinate. Stasis and nucleating factors also may play a role in the development of these stones. Although it has been assumed

that the gallstones associated with distal ileal resection occur as a result of an interruption of the normal enterohepatic circulation with the resultant decrease in the bile salt pool, cholesterol saturation of bile, and cholesterol stone formation, the gallstones noted in children with ileal disorders such as short-bowel syndrome and inflammatory bowel disease who are maintained on TPN are pigment stones.

Sickle Cell Anemia

Approximately 50,000 blacks have sickle cell disease, and 10% carry the gene. The incidence of cholelithiasis in patients with sickle cell anemia has been reported to be 10% to 70%. The incidence of gallstones increases with age, with 12% affected in the 2- to 4-year age group and 42% affected in the 15- to 18-year age group.

Often, it can be difficult to differentiate symptoms of biliary colic from an abdominal crisis in the sickle cell patient. Ultrasound should be performed in all children with sickle cell disease and abdominal pain before labeling them as having a sickle crisis. If signs of acute cholecystitis are noted on ultrasound, biliary scintigraphy can be performed, although there is a high false-positive rate in patients with sickle cell anemia.

There has been an increased risk of complications related to cholelithiasis in patients with sickle cell disease and a significantly lower complication rate associated with elective laparoscopic cholecystectomy in this population. For this reason, prophylactic cholecystectomy for asymptomatic cholelithiasis has been advocated by some investigators. Of previously asymptomatic patients, 50% require operation within 3 years because of significant complications or symptoms of acute cholecystitis. Careful preoperative preparation of a child with sickle cell anemia is essential to avoid perioperative sickling of the abnormal red blood cells. This sickling may be precipitated by hypoxia, hypothermia, acidosis, hypovolemia, and a high level of hemoglobin S. For elective operations, preoperative transfusion can be performed intermittently over 2 to 3 weeks before the operative procedure. This transfusion increases the total hemoglobin level, suppresses the bone marrow, and decreases the reticulocyte count. The sickle cells are cleared as a result of their short half-life, and the percentage of hemoglobin S generally decreases to less than 30% to 40%. For urgent cholecystectomy, simple transfusion to a hemoglobin level of approximately 12 g/dL can allow a safe procedure. A large percentage of the cells can sickle if acidosis or hypothermia occur, however. Another technique in the more urgent setting is exchange transfusion through a large-bore catheter. This procedure results in approximately 90% hemoglobin A cells and 10% hemoglobin S cells. Intraoperatively, it is vital to avoid hypothermia, hypovolemia, and acidosis in these patients.

Hereditary Spherocytosis

The incidence of cholelithiasis in hereditary spherocytosis is 43% to 63% and is slightly more common in girls than boys. Abdominal ultrasound should be performed before elective splenectomy to detect the presence of gallstones. Laparoscopic cholecystectomy is recommended in all patients with hereditary spherocytosis and symptoms and all patients with gallstones who are undergoing laparoscopic splenectomy. Although not used routinely, there have been reports of simple cholecystotomy with removal of the stones at the time of splenectomy with no recurrence of stones after 11-year follow-up. Although there is an increased risk of recurrent gallstones after cholecystotomy and stone removal, with the spleen removed, the level of hemolysis may be low enough to avoid new stone formation.

Thalassemia Major

The incidence of cholelithiasis in children with thalassemia major varies from 2.3% to 23% and increases with age. Gallstones have been observed in 6% of children 6 to 10 years old and 45% of children 11 to 14 years old. The risk of cholelithiasis in this patient population is decreasing, however, as a result of a hypertransfusion therapy that blocks the bone marrow so that the fragile cell of thalassemia major is no longer produced. For all symptomatic patients and for patients undergoing laparoscopic splenectomy in whom preoperative ultrasound shows the presence of gallstones, laparoscopic cholecystectomy is recommended.

CLINICAL PRESENTATION

Neonates and Infants

Cholelithiasis in neonates and young infants frequently results from an associated condition, such as prematurity, ileal resection, cystic fibrosis, chronic prolonged hyperalimentation, and fasting (Fig. 67-1). Other associated conditions include the use of furosemide and phototherapy, polycythemia, and after exchange transfusion. Of children receiving long-term TPN, 43% have been shown to develop gallstones. In approximately 44% of patients, bile sludge has been observed before stone formation. Other factors in this age group responsible for gallstone development may include decreased bile acid output in premature infants, lack of enteral intake, and increased excretion of unconjugated bilirubin into the bile during

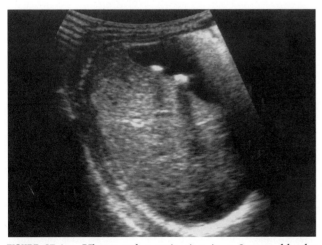

FIGURE 67-1 ■ Ultrasound examination in a 2-year-old who required ileal resection shows two gallstones with acoustic shadowing.

phototherapy used to treat physiologic jaundice. Phototherapy has been implicated in the development of gallstones in the absence of TPN. The shortened red blood cell life in premature infants also may increase bilirubin excretion. Neonatal gallstone formation is probably a multifactorial problem with stasis and the lack of enteral feedings having a significant impact. Choledocholithiasis with obstructive jaundice also can be seen in newborns and is associated more commonly with prematurity and the administration of TPN.

Spontaneous resolution of gallstones in neonates and infants has been observed on serial ultrasound examinations in 20% of patients. It may be difficult to differentiate biliary sludge from cholelithiasis in premature infants, however, and in some cases that resolved, the patients may have had sludge rather than actual stones. It has been shown that resolution of gallstones may occur 2 to 20 days after the cessation of TPN. Many neonates and infants have calcified stones, however, which do not resolve. The recommended treatment in this age group has not been clarified. Nonoperative therapy for noncalcified, asymptomatic TPN-related gallstones for 1 year is not unreasonable, however. Laparoscopic or open cholecystectomy for symptomatic infants with TPN-associated gallstones and for infants with calcified radiopaque stones is reasonable.

Choledocholithiasis with cholestatic jaundice in neonates and infants usually requires operative intervention, although spontaneous resolution also has been reported in some patients. Endoscopic retrograde cholangiopancreatography (ERCP) and endoscopic sphincterotomy with stone removal have been reported in infants, although many endoscopists are not facile with this technique in this age group. If endoscopic sphincterotomy is unsuccessful or if the child is too small for ERCP, an open or laparoscopic procedure with irrigation of the common bile duct through the cystic duct or an open transduodenal sphincterotomy may be required. If bile duct perforation has occurred, early peritoneal irrigation and drainage usually is effective. If the diagnosis is delayed, a severe inflammatory process may result in a common bile duct stricture, which may require operative repair or reconstruction.

Older Children

Most older children and adolescents with cholelithiasis present with symptoms related to biliary colic with abdominal pain, nausea, and vomiting. In acute calculous cholecystitis, patients present with a distended, tender gallbladder, and the pain is localized in the right upper quadrant. The pain is less well localized in younger children. Chronic cholecystitis commonly is characterized by recurrent bouts of right upper quadrant abdominal pain associated with meals. The pain is often vague and rarely is associated with fatty food intolerance as is seen often in adults. In children with chronic cholecystitis and cholelithiasis, the physical examination is often normal. Patients with acute cholecystitis may show elevated temperature, right upper abdominal tenderness, and muscle guarding. If jaundice is noted, the patient may have choledocholithiasis. This is especially true in the absence of hemolytic disease. Patients with acute cholecystitis

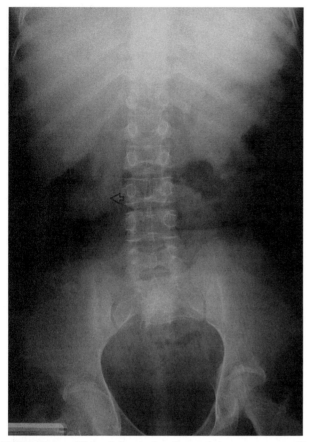

FIGURE 67-2 ▪ Plain abdominal radiograph in a teenager with right upper abdominal pain documents calcified gallstones (arrow).

may have leukocytosis. Elevated serum direct bilirubin, alkaline phosphatase, and γ-glutamyl transferase levels are seen. Because pancreatitis can occur in 10% of patients, serum amylase and lipase levels should be monitored as well.

In patients with suspected gallstones, the most accurate and useful diagnostic test is ultrasound. An abdominal radiograph also may be performed and reveals radiopaque gallstones in 30% of patients (Fig. 67-2). At the time of ultrasound, the assessment of the gallbladder size, wall thickness, and diameter of the common bile duct are important measures. For patients with suspected acute cholecystitis, cholescintigraphy with technetium-99m-labeled iminodiacetic acid (DISIDA) is the most useful test to detect obstruction of the cystic duct. With this study, the gallbladder is not visualized if the cystic duct is obstructed (Fig. 67-3). A false-positive result may occur if the patient has been fasting or has been receiving TPN. In this setting, intravenous morphine can be administered before the scintigram because it causes spasm of the sphincter of Oddi and results in an increase in the common bile duct pressure with enhanced visualization of the gallbladder. This test has a sensitivity close to 100% and a specificity of 95%. Cholescintigraphy is also useful in detecting common bile duct obstruction or choledochal cyst. Computed tomography is not helpful in the initial evaluation of gallstones in children but may be useful in

cases complicated by choledocholithiasis or gallstone pancreatitis.

Biliary Dyskinesia

A distinct clinical entity that occurs primarily in older children and adults is biliary dyskinesia, which is characterized by poor gallbladder contractility and the presence of cholesterol crystals in the gallbladder bile. This condition may be an early stage of cholesterol gallstone formation. Several reports have correlated the presence of biliary dyskinesia in association with chronic cholecystitis in patients who subsequently undergo cholecystectomy. There is often a delay in diagnosis of patients with this condition because ultrasound does not show cholelithiasis. These patients have a history of nausea and intermittent right upper abdominal pain with the onset usually after meals.

Biliary dyskinesia is diagnosed with a technetium-99m DISIDA study during the injection of intravenous cholecystokinin. Patients with this condition have an ejection fraction usually less than 35%. If a child appears symptomatic with this condition and the ejection fraction is less than 35%, laparoscopic cholecystectomy is recommended, although the patient and family should be counseled that there is no guarantee that symptoms will resolve. On histologic examination of the gallbladder, there is often evidence of chronic cholecystitis.

TREATMENT

In the 1980s and 1990s, numerous nonoperative therapies were introduced for the management of gallstones, including dissolution of cholesterol gallstones with oral administration of chenodeoxycholic acid, the use of

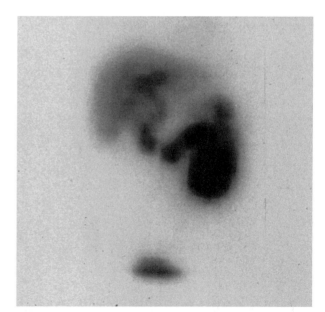

FIGURE 67-3 ▪ A 15-year-old patient with epigastric pain underwent a technetium-99m-labeled DISIDA study. This delayed image after administration of intravenous morphine shows filling of the common bile duct without visualization of the gallbladder. There is significant activity in the intestinal tract on this delayed study.

extracorporeal shock-wave lithotripsy, and percutaneous endoscopic cholecystolithotomy. The dissolution rate for chenodeoxycholic acid was found to be less than 15% after 2 years. Only 15% to 20% of patients with gallstones qualified for extracorporeal shock-wave lithotripsy. No studies have been performed in children with these therapies, and they largely have been abandoned at this time. Percutaneous endoscopic cholecystolithotomy is invasive, has a high risk of gallstone recurrence, and is not suited for infants or young children.

Laparoscopic cholecystectomy has become the preferred standard for management of symptomatic children with cholelithiasis. Preoperatively an ultrasound examination is performed on each patient to confirm the diagnosis of cholelithiasis and to evaluate the presence or absence of common bile duct involvement. Children with stones in the common bile duct present with jaundice, severe pain, or pancreatitis. If there is suspicion of choledocholithiasis on initial evaluation, ERCP and sphincterotomy are recommended before the laparoscopic operation. The primary advantage of proceeding with ERCP preoperatively and, if needed, sphincterotomy is that this approach enables the surgeon to proceed with straightforward laparoscopic cholecystectomy if choledocholithiasis is not present or, if present, the stones will have been removed from the common bile duct. This is important because the expertise to remove these stones endoscopically is not universally available in all children's hospitals. If choledocholithiasis is documented and the stones cannot be removed endoscopically, the surgeon must decide whether to proceed with the laparoscopic cholecystectomy and laparoscopic choledochal exploration or to perform an open operation.

After induction of general and endotracheal anesthesia, the urinary bladder is emptied with a Credé maneuver, and the abdomen is prepared and draped in a sterile fashion. A 10-mm incision is made in a vertical direction through the umbilical skin and carried down through the umbilical fascia with cautery. A 10-mm port is introduced directly into the abdominal cavity. The primary reason that this cannula is 10 mm in diameter is for exteriorization of the gallbladder through the umbilical fascia and skin. The position of the other incisions and ports varies according to the patient's size. It is especially important to place these ports widely in the younger patient because the intra-abdominal working area is reduced (Fig. 67-4). Two 3- or 5-mm ports are placed on the right side of the abdomen, one below the right costal margin and one in the right mid to lower abdomen. The fourth incision is usually 5 mm in length in children (but occasionally may need to be 10 mm if a 10-mm endoscopic clip applier is required), and this is situated just to the patient's right of the midline in the epigastric region in the older child or to the left of the patient's midline in the younger child.

The fundus of the gallbladder is grasped with a grasping forceps that has been introduced through the right lower cannula, and the gallbladder is retracted superiorly and ventrally over the liver. The infundibulum is retracted to the patient's right with the instrument placed through the right upper port, allowing the cystic duct to enter to the common bile duct as close to a 90-degree

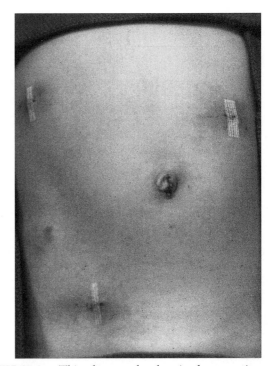

FIGURE 67-4 ■ This photograph taken in the operating room shows wide spacing of the incisions for laparoscopic cholecystectomy in a 2-year-old patient. The right lower incision is placed near the inguinal crease for cosmetic reasons, and the 5-mm epigastric incision is placed in the left epigastrium so as to allow an efficient working space between instruments. The 5-mm umbilical incision used in this young child has been closed with absorbable sutures.

angle as possible (Fig. 67-5). If the cystic duct is not oriented 90 degrees in relation to the common bile duct but is oriented parallel to the common bile duct, the common duct may be misidentified as the cystic duct and clipped and divided.

When the cystic duct has been skeletonized, the decision is made whether or not to perform cholangiography. The primary utility of intraoperative cholangiography currently is the delineation of correct anatomy. When the surgeon has achieved a suitable comfort level with laparoscopic cholangiography, it is not routinely needed unless there is confusion regarding the correct identification of the cystic or common bile ducts. If it is used, an incision is made in the lateral wall of the cystic duct, and a cholangiocatheter is passed through one of the right-sided ports and into the cystic duct. It can be secured with either a suture or a clip, and cholangiography is performed in the standard fashion. The cholangiocatheter is removed, and, assuming the cholangiogram is normal, the cystic duct is doubly clipped and divided. In a similar fashion, the cystic artery is doubly clipped and divided in the triangle of Calot. The gallbladder is dissected free from its liver bed in a retrograde fashion with either hook or spatula cautery (see Fig. 67-5). Before almost complete detachment of the gallbladder from the liver, the area of dissection is inspected carefully and hemostasis is controlled. The gallbladder is detached completely from its liver bed. Assuming a 5-mm epigastric port was placed,

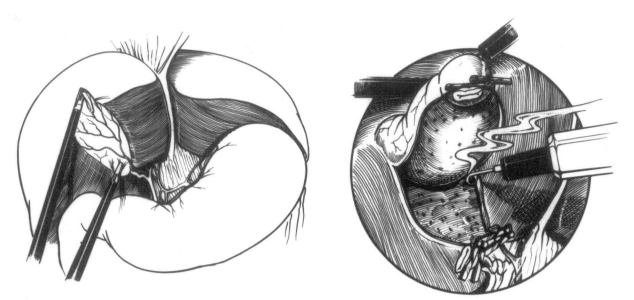

FIGURE 67-5 ■ On the left, the infundibulum of the gallbladder is being pulled laterally to create as close to a 90-degree entry of the cystic duct into the common duct as possible. By orienting the cystic duct transversely in relation to the vertical common duct, misidentification of these two structures is less likely. On the right, the gallbladder is being dissected in a retrograde fashion from the gallbladder bed using the hook cautery. (From Halcomb GW: Laparascopic cholecystectomy. In Holcomb GW: Pediatric Endoscopic Surgery. Appleton and Lange, Norwalk, CT, 1994, by permission.)

a 5-mm telescope is introduced through this cannula, and a 10-mm grasping forceps is placed through the umbilical cannula. The gallbladder is grasped with the forceps and extracted either through the umbilical cannula or through the umbilical fascia after removal of the cannula. Repeat endoscopic visualization is performed to ensure that there is adequate hemostasis. All cannulas then are removed, the incisions are closed, and anesthesia is terminated.

Laparoscopic exploration of the common bile duct is possible either through an enlarged cystic duct or directly through the common bile duct. Exploration through the cystic duct is performed before ligation and division of the cystic duct. Choledochoscopy can be

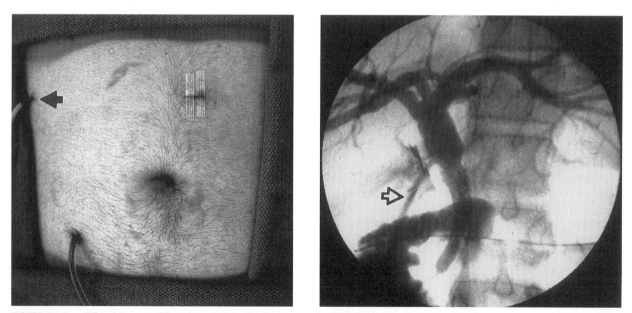

FIGURE 67-6 ■ This 16-year-old patient required a laparoscopic choledochal exploration for obstructive jaundice secondary to impacted stones in the common bile duct. There was extensive inflammation in the area of the gallbladder and common bile duct, and a closed suction drain was placed in the gallbladder bed and exteriorized through the patient's right lower port site. In addition, a T-tube was placed in the common bile duct after the choledochotomy and choledochoscopy and was exteriorized through the patient's right subcostal port site (arrow). On the left, a T-tube study, performed 6 weeks postoperatively, shows a patent common bile duct and no evidence of leak around the T-tube (open arrow).

performed with a flexible choledochoscope introduced through one of the right-sided ports and positioned through the incision in the enlarged cystic duct. Stone retrieval is performed if necessary. With experience, surgeons are becoming more comfortable with performing direct exploration of the common bile duct. This is performed in a similar fashion as with the open operation in that stay sutures are placed on each side of the planned choledochotomy, and the choledochus is sharply incised between the stay sutures. A flexible choledochoscope is introduced through one of the right-sided ports into the common bile duct. Stone retrieval can be performed if required. With this approach, the choledochal incision should be closed with interrupted absorbable sutures around a T-tube, which can be exteriorized through one of the right upper quadrant incisions. A closed suction drain also can be placed, if desired, and exteriorized through one of the right lower incisions (Fig. 67-6). A T-tube cholangiogram should be performed 4 to 6 weeks postoperatively, and the T-tube is removed if the study is normal.

The advantages of the laparoscopic approach for cholecystectomy include less postoperative discomfort, reduced hospitalization, and an early return to full activity. In a study of 100 children undergoing laparoscopic cholecystectomy, Holcomb and colleagues found an average postoperative hospitalization of 1.10 (± 0.4) days for elective operation compared with 1.68 (± 1.2) days for an urgent or emergency procedure (P = .0005). In that study, no complications developed, and two patients underwent laparoscopic choledochal exploration. Six patients underwent preoperative ERCP for evaluation of suspected common duct stones. The study was positive in two patients, and the stones in the common duct were able to be removed successfully endoscopically with sphincterotomy in one. The other patient underwent laparoscopic choledochal exploration and retrieval of the stone.

Significant complications have been reported in the adult literature from patients undergoing laparoscopic cholecystectomy at a higher rate than open cholecystectomy. There is a definite learning curve with a significant decrease in complications with increased operator experience. The conversion rate to an open operation is less than 2%, and injury to the common bile duct is around 1% in the adult literature. In an early report of 1518 laparoscopic cholecystectomies from 20 different centers, there was an occurrence of bile duct injuries in 2.2% of the early cases but only 0.1% of the later cases.

Bile leak is another complication that has been found with laparoscopic cholecystectomy in 1.5% to 2% of patients. These patients often can be treated successfully with ERCP and placement of a stent across the area of leakage in the choledochus. In addition, either a laparoscopic or an open procedure can be performed to close the duct if the leak persists.

SUGGESTED READINGS

De Caluwe D, Akl U, Corbally M: Cholecystectomy versus cholecystolithotomy for cholelithiasis in childhood: Long-term outcome. J Pediatr Surg 36:1518-1521, 2001.

The authors describe 10 patients over a 25-year period who underwent cholecystolithotomy. Of patients, 30% showed recurrent stones within 1 year of the operation. The authors conclude that cholecystolithotomy should not be employed for symptomatic children with gallstones.

Dumont RC, Caniano DA: Hypokinetic gallbladder disease: A cause of chronic abdominal pain in children and adolescents. J Pediatr Surg 34:858-861, 1999.

The authors discuss their experience with 42 patients requiring gallbladder-emptying studies measured by either ultrasonography or scintigraphy with intravenous cholecystokinin for chronic abdominal pain. All 42 patients underwent cholecystectomy, and the response to surgical therapy was excellent in 41 patients with a mean follow-up of 20 months.

Holcomb GW III, Morgan WM III, Neblett WW III, et al: Laparoscopic cholecystectomy in children: Lessons learned from the first 100 patients. J Pediatr Surg 34:1236-1240, 1999.

The authors reviewed 100 consecutive infants and children undergoing laparoscopic cholecystectomy from 1990 to 1998. They discuss their management of 78 patients undergoing an elective operation and 22 children who presented with symptoms requiring hospitalization. In this series, two patients underwent laparoscopic choledochal exploration.

Shah RS, Blakely ML, Lobe TE: The role of laparoscopy in the management of common bile duct obstruction in children. Surg Endosc 15:1353-1355, 2001.

The authors discuss their management of five children with a mean age of 11.6 years who required laparoscopic common bile duct exploration. The authors recommend laparoscopic common duct exploration for obstructing lesions of the common duct and endoscopic sphincterotomy for recurrent lesions after laparoscopic cholecystectomy.

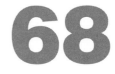

Disorders of the Pancreas

EMBRYOLOGY, ANATOMY, AND PHYSIOLOGY

The pancreas originates as dorsal and ventral outpouchings from the primitive duodenum by 5 weeks' gestation. The ventral bud forms the head of the pancreas, the dorsal bud forms the body and tail, and fusion of the two occurs by rotation of the ventral bud at around 7 weeks' gestation. The pancreas itself ends up lying at approximately the L1-2 level. Its arterial supply is from splenic artery branches, the inferior pancreaticoduodenal artery from the superior mesenteric artery usually supplying the lower border of the pancreas and the gastroduodenal artery from the hepatic artery, which gives off the superior pancreaticoduodenal artery. Venous drainage is to the splenic vein and via a large dorsal vein along the common bile duct. Lymphatic drainage is among the most extensive in the abdomen.

Anomalies in rotation and fusion of the primordial dorsal and ventral buds may produce an annular pancreas. The latter usually is associated with intrinsic webs of the duodenum as well. The duct of Santorini, which drains the dorsal bud, may persist as an accessory pancreatic duct emptying separately into the duodenum; however, the normal fusion of dorsal and ventral ducts results in the duct of Wirsung, which is the main duct of the pancreas, opening into the duodenum by way of the common bile duct. The epithelial cords of the primitive pancreas give rise to the secretory acini and the islets of Langerhans, which separate at an early stage of gestation and differentiate independently.

The head of the pancreas is located to the right of the vertebral column, whereas the body covers the first lumbar vertebra, making it vulnerable to blunt abdominal trauma. The head of the pancreas and the duodenum share a common blood supply from the superior and inferior pancreaticoduodenal arteries so that resection of the head of the pancreas usually, but not always, requires duodenectomy as well.

The pancreas is an organ of major importance to a child's normal growth and development. In the fetus and newborn, the pancreas produces essentially no amylase and negligible lipase until 2 months of age, after which time there is gradual maturation; production of amylase and lipase is at full adult levels by age 2 years. In the newborn, trypsin levels are between 10% and 60% of adult levels, maturing in the same fashion. Pancreatic duct pressures are in the range of 15 cm H_2O, and exocrine secretions have a high proportion of bicarbonate with a pH of 6 to 9. Although there is a poor response to secretin stimulation at birth, this gradually matures to be normal by age 2 years as well.

ACUTE PANCREATITIS

Although children can have many of the pancreatic disorders, including pancreatitis, seen in adults, other conditions are unique to children. Table 68-1 lists the various types of pancreatitis encountered in childhood, divided into acute and chronic forms.

Pancreatitis has been recognized increasingly as a cause of abdominal pain in children varying from mild to severe, involving a spectrum from mild parenchymal edema to severe hemorrhagic pancreatitis with gangrene and necrosis. The typical presentation includes epigastric pain and tenderness accompanied by nausea and vomiting. There also may be back pain and shoulder pain. Approximately 5% to 10% of patients are severely ill presenting with hypotension, metabolic derangements, sepsis, fluid sequestration, and other manifestations of the systemic inflammatory response syndrome progressing to multiple organ failure. Because signs and symptoms are often nonspecific, diagnosis may not be made until laparotomy or autopsy. The usual preoperative diagnosis is acute appendicitis or peritonitis of undetermined etiology, and the difficulty in establishing a correct diagnosis is compounded by the infrequency of pancreatitis in children and the numerous conditions that may simulate pancreatitis.

TABLE 68-1 ■ Types of Pancreatitis in Children	
Acute	**Chronic**
Nonobstructive	Fibrosing
Obstructive	Idiopathic
Hemorrhagic	Familial

Etiology

Acute hemorrhagic pancreatitis is uncommon in children. These patients usually present with poor oral intake, vomiting, diarrhea, abdominal pain, jaundice, and coma. In many patients, the diagnosis of fulminant pancreatitis is not suspected at all. Septic pancreatic infarction has been reported rarely in infants with infections caused by various enteric bacteria, a different presentation from that in adults.

Table 68-2 lists the various causes of pancreatitis in children, which may be divided into obstructive and nonobstructive causes. Approximately half of reported cases are idiopathic. Traumatic causes, infections, and drugs are the next most frequent causes. Although there is some controversy about whether corticosteroids cause pancreatitis, approximately 15% of children with end-stage renal disease develop pancreatitis, and the incidence may increase almost threefold in children with renal disease who receive corticosteroids. There is also an increased incidence of pancreatitis after renal transplantation, but some of the same drugs are used in these patients as well. Secondary hyperparathyroidism and hypercalcemia are causative factors. The pancreas is also known to be a major site of viral localization in patients on immunosuppression or in children with liver disease who receive corticosteroids.

The acute familial/hereditary varieties of pancreatitis tend to become recurrent and chronic gradually, eventually producing pancreatic scarring and calcification. Diffuse pancreatic calcification has been observed in children with cystic fibrosis, chronic familial pancreatitis,

and hyperparathyroidism. Mumps pancreatitis is uncommon in children today, and hyperamylasemia is not diagnostic of concomitant pancreatitis, in contrast to sialoadenitis. Pancreatitis has been reported in children in association with collagen vascular disorders and metabolic problems, such as familial aminoaciduria and hyperlipoproteinemia. Additional causes of pancreatitis include infectious mononucleosis, porphyria, and ulcerative colitis.

Obstructive forms of pancreatitis are less common in children than in adults. Obstruction of the pancreatic duct by *Ascaris lumbricoides* has been reported as a cause of pancreatitis in the United States, but it is much more prevalent in countries where this intestinal parasite is endemic. In contrast to adults, in children extrahepatic biliary tract disease is an uncommon cause of pancreatitis. Congenital anomalies and either congenital or acquired strictures of the common bile duct and pancreatic ducts have been found with increasing frequency in children with recurrent pancreatitis since the advent of endoscopic retrograde cholangiopancreatography (ERCP). Most children with choledochal cysts have a so-called common channel with a high, anomalous communication between the pancreatic duct and the common bile duct with free flow of pancreatic fluid into the cyst. Although there is no direct evidence that bile refluxes into the pancreatic duct, acute pancreatitis occurs in some cases of choledochal cyst. Pancreatitis is extremely rare after excision of choledochal cyst with choledochojejunostomy. Older children with cholelithiasis and choledocholithiasis may develop pancreatitis, but this is uncommon. Septic patients who develop inspissated bile syndrome causing relative obstruction and occasional patients with total parenteral nutrition (TPN) cholestasis may develop acute pancreatitis.

Diagnostic Studies

Pancreatitis can be diagnosed early in the course of the disease by measuring serum amylase and lipase levels, which are often several times normal in children with an acute or fulminating course, although normal in others (Table 68-3). Hyperamylasemia can be observed in children with other clinical disorders, such as renal failure, common bile duct obstruction, parotitis, peptic ulcer disease, intestinal obstruction, intestinal perforation, hepatic trauma, acute salpingitis, ectopic pregnancy, opiate administration, and intestinal infarction. These conditions must be excluded before the diagnosis of acute pancreatitis can be established. Analysis of amylase isoenzymes has

---

TABLE 68-2 ▪ Causes of Pancreatitis in Children

Nonobstructive
  Trauma
    External, operative, postpancreatography
  Drug-induced
    Steroids, adrenocorticotropic hormones, estrogens
      including contraceptives, azathioprine, asparaginase,
      tetracycline, chlorothiazides, valproic acid
  Hereditary/familial
  Renal disease, transplantation
  Metabolic disorders
    Aminoaciduria, hyperlipoproteinemia types I and V,
      hypercalcemia, porphyria
  Inflammatory disorders
    Mumps, ulcerative colitis, mononucleosis, cystic fibrosis,
      scorpion venom
  Collagen vascular diseases
    Polyarteritis nodosa, lupus erythematosus
  Idiopathic
  Alcohol-induced
Obstructive
  Anomalies
    Choledochal cyst with anomalous pancreaticobiliary
      drainage, pancreas divisum
  Choledocholithiasis
  Congenital or acquired bile duct strictures
  Ascaris lumbricoides or other parasites
  Tumors

TABLE 68-3 ▪ Diagnosis of Acute Pancreatitis

Serum amylase, lipase
Amylase isoenzymes
Amylase-to-creatinine clearance ratio
Peritoneal fluid analysis
Abdominal radiograph
Ultrasound
Upper gastrointestinal contrast radiographs
CT
ERCP, MRCP

been of some benefit in distinguishing acute pancreatitis from other disorders that also may cause hyperamylasemia, such as trauma to the parotid gland. Studies of urinary amylase and amylase clearance studies are rarely helpful. On rare occasions, the ratio of amylase to creatinine clearance is a useful study to determine if there is decreased tubular resorption of amylase by the kidney. Ultrasound, computed tomography (CT), and magnetic resonance imaging have been used to document pancreatic size, the presence of pseudocysts, pancreatic duct size, and the status of the biliary tree. Ultrasound has been particularly helpful in pediatric patients, and it is one of the best studies for serial follow-up imaging. CT with thin cuts has been useful for the study of patients with pancreatic trauma and pancreatic ductal enlargement. ERCP has been used effectively in children to delineate ductal anatomy, although its use is contraindicated in the acute phase of pancreatitis, and the procedure itself may induce transient pancreatitis. Magnetic resonance cholangiopancreatography (MRCP) with full reconstruction of all images has been refined to the point where it may be used in place of ERCP because it is essentially noninvasive. Children with the presumptive diagnosis of jaundice secondary to pancreatitis may benefit from a hepato-iminodiacetic acid scan or occasionally from percutaneous transhepatic cholangiography. Peritoneal lavage affords further objective criteria to evaluate acute pancreatitis in children.

Nonoperative Management

Table 68-4 lists the various approaches available for the treatment of acute pancreatitis, but supportive measures are the mainstays of treatment. The primary treatment of acute pancreatitis consists of cessation of oral intake to decrease pancreatic secretory activity by inhibiting secretin and pancreozymin release. Unless pancreatitis is exceedingly mild, nasogastric suction should be instituted

---

TABLE 68-4 ■ Nonoperative Management of Acute Pancreatitis

Supportive measures
  Intravenous fluid therapy
  Electrolyte replacement
  Analgesia
  TPN
  Antibiotics
  Respiratory support
  Nasogastric suction
Pancreatic exocrine secretion suppression
  Histamine receptor antagonists
  Antacids
  Anticholinergics
  Glucagon
  Somatostatin
  Calcitonin
Pancreatic enzyme inhibition
  Protease inhibitors
  Antifibrinolytics
  Fresh-frozen plasma
  Peritoneal lavage to eliminate toxic waste

---

because most patients have vomiting and ileus. Appropriate intravenous fluids should be given to replace losses and correct imbalances. A central venous catheter usually is needed to facilitate parenteral nutrition and fluid and antibiotic administration. Pain can be severe, so narcotics are indicated, but it is probably best to avoid the use of morphine, which causes ampullary spasm. Anticholinergic drugs play a minor role. Prophylactic antibiotics are justified because sepsis may be a lethal complication, but the use of antibiotics in patients with acute pancreatitis is controversial as so few patients are actually infected. Low blood levels of calcium resulting from saponification of necrotic pancreas, glucagon-related thyrocalcitonin release, and hypomagnesemia should be replaced with intravenous calcium gluconate.

In severe acute pancreatitis, extensive losses of plasma and blood from the intravascular space result in major reductions in blood volume, which may require colloid and blood replacement as well. Close monitoring of arterial and central venous pressures and urinary output provides the best guidelines for appropriate fluid and colloid repletion. As pancreatitis progresses in fulminating cases, respiratory demand increases with reduction in pulmonary function. Ascites, retroperitoneal edema, phrenic elevation, extensive pleural effusion, and abdominal splinting from pain may combine to produce lower lobe atelectasis and intrapulmonary arteriovenous shunting. A vicious cycle of increasing metabolic demand, systemic inflammatory response syndrome, and decreasing pulmonary reserve leads to respiratory failure and shock. Control of ventilation and replacement of bicarbonate for maintenance of a near-normal arterial pH may become necessary.

Hyperglycemia and hypocalcemia indicate severe pancreatic inflammation, whereas elevated levels of serum lactate dehydrogenase and aspartate aminotransaminase (AST) reflect continuing tissue necrosis. An elevated hematocrit level reflects initial hemoconcentration, but a subsequent decrease to less than normal indicates retroperitoneal hemorrhage. High fever usually responds to rectal acetaminophen. Steroids are not recommended, but appropriately tailored TPN has been essential in providing adequate nutrition to minimize catabolism during the period of bowel rest.

Surgical Management

Laparotomy is indicated infrequently for acute pancreatitis in children when the diagnosis is known. Operation on a severely ill child with unsuspected pancreatitis secondary to another serious condition, such as renal disease or drugs, can lead to increased morbidity and mortality. Because pancreatitis seldom is suspected in children, the most common preoperative diagnosis is acute appendicitis. At laparotomy, fat necrosis and a large volume of peritoneal fluid with high amylase content usually are found. Complications of pancreatitis, such as pseudocysts and peripancreatic or subphrenic abscess, often require surgical management. The latter problems usually occur 1 or more weeks after the onset of pancreatitis, however, and surgery should be planned carefully.

Peritoneal lavage via a peritoneal dialysis catheter placed under local anesthesia and introduced a few centimeters below the umbilicus has been of benefit when children with pancreatitis experience progressive deterioration of vital signs despite supportive therapy. The usual dialysate is an isotonic electrolyte solution containing dextrose, potassium, and calcium if the serum calcium is low and either ampicillin or cefazolin. The dialysate is infused for approximately 30 minutes, then repeated every 2 to 3 hours as necessary. The volume of dialysate varies depending on the size of the patient, using approximately 20 mL/kg of body weight in smaller children and 1.5 to 2.0 L in adolescents. Smaller volumes are used if abdominal distention induces respiratory distress. Lavage generally is continued for 24 to 72 hours, depending on the clinical status of the patient and the character of the drainage fluid. The initial fluid recovered from dialysis is analyzed for levels of amylase, lactate dehydrogenase, and AST, and Gram stain and culture should be done to evaluate for bacteria. If the fluid contains high amylase levels or blood or both, lavage is continued for its dilutional effect. If only a few gram-negative bacteria are recovered, lavage with antibiotics may be continued, but if many bacteria are recovered, if the peritoneal fluid continues to be bloody, or if the patient's condition continues to deteriorate, laparotomy is probably in order. Ultrasound, CT, and MRCP should be performed first to delineate any lesions likely to be responsive to surgery.

At planned laparotomy, the lesser omental space should be opened widely by dividing the gastrocolic ligament, and the pancreas should be examined under direct vision. In patients with severe pancreatitis the pancreas is usually edematous, thickened, and hemorrhagic with some areas of necrosis. Clearly necrotic tissue should be débrided. If no specific lesions are identified that are amenable to surgical repair, such as biliary obstruction or a tumor, the peritoneal cavity should be lavaged with warm saline to clear debris and dilute the enzyme-containing fluid. Unless a specific lesion has been delineated on imaging study, the ampulla and extrahepatic bile ducts should not be manipulated. Soft Silastic or latex sump-suction catheters should be inserted through separate stab wounds and placed adjacent to the pancreas, under both sides of the diaphragm and into the pelvis. Postoperative irrigation of the catheters is performed at least three times daily to continue to dilute enzymes that may have been activated and to clear debris. Peritoneal lavage has played a major role in saving the lives of children with severe early acute pancreatitis. Gastrostomy has been a useful adjunct, but initially administration of TPN has been useful for maintenance of adequate nutrition.

Mortality from acute pancreatitis in pediatric patients has decreased through the years and is still less than that noted in adults. Death from acute pancreatitis usually stems from a combination of factors, including infection, hemorrhage, and shock leading to systemic inflammatory response syndrome and multiple systems organ failure. The mortality with acute pancreatitis in childhood is less than 5%.

CHRONIC PANCREATITIS

Chronic pancreatitis in children has multiple causes, including congenital, hereditary, metabolic, inflammatory,

and collagen vascular disorders. Most cases are idiopathic. Chronic fibrosing pancreatitis should be considered in children with recurrent abdominal pain of undetermined cause or children with signs of biliary obstruction and only subtle or mild abdominal pain. Patients with chronic fibrosing pancreatitis usually do not have associated biliary or gastrointestinal disease, however, and they are more likely to have a hereditary or familial disorder or to have hyperlipoproteinemia or aminoaciduria, cystic fibrosis, previous trauma, or a combination of factors. Other than recurrent abdominal pain and occasionally obstructive jaundice, the symptoms are usually variable and increase in frequency and severity with the eventual development of pancreatic exocrine insufficiency accompanied by steatorrhea and weight loss. Diabetes may occur late in rare patients.

Laboratory studies are often inconclusive, but occasionally the secretin/pancreozymin test, which directly stimulates and measures pancreatic enzyme levels, may be helpful. Serum levels of lipase, amylase, and calcium; fasting blood glucose; and serum lipid profile should be determined. Duodenal trypsin levels may be abnormally low. Determinations of fecal fat, trypsin, and nitrogen may show enzyme insufficiency. Plain radiographs of the abdomen may show calcification, particularly in long-standing disease. Ultrasound may show pancreatic thickening or ductal enlargement in some instances. ERCP or MRCP may show abnormalities of the pancreatic ducts, although the "chain-of-lakes" appearance often seen in adults is unusual in children. Hyperparathyroidism must be ruled out before one establishes the diagnosis of primary chronic pancreatitis.

If the diagnosis of chronic pancreatitis cannot be established by laboratory studies, and this is usually the case, laparotomy may be needed. The pancreas is found to be diffusely hard and nodular and enlarged. Biopsy, which is usually unnecessary, reveals fibrosis and loss of acini, initially sparing the islets. Intraoperative cholangiograms and pancreatograms are helpful, but if no correctable disease is found, duodenal sphincteroplasty should be performed. Alternately, papillotomy can be performed at the time of ERCP. Careful evaluation should be done for stones or strictures or both of the ampulla; a possible duplication cyst in the duodenal wall; and possible anomalies of the pancreatic ductal system, such as pancreas divisum.

Familial or hereditary pancreatitis is an autosomal dominant mutation of the trypsinogen gene localized to chromosome 7q35. This mutation results in an amino acid substitution in the trypsinogen molecule, which prevents its inactivation and permits autodigestion of the gland, resulting in acute and chronic pancreatitis. This disorder may be seen either with or without associated ductal ectasia, most commonly with it. For symptomatic children with pancreatic ductal ectasia or calculi or both, distal duct drainage by the Puestow method of longitudinal pancreaticojejunostomy (Fig. 68-1) has provided durable relief. Pancreatic duct stenting has been used as a treatment for hereditary pancreatitis, particularly for intrahepatic ductal strictures, but most have found that this is simply a temporizing measure and that surgical drainage usually is needed. For patients with chronic

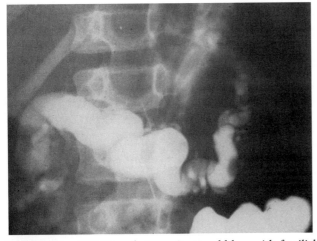

FIGURE 68-1 ■ ERCP study in an 8-year-old boy with familial pancreatitis shows severe ectasia of the pancreatic duct, which responded nicely to longitudinal pancreaticojejunostomy.

fibrosing pancreatitis and normal pancreatic ducts, sphincteroplasty has provided long-term relief of symptoms in most series reported.

CONGENITAL ANOMALIES

Ectopic Pancreas

Pancreatic tissue has been identified in many ectopic locations, most commonly the pylorus, duodenum, or Meckel's diverticulum. More unusual locations are the colon, appendix, gallbladder, and anomalous bronchoesophageal foregut fistulas. In most patients, the accessory pancreatic tissue is functional. Islets of Langerhans are present in about one third of the heterotopic foci in the stomach, but only rarely are they present in other sites of ectopic pancreas. Although most patients with ectopic pancreas are asymptomatic, occasionally obstruction or bleeding may occur. When recognized, local resection usually is recommended; however, pancreatitis or carcinoma rarely develops.

Annular Pancreas

The most frequent pancreatic anomaly is annular pancreas, in which a thin flat band of pancreatic tissue surrounds the second portion of the duodenum and continues on either side into the head of the pancreas. This annular tissue is histologically normal, containing acini and islet cells. Pancreatic tissue often penetrates the muscularis of the duodenum, although it occasionally may be free enough to lift away from the duodenal wall. A large duct is usually present in the annular pancreas that connects with Wirsung's duct or, less often, opens either independently into the common duct or by several orifices into the duodenum. In most cases of annular pancreas, there is coexisting stenosis or atresia of the duodenum at that site. Down syndrome occurs in approximately one fourth of patients. Intestinal malrotation, tracheoesophageal fistula, and congenital heart disease occasionally occur in patients with annular pancreas. Symptoms from annular pancreas usually appear in the neonatal period but

occasionally not until middle age, depending on the degree of obstruction.

Annular pancreas is a cause of high-grade duodenal obstruction in the fetus and may produce maternal polyhydramnios. Antenatal ultrasound may identify the anomaly. The double-bubble sign of air in the stomach and duodenum on abdominal x-ray mimics that seen with duodenal atresia. Otherwise the pattern is one of duodenal stenosis with small amounts of air distally in the intestine.

Operative exposure is accomplished best through a right upper quadrant abdominal transverse incision, unless there is situs inversus. When annular pancreas is identified, duodenoduodenostomy should be performed around the annular obstruction without mobilizing the annular pancreas itself because of the risk of injuring a pancreatic duct within it, which could result in production of a chronic fistula. With this approach, long-term outlook is excellent, and postoperative pancreatitis is exceedingly rare.

Pancreas Divisum

Pancreas divisum results when the dorsal component of the pancreas drained by the duct of Santorini and the ventral component drained by the duct of Wirsung fail to fuse before communicating with the common bile duct. The residual of the dorsal component, the uncinate process, is drained exclusively by the accessory duct of Santorini. The frequency of pancreas divisum is believed to be 5% to 10% of the population, but drainage is normal in most of these individuals without any site of obstruction. It is unclear how many patients with this anomaly ultimately develop chronic recurrent pancreatitis because symptoms may have their onset from early childhood to mid adulthood. ERCP usually shows a short or absent ventral duct of Wirsung (Fig. 68-2). There are many patterns of this anomaly, and pancreatitis does not result unless there is either a stenosis of the accessory ampulla or a stenosis somewhere in the ductal system within the pancreas, usually at the junction point between the two ducts. Occasional patients may develop a central pseudocyst.

For patients who experience recurrent pancreatitis, sphincteroplasty of one or both ducts accompanied by cholecystectomy is recommended because many patients develop bile stasis and stones. Sphincteroplasty should be guided by operative pancreatography unless accurate ERCP or MRCP has been accomplished preoperatively. Although the pancreatic ducts rarely are noted to be dilated, even in symptomatic patients, it is believed that the dilation is transitory and dependent on pancreatic stimulation with eating. Approximately 75% of patients have a good outcome after operation.

PANCREATIC CYST AND PSEUDOCYST

Pancreatic pseudocysts are usually the result of acute pancreatitis or trauma. True pancreatic cysts are uncommon in children and may be classified as congenital and developmental, retention, duplication, neoplastic, and parasitic. This classification is arbitrary because pathologic

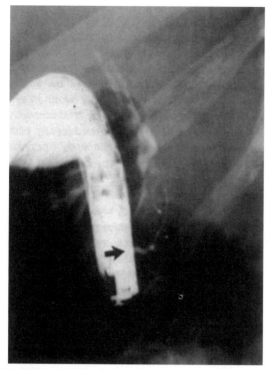

FIGURE 68-2 ■ ERCP study shows pancreas divisum in a 13-year-old girl with recurrent pancreatitis. Note short branching ventral duct of Wirsung (arrow). The duct of Santorini drains 90% of the gland, including the body, tail, and uncinate process. The high-volume flow and relatively small proximal dorsal duct are believed to account for pancreatic enzyme extravasation and recurring pancreatitis.

verification is often difficult when there has been chronic pancreatitis ongoing.

Congenital and Developmental Cysts

True congenital cysts of the pancreas are uncommon but when present usually manifest symptoms before age 2 years. They may be either unilocular or multilocular and may occur spontaneously with cysts in other organs. Von Hippel–Lindau disease is characterized by hereditary cerebellar cysts, hemangiomas of the retina, and cysts of the pancreas and other organs. Developmental cysts are lined by epithelium surrounded by acinar tissue and are most common in the body and tail of the pancreas. They may achieve considerable size and contain cloudy yellow fluid that is sterile, usually with low enzyme activity. Symptoms are uncommon unless the cyst enlarges sufficiently either to exert extrinsic pressure on adjacent organs or to obstruct pancreatic drainage. These cysts rarely are associated with infection or peripancreatic inflammation. When symptomatic, cysts may require surgical treatment, including surgical excision of the cyst with a rim of normal pancreatic tissue or internal drainage.

Retention Cysts

Pancreatic retention cysts are rare in children and are believed to result from chronic obstruction of the ductal system. They may be differentiated from congenital or developmental cysts in that a high concentration of pancreatic enzymes is usually present. Pancreatography is the best guide to performing cyst excision or internal drainage.

Enteric Duplication Cysts

Intrapancreatic or juxtapancreatic gastric duplications separate from the stomach with ductal communications are uncommon anomalies of the pancreas. Symptoms may include failure to thrive, nausea, abdominal pain, and episodes of pancreatitis with elevated serum amylase levels. Intracystic hemorrhage or perforation or both occasionally occur. The lesion may be recognized by ERCP, ultrasound, CT, or MRCP. The lesion is usually small and not palpable. Exploration is necessary to identify the mass and to alleviate recurrent episodes of pancreatitis. Excision should be performed as close to the duplication wall as possible, and any communicating duct should be closed. Occasional patients may require distal pancreatectomy, and a rare patient may require pancreaticoduodenal resection. Most patients are relieved of symptoms after distal pancreatic resection or resection of the duplication and closure of the communicating duct.

Neoplastic Cysts

Papillary neoplastic cysts are rare in childhood but should be presumed to be premalignant. The true nature of the cyst can be established only by microscopic examination, after excision. They are easily ruptured, and the contents are extremely irritating to the peritoneal cavity.

Pseudocysts

Pancreatic pseudocysts account for more than 75% of cystic lesions of the pancreas and are located most often in the lesser sac. The wall is composed of granulation tissue in varying stages of maturity, and the lining is devoid of epithelium. A pseudocyst may or may not communicate with the pancreatic ductal system, but when it does, serum amylase levels frequently exceed 3000 U/L. The cysts are usually unilocular, and volumes greater than 1000 mL are common. Of pancreatic pseudocysts, 70% may result from trauma. Pseudocysts occasionally occur after idiopathic pancreatitis, and rarely a stone impacted in the common duct, a duplication cyst, or mumps may precede the development of a pseudocyst.

Patients with pancreatic pseudocyst often relate a history of blunt abdominal trauma or an illness resembling pancreatitis, followed by a free interval of weeks to months. Epigastric abdominal pain and anorexia progressing to nausea, emesis, and weight loss often ensue. Eventually one is able to palpate a round cystic epigastric mass. The enlarging pseudocyst may displace the stomach superiorly and anteriorly and the colon downward and anteriorly. The C-loop of the duodenum may be widened, and the duodenum in its retroperitoneal portion may be compressed or obstructed. Ascites may develop with markedly elevated pancreatic enzyme levels. Abdominal ultrasound and CT are generally diagnostic (Fig. 68-3).

Small cysts not interfering with gastrointestinal function often can be followed with serial ultrasound or CT until they ultimately disappear. For acute pseudocysts secondary to trauma, percutaneous drainage sometimes is effective. Complications from untreated large pseudocysts

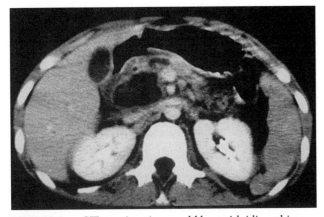

FIGURE 68-3 ■ CT scan in a 6-year-old boy with idiopathic pancreatitis shows a pseudocyst in the head of the pancreas, which responded nicely to Roux-en-Y jejunal drainage.

may include hemorrhage, secondary infection, perforation with peritonitis, and mechanical interference with gastrointestinal, pancreatic, or biliary function. Proper management depends primarily on the age of the cyst and assessment of the thickness of the wall on CT. Of patients with moderately severe acute pancreatitis, including traumatic pancreatitis, who experience pseudocysts, 50% eventually have spontaneous resolution within 3 to 4 weeks when treated conservatively, unless infection supervenes.

When a pseudocyst has achieved chronic status, spontaneous resolution is not to be expected, and persistent nonoperative management may lead to complications. Cysts limited to the tail of the pancreas may be excised by distal pancreatectomy with preservation of the spleen. A large pseudocyst in the body of the pancreas, displacing the stomach, is managed best by cyst-gastrostomy performed either endoscopically via the stomach or operatively. The opening through the posterior gastric wall into the cyst should be constructed sufficiently large so that it will not close before the cyst has collapsed completely. Interrupted nonabsorbable sutures should be placed around the edge of the cyst-gastrostomy to ensure hemostasis because postoperative bleeding is common. Roux-en-Y cyst-jejunostomy is the preferred method of drainage for pseudocysts of the head of the pancreas or for cysts in the body that are not intimately related to the stomach. Postoperative contrast x-ray studies may show the cyst filled with contrast material for weeks or months until the cyst cavity has been obliterated entirely. There are some reports of successful percutaneous drainage of chronic pseudocysts, particularly for traumatic pancreatitis when the pseudocyst has not had any demonstrated connection with the ductal system.

Pancreatic pseudocyst with mediastinal extension is a rare clinical entity that may present with an abdominal epigastric mass with either pleural effusion with high amylase content or a mediastinal mass. CT may reveal the full extent of the pseudocyst above and below the diaphragm. The most successful surgical treatment in these instances has been transabdominal drainage of the major pseudocyst by Roux-en-Y cyst-jejunostomy. Transthoracic drainage of mediastinal pseudocysts

commonly leads to recurrence. Occasionally an isolated congenital mediastinal cyst may contain pancreatic mucosa, in which case the cyst should be excised.

TUMORS OF THE PANCREAS IN CHILDHOOD

Benign and malignant tumors occur in childhood. Most of the benign tumors are endocrine in origin, although some lesions are malignant. Malignant tumors of the pancreas are rare in infants and children, and most are carcinomas. In most patients, by the time the diagnosis is made, a palpable mass can be felt, and jaundice is often present. Patients with malignant pancreatic tumors have been reported ranging in age from 3 months to 16 years with most younger than 10 years old.

The most common malignant tumors reported have been nonfunctioning islet cell carcinomas and adenocarcinomas, although acinar involvement has been present in many instances. Most of the latter lesions occur in the head of the pancreas, and the lesion may be diffuse in occasional patients. Complete surgical resection with an adequate margin is the only therapy that has proved curative, as is the case in adults. Pancreaticoduodenectomy has provided the best long-term results, and lesser operations are best reserved for patients who require palliation. Spread is by lymphatic extension to periportal lymph nodes and subsequently to the liver and lungs. Other than the tumors of endocrine origin, the histologic pattern of pancreatic malignancies in children involving the exocrine pancreas has been pancreaticoblastomas, cystic-papillary tumors, and mixed lesions. Although pancreaticoduodenectomy is the best approach for these patients, the outcome is usually fatal because of delayed diagnosis. The results are better in patients with malignant endocrine tumors; this may be because some of these tumors respond to radiation and chemotherapy with 5-fluorouracil and streptozotocin. Long-term follow-up of children who have had pancreaticoduodenectomy indicates that these children are capable of long-term survival and achieving satisfactory growth and development. Enzyme replacement and insulin usually are required.

Zollinger-Ellison Syndrome

Zollinger-Ellison syndrome is characterized by virulent peptic ulcer disease, gastric hypersecretion, and islet cell tumors of the pancreas. Gastric hypersecretion is the result of excessive secretion of gastrin by the islet cell tumor, which may be shown when the tumor is stimulated by infusion of calcium or secretin by the tumor. A positive calcium infusion study is diagnostic of a gastrinoma. Diarrhea associated with this syndrome in more than a third of patients is related to gastric hypersecretion. Multiple endocrine neoplasia syndrome is a familial disorder characterized by parathyroid, pituitary, and pancreatic endocrine tumors. The initial manifestation of Zollinger-Ellison syndrome may be hyperparathyroidism with the later slow appearance of a pancreatic islet cell tumor.

If the decision is made to operate, the duodenum and pancreas should be explored thoroughly, and if a single tumor is found, it should be resected. Postoperative gastrin levels are monitored to determine the adequacy of resection.

If the tumor proves to be inoperable, if multiple tumors exist, or if no tumor is found, as occurs in half of patients, the recommended treatment is total gastrectomy with Roux-en-Y esophagojejunostomy, preferably with a pouch. Most of the reported cases have been in adults, but 75% of patients with this syndrome treated by total gastrectomy are alive at 1 year, and 40% to 50% are alive at 10 years. More than half of the patients have liver metastases at the time of initial operation. Even so, when metastases are present, the 10-year survival is only slightly less. Although total gastrectomy does not afford permanent cure, it does provide the best overall results for the patient. Streptozotocin and 5-fluorouracil are reported to have some utility in patients with metastatic gastrinomas. The reported involvement of the pancreas by these tumors for the head/body/tail is 4:1:4. Approximately 30% of patients have two or more foci of tumor in the pancreas, and 20% of patients have involvement of the entire gland. Total gastrectomy seems to provide the best results in children, but when children younger than 7 years of age have total gastrectomy, extensive nutritional supplementation is required to ensure adequate growth and development. The use of H_2-blockers such as cimetidine has been beneficial when residual tumor is present.

Other Endocrine Tumors of the Pancreas

Various other endocrine tumors have been reported in children as in adults and include gastropancreatic and enteropancreatic tumors, insulinomas, glucagonomas, apudomas, and vasoactive intestinal peptide tumors. Percutaneous transhepatic venous sampling has proved to be useful in localizing the site of these tumors because the hormone content of the venous effluent in a specific location usually is elevated. Intraoperative ultrasound is also useful in such instances when focal tumors may be small and not easily identified visually. Laparoscopic ultrasound is a useful technique as well.

The definitive diagnosis of these tumors usually is based on the demonstration of an elevated serum level of the specific peptide involved. Preoperative localization is less successful than intraoperative localization as mentioned earlier. In some instances, specific tagged peptide radionuclide studies have proved to be useful. The main approach to treatment is complete surgical excision as with all other pancreatic tumors. Of all the endocrine tumors encountered in children, glucagonomas seem to have the greatest potential for metastasis.

PANCREATIC HYPERINSULINISM AND HYPOGLYCEMIA

Although hypoglycemia may occur in association with many metabolic disorders in children, the three conditions amenable to surgical management are islet cell adenoma, congenital hyperinsulinism, previously called *nesidioblastosis*, and glycogen storage disease.

Congenital Hyperinsulinism

Congenital hyperinsulinism, also called *persistent hyperinsulinemic hypoglycemia*, is a neonatal disorder in which insulin regulation is abnormal, resulting in a low blood glucose level. Patients with this syndrome may have manifestations of hypoglycemia and hyperinsulinism without having hyperinsulinemia, indicating the fact that this is a disorder of regulation.

Congenital hyperinsulinism is a rare disorder of glucose metabolism that has an incidence of 1 in 50,000 live births. Early symptoms include irritability, sweating, tremulousness, and seizures. Patients with repeated seizures invariably have permanent brain damage associated with profound hyperglycemia. The condition is the result of islet cell dysregulation of insulin production with most patients having a recessive genetic mutation of the sulfonylurea receptor (*SUR*) gene or a defect of its associated potassium channel or of the *Kir6.2* gene.

Pathology on resected specimens from infants treated for this disorder has shown numerous abnormalities, including diffuse adenomatosis, occasional focal lesions, and even normal pancreas. Although the response to surgery for focal lesions would be expected to be satisfactory, patients with *SUR* defects seem to require more extensive resection.

Initially at the time of presentation, it is best to restore euglycemia with infusions of concentrated glucose, often exceeding 15 mg/kg/min, to maintain serum glucose greater than 60 mg/dL. Additionally, diazoxide is administered followed by octreotide or glucagon for diazoxide-resistant cases. If all of this does not restore euglycemia and permit the patient to withstand a fast, surgical intervention is indicated. The original surgical approach to this disorder was subtotal pancreatectomy with preservation of the spleen, but subsequent recommendations have favored 95% to 98% pancreatectomy. Some have questioned whether this aggressive approach is worth the potential increased risk of surgical morbidity and exocrine and endocrine insufficiency. Percutaneous transhepatic venous sampling preoperatively is now recommended to distinguish focal cases. In the absence of a discrete nodule felt on exploration or indicated by intraoperative venous sampling, it is usually best to perform 95% pancreatectomy as the initial procedure. In 25% of instances, it may be possible to do intraoperative venous insulin sampling to guide resection, but patients with SUR defects have a more severe form of the disorder and may respond best to extensive resection. Because of the risk of brain damage, most clinicians have believed that extensive resection is in order. In our experience, the risk for diabetes over the long term has been equal with subtotal and near-total pancreatectomy. Patients with the autosomal dominant form of this disease usually can be managed nonoperatively. Patients with *SUR* mutation seem to have disordered glucose metabolism to a greater degree than other patients with this disorder and a higher incidence of diabetes over the long term. The long-term results with resection are usually good in patients who have had extensive resection, although many patients require medical management for 1 year postoperatively. Of infants with this disorder, 20% to 30% have some degree of long-term neurologic impairment, emphasizing the need for early recognition and aggressive treatment.

Glycogen Storage Disease

Infants with glycogen storage disease type I often experience hypoglycemia and seizures, which may result in neurologic impairment. Glycogen storage disease can be distinguished clinically from islet cell adenoma and congenital hyperinsulinism by the presence of hepatomegaly, which is usually impressive. Hypoglycemic seizures may not appear in glycogen storage disease until 3 to 6 months of age or later when nocturnal feedings are discontinued. Hypoglycemia usually is preceded by sweating. In type I glycogen storage disease, glucose-6-phosphatase is deficient or absent, making it difficult for the liver to convert glycogen into glucose. Blood glucose characteristically decreases in these patients 2 to 3 hours after a feeding and may decrease to 5 to 10 mg/dL. Lipids are mobilized as an alternate fuel resulting in high levels of serum triglycerides and the development of xanthomas of the skin. Because of interference with platelet adhesion by the high levels of plasma lipids, bleeding time may be prolonged and present as frequent nosebleeds. These patients are usually acidotic, and there is failure to thrive.

It has been shown that all of the manifestations of glycogen storage disease type I can be reversed by continuous night feedings of glucose. This can be accomplished either with a feeding tube passed by the patient or via a gastrostomy with a continuous infusion pump using 20% glucose solution. Children managed in this fashion have achieved normal height and weight with return of liver size to normal and clearance of plasma lipids. Xanthomas and liver cell adenomas have been noted to resolve, blood glucose returns to normal, and bleeding time normalizes. Liver transplantation is an option for correction of the enzymatic defect in these patients.

PANCREAS TRANSPLANTATION

Pancreas transplantation has been used rarely in children, but it is likely to be used more frequently in the future. This is because more recent improvements in immunosuppression and technique have provided better results with fewer risks, and islet cell transplantation now is being introduced. Pancreas transplantation is performed either as a whole-organ transplantation or simultaneously with kidney transplantation in patients with end-stage renal disease. Enteric drainage has been proved to be preferable to bladder drainage.

Although most children with type 1 diabetes can be managed successfully by implantable insulin delivery systems that mimic physiologic secretion and result in satisfactory glucose control, when patients develop end-stage renal disease, pancreatic transplantation becomes an option. Pancreatic transplantation alone is limited to a small group of patients with insulin-dependent diabetes, including nonuremic patients who have difficult glucose control, patients with end-stage renal disease who need a kidney transplant, and patients with severe complications of diabetes that may be reversed at least partially by successful pancreatic transplantation. Contraindications for pancreatic transplantation generally include the presence of malignancy, active infection, blindness, or severely advanced cardiovascular disease. Successful human islet transplants are now being reported and probably represent the future. Until islet cell transplants are routinely successful, whole-pancreas transplantation with enteric drainage is the best option. A variety of immunosuppressive regimens have been used with 1-year graft survivals reported to be 60% to 80%. The primary purpose of pancreatic transplantation is to reverse or halt the secondary complications of diabetes and to improve the quality of life.

SUGGESTED READINGS

American Society for Gastrointestinal Endoscopy: The role of ERCP in diseases of the biliary tree and pancreas: Guidelines for clinical application. Gastrointest Endosc 50:1-10, 1999.

This consensus statement addresses the role of ERCP alongside all the other options for imaging and concludes that currently ERCP is the best technique for duct visualization and provides the broadest range of therapeutic options.

Cretolole C, Nihoul-Fekete C, Jan D, et al: Partial elective pancreatectomy is curative in focal form of permanent hyperinsulinism in infancy: A report of 45 cases from 1983 to 2000. J Pediatr Surg 37:155-158, 2002.

The use of portal venous sampling as a guide to extent of resection is discussed.

Humar A, Kandaswamy R, Granger D, et al: Decreased surgical risks of pancreas transplantation in the modern era. Ann Surg 231:269-275, 2000.

This article summarizes the current status of whole-organ pancreas transplantation, which will serve as a benchmark for comparison with islet transplantation as it is introduced.

Ky A, Shilyanski J, Gerstie J, et al: Experience with papillary and solid epithelial neoplasms of the pancreas in children. J Pediatr Surg 33:42-44, 1998.

Malignant exocrine tumors of the pancreas are rare in children. This article stresses that long-term survival can be achieved with aggressive surgery.

Lovvorn HN, Nance ML, Ferry RJ, et al: Congenital hyperinsulinism and the surgeon: Lessons learned over 35 years. J Pediatr Surg 34:786-793, 1999.

This article analyzes a large experience with congenital hyperinsulinism from the standpoint of genetics, mode of inheritance, medical and surgical treatment, and long-term risk of diabetes.

Nealon WH, Walser E: Main pancreatic ductal anatomy can direct choice of modality for treating pancreatic pseudocysts (surgery versus percutaneous drainage). Ann Surg 235:751-758, 2002.

This article shows how pancreatic ductal anatomy in patients with complicated pancreatitis should guide the selection of treatment.

Neblett WW, O'Neill JA: Surgical management of recurrent pancreatitis in children with pancreas divisum. Ann Surg 231:899-908, 2000.

Current approaches to diagnosis and treatment of symptomatic pancreas divisum in childhood are described.

69

Disorders of the Spleen

The spleen was long believed to be a nonessential organ that could be removed with little consequence. Important functions of the spleen have now been defined, however, including bacterial clearance, phagocytosis of particulate matter from the blood, antibody formation, and hematopoiesis. In addition, asplenic infants and children are known to be susceptible to life-threatening, overwhelming infections. These observations have changed completely the traditional approach to the management of splenic injuries and disorders in childhood.

The role of the spleen during embryonic development is superseded only by that of the thymus, which is the paramount lymphatic organ in intrauterine life. The spleen is an intrauterine hematopoietic organ. It remains a major site of hematopoiesis during the neonatal period until approximately 5 months of age, at which time the bone marrow takes over all hematopoiesis. During the neonatal period, the spleen and the thymus constitute the major portion of the body's lymphatic tissue.

The microcirculation of the spleen is ideally constituted to provide a relatively prolonged exposure of blood cells and other particulate matter to splenic macrophages. During circulation through the red pulp, splenic phagocytes remove opsonized microorganisms and microorganisms for which there is no preexisting antibody. Although the liver has a larger concentration of phagocytic cells than the spleen and is highly efficient in removing bacteria coated with specific antibody, clearance of bacteria without specific antibody largely occurs in the spleen. This is particularly true of encapsulated bacteria, such as pneumococci, hemophilus, and meningococcus.

Humoral immunity against bacteria is transmitted to the newborn through the placenta. This passive maternal antibody protection dissipates within a few months. Active immunity, defined as the development of immunoglobulins against specific bacteria, develops later in childhood. In the interim, protection against blood-borne bacteria depends largely on the phagocytic ability of the splenic macrophages. During passage through the red pulp, reticulocytes are converted to normal biconcave erythrocytes. Pits and Howell-Jolly bodies are removed from the red blood cells. Acanthotic and old erythrocytes are destroyed and phagocytosed. Spherocytes, fixed sickle cells, and other abnormal erythrocytes are removed in the red pulp.

The germinal centers of the white pulp are important sites of antibody production, particularly against blood-borne bacteria. The bacteria from which the individual has little or no immunity are transported from the red pulp to the white pulp, where specific immunoglobulin M antibody is produced. In the absence of the spleen, this normal antibody response to circulating bacteria is diminished or absent. The proteins tuftsin and properidin are produced by the spleen; these proteins enhance neutrophil phagocytosis and stimulate complement production.

ANOMALIES

Anomalous grooves and divisions on the splenic surfaces are common and generally insignificant. Completely separate or accessory spleens are of clinical importance and are present in approximately 16% of children who undergo splenectomy. Accessory spleens, although generally dark blue, may be difficult to recognize because they closely resemble hypertrophied lymph nodes. They usually are located near the splenic hilum and the tail of the pancreas, along the superior and inferior margins of the pancreas, the greater curvature of the stomach, and less frequently in the splenocolic and splenorenal ligaments, and in the greater omentum. Within a few months after removal of the spleen, accessory splenic tissue may hypertrophy and assume many of the functions of the original spleen. Failure to excise completely all accessory spleens may lead to recurrence of certain splenic disorders.

Congenital absence of the spleen (asplenia) is usually part of a syndrome associated with other serious congenital malformations, primarily cardiovascular. Affected children have an increased susceptibility to infection, occasionally resulting in early fatality. Circulating erythrocytes containing Howell-Jolly antibodies and nucleated erythrocytes also may be found in patients with asplenia.

Polysplenia is characterized by a normally functioning, multilobed spleen. The most common associated anomalies are of cardiac origin. Situs inversus is also a frequent finding. The diagnosis often is made incidentally at laparotomy or laparoscopy. These children often die by the end of the first year of life from cardiac anomalies.

663

SPLENECTOMY

For many years, the most frequent indications for splenectomy in childhood were trauma and hematologic disorders. During the 1980s and 1990s, the importance of preserving the traumatized spleen to maintain the host's immunologic response to bacterial challenge became widely recognized. Complete splenectomy for trauma is rarely performed now. Incidental splenectomy similarly is avoided whenever possible. Splenectomy for hypersplenism and portal hypertension also is performed much less frequently than in previous years. Currently the most common indications for splenectomy in childhood are hereditary spherocytosis, refractory idiopathic thrombocytopenic purpura (ITP), and trauma.

Hemolytic Anemia

When sequestration or trapping and consequent destruction of erythrocytes within the spleen constitute the major cause of anemia, splenectomy often results in partial or complete remission. This splenic hemolysis stems from one of two factors: The red blood cells may be abnormal, or the spleen may be overactive.

Hereditary Spherocytosis

In this hemolytic anemia, usually inherited as an autosomal dominant trait, the red blood cells have an abnormal spherical shape and, as a result, are trapped and destroyed in the spleen at a faster rate than normal. Although the basic abnormality of the red blood cell in this condition is unknown, it is considered to be biochemical in nature and related to a defect in carbohydrate metabolism in the erythrocyte membrane (osmotic fragility). The unusual erythrocyte configuration makes it susceptible to destruction in the slow splenic microcirculation. The mechanism of destruction of the trapped red blood cells is uncertain; however, the spleen seems to exaggerate the metabolic defect of the erythrocytes.

The disorder is characterized by chronic anemia that is usually mild but with occasional "crises" of rapidly developing severe anemia. These crises, usually secondary to intercurrent infection, are caused by temporary failure of bone marrow production to keep pace with the high demand for erythrocytes. Although these crises do not constitute an urgent indication for splenectomy, operation, if necessary, should be performed when bone marrow function is active and hemolysis is minimal. Jaundice is usually mild or absent, tending to parallel the degree of anemia. Rarely a newborn may develop serious hemolytic anemia, however, with bilirubin levels so elevated that splenectomy may be necessary to prevent brain damage due to kernicterus.

The development of biliary tract calculi in patients with spherocytosis increases progressively with age. Although uncommon in infancy and early childhood, the incidence may reach 50% in adolescents and 75% in adults. Ultrasound of the abdomen should be obtained in patients with spherocytosis who have not undergone splenectomy before adolescence. Cholecystectomy for secondary calculi frequently is performed at the time of splenectomy. Cholecystotomy is not generally recommended because recurrent stones can develop.

Children with spherocytosis usually exhibit mild-to-moderate splenomegaly. Pallor and icterus are usually present to a mild degree. Children with long-standing severe symptoms may show some growth failure. Helpful diagnostic laboratory tests include presence of spherocytes and a high reticulocyte count on blood smear examination; increased erythropoiesis on bone marrow study; increased osmotic fragility of the red blood cells in hypotonic saline; increased mechanical fragility of red blood cells in hypotonic saline; increased mechanical fragility of freshly drawn red blood cells; and a negative Coombs' test.

Symptomatic spherocytosis is the most common indication for elective splenectomy in childhood. Splenectomy generally is deferred, however, during the first 5 years of life because of the increased susceptibility to serious infection in this age group. Despite the fact that the erythrocytes remain abnormal after splenectomy, red blood cell survival is prolonged, and the anemia almost always is relieved. If symptoms recur, a missed accessory spleen is likely. The presence of circulating erythrocytes containing Howell-Jolly bodies is evidence that a total splenectomy has been performed. Rarely, Howell-Jolly bodies can be seen, however, when an accessory spleen is still present.

Idiopathic Thrombocytopenic Purpura

ITP is characterized by a persistently low platelet count resulting from the autoimmune destruction of platelets by the reticuloendothelial system. In this disorder, circulating antibodies recognize and bind to specific surface molecules on the platelets, a phenomenon that leads to the premature destruction of the platelets, mainly by the spleen and liver. Affected children usually present with the sudden onset of bruises or petechiae or less frequently with epistaxis, oral mucosal bleeding, or rectal bleeding. Central nervous system hemorrhage is seen in approximately 1% of patients. Nearly 80% of patients give an antecedent history of a nonspecific viral illness within the preceding 3 weeks. Physical examination is usually unremarkable except for the bleeding diathesis. Similarly the complete blood count is normal except for thrombocytopenia. The platelet count may be 5000/mm^3 or lower. Further diagnostic tests, including prothrombin time, partial thromboplastin time, bleeding time, or bone marrow aspirate or biopsy, are not required for evaluating children with acute ITP. Patients presenting with systemic symptoms, lymphadenopathy, or hepatosplenomegaly and children with chronic ITP should undergo bone marrow aspirate or biopsy and a complete immunologic evaluation to exclude malignancy and autoimmune or connective tissue disorders.

Acute Idiopathic Thrombocytopenic Purpura

Nearly 80% of children with acute ITP experience spontaneous remission of thrombocytopenia within 6 months of diagnosis. Only 10% to 20% progress to chronic ITP, which is defined arbitrarily as thrombocytopenia lasting more than 1 year. Treatment of acute ITP consists mostly of limitation of physical activities and avoidance of antiplatelet agents. Pharmacologic treatment of acute ITP is more controversial in view of the high spontaneous remission rate. The most commonly used treatment of acute ITP includes the use of corticosteroids, intravenous gamma globulin (IVGG), and anti-D immune globulin (WinRho). These treatments have not been shown to decrease the incidence of chronic ITP, however. There are many deleterious emotional, psychological, physical, and financial consequences with these medications. Corticosteroids cause mood swings, weight loss, and a cushingoid appearance, whereas IVGG is costly. Pharmacologic treatment is reserved for patients at higher risk for hemorrhage, including patients older than 10 years of age (because of a higher risk of intracranial hemorrhage), patients with a massive cutaneous or mucosal hemorrhage, and patients with evidence of internal bleeding.

Numerous studies have shown the efficacy of corticosteroids in the management of acute ITP, as evidenced by a rise in platelet count during the initial days or weeks of therapy. The typical regimen consists of the administration of oral prednisone, 2 mg/kg/day in divided doses for 1 to 3 weeks. Steroid therapy should be discontinued after this period because its side effects outweigh the likelihood of any further beneficial effects from its use. The principal mode of action of corticosteroids is to inhibit phagocytosis of antibody-coated platelets by the mononuclear phagocytes. In addition, steroids diminish binding of immunoglobulin G (IgG) to the platelet, enhance platelet production, and decrease immunoglobulin (autoantibody) synthesis.

Administration of IVGG leads to a rapid rise in platelet count in children with acute or chronic ITP. This rise is usually faster and reaches a higher peak than that seen with steroid therapy. IVGG causes reticuloendothelial cell blockade by saturating the crystallizable fragment (Fc) receptor binding sites on the mononuclear phagocytes, inhibiting clearance of platelets bound to autoantibodies. The standard dose is 400 mg/kg/day for 5 consecutive days. A sustained rise in platelet count lasting several weeks usually is seen within 1 week of therapy. Despite its efficacy, the exorbitant cost of IVGG administration makes it better suited for the treatment of patients with steroid failure and patients with active bleeding or for prophylaxis in patients undergoing necessary surgical procedures.

Emergency splenectomy rarely is required in acute ITP. It is reserved for patients with intracranial hemorrhage or massive mucosal or internal hemorrhage. These patients probably should receive IVGG and steroids and preoperative and intraoperative platelet transfusions.

Chronic Idiopathic Thrombocytopenic Purpura

Chronic ITP is defined as thrombocytopenia lasting more than 1 year. The symptoms are more insidious than the acute form. Bone marrow biopsy showing normal or increased megakaryocytes has been discussed previously. These patients also should undergo evaluation for other autoimmune or connective tissue disorders including

systemic lupus erythematosus. Most children with chronic ITP do not require special therapy. Contact sports should be avoided. Treatment of chronic ITP should be based on the following considerations: frequency and severity of bleeding diathesis, age of the child (especially children >10 years old or children with menorrhagia), activity level of the child, severity of the thrombocytopenia, the need for elective surgery, and the presence of neurologic symptoms. Corticosteroids and IVGG are the cornerstone of therapy of chronic ITP. The deleterious side effects of corticosteroid therapy make it inappropriate for long-term use, however. Long-term administration of IVGG can postpone (sometimes indefinitely) the need for splenectomy. Newer treatment modalities, such as WinRho, can lead to a rise in platelet count via reticuloendothelial cell blockade. The therapeutic antibody-coated erythrocytes saturate the IgG Fc receptors of the mononuclear phagocyte, resulting in a concomitant increase in platelet survival. Other agents include a monoclonal antibody directed against the immunoglobulin Fc receptor and drugs, such as vincristine, vinblastine, and colchicines, that inhibit microtubular function in the mononuclear phagocyte. Immunosuppressive agents, such as azathioprine, cyclophosphamide, and cyclosporine, have been administered to adults with variable efficacy. Danazol, a synthetic androgen, increased platelet count by downregulating the number of IgG Fc receptors on the phagocytic cells. Response to the drug usually is seen within 2 to 6 months. Interferon alfa also has been used with some success in adults. It probably works by the mechanism of immunosuppression or immunomodulation. Plasmapheresis has been advocated in adults as an adjunct to high-dose IVGG alone; the technique has been used in children also.

The natural history of chronic ITP is relatively benign. Splenectomy for chronic ITP is reserved for patients with symptomatic thrombocytopenia, refractory to corticosteroid and IVGG therapy. Approximately 18% of patients with chronic ITP followed 3 to 37 years required splenectomy for refractory symptomatic ITP. Long-term remission is achieved in 80% of patients undergoing splenectomy. Although they occasionally induce a long-lasting remission in adults with acute or chronic ITP, the cytotoxic immunosuppressive drugs probably should be reserved for patients who do not respond to splenectomy because long-term experience with these new agents in children is limited.

Hereditary Elliptocytosis (Ovalocytosis)

Ovalocytosis is transmitted as a mendelian dominant trait and, similar to spherocytosis, is primarily a defect in erythrocyte structure. The degree of involvement of erythrocytes is relatively constant; however, there is a wide range of severity among affected children. Destruction of red blood cells is usually not sufficiently acute to produce anemia; splenectomy is rarely indicated. As in spherocytosis, the elliptocytes remain and may increase in the peripheral blood flow after splenectomy because only the rate of abnormal cell destruction is altered by removing the spleen.

Thalassemia (Mediterranean Anemia), Sickle Cell Disease, and Hereditary Nonspherocytic Hemolytic Anemia

In thalassemia (Mediterranean anemia), sickle cell disease, and hereditary nonspherocytic hemolytic anemia, there is a defect in the erythrocytes, which causes anemia. Although most children who have any of these conditions do not benefit from splenectomy, in some, an enlarged spleen may trap many red blood cells. When trapping is shown by a progressive shortening of the life span of transfused red blood cells, such as occurs with splenic sequestration, splenectomy may be beneficial.

One form of hereditary nonspherocytic anemia is associated biochemically with a reduction of glucose-6-phosphate dehydrogenase in red blood cells. Neonatal jaundice accompanied by episodes of hemoglobinuria with chronic hemolysis is seen in most of these patients. Although splenectomy fails to achieve a complete clinical remission in these patients, it may reduce the need for blood transfusion and minimize the risk of developing hemoglobinuria.

Hypersplenism

Hypersplenism refers to a group of hematologic disorders characterized by anemia, leukopenia, or thrombocytopenia caused by excessive removal of involved elements by an enlarged spleen. There also are an increased number of the cellular precursors in the marrow. Removal of cells is explained on the basis of circulatory stasis produced by structural alterations in the sinusoids. Inhibited bone marrow release of peripheral blood elements by a humoral splenic factor also has been postulated. Hypersplenism may be primary or secondary to some other disease that results in splenomegaly.

Most pediatric cases of primary hypersplenism stem from other diseases, such as spherocytosis and ITP. Before splenectomy is performed for hypersplenism, the primary disease must be determined. The extent to which the spleen removes deficient cells should be ascertained when possible. In some instances, the spleen may become the site of erythropoietic centers, and its removal may decrease the total body production of erythrocytes. Studies with radioactive chromium–tagged red blood cells support this clinical impression.

In secondary hypersplenism, the primary disease causes splenomegaly, and the enlarged spleen becomes overactive by trapping or destroying one or more normal elements of the blood. This form of hypersplenism rarely causes a patient to become symptomatic and is observed most commonly in portal hypertension regardless of its etiology. Splenectomy is rarely, if ever, necessary under these circumstances. Splenic artery ligation has been shown to reduce the symptoms without increasing the risk of systemic infection that often follows splenectomy. More recently, splenic artery embolization has produced similar results in a few children, although recurrent symptoms may occur as collateral channels develop.

Secondary hypersplenism also occurs in patients with Hodgkin's disease, Gaucher's disease, sarcoidosis, reticuloendotheliosis, certain granulomas, and leukemia.

Some children with massively enlarged spleens, particularly with Gaucher's disease, may benefit from near-total (95%) splenectomy. Although partial splenectomy is effective in the short-term, enzyme therapy has become the standard method of treatment in these patients.

Hyposplenism

Reduced splenic function may result from surgical or congenital absence or from disorders that impair the microcirculation of the spleen, such as sickle cell anemia, or disorders that infiltrate the splenic parenchyma, such as Gaucher's disease. After splenectomy, there may be a precipitous increase in the platelet and white blood cell count. Several disorders can produce functional hyposplenism, including sickle cell anemia, sarcoidosis, chronic ulcerative colitis (rare), celiac disease (rare), and radiation therapy. Affected children are at increased risk for sepsis similar to splenectomized patients.

Technique of Splenectomy

Laparoscopic splenectomy has replaced the open operation as the approach of choice for patients requiring elective removal of the spleen except when the spleen is large. The patient is prepared for the laparoscopic operation in a similar fashion as for the open procedure. Vaccinations are administered at least 3 weeks before the operation, and the platelet count is elevated greater than $20,000/mm^3$, if possible, by administering either IVGG or WinRho or whatever agent the patient best responds to. The patient is placed on the operating table, usually in a 30- to 45-degree right lateral decubitus position with a roll under the left flank. The patient is secured to the operating room table because the operating room table may need to be rotated to a more 90-degree right lateral position or a more 0-degree horizontal orientation. The urinary bladder is emptied with a Credé maneuver or catheter, and an orogastric tube is introduced for gastric decompression.

Placement of the ports can vary by preference among surgeons. A variety of orientations of port positions are possible. Some authors prefer to place 3- and 5-mm incisions in the midline of the epigastric region with a 15-mm incision placed through the umbilicus (Fig. 69-1). Through this 15-mm incision, the stapler is introduced for ligation and division of the splenic hilum and for introduction of the 15-mm endoscopic retrieval bag. The bag is exteriorized at this site and the spleen manually morcellized and extracted piecemeal. Another possible orientation is two small incisions placed in the midline and one in the umbilicus, but the 15-mm incision is placed in either the left mid abdomen or the left lower abdomen (see Fig. 69-1). The advantage of this orientation is that the endoscopic stapler can be advanced at a 90-degree orientation to the splenic vessels and placed more easily across these vessels for ligation and division.

Regardless of the orientation of the cannulas, the essential parts of the operation are as follows: Diagnostic laparoscopy is performed to search for accessory spleens, especially in the patient with ITP (Fig. 69-2). The lieno-colic attachments are divided first, usually with the ultrasonic scalpel, followed by division of the short gastric vessels with this same instrument. The tail of the

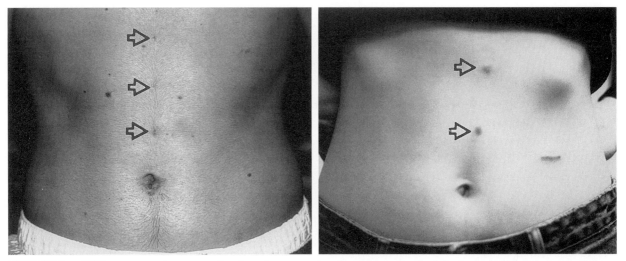

FIGURE 69-1 ■ Different operative approaches for a laparoscopic splenectomy. On the left, three small incisions (arrows) are positioned in the midline. The two most cephalad incisions are stab incisions using a no. 11 blade through which 2.5-mm instruments are introduced directly through the skin. The caudal midline incision is 5 mm and is the site where the telescope is introduced. The largest incision is 15 mm and is placed in the umbilicus. It was through this incision that the spleen was exteriorized. On the right, two epigastric incisions are created (arrows), each measuring 5 mm, and cannulas are introduced through these incisions. A 10-mm incision is made in the umbilicus, and the largest incision, which is 15 mm, is positioned in the left subcostal region. The spleen is removed through this site.

pancreas is separated from the hilum of the spleen using the ultrasonic scalpel followed by division of the lienorenal ligament and the lienodiaphragmatic attachments. When the spleen has been freed completely and is left attached only by its hilar vessels, the endoscopic stapler with the vascular cartilage is placed across these vessels, the stapler is fired, and the vessels are ligated and divided with three rows of staples on each side of the point of division

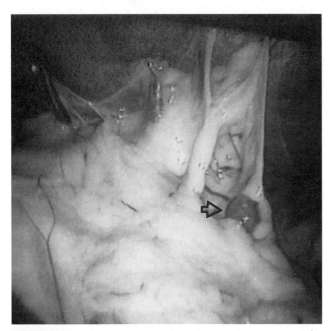

FIGURE 69-2 ■ An accessory spleen (arrow) is seen near the lower pole of the spleen in a child undergoing laparoscopic splenectomy for refractory ITP.

(Fig. 69-3). The splenic artery and vein also can be ligated with endoscopic clips and sharply divided (Fig. 69-4).

Some surgeons prefer initial ligation of the splenic artery with an endoscopic clip with the advantage of reducing the size of the spleen and allowing autotransfusion through the patent splenic vein. If this technique is desired, the splenic artery is dissected after ligation and division of the short gastric vessels. One or two endoscopic clips can be placed across the splenic artery along the superior border of the pancreas (Fig. 69-5). Another advantage of this approach is that there is arterial control of the spleen should there be misfiring of the endoscopic stapler.

When the spleen has been detached completely within the abdominal cavity, a 15-mm endoscopic retrieval bag is introduced through the 15-mm cannula, and the spleen is placed into the bag. The neck of the bag is exteriorized through the 15-mm site. Using either a finger fracture technique or ring forceps, the spleen is morcellized within the bag and extracted piecemeal. Depending on the size of the spleen, morcellization and extraction of the spleen can take 10 to 30 minutes. The bag is completely exteriorized, and repeat endoscopic visualization is performed to ensure adequate hemostasis and that there is no evidence of injury to adjacent organs, particularly the stomach and pancreas. The ports are removed, the incisions are closed, and anesthesia is terminated. Most patients are ready for discharge either the first or second day after the operation.

For children in whom severe splenic rupture is suspected or in whom the spleen is massively enlarged, open splenectomy via a long left subcostal or extended midline incision may be required. When the spleen is actively bleeding after trauma, the splenic pedicle is ligated first to minimize blood loss. Under these circumstances, particular

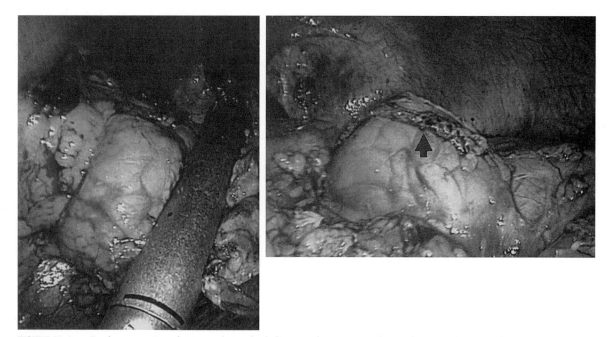

FIGURE 69-3 ■ In the operative photograph on the left, an endoscopic stapler with a vascular cartridge has been placed across the splenic vessels at the level of the splenic hilum. The pancreas is to the viewer's left of the stapler, and the spleen is to the viewer's right. On the right side is seen the staple line across the splenic vessels (arrow) after the spleen has been removed.

caution must be exercised to avoid injury to the tail of the pancreas. An aggressive search should be made for accessory spleens, which should be removed in all patients who undergo splenectomy for hematologic disorders.

When partial splenectomy is performed electively, the lower 35% to 50% of the spleen is removed after the

artery and vein are ligated to the lower splenic segment. The cut edge of the spleen is approximated with interrupted 2-0 absorbable mattress sutures placed over pledgets. The omentum is sutured loosely to the cut surface of the spleen. The appropriate part of the spleen is resected in cases of trauma.

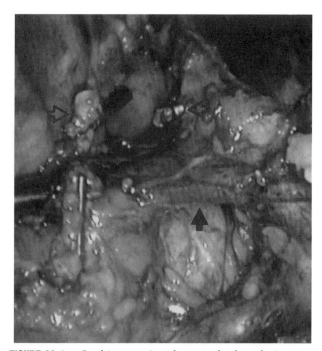

FIGURE 69-4 ■ In this operative photograph, the splenic artery has been divided with endoscopic clips (open arrows). The splenic vein (solid arrow) has been isolated, and clips will be placed across the vein for ligation before division of the vein.

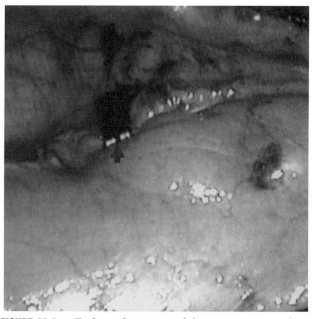

FIGURE 69-5 ■ Early in the course of the operative procedure, the splenic artery has been isolated, and two clips (arrow) have been placed across the proximal aspect of the splenic artery. The advantage of this technique is to reduce the size of the spleen and allow autotransfusion through the patent splenic vein.

POSTSPLENECTOMY SEPSIS AND OTHER COMPLICATIONS

Major complications during the postoperative period generally stem from the primary disease for which splenectomy was performed. Bleeding and infection are rare complications after splenectomy in the pediatric patient. Drainage of the splenic bed is not necessary, unless there has been damage to the tail of the pancreas.

The relationship between splenectomy and subsequent infection has been confirmed by many authors. Typical postsplenectomy infections are rapid in onset, fulminating in course, and fatal in almost 50% of cases. Most cases occur within 2 years after splenectomy, but this complication can be seen many years later. The risk is greatest in children younger than 5 years of age. It remains an uncommon but definite hazard throughout adolescent and adult life. The risk of sepsis is lower for children who undergo splenectomy for spherocytosis, ITP, or traumatic laceration. In disorders that affect the reticuloendothelial system, such as histiocytosis, Wiskott-Aldrich syndrome, and leukemia, the risk of postsplenectomy sepsis is much higher. The risk of sepsis is highest in thalassemia. In the past, nearly 8% of children undergoing splenectomy as part of a staging laparotomy for Hodgkin's disease were found to develop subsequent postsplenectomy sepsis. The mortality is greater than 40% in this group of patients. The risk of infection is as high in adolescents as in younger children who have undergone splenectomy for Hodgkin's disease. In a comprehensive review of the subject, Singer reported an overall postsplenectomy sepsis rate of 4.25% and a mortality rate of 2.52% in a collected series of 2796 patients. The calculated rate of fatal sepsis in asplenic children was 200 times that in normal children.

Pneumococcus is the organism responsible for approximately 50% of postsplenectomy septic episodes. *Meningococcus*, *Escherichia coli*, *Haemophilus influenzae*, *Staphylococcus*, and *Streptococcus* have been implicated less frequently. Active attempts to reduce the incidence of postsplenectomy sepsis have included active immunization against pneumococcus, *Meningococcus*, and *H. influenzae*; prophylactic penicillin therapy; and prompt, aggressive therapy for infections. The polyvalent pneumococcal vaccine (Pneumovax) is commercially available, affords protection against 23 of the serotypes of pneumococci, and is estimated to provide protection against approximately 85% of all pneumococcal infections. The vaccine should be administered before splenectomy whenever feasible or shortly thereafter. The same considerations apply for the other vaccines previously mentioned. Experimental studies have shown that antibody production in response to intravenously administered antigen is impaired after splenectomy, although antibody response to antigen administered by other routes is not affected. In addition, there is a reduced level of immunoglobulin M in patients after splenectomy. Children receiving corticosteroids for treatment of the underlying disease may require a second dose of Pneumovax postoperatively after the steroids have been discontinued. It is estimated that antibody levels persist at satisfactory levels for at least 3.5 years. Because there is an increased risk of reaction to second vaccine injections, booster doses are rarely recommended.

Although opinions vary widely on the subject, it generally is recommended that all children receive prophylactic penicillin after splenectomy until they reach adulthood. Many physicians recommend the administration of penicillin only when the child develops the first symptoms of an infection of any type. Patients with advanced Hodgkin's disease and other serious illnesses who have undergone splenectomy should receive long-term penicillin, regardless of age. The effectiveness of postoperative prophylactic penicillin therapy has not been shown clearly, particularly in view of the difficulty in maintaining patient compliance. Education of the parents and subsequently the child after splenectomy with respect to the significance of infection and the importance of early and aggressive treatment is perhaps one of the most important aspects of managing this problem. Parents are advised to bring the child to the hospital on an emergency basis whenever a fever of up to 102°F develops. The child is evaluated carefully; given an intravenous cephalosporin, such as ceftriaxone; and observed for several hours. If the child shows evidence of aggressive infection, he is admitted to the hospital promptly for treatment.

Postoperative thrombocytosis is not a great concern after splenectomy. All cellular blood elements increase transiently after splenectomy. The platelet count may increase to 1 million/mm^3 or more, and the leukocyte count may reach 30,000/mm^3. The highest counts usually are found approximately 1.5 weeks after splenectomy. Thrombotic complications secondary to this phenomenon are exceedingly rare in children. It is rarely necessary to administer heparin postoperatively because of thrombocytosis.

SUGGESTED READINGS

Al-Salem AH, Naserullah Z, Qaisaruddin A, et al: Splenic complications of the sickling syndromes and the role of splenectomy. J Pediatr Hematol Oncol 21:401-406, 1999.

The authors discuss their management of 113 patients with sickling disorders who underwent splenectomy over a 10-year period. The authors believe that splenectomy was beneficial in these patients in reducing the need for transfusion and its associated risks, in eliminating the discomfort from an enlarged spleen, and in avoiding the risk of acute splenic sequestration crisis.

Hemmila MR, Foley DS, Castle VP, et al: The response to splenectomy in pediatric patients with idiopathic thrombocytopenic purpura who fail high-dose intravenous immune globulin. J Pediatr Surg 35:967-971, 2000.

The authors discuss their experience with patients who were treated with intravenous immune globulin (IgG) before splenectomy. In their experience, a good or excellent response to initial treatment with IgG was associated with a significant probability of a good or excellent response to splenectomy.

Jugenberg M, Haddock G, Freedman MH, et al: The morbidity of pediatric splenectomy: Does prophylaxis make a difference? J Pediatr Surg 34:1064-1067, 1999.

The authors analyzed the incidence of postsplenectomy sepsis, morbidity, and mortality after prophylaxis in children undergoing splenectomy and compared these results with a historical period in which children did not receive prophylaxis. In their experience, the incidence of infection and mortality decreased by 47% and 88% with prophylaxis.

Reddy VS, Phan HH, O'Neill JA, et al: Laparoscopic versus open splenectomy in the pediatric population: A contemporary single-center experience, Am Surg 67:859-863, 2001.

Results are compared in patients undergoing open and laparoscopic splenectomy between 1994 and 1999. In the study, laparoscopic splenectomy seemed to result in longer operative times, but shorter lengths of stay, earlier first oral intake, and significantly fewer requirements for intravenous narcotics.

Rescorla FJ: Laparoscopic splenectomy. Semin Pediatr Surg 11:226-232, 2002.

In this review article, the author describes his experience and operative technique for laparoscopic splenectomy in 127 children. The literature regarding this operation also is reviewed.

Tarantino MD: Treatment options for chronic immune (idiopathic) thrombocytopenic purpura in children, Semin Hematol 37(Suppl 1):35-41, 2000.

This review article discusses salient issues in the treatment of ITP in children.

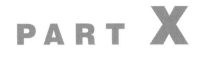

PART X

Kidney, Ureter, and Bladder

Renal Disorders

70

Patients with renal disease requiring surgical intervention most commonly present with a palpable abdominal mass, hematuria (gross or microscopic), flank or abdominal pain, renal failure, or urinary tract infection. As other anomalies are investigated with prenatal ultrasound, renal disease frequently is uncovered as an asymptomatic finding. Among the other anomalies associated with surgical renal disease are imperforate anus, which is evaluated with a voiding cystourethrogram (VUCG) and renal ultrasound, and abnormalities of the external genitalia, including severe hypospadias and urethral duplication.

ABDOMINAL MASS

Incidence and Origin

Figure 70-1 schematically illustrates the types of neonatal abdominal masses. Excluding the palpable bladder caused

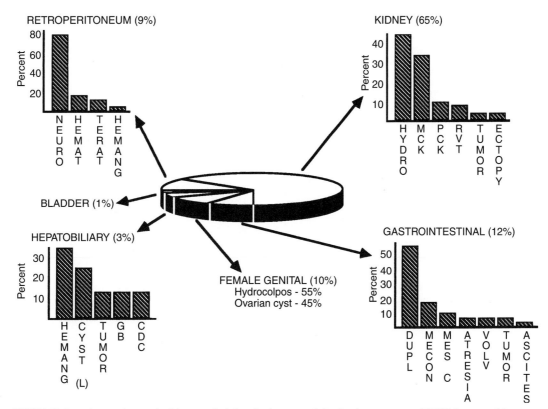

FIGURE 70-1 ■ Approximate incidence of abdominal mass etiologies in neonates. *NEURO,* neuroblastoma; *HEMAT,* hematoma; *TERAT,* teratoma; *HEMANG,* hemangioma; *HYDRO,* hydronephrosis; *MCK,* multicystic kidney; *PCK,* polycystic kidney; *RVT,* renal vein thrombosis; *GB,* gallbladder; *CDC,* coledochal cyst; *DUPL,* duplication; *MECON,* meconium ileus; *MES C,* mesenteric cyst; *VOLV,* volvulus. (Data from Merten DF: Pediatr Clin North Am 32:1397, 1985; Griscome NT: Am J Radiol 93:447, 1967; Wedge JJ: J Urol 106:770, 1971; Raffensperger J: Surgery 63:514, 1968; Wilson DA: Am J Dis Child 136:147, 1982; and Emanuel B: Clin Pediatr 7:529, 1968.)

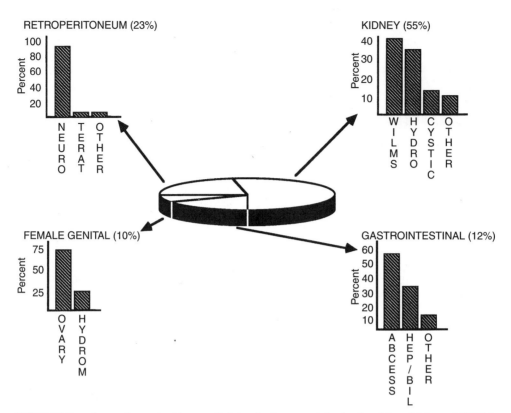

FIGURE 70-2 ■ Approximate incidence of abdominal mass etiologies in older children. *NEURO*, neuroblastoma; *TERAT*, teratoma; *HYDRO*, hydronephrosis; *HYDROM*, hydrometrocolpos; *HEP/BIL*, hepatobiliary. (Data from Merten DF: Pediatr Clin North Am 32:1397, 1985; Griscom NT: Am J Radiol 93:447, 1967; Wedge JJ: J Urol 106:770, 1971; Raffensperger J: Surgery 63:514, 1968; Wilson DA: Am J Dis Child 136:147, 1982; and Emanuel B: Clin Pediatr 7:529, 1968.)

by urinary retention, renal problems are responsible for approximately two thirds of all neonatal abdominal masses. Most relate to hydronephrosis or cystic renal diseases. The most common cystic renal disease is multicystic dysplastic kidney. Autosomal recessive polycystic kidney disease, renal vein thrombosis, and renal tumors are less common but important etiologies. Occasionally an ectopic kidney appears as an abdominal mass because of hydronephrosis, which may be palpable.

The origin of abdominal masses in older children is shown in Figure 70-2. In older children, the kidney accounts for slightly greater than half of abdominal masses, followed by retroperitoneal masses, predominantly neuroblastoma. Wilms' tumor and hydronephrosis are the most common renal masses in this age group, with a decreased incidence of cystic renal disease.

Assessment and Diagnosis

Whether a renal mass initially is detected on prenatal ultrasound or as a palpable abdominal mass, the most appropriate first study is an abdominal ultrasound. Generally the mass can be localized to the kidney with this modality and classified according to its internal sonographic architecture. Definitive radiographic evaluation is performed using computed tomography or magnetic resonance imaging for solid masses and VCUG and renal scan for cystic masses.

Solid Masses

The most common solid renal masses are neoplasms (see Chapter 20), such as Wilms' tumor, renal sarcomas, and renal cell carcinomas. Congenital mesoblastic nephroma (Fig. 70-3) is the most common solid renal mass in neonates.

Occasionally, renal tumors become evident in conjunction with an obvious somatic abnormality. Aniridia, macroglossia (Beckwith-Wiedemann syndrome), and hemihypertrophy occur in association with Wilms' tumor. Adenoma sebaceum occurring with tubular sclerosis may be associated with renal tumors, most commonly angiomyolipomas.

Other important forms of solid renal masses include nephromegaly and pseudotumors. Conditions that mimic neoplasms include prominent columns of Bertin, fetal lobulations, renal abscesses, xanthogranulomatous pyelonephritis, and various pararenal masses. These lesions usually can be distinguished with computed tomography.

Cystic Masses

A cystic mass is either hydronephrosis or cystic renal disease. Usually hydronephrosis is the result of urinary tract obstruction or vesicoureteral reflux of primary or secondary etiology. Bladder dysfunction in the form of bladder outlet obstruction or neurovesical dysfunction may result in bilateral hydronephrotic kidneys. The diagnostic

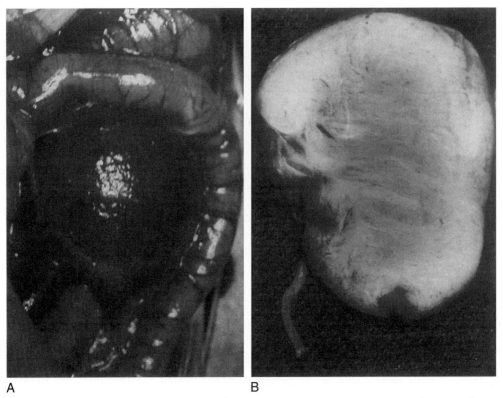

A   B

FIGURE 70-3 ■ Congenital mesoblastic nephroma. **A,** Intraoperative appearance in a newborn. **B,** Appearance on cut surface. The yellow, firm, rubbery, trabeculated appearance resembles that of a uterine fibroid. This mass was detected on antenatal ultrasound. Frequently these lesions present as palpable neonatal masses or possibly as a solid renal mass on prenatal ultrasonography.

evaluation of a cystic mass includes VCUG to detect reflux and bladder disease and renal scintigraphy to evaluate renal function.

Table 70-1 outlines a classification of cystic renal disease. Lesions most commonly requiring surgical evaluation are multicystic dysplasia, autosomal recessive polycystic kidney disease, and autosomal dominant polycystic kidney disease.

Multicystic Dysplasia

Multicystic dysplastic kidney is encountered commonly in newborns (Fig. 70-4A). Prenatal detection by screening ultrasound is common. This lesion is rarely bilateral, in this clinical setting, and usually is caused by ipsilateral ureteral atresia. Concomitant contralateral ureteral pelvic junction obstruction and vesicoureteral reflux is common.

Renal ultrasound (Fig. 70-4B) reveals multiple, variously sized, disconnected cysts that are not associated with any central larger cyst. No identifiable parenchyma is evident. Renal scintigraphy shows total nonfunction of the involved kidney, and VCUG may detect associated reflux with an increased incidence compared with the general population. Contralateral reflux merits careful therapy because of its risk in relation to the solitary functioning kidney.

Complications of multicystic kidney disease include hypertension and infection. Rarely a cystic renal malignancy may be confused with multicystic dysplasia. Concern has been raised with respect to multicystic kidneys developing malignancy from the presence of

TABLE 70-1 ■ Cystic Renal Disease
Cystic renal dysplasia
Multicystic kidney
Obstruction
Genetic polycystic kidney disease
Autosomal dominant (adult)
Autosomal recessive (infantile)
Simple cysts
Acquired cystic disease
Cystic disease of the renal medulla
Juvenile nephronophthisis (autosomal recessive)
Medullary cystic disease (autosomal dominant)
Medullary sponge kidney (rarely inherited)
Malformation syndromes
Chromosome disorders
Trisomy 21, 18, 12, C
Autosomal dominant
Von Hippel–Lindau disease
Tuberous sclerosis
Autosomal recessive
Jeune's, Zellweger's, Meckel's syndromes
X-linked dominant
Oral-facial-digital syndrome
Miscellaneous cystic disorders
Multilocular cyst
Pyelocalyceal cyst

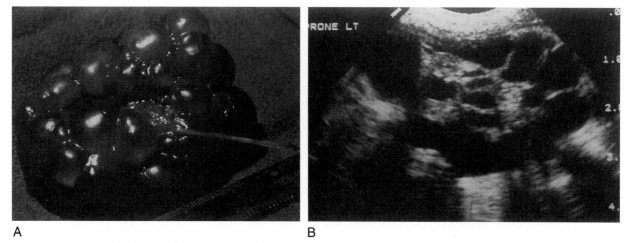

A   B

FIGURE 70-4 ▪ Multicystic kidney disease. **A,** Gross appearance. **B,** Sonographic appearance.

definable nodular renal blastema. The danger of malignancy in this lesion is remote. Multicystic kidney may occur in a hydronephrotic form, which on ultrasound has the appearance of hydronephrosis except the parenchyma is dysplastic and the renogram shows no function. This entity lends credence to the theory that ureteropelvic junction obstruction and multicystic dysplastic kidney may be on the same spectrum of pathophysiology. The degree of obstruction and the timing of obstruction relative to nephron development dictate the outcome.

Polycystic Kidney Disease

The incidence of infantile autosomal recessive polycystic kidney disease is 1 in 6000 to 14,000. The characteristic lesions of this disease are enlarged, radially oriented, microscopic cysts of the collecting ducts (Fig. 70-5). Profound renal insufficiency in infancy commonly occurs, although rarely the abnormality may not appear until later in life. Prenatally, oligohydramnios and pulmonary hypoplasia are often seen.

Ultrasound reveals increased echogenicity of the cortex and medulla. The kidneys are symmetrically enlarged.

Macrocystic changes usually are seen only in older children.

Autosomal recessive polycystic kidney disease may be associated with pulmonary hypoplasia, other stigmata of Potter's syndrome, hepatic cysts, and fibrosis. Complications include renal insufficiency, hypertension, hepatic insufficiency, and urinary tract infection.

Adult or autosomal dominant polycystic kidney disease is characterized by bilateral cystic renal masses with a multitude of fluid-filled cysts involving the cortex and the medulla (Fig. 70-6). The incidence of this abnormality is 1 in 1000 children. Inheritance follows an autosomal dominant pattern with nearly complete penetrance; chromosome 16 has been implicated. Although this lesion usually becomes clinically manifest in adults in their 20s to 30s, it has been seen in infants and even fetuses; consequently this lesion is termed *autosomal dominant polycystic kidney disease.* Associated lesions include polycystic liver, cerebrovascular aneurysms, and pancreatic cysts. Complications include renal insufficiency, hypertension, urinary tract infection, and urolithiasis.

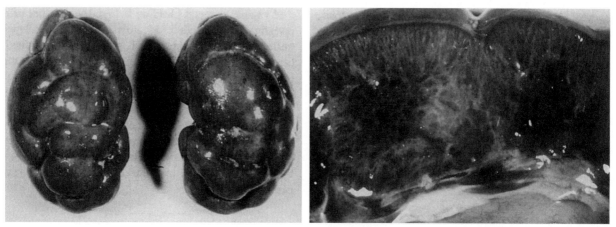

A   B

FIGURE 70-5 ▪ Autosomal recessive polycystic kidney disease. **A,** Gross appearance. **B,** Cut surface.

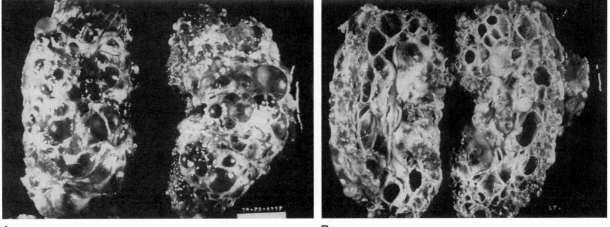

A   B

FIGURE 70-6 ■ Autosomal dominant polycystic kidney disease. **A,** Gross appearance. **B,** Cut surface. The findings are more advanced and prominent than those seen in the recessive form of polycystic renal disease.

HEMATURIA

Hematuria has varied presentations in childhood. It may be found incidentally at the time of routine screening urinalysis or as discolored urine (gross hematuria). Occasionally a discolored diaper or spotting of the underwear is the presenting symptom. Some pharmacologic agents or their metabolites cause urine discoloration or may react with the hypochlorides found in toilet bowel cleaners to produce discoloration. Certain food substances, dyes, and endogenous metabolites can produce urine discoloration. *Serratia marcescens* growth allowed to incubate in wet diapers and urates that occasionally precipitate in the diaper may produce discoloration. Consequently, any urine discoloration must be examined by urinalysis and the red blood cells detected before the diagnosis of hematuria is accepted. Table 70-2 outlines the differential diagnosis of factitious hematuria. Table 70-3 presents the differential diagnosis of true hematuria. Causes generally are classified as collecting system, nonglomerular renal, and glomerular.

Evaluation of the patient with true hematuria begins with a careful history assessing the character of the hematuria. Hematuria should be classified as gross or microscopic and painful or painless. Additionally, gross hematuria should be characterized as to whether it occurs in the initial portion, the terminal portion, or throughout the urinary system.

Voiding symptoms, a history of bleeding disorders, and drug ingestion should be elicited. The presence of arthralgias, rashes, flu-like symptoms, or pharyngitis may be helpful. A family history should be obtained for renal or urologic disease, deafness, hematuria, urolithiasis, and sickle cell disease; hematuria may be encountered with either sickle cell disease or sickle cell trait. Prior instrumentation involving the urethra, percutaneous bladder puncture, or renal puncture indicates an obvious source of hematuria.

Physical examination should include the measurement of blood pressure and examination for abdominal mass. The presence of edema, rashes, arthritis, cutaneous hemangiomas, petechiae, cardiac murmurs, Janeway's

spots, and a central venous line or dialysis shunt should be noted. A rectal examination, including prostate examination, should be performed. The meatus is examined for inflammation and evidence of urethral prolapse and bloody discharge from the urethra, vagina, rectum, and perineum. Bloody discharge may mimic urethral bleeding and present as spotting of the underwear.

Pertinent laboratory studies include urinalysis, urine culture, complete blood cell count, and serum creatinine (Fig. 70-7). A urine calcium-to-creatinine clearance ratio may implicate hypercalciuria as a cause even when a calculus cannot be shown by imaging. Abnormalities in the serum complement profile may implicate glomerular disease. Antistreptolysin O titer elevation and antinuclear antibody assay may yield a specific diagnosis. Hemoglobin electrophoresis is pertinent when sickle cell disease or trait is suspected. Urinalysis of parents may be helpful when

---

TABLE 70-2 ■ **Differential Diagnosis: Factitious Hematuria**

Drugs
  Analgesics
  Phenazopyridine hydrochloride (Pyridium)
  Phenothiazines
  Antimalarials
  Antihypertensives
  Antimicrobials (bacterial, tuberculous)
  Anticonvulsants
  Anthelmintics
Foods
  Beets
  Berries
  Rhubarb
Dyes
Metabolites
  Urobilinogen
  Porphobilinogen
  Melanin
  Homogentisic acid
Urates
  Serratia

TABLE 70-3 ■ Differential Diagnosis: True Hematuria		
Collecting System	**Nonglomerular Renal**	**Glomerular**
Infectious	Systemic	Primary
Bacteria	Sickle-cell trait/disease	Acute poststreptococcal
Viruses	Bleeding disorders: anticoagulants, hemophilia,	glomerulonephritis
Tuberculosis	von Willebrand's disease, idiopathic	Alport's syndrome
Parasites	thrombocytopenic purpura	Benign familial
Neoplastic	Parenchymal	Berger's disease
Rhabdomyosarcoma	Pyelonephritis	Immunoglobulin A
Transitional cell tumors	Obstruction	nephropathy
Other tumors	Nephrolithiasis (hypercalciuria)	Other glomerulonephritis
Chemical	Neoplastic: Wilms' tumor, renal cell carcinoma,	Systemic
Cyclophosphamide	other tumors	Hemolytic uremic syndrome
Methenamine mandelate	Cystic renal disease	Systemic lupus erythematosus
(Mandelamine)	Trauma	Henoch-Schönlein purpura
Trauma	Vascular	Bacterial endocarditis
Urolithiasis	Renal vein thrombosis	Shunt nephritis
Metabolic	Renal artery thrombosis	Goodpasture's syndrome
Infection/obstruction	Renal cortical necrosis	Periarteritis nodosa
Iatrogenic	Papillary necrosis	Other
Needle biopsy	Arteriovenous malformation	
Needle puncture	Hemangioma	
Catheterization	Embolic disease	
Other		

familial hematuria is suspected. Occasionally, audiometry and measurement of serum albumin and total protein levels are useful.

As already noted, spotting of the underwear can be caused by several conditions, including urethral prolapse, urethral or vaginal foreign body, meatitis, idiopathic urethrorrhagia, sarcoma, menses, anal fissure, and other perineal bleeding sources. Idiopathic urethrorrhagia is encountered commonly in pubertal boys. The cause is uncertain, possibly related to irritative voiding symptoms. The course is often protracted and usually self-limited.

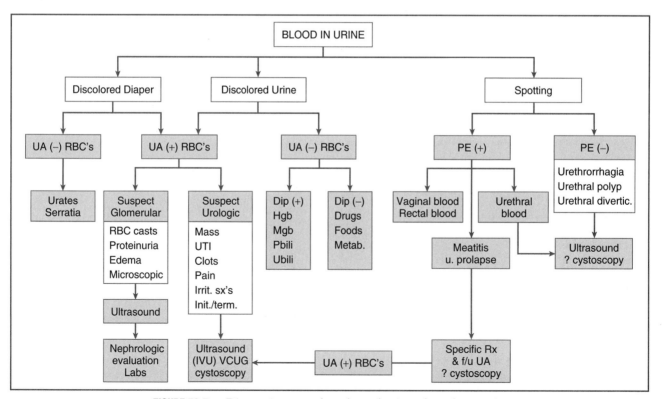

FIGURE 70-7 ■ Diagnostic approach to the evaluation of true hematuria.

TABLE 70-4 ■ Causes of Renal Failure in Children		
Prerenal	**Renal**	**Postrenal**
Dehydration	Congenital anomalies	Posterior urethral
Cardiac	Agenesis	valves
failure	Cystic disease	Ureterocele
Hypovolemia	Hypoplasia/dysplasia	Neurovesical
	Vascular	dysfunction
	Renal artery	Ureteropelvic
	thrombosis	junction
	Renal vein thrombosis	obstruction
	Disseminated	Ureterovesical
	intravascular	junction
	thrombosis	obstruction
	Hemolytic uremic	Anterior urethral
	syndrome	valves
	Cortical necrosis	Other
	Tubular necrosis	
	Metabolic	
	Other	

Serial urinalysis may be necessary. If red blood cell casts or proteinuria is present or if edema is noted, renal ultrasound and nephrologic evaluation are indicated. Patients who have palpable mass, findings of urinary tract infection, passage of clots, renal pain, or irritative voiding symptoms with initial or terminal hematuria should be suspected to have urologic etiology. Investigation begins with ultrasound or intravenous urography, accompanied by VCUG in selected circumstances. Cystoscopy is used in selected cases.

If vaginal or rectal bleeding is found, no further urinary investigation is needed. Meatitis or urethral prolapse is treated directly, and the urine is examined periodically for hematuria thereafter. If the hematuria fails to clear, radiographic and endoscopic evaluation is necessary.

FAILURE TO VOID

Clinicians commonly are asked to evaluate a neonate for failure to void. One must be careful not to overinterpret this finding. Failure to void in the early neonatal period is common. Most neonates void by 12 hours of life, 92% void by 24 hours, and 99% void by 48 hours. Suspicion of an underlying renal or urologic abnormality should begin at 12 hours, and evaluation by physical examination and abdominal ultrasound is undertaken should failure to void continue beyond 24 hours. Table 70-4 outlines the common causes of renal failure that lead to surgical intervention.

ABNORMALITIES OF POSITION, FUSION, NUMBER, AND SIZE

Abnormalities of renal position, fusion, number, and size are encountered frequently in children. Often they occur in isolation, but a prominent correlation occurs with VACTERRL complex (vertebral defects, imperforate anus, tracheoesophageal fistula, and radial and renal dysplasia), Mayer-Rokitansky syndrome, Turner's syndrome, and trisomy 18.

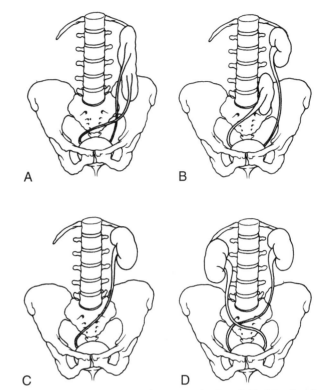

FIGURE 70-8 ■ Crossed renal ectopia. **A,** Fused. **B,** Nonfused. **C,** Solitary. **D,** Bilateral. (From Koff SA, Wise HA: Anomalies of the kidney. In Gillenwater JY, Grayback JT, Howards SS, et al [eds]: Adult and Pediatric Urology, 2nd ed. St. Louis, Mosby–Year Book, 1991.)

Position and Fusion

Abnormalities of renal position include renal ectopia and malrotation. Ectopic kidneys may be simple, crossed, or fused. Approximately 60% of simple ectopic kidneys are pelvic, with the remainder occurring between the pelvis and the usual renal position. Superiorly, malpositioned kidneys as high as the thorax are reported but are extremely rare.

Figure 70-8 illustrates several examples of crossed renal ectopia. Most are fused, but unfused crossed ectopia can occur. Figure 70-9 shows common examples of renal fusion abnormalities. Cross-fused renal ectopia is common in children with multiple congenital anomalies. General guidelines include the following observations:

1. The lower the kidney, the nearer the kidney lies to the midline, and the more ventral the renal pelvis is located.
2. Lower kidneys have a greater number of renal blood vessels.
3. Approximately 10% of unascended kidneys are solitary, a significantly greater percentage than among the general population.
4. Pelvic kidneys have a particularly high incidence of associated abnormalities, including gastrointestinal (about two thirds), skeletal (about half), and cardiovascular (occasionally).

Renal malrotation is closely related to renal ectopia. During development, the renal pelvis begins in a

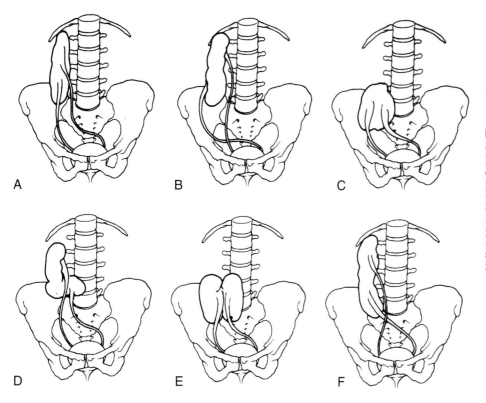

FIGURE 70-9 ■ Crossed renal ectopia with fusion. **A,** Ectopic kidney superior. **B,** Sigmoid kidney. **C,** Lump kidney. **D,** L-shaped kidney. **E,** Disk kidney. **F,** Ectopic kidney inferior. (From Koff SA, Wise HA: Anomalies of the kidney. In Gillenwater JY, Grayback JT, Howards SS et al [eds]: Adult and Pediatric Urology, 2nd ed. St. Louis, Mosby–Year Book, 1991.)

ventral position, and during ascent of the kidney, progressive medial rotation occurs.

There are several important clinical implications. From a diagnostic perspective, unless specifically sought, a small ectopic kidney may be interpreted as absent, allowing a source for infection or hypertension to be missed. These kidneys are missed easily by screening ultrasound and intravenous urography because of overlap of the collecting structures with the bony pelvis or poor function. Renal scintigraphy can help detect these abnormalities, but cystoscopy with retrograde pyelography is diagnostic. Cystoscopy should be done only when the clinical situation dictates further anatomic delineation. The presence of a hemitrigone with no ipsilateral ureteral orifice confirms the diagnosis of renal agenesis or ectopic ureteral insertion.

Renal ectopia has significant surgical implications, altering the type of incision necessary to expose a kidney and possibly requiring an intraperitoneal rather than a retroperitoneal approach, particularly for low fused renal anomalies. In addition, multiple vessels make renal exposure and reconstruction considerably more difficult. Nonrenal surgery, especially of the abdominal aorta, may be compromised significantly by renal ectopia or fusion anomalies, the most notorious being horseshoe kidney in patients requiring surgery for abdominal aortic aneurysms.

Number

Abnormalities in renal number include renal agenesis, either unilateral or bilateral, and supranumerary kidneys. Bilateral renal agenesis is uncommon and occurs in association with Potter's syndrome. The incidence of unilateral renal agenesis is approximately 1 in 1000 children. In 60% of patients, the ureter is absent, and in 10% of patients,

the ipsilateral adrenal is absent. There is a high correlation with reproductive abnormalities, most notably Mayer-Rokitansky syndrome. Absence of the vas deferens in boys may lead one to suspect ipsilateral renal agenesis.

The clinical implications of renal agenesis relate primarily to renal biopsy and renal trauma. Occasionally a renal biopsy, either open or percutaneous, may be required to evaluate azotemia, hematuria, or proteinuria. Images of the kidney must be reviewed before biopsy to avoid attempting to obtain a biopsy specimen of a nonexistent kidney. Every effort to preserve a severely injured kidney during emergent laparotomy for trauma must be made, unless intraoperative or preoperative imaging shows a functioning contralateral kidney.

True supernumerary kidneys are extremely rare. Misconceptions occur in the common mislabeling of duplicated kidneys as supernumerary kidneys.

Size

Abnormalities of renal size include nephromegaly and small kidneys. Table 70-5 lists the most common causes of nephromegaly in patients. Children with bilateral nephromegaly must be evaluated for diabetes, leukemia, lymphoma, glomerulonephritis, and infantile or adult polycystic kidney disease among other important abnormalities. Unilateral nephromegaly represents a diagnostically more difficult situation from the perspective of excluding renal tumors. Pyelonephritis, renal vein thrombosis, and compensatory hypertrophy are commonly encountered causes of unilateral nephromegaly.

Small kidneys may result from hypoplasia/dysplasia or renal atrophy. Hypoplasia/dysplasia is correlated with

TABLE 70-5 ■ Nephromegaly	
Unilateral	**Bilateral**
Pyelonephritis	Diabetes mellitus
Renal vein thrombosis	Leukemia
Compensatory	Lymphoma
hypertrophy	Glomerulonephritis
Tumors and other	Nephrotic syndrome
masses	Amyloidosis
Cystic disease	Glycogen storage disease
Obstruction	Beckwith-Wiedemann
Duplication anomalies	syndrome
	Infantile polycystic kidney
	disease
	Adult polycystic kidney
	disease
	Nephroblastomatosis
	Bilateral involvement of
	conditions listed as
	unilateral

vesicoureteral reflux and urinary tract obstruction at all levels. Renal atrophy also can be associated with obstruction and vesicoureteral reflux and is encountered commonly in patients with a history of urinary tract infection. It also may be associated with ischemia.

VASCULAR DISORDERS
Renal Vein Thrombosis

Renal vein thrombosis is responsible for 20% of cases of neonatal hematuria. The pathogenesis of renal vein thrombosis is related closely to the transitional nephrology of the neonatal kidney. The low renal perfusion pressure in this age group makes these kidneys particularly vulnerable. When complicated by conditions resulting in dehydration, as with an infant with a diabetic mother (osmotic diuresis), diarrheal states, and sepsis, renal vein thrombosis may be precipitated. Sludging has important etiologic implications as well and can be seen with cyanotic congenital heart disease, hemoconcentration, acute hypoxia, sickle cell disease, cytomegalovirus infection, polyhydramnios, toxemia, and perinatal stress.

Of renal vein thrombosis, 65% is diagnosed during the neonatal period. This disorder may be a cause of early postnatal renin-mediated hypertension, and blood pressure must be monitored meticulously.

The typical diagnostic presentation includes a palpable mass (60%), hematuria (70%), and thrombocytopenia (90%). Leukocytosis, proteinuria, anemia, and consumptive coagulopathy are additional diagnostic findings. Ultrasound and renal scintigraphy are the most important imaging modalities and generally provide all the necessary diagnostic information. Occasionally a suggestion of inferior vena caval involvement necessitates computed tomography or magnetic resonance imaging.

The treatment of unilateral renal vein thrombosis concentrates on achieving and maintaining fluid and electrolyte balance. Heparinization or use of thrombolytic agents may be considered, but caution must be exercised in premature or highly stressed neonates, who have a propensity for intracranial bleeding. Patients with bilateral renal vein thrombosis also require hydration, and heparinization is commonly employed. Thrombolytic therapy may be used in selected patients but requires extremely close monitoring. Thrombectomy may be considered in particularly devastating circumstances, but this is only rarely indicated.

The prognosis for patients with bilateral renal vein thrombosis is poor. Unilateral renal vein thrombosis commonly results in a nonfunctioning, fibrosed kidney or a partially fibrosed kidney with decreased renal function. Renin-mediated hypertension is common, as is nephrotic syndrome. Chronic urinary tract infection may be encountered occasionally, as may chronic renal tubular dysfunction. The above-mentioned sequelae may prompt nephrectomy.

PERITONEAL DIALYSIS
Physiology

Peritoneal dialysis for renal failure is accomplished by the simultaneous bidirectional passage of solute and water through the semipermeable membrane. The peritoneal surface approximates the total body surface area. The visceral peritoneum appears more crucial for effective water and solute passage, although there are more capillaries in the parietal peritoneum. The exact route and mechanism by which solutes cross the peritoneal membrane are unknown.

Factors influencing the magnitude of peritoneal transport and the transmembrane solute and water movement in children include molecular size, shape, and charge; surface area of the membrane; transmembrane concentration gradient; swell time; volume of dialysate; and intrinsic membrane permeability. Some of these factors are intrinsic to the dialysis process, whereas others are under the physician's direct control. Water movement occurs by ultrafiltration, which depends on the existing osmotic gradient between blood and dialysate.

Although continuous ambulatory peritoneal dialysis was developed in 1975, it did not gain wide use until 1978, when the procedure was adapted to the use of dialysate solutions in plastic bags. Children first were treated with ambulatory dialysis in 1978. Continuous cycling peritoneal dialysis (CCPD) is an evolution of continuous ambulatory peritoneal dialysis and intermittent peritoneal dialysis. CCPD offers the opportunity for home care with increased mobility during the daylight hours. The development of the Tenckhoff silicone catheter has made it feasible to insert peritoneal dialysis catheters with the anticipation that they will function for prolonged periods (often >1 year), while causing minimal irritation to the viscera and peritoneal surface. Ambulatory peritoneal dialysis has many advantages over hemodialysis in children with end-stage renal disease, including larger dietary intake of calories, maintenance of lower blood pressure, decreased need for transfusion, absence of need for long-term heparin administration, increased mobility,and considerable decrease in cost.

Indications

Indications for peritoneal dialysis in children include focal glomerulonephritis, renal dysplasia, obstructive uropathy, membranoproliferative glomerulonephritis, hemolytic uremic syndrome, and polycystic kidney disease. The criteria used for initiating peritoneal dialysis include creatinine clearance of less than 5 mg/min/1.73 m²; small child or infant (<20 kg); home a long distance from hemodialysis facilities; and preference of the patient, family, and physician. Peritoneal dialysis is considered a preliminary procedure to renal transplantation in children. It permits the patient to achieve optimal metabolic and physical condition for transplantation and provides sufficient time for the appropriate size and type matching of the renal allograft. Approximately 10% of children have had previous renal transplantation with rejection on one or more occasions and required a return to dialysis.

Technique

Complications with peritoneal dialysis are more common in children than in adults, largely because of the need for prompt dialysis after catheter insertion with relatively large volumes into a small abdominal cavity. Although percutaneous insertion of a dialysis catheter may provide immediate relief for children in severe renal failure, the incidence of complications, including viscus perforation, subcutaneous positioning of the catheter, and obstruction as a result of poor positioning, is considerably greater than those after operative insertion of a long-term catheter into the pelvis through a small infraumbilical midline incision. Partial omentectomy is sometimes useful. The percutaneously inserted catheter is useful in an emergency situation but is not often suitable for peritoneal dialysis exceeding several days in infants and young children.

The preferred dialysis catheters are the pediatric or adult Tenckhoff type with one or two Dacron felt cuffs between the peritoneal cavity and the catheter exit site (Fig. 70-10). Fibrous growth into the cuff provides stabilization, minimizes dialysate leak, and reduces the incidence of bacterial migration along the catheter tract. For small infants, a catheter with a single Dacron cuff is used; however, when children are larger, a double-cuffed catheter is preferred. In children older than 2 years of age, a curled loop at the end of the dialyzing portion of the catheter has been used to provide greater surface between the catheter and the lower abdominal cavity. For children younger than 2 years of age, a straight Tenckhoff catheter is used.

For most children, the CCPD routine used involves five exchanges at 2 hour intervals overnight with a portion of an exchange left in the abdomen during the day, 7 days a week. The volume of an exchange is approximately 40 to 50 mL/kg of body weight.

Catheter dysfunction may lead to progressive renal failure; it may take several days to recover function, even after relatively minor dialysis catheter problems. Meticulous care should be taken in the insertion of peritoneal dialysis catheters, with every precaution taken to avoid introducing bacteria into the peritoneal cavity or the subcutaneous tunnel extending to the catheter exit site. Infection may lead to peritonitis and intestinal adhesions,

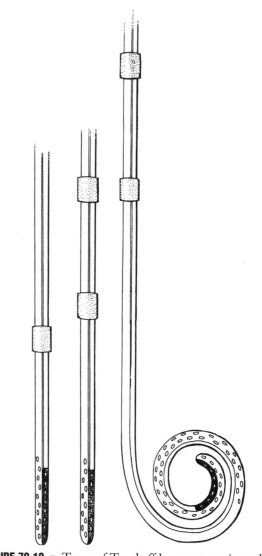

FIGURE 70-10 ■ Types of Tenckoff long-term peritoneal dialysis catheters currently used most frequently in children: straight catheter with one cuff for infants, straight catheter with two cuffs up to age 3 years, double-cuffed catheter with curled tip for older children.

which may make subsequent peritoneal dialysis difficult or impossible. Chronic infection precludes the patient from being considered for a renal transplant.

Complications

The most common reasons for catheter replacement include peritonitis, tunnel infection, obstruction of the catheter, persistent exit-site infection, peritoneal fluid leak, ventral hernia, cuff erosion, migration of the catheter upward in the abdominal activity, and catheter deterioration. With close observation and detailed management of the catheter and dialysis procedure, complications can be avoided.

Approximately 10% of children undergoing dialysis have inguinal hernias first noted after dialysis has been initiated. With standard dialysis volumes, inguinal hernias enlarge and produce discomfort, limiting the function of the dialysis program. Inguinal hernias or hydroceles in dialysis patients should be repaired shortly after the diagnosis is established. The side opposite the clinically apparent hernia or hydrocele should be explored and any hernia sac or patent processus corrected.

Rarely a temporary hydrothorax may develop after several weeks of peritoneal dialysis. The cause is unclear but may be related to diffusion of peritoneal fluid up from the retroperitoneal space via lymphatic absorption. In our experience, patients may be treated effectively without surgery by temporary intermittent peritoneal dialysis, then CCPD with reduced peritoneal dialysate volume.

When the transplant functions well for 3 months without need for dialysis, the catheter is removed. A general anesthetic and sterile operative technique are used for catheter removal with an attempt to remove foreign suture material and to close the muscular defect in the abdominal wall. When low-volume peritoneal dialysis is used for several days after transplant, intestinal adhesions are minimized. If the transplant fails, a new peritoneal catheter may be inserted. The presence of a peritoneal dialysis catheter has not increased patient or renal allograft morbidity rates. Hemodialysis is used primarily for patients older than age 12 or when peritoneal dialysis fails.

SUGGESTED READINGS

Bauer SB: Anomalies of the upper urinary tract. In Walsh PC, Retik AB, Vaughan ED Jr, Wein AJ [eds]: Campbell's Urology 8th ed. Philadelphia, WB Saunders, 2002.

The authors provide a complete description of renal anomalies and the related embryologic considerations and methods of management.

Stephens FD, Smith ED, Hutson JM: The pathogenesis of renal dysplasia. In: Congenital Anomalies of the Urinary and Genital Tracts. Oxford, Isis Medical Media, 1996.

The authors have studied genitourinary embryology and approaches to diagnosis and treatment for many years. This is excellent background reading.

Walker BR, Ellison ED, Snow BW, Cartwright PC: The natural history of idiopathic urethrorrhagia in boys. J Urol 166:231-232, 2001.

Hematuria is a common concern in boys with multiple etiologies, nicely summarized in detail in this article.

Zigman A, Yazbeck S, Emil S, Nguyen L: Renal vein thrombosis: A 10-year review. J Pediatr Surg 35:1540-1542, 2000.

The authors provide a description of renal vein thrombosis and current etiologies; this entity is seen less frequently than previously.

71

Ureteropelvic Junction Obstruction

DEFINITION

Ureteropelvic junction (UPJ) obstruction in children is usually due to a congenital obstruction of urine flow from the renal pelvis to the ureter, resulting in dilation of the intrarenal collecting system with potential damage to renal function and risk of urinary tract infection and stones over time. It is recognized as the most common cause of hydronephrosis in the fetal kidney, occurring in 1 in every 200 pregnancies. Figure 71-1 shows the usual anatomy with a narrowed ureter at the UPJ and marked dilation and blunting of the renal calyces.

UPJ obstruction usually is referred to as *intrinsic* or *extrinsic* and as *primary* or *secondary*. Intrinsic UPJ can be caused by luminal stenosis, fibromuscular polyps, or congenital ureteral folds. The luminal stenosis may be caused by an alteration in the amount or orientation of muscle fibers, fibrous strictures, or kinking of the ureter secondary to the accordion affect of the dilated renal pelvis (Fig. 71-2). The exact cause of this common problem is still unknown. It is hypothesized that in the absence of obvious mechanical factors there may be a functional disturbance in the ability of the pelvis to initiate or conduct peristaltic waves across the UPJ.

Extrinsic UPJ obstruction usually is caused by ureteral angulation or kinking due to abnormal fibrous tissue that tethers the ureter or more commonly due to angulation of the UPJ over an aberrant lower pole vessel (Fig. 71-3). With this anomaly, the renal pelvis protrudes between the middle and lower pole vessel and the ureter, and the UPJ drapes over the lower pole vessel, creating a kink at the UPJ. In a similar fashion, high insertion of the ureter into the renal pelvis may cause an angulation of the UPJ that is accentuated by rapid filling of the renal pelvis. Angulation, kinking, and secondary obstruction can also occur owing to ureterovesical junction pathology, such as high-grade reflux or obstruction.

Primary UPJ obstruction refers to a congenital lesion, and secondary UPJ obstruction results from injury or distortion as a result of open or endoscopic surgery, a recurrent inflammatory process, urinary tract stone disease, an enlarging fibroepithelial polyp, and occasionally vesicoureteral reflux (Fig. 71-4).

PRESENTATION

UPJ obstruction now most commonly presents in the fetal period (Fig. 71-5) because prenatal ultrasound is widely available and almost routinely used during pregnancy. Hydronephrosis seen on prenatal examination has surpassed a palpable renal mass as the most common presentation of urinary tract obstruction. Prenatal hydronephrosis is not always due to UPJ obstruction, however, and can be caused by transient physiologic hydronephrosis, high-grade vesicoureteral reflux, obstruction in the distal ureter, and a misdiagnosed multicystic dysplastic kidney. Occasionally normal echolucent renal pyramids are mistaken for dilated calyces either in utero or in the neonatal period. Any infant born with antenatally diagnosed hydronephrosis should have a complete postnatal evaluation, which is described in detail later in this chapter. There still is controversy regarding the indications and timing of UPJ obstruction when it is found through prenatally detected hydronephrosis. This is due to the difficulty in differentiating transient physiologic hydronephrosis secondary to mild or transient UPJ obstruction from that which may persist well into childhood with resultant symptomatic UPJ obstruction, which later might cause renal damage. Antenatal intervention for rare cases of bilateral hydronephrosis is possible and occasionally indicated, but it is sometimes difficult to differentiate between bilateral UPJ obstruction and reflux, posterior urethral valves, prune-belly syndrome, or cloacal anomalies, which also might present with bilateral hydronephrosis. There is essentially never an indication for antenatal intervention in cases of unilateral hydronephrosis regardless of the severity of the UPJ obstruction. When not identified on prenatal ultrasound, the classic neonatal and pediatric presentation of UPJ obstruction includes flank pain that frequently is associated with nausea and vomiting, palpable flank mass, renal stone, hematuria, and urinary tract infection or hypertension. Occasionally patients are identified incidentally on imaging studies, such as cardiac catheterization, bone scan, or a computed tomography scan for the other symptoms.

PATHOPHYSIOLOGY

In the era of commonly detected prenatal hydronephrosis, decisions and interpretation of diagnostic studies require an understanding of perinatal renal physiology, which has been termed *transitional nephrology*. In utero renal function is primarily through placental dialysis

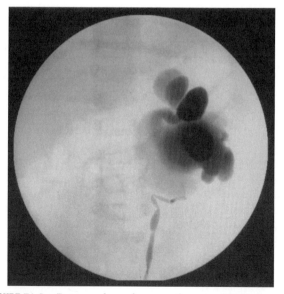

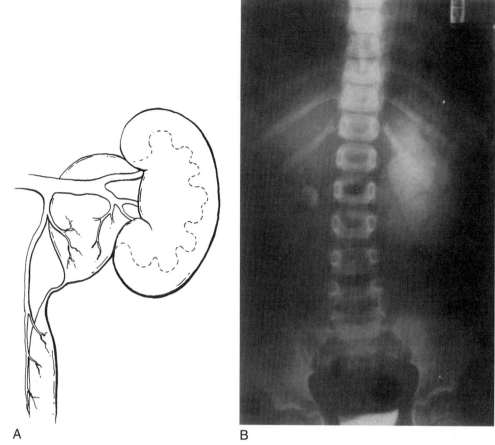

FIGURE 71-1 ▪ Anatomy of UPJ obstruction. **A,** Diagrammatic. **B,** Radiographic.

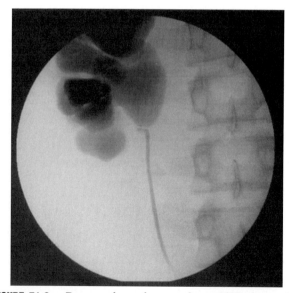

FIGURE 71-2 ▪ Retrograde pyelogram of neonatal UPJ obstruction. Note redundant and angulated ureter and dilated renal pelvis and calyces.

FIGURE 71-3 ▪ Retrograde pyelogram shows UPJ obstruction caused by lower pole crossing vessel. Note vascular impression of vessel at ureteropelvic junction with abrupt angulation of ureter.

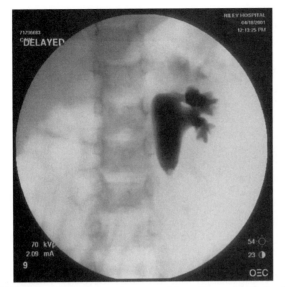

FIGURE 71-4 ■ UPJ obstruction caused by a fibroepithelial polyp causing filling defect at UPJ.

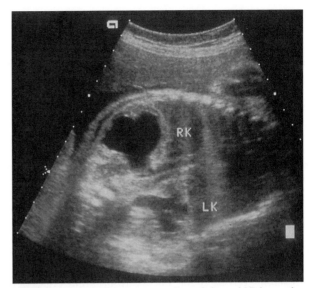

FIGURE 71-5 ■ Prenatal ultrasound shows bilateral hydronephrosis, more severe in right kidney.

despite the fact that the kidney develops early in pregnancy. The fetal kidney is easily visible by 12 to 14 weeks' gestation by ultrasound. Nephrogenesis occurs usually through the first 30 weeks of gestation, but glomerular filtration rate and vascular development of the kidney continue until approximately age 2. The fetal kidney has a fairly high rate of urine output, especially during the later part of gestation. This serves to unmask even mild resistance across the UPJ because the amount of urine overcomes the UPJ and results in dilation of the collecting system. At birth, there is an abrupt decrease in the amount of urine output, which can persist for several days postnatally but eventually stabilizes at approximately 1 to 2 mL/kg/hr. The abrupt change from a fairly high urine output state to a low urine output at birth explains the frequently noted marked improvement on renal ultrasound shortly after delivery despite fairly dramatic in utero hydronephrosis in some children. At birth, the function of water and solid excretion transfers from the maternal placenta and fetal kidney to the neonatal kidney, and this coincides with an increase in renal vascular resistance, decreased renal blood flow, and decreased tubular calyceal gradient. As the neonate matures, these indices normalize; however, early in neonatal development, these changes can have a dramatic impact on the results of imaging studies with either diuretic renal scans or intravenous pyelogram for the first 3 to 4 weeks of life. With in utero primary UPJ obstruction, there is generally a significant increase in the size of the renal pelvis, which dissipates the pressure generated within the collecting system and prevents rapid deterioration of the kidney. Because of this, surgical intervention can be delayed with unilateral UPJ obstruction to allow confirmation of the diagnosis during the first 3 or 4 months of life. Most surgeons currently would recommend earlier intervention with children who present with azotemia or massive hydronephrosis with a palpable hydronephrotic kidney or with children with significant reduced renal

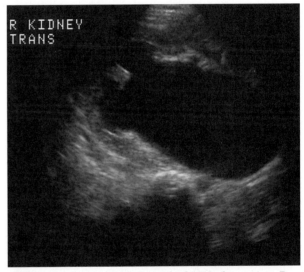

FIGURE 71-6 ■ Neonatal ultrasound of UPJ obstruction. Renal pelvis is markedly enlarged, and calyces are dilated.

function at presentation. In addition, patients with significant bilateral UPJ obstruction or high-grade UPJ obstruction in a solitary kidney also require close observation and intervention if there is no sign of improvement.

DIAGNOSIS

Renal ultrasound is an ideal test for diagnosing and serial evaluation of UPJ obstruction because of its noninvasive nature and ability to identify significant changes in the degree of hydronephrosis and calyceal dilation. Classic findings of UPJ obstruction on ultrasound include a central cystic structure that connects with peripheral cysts, which would represent the dilated calyces (Fig. 71-6). This can be differentiated from the multicystic dysplastic kidney that has disorganized and noncommunicating cysts and poorly defined and more echogenic renal parenchyma. As mentioned earlier, the sonolucent renal pyramids in the newborn and the neonatal kidney may be misinterpreted as hydronephrosis. The traditional standard for evaluating drainage of the kidney was an intravenous pyelogram, but this has been replaced mostly by diuretic nuclear scans. The well-tempered renogram is the best available test for determining differential function and drainage in the obstructed kidney. The most commonly used agents are technetium-99m diethylene-triamine penta-acetic acid (DTPA) or technetium-99m mercaptoacetyltriglycine (MAG III). Both agents allow comparison of the function of the obstructed kidney with the contralateral normal mate. In addition, both agents are excreted into the collecting system, and the degree of obstruction can be assessed by the delay in the drainage curves (Fig. 71-7). If there is evidence of renal pelvic stasis, furosemide (Lasix) is given to create a diuretic effect in an attempt to wash the tracer from the dilated renal pelvis. The half-time drainage time is calculated as the amount of time it takes for half of the tracer to disappear from the dilated collecting system. A half-time greater than 20 minutes is consistent with significant obstruction. Especially in the neonate, it is important that this be done when the child is well hydrated, that the furosemide

be administered after most of the tracer has cleared the renal parenchyma and is within the dilated renal pelvis, and that appropriate drainage is established with a bladder catheter. Because of the early phase of transitional nephrology in the neonate, it is important to obtain serial studies to evaluate for any changes in the function and the drainage of the affected kidney.

The massively dilated kidney with poor function sometimes is managed best with percutaneous drainage. A nephrostomy tube allows decompression to determine whether adequate residual function is present in the kidney. In addition, an antegrade perfusion study (Whitaker test) may provide useful data. This study is performed by placing two catheters within the dilated renal pelvis, one to measure changes in the pressure of the renal pelvis and the second to instill contrast material to delineate the anatomy further. The infusion rate depends on the patient size, and when steady pressure with flow through the UPJ is established, the pressure differential between the kidney and the bladder is calculated. Intrarenal pressure greater than 20 cm H_2O is considered obstructed. Some clinicians also believe that a retrograde pyelogram (usually performed at the time of corrective surgery) confirms the diagnosis of UPJ obstruction and helps to delineate the anatomy of the sometimes tortuous ureter (Fig. 71-8). Others have abandoned retrograde pyelography because of

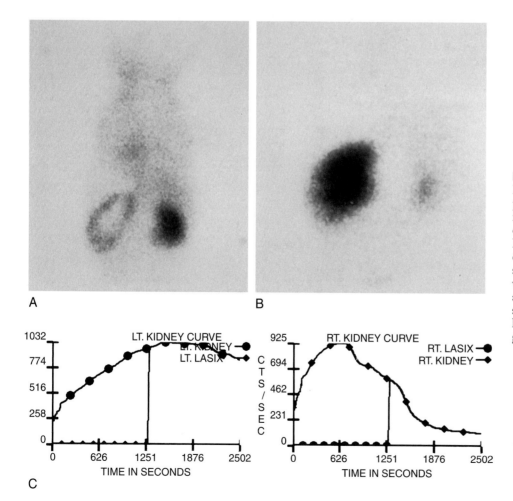

FIGURE 71-7 ■ Renal scan shows left UPJ obstruction. **A,** Early phase with large filling defect in central portion of left kidney owing to hydronephrosis. **B,** Late image shows poor drainage from left collecting system. **C,** Washout curves with normal drainage on right and poor response to furosemide (Lasix) on left (vertical line represents time furosemide given).

the risk of iatrogenic trauma at the ureterovesical junction, which may cause postoperative edema or stricture of the distal ureter.

MANAGEMENT

One management approach to antenatally diagnosed hydronephrosis is depicted in Figure 71-9. There still is controversy regarding timing and necessity for surgical intervention. Some surgeons favor intervening only in the face of significant reduction in renal function, whereas others recommend surgery in the neonatal period or as soon as significant signs of obstruction exist based on either delayed drainage on renal scan or significant hydronephrosis on ultrasound. The protocol outlined in Figure 71-9 favors an approach that allows selective surgical intervention. All patients who are born with the diagnosis of antenatal hydronephrosis undergo renal ultrasound 48 to 72 hours after delivery. Some patients with significant in utero hydronephrosis have normal ultrasound examinations postnatally because of the relatively dehydrated state, and these patients should be re-evaluated in 2 or 3 months with follow-up ultrasound before obstruction can be excluded. At birth, all patients are started on amoxicillin (one third therapeutic dose) for prophylaxis of urinary tract infection. All patients with significant antenatal hydronephrosis should undergo a voiding cystourethrogram as 30% have evidence of vesicoureteral reflux. If the initial ultrasound examination shows hydronephrosis, a diuretic renal scan is obtained. If UPJ obstruction is confirmed with evidence of significant impairment of renal function (differential function <40%), a neonatal pyeloplasty is performed. In addition, if patients have high-grade obstruction with a solitary kidney, bilateral significant UPJ obstruction, or massive hydronephrosis that might impair feeding or respiration, early pyeloplasty is considered. If the early renal scan

shows preservation of ipsilateral renal function, observation is elected. Repeat renal ultrasound and diuretic renal scan is performed in 6 to 12 weeks depending on the degree of hydronephrosis. Patients with continued stable ultrasound findings and differential function (>40%) can be observed safely; however, some data show that if improvement is not seen within 18 to 24 months, surgical intervention should be considered. During observation, if renal function declines or the degree of hydronephrosis worsens significantly, this also would be a relative indication for surgical intervention. In the younger child or adolescent, if symptoms such as flank pain, hematuria, or infection develop, surgery is indicated.

SURGICAL RECONSTRUCTION

Open surgical repair of UPJ obstruction in the child has a 95% to 98% success rate. Complications of surgery include urinary extravasation, pyelonephritis, recurrent UPJ obstruction, and, less commonly, cutaneous fistula. With the advancement of endoscopic and laparoscopic techniques in adults, these procedures have been used in older children. Most surgeons still would opt for open pyeloplasty in the younger child because the success rate is higher than with the minimally invasive techniques and only requires a 1- or 2-day hospital stay at most. In older children and adolescents, endoscopic and laparoscopic techniques have shown success rates in the range of 85% with the advantage of shorter hospital stays and faster return to normal activities. Percutaneous or endoscopic techniques have not been as successful in adolescents with

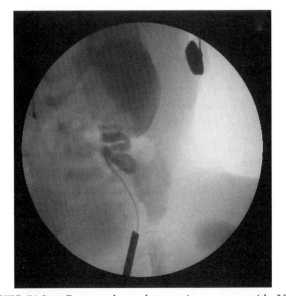

FIGURE 71-8 ■ Retrograde pyelogram in neonate with UPJ obstruction with tortuous ureter caused by accordion effect of dilated renal pelvis.

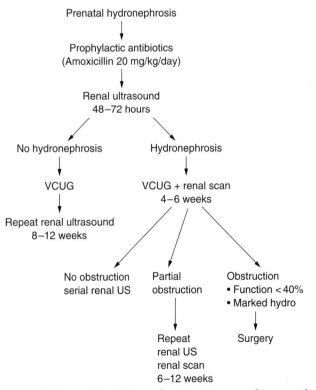

FIGURE 71-9 ■ Algorithm of management of prenatal hydronephrosis.

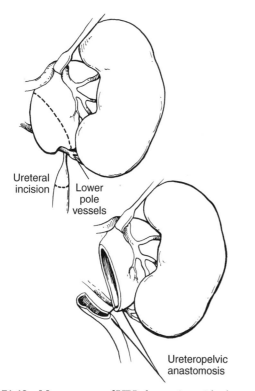

FIGURE 71-10 ■ Management of UPJ obstruction with obstructing lower pole vessels using dismembered pyeloplasty technique.

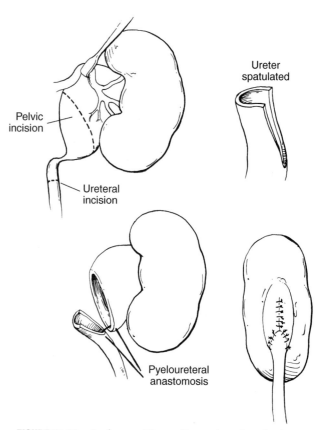

FIGURE 71-11 ■ Anderson-Hynes dismembered pyeloplasty.

extrinsic causes of obstruction (e.g., a lower pole crossing vessel), which accounts for three quarters of the patients presenting with symptoms of pain in later childhood. In these patients, open surgery and laparoscopy have a theoretical advantage in that they allow placement of the renal pelvis and ureter anterior to the aberrant lower pole vessel (Fig. 71-10).

A variety of incisions have been used for open pyeloplasty. The posterior lumbotomy is especially useful in infants and thin children, allowing direct access to the posterior renal pelvis. An extraperitoneal flank or subcostal incision also gives excellent exposure to the retroperitoneal space and allows improved exposure for more complex anatomy or for reoperative pyeloplasty. The retroperitoneal approach is preferred over a transabdominal or transperitoneal approach because there would be expected lower morbidity from adhesions, postoperative ileus, or urinary extravasation.

OPERATIVE TECHNIQUE

Many techniques have been described for open pyeloplasty. The main goals to be achieved are a widely patent anastomosis that allows for dependent drainage from the renal pelvis and a funnel-shaped UPJ, which would allow maximum drainage from the kidney. The Anderson-Hynes dismembered pyeloplasty is the most frequently used procedure because it allows excision of the abnormal segment of ureter and reduction of the dilated renal pelvis (Fig. 71-11). Important technical points include careful preservation of the ureteral blood supply with minimal mobilization of the more distal ureter, complete

excision of the dysplastic ureteral segment and UPJ, and excisional tapering of the redundant renal pelvis that allows dependent drainage of the ureter from the most inferior aspect of the pelvis. The anastomosis can be completed with either a fine interrupted or running absorbable suture.

The Foley Y-V pyeloplasty is an excellent choice when ureteral blood supply is tenuous, such as in reoperative pyeloplasty or for the occasional patient who requires simultaneous distal ureteral reconstruction. The ureter is never completely dismembered from the renal pelvis, and the obstruction is eliminated by creating a flap of renal pelvis that is mobilized down to the ureter (Fig. 71-12). The spiral flap or Culp-DeWeerd pyeloplasty is used less frequently but provides a good option when there is a long segment of abnormal ureter that needs to be replaced (Fig. 71-13).

An 80% to 85% success rate has been reported for endoscopic pyeloplasty using either an antegrade percutaneous technique or a retrograde technique. Because of instrumentation size, these approaches have been primarily used in adults and older children. Both approaches rely on a principle similar to the Davis intubated ureterotomy, in which a full-thickness ureteral incision is made, and a large stent is left across the incision with the intent that the ureter will heal to the size of the stent. This requires a full-thickness ureteral incision deep enough to see the peripelvic fat, and in cases of lower pole crossing vessels this occasionally can result in bleeding.

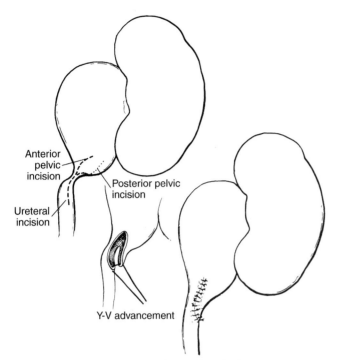

FIGURE 71-12 ▪ Foley Y-V pyeloplasty.

POSTOPERATIVE STENTING

Postoperative intubation is controversial for open pyeloplasty and essentially is left to the surgeon's preference. Multiple reports have documented excellent success with stentless pyeloplasty, especially in younger children. Most surgeons still prefer to leave a Penrose drain in case of urinary extravasation postoperatively. A Foley catheter also is used to provide bladder drainage for 1 or 2 days. There are several specific indications for intubation or stenting, as follows:

1. An inflamed or infected renal pelvis or when there has been a stone or preoperative nephrostomy tube in place
2. A poor-quality or extremely narrow ureter
3. In instances when transabdominal pyeloplasty is required and a risk of anastomotic leakage could result in urinary ascites
4. A long segment proximal stricture or distal ureteral pathology, such as simultaneous ureterovesical obstruction
5. A poorly functioning kidney, which would allow for confirmation of a patent anastomosis postoperatively (a nephrostomy tube would allow a postoperative nephrostogram to provide important information).
6. A solitary kidney or bilateral UPJ obstructions that are corrected simultaneously

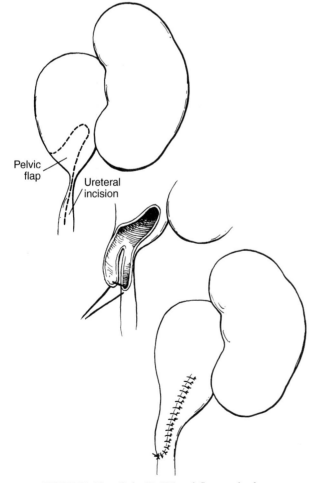

FIGURE 71-13 ▪ Culp-DeWeerd flap pyeloplasty.

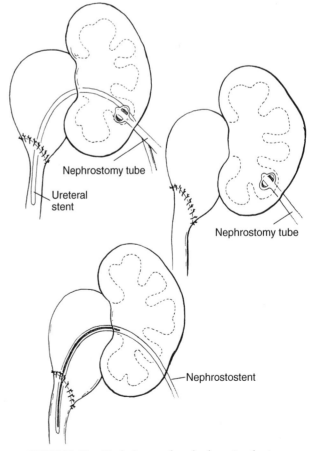

FIGURE 71-14 ▪ Techniques of pyeloplasty intubation.

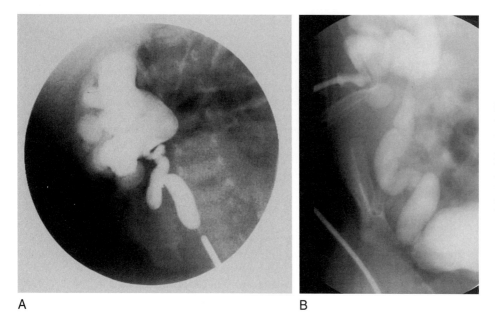

A

B

FIGURE 71-15 ■ Patient with UPJ and ureterovesical junction (UVJ) obstruction. **A,** Retrograde pyelogram before pyeloplasty shows narrowing at UPJ and UVJ. **B,** Postoperative nephrostogram allows pressure measurements to assess further significance of UVJ obstruction.

Figure 71-14 shows options for percutaneous drainage of the kidney. This can be accomplished with the combination of a nephrostomy tube with a separate ureteral stent across the anastomosis or with a special nephrostent that allows splinting of the anastomosis and proximal drainage. In younger children, care must be taken with placement of the ureteral stent so that the stent does not pass across the ureteral vesical junction, which has been associated with early and late stricture formation. Nephrostomy tube drainage alone also has been described with excellent results and still allows for 1 or 2 days of proximal drainage and the ability to perform a nephrostogram to prove ureteral patency. Nephrostomy tube drainage also allows for immediate drainage if any urinary extravasation is noted, which theoretically could prevent the rare case of anastomotic fibrosis and pyeloplasty failure.

In the older child, an indwelling double-J ureteral stent alone sometimes is used. The disadvantage to this type of stent is that a second anesthetic is required to remove the stent 4 to 6 weeks after pyeloplasty. This is particularly helpful, however, with re-operative cases.

SPECIAL PROBLEMS

UPJ obstruction sometimes is seen with high-grade vesicoureteral reflux. With high-grade reflux, when renal function is stable, the reflux is corrected first, and the UPJ obstruction sometimes resolves. With any suggestion of decreased renal function, a pyeloplasty is sometimes necessary as a first surgical procedure, and in these cases, meticulous attention is required to prevent devascularization of the distal ureteral blood supply. In cases in which pyeloplasty is performed in the face of persistent reflux, nephrostomy tube drainage and Foley catheter drainage sometimes are required to ensure effective decompression of the entire collecting system.

Occasionally, UPJ obstruction also exists with a distal dilated ureter and a ureterovesical junction obstruction.

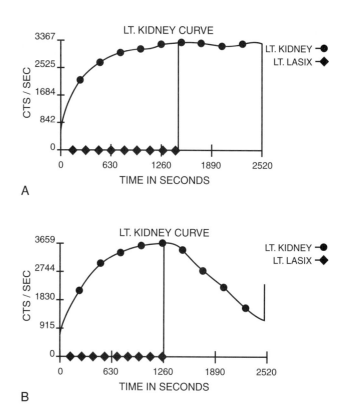

A

B

FIGURE 71-16 ■ Renal scan drainage curves. **A,** Preoperative scan shows no drainage from left kidney. **B,** Renal scan 6 weeks after surgery shows prompt response to furosemide with resolution of obstruction.

In this scenario, the UPJ obstruction usually is repaired first. It is sometimes helpful to leave a nephrostomy tube in place for a postoperative Whitaker test to delineate further the extent of obstruction in the distal ureter (Fig. 71-15).

UPJ obstruction caused by a lower pole crossing vessel usually is found in older children and results in intermittent obstruction during periods of diuresis. The usual presentation is with acute intermittent flank pain that may go undiagnosed for long periods. The important technical point for reconstruction of this anomaly is to transpose the pelvis and ureter anterior to the vessel, leaving the lower pole vessel intact (see Fig. 71-10). This is accomplished best by dismembered pyeloplasty. Simple division of the lower pole vessel frequently results in ischemic renal injury to the lower pole parenchyma and potentially damages the blood supply to the ureter.

In rare cases of failed pyeloplasty or when essentially no extrarenal pelvis is present, a ureterocalycostomy can be used to correct the obstruction. This procedure is facilitated by lower pole partial nephrectomy with removal of the parenchyma to allow a direct anastomosis of the ureter to the lower pole calyx. A stricture at the anastomotic site can occur when the lower pole parenchyma is not adequately removed.

Another atypical presentation of UPJ obstruction is in the case of duplicated collecting system in which the obstruction most commonly is seen in the lower pole. This can be reconstructed in the standard fashion, or if the lower pole ureter is small in diameter with a long stricture, a lower-to-upper pole pyeloureterostomy can be performed.

POSTOPERATIVE CARE

Most patients are discharged home within 1 to 3 days of surgery. After any postoperative drainage tubes are removed, follow-up studies are obtained in 6 to 12 weeks to document stable or improved drainage and function (Fig. 71-16). Follow-up renal ultrasound is obtained 6 to 12 months after surgery, and if the hydronephrosis is improved, follow-up studies are obtained only as needed.

SUGGESTED READINGS

Churchill BM, Feng WC: Ureteropelvic junction anomalies: Congenital UPJ problems in children. In Gearhart JP, Rink RC, Mouriquand PDE (eds): Pediatric Urology. Philadelphia, WB Saunders, 2001.

This chapter is an extensive review of the embryology, anatomy, biophysics, and management of the UPJ obstruction. The biophysical properties of the normal and abnormal UPJ are discussed at length. Evaluation, management, and surgical options are well delineated.

Streem SB (ed): Ureteropelvic Junction Obstruction. Urol Clin North Am 25(2), 1998.

This issue provides an in-depth review of the pathophysiology and management of UPJ obstruction in adults and children. Seven articles by multiple authors specifically cover UPJ obstruction in childhood.

Other Problems of the Upper Urinary Tract

The key to understanding pelviureteral anomalies is an understanding of the embryology of the ureter. Figure 72-1 provides a schematic representation of the ureteral bud theory. At about 4 weeks' gestation, the ureteral bud develops as an outpouching of the mesonephric duct. The ureteral bud then lengthens and extends to the nephrogenic ridge, where it induces the development of the metanephros. As the bladder develops, the proximal portion of the mesonephric duct, called the *common excretory duct*, is incorporated into the portion of the cloaca destined to become the urogenital sinus. The ureter is given off by the mesonephric duct in this process to join the bladder at the trigone. The wolffian duct is given off further distally to terminate into the proximal (prostatic) urethra. Wolffian duct derivatives include the ejaculatory ducts, the seminal vesicles, the vas deferens, and the epididymis.

Figure 72-2 outlines the developmental anatomy pertinent to ureteral ectopia. If the ureteral bud develops too cranially on the mesonephric duct, an ectopic ureter develops. Most commonly, ectopic ureters are found to

insert distally on the trigone; however, they may insert more distally into the bladder neck, urethra, or a wolffian duct derivative in boys. If the ureter inserts into a wolffian duct derivative or into the zone of continence within the bladder neck, the upper urinary tract is obstructed and hydronephrotic.

Figure 72-3 depicts the embryology pertinent to ureteral duplication. Here two ureteral buds develop independently off one mesonephric duct. These independently reach the nephrogenic ridge and induce renal development, resulting in a duplicated system. Each renal moiety drains separately into its respective ureter. If the ureteral buds occur in near-normal position (see Fig. 72-1A), the ultimate ureteral insertions occur in a near-normal position on the bladder trigone (see Fig. 72-1C), and the risk of vesicoureteral reflux or obstruction is low. Because the distalmost ureteral bud (lower pole ureter) is incorporated into the bladder first, it assumes a cranial and lateral position in the urinary tract relative to its proximal counterpart, a principle called the *Weiger-Meyer law*.

If the ureteral buds develop either too far proximally or too far distally on the mesonephric duct (see Fig. 72-1B), their ultimate position is abnormal (see Fig. 72-1D). Here a too-distal ureteral bud results in a lateral and cranial ureteral insertion, which has a high risk of vesicoureteral reflux. The distal ureteral bud may insert ectopically and be obstructed.

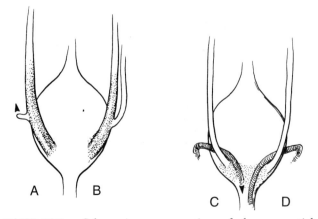

FIGURE 72-1 ■ Schematic representation of the sequential developmental anatomy of the ureter, occurring between approximately 4 and 12 weeks' gestation. At 4 weeks (**A**), 6 weeks (**B**), 8 weeks (**C**), and 12 weeks (**D**) of fetal development. The wolffian duct and the ureter originate from the mesonephric duct. The proximal portion of the mesonephric duct (stippled areas, **A** and **B**) is called the *common excretory duct.*

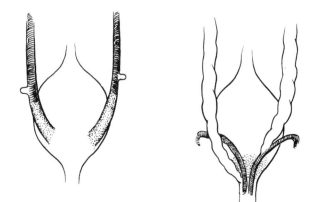

FIGURE 72-2 ■ Development of the ectopic ureter (see text).

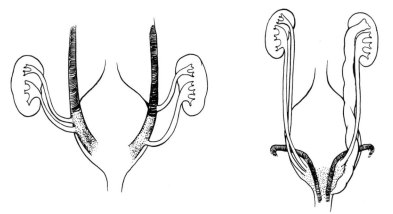

FIGURE 72-3 ■ Development of the duplicated ureter (see text).

Consequently, in duplicated systems, the more cephalad and lateral ureteral insertion generally drains the lower pole renal moiety and is associated most frequently with vesicoureteral reflux, and the distal and medial ureteral insertion drains the upper pole moiety and is associated most frequently with ectopia and obstruction.

Another important upper urinary tract anomaly is ureterocele. The precise embryologic etiology of this lesion is uncertain; however, a persistence of Chwalla's membrane, a primitive thin membrane located over the region of the developing ureteral bud, has been implicated. Failure of this membrane to perforate completely could explain ureteroceles with obstructing orifices. It may not explain fully, however, the development of ureteroceles in the absence of an obstructive orifice. Consequently, dilation of the distalmost portion of the ureteral bud leading to a subsequent ureterocele has been hypothesized.

The ureter is thought to go through a stage of solidification and recanalization between 37 and 40 days' gestation. This stage may have to do with the rapid elongation of the ureter relative to body size. The recanalization process begins in the mid ureter and extends cephalad and caudad, ending at the ureteropelvic junction and ureterovesical junction. Becauses these two sites are the last to recanalize, one may rationalize why these sites are the two most common for urinary tract obstruction.

The nature and the development of the ureteral bud may have a profound influence on the ultimate structure and function of the kidney. The failure of a ureteral bud to develop results in renal agenesis. An ectopic ureteral bud may result in renal injury from hydronephrosis or reflux as previously described. In addition, renal dysplasia has been implicated as an abnormality resulting from an ectopic ureteral bud because of this ectopic ureteral bud interfacing with the nephrogenic ridge in an abnormal position so that normal renal development cannot occur.

URETERAL DUPLICATION

Ureteral duplication occurs with an incidence of approximately 8 in 1000 children. Of cases, 40% are bilateral, and 60% to 70% occur in girls. Ureteral duplication is often an incidental finding. It may be noted on prenatal ultrasound as hydronephrosis, however, or postnatally as urinary tract infection or urinary incontinence. The latter generally implies ureteral ectopia. The clinical implications of ureteral duplication are that associated reflux (lower pole) may be less likely to resolve spontaneously and that obstruction (upper pole) is more likely to be associated with ureteral ectopia.

Ureteral duplication is classified as complete or incomplete. With incomplete duplication, the two ureters join proximal to a common insertion into the bladder. In complete forms of the condition, both ureters drain independently into the bladder. Ureteral ectopia and ureteroceles occur with high frequency in patients with duplicated upper urinary tracts.

ECTOPIC URETERS

Ectopic ureters occur with an incidence of approximately 1 in 2000 children. Of cases, 10% are bilateral, and approximately 85% occur in girls. Of ectopic ureters, 80% are associated with duplicated systems. The most common presentations of ectopic ureters are urinary tract infection, hydronephrosis, and incontinence. Urinary incontinence associated with ureteral ectopia has a characteristic pattern in which the child is continuously damp despite a normal voiding pattern and no associated symptoms.

The diagnosis of an ectopic ureter requires an understanding of the spectrum of ureteral termination as shown in Figure 72-4. In boys (Fig. 72-4A), the ectopic ureter most commonly inserts into the distal trigone, the bladder neck, or the proximal urethra and less commonly into a wolffian derivative, such as the seminal vesicle. In girls (Fig. 72-4B), ectopic ureteral insertion is most likely to be seen within the distal trigone, the bladder neck, the urethra, the vestibule, or the vagina. Ectopic ureteral insertion into the vestibule occurs in the posterolateral aspect of the periurethral tissues, representing the distalmost aspect of Gartner's duct, which shares a common wall with the developing vagina. Rarely an ectopic ureter is encountered more proximally within the uterus or inserting into the rectum.

Diagnosis

Diagnostic evaluation is based on a combination of upper urinary tract imaging by ultrasound, intravenous pyelogram (IVP) or isotope renography, a voiding cystourethrogram (VCUG), and cystoscopy. Figure 72-5 shows the typical radiographic appearance of an ectopic ureter associated with duplication. Characteristically a "drooping lily" picture is seen as shown in the left kidney of the IVP in Figure 72-5. The drooping lily appearance results from nonfunction of a hydronephrotic upper pole with downward and lateral displacement of the lower pole collecting system. A retrograde pyelogram (see Fig. 72-5) opacifies the upper pole system, explaining this mass effect. A typical drooping lily is not always seen if the upper duplicated system has significant function. A VCUG is helpful to rule out the presence of reflux into the nonectopic ureters, which may coexist with ureteral ectopia, but it also may show reflux into the ectopic ureteral segment.

Endoscopic evaluation begins with a careful examination of the periurethral tissues in girls followed by cystoscopic evaluation of the urethra and bladder employing 0-degree and 30-degree lenses. Occasionally, vaginoscopy with magnification reveals the insertion of an ectopic ureter. In boys, a similar evaluation is required, emphasizing the proximal urethra, bladder neck, and trigone. When an ectopic ureteral insertion is encountered, a retrograde catheter injection confirms the diagnosis and facilitates surgical planning.

Figure 72-6 shows the radiographic appearance of an ectopic ureter demonstrated by retrograde contrast injection in a boy. Here a prominent orifice was encountered in the left aspect of the proximal urethra, and its injection not only filled the ectopic ureter but also filled the seminal vesicles and vas deferens, suggesting ectopic ureteral insertion into the seminal vesicle. One should be suspicious of ureteral ectopia when evaluating a young boy presenting with recurrent epididymitis.

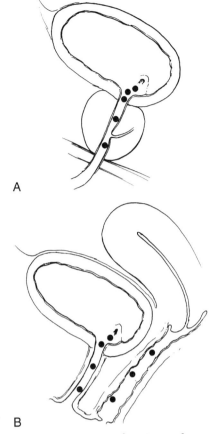

FIGURE 72-4 ■ Most common locations of ectopic ureteral termination in boys **(A)** and girls **(B)**.

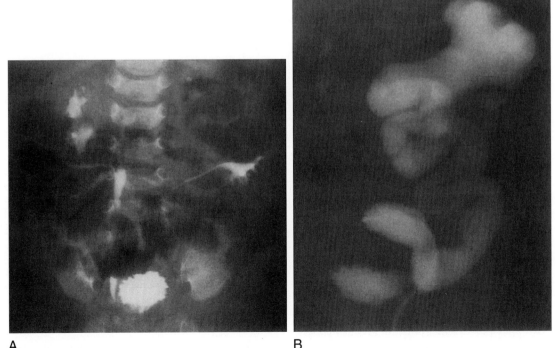

FIGURE 72-5 ■ Ureteral ectopia associated with duplication. **A,** Intravenous urogram shows a "drooping lily" appearance. **B,** Retrograde pyelogram filling the hydronephrotic upper pole system in the same patient.

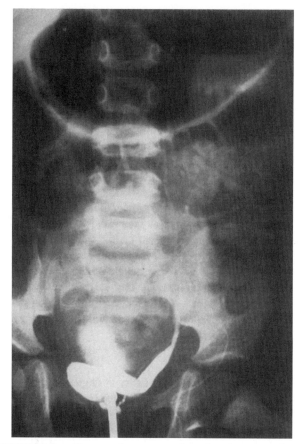

FIGURE 72-6 ▪ Retrograde contrast injection into prominent prostatic ureteral orifice in a boy. Contrast material fills an ectopic ureter and the vas deferens, indicating ectopic ureteral termination into the seminal vesicle.

Treatment

An uncommon but important entity is single ectopic ureter. When unilateral, this condition is treated simply by reimplantation or nephrectomy based on the function of the associated renal moiety. The problem of bilateral single ectopic ureters is more complicated. Characteristically the bladder is underdeveloped and has a small capacity because little urine is stored in it. In addition, the bladder neck may be poorly developed and associated with an incompetent sphincteric mechanism.

Unilateral single ectopic ureters are treated best by ureteral reimplantation when renal function allows. Bilateral single ectopic ureters require a bladder outlet reconstruction in addition to ureteral reimplantation. Bladder neck reconstruction is needed to increase bladder outlet resistance, and bladder augmentation may be needed to increase bladder capacity. Reconstruction of the ectopic ureter associated with duplication is more complex. A detailed assessment must be made of upper pole function. Most commonly the upper pole is found to have poor or no function, and an upper pole heminephroureterectomy is indicated. Figure 72-7 shows the technique of upper pole heminephroureterectomy for a duplicated system. Generally, nephrourecterectomy specimens yield small, scarred, and often dysplastic renal tissue.

The ureter is resected distally as far as possible but at least as low as the iliac vessels through the same flank incision as the upper pole nephrectomy. If the ureter is obstructed distally, the ureter is left open, and the site is drained. If the distal segment is refluxing, the ureteral segment is ligated. These steps help prevent loculated infection or urinary fistula formation in these two situations. The need for reoperation to remove the residual distal ureteral stump is less than 20%. When functioning upper pole renal tissue is shown by isotope renography or IVP, a ureteropyelostomy (Fig. 72-8) is indicated to preserve functioning upper pole tissue.

URETEROCELE

Ureteroceles occur with an incidence of approximately 1 in 4000 children. Of cases, 10% are bilateral, and more than 80% occur in girls. Approximately 80% occur in association with duplication. Ureteroceles have been classified in several different ways, but the most useful is the international ureterocele classification (Fig. 72-9), which divides them into intravesical or ectopic and single or duplicated.

Another more descriptive classification system, described by Stephens (Fig. 72-10), classifies ureteroceles as being stenotic (associated with an obstructed orifice), sphincteric (the ureterocele orifice occurring beyond the bladder neck), sphincterostenotic (the ureteral orifice being stenotic and occurring beyond the bladder neck), and the cecoureterocele—in which case a tongue of the ureterocele extends into the urethra, although the ureterocele orifice drains intravesically. At times, these latter types of ureterocele prolapse through the urethra. A final classification is based on renal function (Table 72-1).

Diagnosis

Ureteroceles most commonly present as hydronephrosis detected prenatally or found incidentally at the time of other diagnostic studies, as urinary tract infection, or rarely as a prolapsing mass. The diagnostic evaluation is best begun with ultrasound, which generally shows a highly characteristic cystic lesion located within the bladder (Fig. 72-11). This lesion may be found to be associated with duplication and often is associated with hydroureter and hydronephrosis. A VCUG most commonly shows a smooth filling defect along the base of the bladder (Fig. 72-12). Occasionally, retrograde eversion of a ureterocele into its associated ureter may give an appearance of a diverticulum rather than a filling defect, which is due to poor muscular backing behind the ureter. An isotope renal scan or IVP is useful to assess the function of the individual renal segments. Cystoscopic examination (Fig. 72-13) must be done with the child well hydrated so that the ureterocele is full but before the bladder is full to maximize the visualization of the cystic mass because progressive bladder filling may compress the ureterocele and make it less obvious to inspection.

Treatment

Multiple treatment options must be considered. Occasionally, endoscopic incision is indicated as shown in Figure 72-13. Endoscopic incision may represent

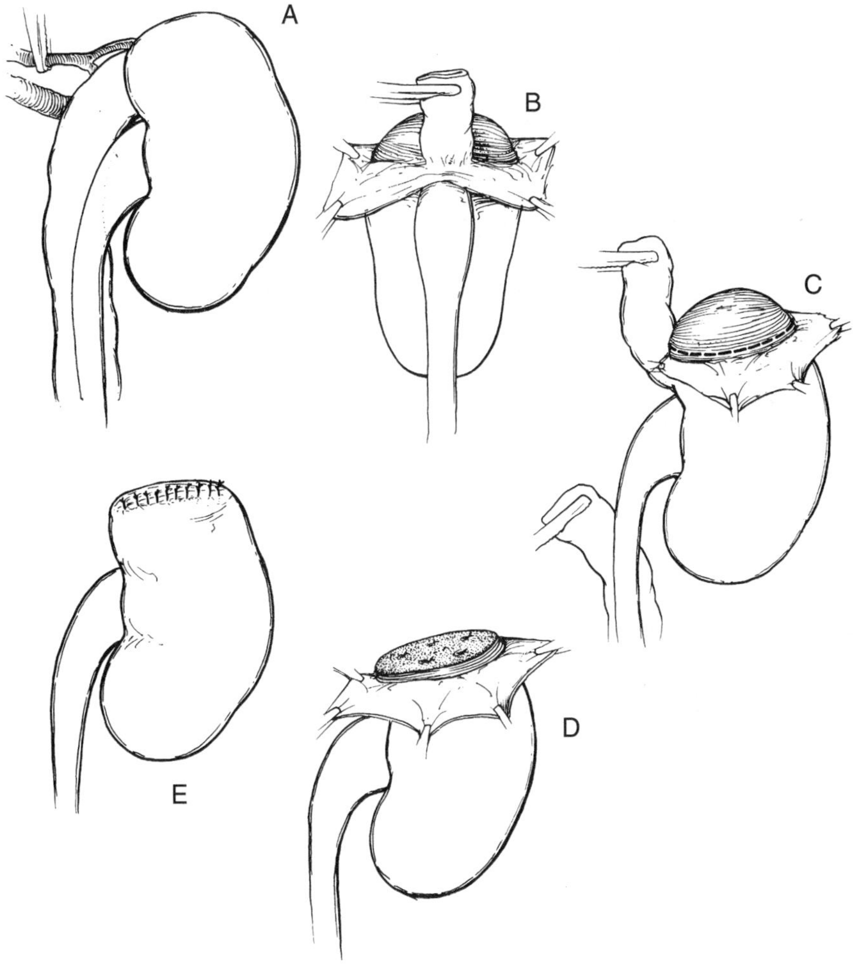

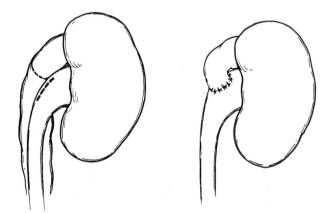

FIGURE 72-7 ■ Upper pole nephro-ureterectomy for complete duplication and upper pole ectopia. **A,** Blood supply to the lower pole is shown and preserved. Blood supply to the upper pole is identified and clamped with a microvascular clamp. If only the upper pole segment becomes cyanotic, these vessels are ligated. **B,** The renal capsule is incised over the upper pole and reflected inferiorly. The upper pole ureter is divided between clamps, and a plane is developed beneath the upper pole ureter by careful blunt dissection. **C,** Dissection is continued to an exit point on the convex surface of the kidney, and a Penrose drain is passed. **D,** The renal substance is divided using a Penrose drain as an end point marker, and vessels are suture ligated with absorbable suture material. **E,** The renal capsule is reapproximated over the remainder of the kidney.

definitive therapy in selected instances, usually intravesical ureteroceles. A low, horizontal endoscopic incision is created to allow full drainage of the ureterocele. Too high or too large an incision may create vesicoureteral reflux. In addition, endoscopic ureterocele incision may be employed diagnostically when indeterminate function of the corresponding renal moiety is encountered.

Improvement in function would favor preservation during reconstruction, and poor function would favor excision. Additionally, endoscopic incision may play a palliative role in children at high risk because of concurrent medical illness, allowing definitive reconstruction to be performed at a more optimal time.

The most frequently performed reconstructive procedure for ureterocele is an upper pole nephroureterectomy for ureterocele associated with obstruction. Occasionally a ureteropyelostomy is indicated and is preferred if its corresponding renal unit is functioning. These procedures are performed in analogous fashion to that described for the ectopic ureter.

Regardless of the upper pole procedure employed, ureteroceles must be drained. Most commonly, this consists of passing a catheter down the divided ureter through which the urterocele is aspirated dry. If no reflux has been shown by the preceding VCUG, the ureteral stump is left open and drained.

Excision of ureteroceles commonly is required and may be performed as a primary, concomitant, or secondary procedure. Primary excision of ureterocele refers to bladder reconstruction without an associated renal procedure. Although this procedure is satisfactory for obstructed ureteroceles associated with good renal function and no other problems, it is generally less

FIGURE 72-8 ■ Ureteropyelostomy for upper pole obstruction. The upper pole ureter is divided and sutured to the lower pole pyelotomy. The distal upper pole ureter is resected.

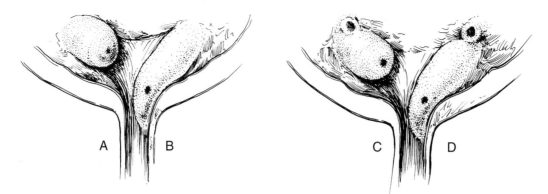

FIGURE 72-9 ■ International ureterocele classification. **A,** Single, intravesical. **B,** Single, ectopic. **C,** Duplicated, intravesical. **D,** Duplicated, ectopic.

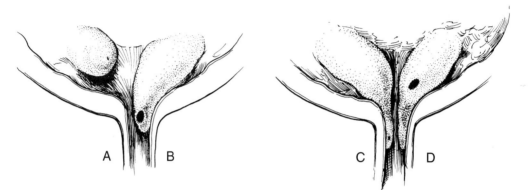

FIGURE 72-10 ■ Descriptive ureterocele classification (Stephens). **A,** Stenotic. **B,** Sphincteric. **C,** Sphincterostenotic. **D,** Cecoureterocele.

applicable in the case of ureteral duplication with upper pole hydroureter.

Figure 72-14 shows the surgical technique for ureterocele excision done as a concomitant procedure. This procedure is done through a second incision, generally a Pfannenstiel incision. This incision allows complete excision of the distal ureter associated with the ectopic ureterocele along with complete excision of the ureterocele itself. Occasionally, simple unroofing may be considered if the muscular backing of the ureterocele is sufficient to prevent subsequent development of a flaccid

bladder segment or a diverticulum, but this is usually unsatisfactory. Any portion of the ureterocele extending into the urethra also must be removed or unroofed. When associated with duplication, the remaining ureter is simply reimplanted into the bladder. In reconstructions of this sort, the blood supply to the remaining ureter draining the lower pole system is tenuous, and preservation is crucial to success. Excision of the entire hydronephrotic upper pole ureter may jeopardize the blood supply of the remaining delicate ureter of a duplicated system. This has been used as an argument against concomitant upper pole and

Grade	Frequency (%)	Definition	Significance
I	25	One renal unit in jeopardy	Only the upper pole parenchyma subtended by the ureterocele shows significant injury. Other renal units are normal, are minimally hydronephrotic, and have low-grade (I or II) reflux.
II	50	Entire ipsilateral kidney in jeopardy	As in grade I. In addition, the lower pole ipsilateral to the ureterocele is significantly hydronephrotic or associated with high-grade (III, IV, V) reflux. The contralateral kidney is normal or has mild hydronephrosis or reflux.
III	25	All renal units in jeopardy	As in grade II. In addition, the contralateral kidney is significantly hydronephrotic or associated with high-grade reflux.

TABLE 72-1 ■ **Functional Classification of Ectopic Ureteroceles**

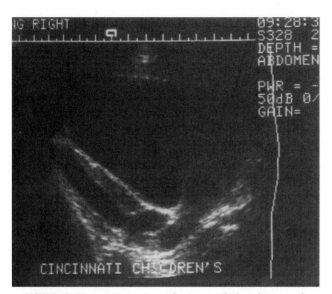

FIGURE 72-11 ■ Appearance of ureterocele by ultrasound.

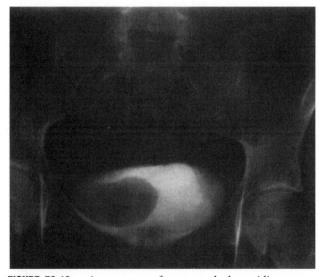

FIGURE 72-12 ■ Appearance of ureterocele by voiding cysto-urethrography.

ureterocele surgery, but careful dissection can obviate this problem. Ureterocele excision as previously described also may be performed as a secondary procedure because of urinary tract infection, voiding disturbance, persistent reflux, or obstruction of a remaining ureter.

Because approximately 90% of patients with grade I ureteroceles never require excision of the ureterocele when it has been defunctionalized by a preceding upper pole procedure, concomitant ureterocele excision is not undertaken. Because 60% to 70% of patients with grade II or III ureteroceles require ureterocele excision, however, it usually is best performed concomitantly. Exceptions include newborns and children who are severely ill in whom the risk of such an extensive procedure is too great. Additionally, simultaneous ectopic ureterocele excision is avoided when concern for the blood supply of the remaining ureter exists.

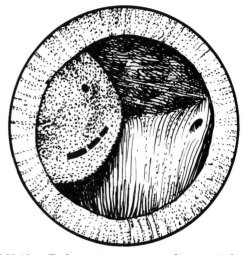

FIGURE 72-13 ■ Endoscopic appearance of intravesical ureterocele. Dashed line shows location of the endoscopic incision.

URETEROVESICAL JUNCTION OBSTRUCTION

Megaureter may be classified (Fig. 72-15) as primary obstructing, primary refluxing, secondary obstructing, secondary refluxing, nonobstructing and nonrefluxing, and refluxing and obstructing. Primary obstructing megaureters are generally associated with an adynamic distal ureteral segment or less commonly may be associated with ureteral valves or a true atretic segment. Primary refluxing megaureters are caused by congenitally incompetent ureterovesical junctions. Secondary obstructing ureters may be associated with posterior urethral valves, neurovesical dysfunction, tumor, inflammation, or consequent to surgical procedures. The nonobstructing, nonrefluxing megaureter requires precise functional diagnostic evaluation because these do not require surgical intervention. The nonobstructing, nonrefluxing megaureter may be either primary (idiopathic or prune-belly) or secondary. Secondary nonobstructing, nonrefluxing ureters are associated most commonly with massive polyuria, severe infection, or previous surgical procedures.

Diagnosis

The patient with megaureter most commonly presents with urinary tract infection, pain, nausea, vomiting, or hypertension. In addition, a newborn may present with prenatal hydronephrosis. Renal ultrasound usually shows hydroureteronephrosis. A VCUG is useful to establish the presence or absence of vesicoureteral reflux or primary bladder pathology. An IVP or antegrade pyelogram as shown in Figure 72-16 usually is diagnostic. Isotope renography allows measurement of renal function and, when associated with diuretic administration, may give functional data supporting the presence or absence of obstruction.

Treatment

Obstructing megaureters are repaired when they present with symptoms such as infection, pain, hypertension, hematuria, stones, or progressive hydronephrosis or when there is a demonstrable reduction in ipsilateral renal

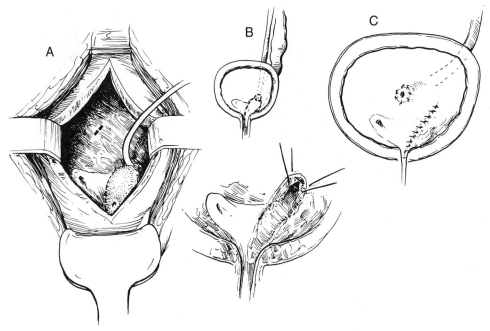

FIGURE 72-14 ■ Technique for excision of the ectopic ureterocele. **A,** Lower pole ureteral orifice is intubated. **B,** Lower pole ureter is dissected from the bladder, and the ureterocele is excised. The detrusor is approximated. **C,** Completion of the bladder closure and reimplantation of the lower pole ureter.

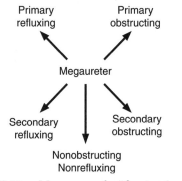

FIGURE 72-15 ■ Megaureter classification (see text).

function as measured by nuclear scan. Obstructing megaureters are managed by dividing them from their insertion into the bladder, excision of the obstructing segment, and ureteral reimplantation. The principle behind a successful ureteral reimplantation is use of a 5:1 ureteral tunnel-to-ureteral diameter ratio and meticulous preservation of ureteral blood supply. These principles may be achieved by the use of tapering or tailoring techniques and the use of a long ureteral tunnel. Excisional tapering generally is preferred over imbrication, and gentle tapering into a long tunnel is preferred over radical tapering techniques. The most frequent complications after megaureter reimplantation are reflux from an insufficient tunnel length and obstruction from excessive tapering or ischemic contracture.

The treatment of the refluxing megaureter is described in Chapter 73. Treatment of the nonrefluxing megaureter may be nonoperative when obstruction is not present.

The patient is followed by serial ultrasound examinations and measurement of differential renal function.

RETROCAVAL URETER

Retrocaval ureter is a rare congenital anomaly based on persistence of the primitive subcardinal veins anterior to the ureter. This lesion is often asymptomatic and nonobstructive, and no surgical intervention is required. When obstruction is encountered, the best approach is ureteral division and reanastomosis, anterior to the vena cava, in the fashion of an Anderson-Hynes dismembered pyeloplasty.

UROLITHIASIS

Urolithiasis is a relatively common childhood problem characterized by pain, hematuria, urinary tract infection, and occasionally azotemia. Urolithiasis or nephrocalcinosis occasionally is asymptomatic. Newborns with stones are usually premature infants who have been treated intensively with furosemide. Urolithiasis in newborns otherwise is caused by renal tubular acidosis, Bartter's syndrome, or other hypercalciuric states. Urolithiasis in older children is most commonly from infection or associated congenital anomalies but is commonly the result of metabolic abnormalities.

Urinary stones are best classified according to their radiographic appearance. Radiopaque stones usually contain calcium in the form of calcium oxalate, calcium phosphate, or struvite calculi. Cystine stones also may be mildly radiopaque. Radiolucent stones usually are composed of uric acid.

Nephrocalcinosis is an important entity that must be distinguished from urolithiasis, but the two problems

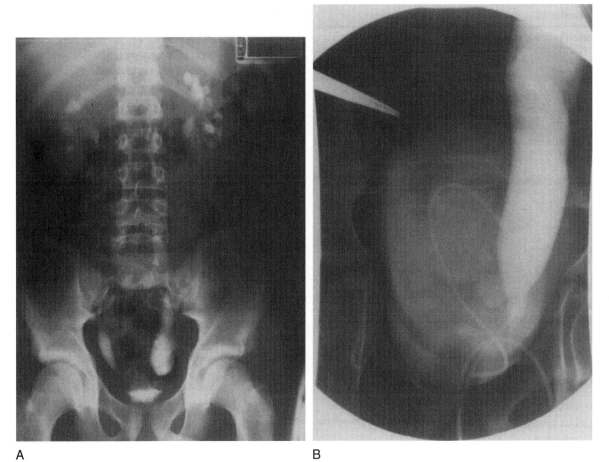

FIGURE 72-16 ■ Appearance of primary obstructed megaureter. **A,** Intravenous urogram. **B,** Antegrade pyelogram.

may coexist. The most common nonmetabolic causes of nephrocalcinosis include cystic renal disease, such as medullary sponge kidney; infectious disease, such as tuberculosis or xanthogranulomatous pyelonephritis; and renal tumors. Vascular abnormalities causing infarction, such as renal vein thrombosis, arteriovenous malformations, and papillary necrosis, may cause stones. Metabolic causes of urolithiasis predominate. Patients presenting with papillary necrosis must be evaluated for sickle cell disease, diabetes mellitus, and drug abuse. The metabolic causes of urinary stone disease are numerous and are listed in Table 72-2. Stone analysis may be helpful in establishing a diagnosis. Routine studies should include urinalysis and culture and levels for urine calcium and creatinine. Urine phosphate, cystine, oxalate, uric acid, citrate, serum calcium, phosphate, uric acid, and parathormone are useful on a selective basis.

Diagnosis

Radiographic evaluation begins with an abdominal film. IVP or computed tomography without contrast is particularly beneficial for the diagnosis of radiolucent stones at the time of acute presentation, and it can show the level of obstruction. Ultrasound is often helpful with radiolucent stones and to assess for hydronephrosis. Noncontrast computed tomography is useful preoperatively for the assessment of calculi either during an acute episode or in planning renal surgery.

Treatment

Although open removal of stones has been standard, advances in ureteroscopy, percutaneous renal lithotripsy, and extracorporeal shock-wave lithotripsy often have obviated the need for open surgery. Patients who have stones require careful follow-up. This includes dietary and hydration instructions. Sequential imaging, usually in the form of plain abdominal radiographs or renal ultrasound, is necessary. In some patients, specific medical therapy proves beneficial. Most commonly, this therapy takes the form of thiazide diuretics for urolithiasis associated with certain types of hypercalciuria. In particular, newborns with furosemide-induced urolithiasis may benefit from switching to a thiazide diuretic.

SHORT URETER

Urinary reconstruction, especially undiversion, frequently requires compensation for short ureteral length. The principles in reconstruction include generous exposure via midline incision, preservation of blood supply, tension-free anastomosis, antirefluxing anastomosis, and avoidance of use of bowel segments when possible.

Technical alternatives include renal, ureteral, and bladder procedures. In some patients, extensive renal mobilization is beneficial. Complete ureteral mobilization should be accomplished with preservation of all

TABLE 72-2 ■ Etiology of Urinary Stone Disease

Metabolic Abnormality	Stone Types
Hypercalciuria	Calcium oxalate
Absorptive	Calcium phosphate
Renal	
Hyperparathyroidism	
Immobilization	
Other	
Hyperoxaluria	Calcium oxalate
Enteric (Crohn's disease, short-bowel syndrome)	
Primary	
Dietary	
Hyperuricosuria	Calcium oxalate
	Uric acid
Hypocitraturia	Calcium oxalate
Chronic diarrhea	
Renal tubular acidosis	
Idiopathic	
Hypermagnesuria	Calcium oxalate
Cystinuria	Cystine
Complex metabolic	Calcium oxalate
Renal tubular acidosis	Calcium phosphate
Bartter's syndrome	
Low urinary volume	Exacerbates all
Infection (urease)	Struvite
Drug induced	
Furosemide	Calcium oxalate
Acetazolamide	Calcium phosphate
Vitamin C	
Vitamin D	
Calcium supplements	
Theophylline	
Calcium channel blockers	
Antacids	
Uricosuric agents	Uric acid

periureteral fibrovascular tissue, including the gonadal vessels. Rarely, autotransplantation to the common iliac vessels may be employed. Another option is transuretero-ureterostomy, in which the short ureter is passed across the midline, spatulated, and anastomosed end-to-side to the recipient ureter.

Bowel interposition with ileum or appendix may provide significant length, but an antirefluxing anastomosis into the bladder generally requires extensive tapering, and significant long-term complications are encountered. Most often, the short ureter is managed by bladder procedures, such as the psoas hitch or the Boari flap. The psoas hitch procedure involves mobilization of the bladder toward the short ureter and fixation to the psoas muscle so that a tension-free tunneled ureteroneocystostomy can be performed. Injury to the genitofemoral nerve must be avoided. More significant ureteral defects may be approached with the use of a Boari flap. In this procedure, a broad-based bladder flap is fashioned toward the ureter to be reconstructed. A tunneled anastomosis is performed into the apex of the Boari flap, and a psoas hitch allows a tension-free anastomosis.

SUGGESTED READINGS

Caldamone AA: Clinical embryology of the urinary tract. In Weiss RA, George NJR, O'Reilly PH (eds): Comprehensive Urology. London, Mosby, 2001.

This chapter focuses on embryology of disorders of the lower urinary tract and the related clinical implications.

Cohen TD, Ehreth J, King LR, et al: Pediatric urolithrosis: Medial and surgical management. Urology 47:292, 1996.

This article provides a complete description of the various aspects of stone disease in childhood.

Cooper C, Snyder HM III: Ureteral duplication: Ectopy, and ureteroceles. In Gearhart JP, Rink RC, Mouriquand PDE (eds): Pediatric Urology. Philadelphia, WB Saunders, 2001.

The authors describe current approaches to various anomalies of the lower urinary tract in childhood.

Husmann D, Strand B, Ewalt D, et al: Management of ectopic ureterocele associated with renal duplication: A comparison of partial nephrectomy and endoscopic decompression. J Urol 162:1406, 1999.

This article describes how to determine which patients with ectopic ureterocele may be treated by endoscopic unroofing.

in a routine setting. If there is a high possibility
atomic abnormalities will produce contamination
atheterization, suprapubic aspiration is advisable.
les include boys with phimosis because careful
preparation cannot be obtained and children with
ital sinus anomalies because preparation of peri-
tissues is not possible. The presence of a
ant degree of bacteriuria with catheterization
e considered as potentially significant. However,
uildren who have a clinically evident UTI have at
,000 colony-forming units (cfu)/mL.

hral catheterization of a child is the most accurate
technique of obtaining urine samples. Greater
0,000 cfu/mL of a single species give approxi-
a 95% level of accuracy in diagnosing a UTI.
than 10,000 cfu/mL makes the diagnosis likely as
pecially in certain clinical settings.

clean-catch voided specimen that yields greater
0,000 cfu/mL in a boy without phimosis is also a
inding. To achieve the same level of accuracy, two
ecimens yielding greater than 100,000 cfu/mL by
tch voiding must be collected in a girl. Young
frequently have a false-positive study. Children
than 18 months old have an accuracy of less than
h this technique, whereas children 3 to 12 years
approximately a 70% accuracy. The presence of
makes this technique unreliable.

itive urine sample obtained by the bag collection
e has only a 10% accuracy level. We consider a
nple obtained with this technique to be mean-
d reliable only if negative. It is ideal to have all
cultures confirmed by a catheterized specimen.
elevance of 100,000 cfu/mL is based on overnight
n in women. Children often do not achieve
t incubation even when uninfected and charac-
y do not achieve overnight incubation when
The risk of a false-negative urine culture in this
significant. Consequently a symptomatic patient
less than 100,000 cfu/mL often may require
t and display the same diagnostic implications as
present with a greater degree of bacteriuria.

e a urine culture cannot provide an immediate
therapy, urinalysis assumes an important role.
begins with a careful microscopic evaluation of
y sediment. The presence of white blood cells,
cells, and various types of casts may have impor-
cations. The presence of white blood cell casts
ignificant infection and implies pyelonephritis.
t, hematuria is a suggestive finding only. Pyuria
t common finding on microscopic examination
to a diagnosis of UTI. One must be aware,
hat false-positive findings of pyuria are encoun-
uently with vaginitis, urinary calculi, chemical
of the perineum, diaper rashes, gastroenteritis,
al immunization, and nonspecific febrile illness.
ly, false-negative findings are common; patients
rent UTIs may have a blunted pyuria response.
oscopic finding of bacteria in the urine is also
owever, this finding in the spun sediment may
tered in the absence of significant bacteriuria.
the finding of bacteria on an unspun urine is
closely to a significant degree of bacteriuria.

A dipstick evaluation commonly is used. Nitrate is normally present and is converted to nitrite in the presence
of most bacteria. The test is based on a colorimetric reaction between nitrite, sulfanilic acid, and α-naphthylamine,
which, if present, indicates a positive result. False-positive
findings are uncommon, whereas false-negative findings
are frequent. Because the conversion of nitrate to nitrite
requires incubation time in the bladder, frequency or
hydration may be a source of a false-negative analysis. In
addition, the child who is extremely ill with a poor oral
intake may have an inadequate dietary source of nitrates,
preventing the reaction from becoming positive.
Occasionally, specific bacteria fail to convert nitrate,
again resulting in a false-negative test.

Classification

To guide treatment, UTI is classified as upper tract
infection (pyelonephritis), lower tract infection, reinfection, and relapse. Pyelonephritis typically is indicated by
a characteristic clinical picture of fever, flank pain, and
flank tenderness. A finding of leukocytosis is helpful, as is
pyuria, particularly with the presence of white blood cell
casts. These clinical findings are not sufficiently accurate.
Renal isotope imaging (discussed later) has proved to be
a helpful indicator of acute pyelonephritis. Pyelonephritis,
especially that encountered in young children, may result
in permanent renal scarring that may be minimized by
the aggressive and prompt administration of parenteral
antibiotics.

Most children who experience recurrent UTIs have
reinfection as the source. This has been proved by careful epidemiologic study. Relapse, in which the recurrent
infection is due to the same bacterial strain, is much less
likely and implies ineffective therapy or a structural
abnormality of the urinary tract, such as is seen with
urolithiasis or urinary tract obstruction.

Pathophysiology

The pathophysiology of UTI is diagrammed in Figure
73-1. Most UTIs begin with colonic colonization by an
organism that is potentially pathogenic with respect to
the urinary tract. The perineum becomes colonized next,
followed by colonization of the urinary tract. When the
bladder is colonized, there are four common outcomes:
(1) The bacteria may be spontaneously cleared; (2) the
patient may develop asymptomatic bacteriuria; (3) clinical cystitis may develop; or (4) ascent into the upper tracts
may occur.

Colonization of the upper urinary tract is facilitated by
the presence of VUR. Some patients who do not show
reflux in the absence of infection develop reflux during
the course of acute infection. Some bacteria may alter the
peristalsis of the ureter, which may facilitate ascent of
bacteria in the absence of reflux or obstruction. The
renal parenchyma becomes infected through a process
termed *intrarenal reflux*. This term refers to the passage
of urine into the collecting ducts and may be either primary
or secondary. Primary intrarenal reflux is diagrammed in
Figure 73-7. Secondary intrarenal reflux may occur
because of distortion of the intrarenal architecture. In
either case, entry of bacteria into the renal parenchyma

Urinary Tract Infection and Vesicoureteral Reflux

Urinary tract infection (UTI) is the most common diagnosis referable to the childhood genitourinary tract. It commonly is associated with voiding dysfunction and anatomic abnormalities, such as vesicoureteral reflux (VUR). Consequently, these abnormalities must be considered collectively because any therapeutic regimen that fails to encompass the management of these disorders is at risk of failure.

URINARY TRACT INFECTION

The presenting symptoms of UTI are well understood in adults; however, these symptoms in children are often misunderstood. Table 73-1 outlines the presenting symptoms in a large series of children and shows the marked variance in symptoms as a function of age. Young children may present with nonspecific symptoms and findings that may be confused easily with gastrointestinal disease. Neonates often present with irritability, temperature instability, lethargy, anorexia, emesis, jaundice, or

failure to thrive. A urinalysis a
tant parts of the evaluation of

Toddlers also may prese
Screaming and irritability are
and vomiting. More specific fi
or cloudy urine, hematuria, an

Older children tend to p
symptoms that are similar
Frequency, urgency, urgency
are prominent. Fever is an in

Specimen Collection

The analysis of a properly c
cornerstone of diagnosis of
error in collection and diag
inappropriate to treat a syn
otics or make the diagnosis (
by urine culture. This appr
a delay in making the corr
necessitate an unwarranted

Inadequately collected c
mens are common, and misi
frequently. Urine collection
ety of techniques, includir
urethral catheterization,
Careful cleansing and appr
vent false-positive results.
be performed only in a chil
has not had previous abdor
imen has been obtained, it
immediately to minimize
The common practice of h
allowing the parent to bri
cian's office creates th
diagnostic error.

Accuracy

Accuracy of urine culture:
collection, the patient's
Hydration and frequenc
accuracy of the test bec;
alter colony counts.

The accuracy of a su
mately 99%. Because
catheterization is also hi

TABLE 73-1 ■ Presenting Symptoms in 200 Children with Urinary Tract Infection				
Symptom	0-1 mo	1-24 mo	2-5 yr	5-12 yr
Failure to thrive, poor feeding	53%	36%	7%	0
Jaundice	44%	0	0	0
Screaming, irritability	0	13%	7%	0
Foul-smelling, cloudy urine	0	9%	13%	0
Diarrhea	18%	16%	0	0
Vomiting	24%	29%	16%	3%
Fever	11%	38%	57%	50%
Convulsions	2%	7%	9%	5%
Hematuria	0	7%	16%	8%
Frequency, dysuria	0	4%	34%	41%
Enuresis	0	0	27%	29%
Abdominal pain	0	0	23%	0
Loin pain	0	0	0	0
Male-to-female ratio	3:1		1:10	1:10

From Smellie J, et al: Br Med J 2:1222, 1964.

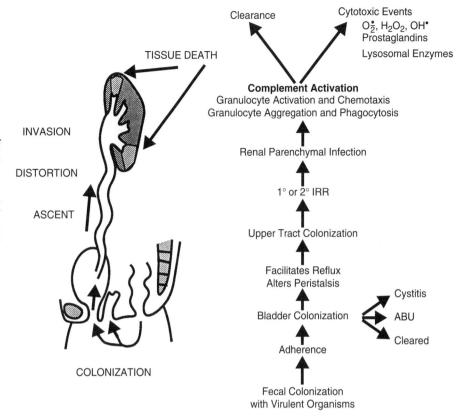

FIGURE 73-1 ■ The pathogenesis of destructive infection. The process is facilitated by, but does not require, defects in the host protective factors, outlined in Figure 73-2. (From Sheldon CA, Wacksman J: Urinary tract infection and vesicoureteral reflux. In Ashcraft KW, Holder TM [eds]: Pediatric Surgery. Philadelphia, WB Saunders, 1993.)

may induce a cascade of events, including complement activation, granulocyte activation, chemotaxis, granulocyte aggregation, and phagocytosis. Although these events may result in clearance of the infection, cytotoxic events may result in permanent destruction of renal parenchyma through the release of free radicals. The degree of destruction depends on the virulence of the organism, the resistance of the host, and the promptness and accuracy of therapeutic intervention.

In general, 10% to 15% of children who experience clinically significant infections go on to develop renal scarring, but most children with renal scarring remain asymptomatic if progression is prevented. Approximately 11% of childhood hypertension is due to renal parenchymal damage from scarring, however. This is more common if scarring is bilateral. In addition, renal insufficiency ultimately may occur. Reflux pyelonephritis continues to be an important cause of end-stage renal disease in children.

Virulence Factors

Several virulence factors have been identified in bacteria that potentiate their ability to cause UTI and promote injury. *P. fimbriae* facilitates the adherence of bacteria to biologic surfaces. K antigens are believed to facilitate adherence but also may help protect the organism from the host immune response. O antigens, which are believed to represent lipopolysaccharides, are an important source of the systemic reactions seen with bacterial infections, such as fever and shock. H antigens, which are associated with flagellae, may relate to bacterial locomotion. Hemolysins may potentiate tissue damage and facilitate

local bacterial growth. Urease, which results in the conversion of urea to ammonium, alkalinizes the urine and facilitates stone formation, which greatly potentiates infection. More invasive infection tends to be associated with a greater incidence of bacterial virulence factors.

Host Defense Factors

Host factors may be protective or may potentiate the development of UTI, as shown in Figure 73-2. Perineal resistance is an important first-line defense. Additionally, uroepithelial cells from healthy individuals have been shown to have antimicrobial activity. These children actively suppress bacterial growth. In contrast, uroepithelial cells from patients with chronic asymptomatic bacteriuria do not show such activity. Maturation of resistance seems to occur in some children as they get older. The presence of chronic infection may reduce the normal resistance of the urinary tract to infection. Many infection-free months are required before resistance returns. Additional important protective mechanisms are the unidirectional flow of urine from the kidneys to the bladder and the unobstructed transport of urine at all levels.

The potentiating host factors also are shown in Figure 73-2. Periurethral colonization is extremely important. Perineal soilage from the presence of a diaper or encopresis facilitates the development of bacteriuria. In addition, perineal inflammation from diaper rashes or from chemical irritants, such as bubble baths or harsh soaps, may be etiologic. Phimosis in boys and labial fusion in girls also may potentiate periurethral colonization.

High intravesical pressure has been implicated in the development of UTI, and the presence of urolithiasis is a

HOST FACTORS vs. URINARY INFECTION

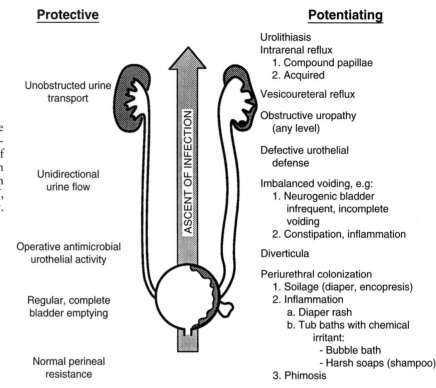

FIGURE 73-2 ■ Host factors that protect the urinary tract from infection and abnormalities that potentiate the establishment of invasive bacterial infection. (From Sheldon CA, Wacksman J: Urinary tract infection and vesicoureteral reflux. In Ashcraft KW, Holder TM [eds]: Pediatric Surgery. Philadelphia, WB Saunders, 1993.)

Protective

Unobstructed urine transport

Unidirectional urine flow

Operative antimicrobial urothelial activity

Regular, complete bladder emptying

Normal perineal resistance

Potentiating

Urolithiasis
Intrarenal reflux
   1. Compound papillae
   2. Acquired

Vesicoureteral reflux

Obstructive uropathy (any level)

Defective urothelial defense

Imbalanced voiding, e.g:
   1. Neurogenic bladder infrequent, incomplete voiding
   2. Constipation, inflammation

Diverticula

Periurethral colonization
   1. Soilage (diaper, encopresis)
   2. Inflammation
     a. Diaper rash
     b. Tub baths with chemical irritant:
       - Bubble bath
       - Harsh soaps (shampoo)
   3. Phimosis

ASCENT OF INFECTION

well-documented potentiating factor. Urolithiasis acts as a foreign body and may entrap bacteria within its matrix, making eradication of bacteriuria difficult.

One of the most important potentiating factors is the presence of VUR. This allows the bacteria access to the upper urinary tracts and results in incomplete voiding. The latter occurs owing to a temporary redistribution of urine into the upper tracts that immediately re-enters the bladder on completion of voiding. As previously noted, either primary or secondary intrarenal reflux is another important potentiating mechanism.

Evaluation

Careful investigation of the child with a UTI is crucial and requires a careful history, physical examination, and selective application of radiographic imaging studies. The number of preceding UTIs and their frequency and associated symptoms (especially fever) are important. Although irritative voiding symptoms are common with infection, the presence of irritative or obstructive voiding symptoms during times when the child is not infected may have important diagnostic implications. Infections associated with instrumentation may have much less significance. Asymptomatic bacteriuria in children on intermittent catheterization who do not have VUR is usually not significant and generally does not require treatment. A history of bowel symptoms is important, particularly the presence of constipation and encopresis. A careful review of perineal hygiene is pertinent, especially the use of bubble baths or submerging baths with harsh soaps.

Lower extremity symptoms, such as pain, weakness, and incoordination, should be analyzed. The combination of lower extremity symptoms, bowel symptoms, and urinary symptoms may suggest a primary neurologic abnormality.

Patients require a careful physical examination with attention to abdominal palpation to detect a mass or distended bladder. The external genitalia are examined, looking for evidence of diaper rash and fecal soiling. In boys, lesions such as phimosis and meatal stenosis may help direct subsequent therapy. Girls should be examined for vaginitis and labial fusion. The child also must be examined in the prone position to assess fully the sacrum and overlying soft tissue structures. The presence of a cutaneous pit (other than pilonidal), lipoma, hair patch, or patch of pigmetation may indicate an underlying spinal anomaly that may be associated with tethering of the spinal cord. The bony sacrum is palpated carefully to detect abnormalities or absence of the sacrum.

There is no controversy that all children younger than 5 years of age or a child with a febrile UTI should be evaluated with ultrasound and a voiding cystourethrogram (VCUG). The evaluation of children older than 5 years of age with an afebrile UTI is controversial. It is usually well accepted, however, that a simple episode of cystitis in a girls older than 5 years of age could be evaluated with an ultrasound alone. Multiple afebrile UTIs require a VCUG, however. Some use the same criteria for boys, whereas others evaluate all boys with a febrile or afebrile UTI with an ultrasound and VCUG. In older children presenting with their first UTI, especially children beyond toilet training years, it is easier to distinguish between upper and lower tract infections, and the incidence of structural abnormalities discovered by radiographic evaluation is significantly lower. The question frequently is asked regarding the necessity of the VCUG if the ultrasound is normal. It has been shown that at least two thirds of patients with reflux have a normal ultrasound. A renal ultrasound is the best screening modality for the upper tracts. This study may reveal hydronephrosis, evidence of renal scarring, or urolithiasis and may be helpful in assessing renal growth. The ureters and bladder should be evaluated. The thickness of the bladder and the presence of ureteroceles, diverticuli, calculi, and foreign bodies can be assessed. A postvoid residual should be estimated if possible.

The other pertinent radiographic evaluation for a child presenting with UTI is a VCUG. The upper tracts are imaged as the bladder is filled via an indwelling catheter, and reflux of contrast material into the ureters or kidney is noted. Care must be taken to use a small catheter, contrast material warmed to body temperature, and a low infusion pressure to prevent false-positive examinations. These studies may be performed using a radioisotope technique (Fig. 73-3) or a formal contrast technique (Fig. 73-4). The radioisotope technique is pertinent for girls in whom underlying neurovesical dysfunction is not suspected based on history and physical examination. It offers a lower radiation dose to the ovaries than does the standard VCUG. Boys require a contrast VCUG, however, to visualize the urethra. This study helps detect abnormalities such as urethral valves and urethral strictures. Girls who have symptoms or physical findings suggesting the possibility of a neurogenic bladder or other bladder abnormality, such as a ureterocele or diverticulum, require a contrast VCUG to detect anatomic abnormalities or evidence of elevated intravesical pressures, such as bladder trabeculation.

Some children benefit from the use of urodynamics. This is discussed in detail in Chapter 74. Urodynamics

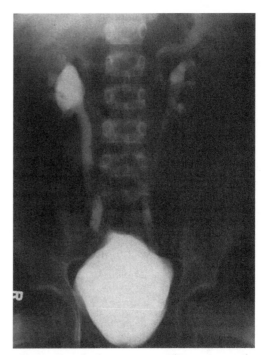

FIGURE 73-4 ■ Standard contrast voiding cystourethrogram with bilateral reflux.

studies are most useful in children who have a significant voiding imbalance that fails to resolve after sterilization of the urinary tract. Lumbosacral spine films (anteroposterior and lateral views) should be performed whenever a sacral abnormality is suspected. Formal spinal imaging using magnetic resonance imaging or computed tomography should be considered if voiding dysfunction has been documented associated with either significant bowel symptoms or lower extremity symptoms.

Treatment

The treatment of UTI is based on the potential for renal injury. The presence of acute pyelonephritis is an indication for admission and parenteral antibiotic therapy if the child is very young, toxic, or unable to tolerate oral antibiotics. The choice of antibiotics is guided by urine culture and sensitivities when these become available. After sensitivities have been determined, an antibiotic is selected that has the least danger of side effects, is the most sensitive, and eventually can be used on an outpatient basis. Oral antibiotics are considered after the child is afebrile for 48 hours, if there is no evidence of bacteremia, and after therapy has been maintained for 10 to 14 days. Infants are extremely vulnerable to renal injury from pyelonephritis and must be treated aggressively. It is prudent to maintain young children on prophylactic antibiotics after a full therapeutic course for treatment of a UTI until the appropriate radiographic evaluation is obtained.

Acute cystitis is seen commonly in children. Although some physicians advocate a short course of therapy, others prefer a 7- to 10-day course of an appropriate antibiotic based on sensitivity testing. The associated dysuria and irritative voiding symptoms may be improved by hydration, phenazopyridine hydrochloride, and, in acute cases,

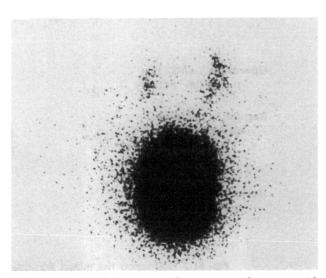

FIGURE 73-3 ■ Radioisotope voiding cystourethrogram with bilateral reflux.

allowing the child to void in a tub of warm water if urinary retention occurs.

Asymptomatic bacteriuria is a controversial subject, and a variety of different approaches are available. An attempt to sterilize the urine, especially in young children, is recommended. The exceptions are older girls who have normal anatomy and children who are on intermittent catheterization and have no VUR.

Recurrent UTI can be a difficult condition to treat. One must maximize perineal hygiene. In general, children who are sufficiently mature may benefit from showers only, in preference to tub baths. Constipation and encopresis must be treated. Adequate hydration is helpful, as is a carefully instructed voiding program. A voiding program is especially important for the infrequent voider, who is managed best with a timed voiding regimen.

Irritative voiding symptoms commonly coexist in children with recurrent UTIs. These children are managed initially only with antibiotics. When their urine has been sterilized, an anticholinergic agent may be administered. The parents must be informed that symptoms generally persist well beyond the attainment of sterile urine and that several months of sterile urine must be achieved before sufficient bladder healing has occurred. The parents should be told that this is to allow relief of irritative voiding symptoms without anticholineric agents and to allow the redevelopment of normal resistance against reinfection.

VESICOURETERAL REFLUX

VUR refers to the retrograde flow of urine from the bladder into the ureters. Most children who are found to have VUR are being evaluated for UTI. Occasionally, children with a history of hypertension, proteinuria, chronic renal insufficiency, prenatally detected hydronephrosis, or a sibling who refluxes undergo screening diagnostic tests and are found to have VUR.

TABLE 73-2 ▪ Secondary Reflux	
Anatomic	**Functional**
PUV	Voiding dysfunction
Ureterocele	Neuropathic bladder
Diverticulum	Myelodysplasia
Ectopic ureter	Sacral agenesis
PBS	
Bladder exstrophy	

International Classification

Figure 73-5 illustrates the international classification for VUR. Grade I VUR refers to partial filling of an undilated ureter. Grade II VUR involves total filling of an undilated upper tract. In grade III VUR, the calyces have become dilated; however, the fornices remain sharp. In grade IV VUR, the fornices have become blunted, and the degree of dilation has become more intense. Children who have massive hydronephrosis with tortuosity of the ureters are classified as grade V VUR.

Occasionally intrarenal reflux is shown radiographically, although this has no bearing on management. One should note whether the reflux occurs during the voiding phase or the filling phase. Primary VUR refers to a congenitally deficient ureterovesical junction, whereas secondary VUR refers to reflux occurring secondary to a primary bladder disease, such as neurogenic bladder or bladder outlet obstruction, or other fixed anatomic defects. Secondary reflux may be functional or anatomic (Table 73-2).

Pathophysiology

Several mechanisms may play a role in VUR, as depicted in Figure 73-6. A short ureteral tunnel diminishes the ability of the ureter to be compressed with bladder filling

GRADE OF REFLUX

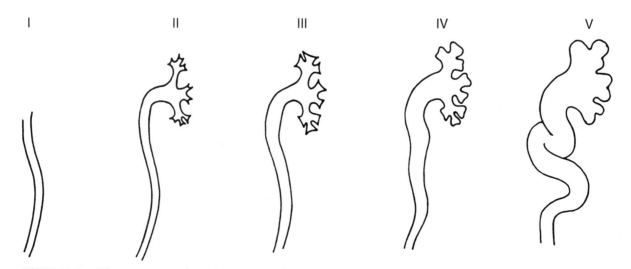

FIGURE 73-5 ▪ The international grading system for vesicoureteral reflux (see text). (From International Reflux Committee: Medical versus surgical treatment of primary vesicoureteral reflux. Pediatrics 67:396, 1987.)

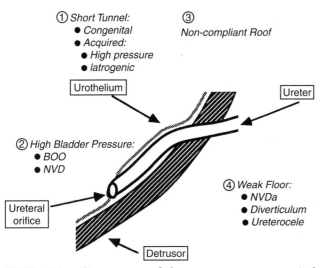

FIGURE 73-6 ■ Components of the competent ureterovesical junction. The abnormalities most often implicated in the cause of vesicoureteral reflux are outlined.

and consequently facilitates reflux. A short tunnel may be either congenital or acquired owing to high-pressure bladder dynamics or iatrogenic injury of the ureteral insertion. A high-pressure bladder may cause VUR even in the presence of an otherwise acceptable ureteral tunnel. A noncompliant roof of the tunnel may promote VUR and is seen in abnormalities such as acute infection and scarring from previous surgery. A weak floor of the ureteral tunnel also may diminish ureterovesical competence and may be seen with neurovesical dysfunction or paraureteral diverticula.

Figure 73-7 shows the concept of intrarenal reflux. Simple papillae receive an oblique insertion of the collecting ducts that prevents reflux. Compound papillae allow intrarenal reflux by the mechanism shown. The fact that compound papillae occur predominantly at the upper and lower poles of the kidneys explains why these regions are predisposed to pyelonephritic scarring. Intrarenal reflux also may be acquired. Chronic injury from hydronephrosis, elevated intravesical pressures, or infection may result in sufficient papillary distortion or compression to cause intrarenal reflux.

Incidence

Screening studies have shown an incidence of reflux in normal children of about 1%. In contrast, children with UTIs have an incidence of reflux ranging between 20% and 50% depending on age at presentation. Girls predominate; boys represent only 14% of children with reflux. Of importance is the familial nature of VUR. The risk of siblings having reflux is approximately 30%. Routine screening seems to be appropriate, especially in children younger than 2 years of age. Important associations with VUR include abnormalities such as bladder exstrophy and imperforate anus.

Evaluation

Radiographic techniques to detect and stage reflux are outlined in the section on UTI. The upper urinary tract must be evaluated. Renal ultrasound gives an excellent estimation of renal size; however, it is less reliable in detecting early scarring. Isotope renography (dimer captosuccinic acid or glucoheptonate) is excellent for detecting renal parenchymal injury as seen with acute pyelonephritis or chronic scarring.

Because high-pressure voiding dynamics have important implications in the cause and management of VUR, urodynamics are indicated in selected patients, such as patients who have an abnormal physical examination that may indicate a neurologic problem, or who have irritative or obstructive voiding symptoms that fail to resolve on sterilization of the urine.

Occasional patients benefit from the endoscopic evaluation of the ureteral insertions. This evaluation may predict the chance of resolution of reflux. The accuracy of this analysis depends on multiple variables and is unreliable.

Natural History

Primary VUR has a progressively increasing prognosis of resolution with decreasing grades of reflux. Patients with grade I VUR have a greater than 90% chance of resolution, whereas patients with grade V VUR have less than a 10% chance of resolution. Grades II, III, and IV VUR fall in an intermediate range (Table 73-3).

Treatment

Formulating a plan for the management of reflux is predicated on two principles. The first principle is that one must

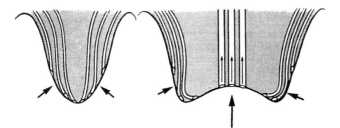

FIGURE 73-7 ■ The normal oblique insertion of the collecting ducts onto the surface of simple papillae prevents intrarenal reflux (left). Collecting duct insertion onto the surface of compound papillae (right) may allow intrarenal reflux. (From Ransly PG: Intrarenal reflux: Anatomic, dynamic, and radiological studies. Urol Res 5:61, 1977.)

TABLE 73-3 ■ Reflux Resolution: 5 Years, Medical Therapy	
Reflux Grade	**Resolution (%)**
I	91.8
II	80.6
III, unilateral, age 0-2 yr*	70
III, unilateral, age 2-5 yr	51.3
III, unilateral, age 5-10 yr	43.6
III, bilateral, age 0-2 yr	49.3
III, bilateral, age 2-5 yr	30.5
III, bilateral, age 5-10 yr	12.5
IV, unilateral	58.5
IV, bilateral	9.9

*Refers to age at presentation. From AUA Reflux Guidelines, 1997.

decide whether the reflux is primary or secondary. The management for secondary reflux must be directed at the underlying cause, be it anatomic or functional. The reflux itself may need to be corrected as well, but only in the context of an overall management plan. A common cause of failure of surgical or medical management of reflux is failure to recognize the reflux as secondary to other anatomic or functional abnormalities. The second principle is preventing UTIs. It is crucial that parents realize surgical correction of reflux does not prevent UTIs but is likely to prevent pyelonephritis. Parents may be disappointed to face postoperative recurrent cystitis after surgically successful ureteral reimplantation.

Medical

Treatment of VUR can be either medical or surgical. Medical management involves careful attention to perineal hygiene as previously discussed, treatment of constipation, and hydration. Selected individuals who have evidence of high-pressure voiding dynamics can benefit from the administration of anticholinergic or spasmolytic agents, as discussed in Chapter 74. Antibiotic suppression is the most important form of medical management. The appropriate dose for antibiotic prophylactics is one third to one fourth of a normal therapeutic dosage given once daily. Renal ultrasound and VCUG usually are done every 12 to 18 months, although this is variable. Patients who have significant reflux nephropathy at presentation may require isotope renal parenchymal imaging to assess accurately whether or not progression of renal injury is occuring.

Surgical

Table 73-4 outlines the indications for surgical correction of VUR. Absolute indications include breakthrough UTIs, progressive renal injury despite suppression, intolerance to suppressive agents, noncompliance with antibiotics, grade V VUR (except in the newborn or young infant), and an anatomic ureterovesical junction abnormality (e.g., a diverticulum). Relative indications include the pubertal age range, failure of resolution after 4 years of suppression, and deficient ureteral insertions by endoscopy.

The principles of ureteral reimplantation for the correction of VUR involve the creation of a ureteral tunnel with a tunnel length-to-ureteral diameter ratio of 5:1, a tension-free anastomosis, and maintenance of good blood supply to the ureter. The last-mentioned consideration is crucial and is often overlooked. The remainder of this discussion reviews ureteral reimplantation of normal or near-normal caliber ureters.

Leadbetter-Politano ureteral reimplantation is one of the commonly applied surgical techniques. The bladder is opened in the midline, and the ureteral orifice is intubated. The ureter is dissected from the surrounding detrusor until it is totally mobilized. The resulting defect in the bladder is examined carefully with the placement of a retractor. Dissection behind the bladder can be performed under direct vision. The peritoneum is visible and may be deflected away from the base of the bladder without injury. When this has been completed, a neohiatus is created by passing a right-angled clamp into the bladder. Thereafter, a suburothelial tunnel is created, and the detrusor defect is closed. The ureter is passed through the tunnel, and the

ureteral orifice is matured as shown in Figure 73-8. The urothelium is closed over the neohiatus. The bladder is closed in the midline, and a paravesical drain is left in place.

The Cohen cross-trigonal procedure also is performed through a midline incision in the bladder. The ureteral orifice is intubated, circumscribed, and mobilized from the detrusor as previously described for the Leadbetter-Politano procedure. In contrast, however, a transtrigonal tunnel is created by sharp dissection, and after this the detrusor is approximated around the ureter to create a normal neohiatal caliber. The ureter is passed through the submucosal tunnel, and the ureteral orifice is matured. The urothelium is closed over the neohiatus, after which the bladder is closed in the midline, and an extravesical drain is placed.

The extravesical detrusorrhaphy is a modification of an earlier extravesical technique, the Lich-Gregoir procedure. The ureter is mobilized for the length of several centimeters with care taken to preserve its blood supply. An incision in the detrusor is carried around the ureteral insertion. When this has been completed, the ureter is left attached only to the underlying bladder mucosa. Two advancing sutures are placed to allow advancement in the distal ureter and fixation of the ureter distally. After this, the detrusor is approximated over the ureter to recreate the tunnel. The advancement sutures are crucial because they allow a relatively longer tunnel to be achieved and allow stabilization of the length of the tunnel by preventing potential retraction of the ureter. Retraction of the ureter would result in the shortening of the effective tunnel length and an increase in the risk of recurrent reflux.

A modification of the Paquin and Leadbetter-Politano techniques is especially valuable when ureteral reimplantation is required as part of a complex urinary reconstruction in which a megaureter is encountered and in which ureteral reimplantation is being performed in a patient with a severely abnormal bladder. The ureter is mobilized, taking care to preserve meticulously its blood supply, then divided at its insertion into the bladder. The insertion site is oversewn with absorbable suture material. The bladder is opened in the midline, and a site of neohiatus is chosen. When the neohiatus has been created, a tunnel is created that is five times the length of the ureteral diameter and is directed toward the trigone. The ureter is passed through the tunnel, and the ureteral orifice is matured. The urothelium is closed over the neohiatus.

A relatively new approach to the management of VUR is the endoscopic technique for correction. A needle is inserted beneath the ureteral orifice under endoscopic control, and a material is injected. This creates a relative increase in the tunnel length in the secure base of the tunnel floor. This procedure may be performed on an outpatient basis with minimal morbidity. Polytetrafluoroethylene (Teflon) paste has been used predominantly and has given good results. Concern with migration of Teflon particles and a demonstrated potential for granuloma formation have made this procedure controversial. Bovine cross-linked collagen has been used with promising results; however, experience with this agent is limited. The only Food and Drug Administration–approved substance to

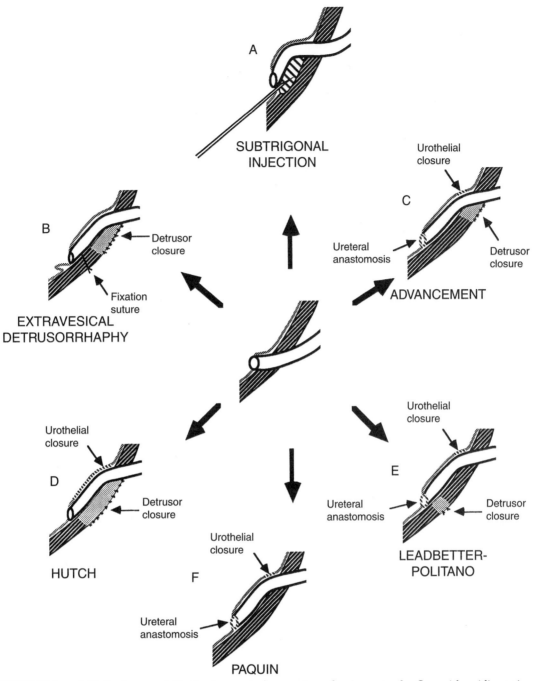

FIGURE 73-8 ■ **A–F,** Options available for the surgical correction of vesicoureteral reflux, with guiding principles to have long length of ureter, strong detrusor backing, and compressible urothelium. (From Sheldon CA, Wacksman J: Urinary tract infection and vesicoureteral reflux. In Ashcraft KW, Holder TM [eds]: Pediatric Surgery. Philadelphia, WB Saunders, 1993.)

date for the endoscopic correction of reflux is dextranomer macrospheres (deflux). Figure 73-8 shows the various surgical options for correction of VUR.

Tables 73-5 and 73-6 outline the considerations pertinent to choosing a procedure for the correction of VUR. A consideration pertinent to any procedure is the distinction between primary and secondary reflux. Any antireflux procedure performed in a patient with secondary VUR has a significant risk of failure, unless high-pressure voiding dynamics have been corrected. This may require

the use of anticholinergic agents, spasmolytic agents, and intermittent catheterization in selected individuals. Patients who fail to show improvements in the high intravesical pressures despite maximum medical management may require bladder augmentation to ensure an effective antireflux procedure.

Table 73-5 outlines the specific advantages and disadvantages of the antireflux techniques in most common use. Table 73-6 outlines the relative success rates of the procedures as reported in literature. The use of various

TABLE 73-4 ■ Guidelines for Consideration of Antireflux Surgery

Absolute	Relative
Breakthrough UTIs	Pubertal age
Progressive renal injury despite suppression	Failure to resolve after 4 yr on suppression
Intolerance to suppression	Grade V VUR
Noncompliance with antibiotics	Deficient ureterovesical insertion by endoscopy
Grade V VUR*	

*Except in young infants and newborns.

TABLE 73-5 ■ Available Options for Antireflux Surgery

Procedure	Specific Advantages	Specific Disadvantages
Subtrigonal injection	Endoscopic procedure	Material injected: Teflon—migration, granuloma formation; Collagen—uncertain durability
Extravesical detrusorrhaphy	Bladder never opened; No hematuria; No ureteral anastomosis; Minimal bladder spasms; Endoscopically accessible ureteral orifices; Avoids complications of neohiatus formation in Leadbetter-Politano reimplantation	
Advancement Cohen (transtrigonal) Glenn-Anderson	Avoids complications of neohiatus formation in Leadbetter-Politano reimplantation	Transtrigonal—difficult to access ureter endoscopically; Glenn-Anderson—limited length of tunnel achievable
Hutch	No ureteral anastomosis; Good alternative with large associated congenital diverticulum	
Leadbetter-Politano	Excellent ureteral tunnel dimensions with endoscopically accessible ureteral orifices	Risk of ureteral obstruction; Risk of sigmoid colon injury with left reimplantation
Paquin	Versatility. Extremely useful during complex reconstructive procedures	

TABLE 73-6 ■ Results of Antireflux Surgery as Reported in Representative Series

Author	Year	Procedure	No. Patients	Success Rate (%)
Endoscopic				
O'Donnell	1986	Subtrigonal injection	61	80
Schulman	1987	Subtrigonal injection	35	88
Kaplan	1987	Subtrigonal injection	28	85
Puri	1987	Subtrigonal injection	31	67
Extravesical				
Zaontz	1987	Extravesical detrusorrhaphy	146	98
Bruhl	1988	Lich-Gregoir	60	91
Linn	1989	Lich-Gregoir	79	93
Wacksman and Sheldon	1990	Extravesical detrusorrhaphy	66	98
Transvesical				
Brannan	1973	Paquin	47	95
Mininberg	1986	Paquin	631	95
Kondo	1987	Transtrigonal	50	100
Brown	1989	Transtrigonal	51	98
Politano	1963	Leadbetter-Politano	100	94
Brannan	1973	Leadbetter-Politano	45	96

intubation techniques with ureteral reimplantation is controversial. A Foley catheter is used routinely after ureteral reimplantation. In general, postoperative epidural analgesia is the limiting factor with respect to the timing of Foley catheter removal. Typically the Foley catheter is removed the morning the epidural catheter is removed.

Ureteral stents only rarely are required. Patients undergoing reoperative reimplantation, a tapered ureteral reimplantation, reimplantation performed with concomitant bladder neck reconstruction, augmentation, or ureterocele excision may require ureteral stenting. In infants undergoing bilateral ureteral reimplantation, temporary obstruction may be encountered owing to edema, and ureteral intubation may be helpful.

A suprapubic tube is used rarely. The exception is a patient who is undergoing a concomitant bladder neck reconstruction or bladder augmentation. In addition, an infant who undergoes significant intravesical reconstruction, such as ureterocele excision, may benefit by placement of a suprapubic tube because the tiny urethral catheter may become occluded by clot. The use of an extravesical approach in this setting is especially rewarding for this reason.

Postoperative follow-up consists of a renal ultrasound and VCUG 3 to 4 months postoperatively. Thereafter, renal ultrasonography is performed annually for 2 to 4 years. Complications of antireflux surgery primarily relate to recurrent or persistent reflux and vesicoureteral obstruction. Recurrent reflux is almost always due to the creation of an inadequate tunnel or failure to recognize or treat high-pressure bladder dynamics.

Causes of ureteral obstruction after reimplantation may be defined as suprahiatal, hiatal, and infrahiatal. Suprahiatal obstruction occurs with kinking or twisting of the ureter, usually owing to failure to mobilize the distal ureter adequately. Prevention may be facilitated by routine division of the obliterated umbilical artery. The Leadbetter-Politano procedure in particular has been associated with a risk of suprahiatal obstruction owing to the fact that the neohiatus in some cases is constructed without direct visualization. The right-angled clamp may be passed through a segment of peritoneum, and cases have been reported in which the ureter has been passed through a segment of bowel. In either case, a constriction of the ureteral lumen may develop.

Hiatal obstructions may occur when the hiatus is too small or when there is kinking of the ureter as it enters the hiatus. The creation of a hiatus too high on the bladder wall may create a situation in which the ureter becomes obstructed owing to kinking as the bladder fills. This problem may be relieved to some degree by frequent bladder emptying but occasionally may require surgical revision. This occurrence has been documented by intergrade pressure-flow studies performed at various levels of bladder filling.

Infrahiatal obstructions may include anastomotic stricture, the creation of a too-narrow tunnel, or ischemic stricture. Technical complications associated with recurrent reflux and postoperative obstruction are readily preventable. Strict adherence to the principles described make the need for surgical revision rare. In contrast to the extravesical detrusorrhaphy procedure, a transient postoperative obstruction may be encountered in any procedure requiring a ureteral-urothelial anastomosis. This obstruction appears to resolve over 2 to 3 weeks, and it is generally relatively minor and not associated with renal injury.

Another surgical complication that always must be considered is postoperative voiding dysfunction. This may occur from excessive extravesical dissection that may interfere with detrusor nerve supply, or it may result from injury of the urethra or bladder neck. The latter is rare unless reimplantation is accompanied by excision of an ectopic ureterocele. The extravesical detrusorrhaphy has a small but real risk of temporary urinary retention owing to the required extravesical dissection. This retention seems to occur primarily when bilateral ureteral reimplantations are done that involve the creation of long tunnels. Consequently, careful patient selection can help minimize this complication. In particular, avoidance of this technique for megaureter repair (especially if bilateral) is indicated.

Reoperative ureteral reimplantation is considerably more difficult than initial reconstruction. Preservation of the blood supply to the ureter is the most crucial concern. Patients undergoing reoperative surgery for recurrent reflux should undergo urodynamics evaluation, and any documented voiding imbalance should be controlled medically before reconstruction is undertaken. If this is not possible, consideration for bladder augmentation is appropriate.

Reoperative reimplantation for ureterovesical obstruction is required most often because of distal ureteral ischemia and contracture. Consequently, this rare occurrence is approached best transperitoneally. This allows optimal preservation of the blood supply of the remaining ureter. Additionally, mobilization of the ureter along with the associated gonadal vessels may help preservation of ureteral blood supply.

COMMON PROCEDURES FOR GENITOURINARY EVALUATION

Urine Collection for Analysis and Culture

Bag

Despite careful skin preparation and placement of a sterile collection bag on the perineum, false-positive urine cultures are frequent and unavoidable. Consequently, this technique is useful only for screening. Results are significant only if the culture is negative. Positive culture results require confirmation or correlation with the urinalysis. This technique is inappropriate for clinically ill children or uncircumcised boys.

Midstream Voiding

After careful sterile preparation and cleansing of the genitalia in either a boy or a girl, the child is instructed to void, then when some urine has been passed, urine is collected in midstream into a sterile container avoiding contamination. Results in cooperative circumcised boys are highly reliable. Positive cultures in girls are suggestive if clinical symptoms are supportive, but consideration should be given to confirmation.

Indwelling Catheter

To collect a specimen from an indwelling catheter, the catheter port should be cleansed with an alcohol sponge and punctured directly with a needle and syringe for collection. Culture results from indwelling catheters are unreliable, however.

Suprapubic Puncture

This technique generally is used only in infants. To ensure a full bladder during urine collection by bladder tap, patients should maintain a high fluid intake. The skin overlying the pubic symphysis is prepared and draped in sterile fashion. A local anesthetic can be used but is not necessary. A sterile 22-gauge, 4-cm-long needle (or a no. 22 spinal needle) fixed to a sterile syringe is advanced through the skin, fascia, and bladder wall in one quick movment, and the specimen is collected (Fig. 73-9).

Previous lower abdominal surgery with resultant adhesions increases the risk of bowel penetration and precludes using this procedure. This technique is useful when an ill child requires prompt and accurate diagnosis and when catheterization is difficult (e.g., phimosis and urogenital sinus anomalies).

Urethral Catheterization

Catheterization is the most reliably accurate method of urine collection and is performed with strict sterile technique and careful cleansing. The catheter should glide smoothly through the urethra. If resistance is encountered, the catheter should be withdrawn. A different size or type of catheter should be used, or the original catheter should be relubricated and passed again. Blood on the catheter or at the meatus implies urethral trauma, which may be worsened by continued attempts. Catheters with balloons should be advanced well into the bladder several centimeters beyond the point where urine is obtained before the balloon is inflated to prevent urethral disruption by intraurethral inflation. Catheters without balloons should not be advanced excessively to prevent intravesical knotting.

A Foley catheter balloon may fail to decompress, making removal difficult. Blood clots or crystalline deposits may clog the tiny balloon port. Initial attempts may involve removal of the valve mechanism and passing a guidewire down the line. Balloons may be ruptured by solvent injection down the injection port or by direct needle puncture. In children, balloon rupture is done under anesthesia so that the bladder may be irrigated immediately and examined endoscopically to ensure that all balloon fragments have been removed.

Most patients can be catheterized with a straight catheter (with or without a balloon). Patients with a prominent bladder neck (e.g., posterior urethral valves) or an irregular urethra (e.g., imperforate anus or reconstructed urethra) may benefit from a catheter with a curved tip (coudé) directed anteriorly (with or without a balloon). Catheters with holes at their tip may be used for passage over a guidewire or filiforms in difficult cases. When the urine specimen has been collected, it should be sent to the laboratory as quickly as possible and cultured immediately after collection or refrigerated.

Radiographic Imaging of the Urinary Tract

Ultrasonography

Ultrasonography is an excellent screening tool used to detect hydronephrosis, renal parenchymal abnormalities, calculi, some bladder abnormalities, and renal size.

Kidney and Ureters

No preparation is required to study the kidney and ureters ultrasonographically, unless there is intestinal distention.

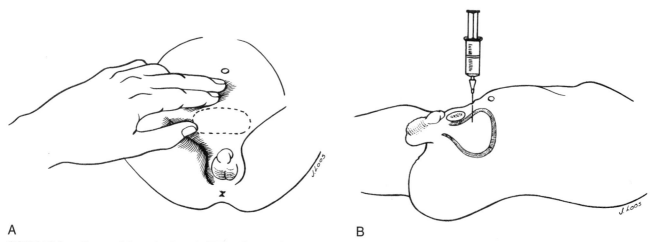

A   B

FIGURE 73-9 ■ Suprapubic aspiration. **A,** The infant is placed in a supine position, and the bladder is palpated. **B,** While withdrawing on the syringe, the needle is advanced from a point just superior to the symphysis pubis directly posteriorly until urine is obtained.

Bladder

Better bladder images are obtained when the bladder is full. Children 3 years old or older are instructed to drink fluids 30 minutes to 1 hour before the scheduled examination and not void.

Voiding Cystourethrogram

A VCUG allows visualization of the lower urinary tract (bladder and urethra) and evaluation of the ureterovesical junctions for reflux. A catheter is introduced into the bladder, and under gravity pressure not to exceed 100 cm H₂O, contrast material is infused until the bladder is full. The catheter is withdrawn, and radiographs are taken as the child urinates (Fig. 73-10).

This study also can be done using radioisotopes (technetium sulfur colloid). After catheterizing the bladder and measuring the residual, the radioisotope is infused with sterile saline until bladder pressure reaches 30 cm H₂O (measured through a manometer attached to the infusion device). The dose of the radioisotope varies with age: 300 μCi for children younger than 2 years old and double that dose for older children. Children are placed upright during the voiding phase of the scanning (Fig. 73-11). The potential advantage of the radionuclide cystogram is reduced radiation exposure and continuous monitoring for reflux. The compromise is, however, that there is a loss of anatomic detail in grading the reflux and evaluating the bladder and urethra. Most clinicians use a radiographic contrast VCUG for the initial evaluation, then selectively use the radionuclide cystogram for follow-up.

Renal Nuclear Scans

Preparation usually is not required. Children younger than 3 years old should not eat or drink for 4 hours before the examination. Sedation may be necessary in some cases. Radionuclide renography may be done for a variety of reasons, and the agent and study protocol should be adapted depending on the clinical situation. DMSA (technetium-99m meso-2,3 dimercaptosuccinic acid) is an excellent parenchymal marker and can be used to detect renal scarring or acute pyelonephritic changes and overall renal function (see Fig. 73-11). Mag-3 and diethylene-triamine penta-acetic acid (DTPA) are used to assess renal function and excretion and are used to evaluate for obstruction (see later).

Excretory Urogram

The excretory urogram is not used frequently in children because improved ultrasound images have largely replaced the anatomic qualities of the urogram, and the diuretic renogram has replaced the functional qualities of the urogram.

Computed Tomography

Patients should not eat or drink for 4 hours before computed tomography (CT) scanning. Chloral hydrate is given to children younger than 18 months old for sedation. Older children who are unable to lie still for the examination also are sedated. Oral and intravenous contrast material is given 30 minutes before the examination. This study is essential for the evaluation of renal masses and renal trauma, and CT is being used with increasing frequency for the evaluation

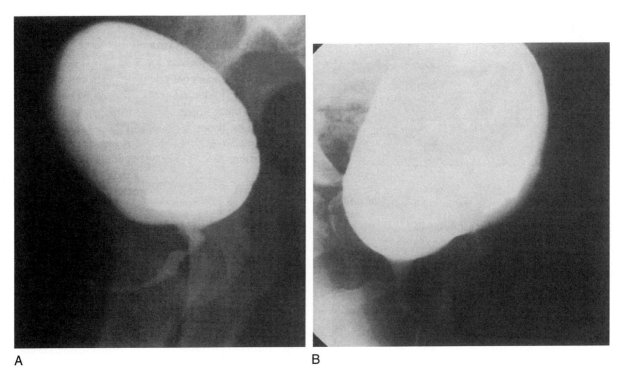

A   B

FIGURE 73-10 ■ Voiding cystourethrogram (VCUG). **A,** VCUG in a boy. Note the smooth wall, absence of intravesical defects, and nondilated urethra. **B,** A normal VCUG in a girl.

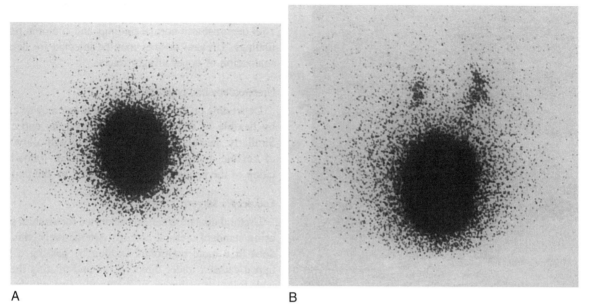

A   B

FIGURE 73-11 ■ Nuclear medicine voiding cystourethrogram (VCUG). **A,** A normal nuclear medicine VCUG. Although no reflux is present, relatively little information regarding the contour of the bladder and the urethra is available compared with the studies shown in Figure 73-10. The radiation exposure is, however, much less. **B,** Nuclear medicine VCUG shows bilateral vesicoureteral reflux.

of urinary calculi, especially in the acute setting. In the latter clinical scenario, no contrast material is given intravenously to maximize stone visualization.

Magnetic Resonance Imaging

If children are younger than 1 year of age, no food or fluids are given for 3 hours before magnetic resonance imaging. General anesthesia often is required. Older patients should avoid solid food for 8 hours and clear liquids for 4 hours before the procedure. Sedation is similar to that for CT. Older patients also can receive sedation if they are anxious. A contrast medium may be injected intravenously. Magnetic resonance imaging provides highly useful imaging data of the great vessels in patients with renal malignancies. It is also useful in the evaluation of pelvic anomalies, such as a cloaca, and can image the spinal cord accurately.

Endoscopic Evaluation of the Urinary Tract

Cystoscopy

After induction of anesthesia, the patient is placed in the lithotomy position. The genital area is cleansed with an antiseptic solution, and the patient is draped. After lubrication with the sterile gel, the endoscope is introduced gently, generally under direct vision, with a 0-degree or 30-degree lens. The urethra is examined under conditions of retrograde and antegrade flow. The bladder and ureteral orifices are examined with the bladder inflated and deflated. Figure 73-12 shows normal findings and common pathologic findings. Ureteral orifices may be injected for detailed visualization of the upper urinary tracts.

Ureteroscopy and Nephroscopy

Depending on the child's age, the ureter may be examined by flexible or rigid ureterscopes over its entire length.

Similarly, percutaneous renal puncture allows passage of flexible or rigid endoscopic equipment after dilation of the percutaneous tract created by the puncture.

Endoscopic Surgery

Urethral dilation can be performed for urethral strictures using standard urethral sounds. Alternatively, this may be done in a more controlled fashion by passing a filiform-tipped catheter under direct vision and dilating the urethra with follower catheters of increasing size attached to the end of the filiform-tipped catheter. Both of these methods may incur a significant amount of renal scarring, and recurrent strictures are common.

Direct visual internal urethrotomy is an excellent way to manage urethral strictures. The stricture is cut under direct vision with a cold knife. Depending on the extent of the incision, an indwelling catheter may be necessary until healing has occurred.

Transurethral incision under direct vision is employed for posterior urethral valves. The valves are divided at the 5 and 7 o'clock positions. Alternatively a single incision at 12 o'clock may suffice.

Endoscopic stone extraction may be performed with a direct grasper or stone baskets. Alternatively, stones may be fragmented for removal with ultrasonic, electrohydraulic, or laser lithotripsy. This can be performed through a cystoscope, ureteroscope, or nephroscope.

Endoscopic ureteropyelotomy for ureteropelvic junction obstruction may be performed under direct vision through a dilated percutaneous tract into the renal collecting system. With a guidewire passed through the ureteropelvic junction, a cold blade is used to cut through the obstructing segment. The incised junction is left stented until healing is documented.

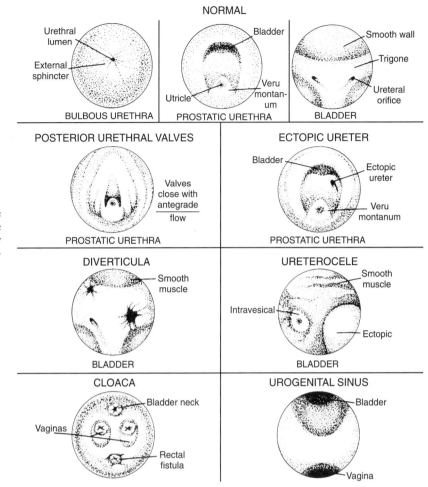

FIGURE 73-12 ■ The endoscopic appearance of the normal urinary tract. Also shown are representative pictures of commonly encountered, endoscopically detected congenital abnormalities.

Functional Evaluation of the Urinary Tract

Noninvasive Urodynamics

The patient is instructed to come to the examination room with a full bladder. Electromyogram electrodes are placed on the inside of the thighs and the buttock to allow measurement of the pelvic floor muscular activity. The patient voids into a receptacle that empties into a flowmeter, providing measurements of flow rate and flow time. A graphic representation of the flow pattern and EMG activity is provided (Fig. 73-13). After voiding, residual urine is measured by ultrasound (see Fig. 73-13B).

Cystometrogram

A cystometrogram measures bladder pressures and can detect inappropriate detrusor activity. Figure 73-14 shows a normal cystometrogram pattern. A dual-lumen catheter is passed into the bladder. One lumen is attached to a pressure transducer for measurement of bladder pressures during bladder filling, and the second lumen is attached to an infusion line. A rectal line is placed and attached to a transducer to allow measurement of abdominal pressure. Patch electrodes are placed to allow measurements of pelvic floor musculature activity. Vesical pressure is monitored as the bladder is being filled by gravity with normal saline solution until there is a leak from the urethra or the patient expresses a strong urge to void (the bladder also may be filled by an infusion pump). A true urge to void usually is accompanied by a mild-to-moderate increase in electromyogram activity, restlessness, or complaint of abdominal discomfort.

Urethral Pressure Profile

A single-lumen 8F urethral pressure profilometry catheter is passed into the bladder. Sterile normal saline solution is infused through the catheter at a low rate, while the catheter is pulled slowly from the urethra at a specific controlled speed. A pressure-monitoring line attached to the catheter allows measurement of pressure within the urethra. Urethral pressure also may be measured during a cystogram with the use of a triple-lumen catheter. This study allows measurement of the urethral resistance exerted by the sphincteric mechanism (Fig. 73-15).

Diuretic Renogram

The patient is placed supine and intravenously hydrated with 10 mL of fluid per kg of body weight; 5% dextrose in 0.25 normal saline is used for infants younger than 12 months old and 5% dextrose in 0.5 normal saline is used for children older than 12 months. A catheter is left

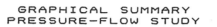

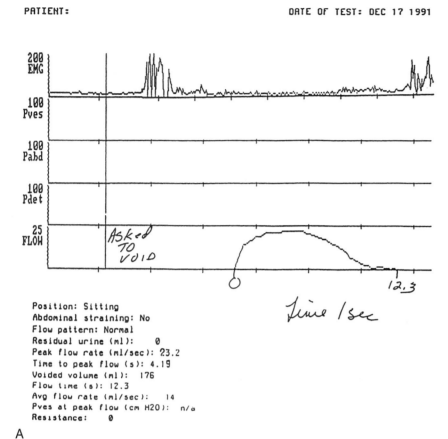

Position: Sitting
Abdominal straining: No
Flow pattern: Normal
Residual urine (ml):   0
Peak flow rate (ml/sec): 23.2
Time to peak flow (s): 4.19
Voided volume (ml):   176
Flow time (s): 12.3
Avg flow rate (ml/sec):   14
Pves at peak flow (cm H2O):   n/a
Resistance: 0

A

FIGURE 73-13 ■ A normal noninvasive urodynamic study. **A,** The patient voids with a normal flow pattern and a normal peak flow rate. There is no interruption of the urinary stream, and the stream is not prolonged. The perineal electro-myographic pattern becomes silent during voiding, indicating appropriate relaxation of the sphincteric mechanism. **B,** Residual urine is being determined employing an ultrasound technique. This technique has proved to be highly reliable and does not require catheterization.

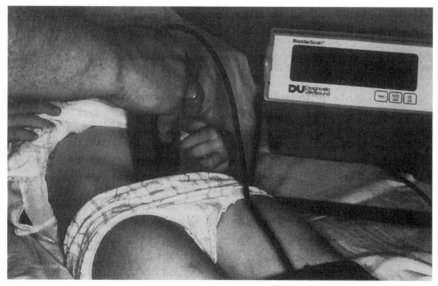

B

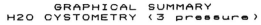

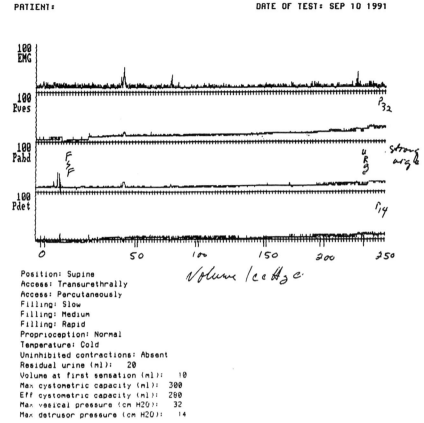

FIGURE 73-14 ■ A normal cystometrogram. Note the maintenance of low intravesical pressure while the bladder fills. Pertinent abnormalities include the development of spikes of pressure that could not be suppressed and the presence of diminished bladder compliance, as indicated by a premature rise in intravesical pressure during filling.

in place for the entire examination to prevent bladder distention and ureteral obstruction in pretoilet-trained children, otherwise the child is asked to empty the bladder. The technetium-99m MAG-3 isotope is injected intravenously, and after scanning for 20 minutes, a diuretic (furosemide) is administered. Scanning continues for another 30 minutes (Fig. 73-16). Half-life analysis is helpful in determining whether or not hydronephrosis is due to obstruction. A half-life less than or equal to 10 minutes is unobstructed, greater than or equal to 20 minutes is obstructed, and 10 to 20 minutes is equivocal. The incidence of false-positive and false-negative studies can be significant.

Technetium-99m DTPA Studies

Technetium-99m DTPA is used mainly for studies of glomerular filtration rate, renal differential function, as well as excretion. Two hours after the injection of technetium-99m DTPA, four blood samples are drawn at 30-minute intervals to estimate glomerular filtration rates. When differential function is being investigated, a higher dose is used.

Whitaker Percutaneous Antegrade Pyelogram

School-age and younger children usually require general anesthesia for this procedure. Older adolescents and young adults may be comfortable with intravenous sedation. A peripheral intravenous line is placed. Pressure and Foley catheters are passed into the bladder. The Foley catheter is attached to gravity drainage. Two needles are placed percutaneously into the affected renal pelvis. One needle is attached to a pressure-monitoring line, and the other needle is attached to an infusion line. Pressure lines are connected to a computer that provides a graphic presentation of the pressure measurements. Bladder pressure is monitored throughout the study. The Whitaker test begins with infusion of contrast material into the renal pelvis, which is visualized by fluoroscopy. Pressure within the renal pelvis is measured continually during the infusion. Infusion rates vary from 2 mL/min to a maximum of 12 mL/min. The rate is increased incrementally throughout the study as the renal pelvic pressure is monitored with the bladder decompressed and full. Renal pelvis pressures greater than 20 cm H_2O above the bladder pressure indicate obstruction. After the study is completed, a nephrostomy tube may be placed to allow continued decompression of the renal pelvis. Otherwise, both needles are removed from the kidney, and the bladder pressure line is withdrawn. The Foley catheter is left indwelling for monitoring urine output and to detect bleeding. Patients may receive parenteral antibiotics before and after the procedure as indicated by their condition. Figure 73-17 shows a normal study.

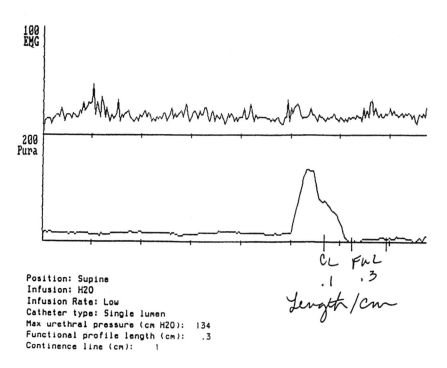

GRAPHICAL SUMMARY
H2O/CO2 PROFILOMETRY (1 pressure)

PATIENT: DATE OF TEST: NOV 26 1991

Position: Supine
Infusion: H2O
Infusion Rate: Low
Catheter type: Single lumen
Max urethral pressure (cm H2O):   134
Functional profile length (cm):   .3
Continence line (cm):   1

FIGURE 73-15 ■ Urethral pressure profile. This normal study reveals a good maximum urethral pressure and an adequate functional profile length. Low maximum urethral pressures and the application of pressure over short distances indicate inadequate sphincter function.

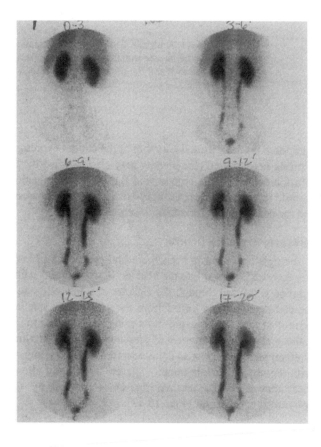

FIGURE 73-16 ■ Lasix (furosemide) renography. This study provides a rough outline of the renal cortex and the collecting system of the upper urinary tracts. An indwelling catheter is placed to ensure bladder drainage. This study allows one to estimate the relative contribution of each kidney to total renal function and gives a good estimate of the adequacy of urine drainage.

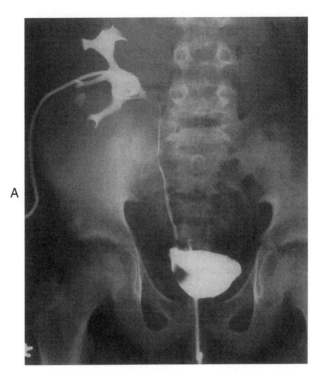

FIGURE 73-17 ■ A normal Whitaker study. **A,** The antegrade pyelogram shows the infusion of contrast medium into a mildly dilated pelvocalyceal system. A nondilated ureter is opacified, and contrast material rapidly fills the urinary bladder. **B,** Pressure measurements taken at intervals throughout the study reveal low renal pelvic pressures at low and rapid rates of infusion.

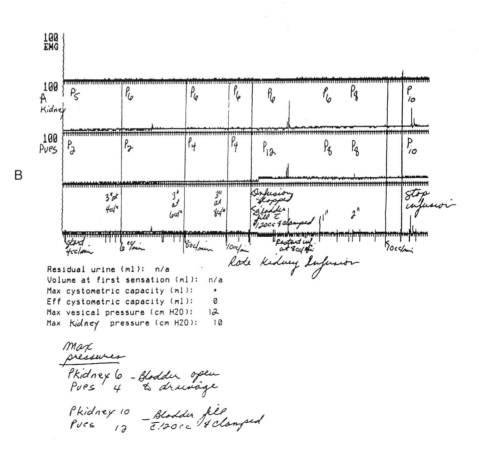

```
GRAPHICAL SUMMARY
H2O CYSTOMETRY (3 pressure)
      Whitaker    Kidney
PATIENT:                    DATE OF TEST: NOV 19 1991
```

Residual urine (ml): n/a
Volume at first sensation (ml): n/a
Max cystometric capacity (ml): *
Eff cystometric capacity (ml): 0
Max vesical pressure (cm H2O): 12
Max Kidney pressure (cm H2O): 10

SUGGESTED READINGS

Close CE: Current surgical trends in ureteral reimplantation. Dialogues in Pediatric Urology 24:11, 2001.

This is an excellent summary of the various technical approaches to vesicoureteral reflux.

Elder JS, Peter CA, Arant BS, et al: Pediatric vesicoureteral reflux guidelines panel summary report on the management of primary vesicoureteral reflux in children. J Urol 157:1846-1851, 1997.

This article summarizes the conclusion of a panel of experts on indications for and approaches to the management of reflux.

Nijman RJM: Urodynamic studies of the lower urinary tract. In Gearhart JP, Rink RC, Mouriquand PDE (eds): Pediatric Urology. Philadelphia, WB Saunders, 2001, p 187.

This chapter outlines all of the details and indications for various urodynamic studies of the lower urinary tract in the pediatric age group.

Piepsz A, Blaufox MD, Gordon I, et al: Consensus on renal cortical scintigraphy in children with urinary tract infection. Scientific Committee of Radionucleids in Nephrourology. Semin Nucl Med 2:160-174, 1999.

This consensus statement on renal scintigraphy presents current thoughts on the interpretation and use of radionuclide studies of the kidney as indicated for various disease states. It is a helpful guide to interpretation.

Pracros JP: Contrast studies in pediatric urology. In Gearhart JP, Rink RC, Mariquand PDE (eds): Pediatric Urology. Philadelphia, WB Saunders, 2001, p 109.

This valuable review discusses not only indications for various contrast x-ray studies for pediatric genitourinary anomalies, but also technique and interpretation as related to the selection of surgical approaches.

Smellie JM, Barratt TM, Chantler C, et al: Medical versus surgical treatment in children with severe bilateral vesicoureteric reflux and bilateral nephrophathy: A randomized trial. Lancet 357:1329-1333, 2001.

This article discusses which patients can be treated with antibiotics effectively and which inevitably require surgical correction of reflux.

Walker RD, Weiss RA: Vesicoureteral reflux 2000. AUA Update Series 37:19.

These authors provide current views regarding vesicoureteral reflux, diagnosis, treatment, and long-term outlook.

74

Bladder Function

Lower urinary tract dysfunction includes problems associated with the bladder, urethra, and periurethral striated muscle. The causes may be neurologic, non-neurologic, or muscular, and temporary functional developmental delay is common. Myelomeningocele is one of the most common entities in this category. Generally, neuromuscular disorders do not affect the upper urinary tract primarily but only secondarily through infection, obstruction, or a sustained increase in intravesical pressure or vesicoureteral reflux. Treatment of lower urinary tract dysfunction is aimed primarily at preventing upper urinary tract damage and secondarily toward providing normal socialization of the child with an adequate cosmetic appearance. The clinical manifestations include voiding disorders, incontinence, and enuresis.

CLINICAL MANIFESTATIONS

Abnormal bladder function may present with urinary tract infection, irritative or obstructive voiding symptoms, incontinence, or renal injury. Table 74-1 lists the most common irritative and obstructive symptoms encountered in children. Frequency, urgency, and urgency incontinence are prominent features. These irritative symptoms commonly coexist with infection, but they should be relieved with successful treatment. The range of urinary incontinence may be simply enuresis or may be represented by incontinence with bladder instability, total urinary incontinence, or postvoid dribbling. Particularly notable is Vincent's curtsy, most often seen in girls. The child assumes a squatting position or sits on her foot to control urgency incontinence, usually as a result of uninhibited bladder contractions (Fig. 74-1).

Urinary Incontinence

Total urinary incontinence may result from bladder, urethral, or sphincteric disorders. Myelomeningocele, sacral agenesis, spinal tumors, trauma, and inflammation are frequent causes of neurologic deficits that result in incontinence. Extreme bladder instability or an extremely small functional capacity, either from congenital or infectious causes, may result in incontinence.

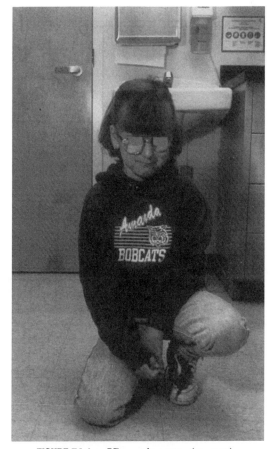

FIGURE 74-1 ▪ Vincent's curtsy (see text).

TABLE 74-1 ▪ Symptoms of Voiding Dysfunction	
Irritative	**Obstructive**
Frequency	Hesitancy
Urgency	Sensation of incomplete voiding
Urgency incontinence	Dribbling
Vincent's curtsy	Nocturia
Suprapubic/perineal pain	Intermittency
Dysuria	Diminished stream
Hematuria	Splayed stream

A primary sphincteric defect, such as exstrophy or denervation as seen with myelodysplasia, can cause incontinence. Postvoid dribbling may result from urethral obstruction caused by posterior urethral valves or strictures. Vaginal pooling in girls, which may be related to labial adhesions, or urethral diverticuli in boys, also may cause postvoid dribbling.

Enuresis

Enuresis may be classified as daytime urinary incontinence, which refers to daytime wetting and incontinence, and nocturnal enuresis, which refers to nighttime wetting. The disorder is primary in children who have always been enuretic and secondary in children who have had a dry interval after toilet training. Most children have urinary sphincter control by age 3 years, and most assume daytime and nighttime continence by age 4. The course of development of continence is generally in this order: nighttime fecal, daytime fecal, daytime urinary, and nighttime urinary. Of children, 15% still wet at night at age 5, but after this age, evaluation and treatment should be considered. Daytime urinary incontinence that persists after toilet training is usually pathologic.

Diagnostic evaluation should start with a detailed history, physical examination, and urinalysis (Fig. 74-2). Important details of history include age and success at toilet training, the pattern of incontinence, and maneuvers used in an attempt to stay dry. Enuresis usually is related to development delay, sleep abnormalities, stress, and psychological disorders and occasionally organic disorders of the urinary tract. Although most children do not have an organic lesion, a potentially harmful and correctable disorder should be identified. Urodynamic testing is reserved for children with suspected organic problems or for those whose initial management has failed.

Additionally, ultrasound for postvoid residual is useful. Parents are instructed to keep a voiding diary to verify incontinence patterns. Small bladder capacity and uninhibited detrusor contractions have been associated with enuresis, but these conditions improve with age and may represent neurophysiologic immaturity rather than a true organic disorder.

After organic causes are excluded, treatment should begin with modifying fluid intake. Typically, children have a low fluid intake while in school, which increases on returning home and is maintained until bedtime. Encouraging high fluid intake in the early part of the day with reduction after dinner may reduce the frequency of nocturnal enuresis. Also, children should be encouraged to void at bedtime. Another option is to awaken the child to void during the night. Additional forms of behavior modification have variable success rates, including retention control training and conditioning with an alarm. Alarm training involves use of a moisture-sensitive alarm in the underpants, and the child is instructed to awaken when the alarm sounds, to stop voiding, and to go to the bathroom.

Medical treatment includes anticholinergic agents, imipramine and antidiuretic hormone (1-deamino-8-D-arginine-vasopressin [DDAVP]). Although the mode of action of the tricyclic imipramine is not known, it has been shown to be effective in many trials. DDAVP (desmopressin) at night decreases urine output and bedwetting, but similar to imipramine, patients usually resume bedwetting when the treatment is stopped. Ultrasound treatment to the bladder has been applied in case of primary nocturnal enuresis for several minutes a day for 10 days. A greater than 80% success rate has been reported of lasting for more than 12 months compared with placebo-treated control patients, who did not show any benefit. Additional studies of this approach are necessary, however.

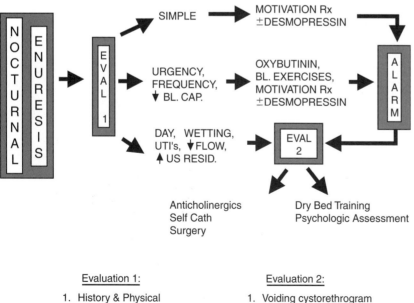

FIGURE 74-2 ■ Evaluation of children presenting with nocturnal enuresis.

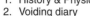

Evaluation 1:

1. History & Physical
2. Voiding diary
3. Voided volumes
4. ±Uroflowmetry
5. Ultrasound residual

Evaluation 2:

1. Voiding cystorethrogram
2. Renal ultrasound
3. Urodynamics

Other Causes of Bladder Dysfunction

Several childhood diseases are associated with underlying bladder dysfunction and usually involve either neurologic or structural deficiencies, including imperforate anus, partial sacral agenesis, central nervous system trauma, cerebral palsy, prune-belly syndrome, posterior urethral valves, bilateral single ectopic ureters, and renal failure.

CLASSIFICATION OF VOIDING DISORDERS

The various forms of voiding dysfunction may be thought of as failure to store and failure to empty, and they may be due to bladder wall, bladder outlet, or urethral disturbances. Bladder wall dysfunction is either myogenic or neurogenic, causing either hypertonia or hypotonia. Urethral or outlet dysfunction is either structural or sphincteric. Structural abnormalities include urethral valves, stricture, diverticula, Cowper's duct cysts, polyps, and meatal stenosis. Sphincteric dysfunction may be caused by an anatomic deficit as with exstrophy or sphincter trauma. Commonly, these children do not have a single discrete storage or emptying failure, and many are combination deficits.

A coordinated set of events between the detrusor muscle and the sphincter is necessary for proper bladder function. Between voiding, the relaxed bladder permits low-pressure storage, in which case the bladder outlet is closed and competent. With voiding, sphincteric relaxation is followed immediately by detrusor contraction, and voiding is carried to completion. Primary or secondary factors can disturb the timing or function of the voiding cycle, and these can compound damage to the bladder or sphincter.

Primary factors affecting bladder function are intrinsic, such as the bladder in patients with prune-belly syndrome and posterior urethral valves. Secondary effects of infection, retention, previous surgery, high urinary output, and calculi add to storing and emptying problems. Involuntary detrusor sphincter dyssynergia is a primary or intrinsic disorder of the bladder outlet caused by a neurologic deficit. Voluntary detrusor sphincter dyssynergia also exists, in which the child actively contracts the urinary sphincter while voiding. Voluntary dyssynergia can result from pain caused by bladder spasms, infection, or previous surgery. Other classifications of bladder dysfunction also are reported.

As mentioned, the primary goal of diagnosing and treating bladder dysfunction is to preserve renal function. Reflux and hydronephrosis are the consequences of urinary retention and high intravesical pressure. Hydronephrosis and retention also may develop, however, from high-output renal failure, and all three may be related in a cyclical fashion (Fig. 74-3). The "valve bladder" illustrates this point. Patients with posterior urethral valves often have a thickened hyperreflexive bladder that may persist after valve ablation and is often the cause of continued renal deterioration and urinary incontinence. Despite adequate valve ablation, these patients have continued high-pressure noncompliant bladders with reflux

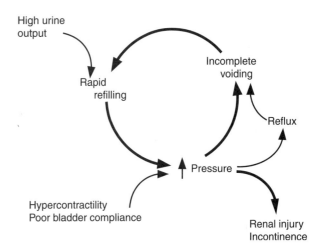

FIGURE 74-3 ■ The renal-bladder axis as illustrated by the "valve bladder."

so that the bladders never truly empty with voiding. Compounding the residual from poor bladder contraction is a diverticulum effect of the upper urinary tract and a large volume of poorly concentrated urine from high-output renal failure. Infection is common because of the high residual, and infection and reflux together are detrimental to renal function.

EVALUATION

Historical details important to evaluation of bladder function include the determination of obstructive or irritable voiding symptoms; bowel symptoms such as constipation or encopresis; and lower extremity symptoms, such as pain, weakness, or incoordination. Birth trauma, daily urine volumes, voiding patterns, positioning during voiding, and social consequences of voiding dysfunction are important areas to question. Physical examination includes palpation of the kidneys and bladder in the abdomen and examination of the external genitalia, sacrum, and overlying soft tissues. Sacral findings, such as a sinus tract, a patch of pigmentation or hair, a lipoma, a palpable sacral defect, or sacral absence, indicate significant underlying spinal disease. Observation of the urinary stream and examination of the underpants also can provide objective information.

Imaging studies should include a voiding cystourethrogram, nuclear scintigraphy, and ultrasound. These studies provide an assessment of anatomy, including trabeculae, diverticula, ureteroceles, strictures, and calculi, and functional data, such as reflux, bladder neck competence, and differential renal function.

Urodynamics testing provides important functional data, including cystometry, uroflowmetry, urethral pressure profilometry, and combined studies. The testing usually begins with the least invasive procedure. Because sensory tests are subjective, integration of clinical data is necessary for successful interpretation. In general, testing should reproduce the child's clinical problem to be most accurate, and the physician should be involved when testing is being performed.

Flowmetry

Flowmetry involves voiding into a measuring device with a pressure transducer recording the volume voided over time. Electromyography (EMG) pads can be placed over the perineum to record electrical activity in the external urinary sphincter. A normal flow study (Fig. 74-4A) is characterized by rapid flow with a short duration of voiding and a silent EMG pattern. An obstructive study (Fig. 74-4B) shows a prolonged voiding time with a low flow rate (volume/time). Striated sphincter dyssynergia typically shows a voided stream interrupted by bursts of sphincteric action (Fig. 74-5). The latter noninvasive test can provide a significant amount of information, particularly when combined with ultrasound for postvoid residual.

Cystometry

Cystometry involves measuring changes in bladder pressure related to changes in volume. During the filling

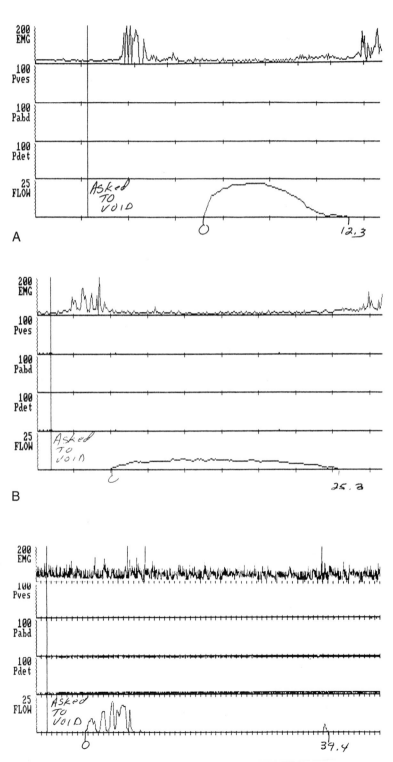

FIGURE 74-4 ■ Uroflowmetry. **A,** Normal—peak flow 23.2 mL/sec; EMG silent. **B,** Urethral obstruction—peak flow 6.75 mL/sec; EMG silent.

FIGURE 74-5 ■ Uroflowmetry: dyssynergia. Intermittent flow is associated with bursts of EMG activity.

phase of cystometry, bladder pressure should remain less than 15 cm H_2O until capacity is reached. The filling phase reflects bladder wall compliance and smooth muscle tone. Bladder wall fibrosis or hypertrophy may cause a steeper curve in the filling phase. At peak capacity, the detrusor and elastic tissues of the bladder have stretched to the maximum, and any increase in volume causes an increase in pressure. In children, bladder capacity in ounces is equal to their age in years plus 2. Variables to be observed include compliance, contractility, sensation, capacity, and leak point pressure (LPP). A normal cystometric study is contrasted with two abnormal studies in Figure 74-6.

The LPP is determined during cystometric filling in which water can escape around the catheter. It has been shown that if LPP in myelomeningocele patients is greater than 40 cm H_2O there is an increased risk of

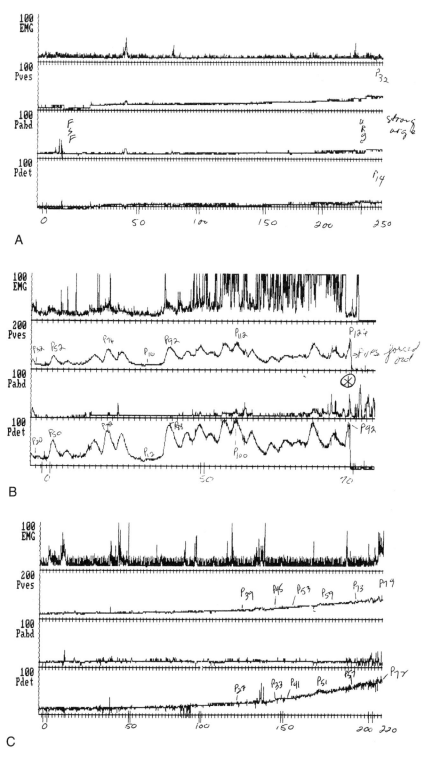

FIGURE 74-6 ■ Cystometrogram. **A,** Normal study shows maximal capacity 300 mL and maximal detrusor pressure 14 cm H_2O. **B,** Abnormal study shows uninhibited detrusor contractions; maximal capacity 70 mL, maximal detrusor pressure 100 cm H_2O, leak point pressure, 92 cm H_2O. **C,** Cystometrogram shows poor bladder compliance; maximal detrusor pressure 72 cm H_2O and maximal capacity 230 mL in a patient with a high-pressure, low-capacity bladder. Treatment is indicated in patients in **B** and **C** to prevent upper tract damage.

upper tract deterioration. Prognostically the LPP is highly useful in young children with increased bladder contractility or decreased compliance.

Urethral Pressure Profile

Static and dynamic urethral pressure profilometry is intended to provide information regarding intraurethral pressures, specifically variations in sphincter closing pressures. Although variables of position and pressure can alter a bladder pressure curve and may be difficult to interpret, evaluation of function of an artificial sphincter and diagnosis and treatment of urinary incontinence may be aided by a urethral pressure profile.

TREATMENT

Treatment goals are to achieve total urinary continence with a 4-hour dry interval and a low-pressure storage organ capable of completely emptying either by voiding or by catheterization. Medical and surgical treatment should restore and use normal anatomy wherever possible but not compromise function in doing so.

Medical Treatment

Table 74-2 outlines the various medications useful in modulating lower urinary tract function, including anticholinergics, antispasmodics, and other drugs. Intermittent catheterization commonly is performed using clean technique, but occasionally sterile technique may be necessary to prevent recurrent infection. In particular, myelomeningocele patients with detrusor hyperreflexia usually are managed with anticholinergic drugs with

TABLE 74-2 ■ Types of Medicines That Modulate Lower Urinary Tract Function

Type	Minimum	Maximum
Cholinergic		
Bethanechol	0.7 mg/kg tid	0.8 mg/kg qid
Anticholinergic		
Propantheline	0.5 mg/kg bid	0.5 mg/kg qid
Oxybutynin	0.2 mg/kg bid	0.2 mg/kg qid
Sympathomimetic		
Phenylpropanolamine	2.5 mg/kg bid	2.5 mg/kg tid
Ephedrine	0.5 mg/kg bid	1.0 mg/kg tid
Sympatholytic		
Prazosin	0.5 mg/kg bid	0.1 mg/kg tid
Phenoxybenzamine	0.3 mg/kg bid	0.3 mg/kg bid
Propranolol	0.25 mg/kg bid	0.5 mg/kg bid
Smooth muscle relaxant		
Flavoxate	3.0 mg/kg bid	3.0 mg/kg tid
Skeletal muscle relaxant		
Diazepam	0.03 mg/kg bid	0.2 mg/kg tid
Baclofen	0.1 mg/kg bid	0.3 mg /kg tid
Other		
Imipramine	0.7 mg/kg tid	1.2 mg/kg tid
Desmopressin	10 μg IN or 200 μg Po at bedtime	40 μg IN or 600 μg Po at bedtime

tid, three times daily; qid, four times daily; bid, two times daily; IN, intranasally; Po, by mouth.

clean intermittent catheterization, and autoaugmentation or enterocystoplasty is a last resort. Another approach has been reported involving injection of botulinum type A toxin into numerous sites of the detrusor muscle. Maximum bladder capacity and detrusor compliance have been shown to be increased with this treatment, but it is likely that the benefits of this approach are only temporary. It should be reserved for patients who do not respond to anticholinergic drugs.

Surgical Treatment

Many patients with organic bladder dysfunction benefit from surgical treatment. After reconstructive procedures on the bladder, patients frequently require laparotomy for a variety of reasons so that an intimate knowledge of reconstructive anatomy is essential.

Augmentation

A segment of gastrointestinal tract is used for bladder augmentation to increase bladder capacity, while keeping intravesical pressure low. In the past, a segment of intact bowel was attached to the bladder, but mass contractions of the augmentation increased intravesical pressure and negated any benefit of the added volume. This led to detubularization of bowel segments, which did decrease intraluminal pressure by interrupting circular muscle contraction and increasing the bladder radius and the volume. According to the formula ($T = pr$), the container with the greater radius and greater wall tension holds greater volumes at a constant pressure. The volume of a sphere ($V = 4/3\ \pi\ r^3$) maximizes volume to surface area as well. These principles hold for construction of a neobladder.

Figure 74-7 shows the technique of bladder augmentation using small or large intestine. The bladder is open in the midline with a clamshell incision, and the detubularized patch of bowel is converted into a cup patch by approximating the two adjacent edges. The base of the cup is anastomosed to the posterior edge of the bladder, and augmentation is completed with a running suture. A second layer is desirable because a watertight closure is necessary. Suprapubic tube and perivesical drainage control the repair until it is healed, and ureteral stents are optional.

Gastrocystoplasty is useful in children with renal failure because the use of gastric tissue has a lower risk of postoperative acidosis than with intestine. Decreased mucus production and a lower infection rate compared with intestinal augments are additional benefits. Avoiding the antrum, a wedge of stomach is harvested based on the right gastroepiploic vessels. The patch is brought retroperitoneally into the pelvis and anastomosed with the opened bladder (Fig. 74-8).

Autoaugmentation involves stripping the muscular layer from the bladder, leaving the epithelium bulging like a diverticulum. Although this technique may result in improved bladder compliance, there is little change in capacity, so it is limited in value.

When necessary, the ureters can be reimplanted into either the native bladder or the gastric augmentation using a nonrefluxing, tunneled technique. When using large intestine, reimplantation should be done into the taenia. The small bowel is not as amenable to performance of a nonrefluxing anastomosis. The bladder also can

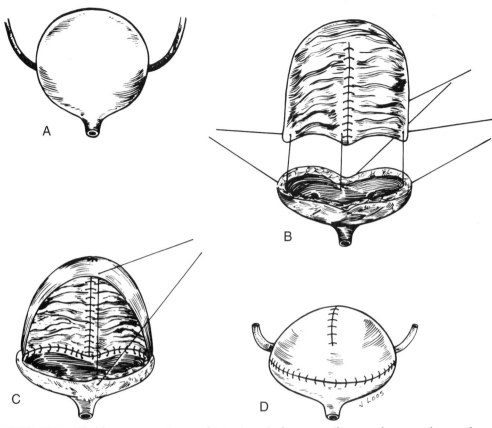

FIGURE 74-7 ■ Bladder augmentation employing intestinal segment: ileocystoplasty or colocystoplasty. **A,** The bladder is opened as a "clamshell." **B-D,** Detubularized bowel is reconfigured side-to-side, then sutured to the opened bladder, using a two-layer, running closure of absorbable suture.

FIGURE 74-8 ■ Bladder augmentation employing gastric segment: gastrocystoplasty. **A,** A wedge of nonantral stomach is isolated, based on the right gastroepiploic vessel. **B,** The bladder is opened as a "clamshell." **C,** The anastomosis is completed with a running double layer of absorbable suture.

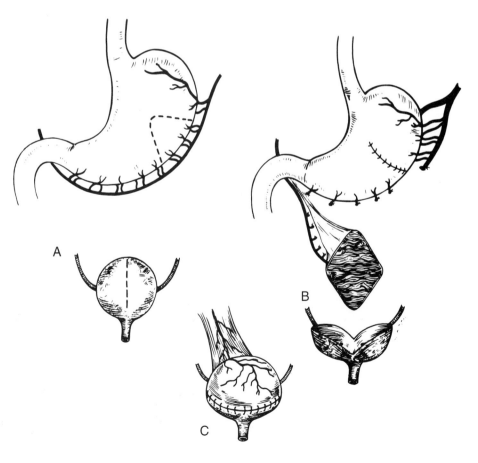

be augmented with the ileocecal portion of the intestine, intussuscepting the ileocecal valve to make it nonrefluxing, but the latter method is not always reliable.

Although bladder augmentation using intestine was thought to be associated with decreased linear growth in bladder exstrophy and myelomeningocele patients in the past, more recent long-term studies have shown that intestinal augmentation is safe and does not interfere with linear growth or bone density in patients with bladder exstrophy or myelomeningocele. Also, gastric augmentation in patients with cloacal exstrophy or metabolic acidosis has been found to be useful. Histamine blockers and proton-pump inhibiters may be needed for the hematuria/dysuria associated with gastric augmentation. Regardless of the form of augmentation, close metabolic monitoring is essential.

Diversion

Diversion can be either continent or incontinent, and incontinent diversion can be either temporary or permanent. Table 74-3 lists various incontinent diversions and their characteristics. Permanent urinary diversion is now infrequent since the introduction of many new reconstructive options. In children who have no bladder or whose bladder is severely damaged, however, continent and incontinent diversions are possible. The ileal and sigmoid conduits have been used for many years, but they have late problems of stomal stenosis, stenosis of the ureterointestinal anastomosis, and stenosis of the intestinal segment itself and deterioration of the upper urinary tract in two thirds of patients.

Ureteral sigmoidoscopy (Fig. 74-9) is the oldest form of intestinal diversion. With this, the ureters are reimplanted directly into the sigmoid colon, and the anal sphincter provides continence. Late development of carcinoma at the anastomotic site occurs in 5% of patients, however, most of whom have had frequent infections, so that close follow-up is necessary. Because carcinoma seems to be enabled by contact of the anastomosis with urine and stool, it is probably best to use one of the modifications of this procedure to separate urine and stool from the anastomotic site. If a patient undergoes undiversion, excision of the ureterocolonic segment should be performed because delayed carcinogenesis can occur.

Continent urinary diversion is preferred. It can be orthotopic or ectopic, including many variations of gastrointestinal reconstruction. The Koch pouch (ileal), Indiana and Penn pouches (ileocolic), and the gastric pouch are some examples (Figs. 74-10 and 74-11), according to surgeon preference.

Aside from catheterization, a vesicostomy is probably the most common temporary diversion technique. A vesicostomy (Fig. 74-12) permits continuous low-pressure drainage of urine into a diaper in children who have renal deterioration from progressive hydronephrosis, sepsis, or severe reflux from a high-pressure bladder. Typical indications for cutaneous vesicostomy include myelodysplasia in which medical therapy has failed, posterior urethral valves, severe prune-belly syndrome, and high-pressure neurogenic bladder that may be associated with imperforate anus. The vesicostomy can be closed after further growth and development of the child, when the primary disorder can be addressed.

TABLE 74-3 ▪ Incontinent Diversions		
Diversion Type	**Advantages**	**Disadvantages**
Permanent		
Ileal conduit	Quick, simple	Refluxing, risks acidosis, infection, stones
Sigmoid conduit	May avoid radiation field with bladder tumors; nonrefluxing	Risks acidosis, infection, stones
Ureterostomy	Quick, simple	Tendency for stenosis
Temporary		
Vesicostomy	Definitive, easily reversed bladder diversion	Prolapse, loss of bladder capacity; prevented to large degree by Blocksom technique
Pyelostomy	Definitive diversion for renal failure caused by bilateral obstruction; easily reversed	Infection; more difficult than vesicostomy

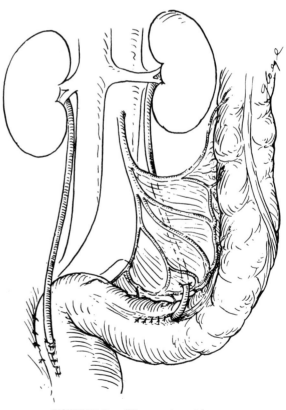

FIGURE 74-9 ▪ Ureterosigmoidoscopy.

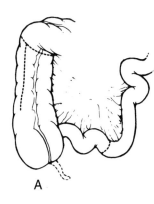

A

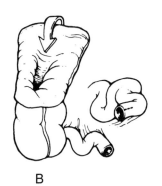

B

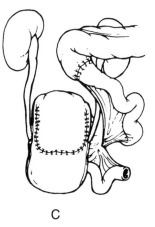

C

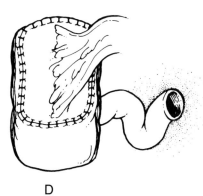

D

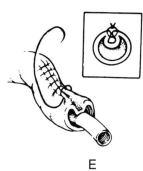

E

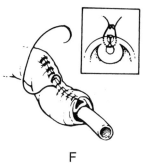

F

FIGURE 74-10 ■ Indiana pouch.

FIGURE 74-11 ■ Penn pouch. Either the appendix (Mitrofanoff) or a segment of tubularized ileum (Monti) may be used as a continent catheterizable stoma on the abdominal wall.

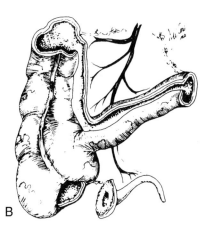

A

B

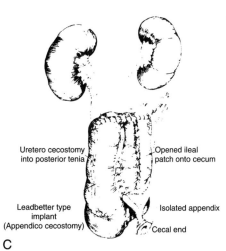

Uretero cecostomy into posterior tenia

Opened ileal patch onto cecum

Leadbetter type implant (Appendico cecostomy)

Isolated appendix

Cecal end

C

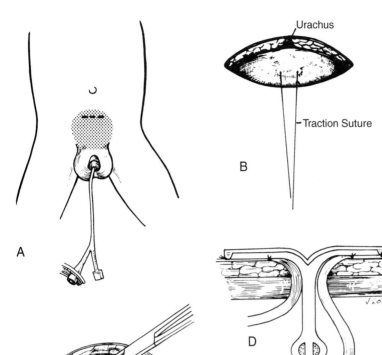

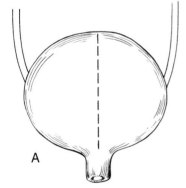

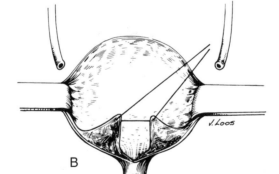

FIGURE 74-12 ■ Cutaneous vesicostomy construction. **A,** After filling the bladder, an incision is made halfway between the umbilicus and pubis. **B,** A traction suture is used to deliver the urachus into the wound. **C,** The urachus is maneuvered gently out of the wound, which ensures the bladder dome being used as the vesicostomy, preventing future prolapse. **D,** After tacking the serosa to the fascia, the bladder mucosa is sutured to the skin. The vesicostomy is stented using a split Malecot catheter for 7 days and drains into the diaper.

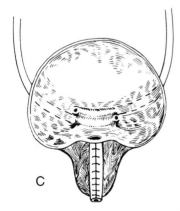

FIGURE 74-13 ■ Young-Dees-Leadbetter bladder neck reconstruction. **A,** The bladder is incised. **B,** Mucosal triangles are excised, the series of muscular incisions relax and lengthen the neourethra, and the edges of the neourethra are approximated. **C** and **D,** Two-layered muscular closure surrounds the neourethra.

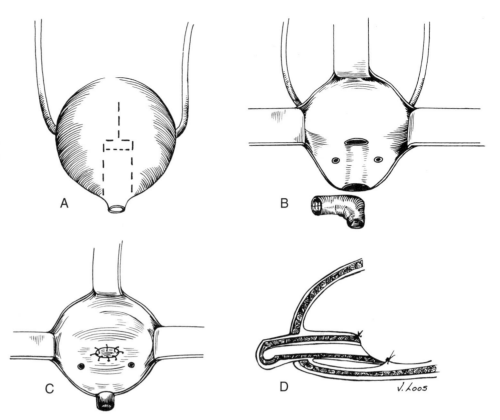

FIGURE 74-14 ■ Kropp bladder neck reconstruction. **A,** Bladder incision creates the urethra-based bladder flap. **B,** The bladder flap is tubularized to create the neourethra; the submucosal tunnel is created in the bladder base. **C,** Neourethral anastomosis is completed. **D,** Functional result—increasing bladder pressure compresses and occludes the neourethra, producing continence.

Continence Procedures

Continence procedures include bladder neck reconstruction, the use of an artificial sphincter, the sling procedure, injection of bulking materials, or construction of nipple or flap valves. The Young-Dees-Leadbetter procedure (Fig. 74-13) is especially useful for reconstruction for bladder exstrophy, in which urethral continence is achieved best by construction of a long (3 to 4 cm) and narrow (8F to 10F) neourethra. The Kropp procedure (Fig. 74-14) entails tubularizing the anterior bladder wall to implant into the bladder base in a nonrefluxing fashion. Spontaneous voiding is achievable with the Young-Dees-Leadbetter procedure, but catheterization is necessary with the Kropp procedure and may be difficult.

The artificial urinary sphincter is appropriate for children with isolated sphincter dysfunction and adequate bladder capacity. The artificial sphincter consists of an inflatable cuff surrounding the bladder neck, a pressure-regulating balloon reservoir, and a pump located in the scrotum or labia (Fig. 74-15). Activation of the pump shifts fluid to the reservoir to the cuff and opens the urethra to allow voiding. Over time, the cuff refills, closing the urethra to a preselected pressure inherent in the balloon. Cuff erosion occurs because of infection, trauma, or pressure necrosis from a high-pressure balloon.

The sling procedure involves using rectus fascia to encircle the bladder neck, suturing the ends of the rectus abdominis muscle. Injection of Teflon (polytef) and collagen to compress the urethra is sometimes useful.

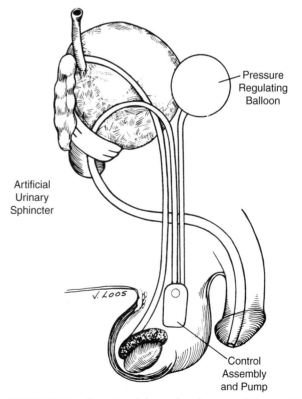

FIGURE 74-15 ■ Functional basis for the use of the artificial urinary spincter (see text).

The Mitrofanoff procedure involves implanting an end of a vascularized tube of intestine into the bladder, while exteriorizing the other end to the abdominal wall. Perineal implantation also can be performed, but over time catheterization may become overly difficult (Fig. 74-16). A flap valve mechanism results in a continent catheterizable stoma, usually made with appendix, ureter, or tapered ileum. Because the appendix is useful in urologic reconstruction, incidental appendectomy should be avoided in children with congenital urologic anomalies. A reconfigured, tubularized piece of ileum as described by Yang and Monti is a currently popular means of providing a catheterizable conduit with an abdominal stoma. The Benchekroun and Koff valves also may be useful in individual situations.

Complications of Bladder Reconstruction

Choosing the appropriate operation for each patient is the best way to avoid complications, taking into consideration preoperative anatomy, physiology, patient ability, and patient motivation. Careful operative technique and regular follow-up may help to prevent complications. Complications specific to urinary tract reconstruction include urinary leaks, perforation of intestinal segments, metabolic derangements, stone formations, diarrhea, and carcinoma.

Leaks can be prevented only with careful technique and appropriate postoperative drainage. Although use of stents may prevent perioperative anastomotic obstruction from edema, they do not prevent leaks. Spontaneous rupture of an augmentation usually occurs late and is located at the suture line or in the intestinal augmentation. Perforation may be associated with impaired sensation but most likely occurs in ischemic watershed areas when the reservoir is overdistended. A high index of suspicion must be maintained when a child presents with signs and symptoms of an acute abdomen because perforation is difficult to diagnose. The contrast cystogram may be diagnostic but not always. Death may result from septic shock caused by the leakage of infected urine so that when the diagnosis is suspected, exploratory laparotomy is in order.

Progressive hypochloremic metabolic acidosis can occur when intestine is used, especially in children with azotemia. Ileal and colonic segments absorb chloride and hydrogen, whereas gastric segments secrete chloride and hydrogen into the urine. Hematuria and dysuria may occur in patients with gastrocystoplasty because of acid irritation of the urethra and bladder. H_2-blockers and proton-pump inhibitors may help to alleviate this problem. A potentially life-threatening complication of augmentation gastrocystoplasty is hypokalemic metabolic alkolosis perpetuated by hypergastrinemia. This can be avoided by

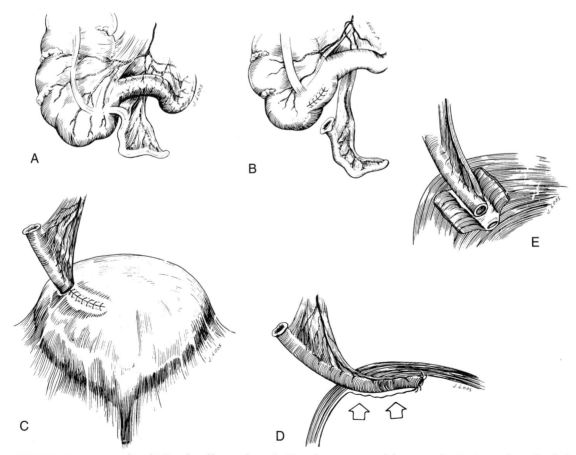

FIGURE 74-16 ■ Appendiceal Mitrofanoff procedure. **A,** Vascular anatomy of the appendix. **B,** Appendix is divided from the cecum and mobilized on the vascular pedicle. **C** and **D,** Appendix is implanted submucosally into the bladder. **E,** Functional basis for Mitrofanoff continence.

TABLE 74-4 ■ Choosing Intestinal Segments

Segment	Advantages	Disadvantages
Jejunum	None	Electrolyte disturbances
Ileum	Easy mobilization to allow bladder augmentation or ureteral replacement; excellent blood supply	Risk of acidosis; difficult to perform nonrefluxing anastomosis; risk of infection
Colon	May perform nonrefluxing ureteral anastomosis; accepts Mitrofanoff neourethra	Risk of acidosis; risk of infection; stone formation
Stomach	Excellent blood supply; easy mobilization; avoids risk of acidosis; nonrefluxing anastomosis;	Technical familiarity with stomach required; small risk of alkalosis; gastric hypersecretion possible
Ileocecal	Technically easy to perform	Loss of ileocecal valve may create incapacitating stool incontinence in children with marginal rectal continence mechanism, e.g., imperforate anus and myelodysplasia

not incorporating antrum into the gastric augmentation and careful long-term metabolic monitoring. Construction of jejunal conduits has been associated with hyponatremic hypochloremic alkalosis, which can be reversed with sodium chloride therapy. Bone demineralization, vitamin B_{12} deficiency, steatorrhea, and long-term growth failure are potential problems. One must be particularly cautious when using an ileocecal segment in reconstruction because loss of the ileocecal valve may cause troublesome diarrhea. This is particularly the case in patients with short-bowel or rectal continence problems,

as seen with myelomeningocele and imperforate anus. In addition, any reconstructive procedure that requires use of a segment of distal bowel should be avoided in patients with neurogenic bladder as a result of imperforate anus because of the risk of devascularizing the distal segment of the pull-through bowel. Table 74-4 summarizes the advantages and disadvantages of the various segments used in urinary reconstructive procedures. Individualization is important. Table 74-5 summarizes how one approaches individualization depending on the problem encountered.

TABLE 74-5 ■ Principles of Pediatric Reconstruction: Operative Strategy

Problem	Principles	Sample Solution
Urine is diverted	Careful assessment of prediversion status Complete preoperative evaluation; consider reflux, obstruction, high-pressure storage, and incontinence Surgical strategy with options prepared before surgery	Preoperative evaluation Renal function assessment (renal scan, GFR) Complete anatomic delineation IVU and VCUG with upright film Retrograde conduit and ureterostomy studies Endoscopy (retrograde injection of ureteral stumps if necessary) Functional assessment CMG UPP or leak pressure Urethroscopy (sphincter) Periurethral EMG Bladder cycling (CIC versus SP tube)
Ureter is too short	Avoid interposed bowel segments if possible Avoid tapered bowel segment implantation into bowel or bladder Uroepithelium-to-uroepithelium anastomosis is best, even if it requires use of much of the bladder	One ureter short: Transureteroureterostomy Psoas hitch/Boari flap Downward renal mobilization Both ureters too short: Psoas hitch/Boari flap Autotransplantation plus ureteropyelostomy Bowel interposition
Ureter is too wide	Two wide ureters often best managed by one long tunnel and transureterostomy Tailored ureteral implantation into bladder preferable to any implantation into bowel Use of ileocecal segment may be preferable to implantation of tapered ureter into bowel Previously tapered ureter should not be retapered because of blood supply concerns (nonresectional tailoring acceptable)	Attempt direct ureteral implantation into bladder No tailoring if 5:1 ratio can be achieved Otherwise excisional tapered or imbricating tailoring bladder implantation If ureter is too short or has been previously tapered, consider ileocecal cystoplasty with modified ileocecal intussusception to create flap valve antireflux mechanism

TABLE 74-5 ■ Principles of Pediatric Reconstruction: Operative Strategy—cont'd		
Problem	**Principles**	**Sample Solution**
Ureterovesical junction is incompetent	Ureterovesical reflux in defunctionalized bladder may resolve after refunctionalization (unless primary reflux is reason for diversion) Ureteral reimplantation into a high-pressure reservoir has a high risk of failure Concomitant upper ureteral undiversion and lower ureteral reimplantation acceptable with meticulous preservation of ureteral blood supply Direct ureteral implantation into bladder if possible is always preferable to bowel interposition	Attempt ureteral implantation into bladder even if augmentation is necessary With concomitant proximal diversion and distal refluxing ureteral stump: Single-stage undiversion Ureteroureterostomy Detrusorrhaphy reimplantation Staged undiversion Avoid dry reimplant Do undiversion first
Bladder too small	Persistent noncompliant or hypertonic CMG curve or inadequate capacity <40 cm H_2O pressure indicates need for augmentation Intermittent catheterization is always anticipated with bladder augmentation Liberal use of bladder augmentation increases chance of success with major reconstruction Avoid tubular bowel segment for augmentation	A detubularized bowel segment is always used for augmentation (e.g., small or large bowel cup patch) Gastrocystoplasty has several metabolic and technical advantages over intestinocystoplasty Bladder cycling may enlarge bladder, facilitating reconstruction and negating need for augmentation (CIC, SP tube, undiversion)
Bladder absent or small	If urethra and continence mechanism intact, attempt to re-establish urethral continuity Creation of alternate Mitrofanoff neourethra provides a source of continent bladder drainage if native urethra fails	If neurologically normal and rectal continence proved by 500 mL saline solution enema, consider internal diversion (nonrefluxing colon conduit, staged colocolostomy) Gastric or colonic neobladder with Mitrofanoff neourethra (may be isotopic) or total bladder "Kropp neourethra"
Urethra incompetent	UPP or leak pressure <40 cm H_2O, quiet EMG, and incompetent bladder neck on upright cystogram—likely incompetent Success of urethral reconstruction without concomitant bladder augmentation is low if low-volume or high-pressure reservoir used Suspension procedures alone are rarely successful in pediatric reconstruction Benefits of AUS consistently outweigh risks only if spontaneous voiding is likely, if no previous bladder neck reconstruction has been performed, and no concomitant bladder augmentation is necessary Anticipated need for CIC is not contraindicated	Young-Dees-Leadbetter urethral lengthening especially applicable to exstrophy; neourethra should be long (>3.5-4 cm) and narrow (10F) for adequate hydraulic resistance Kropp procedure most applicable for neurovesical dysfunction Keeling procedure for iatrogenically divided bladder neck Concomitant Mitrofanoff or Yang-Monti procedure with urethral reconstruction maximizes success: Appendix, extended appendix Ureter, tapered ileum A motivated and functional patient able to empty bladder spontaneously through an intact native urethra is ideal candidate for AUS Selected instances—urethral division and Mitrofanoff neourethra creation
Urethra is inaccessible or nonreconstructable	Successful reconstruction directly dependent on frequent CIC of continent catheterizable channel Compliance directly dependent on patient convenience and potential for self-care	Mitrofanoff procedure: Appendix available—appendiceal Mitrofanoff Appendix unavailable: Ureter Tapered ileum
Patient has ventricular peritoneal shunt	Risk of shunt contamination is present Morbidity of shunt contamination is high Postoperative shunt malfunction may occur	Avoid opening bowel if possible If augmentation is necessary, gastrocystoplasty preferred to intestinocystoplasty Closed suction drainage only Effective temporary urinary diversion (stents or nephrostomy) important to avoid urinary leakage Antibiotic coverage essential
Patient has imperforate anus	Blood supply to previously reconstructed anus is primarily descending	Avoid use of colon segments for urinary reconstruction

TABLE 74-5 ■ Principles of Pediatric Reconstruction: Operative Strategy—cont'd		
Problem	**Principles**	**Sample Solution**
Patient has marginal fecal continence	All patients with myelodysplasia or imperforate anus assumed to have marginal fecal continence Removal of ileocecal segment may produce intractable incontinence	Use of ileocecum for reconstruction
Patient has chronic renal failure	Incorporation of intestine into urinary tract may result in metabolic disturbances (acidosis) Pretransplant augmentation needed in some patients and is much preferable to post-transplant augmentation	Gastrocystoplasty is augmentation modality of choice

GFR, glomerular filtration rate; IVU, intravenous urography; VCUG, voiding cystourethrogram; CMG, cystometrogram; UPP, urethral pressure profile; EMG, electromyogram; CIC, clean intermittent catheterization; SP, suprapubic; AUS, artificial urinary sphincter.

Modified from Sheldon CA, Snyder HM: Principles of pediatric urinary reconstruction. In Gillenwater JY, Grayhack JT, Howards SS, et al (eds): Adult and Pediatric Urology, 2nd ed. St Louis, Mosby-Year Book, 1991.

SUGGESTED READINGS

Atala A: Future perspectives in reconstructive surgery using tissue engineering. Urol Clin North Am 26:157-165, 1999.

This article describes how bladder augmentation may be approached in the future.

Borer JG, Retik AB: Improving outcome in pediatric bladder replacement surgery. Contemp Urol 13:75-91, 2001.

This article presents an excellent summary of necessary monitoring and aftercare in patients.

Glassberg KI: The valve bladder syndrome: 20 years later. J Urol 166:1406-1414, 2001.

This article presents long-term data on the problem of high bladder pressures despite relief of urethral valve obstruction, why the problem must be followed, and available solutions.

Koff SA, Wagner TT, Jayanthi VR: The relationship among dysfunctional elimination syndromes, primary vesicoureteral reflux and urinary tract infections in children. J Urol 160:1019-1022, 1998.

A good description is provided of the relationship between bladder dysfunction and upper tract damage.

Mingin GC, Nguyen HT, Mathias RS, et al: Growth and metabolic consequences of bladder augmentation in children with myelomeningocele and bladder exstrophy. Pediatrics 110:1193-1203, 2002.

This is an encouraging follow-up study of outcome after bladder augmentation, which stresses the value of close follow-up.

Monti PR, Lara RC, Dutra MA, de Carvalho JR: New techniques for construction of efferent conduits based on the Mitrofanoff principle. Urology 1997; 49:112-115, 1997.

This article describes how reconfigured tabularized ileum may be used as a continent catheterizable stoma.

Bladder Exstrophy

75

Bladder exstrophy is an abnormality of bladder and abdominal wall development in which the anterior wall of the bladder and the overlying abdominal musculature is displaced. The bladder, urethra, and ureteral orifices are exposed on the surface of the open bladder. The pubic bones are widely displaced laterally with incomplete formation of the pelvic floor muscles and urinary sphincters. In the complete complex, this musculoskeletal abnormality also is associated with complete epispadias.

Isolated epispadias is a closely related abnormality that occurs in boys and girls. The bladder and abdominal wall are closed in this anomaly. In boys, it involves transposition of the urethra to the dorsal part of the penis with exposure of the urethra on the penile shaft. This is associated with foreshortening of the forward extension of the penis and dorsal chordee or upward curvature of the penis. Depending on the severity of the defect, the urethral meatus can be anywhere on the dorsal aspect of the penis. More proximal lesions are associated with urinary incontinence resulting from sphincter insufficiency. Epispadias in girls is associated with a patulous urethra, which often is displaced anteriorly and associated with incontinence. Female epispadias and exstrophy are associated with anterior displacement of the vaginal introitus and the anus.

Cloacal exstrophy is the most severe form of the spectrum of exstrophy. In this anomaly, the bladder and a large portion of the hindgut are exposed on the anterior abdominal wall. Omphalocele is usually present.

EMBRYOLOGY

The embryogenesis of exstrophy is controversial. The abnormality is thought to develop at 4 to 10 weeks' gestation. The most widely held theory speculates abnormal overdevelopment of the cloacal membrane. The variability and extent of the defect depend on the timing of rupture of this membrane. Classic bladder exstrophy results from a rupture of the membrane after complete division of the cloaca into the urogenital sinus and rectum. Cloacal exstrophy would develop when the rupture of the membrane occurs before cloacal division.

CLINICAL FEATURES AND DIAGNOSIS

Figure 75-1 shows the wide spectrum of the exstrophy complex. Diastasis pubis is associated with a laterally separated pubis and rectus abdominis muscle. This can be seen on physical examination with palpation or on radiographs. The bladder, genitalia, and remainder of the abdominal wall are intact with this anomaly.

Isolated male and female epispadias are two additional forms of the exstrophy complex evident on physical examination. Only the urethra and genitalia are involved (Fig. 75-1B and C). Classic exstrophy (Fig. 75-1D) with the combination of bladder exstrophy and epispadias and diastasis pubis is the most common form of the complex.

Supravesical fissure is much less common and is not associated with genital anomalies or urinary incontinence (Fig. 75-1E). This abnormality is associated with an isolated plate of bladder mucosa that is exposed ventrally in an infraumbilical position. There is usually a small bladder fistula and diastasis pubis. One may or may not be able to show communication between the fissure and the bladder. Exstrophy also can occur with a duplicate bladder in which one hemibladder may be exposed and one covered. If present, the associated epispadiac urethra almost always is connected to the underlying bladder. Careful examination to identify both ureteral orifices that may enter the separate hemibladders is necessary to avoid missing a diagnosis.

EXSTROPHY OF THE URINARY BLADDER

Classic bladder exstrophy has an incidence of approximately 1 in 30,000 to 40,000 live births. Boys predominate over girls by a ratio of 3:1 or 4:1. Figure 75-2 shows the appearance of a girl and a boy presenting with classic exstrophy.

Diagnosis

Bladder exstrophy can be recognized on prenatal ultrasound. Key elements of the diagnosis include absence of cyclical bladder filling, a low-set umbilicus, widened pubic bones, small genitalia, and an echogenic mass in the lower abdomen representing the exstrophic bladder.

The initial diagnostic evaluation at birth consists of renal ultrasound and physical examination. One attempts to estimate the size of the bladder plate and identify a ureteral orifice that would drain each of the kidneys identified by ultrasound.

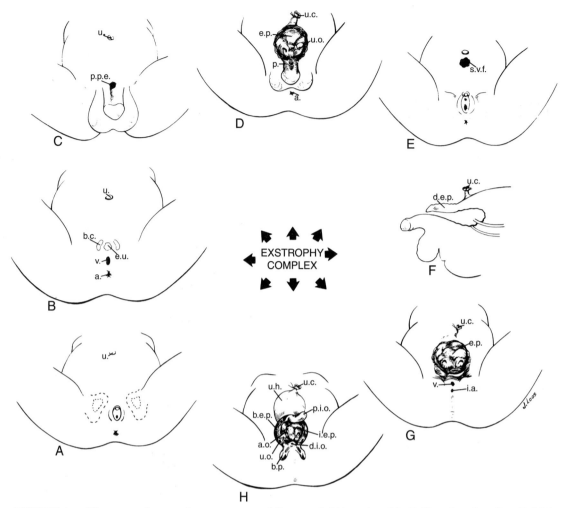

FIGURE 75-1 ■ The exstrophy complex: a spectrum of diseases. **A,** Diastasis pubis. **B,** Female epispadias. **C,** Male epispadias. **D,** Classic bladder exstrophy. **E,** Supravesical fissure. **F,** Duplex exstrophy. **G,** Bladder exstrophy with imperforate anus. **H,** Cloacal exstrophy. u., umbilicus; b.c., bifid clitoris; e.u., epispadic urethra; p.p.e., penopubic epispadias; a., anus; p., penis; u.o., ureteral orifice; e.p., exstrophic plate; u.c., umbilical cord; s.v.f., supravesical fistula; d.e.p., duplicate exstrophic plate; v., vagina; i.a., imperforate anus; u.h., umbilical hernia; p.i.o., proximal intestinal orifice; i.e.p., intestinal exstrophic plate; d.i.o., distal intestinal orifice; b.p., bifid penis; b.c.p., bladder exstrophic plate; d.o., appendiceal orifice.

Treatment

Management begins at birth. With recognition of exstrophy, the umbilical cord should be sutured and the umbilical clamp removed to avoid trauma to the exposed bladder plate. A nonadherent plastic wrap dressing (e.g., Saran wrap) should be applied, and great care must be taken to prevent abrasion of the exposed bladder mucosa until the time of bladder closure.

The first reconstructive procedure is best performed in the immediate neonatal period. In rare cases, the bladder is small and fibrotic and may not be amenable to neonatal closure. The benefit of neonatal reconstruction is the relative ease of pelvic and bladder closure because of the pliability of the pelvic ring in the neonate. Although the use of bilateral iliac osteotomy at this age is still controversial, many find that its routine use optimizes early and late results. Early reconstruction also results in a bladder plate that is less fibrotic and more pliable. In addition, the intestinal tract contains only meconium and has been colonized minimally by bacteria, lowering the risk of postoperative infection.

Many surgeons have found that osteotomy assists with closing the symphysis pubis. There are several benefits to osteotomy, including a more anatomic positioning of the bladder, bladder neck, and urethra in the pelvis. Osteotomy also brings the proximal corpora cavernosa together as they insert into the ischial tuberosity, which is widely separated in exstrophy patients (Fig. 75-3). This procedure also provides for additional penile lengthening. Most surgeons would agree that infants more than 72 hours old, newborns with a wide pubic diastasis, and patients who have had a previously failed bladder exstrophy closure are excellent candidates for osteotomy. This procedure helps secure the midline closure and prevents dehiscence. Some surgeons also use osteotomy in a more routine fashion in an attempt to restore more normal musculoskeletal anatomy.

Several techniques are described for osteotomy, including an anterior and posterior approach to iliac osteotomy. There has been a large experience from Johns Hopkins University using combined anterior innominate and vertical iliac osteotomies, which have produced improved

FIGURE 75-2 ■ Bladder exstrophy. **A,** Girl with a large bladder plate. Note the ureteral orifices and vagina. **B,** Boy with a small bladder plate.

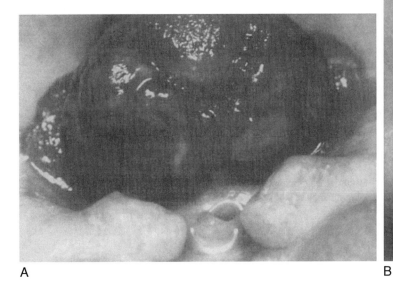

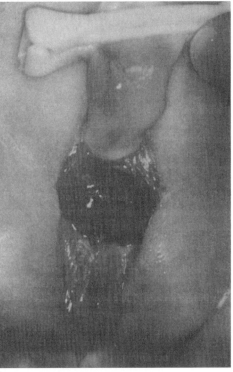

A   B

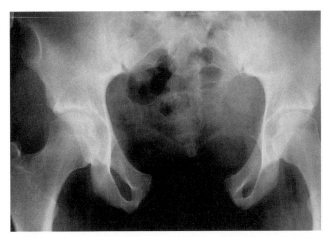

FIGURE 75-3 ■ Radiograph shows wide pubic diastasis in an adolescent with exstrophy.

long-term results with regard to continence and pelvic stability.

There are currently two schools of thought regarding technique for closure of bladder exstrophy. The more traditional approach involves a planned staged repair beginning with an initial neonatal bladder closure (Fig. 75-4). This is followed by epispadias repair, usually performed at 12 to 18 months of age in an attempt to increase outlet resistance to provide a larger bladder volume for later reconstruction. The epispadias repair also can be combined with the initial bladder closure, although this is a technically demanding procedure even in the hands of an experienced surgeon. The traditional third stage is bladder

neck reconstruction, which usually is performed at 4 or 5 years of age or when there is adequate bladder capacity to tubularize the posterior bladder neck. Alternatively, complete primary repair for exstrophy can be performed in the neonatal period. This repair involves complete bladder closure, repositioning of the bladder and bladder neck posterior to the pelvis within the pelvic diaphragm, and total penile disassembly with transposition of the urethra to the ventral aspect of the corporeal bodies (Fig. 75-5). Whichever technique is employed, the initial closure has the greatest impact on the ultimate ability to obtain continence.

The staged approach to bladder exstrophy closure begins with circumferential body preparation to allow movement of the infant from the prone to supine position if needed for pelvic osteotomies. A traction suture is placed through the glans penis, and 3.5F ureteral stents are placed in each ureter. An incision outlining the exstrophic bladder plate is made. The umbilical cord can be excised, which theoretically would reduce the risk of infection, or alternatively it is left attached to one of the umbilical arteries and transposed superiorly to allow a more normal anatomic position above the iliac crest. If the umbilicus is resected, several procedures are described to reconstruct the umbilicus at a later date. The bladder must be completely mobilized deep into the pelvis with a great deal of attention directed to preserving its lateral blood supply. The peritoneum must be reflected intact off the posterior bladder wall. Previously the bladder plate would be divided from the penis and urethra and paraexstrophy flaps used to bridge this gap created between the prostate and the penile urethra. More recent techniques have avoided the need for paraexstrophy flaps

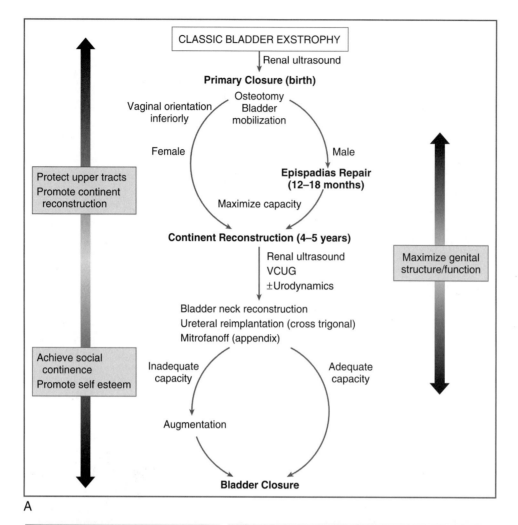

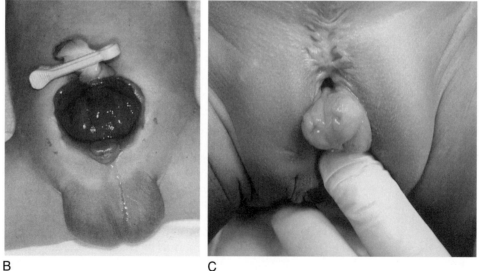

FIGURE 75-4 ■ Traditional staged bladder exstrophy repair. **A,** Conceptual approach to classic bladder exstrophy reconstruction. **B,** Neonate before closure. **C,** Penopubic epispadias created after initial bladder closure. The epispadias repair is performed at 1 to 2 years of age.

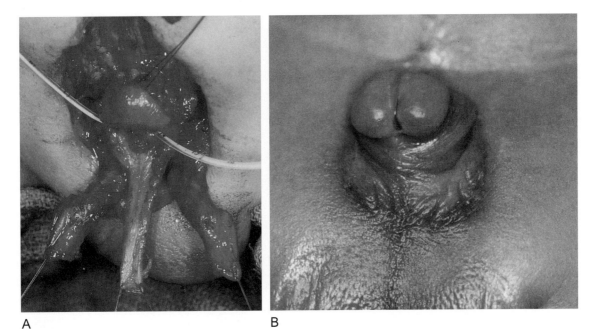

A   B

FIGURE 75-5 ■ Complete penile disassembly to correct epispadias. **A,** The urethral plate is separated from the two corporeal bodies, and the glans is divided in the midline, completely separating each corporeal body. **B,** Early postoperative result, with correction of severe dorsal chordee and ventally placed urethra.

by more aggressive bladder dissection at the bladder neck to allow posterior positioning of the entire bladder and bladder neck. Dissection of the corpora cavernosa off the inferior pubic rami must be done carefully to preserve their blood supply because vascular injury during this step leads to atrophy or complete ischemia of one or both corporeal bodies. The bladder and urethra are tubularized after exteriorizing the ureteral stents and placing a suprapubic tube.

In boys and girls, closure of the pelvic ring is performed by reapproximating the pubic bone over the closed urethra. This reapproximation should be done with one or two nonabsorbable monofilament sutures with care taken to place the sutures so that the knot remains anterior to the approximated pubis and urethra. This avoids the complication of erosion into the neourethra, creating a fistula and possible late stone formation and urinary tract infection.

The technique for staged reconstruction of a girl with bladder exstrophy is similar with aggressive dissection of the lateral bladder to allow positioning into the deep pelvis. In addition, the vagina must be mobilized to allow more posterior positioning at this time. This can be performed using a total urogenital sinus mobilization technique with movement of the urethra and vaginal introitus posterior in the perineum (Fig. 75-6).

Postoperatively, patients are maintained on prophylactic antibiotics. An elastic dressing is placed around the pelvis and lower extremities, and lower extremity traction is maintained for 3 weeks to prevent distractive forces on the pubic closure. Occasionally, mechanical ventilation and sedation are required. Parenteral nutrition is used as needed until gastrointestinal function returns.

Careful follow-up after discharge includes evaluating for postvoid residual urine, renal ultrasound to ensure

that upper tract deterioration does not occur, and antimicrobial suppression for vesicoureteral reflux. Urinary retention can occur due to stenosis of the neourethra. Obstruction with urinary tract infection and reflux pyelonephritis can be a devastating complication, so every effort must be made to avoid infection.

Girls require no further reconstruction until approximately 4 years of age. Boys who did not undergo complete exstrophy and epispadias repair should undergo penile reconstruction at approximately 1 to 2 years of age. Bladder outlet reconstruction is performed at approximately 4 years of age. Before performing continent reconstruction, complete diagnostic evaluation of the kidneys and urinary tract is necessary. This would include renal imaging by ultrasound and nuclear renal scan, voiding cystourethrogram, formal urodynamic studies, and cystoscopy.

Continent reconstruction of the bladder outlet has the basic goal of restructuring the functional bladder outlet to provide urethral lengthening to increase the outlet resistance. This also is a technically demanding procedure because it requires making a long enough and tight enough bladder outlet not only to create social continence, but also to allow the child to void through this controlled stricture of the urethra. This procedure is essentially always necessary and usually takes the form of Young-Dees-Leadbetter procedure or one of the variations described in Chapter 74. Because almost all patients with bladder exstrophy have vesicoureteral reflux, the ureters can be moved away from the bladder neck during ureteral reimplantation, allowing space for bladder neck tubularization. The cross-trigonal ureteral reimplantation technique maximizes the amount of space available for urethral lengthening.

Urethral lengthening procedures are designed to achieve three goals to be considered successful: adequate patency to permit voiding, continence, and, as an

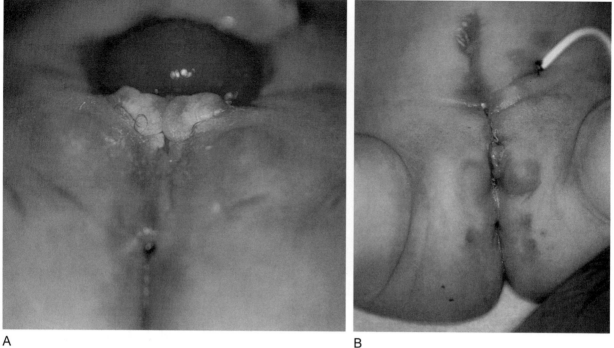

A   B

FIGURE 75-6 ■ Repair of female epispadias. **A,** Anterior orientation of vagina and anus and bifid clitoris. **B,** Initial result at 4 weeks. The suprapubic tube is left in place until residual urine is minimal.

alternative to continence, ability to catheterize to empty the bladder. Use of the Mitrofanoff procedure has simplified these requirements for urethral reconstruction, allowing a more aggressive bladder outlet tightening procedure for urinary continence, while providing an alternate route for bladder catheterization if needed. Occasionally, bladder augmentation using intestine is required in patients with small bladder plates.

Children and parents require medical, social, and psychological support to deal with this severe anatomic abnormality. This support involves efforts to obtain social urinary continence and to normalize the appearance of the external genitalia. In girls, delayed monsplasty and umbilicoplasty are performed at the time of continent reconstruction to allow a more normal appearance of the external genitalia and lower abdomen.

Occasionally, patients are encountered in whom previous attempts at bladder reconstruction have resulted in loss of the bladder plate. These patients frequently require complete urinary diversion to control infections, stones, and azotemia.

Complications of bladder exstrophy reconstruction include hydronephrosis, urinary tract infection, and incontinence. Hydronephrosis generally is caused by bladder outlet obstruction. Bacteria frequently are related to stasis of urine owing to urinary retention and occasionally contamination by intermittent catheterization.

Incontinence results from inadequate urethral length or a bladder that is too small with poor compliance. The reported incidence of incontinence varies considerably in the literature. Mild incontinence almost always improves with age, especially in boys with growth of the prostate. Recapturing continence is more difficult than achieving it at the time of the staged reconstruction.

Depending on severity, alternatives include administration of anticholinergic medications, intermittent catheterization, repeat urethral lengthening procedures, and use of an artificial urinary sphincter. As a last resort, bladder augmentation with intestine is sometimes necessary for the small scarred bladder plate. Urolithiasis and renal failure are usually complications of obstructed hydronephrosis and repeat urinary tract infections. When urolithiasis has been managed or azotemia reversed, repeat reconstruction may be required to prevent recurrent episodes.

The strategy for staged surgical reconstruction of bladder exstrophy begins with primary bladder closure at birth. Attention is directed at protecting the upper urinary tract, promoting subsequent continent reconstruction, and maximizing genital structure and function. The upper urinary tract is protected by early bladder closure, suppressive antibiotics, avoidance of emergence baths, and careful follow-up. Continent reconstruction is attempted when the bladder capacity has been maximized in childhood. An alternative to the classic three-stage surgical approach would be to combine the exstrophy closure with epispadias repair in the neonatal period. This is a challenging surgical procedure and adds the potential complications of injury to the corporeal bodies, which are much smaller and more delicate in the neonatal period.

Genital structure and function are maximized by posterior repositioning of the vagina in girls and by early epispadias repair by 1 or 2 years of age in boys. A final goal is achievement of social continence and promotion of self-esteem. This necessitates a realistic and aggressive continent reconstruction with attention to cosmetics of the lower abdomen, including neoumbilicus and monsplasty is some patients.

EPISPADIAS

Isolated epispadias occurs in approximately 1 in 100,000 live births. Boys are affected four times more often than girls. Figure 75-7 shows the spectrum of epispadias, which can range from balanic (glanular) epispadias, which occurs in less than 5%, to mid penile epispadias (occurring in about 20%), with the remainder penopubic or more proximal epispadias. Reconstruction of penile epispadias focuses on the crucial element of penile lengthening, correction of the upward or dorsal curvature of the corporeal bodies, and complete reconstruction of the deficient urethra. This employs a variety of adjunctive surgical techniques that usually are used for repair of hypospadias. A more recent technique described employs complete penile disassembly with proximal and distal corporeal rotation and placement of the urethra completely on the ventral aspect of the penile shaft. This type of urethral disassembly and reconstruction risks creation of hypospadias if the urethra is not of adequate length to reach the ventral glans. This problem is not encountered with the more traditional Cantwell-Ransley approach, in which the urethral plate is left in continuity with the distal glans.

CLOACAL EXSTROPHY

Cloacal exstrophy has an incidence of approximately 1 in 200,000 live births. Boys are affected more commonly than girls. Figure 75-8 shows the usual anatomy of the

FIGURE 75-7 ■ Male epispadias. **A,** Glanular epispadias. **B,** Penopubic epispadias.

A

B

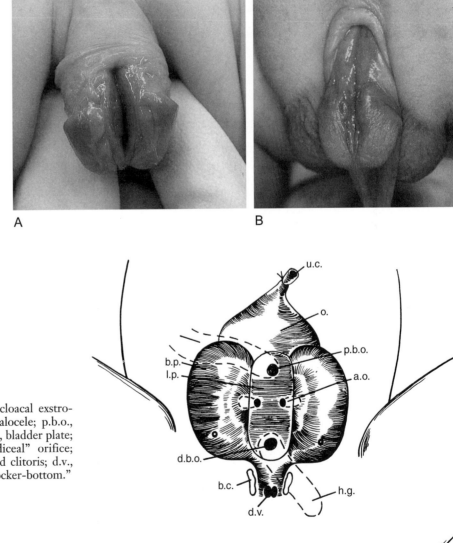

FIGURE 75-8 ■ Topical anatomy of cloacal exstrophy. u.c., umbilical cord; o., omphalocele; p.b.o., proximal bowel orifice; i., ileum; b.p., bladder plate; i.p., intestinal plate; a.o., "appendiceal" orifice; d.b.o., distal bowel orifice; b.c., bifid clitoris; d.v., duplex vagina; h.g., hindgut; r.b., "rocker-bottom."

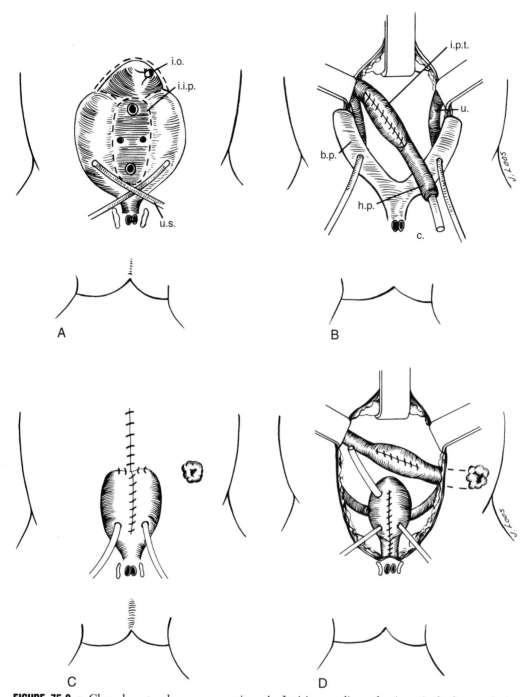

FIGURE 75-9 ■ Cloacal exstrophy reconstruction. **A,** Incision outlines the intestinal plate and the omphalocele. **B,** Intestinal plate tubularized and hindgut preserved. **C,** Bladder plates are approximated in midline, and the abdomen is closed with creation of hindgut stoma. **D,** When possible, the bladder may be tubularized along with paraexstrophy flap neourethral construction at the same setting. Otherwise, this is performed at a separate setting. i.o, incision outlining omphalocele; i.i.p., incision outlining intestinal plate; u.s., ureteral stent; i.p.t., intestinal plate tubularized; u., ureter; b.p., bladder plate; h.p., hindgut preserved; c., catheter.

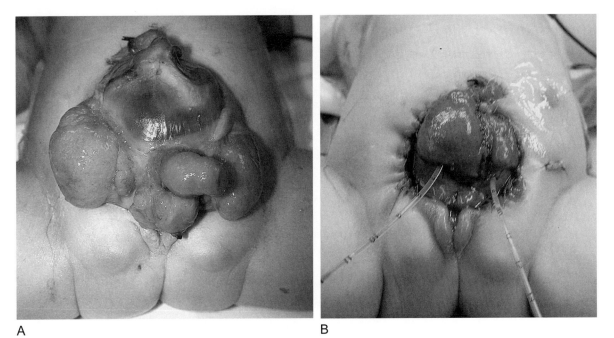

FIGURE 75-10 ■ Cloacal exstrophy in genetic female. **A,** Initial presentation with prolapsed terminal ileum and moderate omphalocele. **B,** Initial closure with creation of midline exstrophic bladder plate because abdominal wall could not be closed safely.

cloacal plate. Two laterally placed hemibladders are divided by a midline intestinal plate. Careful examination of the intestinal plate reveals a proximal bowel orifice that leads to the terminal ileum. This portion of the ileum frequently is prolapsed. A distal bowel orifice leads to the hindgut, which can be extremely short in some patients. One or two additional orifices usually represent a single or duplicate appendix. The ureteral orifices to both hemibladders may be identified when two kidneys are present.

Cloacal exstrophy is associated much more commonly with additional severe abnormalities. Intestinal abnormalities include cecal exstrophy, a blind-ending hindgut, and a foreshortened midgut. This condition results in a predisposition to malabsorption and failure to thrive. Spinal abnormalities are common and include vertebral anomalies, myelomeningocele, spinal cord tethering, and a "rocker bottom," which is generally predictive of an extremely poor prognosis for functional pelvic floor musculature reconstruction.

Renal anomalies are common and include renal agenesis, renal ectopia, and fusion anomalies. Omphalocele is a common finding with cloacal exstrophy and may complicate surgical reconstruction because of the deficiency of the abdominal wall musculature. Boys generally have a small bifid penis, and girls frequently have duplication of the vagina but also may have vaginal atresia or agenesis. Almost 50% of patients with cloacal exstrophy are premature.

Management

Management begins with stabilization and gender assignment. Traditionally, all patients were given a female gender assignment because the phallic structures in most males were considered inadequate for male reconstruction. Psychosexual development of gender-converted genetic males has become a controversial issue, and the decision to assign the female gender should be made only after chromosome analysis and extensive parental counseling with input from a pediatric endocrinologist, psychiatrist, urologist, and surgeon. With improvements in male phallic reconstruction, most genetic males can be reconstructed successfully. Figure 75-9 outlines the initial steps directed at reconstruction. Closure of the omphalocele is completed first; this may be performed with or without simultaneous bladder closure. Intestinal reconstruction is performed beginning with an incision that encompasses the entire intestinal plate and that allows tubularization of the plate over a large catheter. This allows careful evaluation of the internal structure of the hindgut in which obstructive lesions may be encountered. The hindgut is brought out as a stoma. Only rarely is anal reconstruction subsequently entertained because of the poor muscular support of the pelvis.

Bladder closure is performed as previously described for exstrophy. In some cases, this is not possible because the abdominal wall deficiency is too great to allow closure of the omphalocele and the bladder. In this case, the bladder plates are approximated in the midline, leaving the exstrophic bladder to replace a portion of the anterior abdominal wall (Fig. 75-10). Subsequent reconstruction and bladder augmentation, and genital reconstruction as appropriate, are performed.

Figure 75-11 outlines the surgical strategy for cloacal exstrophy reconstruction. The concerns are the same as those described for bladder reconstruction for classic exstrophy. Additional concerns center around genital reconstruction and preservation of intestinal length.

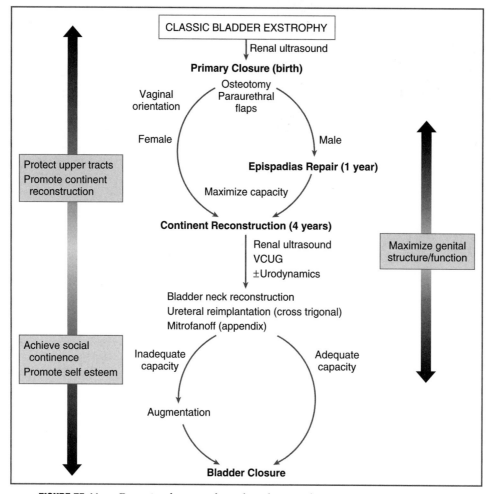

FIGURE 75-11 ■ Conceptual approach to cloacal exstrophy reconstruction (see text).

Most cloacal exstrophy patients have a tendency for short gut physiology initially but eventually recover. Every effort must be made to preserve the entire hindgut and intestinal plate. The surgeon should never sacrifice these structures to facilitate bladder closure. The use of gastrocystoplasty, if augmentation or neobladder creation is required, makes this sacrifice unnecessary.

SUGGESTED READINGS

Gearhart JP: The bladder exstrophy-epispadias-cloacal exstrophy complex. In Gearhart JP, Rink RC, Mouriquand PD (eds): Pediatric Urology. Philadelphia, WB Saunders, 2001, pp 511–546.

The author presents a detailed description of urinary reconstruction and the principles involved in patients with cloacal exstrophy.

Gearhart JP, Jeffs RD: Techniques to create urinary continence in the cloacal exstrophy patient. J Urol 146:616–618, 1991.

The staged procedures necessary to promote urinary continence in patients with this extreme form of bladder exstrophy are described.

Grady R, Mitchell ME: Complete repair of exstrophy. J Urol 162:1415, 1999.

The authors describe current approaches to bladder closure, pelvic approximation, and subsequent epispadias repair and subsequent management.

Mitchell ME, Bagley DJ: Complete penile disassembly for epispadias repair: The Mitchell technique. J Urol 155:300 1996.

This article provides a thorough description of how to deal with severe forms of epispadias, including urethral reconstruction.

76

Prune Belly Syndrome

Prune belly syndrome also is called the *triad syndrome* because when fully expressed, three classic manifestations are present: (1) absence or deficiency of the musculature of the abdominal wall; (2) bilateral cryptorchidism; and (3) urinary tract malformation, specifically a dilated collecting system and distal ureters and an enlarged bladder (Fig. 76-1). In some instances, not all of the three classic criteria of the syndrome are present. Absence of the abdominal musculature together with urinary tract dilation occasionally occurs in girls and boys without undescended testicles. Under these two circumstances, the term *pseudo–prune belly syndrome* has been used.

The overall incidence of prune belly syndrome is 1 in 35,000 to 40,000 live births. It occurs more commonly in twin pregnancies, blacks, and children of younger mothers. The clinical outcome varies dramatically from neonatal mortality due to renal failure and pulmonary

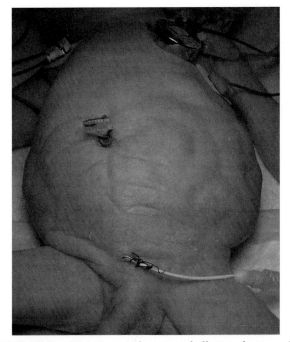

FIGURE 76-1 ■ Neonate with prune belly syndrome with distended bladder and abdomen, flared lower rib cage, and undescended testicles.

hypoplasia to stable long-term renal function and normal life expectancy.

EMBRYOLOGY

Although no specific genetic basis has been found for prune belly syndrome, the male predominance has suggested a sex-linked inheritance. Only rarely have any definable chromosomal anomalies been found, however. With regard to embryology, several theories have been offered. None of them fully explain the genitourinary manifestations of this syndrome. One theory suggests that the primitive yolk sac does not resorb but persists after the abdominal wall closes around it during early stages of gestation; this leaves the abdominal wall musculature highly redundant. Persistence of the yolk sac also partly could explain the abnormalities of the urachus, bladder, and prostatic urethra seen in this syndrome.

Transient in utero bladder outlet obstruction with massive bladder distention also has been postulated as the cause of the urinary tract dilation and the severe stretching and maldevelopment of the abdominal wall. The distended bladder also could cause mechanical obstruction of the normal pathway of testicular descent, leaving the testis intra-abdominal. This theory relies on severe obstruction with massive dilation of the urinary tract early in gestation with spontaneous relief later in gestation because most patients do not have any demonstrable evidence of outlet obstruction at birth. Another argument against this theory is the fact that most infants with posterior urethral valves or other causes of obstruction of the bladder outlet do not tend to have significant abdominal musculature problems.

A third theory to explain prune belly syndrome is known as the *mesodermal defect theory*, which suggests an arrest or deficiency in mesenchymal migration of the thoracic somites forming the lateral plate of the abdominal wall. This theory also could explain deficiencies in development of the genitourinary tract, which are derived in part from the lateral plate of the mesoderm. If these mesenchymal components are deficient and unresponsive to hormonal stimuli, cryptorchidism and hypoplasia of the prostatic urethra could occur. A poorly supported membranous urethra may cause angulation and obstruction of the bladder outlet. This theory would

751

combine a defect in the development of the mesoderm and transient outlet obstruction of the bladder with regard to overall etiology.

CLINICAL MANIFESTATIONS

Table 76-1 summarizes clinical manifestations.

Genitourinary

Regardless of the organ system involved, the severity of the various manifestations of prune belly syndrome is highly variable. This is particularly true of the genitourinary tract, and for the most part, this is the limiting factor in terms of morbidity and mortality. There is no correlation between the degree of deficiency of the abdominal musculature and the status of the genitourinary tract. Renal dysplasia or even full-fledged Potter's syndrome occasionally may be present, under which circumstances maternal oligohydramnios usually is seen.

Kidneys

The kidneys in patients with prune belly syndrome are normal in approximately 50% of cases, and in the remaining 50%, some degree of renal dysplasia is present.

TABLE 76-1 ■ Clinical Manifestations of Prune Belly Syndrome

Site	Finding
Abdominal wall	Absence or deficiency of abdominal musculature
Kidney	Some degree of dysplasia in 50% Pelvic dilation without obstruction Abnormalities of rotation and internal structure
Ureters	Asymmetrically dilated, tortuous ureters, typically marked in the lower third
Bladder	Large, thick-walled nontrabeculated, irregular in shape; urachal diverticulum, cyst, or patent urachus
Prostate and urethra	Prostate hypoplastic, prostatic urethra excessively dilated Penile urethra may be mildly dilated, scaphoid megalourethra with deficiency of corpora spongiosa; severe fusiform megalourethra with deficiency of corpora cavernosa Urethral atresia rare
Testes	Abdominal cryptorchidism Deficient spermatogenesis, normal hormonal production
Cardiovascular	10% incidence including ventricular and atrial septal defects, patent ductus, tetralogy of Fallot
Pulmonary	Hypoplasia of lung and chest wall, cystic adenomatoid malformation
Gastrointestinal	Malrotation, omphalocele, imperforate anus
Musculoskeletal	Talipes equinovarus, arthrogryposis multiplex, hip dislocation, polydactyly, limb absence

Dysplasia is a histologic diagnosis, and currently available information suggests that dysplasia is present on a developmental basis rather than resulting from obstruction. The two kidneys may have different degrees of hydronephrosis, function, and dysplasia. Functional impairment shown on nuclear glomerular filtration studies may indicate the degree of renal dysplasia.

Hydronephrosis is seen commonly in patients with prune belly syndrome, but ureteropelvic junction obstruction is uncommon. The character of the renal parenchyma with prune belly syndrome is usually much better than might be expected considering the degree of dilation of the renal pelvis. Some patients with prune belly syndrome have associated urethral atresia. In this subset of patients, small dysplastic kidneys with little or no function frequently are found, leading to a high mortality.

Ureters

The most common genitourinary manifestation of prune belly syndrome is ureteral dilation. Characteristically the ureters are elongated and tortuous, although the degree of involvement varies from patient to patient, and the two ureters frequently are asymmetrically involved. Histologic studies of the ureters have shown fibrosis and deficiency of the smooth muscle of the ureteral wall. The degree of ureteral dilation is usually segmental, with the lower third of the ureter involved more significantly. Occasionally the more proximal one third of the ureter is almost normal in caliber. As would be expected with the degree of dilation, ureteral peristalsis is impaired with significant retention of urine in the upper urinary tract. Vesicoureteral reflux is present in approximately 80% of patients and is associated with lateral placement of the ureteral orifices in the bladder trigone. With long-term observation, the tortuous ureters tend to straighten as the child grows, and generally ureteral peristalsis would be expected to improve. This sometimes can take several years of observation. Prevention of urinary tract infection during this observation period is crucial to prevent upper urinary tract deterioration. Another important point to remember is that the degree of dilation of the urinary tract does not behave similar to and should not be treated similar to urinary tract dilation that is secondary to distal obstruction.

Bladder

The urinary bladder in patients with prune belly syndrome typically is enlarged with a thickened wall and irregular configuration (Fig. 76-2). Trabeculation within the bladder is seen less commonly. Similar to the histology of the renal pelvis and ureter, the bladder wall is thickened, with deficient muscle fibers that have been replaced with excess collagen and fibrous tissue. This leads to abnormal bladder contractility with urinary retention. The ureteral orifices tend to be lateral and asymmetric in location in the bladder.

Despite the abnormal histology of the bladder, most patients with prune belly syndrome have relatively normal urodynamics with normal filling pressures, absence of hypercontractility, and relatively normal compliance. In many patients, bladder sensation during filling is abnormal, however, and with the large-capacity

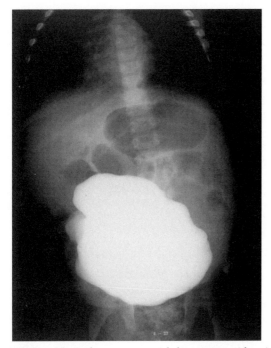

FIGURE 76-2 ■ Typical cystogram with large postvoid residual, with a smooth but irregular contour of the bladder wall.

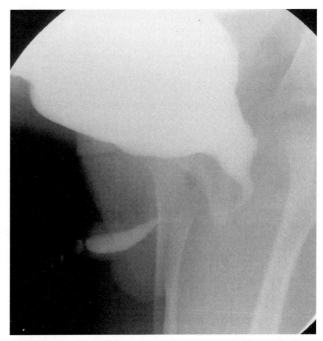

FIGURE 76-3 ■ Voiding cystourethrogram with classic findings of widened prostatic urethra without obstruction, slightly dilated anterior urethra, and urachal diverticulum.

bladder, they develop urinary retention over time. This situation is compounded further by high-grade reflux with constant refilling of the bladder after voiding. These patients are particularly at increased risk for infection so that efforts must be made to keep the urine sterile with the combination of prophylactic antibiotics, timed voiding with occasional double voiding, and intermittent catheterization as required.

At the apex of the dome of the bladder, it is common to see an urachal remnant or diverticulum. In cases of urethral atresia, the urachus may be patent, which provides a pressure pop-off valve and protects the kidney during development in utero.

Prostate and Urethra

Prostatic hypoplasia is characteristic of prune belly syndrome, as is the associated posterior bulging and enlargement of the prostatic urethra (Fig. 76-3). The verumontanum is usually small, as are the ejaculatory ducts. Significant enlargement of the prosthetic urethra compared with the adjacent membranous portion of the urethra would suggest obstruction; however, this is usually not seen. Occasionally an anterior fold of tissue, sometimes called a *pseudovalve*, is seen in the prostatic urethra and can be associated with poor emptying.

The membranous urethra is usually normal, but in some cases of prune belly syndrome, severe stenosis or atresia of the membranous urethra also may be present. These patients generally have small dysplastic kidneys with poor function, and survival is limited in this patient population unless a patent urachus is present. A few case reports have shown improved chance for survival with urethral atresia with in utero vesicoamniotic shunting, when it is established early in pregnancy.

Although the anterior or penile urethra is usually normal in patients with prune belly syndrome, mild urethral dilation is present in at least two thirds of the patients, although usually of little clinical significance. Significant megalourethra also can occur, but this is less common. In severe forms of megalourethra, stasis of urine and subsequent infection can occur, and reconstruction of the urethra would be warranted.

Cryptorchidism

Undescended testes are an essential part of the diagnosis of prune belly syndrome. The testes usually are located within the abdomen overlying the ureters at the level of the iliac arteries. This is thought to be due to mechanical obstruction of the massively dilated bladder in utero, the decrease in abdominal pressure secondary to the absent abdominal musculature, or a combination of both. Although the testes in infants with prune belly syndrome are similar to the testes of normal age-matched controls, over time germ cell maturation is poor even when orchiopexy is performed early. In addition, the peritesticular ductal structures are frequently abnormal, including detachment of the epididymis and irregular tortuosity of the vas deferens, as can be seen with isolated cryptorchidism. Histology of the testis itself is also abnormal, with decreased spermatogonia and Leydig cell hyperplasia frequently identified in the older child. Although it is currently common practice to perform early orchiopexy in these children for psychological reasons, all patients with prune belly syndrome have poor fertility but normal potency. This situation is due to a deficiency of prostatic fluid and inadequate spermatogenesis. Retrograde ejaculation is also common because of the markedly dilated prostatic urethra and open bladder neck.

Sperm has been collected in postejaculate urine specimens in a few patients, with at least one reported pregnancy. The risk of testicular malignancy in patients with prune belly syndrome is similar to that seen in normal patients with abdominal cryptorchidism. Several cases of cancer have been documented, and these patients should undergo lifelong surveillance with testicular self-examination after successful orchiopexy.

Abdominal Wall

As is the case with all organ systems affected with prune belly syndrome, the degree of deficiency of the musculature of the lateral and ventral abdominal wall is diffuse and in a variable pattern, which can be patchy and asymmetric. The primary deficiency in most patients is in the lower abdomen, including the lower portions of the rectus abdominis and the internal and external oblique muscles. The abdominal wall characteristically has a wrinkled and redundant appearance and often the thin abdominal wall allows observation of peristalsis of the intestinal tract. The wrinkled prune-like appearance of the abdomen becomes less evident after the first year of life as more subcutaneous fat is deposited. As children get older, the prominent bulge in both flanks is replaced by a more potbellied appearance consistent with the poor muscle tone in the midline of the lower abdomen. This deficiency in the lower abdominal musculature can cause difficulty in bladder and rectal emptying and difficulty in the ability to sit up, especially early in life.

Another problem that is usually more evident in the neonatal period that is related to the deficiency of the abdominal musculature is the secondary pulmonary effects with retention of pulmonary secretions and increased risk of pneumonia because of the poor abdominal component of coughing and pulmonary toilet. This problem increases the risk of anesthesia in the neonatal period significantly.

Other Associated Malformations

Cardiovascular

Approximately 10% of patients with prune belly syndrome are estimated to have cardiac defects. Most commonly reported are patent ductus arteriosus, ventricular and atrial septal defects, and tetralogy of Fallot, all of which usually present with a heart murmur or cyanosis.

Pulmonary

In patients with renal hypoplasia associated with significant maternal oligohydramnios, pulmonary hypoplasia is common. This is associated with a high neonatal mortality rate and neonatal pneumothorax and pneumomediastinum. The combination of chest wall deformity and abnormal abdominal wall musculature results in increased risk of pneumonia and atelectasis that persists throughout childhood. This risk is critical in the perioperative period because patients require aggressive pulmonary toilet and careful monitoring of postoperative pain medication.

Gastrointestinal

Reported abnormalities of the gastrointestinal tract include malrotation with midgut volvulus and duodenal bands. In severe forms of prune belly syndrome, anorectal atresia can be seen. Constipation is a common problem in prune belly syndrome and usually is attributed to poor abdominal muscle tone.

Skeletal

Numerous musculoskeletal abnormalities have been reported, and many appear to be the result of intrauterine compression of the limbs and thorax related to oligohydramnios. The reported orthopedic abnormalities include dislocation and dysplasia of the hips, absence of a limb, polydactyly, arthrogryposis multiplex, and talipes equinovarus. Flaring of the lateral rib cage also commonly is seen as a result of the marked abdominal distention in utero.

DIAGNOSTIC EVALUATION

The clinical manifestations described in the foregoing section describe all of the many physical characteristics of infants with prune belly syndrome. The cardinal physical findings are, however, absence of the musculature of the abdominal wall, enlarged bladder and urinary tract, cryptorchidism, and occasionally a patent urachus and megalourethra. Infants with typical manifestations of prune belly syndrome initially should be observed and monitored as opposed to resorting to emergency and unnecessary operative intervention.

Prenatal Diagnosis

Prune belly syndrome has been recognized on prenatal ultrasound; however, the antenatal findings may be confused easily with those seen in association with posterior urethral valves, high-grade vesicoureteral reflux, megacystis-microcolon syndrome, omphalocele, and several other congenital anomalies. In addition, because the dilation of the urinary tract seen in patients with prune belly syndrome usually is not associated with obstruction in most cases, antenatal intrauterine intervention with vesicoamniotic shunting usually is not indicated. Several case reports have documented survival in patients without a patent urachus with the usual lethal variant of prune belly syndrome associated with urethral atresia that had early vesicoamniotic shunting, but all of these cases were associated with fairly severe oligohydramnios as an indication for intervention. The prime value of making the diagnosis on a prenatal ultrasound study is to anticipate care that might be needed immediately after birth. Because of the common pulmonary and cardiac complications, these infants should be delivered at high-risk centers with a neonatal intensive care unit. Studies also have indicated that prenatal diagnosis has had a large role in the increasing incidence of elective termination for prenatally diagnosed prune belly syndrome and other severe congenital anomalies.

POSTNATAL DIAGNOSTIC STUDIES

Laboratory Studies

During the first few days of observation after birth, serial measurement of serum electrolytes, blood urea nitrogen, and creatinine should be made to determine if there is evidence of renal functional impairment that may be related to severe dysplasia.

Imaging Studies

The most helpful initial study is ultrasound of the kidneys, ureters, and bladder. This study is capable of visualizing the degree of dilation of the renal collecting system and the thickness of the renal cortex (Fig. 76-4). Ultrasound also is able to show bladder wall thickness and the degree of urinary retention. Unless there is evidence of urinary tract obstruction, any additional imaging studies, especially voiding cystourethrogram, should be deferred for several weeks because of the risk of early infection from instrumentation of the dilated urinary tract. In addition, the results of functional studies often are improved after several weeks have passed when renal physiology has matured. A voiding cystourethrogram often is obtained after approximately 2 to 4 weeks of life when renal function has been stable. It is important to initiate prophylactic antibiotics before obtaining this study. The voiding study usually confirms the presence of vesicoureteral reflux and can give secondary information with regard to bladder contractility and ability to empty. In addition, it provides imaging of the urethra to rule out the rare case of obstruction or dilation of the anterior urethra. Provided that the infant has stable renal function, functional renal radionuclide scans usually are obtained at 1 to 2 months of age. Initial renal scans show the dilated ureters with slow drainage. This usually improves with observation (Fig. 76-5).

At the time the infant with prune belly syndrome is born, rapid assessment of all potentially affected organ systems should be performed. This assessment should include chest films, abdominal films, and echocardiography. If malrotation is suspected, an upper gastrointestinal series should be performed. All infants also should be screened for the possibility of congenital hip dislocation.

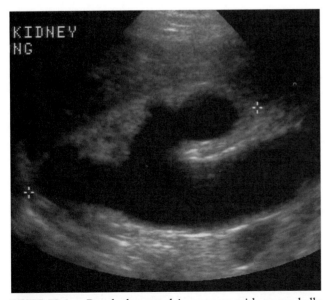

FIGURE 76-4 ■ Renal ultrasound in neonate with prune belly syndrome. Renal parenchyma has increased echogenicity compared with liver suggesting dysplasia. Renal pelvis and proximal ureter are dilated.

MANAGEMENT

The limiting factor in survival is generally the status of the renal function; however, pulmonary and cardiac abnormalities may be severe and require immediate attention after delivery as well. Urinary tract infection is a prime concern throughout the lifetime of these patients. Prophylactic antibiotics should be initiated in the neonatal period, usually with oral amoxicillin followed by trimethoprim-sulfamethoxazole after 2 or 3 months. For specific infections or urosepsis, culture-specific antibiotics should be administered immediately because undetected or incompletely treated infection can result in significant decrease of renal function. Severe infection in the urinary tract may be an indication for drainage of the urinary tract even if this was not indicated initially. Patients with persistent ureteral dilation who have recurrent infections later in life should undergo reconstruction.

Historically, there have been two schools of thought regarding surgical management of the prune belly syndrome patient. Some advocate aggressive surgical reconstruction of the urinary tract in all patients, which is based primarily on experience with other disorders, which shows that eliminating persistent reflux and urinary tract stasis reduces the risk of infection and progressive renal damage. Reconstruction in these patients is technically demanding and is associated with a higher risk of complications even in experienced hands.

The alternative school of thought advocates a nonoperative approach, resorting to surgical intervention only when persistent infection or progressive deterioration in renal function or both occur. With observation and advancing age, ureteral peristalsis and emptying of the upper urinary tract seem to improve, as does bladder emptying. It has been shown that surgical intervention has not improved renal function because this usually is related to underlying preexisting renal dysplasia. Because the results with the nonoperative approach seem to be equal and, in some cases, better than the results with early operation, most clinicians today prefer a nonoperative approach initially.

Urinary Diversion

Initial urinary diversion in the neonatal period is indicated only for the rare infant with a demonstrated site of obstruction. In cases of early deterioration of renal function, obstruction should be suspected rather than dysplasia, which usually takes longer to manifest itself as diminished renal function. The site of external urinary drainage must be selected carefully to avoid injury to the blood supply of the ureter, which may be necessary for later reconstructive procedures.

The simplest and most helpful initial approach to drainage for an obstructed upper urinary tract is placement of percutaneous nephrostomy tubes. A more permanent form of upper tract diversion should be considered only in the case of improved renal function after proximal decompression. If the renal pelvis is markedly dilated compared with the rest of the urinary tract, and percutaneous nephrostomy has shown improvement in renal function, cutaneous pyelostomy would be the best procedure to perform. This is relatively uncommon in

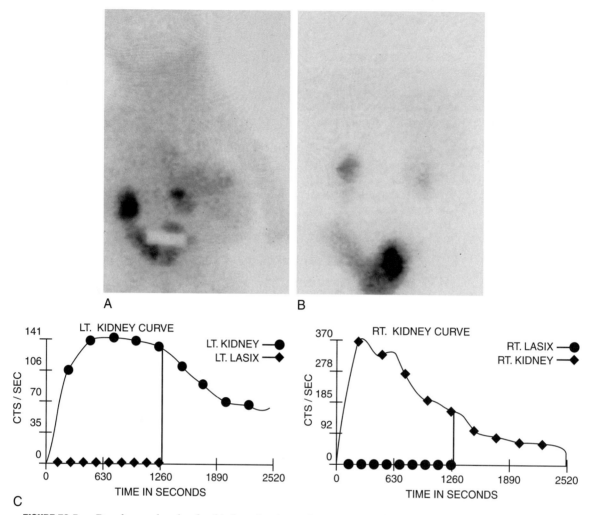

FIGURE 76-5 ■ Renal scan shortly after birth and at 1 year in a patient with prune belly syndrome. **A,** Marked bilateral hydroureteronephrosis with poor drainage. **B,** Significant improvement in drainage with persistent ureteral dilation at 1 year with observation only. **C,** Drainage curve from renal scan at 1 year shows good washout with furosemide (Lasix) in both kidneys.

prune belly syndrome because the upper urinary tract is usually not as dilated as the more distal ureter.

If the renal pelvis is small or only moderately dilated and the ureter is large, cutaneous ureterostomy would be indicated. Great care should be taken in performing this procedure because ureteral vascularity can be compromised, making later reconstruction more difficult. Most commonly, the entire urinary tract is uniformly dilated, and cutaneous vesicostomy provides excellent drainage. Cutaneous vesicostomy is best performed at the dome of the bladder regardless of the site on the abdominal wall. In addition, a large stoma should be created to avoid stenosis (some suggesting a stomal size 30F). One should not expect the dilated upper urinary tract to decrease in size a great deal despite adequate diversion because of the deficiency of the smooth muscle in the wall of the urinary tract.

Alternative to Urinary Diversion

Some clinicians have focused on the poor bladder emptying as the source of urinary stasis and increased risk of infection. Chronic intermittent catheterization has been used but also can lead to bladder contamination and persistent recurrent infections. In addition, these patients frequently have difficulty with urethral catheterization because of the normal sensation in the urethra and occasional abnormalities in the proximal urethra. The Mitrofanoff procedure has provided an excellent alternative channel for bladder emptying in these patients, most commonly by creating an appendicovesicostomy.

Reduction cystoplasty has been recommended in the past with the thought that decreasing the size of the bladder would improve emptying. This is helpful in cases in which there is a large urachal pseudodiverticulum. In most cases, reduction cystoplasty has resulted in late failure, however, due to the gradual re-enlargement of the bladder secondary to poor emptying. If reduction cystoplasty is to be performed, it is probably best done in association with ureteral reconstruction and reimplantation.

Urethral sphincterotomy also has been recommended to improve bladder emptying. This procedure should be used judiciously because most patients have an incompetent bladder neck and depend on the external sphincter for urinary continence.

Urinary Reconstruction

Urinary reconstruction is indicated after diversion when renal function has stabilized or improved. As mentioned earlier, surgical reconstruction in these patients who have a deficiency in peristalsis and the musculature of the urinary tract is exceedingly difficult. It is uniformly agreed on that it is best to discard the poorly functioning redundant distal third of the ureter that tends to have more significant disease, allowing reimplantation of the more healthy proximal ureter. The dilated ureter can be addressed with standard excisional tapering; however, ureteral imbrication also has been used successfully. This avoids the complication of stenosis related to ischemia because the blood supply to the distal dilated structures may be marginal. Ureteral reimplantation is not indicated based on presence of reflux or dilation of the ureter when infection is under control. As previously stressed, the conservative approach to urinary reconstruction is most likely the best solution in most cases.

Abdominoplasty

Either with or without surgical reconstruction, some form of corset or abdominal binder is helpful, particularly early in life, to maximize function of the abdominal wall. The timing of abdominoplasty should be based on the timing of other surgical procedures either for reconstruction of the urinary tract or for orchiopexy. In most instances, this is sometime between 1 and 2 years of age (Fig. 76-6). Several techniques for abdominoplasty have been described using a midline incision with preservation of the umbilicus (this provides optimal exposure for urinary tract reconstruction and transabdominal orchiopexy) or via a low curved abdominal incision.

Orchiopexy

As mentioned previously, the benefit from orchiopexy may be more psychological than physiologic because

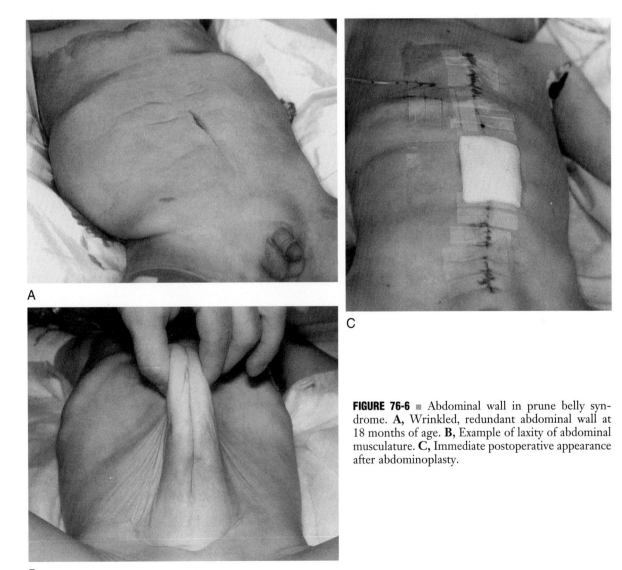

FIGURE 76-6 ■ Abdominal wall in prune belly syndrome. **A,** Wrinkled, redundant abdominal wall at 18 months of age. **B,** Example of laxity of abdominal musculature. **C,** Immediate postoperative appearance after abdominoplasty.

virtually all patients with prune belly syndrome are sterile. Current data suggest, however, that there is some advantage to potential gonadal development with early orchiopexy. In addition, placement of the testis in the scrotum would allow observation for the potential of malignant changes in the testis later in life. Orchiopexy can be performed if any abdominal surgery is required as early as the neonatal period in a stable patient. When orchiopexy is done in the first 6 to 12 months of life, it is frequently possible to mobilize the testis without dividing the primary vascular supply. As the patient gets older, a Fowler-Stevens orchiopexy may be required. With this approach, both spermatic vessels are divided, and the blood supply of the testis is based on the wide peritoneal mesentery surrounding the vascular supply of the vas deferens. This procedure can be performed in either a single or a staged approach in which the vessels are divided in the initial operation, and the testis is brought down at a later stage, allowing maturation of the vasal blood supply. Laparoscopic single-stage and two-stage orchiopexy has been successful and is advantageous when additional abdominal surgery is not required.

PROGNOSIS

The outlook for infants with prune belly syndrome has improved remarkably over the last several decades, although the ultimate outcome is based on the development of the lungs and kidneys and whether dysplasia is present. Renal transplantation and peritoneal dialysis is possible in situations even when renal failure occurs early in life. Previous mortality rates in the first 2 years of life were 50%; however, with improvement in respiratory care, the neonatal mortality rate has improved. Current survival with a conservative surgical approach to management exceeds 70%.

SUGGESTED READINGS

Fallat ME, Skoog SJ, Belman AB, et al: The prune belly syndrome: A comprehensive approach to management. J Urol 142:802-805, 1989.

This excellent review was one of the first to discuss timing of urinary reconstruction and abdominoplasty.

Noh PH, Cooper CS, Winkler AC, et al: Prognostic factors for long-term renal function in boys with the prune belly syndrome. J Urol 162:1399-1401, 1999.

This article provides information on long-term renal function as related to renal dysplasia in patients with prune belly syndrome.

Smith CA, Smith EA, Parrott TS, et al: Voiding function in patients with the prune belly syndrome after Monfort abdominoplasty. J Urol 159:1675-1679, 1998.

This article discusses the urodynamics of the bladder in patients with prune belly syndrome. (See also editorial by Woodard, page 1680.)

Woodard JR, Zucker I: Current management of the dilated urinary tract in prune belly syndrome. Urol Clin North Am 17:407-418, 1990.

A conservative early approach to these patients with close follow-up is discussed.

PART XI

Genitalia

Male External Genitalia

Common considerations related to the male external genitalia are discussed in this chapter, including circumcision, hypospadias, urethral obstruction, and trauma. Genital trauma also is discussed in part in Chapter 13.

CIRCUMCISION

Attitudes toward routine circumcision have varied a great deal through the years because of questions regarding the risks and benefits of the procedure. The American Academy of Pediatrics has published several task force reports on circumcision, and the recommendations have varied widely. In 1971, 1975, and 1983, the American Academy of Pediatrics' official statements concluded that there was no absolute medical indication for routine circumcision. In 1989, additional longitudinal research related to circumcision and its association with urinary tract infection and sexually transmitted disease prompted a change in the recommendation with the publication of a new statement indicating that newborn circumcision has potential medical benefits and advantages as well as disadvantages and risks. After this, other organizations published conflicting statements, some recommending routine circumcision and others not. In 1999, the American Academy of Pediatrics established a task force on circumcision using an evidence-based approach and an extensive meta-analysis. On this basis, they now have recommended that existing scientific evidence shows potential medical benefits of newborn circumcision but that the data are not sufficient to recommend routine neonatal circumcision. They further recommend that with regard to circumcision, in which there are potential benefits and risks, the immediate condition and well-being of the infant be considered when making the decision.

One of the issues related to the perceived need for circumcision is a lack of knowledge about appropriate neonatal care that has resulted in complications, which has supported the concept of routine circumcision. Many male infants today remain uncircumcised, and appropriate management of the foreskin in the newborn must be taught to new parents. Developmentally the interepithelium of the prepuce and the epithelium of the glans are stratified squamous epithelium and initially are fused to one another. The foreskin undergoes a separation process over time that begins at birth and continues throughout childhood. The prepuce is generally not retractable in the newborn; by 6 months, it can be retracted completely in 20% of boys; and by 6 years of age, approximately 40% of boys have total separation of the prepuce from the glans. By adolescence, virtually all males have retractable foreskins. Most errors are a result of inappropriate aggressive attempts at early retraction of the foreskin. Attempts to do so result not only in pain, but also lacerations and abrasion, which leads to progressive scarring at the tip of the prepuce. The resulting ring of scar tissue creates true phimosis, which may be associated with infection or difficulty voiding.

External cleansing of the penis is all that is required in the prepubertal boy. As the attachment between the prepuce and the glans gradually resolves, normal hygienic cleansing should include gentle retraction of the foreskin, but this should not be attempted until at least 12 to 18 months. Use of harsh soaps or abrasive clothing may potentiate further the development of phimosis.

Three approaches to circumcision are generally in use—the Gomco clamp (Allied Healthcare, St. Louis), the Plastibell (Hollister, Inc. Libertyville, FL), and the Mogen clamp (Mogen Care Instruments Ltd., Brooklyn, NY), all applicable to the newborn. After the newborn period, freehand circumcision is indicated. In general, neonatal circumcision is performed approximately 2 hours after the last feeding and after performance of a dorsal penile nerve block. The procedure begins with a thorough sterile preparation, complete separation of the glanular adhesions, sometimes followed by a dorsal slit. It is important to dilate the preputial orifice so that the urethra can be visualized and protected. The clamp is placed with the tension directed at avoiding torsion or tension of the penile shaft skin so that an appropriate amount of preputial skin is removed. When the Gomco or other clamp is secured for 10 minutes, the redundant foreskin is excised, and the clamp is removed, ensuring that hemostasis is secure. If a Plastibell is used, a cotton tie is placed around the clamp, the foreskin is excised, the clamp handle is broken off, and the remainder of the device is permitted to separate over time. The area of junction between the skin and the inner epithelium of the glans is covered with either an antiseptic ointment or a strip of petrolatum gauze. In older patients in whom a freehand technique is necessary, after excision of the redundant foreskin, careful hemostasis is achieved with

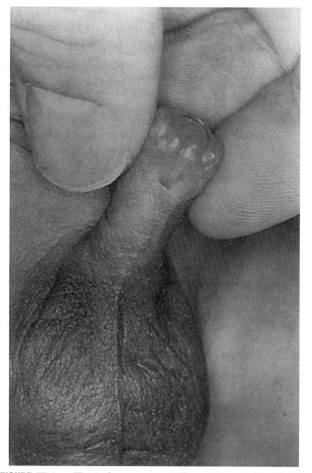

FIGURE 77-1 ▪ Typical appearance of a patient with midshaft hypospadias with excess dorsal prepuce. (From Duckett JW, Baskin LS: Hypospadias. In Gillenwater JY, et al (eds); *Adult and Pediatric Urology*, 3rd ed. St Louis, Mosby-Year Book 1996.)

electrocautery, and the apposing skin edges are approximated with interrupted sutures of fine absorbable suture, which separates in a week or so.

The complications associated with retention of the foreskin are significant and include phimosis; paraphimosis, which may result in the need for an emergency dorsal slit procedure; balanitis; urinary tract infection; a higher risk of sexually transmitted disease; and late occurrence of penile cancer. Virtually all of the latter complications are related to local infection and chronic inflammation, much of which is preventable.

The exact incidence of complications after newborn circumcision is unknown, but various reports indicate that the complication rate may be 1%. Although most complications are minor, serious complications can occur, including persistent bleeding, secondary infection, recurrent phimosis, poor healing, and either inadequate or excessive skin excision. Less common complications include devastating skin and subcutaneous infections, meatal stenosis, urethral fistula, and either amputation or necrosis of all or a portion of the penis or glans.

HYPOSPADIAS

Hypospadias anomalies are understood best through an understanding of the embryology of the male external genitalia. The penis and its associated urethra develop from at least three primordial structures. The glans forms from the genital tubercles, the urethral folds fuse to form the penile urethra, and the scrotum is formed from the primitive genital swellings. Hypospadias includes a spectrum of penile anomalies associated with varying degrees of proximal placement of the urinary meatus. Hypospadias may be associated with ventral curvature of the penis, called *chordee*, which is accentuated by erection. The incidence of hypospadias in newborn boys is 1 in 300 to 500 and appears to be increasing.

Hypospadias is classified best according to the location of the meatus and the presence or absence of chordee (Fig. 77-1). Figure 77-2 outlines one of the many classification systems that have been developed for hypospadias.

An important initial consideration is that circumcision must be avoided and appropriate counseling provided to parents in the newborn period. Circumcision may eliminate more straightforward reconstruction. It is important to council parents that even children with severe hypospadias anomalies are capable of achieving normal voiding and sexual function and that postoperative complications are minimal today.

Many procedures are available for reconstruction of hypospadias depending on its degree as outlined in Table 77-1. The meatal advancement and glanuloplasty (MAGPI) procedure (Fig. 77-3) is appropriate for children with no chordee other than skin tethering and who have a glanular meatus or an extremely mobile subglanular meatus. The Mathieu procedure (Fig. 77-4) is useful for subglanular hypospadias not associated with chordee. Also, it is suited best for patients with good-quality perimeatal skin. The pyramid procedure is useful for indications similar to those described for the Mathieu procedure. It is particularly useful in a patient who has a deep urethral groove or a megameatus. The island flap

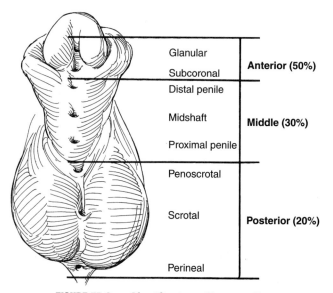

FIGURE 77-2 ▪ Classification of hypospadias.

onlay procedure (Fig. 77-5) is useful in patients who have no chordee but have poor-quality perimeatal skin, deficient ventral shaft skin, significant meatal stenosis, or proximal shaft meatal position, characteristics that make the Mathieu procedure less effective. The tubularized

incised plate (TIP) urethroplasty combines modifications of the previously described urethral plate incision and tubularization. In the TIP technique, a midline longitudinal plate relaxing incision is used as an adjunct to hypospadias repair to permit tension-free neourethral tubularization (Fig. 77-6). The tubularized pedicle flap (Fig. 77-7) is an extremely versatile technique that can be used as a single-stage procedure for severe hypospadias associated with chordee. A variety of variations also are available. Patients who have insufficient foreskin may undergo single-stage reconstruction employing a tubularized free graft of buccal or bladder mucosa. In general, well-vascularized flaps of non–hair-bearing skin are the best options for hypospadias reconstruction and minimize the risk of subsequent urethral contracture, failure of urethral growth, and hair growth within the urethra. The various factors to be considered when selecting a reconstructive procedure for hypospadias are outlined in Table 77-1.

Abnormalities associated with hypospadias, particularly the more proximal forms, include chordee, mentioned earlier, and torsion. Torsion is correctible by complete mobilization of the penile shaft skin with cutaneous anastomosis after detorsion. Chordee (Fig. 77-8A) is more complicated and is best shown by intraoperative artificial erection at the time of repair (Fig. 77-8B). The problem of chordee may be related to skin tethering, the presence of a fibrous band adjacent to the urethra, corporal disproportion, or a short urethra. Skin chordee is treated easily by mobilization of the penile shaft skin. After penile shaft straightening, however, there is a ventral skin defect that must be compensated for by the creation of Byars flaps developed from the dorsal hood of the foreskin following a midline incision. Fibrous chordee requires

TABLE 77-1 ▪ Choosing Hypospadias Repair		
Procedures	**Favors**	**Disfavors**
MAGPI	Distal meatus; mobile urethra	True chordee
Mathieu	Furrowed flans; distal meatus	True chordee; poor-quality perimeatal skin; deficient ventral shaft skin
Pyramid urethral	Megameatus	True chordee; native hypoplasia
Island onlay	Poor-quality perimeatal skin; native urethral hypoplasia	True chordee
Preputial tube	True chordee	Deficient ventral shaft skin; insufficient prepuce
Double-faced tube	Deficient ventral shaft skin	Insufficient prepuce
Free bladder mucosal graft	Reoperative repair; deficient skin	—
Rickettson	Reoperative repair	—
Mustarde	Reoperative repair	—

MAGPI, Meatal advancement and glanuloplasty.

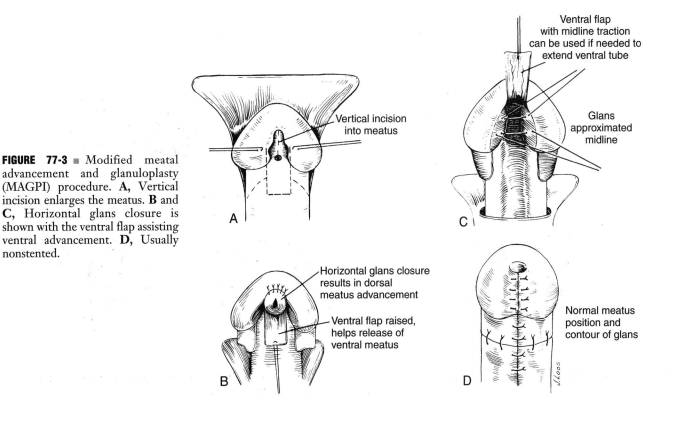

FIGURE 77-3 ▪ Modified meatal advancement and glanuloplasty (MAGPI) procedure. **A,** Vertical incision enlarges the meatus. **B** and **C,** Horizontal glans closure is shown with the ventral flap assisting ventral advancement. **D,** Usually nonstented.

Vertical incision into meatus

Ventral flap with midline traction can be used if needed to extend ventral tube

Glans approximated midline

Horizontal glans closure results in dorsal meatus advancement

Ventral flap raised, helps release of ventral meatus

Normal meatus position and contour of glans

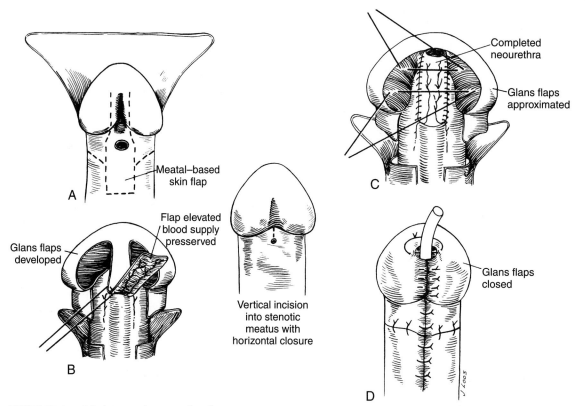

FIGURE 77-4 ■ Mathieu technique (flip-flap). **A,** Perimeatal-based skin flap is flipped distally, with the vascular mesentery intact. **B,** The glans incisions are deepened and glans flaps developed. **C,** The meatal-based flap is sutured to the urethral plate and the glans approximated. **D,** May be stented or unstented.

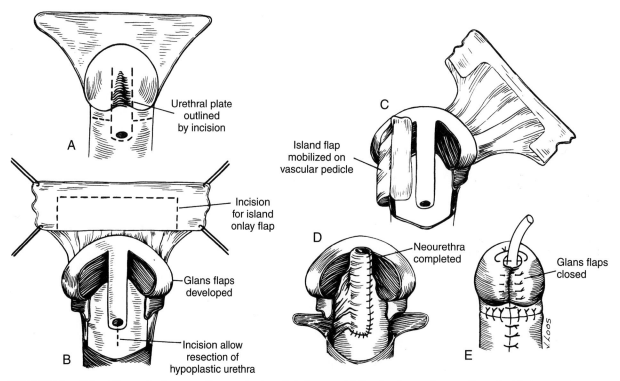

FIGURE 77-5 ■ Island flap onlay hypospadias repair. A pedicled preputial flap is advanced ventrally and added as patch. Some workers may use a free graft for better cosmesis, but this has a higher complication rate.

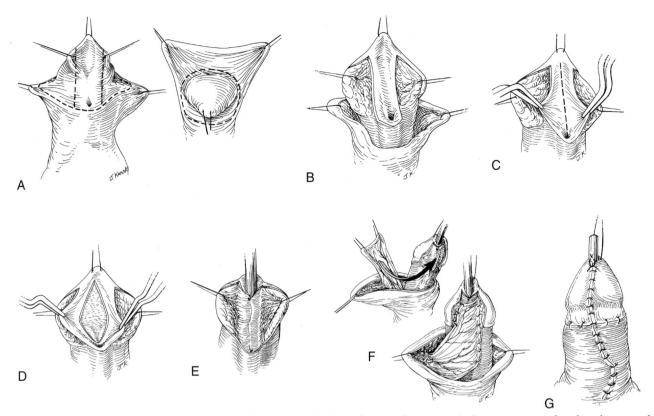

FIGURE 77-6 ■ Tubularized incised plate urethroplasty in distal primary hypospadias repair. **A,** Stay sutures are placed, and proposed urethral plate demarcating and circumferential incisions are marked. **B,** Parallel longitudinal and circumferential incisions have been made. **C,** Proposed longitudinal line of incision in the midline of the urethral plate. **D,** Urethral plate has been incised. **E,** Urethral plate is tubularized over a 6F Silastic catheter. **F,** Subcutaneous tissue flap is harvested from lateral or dorsal penile shaft and repositioned over the neourethra as second layer coverage. **G,** Glans penis is approximated in two layers, redundant skin is excised, and indwelling bladder catheter is secured.

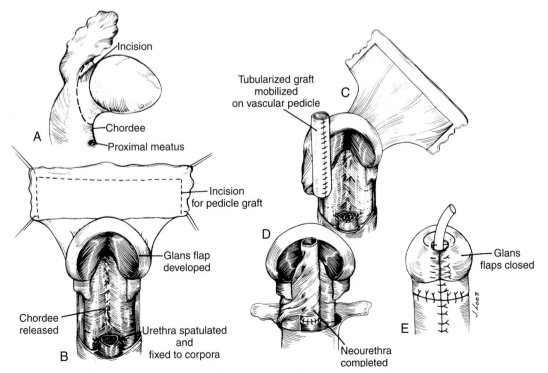

FIGURE 77-7 ■ Tubularized preputial pedicle flap. A pedicled preputial skin tube is advanced ventrally. Some workers do not split the glans but tunnel a new urethra to insert the tube.

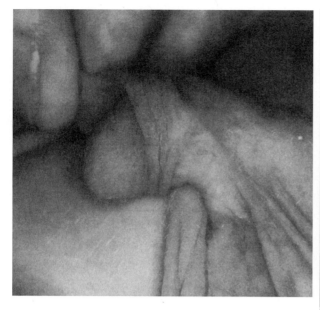

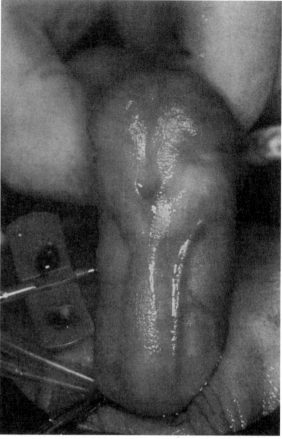

FIGURE 77-8 ■ **A,** Penile chordee. **B,** Absence of chordee is documented by intraoperative artificial erection.

complete excision of the fibrous tissue, which has its greatest density beneath the distal hypospadic urethra and between the hypospadic meatus and the glans. After excision, a repeat artificial erection is performed to show complete correction. *Corporeal disproportion* refers to a length discrepancy between the dorsal and ventral aspects of the corpora cavernosa. When the penis is sufficiently large, this can be managed by dorsal plication, but otherwise ventral excision of the defective segment of tunica albuginea followed by grafting is performed. The resulting short urethra is managed by urethral division. Interposition of a pedicle tube graft fashioned according to the individual case for a single staged repair or alternately a two-stage repair can be done.

MEATAL STENOSIS

Meatal stenosis may be primary or developmental, or it may be secondary to chronic inflammation or present as a complication of circumcision. Meatal stenosis may present with obstructive symptoms, such as straining, hesitancy, dribbling, and intermittency, but most commonly presents with an anteriorly directed urinary stream. Diagnosis depends on observation of voiding. Usually a thin, forceful, and often deflected urinary steam is noted. Treatment consists of meatoplasty, and whenever the symptoms seem out of proportion to the degree of meatal stenosis, urethroscopy is performed to rule out other possibilities such as urethral stricture or posterior urethral valves.

URETHRAL VALVES

The most common life-threatening anomaly of the male external genitalia is posterior urethral valves, which cause urinary obstruction in the newborn. Figure 77-9 depicts the pathology. Because of the extreme degree of obstruction associated with the commonly encountered type I posterior urethral valves, both kidneys may be affected prenatally. The anomaly requires urgent diagnosis and aggressive treatment. In the fetus and newborn, renal injury may be evident in the form of dysplasia, obstructive hydronephrosis, or reflux nephropathy that is progressive. Bladder trabeculation is often extreme, and the proximal urethra and bladder neck are enlarged and may be associated with high-grade vesicoureteral reflux. Even after valve ablation, severe bladder dysfunction often persists along with vesicoureteral reflux and the risk of ongoing renal injury. This is called *valve bladder* and is described further in Chapter 74. Figure 77-10 shows the appearance of posterior urethral valves on voiding cystourethrogram. Occasional patients may require a temporary urinary diversion to preserve renal function, including patients with prune-belly syndrome. In the fetus, if bladder decompression occurs, renal damage may be less severe. Severely obstructive posterior urethral valves in the fetus may result in oligohydramnios or Potter's syndrome associated with pulmonary hypoplasia. By now, fetal intervention for urinary anomalies has been

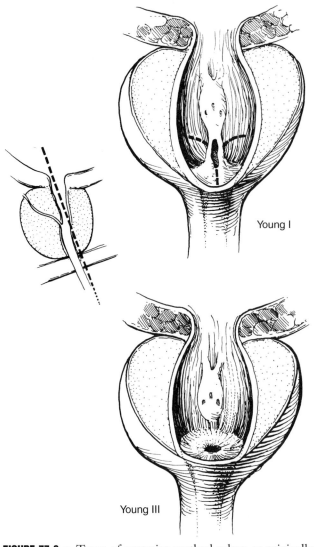

Young I

Young III

FIGURE 77-9 ■ Types of posterior urethral valves, as originally described by Young. Type I extends distally from the veru montanum. Type III appears as a perforated diaphragm. Type I is the most common, and there is no type II as originally described.

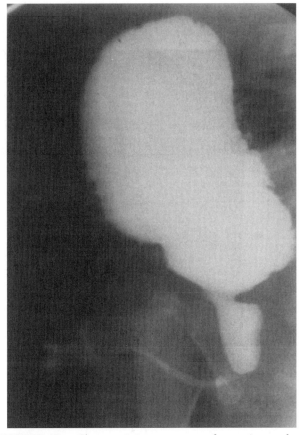

FIGURE 77-10 ■ Characteristic appearance of posterior urethral valves on voiding cystourethrogram.

abandoned almost completely because renal damage occurs so early that fetal intervention is ineffective. The one exception may be relief of posterior urethral valves in utero. This situation is still debatable, and the current consensus is that only rare conditions should be recommended for intervention, including oligohydramnios with suspected favorable renal function and the absence of other life-threatening congenital anomalies. Fetal cystoscopic ablation of posterior urethral valves currently is being investigated, but the long-term outcome in terms of renal function is not yet known.

With regard to diagnosis, voiding cystourethrogram, as mentioned earlier, is the best screening study. Cystoscopy is the definitive diagnostic test, however, and allows valve ablation. Endoscopic evaluation must be performed carefully because minimal urethral valves may be missed easily. It is important to examine the urethra under conditions of retrograde and antegrade

TABLE 77-2 ■ Posterior Urethral Valve Treatment Options	
Procedure	**Indications**
Valve fulguration	
Retrograde	Preferred whenever available
Antegrade	Urethra too small to allow endoscopic fulguration
Vesicostomy	Severe reflux; azotemia; urethra too small to allow endoscopic fulguration
Ureterostomy	Avoid
Pyelostomy	Azotemia not responding to direct bladder drainage
Percutaneous nephrostomy	Azotemia; sepsis in infant too ill to allow surgical procedure

urethral flow because the valves tend to appose each other during antegrade urethral flow and separate during retrograde flow.

Table 77-2 outlines the various treatment options available and their indications, but treatment most commonly takes the form of valve fulguration using a Bugbee or similar electrode. At times, vesicostomy or pyelostomy may be useful temporizing procedures for children with severe obstructive manifestations. Ureteral reimplantation and bladder augmentation subsequently may be required, as may renal transplantation in the latter instances. Renal insufficiency, urinary incontinence, and urinary tract infection are the most important long-term complications of valve disease.

It is also important to be aware of anterior urethral valves, more appropriately termed diverticula, which may cause severe obstructive uropathy. These may be difficult to diagnose. Voiding cystourethrography is the best screening procedure. In addition to the anatomic forms of urethral obstruction mentioned earlier, functional obstruction may exist in the form of detrusor sphincter dyssynergy as discussed extensively in Chapter 74.

URETHRAL STRICTURE

Urethral stricture is relatively uncommon in childhood, and it is usually secondary to trauma, infection, or urethral instrumentation, including catheterization.

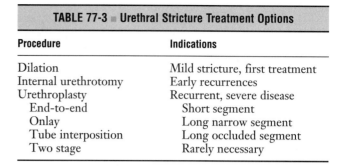

TABLE 77-3 ■ Urethral Stricture Treatment Options	
Procedure	**Indications**
Dilation	Mild stricture, first treatment
Internal urethrotomy	Early recurrences
Urethroplasty	Recurrent, severe disease
End-to-end	Short segment
Onlay	Long narrow segment
Tube interposition	Long occluded segment
Two stage	Rarely necessary

Congenital urethral strictures are rare but when present may be associated with urinary tract infection and either obstructive or irritative voiding symptoms.

Diagnosis is made by retrograde urethrography or voiding cystourethrography. Cystoscopic examination is diagnostic. Table 77-3 outlines the treatment options available. Uncomplicated strictures can be managed by simple urethral dilation or internal urethrotomy. Formal urethral reconstruction is reserved for recurrence after less invasive treatment. Formal reconstruction involves excision with end-to-end anastomosis or onlay urethroplasty. At times, a staged procedure is required (Figs. 77-11 and 77-12).

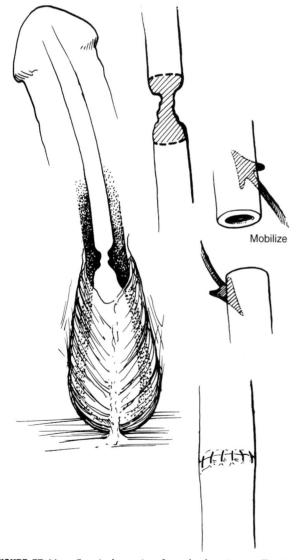

FIGURE 77-11 ■ Surgical repair of urethral stricture. Excision and end-to-end anastomosis are shown (see text).

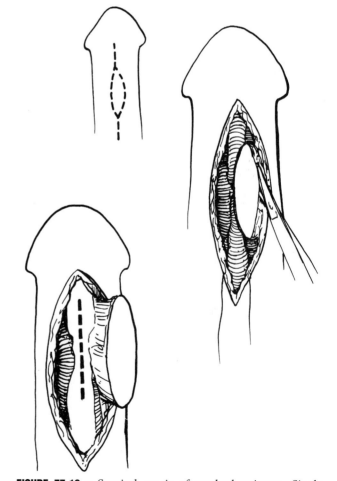

FIGURE 77-12 ■ Surgical repair of urethral stricture. Single-stage onlay urethroplasty is shown (see text).

OTHER CAUSES OF URETHRAL OBSTRUCTION

Urethral obstruction from Cowper's duct anomalies is rare and often difficult to diagnose. Children present either with infection or with obstructive voiding symptoms.

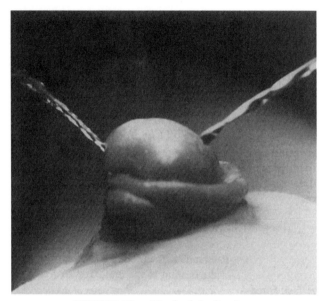

FIGURE 77-13 ■ Urethral duplication.

The usual screening studies of ultrasonography and voiding cystourethrography often fail to detect a Cowper's duct anomaly. Occasionally a filling defect in the bulbous urethra may be shown. Diagnosis is made at the time of cystoscopic evaluation for persistent symptoms. Treatment consists of endoscopic unroofing. Urethral polyps are additional rare abnormalities that may cause urethral obstruction and can be treated by cystoscopic ablation.

TRAUMA

Penile trauma generally is not severe in childhood, but severe injuries do occur. The trauma may be caused by sharp or blunt forces, and amputation may be encountered. Sharp trauma with laceration of the skin or glans is repaired easily. Corporeal lacerations require accurate reapproximation of the tunica albuginea. Interruption of the neuromuscular bundle always must be considered in corporeal lacerations, and microsurgical repair is required.

Blunt penile trauma usually consists of a contusion, and patients may have voiding difficulties related to glanular congestion and hematoma. Meatal stenosis is a common late complication. Corporeal rupture and urethral disruption are rare problems in childhood but when encountered are usually secondary to straddle injuries or severe pelvic fractures. The diagnosis should be suspected if blood appears at the urinary meatus or if

FIGURE 77-14 ■ Urethral duplication. **A,** Incomplete. **B,** Complete.

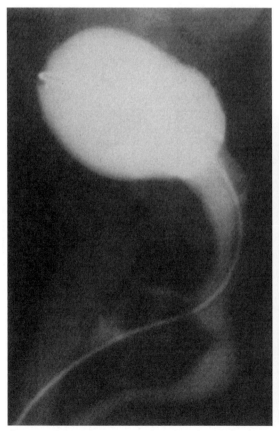

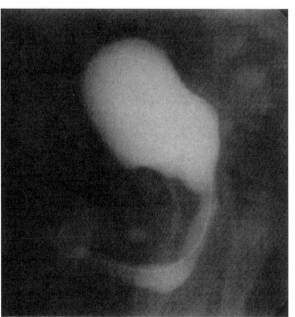

A   B

there is gross hematuria after an injury. Rectal examination may reveal a floating prostate or a perioprostatic hematoma. Retrograde urethrography should be performed before attempting to pass a urethral catheter to avoid a false passage. Mild injuries often permit passage of a catheter when the presence of an injury is known, under which circumstances several days of catheter drainage is sufficient treatment. Severe urethral disruption is managed best by placement of a suprapubic tube followed by definite urethral reconstruction when the patient has completely stabilized.

Entrapment of the penis by hair or clothing threads may cause tourniquet injuries. Zipper injuries are encountered frequently and usually involve the foreskin. Initial management consists of removing the clothing by cutting the zipper free of the clothing and leaving it attached to the penile foreskin, from which it can be removed by dividing the fastening clasp at the bottom of the zipper after placement of a dorsal penile nerve block.

Scrotal trauma may include soft tissue injury with or without testicular or epididymal injury. Significant trauma should be evaluated by ultrasound. If there is any suggestion of testicular disruption, scrotal exploration, débridement, and reapproximation of the tunica albuginea are in order.

DUPLICATION ANOMALIES

Duplication anomalies of the penis are rare but easily diagnosed. Urethral duplication is more common and requires definitive evaluation. Figure 77-13 shows the typical appearance of this anomaly consisting of a dorsal and a ventral penile meatus. Regardless of where the two openings are, the more ventral urethra is usually the more functional urethra containing the verumontanum and ejaculatory ducts. Urethral duplication may be complete (Fig. 77-14A) or incomplete (Fig. 77-14B). Voiding cystourethrography and retrograde urethrography are the best diagnostic tests. It is important to evaluate the upper urinary tracts in patients with urethral duplication because of the frequency of associated upper tract anomalies, so renal ultrasound is indicated. Treatment depends on the anatomy and severity of the anomaly and usually consists of excision of the nondominant urethra, which is usually the dorsal one.

OTHER ANOMALIES OF THE MALE EXTERNAL GENITALIA

Penoscrotal transposition and penoscrotal webbing may be encountered in the presence or absence of hypospadias. The latter anomalies are usually readily reconstructible. Penile agenesis is difficult to reconstruct, and sometimes gender conversion is necessary. Utricular cysts may occur in isolation but usually are associated with hypospadias or intersex. They are usually not symptomatic, and treatment often is not needed, unless there is sufficient degree of urinary stasis to cause recurrent infection. When repair is needed, it usually is performed through a transvesical or retrovesical approach. Megalourethra usually is associated with prune-belly syndrome but may occur as a primary anomaly. Repair of megalourethra is varied according to the severity of the malformation.

SUGGESTED READINGS

American Academy of Pediatrics Taskforce on Circumcision: Circumcision policy statement. Pediatrics 84:388, 1989.

This is consensus statement on neonatal circumcision for the first time is evidence-based so that the recommendation is likely to endure.

Borer JG, Retik AB: Current trends in hypospadias repair. Urol Clin North Am 26:15-37, 1999.

This article updates and summarizes the technical enhancements that have improved the operative approaches to hypospadias.

Duckett JW: MAGPI: A procedure for subcoronal hypospadias. Urol Clin North Am 8:513, 1981.

This issue of the Urologic Clinics *describes all of the currently used procedures for hypospadias, including the commonly performed MAGPI procedure.*

Duckett JW: Hypospadias. In Walsh PC, Retik AB, Vaughn ED, Wein AJ (eds): Campbell's Urology, vol 2, 7th ed. Philadelphia, WB Saunders, 1998, p 2093.

This is a nice summary of embryology, classification, various approaches to treatment, outcomes, and management of complications. This in-depth discussion of hypospadias by the expert in the field is invaluable reading.

Psihramis KE, Colodny AH, Lebowitz RL, et al: Complete duplication of the urethra. J Urol 136:63, 1986.

A 40-year review of all types of duplications and approaches to diagnosis and treatment.

Female Genital Tract

VAGINAL ANOMALIES

Embryology

The course of development of the human genital tract is indifferent up to approximately 9 weeks' gestation, during which time the wolffian (mesonephric) and the müllerian (paramesonephric) ducts are present as symmetric paired structures. The latter, together with the urogenital sinus and the metanephric ducts, which become the ureters eventually, provide the tissue origins for the internal genital and urinary structures. The final anatomy of the female genital tract results from pairing, fusion, and recanalization of the müllerian ducts, which grow caudally to join the cloaca. The proximal müllerian ducts remain unfused and form the fallopian tubes, whereas the distal ducts fuse to form the uterus and the proximal vagina. The lower vagina arises from the urogenital sinus, and in general, the upper two thirds of the vagina are of müllerian origin, and the lower third is of urogenital sinus or cloacal origin. In support of this statement is the situation with congenital androgen insensitivity syndrome, in which individuals have bilateral cryptorchid testes that elaborate normal müllerian inhibitory substance such that only the distal third of the vagina forms without any müllerian derivatives. The clitoris arises from the genital tubercle, and the labial majora arises from the genital swellings.

Urogenital sinus and cloacal malformation are in the category of caudal regression syndromes, which can present with a variety of vaginal, bladder, renal, and rectal anomalies. If the müllerian ducts do not fuse to form the müllerian tubercle, the vaginal plate does not form and join with the distal vagina, resulting in the formation of a urogenital sinus.

Vaginal Atresia

Vaginal atresia can be complete, proximal, or distal (Fig. 78-1; see Fig. 78-3). Complete vaginal atresia results from failure of the müllerian ducts to reach the urogenital sinus, as mentioned previously. In this situation, the fallopian tubes are normal, but the uterus is bicornuate and rudimentary. The ovaries are always normal. Proximal vaginal atresia is a result of the müllerian duct fusing to form the müllerian tubercle. In this case, the fallopian tubes and the uterus and cervix are hypoplastic or absent. If the sinovaginal bulbs, which originate from the urogenital sinus to form the vaginal plate, do not proliferate, distal vaginal atresia results, and the cervix, uterus, and fallopian tubes above are normal.

Hydrocolpos or hydrometrocolpos may occur in infancy if the vagina or uterus or both fill with mucus because of maternal estrogen stimulation of the uterine and vaginal glands. At menarche, hematocolpos or hematometrocolpos can occur when the obstructed vagina becomes filled with blood. In either of these situations, patients can present with a large midline abdominal mass. In distal vaginal atresia, the proximal vagina and the uterus are normal, and sharp, intermittent abdominal pain occurs at menarche. This sort of cyclical pain does not occur in patients with proximal vaginal atresia, vaginal and uterine hypoplasia, or agenesis. Hydrocolpos, hydrometrocolpos, hematocolpos, and hematometrocolpos associated with distal vaginal atresia

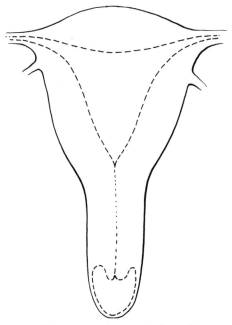

FIGURE 78-1 ■ Low vaginal atresia.

can be managed with a perineal repair. If these abnormalities are secondary to an imperforate hymen (Fig. 78-2), drainage with or without a formal vaginoplasty is appropriate. If these entities are associated with proximal vaginal atresia, laparotomy is required to drain the uterus and connect it to the distal vagina. The combination of congenital absence of the vagina and some form of abnormal uterus or absent uterus constitutes the Meyer-Rokitansky syndrome. The principal features of this syndrome include primary amenorrhea associated with congenital absence of the vagina; a 46,XX karyotype; a uterus that varies from anatomically complete to rudimentary bicornuate cords to complete absence; normal ovarian function and ovulation; normal breast development and body configuration; and frequent association of renal, skeletal, and other congenital malformations. A common presentation is an adolescent girl with an apparently normal vagina with an obstructed or absent duplicated vagina and a rudimentary, bicornuate uterus filled with mucus and blood. In the latter instances, there is usually renal agensis on the side of the anomalous vagina.

Vaginal agenesis requires vaginal replacement, preferably with vascularized intestine, although skin graft tubes have been used. Sigmoid colon is probably the best substitute for vaginal reconstruction because of its size and the ability to bring it down to the perineum for anastomosis. Vaginoplasty with sigmoid colon provides an excellent appearance and long-term function. A persistent vaginal septum is repaired by division transvaginally.

Urogenital Sinus Defects

Urogenital sinus malformations occur in normal females because of failure of the urethra and the vagina to separate (see Chapter 79). In these cases, the rectum is normal, and the uterus is bicornuate. This anomaly results from failure of fusion of the müllerian ducts to form the müllerian tubercle and the vaginal plate, which takes place after the urorectal septum has separated the rectum from the urogenital sinus. Most urogenital sinus anomalies can be repaired with a perineal wide-V vaginoplasty, but occasionally in more masculinized versions of this malformation, a high insertion of the vagina into the sinus requires a pull-through procedure.

Cloacal Malformations

Female infants with cloacal malformations have a single opening on the perineum with no separate opening for the vagina or the anus (see Chapter 61). The labia are often flat, and the phallus is small. These infants can be genetic males or females; the sex of rearing depends on the size of the phallus and whether it can be reconstructed. In general, most of these individuals are reared as females. Various forms of vaginal atresia are associated with cloacal malformations, and their surgical management depends on whether there is vaginal agenesis, proximal vaginal atresia, or distal vaginal atresia. In more recent years, the posterior sagittal approach with extensive mobilization of the internal structures has been used to repair simultaneously the rectal, vaginal, and urinary abnormalities in these children.

UTERINE ANOMALIES

Uterine anomalies are generally not symptomatic during childhood, and few are symptomatic during adolescence. Most of the problems created by uterine anomalies are related to infertility or are complications of pregnancy. Uterine anomalies are common in females with either ischiopagus or pygopagus conjoined twinning.

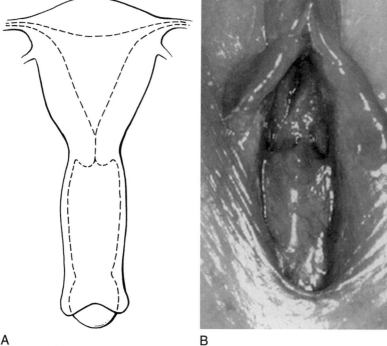

A   B

FIGURE 78-2 ■ A, Imperforate hymen. **B,** Imperforate hymen in a newborn.

Cervical Atresia

Atresia of the cervix, a rare anomaly, is the result of failure of development and canalization of the cervical portion of the fused paranephric ducts. The atretic cervix forms a solid cord of tissue between the uterine corpus above and the proximal vagina below. When menses begin, a hematometra forms above it with marked dilation of the uterine cavity associated with pain. Treatment consists of transvaginal incision into the atretic cervix with dilation to obtain adequate drainage of the hematometra. Hysterectomy rarely is required. Occasionally the vaginal approach is unsuccessful, in which case the uterus must be opened from above and an opening made into the proximal vagina from that approach. Congenital cervical stenosis occurs but is even more rare than atresia.

Hypoplasia of the Uterus

True hypoplasia, which is rare, is characterized not only by failure to achieve normal size, but also by a greater proportionate length and development of the cervical canal compared with the shorter and relatively smaller corpus (Fig. 78-3). Severe hypoplasia results in failure of growth beyond an early fetal stage, in which case the uterus ends up as a small cord of tissue, usually without a cavity.

The few females with hypoplastic uteri and who are amenorrheic have normally functioning ovaries as evidenced by well-developed female characteristics and cyclical breast changes. Hormonal therapy is not effective in promoting growth in this condition. The best clinical indication of a truly hypoplastic uterus is the absence of menses. Some uteri that seem hypoplastic do not grow, however, because of lack of ovarian stimulation.

Hormonal therapy in this situation causes an increase in the size of these organs, and menses are initiated.

Uterine Aplasia

Complete aplasia of the uterus is exceedingly rare. Although the uterus seems to be absent, inspection usually shows thin cords extending from the ends of the uterine tubes medially along the superior surface of the broad ligaments. A medial remnant of the fused paramesonephric ducts creates a firm strand between the bladder and rectum. The ovaries are usually normal but may be displaced laterally toward the pelvic brim. Aplasia of the uterus is accompanied by poorly developed or aplastic fallopian tubes. Vaginal agenesis is always associated if there is a true agenesis of the uterus, and associated anomalies of the lower urinary tract are usually present. A unicornuate uterus results when there is aplasia of part or all of one paramesonephric duct, and the accompanying fallopian tube is usually absent or rudimentary.

Uterine Duplication

Partial or complete duplication of the uterus is caused by abnormal fusion of the paramesonephric ducts. The genital folds fail to unite normally, and the result is either a complete bicornuate uterus with two cervices or duplication of the uterine horns (Fig. 78-4).

Uterine Tube Malformations

Anomalies of the uterine tube are not significant in childhood or adolescence, but they are suspected of causing sterility or abnormal pregnancy. Small supernumerary or accessory tubes attached to the fimbriated ends or communicating with the isthmic or ampullar portions of the tube are relatively common and may be seen at the time

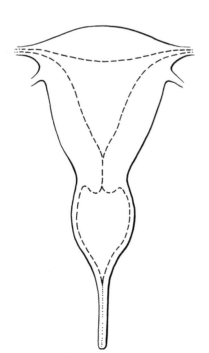

FIGURE 78-3 ■ High vaginal atresia with associated cervical atresia and uterine hypoplasia.

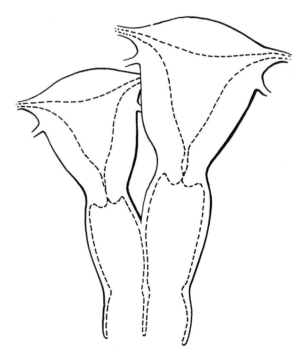

FIGURE 78-4 ■ Duplication of the vagina and uterus.

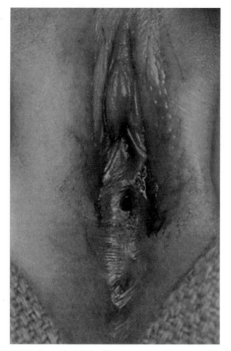

FIGURE 78-5 ■ Labial adhesions in a 7-year-old girl.

a child is operated on for some other condition. Accessory tubes of this type cause no problems and need not be dealt with.

LABIAL FUSION

Two forms of fusion of the labia minora are normally encountered. The most common is labial adhesions seen predominantly in girls 1 to 6 years old, which are due to synechiae formation (Fig. 78-5). The cause of labial adhesions is not known but is thought to be related either to chronic irritation or to a relative lack of estrogen stimulation. At times, labial fusion is primary and consists of an actual skin bridge. This entity is usually asymptomatic, but occasionally difficulty with urination and urinary stasis in the vagina may occur associated with secondary infection.

The diagnosis is made easily by inspection on spreading the labia majora. The hymen is not visible, and only the urethral opening is visible. In patients with labial adhesions, the thin membrane frequently can be separated in an outpatient setting or occasionally requires an anesthetic. Anesthesia with formal incision is necessary for patients with a true skin bridge. After division of either labial adhesions or fusion, it is useful to apply estrogen cream once a day to the area for 1 month. Labial adhesions may recur unless careful hygiene is ensured.

VAGINITIS

At the time of birth, the vaginal mucosa is similar to that seen in adults because of maternal estrogen stimulation during gestation. The pH at this time is 5.7. Several weeks after birth, the vaginal mucosa thins, however, and is susceptible to infection. At puberty, the mucosa thickens again from estrogen stimulation, and normal vaginal flora is established, raising the pH to the 6.0 to 8.0 range.

The most common cause of vaginitis in prepubertal girls is secondary to bubble bath, soap, or laundry detergent. The next most common cause is the presence of a foreign body, in which case there is an associated foul discharge that occasionally can progress retrograde up the fallopian tubes and cause peritonitis. If a foreign body is suspected, vaginoscopy is required under general anesthesia using either a nasal speculum or a panendoscope. Primary infections with bacteria, fungi, viruses, or parasites are uncommon. The most common infectious agents are gonococci, streptococci, *Haemophilus influenzae*, *Shigella*, *Escherichia coli*, *Candida albicans*, herpes simplex virus, pinworms, and *Trichomonas vaginalis*; infections should be treated with the appropriate antibiotic. The latter organisms easily may contaminate a "clean voided urine" sample obtained for culture, so a catheterized specimen is preferable. Occasional vaginal infections indicate child abuse. Treatment is by eliminating the offending allergen or irritant, removing the foreign body, or treating the specific infection to relieve the clinical manifestations of purulent discharge, local erythema, pain, itching, and dysuria.

SUGGESTED READINGS

Hendren WH: Cloaca, the most severe degree of imperforate anus: Experience with 195 cases. Ann Surg 228:331-346, 1998.

This is the most complete description of cloacal malformations, their classification, and treatment.

Martinez-Mora J, Isnard R, Castellvi A, Lopez-Ortiz P: Neovagina in vaginal agenesis: Surgical methods and long-term results. J Pediatr Surg 27:10-14, 1992.

These experienced authors present a thorough analysis of this subject and how to approach it and when.

Skandalakis JE, Gray SW: Embryology for Surgeons, 2nd ed. Baltimore, Williams & Wilkins, 1994, pp 827-847.

The embryology of the female genital tract, related malformations, and their clinical malformations are described.

Ambiguous Genitalia

Reference has already been made to abnormalities of the male and female genitalia in the Chapters 77 and 78. *Ambiguous genitalia* refers to a condition of the external genitalia in which there is a question about whether the sex of the child is male or female. Proper gender assignment to a neonate born with ambiguous genitalia should be expeditious and timely, but it is crucial that gender assignment be proper and accurate. Proper gender assignment should entail a multiple disciplinary approach that includes, but is not limited to, input from pediatric endocrinology, surgery, urology, psychiatry, and radiology consultants and the parents. When an appropriate sex assignment has been made, it is possible to proceed with a reconstructive procedure in a timely fashion, if one is required.

EMBRYOLOGY

Normal sexual development during gestation (Fig. 79-1) requires a coordinate interplay among the following factors: the correct chromosome complement and composition, proper migration of germ cells from the yolk sac to the urogenital ridge for initial induction of the gonad, appropriate hormone production by that gonad, and proper response by the target organs to the secreted hormones. A defect or imbalance in any one of these steps can result in the development of a child with a broad spectrum of ambiguous genitalia.

The Y chromosome of the male leads to formation of a testis, and the SRY antigens (sex-determining region of the Y chromosome) of the primitive gonad initiates differentiation into a testis. Although the SRY antigens can be found on all male cells, the only cells that have receptors for SRY antigens are those of the genital ridge. SRY antigens binding to these receptors on the genital ridge tissue are responsible for differentiation into a testis. Factors produced by the SRY antigens lead to the differentiation of the medullary cords of the primitive gonad into seminiferous tubules. Next, Sertoli cells of the

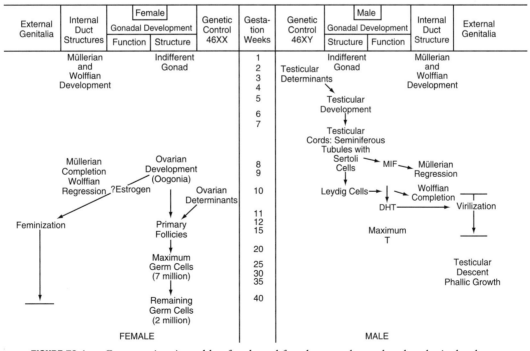

FIGURE 79-1 ■ Comparative timetable of male and female normal sexual embryologic development.

seminiferous tubules develop and begin to produce müllerian inhibitory substance, which causes regression of the müllerian ducts. The next step is the differentiation of interstitial cells of the testis into Leydig cells, which then begin to produce testosterone. Testosterone stimulates the development of the wolffian duct system to form the vas deferens, seminal vesicles, and epididymis. In addition, testosterone is reduced at the site of the external genitalia to dihydrotestosterone, which regulates the development of the external genitalia in the male.

In the absence of the Y chromosome and the SRY antigens, the primitive gonad differentiates into an ovary. Female development of the müllerian duct system and external genitalia is also an autonomous process. The normal female is not exposed to müllerian inhibitory substance so that the müllerian ducts form the fallopian tubes, uterus, cervix, and upper portion of the vagina. Simultaneously, in the absence of testosterone, the wolffian ducts regress. The genital tubercle, genital folds, genital swellings, and urogenital sinus develop into the clitoris, labia minora, labia majora, and lower vagina when dihydrotestosterone is not present.

DIAGNOSTIC EVALUATION

The long-accepted classification of ambiguous genitalia includes female pseudohermaphroditism, male pseudohermaphroditism, true hermaphroditism, and gonadal dysgenesis. During the initial evaluation of an infant with ambiguous genitalia, it is often possible to differentiate these four entities accurately by noting the symmetry of the gonads. Preliminary karyotypic analysis is best performed by fluorescent in situ hybridization (FISH) before having full karyotypic analysis available. FISH generally permits appropriate gender assignment. Asymmetric gonads in a karyotypic female frequently indicate a true hermaphrodite, and asymmetric gonads in a karyotypic male usually indicate the presence of mixed gonadal dysgenesis (Fig. 79-2). It should be determined

initially if other family members have a history of ambiguous genitalia, whether apparent female relatives died in infancy suggestive of congenital adrenal hyperplasia, or whether there is infertility in the family. A detailed evaluation of drug ingestion during pregnancy is important, especially for androgenic agents such as progesterone. Initial FISH analysis, full karyotype, urinary mineralocorticoid and glucocorticoid steroid measurements, and serum electrolyte levels should be obtained. Pelvic ultrasound, endoscopy, and contrast genitography are performed to clarify the status of the internal genital structures and to show the vaginal entrance into the urogenital sinus (Fig. 79-3). Occasionally, laparoscopy is required for definitive sex identification, particularly with true hermaphrodites.

In general, most infants with ambiguous genitalia are best reconstructed as females because of the practicality of surgical reconstruction based on the size of the phallus. Although there is a great deal of discussion of the subject, it generally is agreed that regardless of genotype, if an inadequate phallus cannot be corrected surgically, the patient will fare better in the female gender role. The matter of testosterone imprinting on the brain requires careful consideration and more research than is available at present. Genetic males with severe penoscrotal hypospadias and bilateral undescended testes frequently may be reconstructed successfully, however, so they usually are reared as males.

SPECIFIC DISORDERS
Female Pseudohermaphroditism (Adrenogenital Syndrome)

Infants with congenital adrenal hyperplasia (Figs. 79-4 through 79-6) have a 46,XX karyotype, but they have ambiguous genitalia because they have been exposed to excessive levels of endogenous androgens in utero as a result of one the following three recognized enzymatic

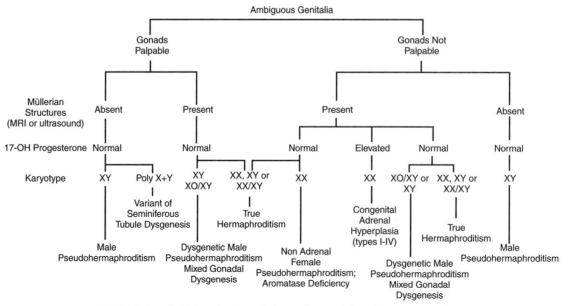

FIGURE 79-2 ■ Initial evaluation of the newborn with ambiguous genitalia.

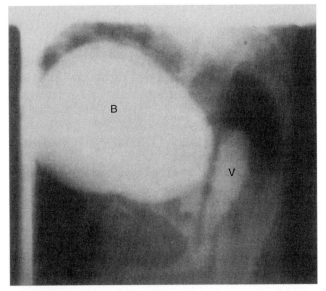

FIGURE 79-3 ■ Retrograde genitogram in a patient with congenital adrenal hyperplasia. This procedure is performed with a Foley catheter inserted just inside the perineal opening with the balloon inflated. Note the low insertion of the vagina into the urogenital sinus. V, vagina; B, bladder.

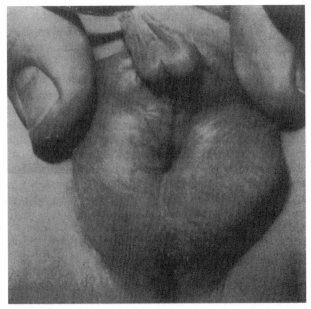

FIGURE 79-5 ■ More masculinized female pseudohermaphrodite with congenital adrenal hyperplasia and severe clitoral hypertrophy, urogenital sinus, and fusion of the labia to form a scrotum. A high insertion of the vagina into the urethra was seen on endoscopy and contrast genitography.

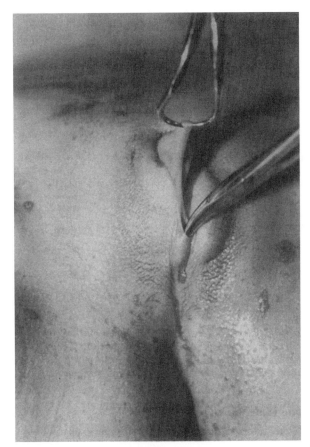

FIGURE 79-4 ■ Female pseudohermaphrodite with congenital adrenal hyperplasia with moderate clitoral hypertrophy (towel clip) and urogenital sinus (hemostat).

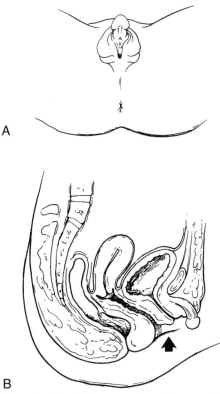

FIGURE 79-6 ■ **A,** Clitoral hypertrophy and urogenital sinus in the common form of congenital adrenal hyperplasia. **B,** Low insertion of the vagina into the urogenital sinus (arrow).

deficiencies: 21-hydroxylase, 11-hydroxylase, and 3β-hydroxysteroid dehydrogenase. Each of these enzyme deficiencies results in overproduction of adrenal intermediary steroid hormones with androgenic properties that masculinize the external genitalia of the female XX fetus. The phenotypic picture is variable, from mild clitoral enlargement alone to complete masculinization of the urethra with a normal-appearing but small male phallus and the urethral meatus at the glans penis. This usually is associated with complete fusion of the labia and a high insertion of the proximal vagina into the urogenital sinus.

Because of the proximal defect in glucocorticoid synthesis, these patients all require cortisol replacement. Additionally, patients with mineralocorticoid deficiency and the salt-losing form of the adrenogenital syndrome require fludrocortisone acetate replacement. All of these children are reared as females and should have normal fertility because they have normal internal genitalia. Surgical treatment is designed to correct the appearance of and functional deformities of the external genitalia, primarily the hypertrophy of the clitoris and the malformation of the vaginal introitus. In the usual form of this malformation, reconstruction is by flap or wide-V vaginoplasty and clitoral recession, usually performed at 3 to 6 months of age. In infants with the more masculinized form of congenital adrenal hyperplasia in which the vagina inserts into the urethra proximal to the external sphincter, vaginoplasty is delayed until at least 2 years of age so that a pull-through of the vagina to the perineum can be performed safely. This has been corrected at an earlier age with a posterior sagittal approach or a total urogenital sinus mobilization technique.

Mixed Gonadal Dysgenesis

The syndrome of mixed gonadal dysgenesis (Fig. 79-7) is associated with dysgenetic gonads and retained müllerian structures. Most commonly, there is a streak gonad on one side with müllerian structures and a testis on the opposite side with a vas and epididymis. In general, these individuals have 45,XO/46,XY mosaicism. Half of these individuals eventually develop malignancy in their dysgenetic gonads. Gonadoblastoma is the most common malignancy overall, but seminoma and dysgerminoma may occur in streak gonads. For this reason, gonadectomy of the streak gonad is recommended in all patients with mixed gonadal dysgenesis early in childhood. Surgical reconstruction is similar to that for congenital adrenal hyperplasia. Those with adequate virilization may be raised as males and reconstructed accordingly with careful surveillance of the scrotally placed testis.

Male Pseudohermaphroditism

Male pseudohermaphroditism occurs in infants with an XY karyotype but deficient masculinization of their external genitalia. This disorder used to be called *testicular feminization syndrome*, but it is best referred to as *androgen insensitivity syndrome*, which is more descriptive of the pathophysiology. This condition can result from inadequate testosterone production caused by deficiencies of the enzymes necessary for its synthesis, inability of the external genitalia to convert testosterone to dihydrotestosterone because of 5α-reductase deficiency, müllerian inhibitory

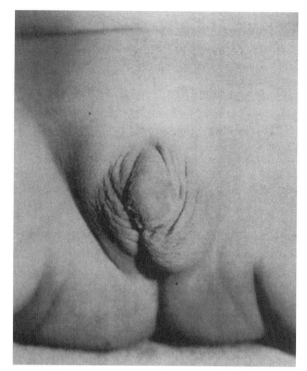

FIGURE 79-7 ■ Infant with mixed gonadal dysgenesis (46,XO/46,XY) with significant clitoral hypertrophy, asymmetric gonads, and a gonad in the left labioscrotal fold.

factor (MIF) deficiency, and deficiencies in androgen receptors. Although each form may be specifically named, the most common and well-known condition is androgen insensitivity or receptor deficiency, which is inherited as an X-linked recessive trait. The sex of rearing is dependent on the degree of external genital virilization.

In many of these children, the diagnosis is made at the time of routine inguinal herniorrhaphy in a phenotypic female who has palpable gonads within the inguinal canals. Given the risk of eventual malignant degeneration to gonadoblastoma or seminoma of the intra-abdominal gonads, removal is required. There is some discussion as to whether this is best done at the time of discovery or whether gonadal removal should be delayed until puberty because these gonads can induce breast development. The best answer to this question probably is based on determination of urinary steroid levels because individuals with high androgen levels probably should have early gonadectomy to prevent masculinization during puberty. The current opinion is that it is probably best to perform gonadectomy early in these patients. Occasionally a patient does not present until puberty with amenorrhea. Under these circumstances, when the diagnosis is confirmed, bilateral gonadectomy and vaginal reconstruction should be performed if needed. All patients with androgen insensitivity syndrome have a short vaginal vault because they have a deficiency in the proximal two thirds of the vagina. Most can be treated with vaginal dilation, however, to produce a functionally adequate vaginal cavity, but some require vaginal augmentation with sigmoid colon. Although most of these individuals do not have clitoral hypertrophy, a few require clitoral reduction.

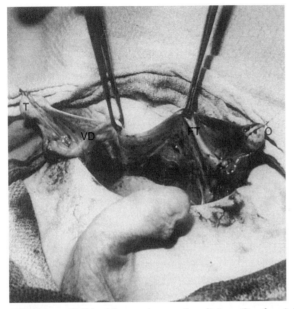

FIGURE 79-8 ■ Child with true hermaphroditism. On the right side of the picture (the patient's left) are a fallopian tube (FT) and ovary (O). On the left side, a vas deferens (VD) and a testis (T) are present. Note the large phallus. This patient was raised as a male.

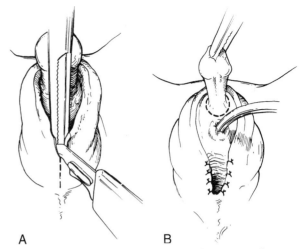

FIGURE 79-9 ■ **A,** Cutback vaginoplasty done over a hemostat. **B,** Completed cutback vaginoplasty with vagina marsupialization to the perineal skin. The clitoris is being mobilized for the clitoral recession (dashed circle).

True Hermaphroditism

The rarest form of ambiguous genitalia is true hermaphroditism (Fig. 79-8). These patients have normal male and female gonadal tissue with an ovary on one side and a testis on the other or an ovotestis on one or both sides. Streak ovaries are common. Of these patients, 80% have a 46,XX karyotype, and others have a mixed karyotype. Most of these children have an inadequate phallus and are raised as females. In these patients, the testis and the testicular portion of the ovotestis should be removed, leaving the ovarian tissue in place. The surgical goals of reconstruction are similar to those for children with other forms of ambiguous genitalia. When the phallus is adequate for the male gender role, all ovarian and müllerian structures are removed, and a hypospadias repair is performed. Occasionally, exogenous testosterone treatment is needed for these patients. After puberty, a testicular prosthesis may be inserted in individuals to be raised as male.

SURGICAL RECONSTRUCTION

The timing of surgical reconstruction for patients with ambiguous genitalia represents a balance between the desirability of early reconstruction and the technical limitations imposed by the small size and delicacy of the structures involved. The earlier reconstruction can be performed safely, the better. One of the most common considerations has to do with clitoral hypertrophy. Because the clitoris is essential for normal female sexual function, all procedures are designed to preserve all or part of that organ with its nerve supply. Reconstruction ranges from recession of the entire clitoris beneath the pubic symphysis to a clitoral reduction procedure in which the glans is preserved with its neurovascular bundle and

the corpora are partially or completely resected. The latter procedure may permit the clitoris to be recessed underneath the symphysis in patients with extreme clitoral hypertrophy. Experienced evaluation of each individual patient determines the best approach to clitoral hypertrophy. Either way, long-term functional evaluations are needed to indicate which is the preferred approach to this problem.

Figure 79-9 describes one approach to vaginoplasty for the common form of congenital adrenal hyperplasia with minimal to moderate masculinization. At times, simple cutback vaginoplasty is inadequate, and a Y-V plasty is needed with a posterior advancement flap. At other times, more extensive lateral flap mobilization is required along with labial reconstruction. Instances of high insertion of the vagina into the urethra require a pull-through vaginoplasty as described by Hendren. The high vagina has been approached via a posterior sagittal technique or total urogenital sinus mobilization.

PENILE AGENESIS

Penile agenesis is a rare anomaly in which the urethral opening may lie anterior to the rectum on the perineum or be located anterior to the scrotum or pubic symphysis. The testes and scrotum are usually normal. Prostatic hyperplasia and aplasia, cryptorchidism, polycystic kidneys, and agenesis of the kidneys frequently are associated anomalies. Imperforate anus frequently is associated. Because penile reconstruction is not feasible, gender conversion to female is the most practical approach. It is best to remove the testes in infancy to reduce androgen imprinting and masculinization, and a vagina should be constructed from the scrotal skin or intestine. Revision of these vaginoplasties performed in infancy frequently is required after puberty, in which augmentation with sigmoid colon may be a desirable approach. Exogenous estrogen administration should be initiated at 10 to 12 years of age to promote breast development and development of secondary sex characteristics.

MICROPENIS

If the phallus is determined to be inadequate for adequate male function after testosterone stimulation, these infants are best converted to female gender. Average penile length in the term infant is 3.5 ± 0.4 cm with the size being smaller for premature infants depending on length of gestation. A phallus more than 2 standard deviations below the mean is inadequate. In the presence of hypospadias with chordee, length may be greater than apparent. In borderline cases, testosterone administration may result in adequate growth of the penis; this usually takes 8 to 12 weeks of treatment to determine whether male gender assignment is appropriate in these marginal cases.

SUGGESTED READINGS

Baskin LS, Erol A, Li YW, et al: Anatomical studies of the human clitoris. J Urol 162:1015-1020, 1999.

This article provides detailed anatomic information related to the clitoris and can serve as a basis for determining approaches to surgical procedures to correct clitoral hypertrophy.

Diamond DA: Sexual differentiation—normal and abnormal. In Walsh PC, Retik AB, Vaughan ED Jr, Wein AJ (eds): Campbell's Urology, 8th ed. Philadelphia, WB Saunders, 2002.

This chapter provides an in-depth description of the embryology of sexual differentiation and development and serves as an excellent guide to understanding ambiguous genitalia and approaches to treatment.

Donahoe PK, Hendren WH: Perineal reconstruction of ambiguous genitalia in infants raised as females. Ann Surg 200:363, 1984.

Hendren WH, Donahoe PK: Correction of congenital abnormalities of the vagina and perineum. J Pediatr Surg 15:751, 1980.

These two articles by Donahoe and Hendren are classic in that they represent one of the largest series ever reported, and they provide information on appropriate reconstructive approaches to all of the various forms of ambiguous genitalia.

Newman K, Randolph J, Anderson K: The surgical management of infants and children with ambiguous genitalia: Lessons learned from 25 years. Ann Surg 215:643-653, 1992.

The value of this article is that it not only provides current information on approaches to diagnosis and treatment, but also it emphasizes the need for an ongoing care program encompassing the physical, endocrinologic, and psychological needs of each patient and each parent involved so that late maladjustment, sexual failure, and psychic distress can be avoided.

PART XII

Skin, Soft Tissue, and Blood Vessels

Hemangiomas and Vascular Malformations

Vascular anomalies, specifically hemangiomas, are the most common human birth defects. The clinical importance of these lesions arises from their wide prevalence and their sometimes shocking cosmetic effects. More recent work has provided clinical and scientific insights into the fundamental biologic nature of vascular anomalies and an improved understanding of their natural history and treatment.

In 1982, Mulliken and colleagues proposed a classification dividing vascular anomalies into two broad categories—vascular tumors and vascular malformations. While simplifying an archaic array of semidescriptive terms and eponyms that dated to the late 19th century, the new nomenclature also recognized the fundamental clinical and biologic differences between the two entities, vascular tumors and vascular malformations. Endothelial hyperplasia characterizes vascular tumors, typified by hemangiomas. Vascular malformations represent errors of development and morphogenesis of vascular structures, and they usually have normal endothelial turnover. The predominant vessel represented (capillary, arteriole, vein, lymphatic, or combinations thereof) and the relative rate of flow of blood through the lesion (fast flow and slow flow) differentiates these lesions further. This classification was adopted officially by the International Society for the Study of Vascular Anomalies in 1996.

HEMANGIOMAS

Hemangiomas are the most common human birth defects, occurring in approximately 1% of newborns and 10% of infants. They affect female infants more frequently than male infants, with a sex ratio of 3:1 to 5:1. Of hemangiomas, 60% occur in the head and neck region, 25% occur in the trunk, and 15% occur in the extremities. One third are present at birth. Most appear during the first weeks of life. Deeper lesions located in the subcutaneous tissue or visceral hemangiomas may not become manifest until later in infancy. Of lesions, 80% are solitary. The 20% that are multiple often affect the viscera, typically the liver, gastrointestinal tract, lungs, and brain.

Pathophysiology

Mitotically active endothelial cells and pericytes line masses of microvessels that compose hemangiomas.

Hemangiomas usually appear a week or so following birth, then undergo a period of rapid postnatal growth for 8 to 12 months, called the *proliferating phase*. Superficial lesions are raised, bright red, and bosselated. Deeper lesions appear as a raised blue-to-purple lesion that may be mistaken for a vascular malformation. Superficial hemangiomas reach their maximal size by about 8 months of age. Deeper lesions may continue to grow until age 2 years. The involuting phase follows, in which the lesion regresses in a slow process lasting 1 to 5 years. The endothelial cells undergo apoptosis, and the lesion is replaced by fibrofatty tissue and scar. With the onset of involution, the bright red surface of the lesion begins to dull, and gray patches appear. Over time, the lesion appears to deflate and becomes less turgid. The end of involution occurs in 50% by age 5 years and 70% by age 7 years. Involution leaves nearly normal skin in half of patients. The remaining patients have damaged skin, with tissue-paper consistency, yellow discoloration, patches of scar, and telangiectasias over the surface.

Folkman first hypothesized that hemangiomas represented disorders of angiogenesis, referring to the process by which cellular mediators initiate the formation of capillary networks. Supporting this view was the discovery that proliferating hemangiomas had high expressions of the proteins proliferating cell nuclear antigen, reflecting the S phase of the cell cycle, and vascular endothelial growth factor, a specific mitogen for endothelial cells. Involuting lesions express a tissue inhibitor of metalloprotease, an inhibitor of new blood vessel formation.

Clinical Manifestations

Hemangiomas have typical appearances on radiographic examinations so that distinguishing them from solid tumors and vascular malformations is straightforward. Ultrasound shows the vascular nature of the tumor and the rapid transit of blood through the lesion. Computed tomography reveals the early contrast enhancement of the lesion, followed by late clearance of contrast material in scattered pools. Magnetic resonance imaging shows these tumors as well-circumscribed, densely lobulated masses with an intermediate signal intensity on T1-weighted images and a moderately hyperdense signal on T2-weighted images.

The location of a hemangioma dictates the urgency of treatment. One in the upper airway may interfere with breathing. Hemangiomas that involve wide areas of the face, particularly in a beard distribution over the lower face and jaw, signal the possible presence of other significant hemangiomas in the upper airway. Hemangiomas positioned in the periorbital region pose a risk to vision. Amblyopia may result from a hemangioma that covers the visual axis. The tumor may compress the globe from the side or behind and cause astigmatism. Conductive hearing loss may result from a hemangioma in the external auditory canal and lead to delayed or impaired speech development.

Ulceration is the most common complication. Rapidly proliferating lesions, typically lesions that are large and deep, may become necrotic. Painful ulcers may develop and require analgesics. Ulcers may bleed, an alarming event to parents, but usually not to any significant degree. Superinfection may occur and lead to cellulitis but rarely to septicemia and death. Small superficial ulcers in small hemangiomas respond to the application of topical antibiotic and thin hydrocolloid dressings. Large ulcers may demand more aggressive treatment to speed the involution of the lesion, such as oral steroids, pulsed-dye laser therapy, or surgical excision. Established soft tissue infections arising from an ulcerated hemangioma require intravenous antibiotics. Bleeding ulcers nearly always respond to direct compression. Rarely needed, topical hemostatic agents or fibrin glue may be used to control troublesome bleeding.

Kasabach-Merritt phenomenon describes patients with rapidly enlarging vascular lesions who develop hemolytic anemia, thrombocytopenia, and coagulopathy. The lesions that produce this syndrome differ from classic infantile hemangiomas. Most patients who develop this syndrome have kaposiform hemangioendothelioma or tufted angiomas that differ from patients who have classic infantile hemangiomas. The lesions associated with the Kasabach-Merritt phenomenon appear red-purple in color, grow rapidly to a large size (>5 cm in diameter), and are single, never multiple. An advancing rim of ecchymosis, redness, and induration surrounds the lesion. Lesions do not respond completely to corticosteroids, chemotherapy, radiation, or embolization. Approximately 50% regress in response to interferon alfa-2a. Chemotherapeutic agents have been tried, including cyclophosphamide and vincristine, in combination with interferon with some additive effect. Supportive therapy may allow nonresponders ultimately to survive, but mortality remains 25%, particularly among patients with retroperitoneal lesions.

Multiple cutaneous hemangiomas identify the patient at risk for visceral involvement. Although rare, visceral hemangiomas have a high mortality so that identification of affected children is important. Visceral hemangiomas follow the same natural history of proliferation and involution as cutaneous hemangiomas, a feature that may affect therapeutic decision making.

The liver is the most common site of visceral hemangiomas. Small tumors may remain without symptoms and be incidental findings during abdominal exploration or radiographic examinations for other conditions. Large hepatic hemangiomas (hemangioendotheliomas) may cause hepatomegaly, anemia, coagulopathy, high-output

cardiac failure, and enlargement of the liver to the point where abdominal compartment syndrome develops and ventilation becomes impossible. Tumors that remain small and asymptomatic do not require intervention. Large hemangiomas that cause heart failure or abdominal distention should be treated. First-line therapy is the administration of systemic corticosteroids or cyclophosphamide. Patients who do not respond to the latter should receive interferon alfa-2a. Therapeutic embolization is most effective if identifiable vessels feed the lesion. Surgical resection is almost never indicated or necessary. Liver transplantation is reserved for the rare unresponsive case of massive hepatomegaly associated with abdominal compartment syndrome.

Hemangiomas of the stomach or intestine cause gastrointestinal bleeding that may be mild or massive. Solitary lesions are unusual; an isolated tumor can undergo endoscopic banding or injection with intralesional steroids. More often the gastrointestinal tract has diffuse involvement with numerous lesions. Bleeding requires systemic therapy with steroids or interferon. Because these lesions usually ultimately regress, aggressive support with multiple transfusions is in order.

Facial hemangioma is also part of the PHACE syndrome (*p*osterior fossa malformations, *h*emangioma of the face, *a*rterial anomalies, *c*oarctation of the aorta, *c*ardiac anomalies, and *e*ye abnormalities). Lumbosacral hemangiomas may be associated with spinal dysraphism and anorectal and urogenital anomalies. Patients with lesions in the lumbosacral region require imaging of the spine and cord.

Large lesions may express type 3 iodothyronine deiodinase and cause hypothyroidism by the inactivation of circulating thyroxine. Patients who develop this complication often require large doses of thyroid hormone to become clinically euthyroid.

Treatment

Hemangiomas with immediate treatment priority are those that threaten life by airway obstruction, massive hepatomegaly, or high-output congestive heart failure. Threatened loss of vision or hearing also justifies aggressive intervention. Most hemangiomas have trivial cosmetic effects and no physiologic consequences. A significant number cause disfigurement, scarring, and other troublesome complications, however, that require medical or surgical attention. Lesions that have the highest risk of scarring are large facial lesions; lesions that involve the lips, nose, ears, and glabella; lesions with prominent dermal components; and ulcerated lesions.

Many treatment options exist: "active nonintervention," or awaiting involution of the tumor; laser therapy; intralesional corticosteroids; systemic corticosteroid therapy; interferon alfa-2a; excisional surgery; and other pharmacologic agents, such as cyclophosphamide, vincristine, and bleomycin. Selection depends on the location of the hemangioma, the depth of the lesion within the skin, the age of the patient, the presence or likelihood of complications, the availability of certain treatments, the expertise of the physician, and parental preference. Radiation no longer is used because long-term complications do not justify the minimal response.

Hemangiomas themselves may be at risk for carcinogenesis that may be induced by the therapeutic use of gamma radiation.

Active nonintervention is a term used by Frieden to describe the close monitoring of lesions that do not require immediate pharmacologic or surgical treatment. Although hemangiomas undergo involution, they often leave abnormally colored, damaged, and scarred skin and residual deformities. It is nearly impossible to predict the future growth of a small hemangioma in a newborn or young infant so that patients must be monitored frequently and treatment strategy modified when troublesome features become manifest. With the presence of a tracheotomy, obstructing lesions of the upper airway also can be observed. Active interventions may compromise the airway acutely: Intralesional steroid injections distend the lesion, and laser treatment causes mucosal edema and late scarring. Tracheotomy alone, without pharmacologic intervention, allows the lesion to regress spontaneously.

A pulsed-dye laser system has limited depth of penetration (1 mm) and finds its greatest utility in the ablation of superficial lesions and residual telangiectasias that remain after involution. Pulsed-dye laser therapy is appropriate treatment for ulcerations, decreasing pain and fostering re-epithelialization. Continuous-wave lasers (argon, neodymium:yttrium-aluminum-garnet, and potassium titanyl phosphate) deliver deeper thermal energy to tissues and have been applied to deeper lesions or those destined to become deep lesions. The risk of scarring is higher, the result of larger lesions and deeper tissue damage. Outcomes with continuous-wave systems seem to be more operator dependent. Carbon dioxide lasers have been used to ablate subglottic hemangiomas, primarily small, solitary lesions. Scarring and laryngeal stenosis may result in laser treatment of more extensive airway lesions, particularly circumferential subglottic lesions. Pretreatment with dexamethasone is essential to control post-treatment airway edema that may compromise the airway acutely. To limit the risk of stricture, most authorities limit a patient with an airway hemangioma to two laser treatments.

Intralesional injection with triamcinolone (maximum, 3 to 5 mg/kg/session) or betamethasone (maximum, 6 mg/session) is most effective in small cutaneous lesions. Multiple injections are usually necessary to achieve uniform distribution of steroids throughout the lesion. Injections of periocular hemangiomas are contraindicated because of the risk of atrophy of the skin, necrosis, central retinal artery occlusion, and blindness. Class 1 topical corticosteroids (clobetasol) have been used for small superficial tumors. Their use is not recommended for larger tumors or tumors that threaten sight.

Systemic corticosteroids are the mainstay of treatment of hemangiomas that threaten life, patency of the airway, or vision. Oral prednisone (2 to 5 mg/kg/day) is the first line of treatment. Patients with massive hepatomegaly or Kasabach-Merritt phenomenon should receive intravenous steroids. In approximately one third of cases, dramatic shrinkage of the tumor occurs within days. This response is not universal. In another one third, growth of the tumor ceases, and the size of the hemangioma stabilizes; one third fail to respond to prednisone therapy.

Clinical response may be partially dose dependent, leading some authorities to recommend that the higher end of the dose range be used (4 to 5 mg/kg/day). Duration of therapy ranges from weeks to months and depends on the age of the child, indications for treatment, and the growth phase of the tumor. A tumor in the proliferating phase of growth may rebound on premature discontinuance or too-rapid tapering of steroid dosages. Side effects from high-dose steroid therapy occur but are well tolerated. "Catch-up" growth rapidly corrects steroid-induced growth retardation. Other side effects are those commonly associated with steroid exposure, including irritability, gastrointestinal upset, immunosuppression, and hypertension.

Interferon alfa-2a, an inhibitor of angiogenesis, has proved to be effective in the treatment of life-threatening or function-threatening hemangiomas that do not respond to steroid therapy. The patient receives the compound as a subcutaneous injection, 2 to 3 million U/m^2 body surface area. Duration of therapy is variable, similar to that of steroids, lasting weeks to months. Interferon alfa-2a and interferon alfa-2b seem to be effective. Regression of the lesion by more than 50% occurs in 71% to 90% of patients. Spastic diplegia is the most significant side effect, affecting 20% of patients. Not all patients recover neurologic function after discontinuance of the drug. Appearance of interferon-associated neurotoxicity has led some to recommend the use of the lower end of doses (2 million U three times weekly for 6 months). Other side effects include irritability, neutropenia, and elevations of serum levels of liver enzymes.

Mulliken summarized the indications for surgical excision depending on the growth phase of the tumor and age of the patient. Excision in infancy during the proliferating phase of growth is indicated for failure of pharmacologic therapy for (1) visual or subglottic obstruction, (2) compression of the globe that risks astigmatic amblyopia, (3) bleeding, (4) ulceration, and (5) lesions at high risk for scarring. Indications for surgical removal before school attendance during the involuting phase are (1) postulcerative scarring, unalterably expanded skin, or a high probability of fibrofatty residuum; (2) same scar length or appearance if excision were postponed; (3) scar easily concealed in relaxed cutaneous tension lines or border of a facial esthetic unit; and (4) the need for staged resection or reconstruction. For lesions that have completed involution, excision is indicated if damaged skin or residual effects affect cosmetic appearance or have caused anatomic distortion or destruction.

VASCULAR MALFORMATIONS

Vascular malformations arise from faulty development of vascular structures. The classification scheme identifies lesions according to the predominant malformed vessel and the rapidity of blood flow through it. Capillary, lymphatic, and venous malformations (CMs, LMs, VMs) are slow-flow lesions, whereas arterial malformations are fast-flow lesions. Combined lesions occur, identified as acronyms of the abnormal vessel that are present (i.e., capillary [C], lymphatic [L], venous [V], and arterial [A]).

Standard terms replace archaic eponyms and misleading descriptive names. Vascular malformations typically grow proportionately with the patient, although fast-flow arterial malformations and certain mixed lesions are associated with overgrowth of soft tissue and bone.

Capillary Malformations

CMs are pink-to-red macular lesions that occur most often in the head and neck region, although they can occur anywhere in the body. Old terms include *port-wine stain* and *nevus flammeus*. The location is deep within the dermis, often in the distribution of various sensory nerve branches. Facial involvement corresponds to the distribution of branches of the trigeminal nerve. In contrast to hemangiomas, CMs neither enlarge nor regress, but they may darken with age. Hyperkeratotic nodules and eczema may develop over the surface of the CM. Cosmetic makeup covers mild lesions, but disfiguring CMs require surgical excision and skin grafting from color-matched donor sites. Some lesions may respond to pulsed-dye laser therapy.

CMs are considered distinct from neonatal staining—pink macular lesions that occur in the midline of the base of the posterior neck, over the forehead, and over the sacrum. These discolorations fade spontaneously within several months and require no specific treatment. Sturge-Weber syndrome includes CMs of the upper trigeminal dermatomes, ocular choroids, and leptomeninges.

Lymphatic Malformations

LMs are discussed more fully in Chapter 81. Old terms for variants that occur in the skin and subcutaneous tissue include *lymphangiomas* and *cystic hygroma*. The most common locations are the skin and subcutaneous tissue of the head and neck, axilla, and trunk, but other body regions and organ systems may be involved. LMs may appear as a localized mass, diffuse infiltration of tissues, chylous fluid accumulation in a body cavity, or a lymphedematous limb. The malformation disturbs lymphatic clearance of bacteria so that infection is the primary complication of LM. Bleeding may occur, leading to acute pain and swelling of the lesion in many instances. Principles of therapy are discussed in Chapter 81.

Venous Malformations

VMs range from congenital varicose veins and venous ectasias to spongy masses and complex vascular channels that may be localized or spread diffusely in an entire body region or organ system. They usually are evident at birth, in contrast to hemangiomas, which more often are not recognized for weeks. An old term, *cavernous hemangioma*, causes confusion with the current meaning of the term that describes a vascular tumor that undergoes proliferation and regression. Another term, *circoid angioma*, inadequately describes the predominance of venous structures that compose these lesions. VMs do not regress. Pain and swelling are common complaints and may signal phlebothrombosis from venous stasis. Phleboliths may form within the lesion. Intramuscular VMs may create a mass that may be mistaken for cancer. Extensive VMs may cause localized or disseminated intravascular coagulopathy. Visceral VM (blue rubber bleb nevus syndrome) is the most common vascular anomaly that causes gastrointestinal bleeding.

Persistently swollen limbs may respond to compressive garments. Localized lesions may be treated with excision and ligation of adjacent communicating veins. Injection of sclerosing solutions is considered first-line therapy, using agents such as sodium morrhuate and sodium tetradecyl sulfate (Sotradecol) in repeated doses followed by compression. Patients with extensive VMs are often coagulopathic after sclerotherapy. Sloughing of the overlying skin may occur. If the limb requires improvement of contour or function, resection should follow 6 to 8 weeks after sclerotherapy to allow swelling to recede and before recanalization can occur. VMs that extensively involve limbs or VMs in anatomically complex regions may undergo staged resections.

Arteriovenous Malformations

Arteriovenous malformations (AVMs) are high-flow lesions that occur in the cranium, extracranial head and neck, extremities, and viscera. *Arterial hemangioma* is an old term for AVM. Although present at birth, AVMs become manifest later in life as they expand and as the flow through the lesion increases. Complications include bleeding, ischemia to downstream regions, and high-output cardiac failure. Cutaneous AVMs are bright red, have an increased skin temperature, and may create an audible bruit. Elevated venous pressure may lead to venous varicosities and distention. An AVM may erode neighboring bone and cartilage. Arteriography reveals multiple tiny arteriovenous shunts in the region.

An occasional patient has marked regional gigantism of the involved body region, typically an extremity, lower jaw, or lip. The AVM increases flow to the part and stimulates growth of bone and soft tissues. Bone may become rarefied and radiolucent where AVMs exist, typically in the shafts of long bones. The overlying skin becomes violaceous.

Management depends on the extent of disease and the proximity of other vital structures. All patients should receive compressive hose to control the size of the extremity and enlargement of the AVMs. Intermittent pneumatic compression may provide added benefit. Surgical removal must eliminate all arteriovenous shunts because the lesion recurs if an appreciable number of shunts remain. Proximal arterial occlusion is not recommended because it precludes access to the lesion for therapeutic or preoperative embolization and may cause distal ischemia with pain, ulceration, and possibly gangrene. Peripheral ligation of feeding vessels, injection of sclerosants, and therapeutic embolization have been used with variable success. Wide local excision, guided by angiography, frozen section of margins, and clinical observation of bleeding at the margin of resections help guide the extent of resection. Preoperative embolization or sclerotherapy may assist wide local excision, which should follow 48 to 72 hours after interventional angiography. Poor wound healing frequently complicates resection because of chronic inflammation and venous stasis. Extensive disease and recurrence of disabling AVM may justify amputation.

Combined Vascular Malformations

Because of confusion of what constitutes a given condition described by an eponymous diagnosis, the current nomenclature emphasizes the combinations of vascular malformations that are present in a given patient. Klippel-Trenaunay syndrome is a combined capillary-lymphatic-venous malformation that causes soft tissue and skeletal overgrowth in a limb or thorax. High flow through the extremity dilates deep veins and causes varicosities, but the venous malformation is not thought to cause the spectrum of vascular malformations. Parkes-Weber syndrome is a combined capillary-arteriovenous malformation (capillary-arterial-venous malformation or capillary-lymphatic-arterial-venous malformation) involving a limb and proximal trunk.

Grossly enlarged extremities may require amputation. Staged resection of skin and subcutaneous tissue improves the contour of enlarged extremities. Annual radiographic measurements of limb length help to detect increasing differences in lower limb length that would require epiphysiodesis. Differences in upper limb length do not require orthopedic correction. Venous malformations are managed with compressive garments. Patency of the deep system allows removal of superficial venous varicosities and ligation of incompetent perforators. Injection of sclerosants, ligation of underlying veins, and excision with skin grafting treat areas of intermittent drainage and oozing from abnormal hemolymphatic vessels.

SUGGESTED READINGS

Drolet BA, Esterly NB, Frieden IJ: Primary care: Hemangiomas in children. N Engl J Med 341:173-181, 1999.

This is a concise review of the diagnosis and treatment of hemangiomas.

Fishman SJ, Burrows PE, Leichtner AM, et al: Gastrointestinal manifestations of vascular anomalies in childhood: Varied etiologies require multiple therapeutic modalities. J Pediatr Surg 33:1163-1167, 1998.

This is a valuable review of the spectrum of visceral vascular anomalies and their treatment.

Greinwald JH Jr, Burke DK, Bonthius DJ, et al: An update on the treatment of hemangiomas in children with interferon alfa-2a. Arch Otolaryngol Head Neck Surg 125:21-27, 1999.

This is a detailed analysis of the treatment of massive and life-threatening hemangiomas with interferon alfa-2a. The authors attempt to use the lowest effective doses of interferon alfa-2a to minimize neurotoxic effects (which occurred in 28% of patients).

Mulliken JB, Fishman SJ, Burrows PE: Vascular anomalies. Curr Probl Surg 37:517-584, 2000.

This monograph summarizes the current state of the art in the diagnosis and management of vascular anomalies, based on the modern Mulliken-Glowacki classification.

Sakar M, Mulliken JB, Kozakewich HPW, et al: Thrombocytopenic coagulopathy (Kasabach-Merritt phenomenon) is associated with Kaposiform hemangioendothelioma and not with common infantile hemangioma. Plast Reconstr Surg 100:1377-1386, 1997.

This life-threatening complication is associated with kaposiform hemangioendothelioma, a lesion distinct from infantile hemangioma, and is resistant to pharmacologic therapies (corticosteroids, interferon alfa-2a) that otherwise are effective in the treatment of complicated cases of infantile hemangioma.

Takahashi K, Mulliken JB, Kozakewich HP, et al: Cellular markers that distinguish the phases of hemangioma during infancy and childhood. J Clin Invest 93:2357-2364, 1994.

Proliferating and involuting hemangiomas underwent immunohistochemical analysis. A high expression of tissue inhibitor of metalloproteinase, an inhibitor of angiogenesis, was found exclusively in involuting tumors.

Lymphangiomas and Lymphatic Malformations

Lymphatic vessels remove excess fluid and small molecules and macromolecules from interstitial tissues. Lymphatic capillaries lack an intact basement membrane and so are permeable to large molecules and cells. The lymphatic system develops in close relationship to venous structures. By 6 weeks' gestation, paired jugulolymphatic sacs can be identified in the developing neck, and iliac sacs can be seen in the lumbar region (Fig. 81-1). By 8 weeks' gestation, a retroperitoneal lymph sac can be identified at the base of the mesenteric root. The cisterna chyli develops dorsal to the abdominal aorta. Paired thoracic ducts course cephalad through the chest and connect the abdominal lymphatics with the jugular system in the neck. The final configuration of the thoracic duct leaves one duct that courses cephalad in the right side of the neck, then crosses over to the left side to enter the venous system at the left jugular-subclavian junction.

Lymphatic malformations originate during fetal development as a result of lymphatic obstruction, hypoplasia, dysplasia, or aplasia. Interference with lymphatic drainage may result from excessive fluid or a deficient drainage system. Lymphatic obstruction results in dilated endothelium-lined spaces that range from small microscopic channels with small cysts to large unilocular cysts. A unifying concept links disturbed lymphangiogenesis with the different manifestations of lymphatic disease—lymphangiomas, lymphangiectasia, and lymphedema. *Lymphangiomas* are a contiguous mass of dilated lymphatic channels. *Lymphangiectasia* is a dilation in the course of a lymphatic caused by obstruction or hypoplasia in parenchymal or solid structures. *Lymphedema* is the term that describes the same phenomenon that results in lymphatic obstruction or hypoplasia in the limbs. Cystic lymphangiomas are thought to be dysplastic sequestrations of

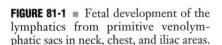

FIGURE 81-1 ■ Fetal development of the lymphatics from primitive venolymphatic sacs in neck, chest, and iliac areas.

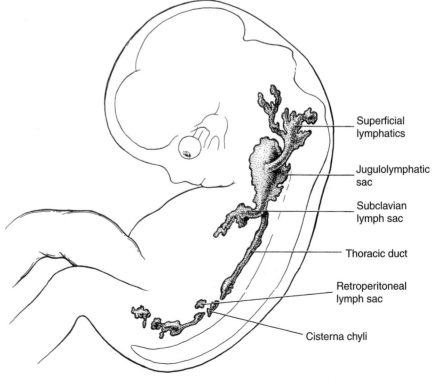

Superficial lymphatics

Jugulolymphatic sac

Subclavian lymph sac

Thoracic duct

Retroperitoneal lymph sac

Cisterna chyli

lymphatic tissue that fail to communicate with the rest of the lymphatic system.

LYMPHANGIOMAS

Lymphangiomas are benign lymphatic tumors that occur in nearly all regions of the body (Fig. 81-2). More than two thirds of lymphangiomas are apparent at birth. Often prenatal ultrasound documents the presence of

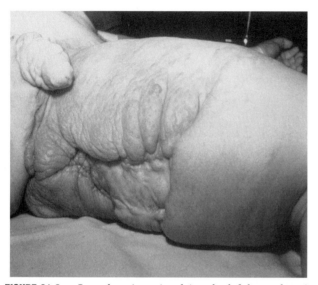

FIGURE 81-2 ■ Lymphangioma involving the left leg and genitalia of a 3-year-old boy who was undergoing staged resection of this lesion involving skin and subcutaneous tissue.

lymphangiomas in the fetus. Most lymphangiomas are evident at birth. In contrast to hemangiomas, spontaneous regression rarely occurs in lymphangiomas. The most common complications of lymphangiomas are infection and inflammation causing pain, fever, redness, and swelling. Lymphangitis and sepsis may follow. Clinically, two forms exist: infiltrative forms that have a firm consistency and cystic forms that are soft and compressible.

Infiltrative lymphangiomas consist of tiny lymphatic spaces (microcysts) within a dense stroma of connective tissue and lymphatic channels. They tend to involve the tongue, floor of the mouth, cheek, thorax, retroperitoneum, and extremities but may occur in bone. Lesions of the tongue infiltrate the floor of the mouth and cause bilateral submandibular swelling. Enlargement of the tongue may prevent closure of the mouth, making it subject to trauma, bleeding, and infection. Antibiotics are helpful in the resolution of infection, commonly caused by streptococcus and staphylococcus, and protracted maintenance administration may be helpful when infections are recurrent.

Cystic lymphangiomas are soft and compressible and glow with transillumination. Cystic lymphangiomas may be single or a mass of multiple noncommunicating loculations. Cystic variants appear most commonly in the neck (where it is called a *cystic hygroma*), axilla, mediastinum, groin, and lower abdomen (Fig. 81-3). In some patients, the mass involves the neck and mediastinum or the neck and axilla. Rarely, cystic lymphangiomas arise in the liver, spleen, and kidney. Cystic and infiltrative forms may coexist, particularly in the neck. A lesion may have cystic components in the lateral neck and blend into an infiltrative lesion as it approaches more medial structures near the pharynx, trachea, and esophagus.

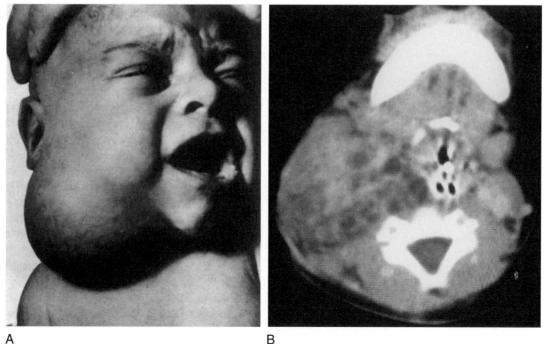

A   B

FIGURE 81-3 ■ **A**, Cystic hygroma in the right anterior triangle of the neck in a 3-week-old infant. **B**, CT scan of an infant with a macrocystic and microcystic hygroma infiltrating the tissues of the neck.

The treatment of choice for lymphangiomas is excision when possible. These lesions are benign, so vital structures, including blood vessels and major nerves, should not be sacrificed during surgical removal. Resection of cystic lymphangiomas of the neck puts important structures at risk, such as the brachial plexus, spinal accessory nerve, and marginal mandibular branch of the facial nerve. At the time of operation, the patient should not receive neuromuscular blockade so that a nerve stimulator can be used to identify motor nerves during operation. The surgeon sometimes may opt to unroof cysts in the region of vital structures and nerves rather than excise the cyst and risk damage. Infiltrative lymphangiomas surround tissues by local extension and encase normal structures, usually splaying out and thinning nerve branches, making excision difficult. Dissections may be lengthy and technically tedious. Familiarity with the regional anatomy is mandatory in anatomically complex areas, such as the head and neck, axilla, mediastinum, and pelvis. At time, it is prudent to stage resections.

Immediate postoperative complications include protracted postoperative drainage, hematoma, and cellulitis. A localized fluid collection may have to be aspirated or drained repeatedly to allow cutaneous flaps to adhere. Physical examination and radiographic imaging may show far greater lymphatic tissue remaining after resection than originally estimated at operation. Recurrence from regrowth and re-expansion of residual lymphatic tissue occurs in 5% to 15% of patients and may require reoperation. Other late complications include recurrent cellulitis and the emergence of warty vesicles (lymphangioma circumscripta) in the surgical scar and surrounding skin. Topical desiccation with dry ice or laser ablation is effective in areas where skin becomes involved.

Treatment of unresectable cystic lesions or recurrent lymphangiomas with radiation, steroids, and sclerosing agents has not been effective. Some reports have indicated that intralesional injection of OK-432 (Picibanil), a lyophilized mixture of low-virulence steptococci and penicillin, has better rates of success (60% response rate). Giant cystic lymphangiomas of the head and neck, lymphangiomas with a significant microcystic component, and residual tumors that persist after surgery tend not to respond. Injection of fibrin sealant also has been used with success; 17 of 19 cases in one report showed complete remission.

Fetal Cystic Hygroma

The prenatal diagnosis of cystic hygroma requires careful investigation for other chromosomal and structural anomalies. Affected fetuses frequently have Turner syndrome (45,XO) or autosomal trisomies. Only 22% have normal karyotypes. Hydrops fetalis complicates more than 60% of cases. The presence of a chromosomal anomaly, hydrops fetalis, or an associated structural anomaly identifies a fetus at risk for intrauterine fetal demise. Survival to birth is less than 10%. Surviving newborns with cystic hygroma and hydrops remain at risk for early postnatal death from circulatory failure or airway obstruction. Infants free from hydrops and chromosomal anomalies can survive, but some authorities recommend prenatal magnetic resonance imaging of the fetal airway

to confirm patency before birth. Evidence of airway occlusion by the lesion requires that a surgical team be prepared to control the newborn's airway in the delivery room, either immediately after birth or as part of a planned ex utero intrapartum treatment procedure. There have been case reports of successful intrapartum ultrasound-guided injection of OK-432 in fetuses with large cystic hygromas free from other anomalies.

Mesenteric and Omental Cysts

See Chapter 43 for a discussion of mesenteric and omental cysts.

LYMPHANGIECTASIA

Lymphangiectasia refers to a lymphatic malformation that affects solid and hollow organs, including intestine, lung, and bone. Intestinal lymphangiectasia usually occurs in children younger than age 3 years. Protein-losing enteropathy, which may be mild or severe, results, and affected patients have diarrhea, vomiting, and growth failure. Small bowel biopsy showing dilation of lymphatics in the intestinal villi establishes the diagnosis. The lesion may extend through all layers of the intestine and include the mesentery. One variant involves the mesenteric lymphatics alone. Pitting edema may result from hypoproteinemia. Lymphopenia and hypogammaglobulinemia also occur. Obstruction of intestinal and mesenteric lymphatics also causes fat malabsorption. Treatment of intestinal lymphangiectasia includes a high-protein, low-fat diet with supplemental medium-chain triglycerides and vitamin supplementation. This dietary plan usually reduces diarrhea and alleviates hypoproteinemia. Lymphangiectasia of the intestine is usually too extensive for resection to be an option, but often the symptoms resolve over time.

Pulmonary lymphangiectasia is a condition that presents with respiratory distress during the newborn period or early infancy. Obstruction of pulmonary lymphatics causes pulmonary edema and pleural effusion. The condition is usually bilateral and affects both lungs diffusely. The condition has been associated with congenital heart disease, and a familial form has been reported. Some cases resolve spontaneously, but many patients have rapidly progressive respiratory failure that ends in death. Older patients have clubbing, dyspnea, and hemoptysis. Chest film reveals interstitial edema, with or without pleural effusion. Lung biopsy confirms the diagnosis. Treatment is supportive, with drainage of pleural fluid performed as necessary. Chemical pleurodesis to prevent recurrent accumulation of pleural fluid may assist in overall management.

Lymphangiectasia of bone causes pain, deformity, and pathologic fracture. The lesion causes a lytic lesion visible on radiographs. Lesions may affect nearly all bones except for the cranium and phalanges. Bone lesions may coexist with lymphatic malformations in other body regions, including lymphangiomas of the trunk and chylothorax. The lesion gradually increases in size until it begins to destroy bone. Curettage and filling the defect with autologous bone chips is usually helpful. Collapse of a cervical vertebra may cause death.

LYMPHEDEMA

The most common cause of lymphedema (Fig. 81-4) in children is a primary congenital abnormality affecting the lymphatics of the lower extremities. Girls are predominantly affected (65% to 70%). Upper extremity lymphedema is exceptionally rare in children. Other causes of lymphedema may occur but are uncommon— chronic lymphangitis (including filariasis), insect bites, neoplasms, inguinal or axillary surgery and irradiation, and trauma. Unilateral leg swelling may arise from a retroperitoneal tumor or lymphoma resting on the iliac vein. Bilateral lower extremity edema should lead to a work-up to exclude the various causes of hypoalbuminemia, such as nephritic syndrome and bilateral venous obstruction as from intracaval Wilms' tumor.

Lymphedema has been classified into three categories based on the age of onset: (1) congenital lymphedema,

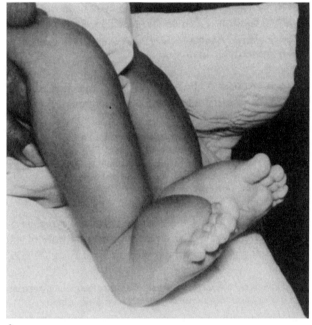

A

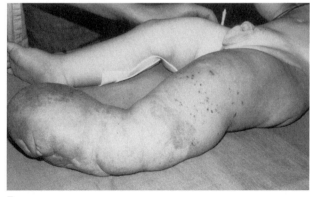

B

FIGURE 81-4 ■ **A**, Congenital lymphedema affecting both lower extremities (dorsum of the feet and calves) in a 2-month-old infant. **B**, This 2-year-old boy has the typical appearance of lymphedema with associated venous and capillary vascular malformations.

present at birth and also called *Milroy's disease*; (2) lymphedema praecox, which appears in early adolescence; and (3) lymphedema tarda, which occurs spontaneously after 35 years of age. Congenital lymphedema has a strong family association, with 35% of patients having a positive family history with an autosomal single-gene inheritance pattern. In contrast to primary lymphedema, boys and girls are affected equally. Genetic linkage analysis has uncovered a possible genetic basis for familial lymphedema. Affected families have single nucleotide substitutions at the chromosomal locus 5q35.3. The gene for vascular endothelial growth factor receptor 3 (*VEGFR3*) maps to the locus. Only lymphatic endothelium expresses *VEGFR3*, giving further support that the gene is responsible for familial lymphedema. Lymphedema also may complicate Turner and Noonan syndromes.

The underlying pathology in most cases of lymphedema is an absence, aplasia, or hypoplasia of the lymphatic channels of the lower extremities. Hormonal factors may influence lymphatic development, accounting for the development of lymphedema praecox in adolescent girls. The 'yellow nail' syndrome arises from inadequate lymphatic drainage in the nail beds, resulting in discoloration and dystrophic changes. Children with pulmonary lymphangiectasia associated with chronic bronchitis and bronchiectasis also may develop nail bed changes associated with clubbing of the fingers. Complications of lymphedema include brawny edema with skin thickening and discoloration, cellulitis, and lymphangitis. Recurring episodes of lymphangitis require long-term prophylactic gram-positive antibiotic coverage.

Clinical examination establishes the diagnosis of lymphedema. Doppler studies and plethysmography rule out arterial and venous malformations. Computed tomography and ultrasonography assess the abdomen and retroperitoneum. Magnetic resonance imaging provides delineation of the extent of lymphedema, the presence of other associated vascular malformations, and the presence of lesions that might obstruct venous or lymphatic return. Radionuclide imaging using antimony technetium-99m sulfur colloid usually shows lymphatic channels and sites of obstruction. Lymphangiograms are no longer done because of the risk of lymphangitis.

The treatment of lymphedema of the lower extremity includes a program of careful foot care and hygiene, the use of graduated compressive support stockings and pants during the day, and elevation of the legs at night. Pillows do not provide adequate lower extremity elevation. Shock blocks, 10 to 12 inches, that elevate the lower end of the entire bed give better results. Pneumatic sequential pumping systems (Jobst, Wright linear pump) reduce the degree of lymphedema that accumulates during the day and help mobilize fluid in the legs at night. Compressive hose reduces the amount of edema accumulation and diminishes the psychological impact of unsightly swollen legs.

Warfarin (Coumadin) seems to have a beneficial effect in the treatment of lymphedema, with a mean decrease in edema volume of about 55%. The action of warfarin in the treatment of lymphedema may be based on its stimulatory effect of cutaneous macrophages and local proteolysis and protein absorption. Some advocate increasing dietary flavonoids and restricting long-chain triglycerides in an effort to protect vascular endothelium and to improve microcirculation.

About 85% of patients with lower extremity lymphedema have distal disease and normal iliac and pelvic lymphatics. Severe problems seldom arise in this group. Of patients, 15% have proximal obstructive hypoplasia and develop more severe lymphedema that may require surgical intervention. Surgical therapy involves the excision of excess skin and subcutaneous tissue and depends on the concept that subfascial lymphatics are normal. Venous imaging of the involved extremity is useful to ascertain that venous drainage is adequate for the remaining skin flaps. Radionuclide lymphangiogram is recommended before the procedure to confirm that subfascial lymphatic clearance is normal. Resection of subcutaneous lymphatics reduces the edema and improves the cosmetic appearance of the affected extremity. Resectional operations are usually staged, with the medial side of legs being excised first and the lateral portion at a second procedure. Prolonged postoperative lymphatic drainage despite the use of drainage catheters may require several weeks to resolve. More recent approaches have used liposuction to remove subcutaneous tissue, followed by compressive dressings. Other experimental surgical procedures have been devised to enhance lymphatic drainage, including implanting omentum, a small bowel pedicle stripped of mucosa, and the creation of new lymphaticovenous connections with microvascular anastomosis. None have resulted in significant success.

SUGGESTED READINGS

Alguahtani A, Nguyen LT, Flageole H, et al: 25 years' experience with lymphangiomas in children. J Pediatr Surg 34:1164-1168, 1999.

This article presents the general strategy for surgical management of lymphangiomas.

Greinwald JH Jr, Burke DK, Sato Y, et al: Treatment of lymphangiomas in children: An update of Picibanil (OK-432) sclerotherapy. Otolaryngol Head Neck Surg 121:381-387, 1999.

In a prospective study using OK-432 in newborns and infants with cystic lymphangiomas, 42% had a complete response; 16%, an intermediate response; and 42%, no response. Factors thought to contribute to failure of sclerotherapy with OK-432 include significant microcystic component to the malformation, massive craniofacial component, and previous surgical resection.

Irrthum A, Karkkainen MJ, Devriendt K, et al: Congenital hereditary lymphedema caused by a mutation that inactivates VEGFR3 tyrosine kinase. Am J Hum Genet 67:295-301, 2000.

This article establishes a possible molecular basis for the development of familial lymphedema.

Mulliken JB, Fishman SJ, Burrows PE: Vascular anomalies. Curr Probl Surg 37:517-584, 2000.

This authoritative monograph covers the spectrum of vascular malformation in children.

Ogita K, Suita S, Taguchi T, et al: Outcome of fetal cystic hygroma and experience of intrauterine treatment. Fetal Diagn Ther 16:105-110, 2001.

This article identifies chromosomal anomalies, hydrops fetalis, and other structural anomalies as being risk factors for intrauterine fetal demise with prenatal diagnosis of cystic hygroma. The authors attempted sclerotherapy in two fetuses, with one responding.

Padwa BL, Hayward PG, Ferraro NF, et al: Cervicofacial lymphatic malformation: Clinical course, surgical intervention, and pathogenesis of skeletal hypertrophy. Plast Recontr Surg 95:951-960, 1995.

The management of cystic hygroma and other lymphatic malformations of the head and neck is described.

Rockson SG: Lymphedema (review). Am J Med 110:288-295, 2001.

A review is presented of the pathophysiology, natural history, and treatment of lymphedema.

82

Venous Disorders

EMBRYOLOGY

Venous disease in children is most commonly congenital. An understanding of the embryogenesis of the venous system is essential to understanding venous anomalies. The best-accepted theory of the embryogenesis of the vascular system is that multiple separate foci of mesodermal cells give rise to the various components of the arterial and venous systems. The yolk sac is the site of formation of the first blood vessels. Mesodermal cells differentiating into hemangioblasts form clusters that develop into blood islands. The hemangioblasts are precursors to vascular endothelium and cellular components of the blood. In the yolk sac and in other mesenchymal locations, blood islands coalesce to form multiple plexus of small channels or spaces. As some of these endothelial vascular channels enlarge and acquire an adventitia, they form definite vessels, whereas other channels atrophy.

The venous system arises from three paired groups of veins: (1) cardinal, (2) vitelline, and (3) umbilical (Figs. 82-1 through 82-4). These three systems allow venous return from the embryo, yolk sac, and placenta to the developing heart. The initially symmetric blood-collecting system develops asymmetrically; the right half persists and the left half atrophies.

ARTERIOVENOUS MALFORMATIONS

An arteriovenous fistula is an abnormal communication between an artery and vein, bypassing the normal capillary bed (see Chapter 83). Acquired arteriovenous communications are usually the connection of a relatively large artery to a vein via a single channel, which is corrected easily by dividing the channel between the vein and the artery. The term *arteriovenous fistula* is best reserved for these lesions. Congenital communications are more complex lesions always having multiple connecting channels and, as a result, are resistant to treatment. The artery and vein are joined by many vessels varying in size from capillaries (microfistulas) to vessels several millimeters in diameter (macrofistulas). These lesions are best termed *arteriovenous malformations*.

The clinical presentations of arteriovenous malformations are the result of variations in the various embryologic anomalies that develop during formation of the vascular system. Embryologic maturation begins as a capillary network. These vessels enlarge and coalesce to form larger vessels, assuming a retiform configuration (retiform stage). Through a process of selective enlargement and atrophy, the mature arterial and venous systems emerge. This is the mature vascular stem stage. Developmental arrest at the capillary stage or unregulated angiogenic signals are believed to result in hemangiomas. During the retiform stage, early arrest results in microfistulous communications, whereas later arrest results in macrofistulous ones.

Two major groups of arteriovenous malformations are seen:

1. *Truncal* lesions arise from major arterial branches and are hemodynamically active and progressive. The communications are large and can be identified by arteriography. They are more common in the upper extremities, head, and neck.

2. *Diffuse* arteriovenous malformations are most common in the lower extremities. The communications are small in size and large in number. The communications may not be visualized on angiography and are seldom hemodynamically active. A bruit and increased temperature on palpation are often present. The combination of superficial capillary malformations, arteriovenous malformations, and limb hypertrophy constitutes Parkes-Weber syndrome. Klippel-Trenaunay syndrome, a complex group of abnormalities, also has cutaneous lesions, venous varicosities, and limb hypertrophy but is distinct from Parkes-Weber syndrome. The vascular lesions in Klippel-Trenaunay syndrome, although clinically similar, are venous and do not consist of arteriovenous malformations. Table 82-1 lists the characteristics of these two commonly encountered vascular syndromes.

Treatment

Treatment of an arteriovenous malformation can be frustrating and disappointing. In the rare instance when the lesion is well localized in a nonvital area, it can be totally excised with good results. This is seldom the case, however. At times, therapeutic embolization is helpful, but it often must be repeated. Nonetheless, embolization may provide

Text continues on page 800

Cardinal Veins: Origin of the Superior Vena Cava

The anterior cardinal veins form the primary drainage for the cephalad portion of the embryo

→

They connect with the posterior cardinal veins to form the common cardinal veins, which drain into the sinus venosus (SV)

→

Anastomoses between the paired anterior cardinal veins form as the thymico-thyroid veins

→

This anastomotic channel enlarges and becomes the left brachiocephalic vein

→

The subclavian veins originate separately in the limb buds and join the anterior cardinal veins

→

The distal left anterior cardinal vein forms the left internal jugular vein, and a remnant of the proximal left anterior cardinal vein forms the highest intercostal vein

→

The most proximal remnant of the left common cardinal vein forms the coronary sinus

The right anterior cardinal vein (forming the right internal jugular vein distally) receives the left brachiocephalic vein and right subclavian vein and continues into the right common cardinal vein to form the superior vena cava

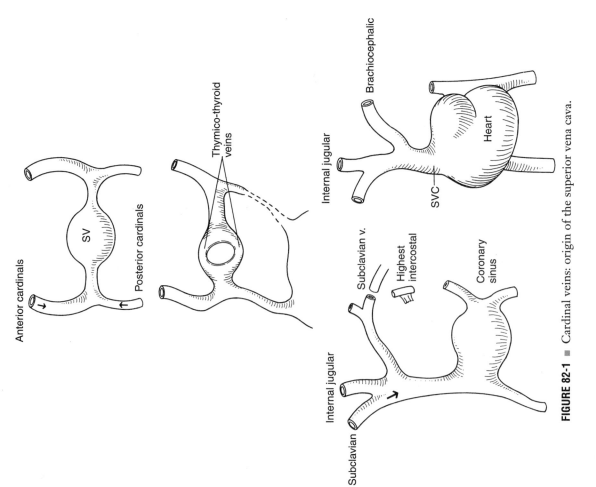

FIGURE 82-1 ■ Cardinal veins: origin of the superior vena cava.

Cardinal Veins: Origin of the Inferior Vena Cava

1. Paired posterior cardinal veins—initial (wk 1-4) drainage of blood from the caudal portion of the embryo, to be replaced by subsequent paired veins
2. Paired veins (wk 5-7)
   A. Subcardinal veins drain the kidneys
      Anastomosis is formed, and the proximal left subcardinal vein disappears
      The anastomosis becomes the left renal vein
      The distal left subcardinal vein becomes the left gonadal vein
      The right subcardinal vein becomes the renal segment of the inferior vena cava (IVC)
   B. Sacrocardinal veins drain lower extremity
      Anastomosis is formed, and the left common iliac vein disappears
      The proximal left sacrocardinal vein disappears
      The right sacrocardinal vein becomes the sacrocardinal IVC
      The right sacrocardinal vein joins the right subcardinal vein, which joins the right vitelline vein (which also receives the right hepatocardiac channel), and the IVC is established
   C. Supracardinal veins drain the body wall via intercostal veins into the posterior cardinal veins
      The distal posterior cardinal veins obliterate, and connection with the supracardinal veins remains with increasing flow
      Anastomosis forms between the supracardinal veins
      The right supracardinal vein becomes the azygos system
      The proximal left supracardinal vein separates to become the left superior intercostal vein
      The distal left supracardinal vein becomes the hemiazygos system

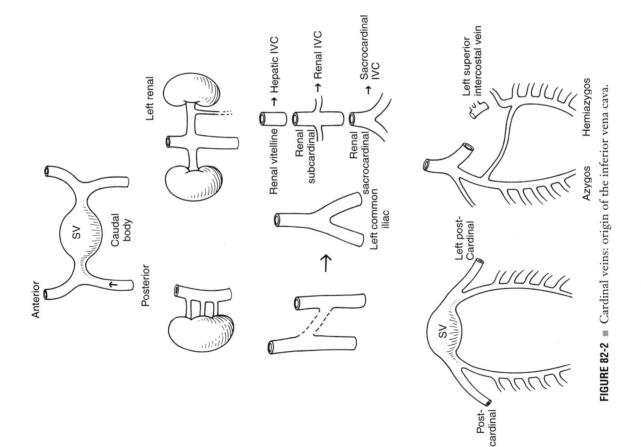

FIGURE 82-2 ■ Cardinal veins: origin of the inferior vena cava.

Vitelline Veins: Origin of the Portal Vein

The paired vitelline veins transport blood from the yolk sac → sinus venosus

→

The growing hepatic bud envelops the vitelline veins

→

Anastomoses between the vitelline veins occur (1) within parenchyma → sinusoid and (2) around the primitive duodenum

→

The proximal right vitelline vein becomes the hepatic portion of the IVC. Intraparenchymal anastomoses coalesce to form the right and left hepaticocardiac channels (to become hepatic veins). The right hepaticocardiac channel predominates

→

With normal rotation and fixation, the duodenal loop swings to the right and the superior anastomosis between the vitelline veins remains posterior to the duodenum, and the inferior anastomosis remains anterior to the duodenum

→

The left vitelline vein becomes the primary inflow to the hepatic sinusoids as portions of the right vitelline vein regress

→

The left vitelline vein ultimately receives blood from the superior mesenteric vein and splenic vein to become the portal vein

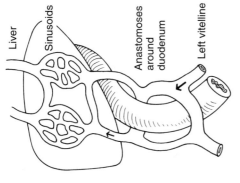

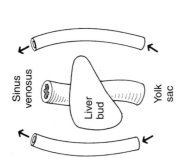

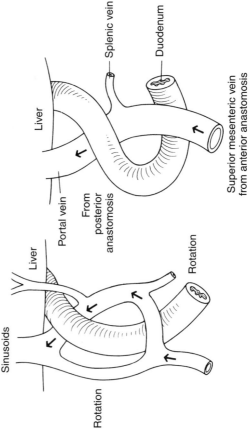

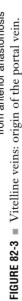

FIGURE 82-3 ■ Vitelline veins: origin of the portal vein.

Fate of Umbilical Veins

Paired umbilical veins transport blood from the placenta → sinus venous

→

The hepatic bud grows and envelops both umbilical veins and both vitelline veins

→

The vitelline veins form sinusoids and establish outflow via the hepaticocardiac channels to the sinus venosus

→

The proximal portion of both umbilical veins disappears, and inflow from the umbilical veins goes through the sinusoids and out via the hepatocardiac channels

→

The distal right umbilical vein disappears

→

Large inflow from the left umbilical vein establishes a direct route to the right hepaticocardiac channel and forms the ductus venosus

→

The right hepatocardiac channel receives oxygenated blood via the ductus venosus and unoxygenated blood from liver sinusoids from the vitelline veins, which later form the portal vein

→

At birth, umbilical flow ceases (the umbilical vein becomes the ligamentum teres hepatis), and the ductus venosus closes (forms the ligamentum venosum)

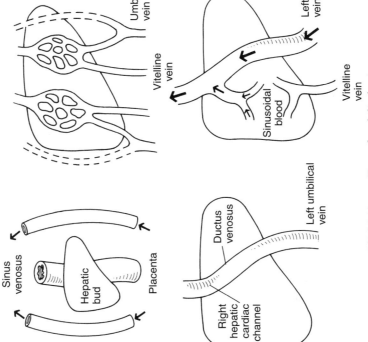

FIGURE 82-4 ■ Fate of umbilical veins.

					Lymphatic	Arteriovenous	
Syndrome	Cutaneous Vascular Lesions	Venous Lesion	Limb Enlargement	Limb Length	Lymphatic Involvement	Arteriovenous Malformation	Prognosis
Klippel-Trenaunay	Almost all cases	Deep venous blockage by bands Deep vein agenesis with femoral vein obstruction Varicosities often lateral; venous anomalies run length of extremity	Much of enlargement from thickening of subcutaneous tissue and skin; toes often grossly enlarged	Usually no major lengthening	Cutaneous lymphatic vessels Lymphedema Reduction in lymphatic vessels	No	Good May require opening of obstructed veins or limb reduction operations; disease not progressive; self-limited
Parkes-Weber	Frequent, usually hemangioma type	Varicosities	Hypertrophy of bone and muscle	Major lengthening	No	Yes	Poor May be progressive Difficult to interrupt arteriovenous communications

TABLE 82-1 ■ Parkes-Weber Syndrome Versus Klippel-Trenaunay Syndrome

significant pain relief. The emboli are placed in small arterial branches, never in a major artery. Major complications are neurologic damage caused by escape of an embolus or distal ischemic necrosis. Embolization is often helpful as a preliminary step before surgery to control operative bleeding and reduce the extent of the operative dissection. Communications are diffuse and multiple, often arising from several arterial branches over a long length of the involved area. Recurrence rates are high because unrecognized channels that are not excised or embolized enlarge and again shunt increasing amounts of blood.

Nonoperative therapy by compression garments and elastic stockings reduces venous hypertension in the extremity and may alleviate pain and promote healing of ulcers. Surgery is dangerous because of bleeding and is seldom successful because of the difficulty in delineating the lesion and the need to preserve the blood supply to adjacent structures. Ligation of major vessels is contraindicated because it frequently makes the situation worse. Proximal ligation does not eliminate flow through the shunts but can reduce distal perfusion and intensifies any distal ischemia. Multiple small feeding arteries frequently are ligated in an attempt to reduce the flow into the arteriovenous communications. When ligation and division of the fistulous tracts themselves are not possible and the lesion cannot be excised, but there are progressive changes including distal ischemia and intractable pain, amputation may become necessary. Of patients, 10% to 30% eventually require amputation.

VENOUS DISORDERS

Venous disorders may be classified into four groups: (1) congenital abnormalities of the central veins, (2) acquired abnormalities of the central veins, (3) congenital abnormalities of the peripheral veins, and (4) acquired disorders of the peripheral veins. Table 82-2 describes some of the characteristics of congenital anomalies of the central veins. Table 82-3 contains the Smith classification for acquired abnormalities of the central veins, congenital abnormalities of the peripheral veins, and acquired disorders of the peripheral veins.

VENOUS THROMBOSES

The most commonly encountered venous thromboses are those related to indwelling intravenous catheters used for monitoring, administration of drugs, or intravenous nutrition. Although the use of intravenous catheters has provided life-saving advantages to innumerable infants and children, thrombotic events have become much more common. In the case of most catheter-related venous thromboses, the catheter simply can be removed, and collateral circulation takes care of the problem. Frequently, infection is involved and must be treated appropriately. At other times, major central veins are thrombosed, such as the superior vena cava, which may lead to cerebral edema or other problems.

Peripheral venous thromboses generally occur in association with peripheral intravenous catheters, surgical or accidental trauma, soft tissue infection, paralysis, or tumors. The same risk factors that are involved in spontaneous arterial thromboses relate to the venous system. Neonates, particularly premature infants, are particularly prone to low-flow states associated with shock, sepsis, birth events, and polycythemia. The relative immaturity of the coagulation system in the newborn compared with the adult results in a higher risk of thrombotic events (see Chapter 9). Congenital disorders involving deficiencies of anticoagulant factors, including antithrombin III,

TABLE 82-2 ■ Congenital Anomalies of Central Veins				
Lesions	**Anatomy**	**Derived from**	**Clinical Significance**	**Comments**
Duplication of superior vena cava	Right vena cava drains into right atrium Left vena cava drains into coronary sinus to right atrium	Left anterior cardinal vein and common cardinal vein do not form highest intercostal vein and vein of Marshall	Problems with cannulation during cardiopulmonary bypass	Diagnosed at cardiac catheterization or open-heart operation
Left superior vena cava	Right vena cava absent—sole return via left superior vena cava into coronary sinus	Left anterior cardinal vein and common cardinal vein do not form highest intercostal vein and vein of Marshall	Problems with cannulation during cardiopulmonary bypass	Diagnosed at cardiac catheterization or open-heart operation
Anomalous venous return to heart	Many variations significant; has left superior vena cava shunting desaturated blood into left atrium	Left anterior cardinal vein and common cardinal vein do not form highest intercostal vein and vein of Marshall, and failure of left horn of sinus venosus to become part of the coronary sinus	Cyanotic at birth Right-to-left shunting Associated frequently with intracardiac defects (atrial septal defects most common)	Diagnosed by wide mediastinum on film—cardiac catheterization Ligation if right superior vena cava present Transplant into right atrium Placement of intra-atrial baffle
Venous aneurysm	Described in internal and external jugular veins, azygos veins, and superior vena cava		Usually not significant, does not rupture Can be injured during surgery	Wide mediastinum Venogram
Absence of inferior vena cava	Venous drainage through azygos system Hepatic veins drain directly into liver	Failure of formation by subcardinal system	Completely asymptomatic unless azygos veins ligated	More common with situs inversus, asplenia-polysplenia syndrome, and congenital heart disease Suspected by lateral chest film Venacavogram
Duplication of inferior vena cava	Can occur at several levels	Failure of disappearance of paired embryonic venous channels	No significance unless ligation attempted	May be a problem if caval interruption attempted to treat thrombophlebitis
Left inferior vena cava	Crosses at the renal vein and runs on right to atrium	Failure of disappearance of paired embryonic venous channels	May cause trouble during aortic surgery	
Congenital obstruction of inferior vena cava	Intracardiac because of persistent eustachian valve Web in suprahepatic vena cava		In older children swelling of legs and edema; hepatosplenomegaly can be fatal with hepatic failure	Diagnosed by cavogram Treat by excising obstruction or bypass
Absence of portal vein	Drainage by mesocaval and mesorenal channels	Failure of vitelline veins to connect to hepatic capillary plexus		
Preduodenal portal vein		Failure of vitelline regression with persistence of collaterals in anterior portal vein	Presents danger at time of operation; may be injured	Can be associated with duodenal anomalies, malrotation, situs inversus; 83% of patients have associated anomalies
Congenital portasystemic connections Duplication of portal vein		Failure of vitelline regression	May be injured at surgery	Dangerous at surgery or liver transplantation

Based on data from Smith BM, Wolfe WG: Venous disease in childhood. In Dean RH, O'Neill JA: Vascular Disorders of Childhood. Philadelphia, Lea & Febiger, 1983.

TABLE 82-3 ■ Venous Disorders

Acquired abnormalities of central veins
  Superior vena cava obstruction
  Inferior vena cava obstruction
  Renal vein thrombosis
Congenital abnormalities of peripheral veins
  Varicose veins
  Absence of valves
  Familial thromboses: antithrombin III deficiency
  Congenital aplasia/hypoplasia of deep veins
    (Klippel-Trenaunay syndrome)
  Iliac compression syndrome
  Axillary vein obstruction
  Duplications and anomalies
Acquired disorders of peripheral veins
  Effort thrombosis
  Catheter-related thrombophlebitis
  Spontaneous deep venous thrombosis
  Pulmonary embolism

Based on data from Smith BM, Wolfe WG: Venous disease in childhood. In Dean RH, O'Neill JA: Vascular Disorders of Childhood. Philadelphia, Lea & Febiger, 1983.

protein C, and protein S, may manifest themselves at the time of birth, but most often these rare deficiencies present as peripheral or visceral venous thrombotic events in mid to late childhood, often in devastating fashion. Hereditary deficiencies in plasminogen formation also increase the tendency toward thromboembolism.

Venous thrombosis in childhood traditionally has been considered to be less of a risk for pulmonary embolism than in adults. Evidence has accumulated, however, that indicates pulmonary embolism associated with venous thrombosis is common; it seems that death results less often in children with this problem than in adults.

Diagnosis

Clinically the signs of peripheral venous thrombosis involve limb edema and sometimes pain. In the case of sudden thrombosis of a major vein, such as the femoral or iliac vein, a lower extremity may swell suddenly and have a deep blue discoloration threatening gangrene, a condition referred to as *phlegmasia cerulea dolens*.

In the case of children with lower extremity fractures, whenever venous thrombosis is suspected, compression duplex or color Doppler ultrasonography constitutes an excellent screening study. With this technique, it is possible to record venous blood flow velocity and volume within the suspected vessel. The technique is useful for the survey of any major vein in the body. The study is highly operator dependent but 95% accurate in good hands. For this reason, venography is not used much now. The case is the same with impedance plethysmography. Magnetic resonance angiography also has been used to survey the venous system, particularly major veins, and it is a highly accurate technique, but its use in small children frequently requires a general anesthetic so that color Doppler ultrasound studies have been the mainstay of diagnosis in these subjects. Abdominal duplex Doppler ultrasound or magnetic

resonance angiography of the abdomen may be used to survey thromboses of major veins in the abdomen, particularly the inferior vena cava, renal vein, and branches of the portal venous system.

In instances of suspected pulmonary embolism, as with adults, the diagnosis usually may be indicated on a ventilation-perfusion scan of the lungs. Only occasionally is a pulmonary arteriogram necessary, but it may be useful if thrombolytic agents are to be infused into the pulmonary artery in these cases.

Treatment

The methods used to treat venous thromboses in adults are the ones used for children. The main approach is treatment with anticoagulant, but occasionally thrombolytic therapy with tissue plasminogen activator is useful, as it may be in cases of arterial thrombosis.

For anticoagulation, the process is started by administration of heparin with a loading dose of 75 U/kg followed by a continuous infusion of 20 U/kg/hr. Anticoagulation is monitored by determination of partial thromboplastin times to achieve levels between 55 and 80 seconds. Adjustments are made accordingly with partial thromboplastin time determinations being done approximately every 8 hours. Children younger than age 1 year usually require higher doses up to 30 U/kg/hr with closer partial thromboplastin time monitoring at first. Heparin usually is administered for 5 to 7 days depending on symptoms and the condition of the patient, after which, if indicated, oral anticoagulation with warfarin (Coumadin) is initiated at doses of 0.1 to 0.2 mg/kg/24 hours to achieve an international normalized ratio of 2.1 to 3.2. The length of oral warfarin therapy is variable depending on the indication but is 3 months in most instances.

In situations in which there has been acute thrombosis of major veins that is organ-threatening or life-threatening, thrombolytic treatment either directly into the clot or systemically may be useful. The latter technique as used for arterial thromboses is described in Chapter 83. For systemic tissue plasminogen activator therapy, a continuous infusion of 0.1 to 0.5 mg/kg/hr over 1 to 2 days while monitoring the coagulation profile has been found to be helpful.

SUGGESTED READINGS

David M, Andrew M: Venous thromboembolic complications in children. J Pediatr 123:337-342, 1993.

This excellent article describes the common problems related to venous thrombosis in children, their diagnosis, and treatment.

Downey RS, Sicard GA, Anderson CB: Major retroperitoneal venous anomalies: Surgical considerations. Surgery 107:359, 1990.

This article provides a practical description of how major venous anomalies affect the conduct of surgical procedures in the abdomen.

Dubois JM, Sebay GH, DeProst Y, et al: Soft-tissue venous malformations in children: Percutaneous sclerotherapy with Ethiblock. Radiology 180:195-198, 1991.

This report of 38 children with venous malformations that were accessible describes a useful approach to venous anomalies that do not have immediate access to large central veins.

Merr J, DeJonghe B, Golliot F, et al: Complications of femoral and subclavian venous catheterization in critically ill patients. JAMA 286:700-701, 2001.

This article points out the greater risk with femoral vein catheterization and the value of compression Doppler ultrasonography.

Smith BM, Wolfe WG: Venous disease in childhood. In Dean RH, O'Neill JA: Vascular Disorders of Childhood. Philadelphia, Lea & Febiger, 1983.

This chapter gives an excellent classification of congenital and acquired venous diseases.

Arterial Disorders

83

A variety of arterial disorders may affect children. These disorders are categorized as congenital malformations, connective tissue disorders, acquired disorders, and various occlusive syndromes (Table 83-1). Although diagnosis is fairly straightforward, treatment is challenging in most patients. Frequently a great deal of judgment must be exercised in the selection of operative versus nonoperative therapy depending on the natural history of the problem.

CONGENITAL MALFORMATIONS

Arteriovenous Malformations

Arteriovenous malformations (AVMs) may be classified into microfistulous or macrofistulous types depending on the degree of embryologic differentiation. A microfistulous AVM may constitute only a small portion of a vascular malformation, and frequently this variety is difficult to show clinically or angiographically. Patients with macrofistulous AVMs usually have clear-cut clinical and angiographic manifestations.

Congenital AVMs are common, but extensive, life-threatening types are unusual. Most AVMs are peripheral and localized and amenable to eradication. Approximately half of congenital arteriovenous fistulas occur in the extremities, and two thirds of these are in the lower limbs. AVMs of the upper extremity are more likely to be significant. Rarely, symptomatic AVMs may be seen in infants younger than 6 months of age, and sometimes these are evident at birth associated with high-output congestive heart failure, which is exceedingly difficult to manage because of myocardial strain in utero (Fig. 83-1). AVMs also may present as vascular nevi, variants of hemangiomas, or aneurysmal varices on an extremity or the scalp. In Parkes-Weber syndrome, microfistulous AVMs are associated with limb overgrowth, but these two manifestations probably are independent manifestations of this congenital disorder. Isolated macrofistulous AVMs on an extremity frequently are associated with late overgrowth of the limb, which most likely is related to the effect of increased temperature on the epiphyseal growth plates. Most commonly, AVMs also may be encountered on the face and neck, intestinal tract, liver, lung, and brain. In the brain, these lesions are often difficult to treat.

Signs and symptoms of AVMs are related to their location and extent and the size and number of fistulous connections. Most frequently the problem is one of disfigurement of the skin or limb swelling and pain. Patients may present with large varicose veins with pulsation, skin ulceration, and bleeding and overgrowth of the involved extremity. The most common manifestation of an intestinal AVM is bleeding, and usually the lesions are widespread. Refractory congestive heart failure may be the first sign of liver AVMs in newborns. AVMs of the lung may be asymptomatic or associated with infectious complications, bleeding, or stroke. AVMs of the central nervous system produce symptoms by compression of associated structures or by intracranial hemorrhage.

The diagnosis of a physiologically significant AVM is usually evident on physical examination. These patients tend to have increased warmth and swelling over the lesion associated with pulsating varicosities under or within the skin. At times, deep AVMs are associated only with small hemangiomatous skin lesions. Color flow duplex Doppler sonography is a helpful tool, ordinarily showing a continuous signal characteristic of a macrofistulous AVM. With conventional angiography or magnetic resonance

---

TABLE 83-1 ■ Classification of Arterial Disorders

Congenital malformations
  AVMs
  Visceral artery aneurysms (renal most common)
Connective tissue disorders—aneurysms
  Marfan syndrome
  Ehlers-Danlos syndrome
  Familial cystic medial necrosis
  Turner syndrome
  Cystinosis
Acquired disorders
  Kawasaki disease with aneurysm formation
  Spontaneous thrombosis
  Embolization
  Mycotic aneurysm
Occlusive syndromes—arteriopathies
  Small-vessel disease: cranial, visceral, extremity
  Mid aortic syndrome
  Renovascular hypertension

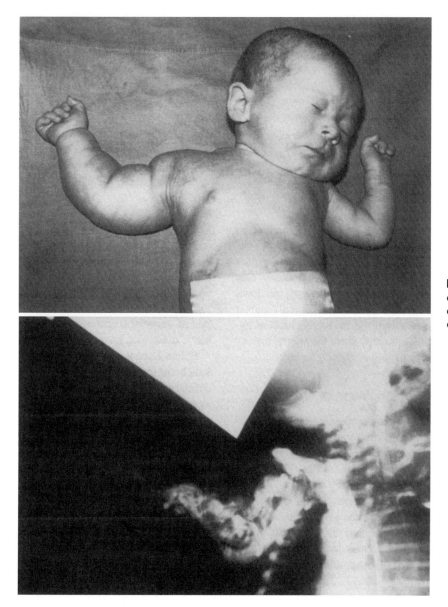

FIGURE 83-1 ■ A newborn boy with severe congestive heart failure secondary to an extensive AVM of the right arm and shoulder shown on the adjacent angiogram.

angiography, the characteristic features include arterial dilation and tortuosity, demonstration of arteriovenous connections, early venous filling, and associated dilation of venous channels. Not all patients show these features, particularly if a significant portion of the AVM is microfistulous. Under the latter circumstances, comparative venous blood oxygen saturation determinations may be required. Magnetic resonance angiography is particularly helpful because it may not otherwise be possible to determine the full extent and depth of an individual AVM.

A variety of therapeutic approaches must be used for the management of patients with congenital AVMs, depending on the location and extent of the lesion and the severity of associated physiologic derangements. It is not always possible or even desirable to perform total resection of every AVM. Many AVMs of the extremities can be treated nonoperatively with compression garments, and frequently the long-term functional result is better than if radical resection had been performed, resulting in the loss of normal tissue. Operative removal of an AVM is

desirable, however, for lesions capable of complete excision without affecting normal function. At times, partial excision or therapeutic embolization may be needed to manage painful skin ulceration and bleeding, and at other times repeated surgical intervention over time may be necessary to manage periodic problems that limit normal activities. Under the latter circumstances, postoperative use of compression garments is an important component of therapy.

AVMs of the head and neck, intestine, and lung occasionally may be treated surgically, but more commonly complete resection is impossible. Under these circumstances, angiographic embolization is a valuable treatment adjunct. The goal is not to eradicate the AVM completely but rather to diminish flow through fistulous connections to the point where the lesion is less painful or is no longer physiologically capable of producing high-output congestive failure. When angiographic embolization is successful in newborns, recurrence of symptoms is unusual, but this is not always the case in older children, who may require repeated embolization procedures.

Congenital Aneurysms of Visceral Arteries

Congenital aneurysms of various visceral arteries are rare. Aneurysms of the renal artery branches are the most common site. In late childhood, the splenic artery may be involved. The natural history of these congenital aneurysms is not known because most are discovered incidentally, but rupture during childhood is uncommon. Aneurysms of the branch vessels of the renal artery usually are discovered when patients are evaluated for hypertension. The pathology seems to be medial dysplasia without obvious cause. Most individuals believe that resection and anastomosis are needed for patients with aneurysms larger than 2 cm, particularly if they are enlarging. The long-term outlook is good after treatment, and subsequent aneurysm formation does not seem to be a problem.

CONNECTIVE TISSUE DISORDERS

The basic constituents of the vascular system are collagen, particularly type III; elastin; and glycoproteins. The various genetic disorders involved affect one or more of these components. Connective tissue disorders that frequently present with arterial manifestations include Marfan syndrome, Ehlers-Danlos syndrome, familial cystic medial necrosis, Turner syndrome, and cystinosis. The most common of these conditions is Marfan syndrome, a hereditary dominant disorder. Affected individuals characteristically are tall and slender with hyperextensibility of the joints with arachnodactyly, dislocation of the lenses of the eye, inguinal hernias in infancy, and pectus carinatum. Additional manifestations include spontaneous pneumothorax and aneurysms of the ascending aorta. The pathology that affects the ascending aorta is degenerative cystic medial necrosis with rupture of the intima and gradual dissection within the vessel wall. Sudden aortic valvular insufficiency is a frequent early manifestation. Numerous reports of successful management of Marfan syndrome patients with ascending aortic dissection have been published.

Ehlers-Danlos syndrome is a group of disorders classified according to their presenting clinical manifestations. So far, 10 forms of Ehlers-Danlos syndrome have been described, but almost all of them are associated with excessive elasticity, laxity, and delicacy of the skin and joint hypermobility. Type IV, which comprises approximately 5% of all cases, also referred to as the *arterial-ecchymotic type*, involves a defect in the collagen III gene on chromosome 2. Although the diagnosis may be made clinically, the definitive diagnosis may be made from culture of fibroblasts from a skin biopsy specimen subjected to molecular studies of the collagen III gene. It is primarily a dominant genetic disorder, but recessive variants have been encountered. Type IV patients, who have complete penetrance of the syndrome, have low birth weight, prematurity, small joint hypermobility, congenital hip dislocation, thin skin, easy bruising, inguinal hernias, spontaneous rupture of the colon, and spontaneous rupture of aneurysms of large arteries. The defect in formation of type III collagen interferes with normal tissue strength, and this is particularly true of arteries. In this syndrome, aneurysms may develop in any artery, but the most serious is progressive aneurysmal dilation and rupture of the ascending or abdominal aorta or any of its major branch vessels. Intestinal rupture also may be associated with this form of the disorder. Noninvasive approaches to the diagnosis of possible aneurysms in patients with Ehlers-Danlos syndrome type IV are the best approach because there is considerable risk with conventional transfemoral angiography. Its use should be reserved for interventional procedures designed to be life-saving because ligation of the femoral artery used under these circumstances is likely to be needed. Suturing and clamping of affected vessels often result in progressive disruption of the vessel wall, making operative management difficult or impossible. When operation is performed for the management of aneurysms in these patients, ligation is probably the most successful approach, but if clamping of the aorta is necessary, vascular occlusion is accomplished best with tourniquets or intraluminal balloon occlusion. If suturing is required for anastomosis, synthetic or fascial pledgets should be used, and an interrupted technique should be used. Also, it is useful to cover all suture lines with an external cuff of synthetic material to reinforce the repair. Use of endovascular stents has been reported, although there have been associated serious complications related to the arterial puncture site. Most patients with Ehlers-Danlos syndrome type IV die before middle age, and most die from spontaneous arterial hemorrhage.

Familial cystic medial necrosis, Turner syndrome, and cystinosis also may result in aneurysm formation anywhere in the arterial tree. Successful management depends on early treatment before rupture. It usually takes some time for aneurysms to develop in patients with connective tissue disorders so that most vascular problems present in later childhood, after age 10 years.

ACQUIRED DISORDERS

Aneurysms

The most common disorder that results in aneurysm formation is Kawasaki disease, which is of unknown origin and is characterized by rash, erythema, and edema of the hands and feet; conjunctivitis; arthritis; and cervical adenopathy. About 15% of patients may develop coronary artery aneurysms, which are diagnosed best by echocardiography and coronary artery angiography. Other peripheral vessels, including the iliac, femoral, brachial, and radial arteries, may be involved (Fig. 83-2). These peripheral artery aneurysms do not appear to enlarge progressively when discovered but occasionally are large enough to warrant resection, or they may be associated with thrombosis. Patients with coronary artery aneurysms related to Kawasaki disease occasionally require ligation and bypass, depending on the symptoms involved. Close follow-up is important. Traumatic abdominal aortic and other aneurysms are discussed in Chapter 15.

Mycotic aneurysms are most commonly the result of bacterial endocarditis and are described in the following section. Other conditions reported to be associated

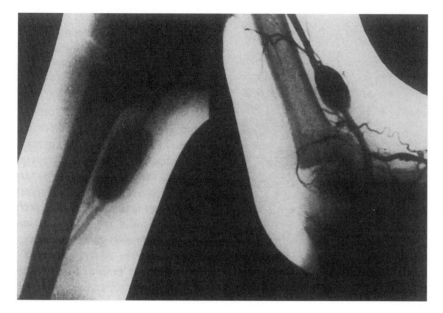

FIGURE 83-2 ■ Patients with Kawasaki disease tend to develop arterial dysplasia resulting in aneurysm formation. Angiograms of this patient show two of five aneurysms. Small aneurysms do not usually enlarge. Larger visceral and coronary artery aneurysms may enlarge, however, so they must be followed closely by periodic Doppler imaging studies.

with aortic aneurysms include tuberous sclerosis and cystinosis.

Thrombosis and Embolism

Septic newborns are susceptible to prolonged low-flow states and may develop spontaneous arterial thromboses. Polycythemic infants and infants born of diabetic mothers with severe hyperviscosity may develop visceral or aortic branch artery thromboses. At times, newborns may develop spontaneous arterial thromboses for no obvious reason. The external iliac, brachial, and various visceral arteries are the ones most commonly involved. The clinical signs of thrombosis are related to manifestations of arterial occlusion, which include limb ischemia, peripheral skin necrosis, and intestinal infarction. Multiple arterial and venous thromboses may be associated with antiphospholipid syndrome. Most infants with arterial thromboses of the extremity vessels may be treated with heparin, management of the hyperviscosity state, and expectant therapy. At times, intra-arterial infusion of tissue plasminogen activator may be used when an extremity is threatened, but care should be taken if there is concern about intracranial hemorrhage. On rare occasions, thrombectomy may be needed, but most newborns with extremity thromboses do not require operative intervention. In older children, spontaneous thromboses may be seen in patients with sickle cell disease, leukemia, protein C deficiency, and other disease states associated with hypercoagulability.

Newborns who require umbilical artery catheters for monitoring and infusion therapy are at risk for aortoiliac; visceral, particularly renal; or peripheral artery embolism or thrombosis. The manifestations are usually those of peripheral ischemia, but with aortic thrombosis, clinical signs include severe congestive failure and extreme hypertension, particularly when the renal vessels are affected. The mainstay of treatment is thrombectomy and heparinization, but occasionally infusion of tissue plasminogen activator is an option. Death usually results

if aortoiliac thrombosis is not corrected. Umbilical artery catheters also may cause peripheral embolization, but no treatment is usually necessary other than catheter removal.

Patients with congenital heart disease and bacterial endocarditis caused by *Staphylococcus aureus* or *Candida albicans* are at great risk for release of septic emboli. The clinical manifestation is that of sudden peripheral ischemia of one or both legs. This is confirmed best by aortography. Prompt embolectomy is needed because otherwise the associated arterial wall may degenerate, and a mycotic aneurysm develops. The incidence of rupture with infected aneurysms is extremely high. Initial vascular ligation and delayed reconstruction are usually successful, provided that the cardiac source is managed promptly.

OCCLUSIVE SYNDROMES

Intracranial and Extracranial Arteries

Stroke is a rare but devastating problem in children. Sickle cell disease is the most common cause, but other causes include neurofibromatosis, congenital heart disease, and arteritis with occlusion of unknown cause. Moyamoya disease, an intracranial occlusive process, has been described in Japanese and occasionally white children as a cause of stroke. If the proximal intracranial vessels are involved, at times superficial temporal-to-middle cerebral artery anastomosis may be therapeutic.

With regard to extracranial arteries, the most common disorder is Takayasu's disease, which is a progressive occlusive disorder of all of the branch vessels of the aortic arch associated with occlusion of the central retinal vessels. At times, it is associated with aneurysm formation. Occasionally, abdominal vessels also are involved in Takayasu's disease and manifest by fibrous dysplasia associated with inflammatory arteritis. This condition also has been called *Williams syndrome*. There is no known

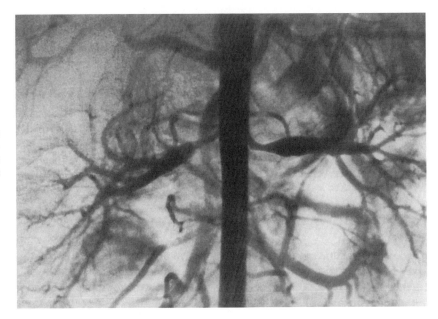

FIGURE 83-3 ■ Aortogram performed on a 6-year-old boy with malignant hypertension. These angiographic findings are diagnostic of bilateral renal artery stenosis from fibromuscular hyperplasia.

etiology or pharmacologic treatment, and revascularization is not often successful long-term.

Mid Aortic Syndrome and Renovascular Hypertension

High blood pressure may occur in 2% of children and 10% of adolescents, but the exact incidence is not known because routine screening of blood pressure generally is not performed in children. Hypertension (Fig. 83-3) may be caused by many conditions; the incidence of surgically correctable hypertension is approximately 75% before age 5 years, 45%, between ages 5 and 10 years; and 20%, between ages 10 and 20 years. Renovascular hypertension is second only to coarctation of the thoracic aorta as a surgically correctable form of hypertension. The basic pathophysiology involved with critical renal artery stenosis from all causes is ischemia-related activation of the renin-angiotensin system. Causes include previous trauma to the vessel, stenosis of the renal artery in a transplanted kidney, nonspecific arteritis, and fibromuscular hyperplasia or dysplasia. Some refer to fibromuscular hyperplasia as Takayasu's arteritis of the abdominal aorta. There is some evidence indicating that it is an autoimmune disorder.

With fibromuscular dysplasia, bilateral renal artery involvement occurs 60% of the time either simultaneously or sequentially over many years. At times, the abdominal aorta and origins of the visceral vessels also are narrowed, constituting an arteriopathy referred to as *mid aortic syndrome*. Fibromuscular dysplasia presenting in childhood affects both sexes equally and may become evident at any age, but the average is around 6 years. It has been seen in newborns, under which circumstances the lesion may be congenital. The signs and symptoms of renal artery stenosis from fibromuscular dysplasia and related mid aortic syndrome depend on the degree and location of vascular narrowing. The signs of renovascular hypertension include headache, ocular disturbances, severe congestive heart failure, and, rarely, oliguric renal failure.

In patients with mid aortic syndrome, there may be additional symptoms of leg claudication. Patients with visceral artery narrowing rarely have symptoms because they seem to compensate with collateral circulation. If hypertension is extreme and long lasting, a stroke may occur. Patients with neurofibromatosis may present with renal artery narrowing and a clinical picture undistinguishable from fibromuscular dysplasia, but histology shows neural and fibrous involvement of the renal artery orifice in neurofibromatosis.

Physical findings in addition to hypertension may include cardiac enlargement, retinopathy, and diminished peripheral pulses. The work-up of patients with renovascular hypertension is detailed in Table 83-2. The studies are designed to rule out causes of hypertension related to hormonally active tumors in children in addition to localizing the site of renal artery narrowing when present. Aortography with selective renal angiography is the most important diagnostic study with 98% accuracy. Computed tomography angiography and magnetic resonance angiography are useful but not yet capable of yielding precise anatomic detail. Although intravenous urography may suggest the diagnosis in patients with unilateral renal artery stenosis, it is abnormal only in about 40% of patients with bilateral lesions. Intravenous urography is more helpful as an indication of the status of renal function and whether parenchymal disease is present (as with glomerulonephritis). Renal vein renin levels may be helpful to determine the physiologic significance of segmental lesions and unilateral lesions and in patients with recurrent hypertension after revascularization procedures. They are not as useful, however, in children as in adults because all children with hypertension associated with renal artery stenosis should have correction performed.

Treatment of patients with mid aortic syndrome, renal artery stenosis, and other similar arteriopathies is best deferred until the active phase of arteritis has abated. The fact that fibromuscular dysplasia "burns out" in the

TABLE 83-2 ■ Diagnosis of Renovascular Hypertension
History and physical examination
Urinalysis and culture, serum electrolyte and potassium levels, blood cell count
Chest film, ECG
24-hr urine to determine values for creatinine clearance, electrolytes, catecholamines, VMA, 17-OH, and 17-KS
Aortography and selective renal vein renin determination for branch vessel lesions or recurrence after renal revascularization

ECG, electrocardiogram; VMA, vanillylmandelic acid; 17-OH, 17-hydroxycorticosteroids; 17-KS, 17-ketosteroids.

abdominal aorta is what distinguishes it from the progressive form of Takayasu's arteritis seen in the aortic arch. Preoperatively, hypertension should be vigorously controlled with β-blockers and diuretics, and angiotensin-converting enzyme inhibitor drugs should be avoided or used cautiously with careful monitoring of renal function.

Percutaneous transfemoral balloon dilation of renal artery narrowing seems to be effective when branch vessels are involved, but it does not produce a long-lasting beneficial effect when the narrowing involves the renal artery orifice within the wall of the aorta. Under the latter circumstances, it is best to perform either reimplantation of the distal renal artery into the wall of the aorta or, more commonly, revascularization with a segment of hypogastric artery or saphenous vein from the side of the descending aorta to the end of the distal renal artery. Balloon angioplasty with stenting is probably unwise in small children because of growth considerations. If reliable absorbable stents are available in the future, however, this policy might be reconsidered. In patients with mid aortic syndrome, it may be necessary to place a synthetic graft from the proximal descending aorta within the thorax or upper abdomen to the bifurcation below; then place grafts to the involved renal arteries from that conduit. An alternate approach is long patch angioplasty.

The long-term results after revascularization procedures are excellent, with complete resolution of hypertension and elimination of need for medication in more than 80% of patients. Occasionally, nephrectomy is necessary, particularly in infants with renal artery narrowing, but revascularization should be performed whenever possible. The long-term results justify an aggressive surgical approach to patients with renovascular hypertension and mid aortic syndrome. There seems to be good compensatory collateral circulation for patients who have narrowing of the celiac axis or superior mesenteric artery so that revascularization of these vessels is not always required. In all these cases, long-term follow-up is in order because arteritis may reactivate years later.

Occlusive Disease of Small Arteries

Occlusive lesions of small arteries in children not related to atherosclerosis or antiphospholipid syndrome usually are related to collagen vascular disorders, including scleroderma, lupus erythematosus, dermatomyositis, and juvenile rheumatoid arthritis. The initial presentation is that of vasoactive symptoms typical of Raynaud's phenomenon, later followed by signs of progressive occlusion of small arteries to the distal fingers and toes as evidenced by spotty areas of erythema and necrosis of the skin. This usually is associated with atrophy of the tufts of the tips of the fingers and toes. Anti-inflammatory drugs may be useful during active phases of vasospasm, and occasionally vasodilator drugs and sympathectomy may be helpful. In many instances, the disease seems to burn out, and patients stabilize. Juvenile diabetics also may present with signs of peripheral ischemia, but none of the measures used for patients with collagen vascular disease seem to help diabetics, and amputation is usually required eventually.

SUGGESTED READINGS

Iglesia KA, Fellows KE: Contemporary interventional procedures for vascular disorders in children. J Pediatr Surg 3:87-96, 1994.

In a monograph on pediatric vascular disorders, this is an excellent summary of techniques and appropriate use of interventional procedures and approaches to imaging.

O'Neill JA: Long-term outcome with surgical management of renovascular hypertension. J Pediatr Surg 33:106-111, 1998.

This article describes the clinical features of renovascular hypertension in childhood, appropriate diagnostic and therapeutic approaches, and long-term results in one of the largest series of such patients in the literature.

Ouriel K: Thrombolytic therapy for acute arterial occlusion. J Am Coll Surg 194:32-39, 2002.

This authoritative review details the techniques and agents available for the relief of acute arterial thrombosis.

Peppin M, Schwartz V: Clinical and genetic features of EDS type IV: The vascular type. N Engl J Med 342:673-680, 2000.

This article presents current information on the genetics of Ehler-Danlos syndrome and its biochemical consequences.

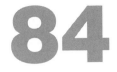

Miscellaneous Skin Lesions

CONGENITAL DEFECTS OF THE SKIN

Congenital Absence of the Skin

Congenital absence of the skin (aplasia cutis congenita) is an extremely rare disorder that may involve portions of the skin, subcutaneous tissue, muscle, and bone. The condition is most common on the scalp, trunk, or extremities and often occurs in a symmetric distribution. Infants may be born with areas of granulation tissue or dark discoloration on the surface. Others may be covered by thin, tight scar tissue. Small areas of involvement rapidly epithelialize, whereas large areas may require split-thickness skin grafting. Unstable scars should be excised and resurfaced because of the possibility of malignant change many years later.

Congenital Agenesis of the Scalp

Congenital agenesis of the scalp is a rare condition involving the vertex of the scalp in which there is a non–hair-bearing patch covered by a thin membrane or dry scabbed area that granulates, epithelializes, and scars. Small areas may be corrected by rotation flaps with or without the use of skin expanders or elliptical excision with direct suture. Mortality of patients with large defects is high. Many require skin grafting. Occasional patients may have an underlying bone defect. Associated congenital anomalies are frequent.

PIGMENTED NEVI

Nevi orginate from melanoblasts and may be of several varieties. The epidermal or marginal nevus of childhood is flat and moderately brown, varies greatly in size, and may cover large areas of the body. Overproduction of melanoblasts and melanin occurs in the basal layers, which may separate the malpighian cells from the basement membrane. Compound nevi are slightly more raised and rougher externally. Microscopically, groups of melanoblasts penetrate the basement membrane into the dermis. The intradermal nevus is the typical mode or nevus of adults, often present during childhood. It is raised and frequently hairy (Fig. 84-1). Histologically, melanoblasts are situated entirely in the dermis. The juvenile melanoma may appear malignant clinically and histologically,

yet usually remains localized until puberty. Local excision is indicated. The blue nevus may be related to the mongolian spot and consists of interlacing extensions of fibroblasts in which pigment cells are interspersed. This lesion does not become malignant.

Nevi on exposed areas and nevi subject to trauma from clothing, belts, or straps should be excised. Nevi with recent appearance or nevi that have undergone recent change in size or development of irregular margins, satellite areas, or increased pigmentation should be removed with wide complete excision. Large lesions may be excised by multiple excision or excision with resurfacing by local rotation flaps or free split-thickness skin grafts. Use of skin expanders in the subcutaneous space may expedite excision of large lesions. The risk of malignant change in giant and bathing trunk nevi is less than 10% during childhood years, but the risk increases with age (Fig. 84-2). Generally speaking, it is useful to consider congenital nevi (i.e., nevi that have been present

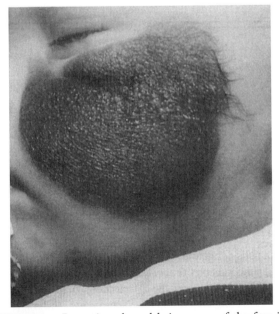

FIGURE 84-1 ■ Large intradermal hairy nevus of the face in a 2-month-old girl. The lesion was resected completely in three stages without grafting.

from the time of birth) as potentially malignant with an approximate risk of 10%, whereas acquired nevi in childhood have little or no risk, unless they undergo the sorts of changes mentioned previously over time.

Malignant Melanoma

Melanoma accounts for 2% of all cancers, and the incidence doubles every 8 to 10 years. There are approximately 40,000 new cases per year. Of all melanomas, 1% to 4% occur before 20 years of age, and 0.3% to 0.4% occur before 12 years of age. In prepubertal children, childhood melanomas tend to occur on the scalp, whereas in postpubertal individuals, lesions tend to occur on the back or neck. Of melanomas, 40% to 80% develop without a known risk factor, and there has been no documentation that a melanoma has developed before 1 year of age. Two risk factors include xeroderma pigmentosum and immunosuppression.

Moles that may be of concern for the development of melanoma include those that are *a*symmetric, have *b*order notching, have *c*olor variegation, have a *d*iameter greater than 60 mm, and have *e*levation (*ABCDE*).

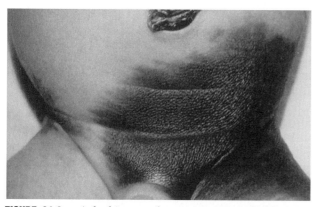

FIGURE 84-2 ■ A bathing trunk nevus is seen on this infant shortly after birth.

A change in the morphology and new onset of bleeding or pruritus are concerning symptoms for the development of a melanoma within a mole. Lesions that are on the scalp or new lesions greater than 6 mm (size of a pencil eraser) are also candidates for a biopsy. An excisional biopsy is preferred, and a shaved biopsy should be avoided. The surgical treatment of malignant melanoma in children is the same as in adults based on depth of penetration as determined on biopsy, clinical stage, and sentinel lymph node mapping (Fig. 84-3).

Xanthoma

Infants may develop yellow plaque-like patches or nodules on the skin, usually around the face, with or without a disturbance of cholesterol metabolism. The lesions are characterized by areas of tissue destruction with pale, swollen "foam cells" and giant cells. Only symptomatic or disfiguring lesions should be excised, and spontaneous disappearance is usual.

Epidermolysis Bullosa

Epidermolysis bullosa is characterized by vesicles and bullae in the skin and a defect in the elastic fibers. The congenital variety is present at birth or appears shortly thereafter and may have a family history. The spontaneous form occurs later in childhood, usually after mild trauma or exposure to sun. Simple lesions are small and usually situated on the extensor aspect of the extremities or the trunk and resolve spontaneously.

The complex form of epidermolysis bullosa usually has considerable dystrophy of the skin and often of the underlying soft tissues and bone. This form frequently requires replacement with more stable soft tissue. There may be involvement of oral, pharyngeal, and tracheal mucosa, making oral and dental hygiene and endotracheal anesthesia difficult. Esophageal stricture is common, and occasional patients may require esophageal replacement. Contracture of the digits of the hand and foot is common. Patients with extensive involvement eventually may develop areas of epidermoid carcinoma.

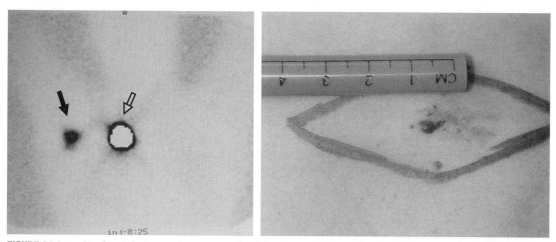

FIGURE 84-3 ■ On the right is a melanoma on the right chest wall in a 15-year-old boy. On the left is a nuclear medicine scan after injection of the lesion (open arrow). A sentinel node is visualized in the right axilla (closed arrow). At operation, no melanoma was found within the axillary node. This patient continued to recover nicely without evidence of metastatic disease.

The condition should be differentiated from Ritter's disease, Leiner's disease, impetigo neonatorum, and congenital syphilis.

Other Cutaneous Anomalies

Nevus sebaceous is a well-circumscribed, plaque-like, waxy lesion without hair growth that usually is found on the scalp or preauricular region. It is seen sporadically in children and occasionally is found at birth. On histologic examination, there is hypoplasia of the hair follicles and sebaceous glands. Over time, the sebaceous glands can become hyperplastic. Of large linear lesions, 10% can be associated with a seizure disorder. In 15% to 20% of lesions, there is malignant degeneration to basal cell carcinoma. These lesions should be excised and may require a Z-plasty for closure of large lesions (Fig. 84-4).

Congenital bands formerly were believed to be the result of amniotic bands, umbilical cord slings, other uterine space–narrowing processes, and various maternal constitutional deficiencies. These bands now are believed to be caused by an endogenesis germ cell deficit or defectively developed tissues.

Transverse or circular, partial or complete soft tissue defects of varying depth and tightness may involve any or all layers of the skin and soft tissues. Severe degrees of congenital bands may involve bone or present as congenital amputation. Edema of the tissue distal to the band should be distinguished from congenital lymphedema.

Circumferential lengthening of the bands by means of serial Z-plasty maneuvers should be initiated by the age of 3 months. Excision of edematous areas may be necessary, with direct closure or conversion of the overlying skin to thick, free skin grafts. If a gross motor or sensory deficit is seen in the extremity distal to the band, early amputation and fitting of a prosthesis is recommended.

Congenital webs are common in the neck (pterygium colli), although they may occur in the anterior axillary folds and in the crural regions. In the neck, the webbing is frequently a manifestation of Turner syndrome. If the webs produce cosmetic or functional disability, they should be lengthened by Z-plasties when patients are 1 to 5 years old. Congenital webs across the cubital and popliteal fossae usually contain misplaced or aberrant tendons and nerves and should be treated by serial Z-plasties, with occasional lengthening or excision of aberrant muscles or tendons.

CONGENITAL DEFECTS OF THE FINGERS

Hyperphalangia refers to an excessive number of phalanges in the longitudinal axis. Simple excision and plaster immobilization are all that is required. In polyphalangia, an increased number of phalanges is present in the transverse direction, usually with an extra metacarpal, which should be excised. *Symphalangia* refers to end-to-end fusion of the phalanges and usually is associated with gross

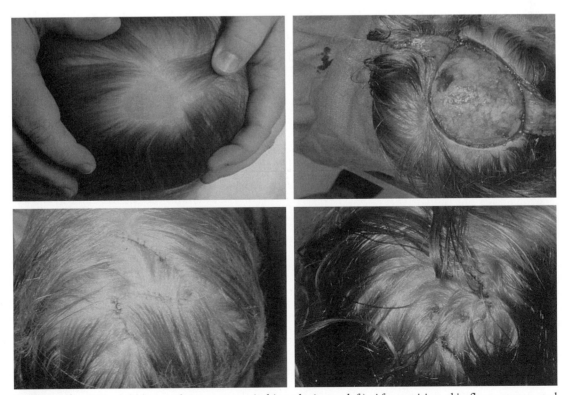

FIGURE 84-4 ■ This child has a sebaceous nevus in his scalp (upper left). After excision, skin flaps were created to close the resulting defect (upper right). In the lower two photographs taken after the operation, the incision is nicely hidden by the child's hair.

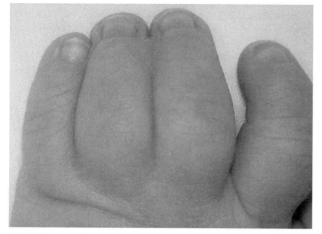

FIGURE 84-5 ■ This infant has syndactyly between the third and fourth digits.

digital deformities. Surgical separation provides improvement. *Acrosyndactyly* refers to fusion of the distal portions of digits. Proximal clefts or sinuses may be present. Treatment is by separation of the phalanges and resurfacing of the uncovered areas.

Adactyly, or absence of the fingers, requires no treatment unless the digit involved is the thumb, in which case pollicization of the index finger is indicated. Ectrodactyly, or partial absence of a digit or portion of fingers, and brachydactyly, or abnormal shortness of fingers, usually require no treatment unless the abnormal digit obstructs function of contiguous digits, in which case amputation is indicated. Polydactyly is an increase over the normal number of fingers or toes. Rudimentary or well-formed extra parts may be present. The accessory thumb is the most common lesion. Treatment is excisional but must be performed cautiously, defining the anatomy clearly. *Megalodactyly* refers to giant digits and may occur as an isolated anomaly or associated with a soft tumor, as in neurofibromatosis, lipomatosis, or hemangiomatosis. Surgical reduction of milder cases is helpful, although if the digit is grossly enlarged, it should be amputated. *Arachnodactyly* refers to abnormally long digits that often are associated with congenital heart disease (Marfan syndrome).

Syndactyly refers to fused digits (Fig. 84-5). Commonly, only skin is involved, but any of the previous digital anomalies also may be present or bony fusion of transversely placed bone or synonchia (fusion of fingernails), so x-ray evaluation is important. Repair for syndactyly is performed best when patients are 6 to 36 months of age with separation of the fused digits and covering of unsurfaced areas with grafts or skin flaps. The normal web spaces at the base of the fingers are reconstructed to prevent secondary tenting of this region. If the webbing involves many digits, as in Apert's deformity, partial-thickness skin may be used. Otherwise, free full-thickness skin grafts produce a better surface. Syndactyly of the thumb requires special consideration because even a highly hypoplastic thumb is worth reconstructing. Syndactyly of the toes is a common anomaly that does not require correction.

CONGENITAL TUMORS

Tumors of the soft tissues in children may be of various types, with tumors originating from mesoderm being more common than tumors from ectoderm. Benign lesions are more common than malignant ones. Malignant lesions may be present at birth, but usually develop later in childhood, either spontaneously or through changes in previously existing benign lesions. Histologic malignancy may not correlate with clinical malignancy. Low-grade malignancies present difficulties to the pathologist because normal tissues and benign tumors of childhood contain many large active young cells that stain hypochromatically and exhibit mitoses. A classification of cutaneous and soft tissue tumors in children is presented in Table 84-1.

Epithelial Lesions

Epidermal or dermoid cysts occur most frequently in the region of embryologic fusion. They are common at the corners of the eye; over the midline of the nose; along the line of the sternomastoid muscle, where they are to be differentiated from branchial cysts; and in the midline of the neck, where they should be differentiated from thyroglossal duct anomalies (Fig. 84-6). They are usually freely mobile in the subcutaneous tissues or are attached to the skin. Occasionally, they arise from the midline of the roof of the mouth, where they are associated with a cleft palate. They contain keratin and occasionally hair within a well-circumscribed but thin wall that contains epidermal elements. The preauricular epidermal cyst usually has a deep attachment to the helix cartilage. A mucous cyst may be present at birth or occur later during childhood and is common in the labial mucosa. Treatment is by excision.

Papillomas resemble skin tags of mucous membrane and, when more sessile, are called *verrucae*. Anal papillomas are common. They may be present at birth or appear at any time in childhood. Simple excision is recommended.

Warts are common from age 4 years throughout childhood. They are most common on the hands but may occur around the mouth and genitalia. They are caused by a virus and tend to spread to other sites and throughout the family. Electric or chemical cauterization or excision of the larger lesions is indicated for esthetic reasons, although they tend to recur until they eventually disappear spontaneously. The plantar wart occurs as a solitary lesion on the transverse arch of the foot. It may occur elsewhere on the sole of the foot and even on the palmar skin. It is also mildly infectious and is located in or immediately deep to the dermis, has a dark central nidus surrounded by callus, and is exquisitely tender. Treatment is with fine-tipped electrocautery or by chemical agents, such as trichloracetic acid crystals, followed by curettage. Recurrences may require excision, but neuromas can develop after excision and be difficult to treat. Basal cell and squamous cell carcinomas of the skin are rare in young children and uncommon in older children.

NEURAL TUMORS

A neuroma is an overgrowth of all nerve elements after division of a nerve. Isolated overgrowth of all nerve elements without nerve division is termed *neurofibroma*.

TABLE 84-1 ■ Classification of Cutaneous and Soft Tissue Tumors in Children		
Tissue	**Benign**	**Malignant**
Epithelial tissue		
Epidermis	Papilloma, verruca, wart, epidermoid (dermoid) cyst, calcifying epithelioma of Malherbe	Basal cell and epidermoid carcinoma
Sweat gland	Spiradenoma, hidradenoma	Adenocarcinoma
Sebaceous gland	Sebaceous cyst	Epidermoid carcinoma
Nerve tissue	Neurofibroma, neurilemoma	Neurofibrosarcoma, malignant schwannoma
Pigmented tissue	Nevus: epidermal, intradermal, junctional, compound, blue, juvenile (pubertal) melanoma, xanthoma	Malignant melanoma, melanotic sarcoma
Mesenchymal tissue		
Undifferentiated mesenchymal	Mesenchymoma, myxoma	Malignant mesenchymoma
Fibrous tissue	Fibroma: hard, soft, calcifying, ossifying Epulis Fibromatosis Keloid	Fibrosarcoma
Vascular tissue	Hemangioma Lymphangioma (cystic hygroma) Glomus	Hemangioendothelioma or sarcoma
Adipose tissue	Lipoma Lipomatosis	Liposarcoma
Muscle tissue	Rhabdomyoma, myofibromatosis	Rhabdomyosarcoma
Synovial tissue	Giant-cell synovioma	Malignant synovioma

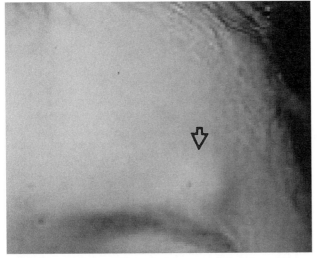

FIGURE 84-6 ■ This child has a left supraorbital dermoid cyst, which was excised in an outpatient setting. The supraorbital region is the most common location for a dermoid cyst.

Neurofibromatosis (von Recklinghausen's Disease)

There are two genetic forms of neurofibromatosis. Neurofibromatosis 1 must have two or more of the following characteristics: six or more café-au-lait spots, two or more neurofibromas or one plexiform neurofibroma, freckling of the axilla or groin regions, optic nerve glioma, a distinctive bony lesion, or a close family history of neurofibromatosis. Neurofibromatosis 2 is less common than type 1 and includes bilateral vestibular schwannomas; a first-degree relative with neurofibromatosis 2; and a unilateral eighth nerve tumor or a dermal or subcutaneous neurofibroma, a plexiform neurofibroma, a glioma, or a juvenile subcapsular cataract. Neurofibromatosis occurs in approximately 1 in 3000 births. Half of the cases result from spontaneous mutations, and the rest are transmitted in an autosomal dominant fashion on chromosome 17.

The most common nerve tissue tumor in childhood is neurofibromatosis (von Recklinghausen's disease). Lesions may present at birth or sometime later, involving any anatomic region and tissue of the body. Café-au-lait spots in the region of the lesion or elsewhere usually are present at birth. The size and number of café-au-lait spots tend to increase throughout puberty. The tumors arise in the Schwann cells, originating in the neural crest. Bony lesions associated with von Recklinghausen's disease may occur without any neurofibromatous elements. Approximately 45% of children with von Recklinghausen's disease have had physical evidence of it from birth, and 65% have manifestations by age 1 year. The congenital giant bathing trunk nevus may occur in association with von Recklinghausen's disease.

Neurologic signs are unusual, but pain may be present from pressure on a nerve in an enclosed space. Neurofibromatosis carries a considerable risk of sarcomatous degeneration. There is also an increased incidence of nonfibromatous malignant tumors and leukemias. Boys are at higher risk of developing malignancy than are girls.

The clinical forms of von Recklinghausen's disease may be divided into several groups: (1) fibroma molluscum, (2) plexiform neurofibroma, (3) elephantiasis nervorum and neurofibromas of the extremities, (4) mediastinal and thoracic neurofibromas, (5) visceral involvement, (6) skeletal manifestations, (7) central neurofibromatosis, (8) endocrine manifestations, (9) cardiovascular manifestations, and (10) neurofibrosarcoma.

Fibroma Molluscum

Fibroma molluscum represents the clinical pattern of neurofibromatosis in which hundreds of small sessile or pedunculated nodules occur in the skin and subcutaneous tissue. They may be firm or so soft as to suggest lymphangiomas. They appear after age 10 years and increase in number and size throughout life. Clinical symptoms are uncommon in childhood, and their sheer number may make cosmetic excision not feasible.

Plexiform Neurofibroma

Plexiform neurofibroma often occurs on the face and scalp, particularly the parotid region, and is characterized by thickened, frequently pigmented skin, beneath which runs a mass of tangled and branching fibers and bundles of tumor nerves. More than one third of children with neurofibromatosis have these lesions. Cranial and facial bony deformity occurs from pressure erosion by the lesion. The disfiguring plexiform neurofibromas of the parotid and scalp should be resected in stages, if necessary. Each of the plexiform extensions may be accompanied by large vessels. Functional nerves and major vessels often intertwine with the tumor projections. After resection of the bulk of the tumor, much of the overlying redundant skin often can be excised. No child should be permitted to develop a grotesque deformity even though the tumor cannot be totally extirpated.

Oral tumors can cause bleeding or difficulty with feeding. The tongue is the most frequently affected intraoral site. Partial glossectomy may improve speech and eating. Lesions may occur on the gingiva, palate, or retropharynx. Tumors of the larynx may cause obstruction and complicate anesthesia. Excision is recommended before they enlarge to unwieldy proportions.

Neurofibromas of the soft tissues of the trunk, scrotum, or vulva can achieve great size. Resection is recommended for painful or excessively bulky tumors.

Elephantiasis Nervorum and Neurofibromas of the Extremities

Elephantiasis nervorum consists of numerous small and large tumors along the nerves of the scalp together with large areas of thickened and involved skin. The disorder also may occur on the extremities and be confused with hemihypertrophy. Large unsightly lesions that impair function should be resected. Unless malignancy is suspected, every effort is made to spare the principal nerves. Procedures to arrest growth or lengthen bones frequently are required to minimize abnormalities in gait or posture caused by discrepancy in limb length.

Mediastinal and Thoracic Neurofibromas

Mediastinal and thoracic neurofibromas may arise from any intrathoracic nerves or spinal nerve root and usually are detected incidentally on chest radiographs. They may grow to sufficient size, however, to cause respiratory impairment. It is better to excise them before this stage. These lesions frequently have an intraspinal extension and must be differentiated from intrathoracic meningocele. Computed tomography (CT) and magnetic resonance imaging (MRI) are useful in delineating the extent of involvement within the spinal canal. Myelography may

be indicated if there are neurologic signs. Small extensions may grow from the surface of the tumor mass at operation. Malignant degeneration may occur in 5% to 40% of these lesions. Resection of the bulk of the tumor is recommended; repeated excision may be necessary.

Visceral Involvement

Symptomatic involvement of the intestinal tract is rare in children, with neurofibromas arising from neural elements in the intestinal wall or mesentery. Anemia, acute bleeding, or intestinal obstruction may occur. Accessible polyps of the small intestine or colon should be removed endoscopically when feasible. Other abdominal masses should be resected when discovered. Larger tumors seem to predispose to malignant degeneration.

The kidney rarely is affected with von Recklinghausen's disease except for renovascular problems. Bladder involvement is more common than is involvement in the upper genitourinary tract. Symptoms are produced by the mass causing decreased bladder capacity or obstruction. Resection and bladder reconstruction are usually necessary and should be undertaken before upper genitourinary tract damage occurs. Occasional lesions may be resected locally and, if malignant, followed by radiation therapy.

Skeletal Manifestations

Kyphoscoliosis with von Recklinghausen's disease may vary in severity, usually related to bony erosion from the pressure of tumor masses. Scoliosis should be corrected early by straightening and fusion procedures in an attempt to avoid further rapid progression and pulmonary insufficiency.

Unilateral bowing or pseudarthrosis of the tibia appears early without apparent cause; the bone is not involved by tumor. The bowed tibia is treated by successive castings, although many patients develop fracture and nonunion.

Central Neurofibromatosis

Meningiomas, gliomas of the cerebral substance, optic gliomas, and acoustic neuromas may occur. When brain lesions are diagnosed early in life, the prognosis is poor. Lesions that first appear in older children have a less dismal outlook. CT or MRI is essential in the evaluation of any of these patients with central nervous system symptoms. Blindness in von Recklinghausen's disease usually is caused by optic nerve glioma. The child with a neurofibroma rather than a glioma of the orbit usually has other facial or cervical neurofibromas. Acoustic neuromas, often bilateral, occur in children after age 10 and often show erosion of the internal auditory canal on skull radiographs.

Occasional children with neurofibromatosis develop gradual or sudden paraplegia as a result of vertebral angulation with kyphosis or occasionally as a result of an intraspinal tumor. Expeditious CT or MRI and possibly myelography are imperative in any child who develops motor weakness. Laminectomy with fusion is often only partially successful; microsurgical techniques offer an improved outlook. Mental retardation or low intelligence is common.

Endocrine Manifestations

The association of von Recklinghausen's disease with pheochromocytoma and medullary carcinoma of the thyroid is well established. The relationship between von Recklinghausen's disease and the syndromes of multiple endocrine adenomatosis is not clear, although frequently there is a familial occurrence of tumors of neuroectodermal origin. Disorders of sexual development may occur, with sexual precocity being most frequent. Developmental retardation is a frequent accompaniment.

Cardiovascular Manifestations

The heart is rarely involved with neurofibromas but may cause symptoms because of interference with contractility, outflow, valvular function, or electric conduction. Occasional lesions may be resected using cardiopulmonary bypass. Hypertension is common and often is caused by unilateral or bilateral renal artery stenosis, sometimes in association with pheochromocytoma.

Neurofibrosarcoma

Larger neurofibromas have a propensity for malignant degeneration, with rapid growth and large size of the tumor being ominous signals. Chemotherapy and radiation therapy are of limited benefit in this otherwise lethal sarcoma.

Patients with von Recklinghausen's disease require a lifetime of close observation with periodic complete physical examinations, including blood pressure, examinations to detect optic or acoustic nerve tumors, and repeated chest films to search for posterior mediastinal tumors and evaluate for spinal deformity. Individual tumors that are large or growing or cause pain or disfigurement should be removed. The implications of the disease are serious, and the ultimate outcome is uncertain; nonetheless, careful observation and judicious operation at an early stage may make a difference in the quality and the duration of life.

Neurofibrosarcoma may occur spontaneously as a solitary lesion but is rare in childhood. When present, it must be treated by radical excision of the involved nerve and surrounding tissues.

NEURILEMOMA (SCHWANNOMA)

When a neurofibroma occurs as an isolated tumor of a peripheral nerve, it is considered a neurilemoma, although it is difficult to differentiate from neurofibroma. Occasional tumors may produce pressure signs and require resection. Excision should be performed cautiously to avoid causing motor disability.

FIBROUS TISSUE TUMORS

Fibrous tissue proliferation may occur in the hand or foot as palmar or plantar fibromatosis. These lesions are not as common in children as in adults. Wide excision is necessary because of the propensity for recurrence.

Keloids are characterized by massive scar tissue in and deep to the skin after any trauma (which often may be trivial). The condition is differentiated from hypertrophic scar, which resolves with time and is not associated with prolonged pruritus. Keloids tend to recur after excision. Children tend to form and reform keloids more than do adults. Severe keloids warrant one attempt at excision, leaving a thin margin or scar on the edges. Injection of triamcinolone (40 mg/mL), 20 to 80 mg directly into the entire scar, may produce some keloid resolution, although the injection is usually painful and often requires general anesthesia.

Fibromas may occur anywhere in the somatic soft tissue, may be firm or soft, and are usually small. The soft fibroma contains young fibrous tissue and little collagen. It may be present at birth or occur later in life. When located near synovial tissue, the lesions are termed *giant cell tumors*. The dermatofibroma is a hard nonencapsulated lesion of the corium, which usually occurs after a surface break and contains dense masses of fibrous tissue.

Fibromatoses are connective tissue hyperplasias that infiltrate locally, do not metastasize, and tend to recur if not adequately excised. They may occur at any age, from infancy to young adulthood. They are circumscribed, but not encapsulated, and usually arise from fascia. Examples of fibromatoses included desmoid, nodular, or pseudosarcomatous fasciitis and plantar fibromatosis.

Aggressive fibromatosis is the term used to better define the marked cellularity and aggressively local behavior of this lesion. Infants and young children are primarily affected. Adequate surgical excision is the treatment of choice for each of these lesions. Recurrence is common, so close follow-up is needed. In some patients with recurrences, chemotherapy may be helpful.

Fibrous tissue tumors may exhibit all degrees of histologic malignancy and are highly invasive locally. They metastasize to regional lymph nodes and lung. Incomplete surgical excision is usually followed by local recurrence. The less well-differentiated types offer a poor prognosis. Wide local excision combined with radical en bloc dissection of the involved lymph nodes is the preferred treatment, with occasional patients requiring quarter amputation. Radiation therapy may enhance survival.

ADIPOSE TISSUE LESIONS

An isolated subcutaneous tumor of fatty tissue, the lipoma, is not as common in children as in adults. Liposarcoma rarely occurs by itself, being seen more often in combination with mesenchymal tissues.

TUMORS OF MUSCLE ORIGIN

Leiomyoma and leiomyosarcoma are rare in soft tissues of infants and children. Rhabdomyoma and granular cell myoblastoma are rare in childhood and have a predilection for the upper respiratory and digestive passages. Treatment is complete surgical excision with careful follow-up.

Infantile myofibromatosis consists of a proliferation of heterogeneous vascular spindle cells with ultrastructural features compatible with myelofibroblastic origin. It is benign when occurring as a single lesion, and treatment is local excision.

SYNOVIAL TISSUE TUMORS

The ganglion cyst is the most common subcutaneous lesion occurring on fingers, hand, and wrist and may be presented on the foot. This cystic lesion is associated with a tendon sheath or joint synovium. Certain movements may cause pain. The capsule consists of thin or dense fibrous tissue that is continuous with the surrounding connective tissue and contains clear jelly-like mucoid material rich in hyaluronic acid. Some lesions disappear spontaneously after direct trauma. Symptomatic ganglion cysts or cysts present for more than several months should be excised, ligating the base of the sinus communicating with the tendon.

SUGGESTED READINGS

Cribier B, Scrivener Y, Grosshans E: Tumors arising in nevus sebaceous: A study of 596 cases. J Am Acad Dermatol 42:263-268, 2000.

The authors have analyzed 596 cases in children over 66 years and describe all the associated epithelial and nonepithelial changes in these lesions. They found that the rate of malignant tumors arising in these congenital lesions was low (1%).

Ho PC, Griffiths J, Lo WN, et al: Current treatment of ganglion of the wrist. Hand Surg 6:49-58, 2001.

The authors describe their thoughts about current treatment of ganglion cysts at the wrist.

Keswani SG, Johnson MP, Hori S, et al: In utero limb salvage: Fetoscopic release of amniotic bands for threatened limb amputation. J Pediatr Surg 38:848–851, 2003.

The authors report advances in fetoscopic release of amniotic bands in an attempt to salvage threatened limbs.

Makkar HS, Frieden IJ: Congenital melanocytic nevi: An update for the pediatrician. Curr Opin Pediatr 14:397-403, 2002.

This review article suggests that melanoma is increasing in incidence in the pediatric population and identifies risk factors for this diagnosis.

Schmid-Wendtner MH, Berking C, Baumert J, et al: Cutaneous melanoma in childhood and adolescence: an analysis of 36 patients. J Am Acad Dermatol 46:874–879, 2002.

This review stresses diagnosis and modern approaches to management which closely parallel current methods for adults.

Seymour-Dempsey K, Andrassy RJ: Neurofibromatosis: Implications for the general surgeon. J Am Coll Surg 195:553-563, 2002.

This is a complete review article regarding neurofibromatosis and its impact on general surgery practice.

85

Conjoined Twins

Conjoined twinning is rare and one of the most challenging of congenital malformations in terms of reconstruction. Historical references date back to Roman times. It is characteristic of this monozygotic anomaly that one or both of such twins have other organ system anomalies. This type of developmental asynchrony has been suggested to be an indication that conjoined twinning itself is a malformation and that other discordant malformations represent individual anomalies in individual twins, which is seen about half the time. To date, approximately 250 successful separations in which one or both twins have survived over the long-term have been reported.

INCIDENCE AND EMBRYOLOGY

The typical form of monozygotic twinning occurs at a relatively constant rate of 4 in 1000 live births. The incidence of dizygotic, fraternal twins is approximately 10 to 15 in 1000 live births. Overall, twin births occur in approximately 1 in 90 births. Parasitic or heterotopic conjoined twins are exceedingly rare, occurring in about 1 or 2 per 1 million live births; this form of twinning also has been shown to be monozygotic. Conjoined twinning probably occurs with a frequency of approximately 1 in 50,000 to 100,000 live births.

Conjoined twins who survive to the point of being candidates for separation are mostly female with a female-to-male ratio of approximately 3:1. In reports of stillborn conjoined twins, however, males predominate. This is consistent with conventional monozygotic twins, which are more frequently male.

By 6 days after fertilization, the cellular zygote cluster becomes the blastocyst. The inner cell mass from which the embryo, amnion, and yolk sac develop forms from an aggregation of cells at one pole of the blastocyst. During this first week of gestation, the cells of the inner cell mass seem to be totipotent and able to split to form two germinal disks. These disks can develop into two identical persons so that division of the zygote within the first 7 days of gestation yields monozygotic identical twins. These twins are identical in sex and karyotype, and they share an amnion and yolk sac. Dizygotic twins result from fertilization of two separate ova, and each fetus has its own amnion, yolk sac, and umbilical cord. Dizygotic twins

may be of the same or opposite sex and have different karyotypes.

The classic theory on the embryology of conjoined twins suggests that they result when the inner cell mass incompletely divides after the first 7 days of when monozygotic twinning is thought to occur (somewhere between 13 and 16 days of gestation). The exact reason that complex fusion results from this late division is still unknown. The range of complex fusion is broad, and incomplete division of the embryo seems to be associated with inhibition of complete differentiation of the various organ systems. Conjoined twins with fused organs usually have incomplete development, as manifested in conjoined hearts, liver, and gastrointestinal (GI) and genitourinary tracts.

CLASSIFICATION

Although various classifications of conjoined twins have been based on the interpretation of the most prominent site of connection, all use the term *pagus* (that which is fixed). The most commonly applied classification in the literature is clinical, simplified to include the most commonly encountered types of twins. The details of each are described subsequently. Table 85-1 and Figure 85-1 provide information on incidence and organ involvement. In the order of frequency, the types of conjoined twinning are thoracopagus, omphalopagus, pygopagus, ischiopagus, craniopagus, and heteropagus. Another commonly used classification system combines the first two as thoraco-omphalopagus because they commonly occur together. Heteropagus twinning is described in a separate section later.

TABLE 85-1 ■ Classification of Conjoined Twins		
Type	Incidence, %	Organs Potentially Involved
Thoracopagus	74	Heart, liver, intestine
Omphalopagus	1	Liver, biliary tree, intestine
Pygopagus	17	Spine, rectum, genitourinary tract
Ischiopagus	6	Pelvis, liver, intestine, genitourinary tract
Craniopagus	2	Brain, meninges

ANTENATAL DIAGNOSIS AND OBSTETRIC MANAGEMENT

Prenatal ultrasound has been shown to be capable, although not universally reliable, of making the diagnosis, at least after 20 weeks' gestation. Other techniques, such as magnetic resonance imaging (MRI), have been used for specific purposes, particularly for evaluation of the heart. Prenatal ultrasound, echocardiography, and three-dimensional cardiac MRI usually provide sufficient information to help families decide whether or not to continue the pregnancy. Conjoined twins are being identified antenatally more often because of the frequency of prenatal ultrasound when the mother is large for gestational age or when polyhydramnios is present.

Prenatal ultrasound is particularly important in planning obstetric management of such complicated fetuses, who frequently have breech presentation. Cesarean section seems to be the safest and preferable approach to delivery. Intrauterine distress, causing premature labor, is common in conjoined twins, so efforts must be made to inhibit labor to permit the fetuses to become as mature as possible. Amniocentesis for analysis of lecithin:sphingomyelin ratios to evaluate pulmonary maturity is useful in determining the timing of cesarean delivery. At the time of birth, the condition of the infants determines just how aggressive supportive care must be to permit the infants to undergo the necessary series of diagnostic evaluations.

PREOPERATIVE DIAGNOSTIC STUDIES

Preoperative evaluation is best directed at the individual organ systems involved because the reconstructive approaches used are generally standard ones for the various individual anomalies encountered. They are modified to the degree the involved structures are shared and incompletely developed. Although simple diagnostic studies, such as conventional radiography, may be performed immediately after birth, the performance of invasive procedures must be timed according to the infant's condition and ability to withstand stress. Another consideration concerns the anticipated timing of separation because diagnostic studies performed later may be more accurate and associated with less physiologic insult than if performed in the immediate perinatal period.

Almost every organ system must be investigated thoroughly in every case unless obviously understood. Table 85-2 details the most useful types of diagnostic studies. In all conjoined twins, one twin is smaller than the other; half the time, one infant has more anomalies than the other. These distinctions should be identified because it is generally best to favor the more normal of the two infants when performing reconstruction, particularly when structures cannot be distributed equally.

Preoperative evaluation of the cardiovascular system is essential in all conjoined twins, whether or not the hearts are conjoined as determined from prenatal studies. Echocardiography and electrocardiography are performed to determine the presence of anomalies in the case of separate hearts and to determine the site of cardiac junction and the presence of intracardiac and extracardiac anomalies in the case of conjoined hearts. Cardiac catheterization was previously the mainstay for diagnosis for definition of complex intracardiac anomalies, but now three-dimensional cardiac magnetic resonance angiography (MRA) is used. MRA provides precise anatomic information that may serve as the basis for deciding whether or not cardiac separation should be attempted. The presence of a single QRS complex on electrocardiography usually indicates that successful cardiac separation would not be possible, but the presence of two separate complexes does not indicate a better outcome.

Another study used to avoid physiologically demanding invasive studies is radionuclide cardioangiography, which provides information on direction of flow and the degree of shared cross-circulation. Because most conjoined twins share a liver that must be separated, it is important whether one or two inferior cavae are present. In many instances of conjoined hearts, one inferior vena cava drains both livers, a key element in planning separation. At this time, three-dimensional MRA is probably the most useful diagnostic study for the evaluation of conjoined hearts and livers after birth.

Because of the high incidence of early gestational births in conjoined twins, impaired pulmonary function is common. Oxygenation may be deficient in the case of intracardiac or extracardiac shunts, if portions of the thorax are shared, and if one twin's chest is smaller than the other's. In addition to cardiac studies, chest radiography, measurement of arterial blood gasses, differential oximetry, and thorough evaluation of physical

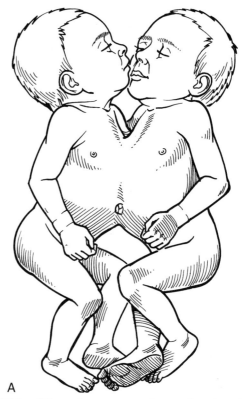

A

FIGURE 85-1 ■ The various common forms of conjoined twins. **A,** Thoracopagus.

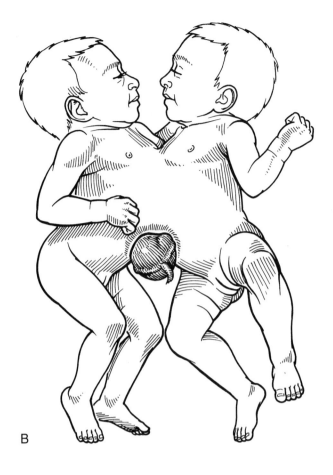

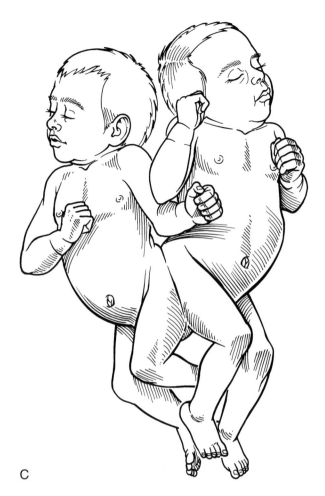

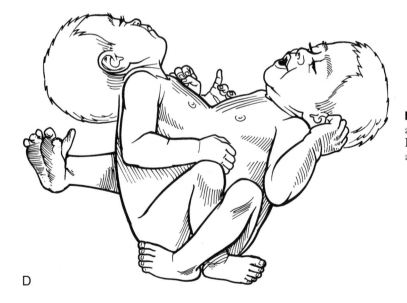

FIGURE 85-1—cont'd ■ **B,** Omphalopagus, sometimes also called *thoraco-omphalopagus*. **C,** Pygopagus. **D,** Ischiopagus tripus; a more common tetrapus form also occurs.

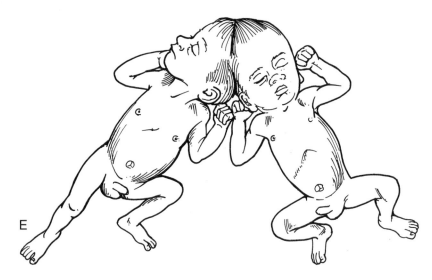

FIGURE 85-1—cont'd ■ **E,** Craniopagus.

findings are important in the evaluation of pulmonary function.

Most conjoined twins share a liver and may share a pancreaticobiliary system, particularly when duodenal junction is present in omphalopagus twins. Ultrasound, three-dimensional MRA, and radionuclide biliary scanning with separately timed injections into each twin are the most helpful studies.

Except for craniopagus twins, all other forms of conjoined twins may share portions of the GI tract. This is evaluated best by upper and lower GI contrast studies; differential injections frequently are needed to define precisely which structures are shared. In thoracopagus and omphalopagus twins, the GI junction is frequently at the level of the duodenum, in which case only one pancreas and extrahepatic biliary system may be present. In ischiopagus and pygopagus twinning, the site of intestinal

junction is usually in the terminal ileum, in the region of Meckel's diverticulum. In the latter case, a single colon and terminal ileum may be shared.

Genitourinary evaluation is best approached by ultrasonography, cystography, computed tomography (CT) with contrast enhancement, radionuclide studies, and endoscopy. The information that must be gathered from these studies includes the status of renal function and the number and location of the kidneys, ureters, and bladders. Because most conjoined twins are female, accurate vaginal or urogenital sinus examinations are crucial to determine whether there is a single vagina or duplex vaginas and the presence or absence of a cervix, urogenital sinus, or hydrocolpos. Determination of the number, size, and location of these cavities is crucial to planning the staged reconstructive procedures required in these cases of complex caudal junction. In males, it is important to evaluate the penis, scrotal structures, and gonads before separation to determine whether sex change is required.

With caudal junction, as seen with ischiopagus and pygopagus twinning, degrees of sharing of the vertebral column, pelvis, and lower extremities vary. Conventional radiography, three-dimensional CT, and MRI are needed (Fig. 85-2). When a lower extremity is shared, as in ischiopagus tripus twins, aortography may be needed to determine the exact nature of the blood supply to the shared limb, the twin to which it primarily is related, and to what degree the limb can be salvaged or possibly shared by the infants. This is another area in which the twins may be discordant. The evaluation of skin territories is less crucial now that skin expanders are used commonly.

ETHICAL CONSIDERATIONS

Mention already has been made about the accumulation of information based on prenatal MRI, ultrasound, and echocardiography, which are known to be reliable. The pediatric surgeon who is experienced with separation of conjoined twins is probably the best person to counsel the prospective parents about the likelihood of successful separation and what the outcome for the twins is likely

TABLE 85-2 ■ Useful Diagnostic Studies in Conjoined Twins	
Type of Conjoining	**Studies**
Thoracopagus	Chest radiography, electrocardiography, echocardiography, three-dimensional MRA, radionuclide cardiography, measurement of blood gases
Omphalopagus	Chest and abdominal radiography, upper gastrointestinal series, DISIDA liver scanning
Pygopagus, ischiopagus	Chest, abdominal, and limb radiography; upper and lower gastrointestinal series; cystoscopy; cystography; renal scanning; vaginography; CT with three-dimensional reconstruction of the pelvis; spinal MRI; aortography or MRA
Craniopagus	Ultrasound, CT with three-dimensional reconstruction, three-dimensional MRA
Heteropagus	Chest and abdominal radiography, gastrointestinal contrast studies, echocardiography

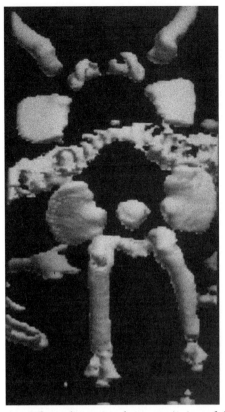

FIGURE 85-2 ■ Three-dimensional reconstruction of the pelvic CT scan in ischiopagus tripus conjoined twins shows the usefulness of this technique in planning separation. The inferior two femurs are part of a single shared lower extremity.

to be given the many advancements that have been made in surgical technique, postoperative care, reconstruction, and rehabilitation. This information puts the parents in the best position to determine whether or not they wish to continue the pregnancy. Before and after the infants are born, the family's right to privacy should be respected. The pediatric surgeon must develop a close and trusting relationship with the family because of the nature of the complicated decisions that must be made and the need for informed consent. Particularly detailed and repeated discussions are necessary if, after the preoperative evaluations are performed, it is evident that only one twin can survive or if one of the two probably would be left with a serious disability. Only solitary survivors may be possible in twins with conjoined hearts, twins with only one inferior vena cava draining shared livers, and twins with a single extrahepatic biliary tree. These difficult decisions can be aided by knowledge that both children usually die without separation under these circumstances, and the situation has been made more rational with the understanding that the operation itself does not determine which twin would survive but rather the nature of the anatomy involved. If high-quality survival is possible, most recommend that twins be separated, even if only one twin can survive, rather than allowing inevitable early death of both infants.

Organs and shared structures usually are allocated individually on the basis of the anatomy and available data with the intent of maximizing both twins when there are no medical differences between the two. If one twin is significantly mentally or physically impaired, allocation may be directed best toward the healthier twin. In the end, the parents have the ultimate right to accept or refuse surgical separation. Every case is different and must be approached with utmost sensitivity for the rights and feelings of the parents and their children.

TIMING OF SEPARATION

Almost all reports suggest that, when possible, separation is best performed on an elective basis when the twins are 9 to 12 months old because emergency separation before 6 months of age is associated with higher mortality. Anesthetic management is easier, and blood loss and physiologic derangement are tolerated better at this time than in the immediate postnatal period. Some of the increased mortality is related, however, to postnatal conditions, such as prematurity and related problems. If operation is delayed much beyond 1 year of age, conjoined twins may have difficulty developing an independent personality for a few months. Emergency conditions that may force emergency separation include the presence of a stillborn twin, intestinal obstruction, rupture of an omphalocele, heart failure, obstructive uropathy, and respiratory failure. Undertaking separation when conjoined infants are 9 to 12 months old also provides time to permit thorough preoperative assessment and integration of all of the specialists who are required for successful separation.

PREOPERATIVE PLANNING AND ANESTHETIC MANAGEMENT

Successful separation of conjoined twins is performed best by an experienced team of pediatric surgical specialists and anesthesiologists who know how to integrate their efforts. Team conferences, including preoperative and postoperative caretakers; all surgical, anesthetic, and diagnostic specialists; and nurses and others involved in the operation and the care of the infants, are necessary and valuable for review of all gathered information. A mock preoperative drill involving all team members expedites the procedure so that everyone knows what the next step will be. Some decisions must be made during the separation, but preoperative drills help the team to anticipate most issues ahead of time.

Because exsanguinating hemorrhage and hypovolemia are the primary risks that the anesthesiology teams must handle, the placement of radial artery and central venous catheters and additional intravenous access lines in both twins is in order. Depending on the degree of shared circulation, judiciously modified doses of intravenously administered sedatives and paralytic agents are used, particularly because it is generally possible to perform endotracheal intubation in only one twin at a time. Short-acting inhalation anesthetics with high concentrations of oxygen are the easiest to manage.

When all monitoring and intravenous lines and the endotracheal tubes have been secured carefully, the two anesthesiology teams can lift the infants into the air so that a thorough total-body sterile preparation and draping can be performed. Although it is permissible to have one operative nursing team for the initial part of the separation, two nursing teams are required when the separation has been accomplished. The nature of the reconstruction anticipated in each twin before surgery governs the instruments and set-up provided to each of the operative nursing teams. Each surgical specialty team is integrated into the operation at the appropriate time as the separation proceeds as determined by the lead surgeon, who must remain available throughout the entire separation procedure.

APPROACHES TO ORGAN SYSTEM RECONSTRUCTION

In general, standard approaches to organ reconstruction are in order when decisions have been made relative to the distribution of the various structures. At times, innovative techniques or specially tailored standard reconstructive techniques are needed. This is particularly true with regard to management of the skin, heart, biliary tree, and genitourinary tract.

Skin

Whenever there is extensive sharing of skin, it is helpful to use skin expanders to increase the amount of skin available for coverage. The chest and abdominal wall, the extremities, and the perineum usually pose a problem for skin coverage and body cavity closure. Most surgeons prefer to use subcutaneous skin expanders, placing as many as possible on the dorsal and ventral surfaces of the body and on the upper part of the lower extremities. Placement of skin expanders in the subcutaneous position in the early postnatal period frequently is complicated by erosion through the skin, even if the expanders are placed under the skin from remote small incisions. They are tolerated better after 4 weeks of age. It takes approximately 6 to 8 weeks or longer to gain the maximum advantage of skin expansion; their placement is best timed according to the scheduled time of separation.

Central Nervous System

Two forms of central nervous system sharing are the craniopagus form, in which there are varying degrees of brain and vascular connection, and forms in which portions of the spinal cord are shared. Craniopagus twinning occurs in only about 2% of conjoined twins. They are classified into partial and complete forms. A practical classification is based on the site and degree of fusion of the brain tissue and the venous structures involved that would require interruption at operation and whether the union is at the vertex, occiput, or parietal portions of the skull. Numerous attempted separations have been reported, but long-term outcome so far has been satisfactory only when minimal brain tissue (partial forms) has been shared and the superior sagittal sinus has not been involved.

Pygopagus and some ischiopagus twins may share varying portions of the vertebral column and the spinal cord. These instances may indicate staging separation with division of the spinal cord structures initially.

Liver and Pancreaticobiliary System

The liver is shared in almost all anterior forms of conjoined twinning except craniopagus. The most crucial preoperative determination is whether each liver has an outflow to its own heart or whether a single inferior vena cava drains both livers. Survival is not possible without hepatic venous drainage. When it has been determined that each twin has its own hepatic venous drainage, separation of the livers is usually feasible. The central area of the livers selected for division first is dissected free circumferentially over a sufficient distance so that Penrose drains can be placed as tourniquets and tightened down. A double row of large overlapping, horizontal mattress absorbable sutures is placed so that the division can be performed between them. As the division proceeds, individual bleeding vessels and bile ducts can be suture ligated, and excessive bleeding can be controlled.

Two pitfalls may be encountered during hepatic division. Although most shared livers have only one or two large portal venous connections, it may be that they take the form of a lacework of multiple venous channels that can be difficult to control. The second pitfall occurs when there is a single extrahepatic biliary tree; this must be determined ahead of time to decide where the liver should be divided on its undersurface. In twins with one extrahepatic biliary tree, operative cholangiography may be necessary to determine which infant should be given the extrahepatic bile duct and which should be left with a single hepatic duct, which may be drained externally into a Roux limb of jejunum (Fig. 85-3). If these twins share a pancreas, the pancreas is best left with the extrahepatic biliary tree. If there are two small pancreatic anlagen, each infant should receive one. The latter consideration determines how the shared duodenum should be reconstructed. In a few cases with a single extrahepatic biliary tree, nothing is available for one of the twins.

Gastrointestinal Tract

Intestinal sharing generally follows two patterns, although there are some variations of each. The first pattern is sharing of the duodenum at the second or third portions; the fourth portion of the duodenum and the rest of the GI tract are separate. Reference already has been made to the pancreatic and biliary considerations with duodenal fusion. If the biliary structures are separate, the method of duodenal reconstruction must be based on preserving an ampulla of Vater for both infants, sometimes requiring duct reimplantation.

The second type of GI sharing is ileocolonic or colonic. The primary point of conjunction is at the level of Meckel's diverticulum with sharing of the terminal ileum and colon. A dual blood supply almost always comes from each twin. It is preferable to provide one twin with the ileocecal valve and the other with the anus, which is usually singular, with both infants getting half of the shared colon. Colostomy no longer is needed routinely because immediate anorectal reconstruction usually can be accomplished. The overall functional results with this approach have been good, and it has made skin closure less of a problem than when colostomy was used.

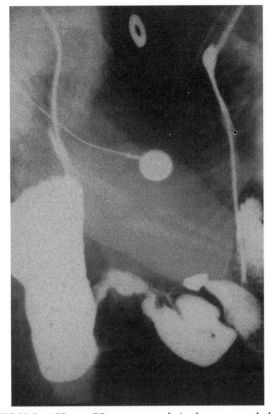

FIGURE 85-3 ■ Upper GI contrast study in thoraco-omphalopagus conjoined twins shows a duodenal fusion, and because soluble contrast material was used, it fortuitously showed the presence of a single extrahepatic biliary tree.

Heart

A variety of approaches have been used for infants with shared hearts. Preoperative studies have shown that most conjoined hearts cannot be separated. The few successes have involved survival of only a single individual who was provided with the cardiac tissue of both twins. All conjoined hearts have complex anomalous development. Cardiac allotransplantation for conjoined twins is probably not a reasonable option to offer families.

Genitourinary System

In ischiopagus and pygopagus forms of conjoined twins, numerous anatomic variations occur, and reconstruction is either immediate or staged, primarily depending on whether two bladders are available. Many infants require bladder augmentation and staged reconstructive procedures to promote continence and vaginal and genital reconstruction. If one bladder is present but there is a urogenital sinus, the latter structure can be used as a substitute bladder, and a new vagina can be made. In the case of a single urinary bladder shared by the two infants, the decision regarding giving each infant a portion of the bladder is made on the basis of the nerve and blood supply to the bladder base. If a shared bladder cannot be divided into two equal parts because of trigonal anatomy, one twin is given the major part of the bladder with satisfactory volume, and the other receives a small part

that is brought out as a temporary vesicostomy with subsequent augmentation cystoplasty.

Most female ischiopagus or pygopagus twins have single external genitalia and double vaginas. Fertility may be preserved in both female twins. Male conjoined twins may have one or two sets of external genitalia that must be separated appropriately. Hypospadias is common and amenable to standard repair. In cases with only one phallus, one twin undergoes male reconstruction and the other undergoes female reconstruction, during which labia are created from available scrotal tissue.

Urinary reconstruction of ischiopagus twins usually requires multiple stages and close long-term follow-up if complications are to be avoided. With careful observation and judicious but aggressive intervention, it is generally possible to maintain normal renal function and reasonable bladder continence. Normal sexual activity and fertility are reasonable and achievable goals.

Skeletal System and Rehabilitation

The most common consideration in long-term follow-up of ischiopagus and pygopagus twins is orthopedic. Whether there is anterior, face-to-face apposition of the twins, lateral connection, or posterior junction, the potential for kyphosis and scoliosis deformities exists. At times, one twin or the other may have a small or asymmetric chest wall that may potentiate scoliosis. If gait disturbances are related to absent limbs or pelvic deficiencies, scoliosis may be a further consideration. Because the potential for scoliosis exists throughout childhood, these children, when separated, must be followed yearly until they are fully grown. Whenever there is any degree of thoracic cage sharing, later revision of initial chest wall closure is required.

The main orthopedic challenges are related to the management of ischiopagus conjoined twins, although some pygopagus twins require orthopedic and neurosurgical involvement because of problems related to sacral sharing. Ischiopagus patients can be divided according to the number of legs into bipus, tripus, or tetrapus. The first challenge is a thorough evaluation of the pelvis and a shared lower extremity. Since the advent and use of skin expanders, it has been possible to consider preserving as much of that extremity as possible for better function. Only after thorough evaluation of three-dimensional reconstruction of a CT scan of the pelvis can the appropriate site for division of the pelvis be determined (see Fig. 85-2). This method also facilitates the decision about whether the acetabulum of a third shared leg would be given to one or a portion to both twins; this decision depends on whether the shared extremity can be split or necessarily must be given to only one of the twins. As mentioned earlier, a crucial part of the evaluation and the separation procedure is evaluation of the blood supply to the extremities whether shared or not because this evaluation determines whether one or both twins provides the main vascular supply.

In these situations in which the pelvis is wide open after completion of the separation procedure, it is best to make some attempt to close the pelvis as much as possible. In this regard, it is probably best to perform posterior iliac osteotomies at the time of the initial separation.

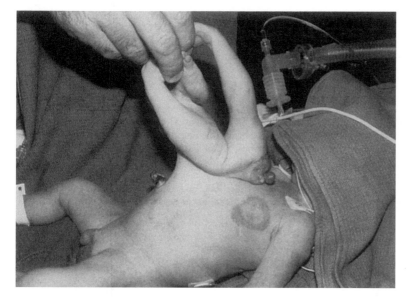

FIGURE 85-4 ■ Heteropagus twin has characteristics typical of this anomaly such as venous drainage into the suprahepatic inferior vena cava.

Not only does iliac osteotomy provide some opportunity to close the pelvic ring, but also it potentiates better skin closure and stability of the perineum. Because one twin in a set of ischiopagus tripus twins often has only one lower extremity, better pelvic closure improves the eventual ability to fit an appropriate bucket-type prosthesis.

Careful orthopedic follow-up is crucial for appropriate long-term rehabilitation and function. The most common and the most difficult issues that must be addressed over time include problems related to the deformed shared leg and to the normal leg, such as recurrent hip dislocation and foot deformities. Typically, repair considerations are staged in multiple procedures over a long period. Although standard orthopedic corrective procedures have been used and for the most part have been successful, innovative reconstructions of the acetabulum and various types of fusions have been needed. Careful prosthetic fitting is essential to providing good long-term function. In most instances, with persistence and close observation, good long-term ambulatory function can be achieved. Although many more improvements are needed in the management of children with shared pelvic structures, the current, acceptable results are related to modern rehabilitation techniques, excellent prosthetic appliances, improved preoperative imaging, and increased surgical experience. It also has been possible to preserve a longer and more functional shared leg with a functional knee for these patients because of the use of skin expanders.

HETEROPAGUS TWINNING

Heteropagus twins, also called *parasitic*, are incomplete. They are attached most commonly to the lower chest and epigastrium (Fig. 85-4), but they also may take the form of caudal duplication, so-called dipygus, or fetus in fetu, in which the duplication is inside the abdomen of the dominant twin. A rare additional type of asymmetric twinning is parapagus, in which there is a laterally oriented axis. Generally, heteropagus twins involve duplication of extra portions of a pelvis and lower extremity, duplicated genitalia, and duplication of portions of the GI tract. An omphalocele is frequently associated. In contradistinction to symmetric conjoined twins, in which delayed separation is preferred, separation shortly after birth is ordinarily possible in heteropagus twins. With a common epigastric point of junction, a prominent feature important to the surgical procedure is that the vascular connections almost always are located adjacent to the falciform ligament with venous drainage passing either directly into the liver substance by way of the ligament or via a large venous channel draining into the suprahepatic inferior vena cava adjacent to the hepatic veins. Complex cardiac malformations are usually present in the autosite.

OUTCOMES

Unless limiting, associated congenital anomalies are present, survival is generally possible in both sets of omphalopagus, ischiopagus, and pygopagus twins and heteropagus twins. Separation is not currently possible in most thoracopagus twins with conjoined cardiac ventricles, although survival has been achieved in a few rare instances. The same is true of craniopagus twinning, in which the only survivors after separation have minimal degrees of conjunction, and even then, long-term neural impairment is a continuing consideration.

SUGGESTED READINGS

Albert MC, Drummond DS, O'Neill JA, Watts H: The orthopedic management of conjoined twins: A review of 13 cases and report of 4 cases. J Pediatr Orthop 2:300-307, 1992.

This article summarizes the various short-term and long-term orthopedic considerations in conjoined twins with pelvic junction.

Cywes S, Millar AJW, Rode H, et al: Conjoined twins—the Cape Town experience. Pediatr Surg Int 12:234-248, 1997.

This is one of the most extensive surgical experiences in the literature; much useful information is provided.

Hsu H-S, Duckett JW, Templeton JM, O'Neill JA: Experience with urogenital reconstruction of ischiopagus conjoined twins. J Urol 154:563-567, 1995.

Although this report refers to ischiopagus twins, the principles described apply to genitourinary considerations in all conjoined twins. The approach to decision making in reconstruction is timely.

O'Neill JA: Conjoined twins. In O'Neill JA, Rowe MI, Grosfeld JG, et al: Pediatric Surgery, 5th ed. Philadelphia, Mosby, 1998, pp 1925-1938.

This chapter provides a thorough description of all aspects of evaluation and treatment of the various forms of conjoined twins based on the largest surgical experience reported.

PART XIII

Additional Miscellaneous Surgical Disorders

86

Neurosurgical Disorders

Brain tumors, central nervous system (CNS) trauma, spinal dysraphism, hydrocephalus, and craniosynostosis are neurosurgical conditions that have important pediatric surgical implications. Trauma and tumors are discussed in Chapters 16 and 19, respectively, but brain tumors are more fully addressed in other texts. The relationship between intraventricular hemorrhage and hydrocephalus is detailed in Chapter 1. Three conditions—spinal dysraphism, hydrocephalus, and craniosynostosis—are discussed here. Because of the frequent association of hydrocephalus with myelomeningocele, these two abnormalities are discussed together.

SPINAL DYSRAPHISM (SPINA BIFIDA)

Primary neural tube defects represent 95% of all cases of spinal dysraphism and are believed to result from failure of neural tube closure during the fourth week of gestation. The most common primary neural tube defect is myelomeningocele. Failure of neural tube closure results in exposure of the neural plate or neural placode along the midline of back, bony and skin defects, and neural abnormalities, such as the Arnold-Chiari II malformation and hydrocephalus. In the most severe form, craniorachischisis, the neural placode has no covering over the entire length of the spinal cord and there is anencephaly.

Secondary neural tube defects (i.e., postneurulation defects) comprise 5% of neural tube defects and result from abnormal development after closure of the primary neural tube. Unlike primary neural tube defects, these lesions usually are skin covered or closed and typically are not associated with hydrocephalus or Arnold-Chiari II malformations. This group of defects includes meningocele, lipomyelomeningocele, cutaneous manifestations of spina bifida, diastematomyelia (split cord malformations), and congenital dermal sinus.

Myelomeningocele

Myelomeningocele is the most common primary neural tube defect. By definition the lesion contains both meningeal and neural components and, therefore, is differentiated from meningoceles, which do not contain neural elements. Myelomeningocele involves the entire CNS. Affected infants are born with an exposed neural placode in the midline, commonly in the lumbosacral or sacral area. The dura is deficient and in the midline is attached to the lateral edges of the neural placode. Cerebrospinal fluid (CSF) either is contained within an intact fluid-filled sac or leaks from the central canal in cases in which the sac has ruptured. The bony canal is malformed and deficient. Almost all patients have an associated Arnold-Chiari II malformation, and the majority have or will develop hydrocephalus. In addition, these patients often have other associated CNS and systemic abnormalities and frequently suffer from multiple neurologic, urologic, and orthopedic problems as they mature.

Incidence, Epidemiology, and Genetics

Myelomeningocele is more common in whites than in African Americans or Asians, and there is a slight predominance of the disorder in girls. The incidence in the United States is 0.4 to 1 per 1,000 live births. It is more common in Ireland and Wales, where the incidence is as high as 4.2 to 12.5 per 1,000 live births. Genetic transmission is multifactorial. Ninety-five percent of children with myelomeningoceles are born to couples with no history of neural tube defects. Having a child with a myelomeningocele can increase the risk that a second child will have a lesion to 2% to 3%. In some studies the recurrence rate if there is one affected sibling is 1 in 33, but this rate rises to 1 in 10 if two offspring are affected. If a close relative has had an infant with myelomeningocele, the risk is 0.3% to 1%. Moreover, mothers with insulin-dependent diabetes and those with seizures who are taking valproic acid or carbamazepine during pregnancy have a risk of approximately 1%.

Etiology and Prevention

Evidence is mounting that folic acid deficiency is directly related to failure of neural tube closure and the occurrence of primary neural tube defects. Administration of supplemental folic acid in the periconceptual period in randomized, placebo-controlled studies decreased the recurrence rate of neural tube defects in women with a previously affected pregnancy as well as the incidence of neural tube defects in women who never had an affected pregnancy. Based on various studies, in 1993 the Committee on Genetics of the American Academy of Pediatrics published its recommendations for folic acid for the prevention of neural tube defects: (1) mothers who have had a fetus with a neural tube defect should take 4.0 mg of folic acid daily starting 1 month before a planned pregnancy through the first trimester of the pregnancy and (2) all women of childbearing age capable of becoming pregnant should take 0.4 mg of folic acid daily to prevent the first occurrence. There is evidence that if all women in the childbearing age capable of becoming pregnant take 0.4 mg of folic acid daily, the occurrence could be reduced by 50%.

Prenatal and Obstetrical Considerations

Neural tube defects are detected by prenatal ultrasonography in 90% to 95% of cases, and measurements of maternal serum α-fetoprotein (AFP) can detect 50% to 90% of open neural tube defects but are falsely positive in 5%. Screening for neural tube defects is initiated in the early part of the second trimester with the determination of maternal serum AFP and high-resolution fetal ultrasonography. If these studies suggest the presence of a neural tube defect, then amniotic AFP and acetylcholinesterase levels should be obtained by amniocentesis because these studies increase the diagnostic accuracy of a neural tube defect to more than 97%.

The safest route of delivery is still controversial. In the past it was believed that labor and vaginal delivery adversely affected neurologic outcome. However, more recent studies suggest that there are no differences in neurologic deficits in infants delivered vaginally or by cesarean section. It is generally agreed that pregnancy should be maintained for at least 34 to 36 weeks before delivery to ensure adequate fetal lung maturation.

Anatomic and Clinical Characteristics

In 85% of patients with myelomeningocele, the defect involves the lumbar area, the caudalmost region of the primary neural tube to close. The patient presents with a cystic mass of the back. The mass is made up of the neural placode, arachnoid, dura, nerve tissue and roots, and CSF (Fig. 86-1). The arachnoid runs from the neural placode laterally to fuse with the skin, forming a subarachnoid space containing CSF.

Neurologic involvement and urologic complications generally correlate with the level of the spinal lesion. Therefore, some generalizations can be made, which are outlined in Table 86-1.

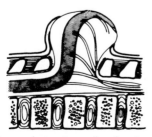

FIGURE 86-1 ■ In myelomeningocele, the tissues of the spinal cord form part of the sac wall and its contents.

TABLE 86-1 ■ Level of Lesion Versus Pathophysiologic Effects		
T1	Some ambulation but only with full braces	Neurogenic bladder
L1	Wheelchair necessary	Upper and lower neuron lesions
L2	"	
L3	Ambulatory with full braces and crutches	
L4	"	
L5	Ambulatory with short-leg braces	
S1	Walks unaided	
S2	"	
S3	"	
S4	"	

Management

There has been considerable controversy concerning the decision to treat infants with extensive myelomeningoceles. Studies suggest that mental retardation is not intrinsic to the lesion but is due to the postnatal events resulting from untreated hydrocephalus and recurring infections. Aggressive treatment of hydrocephalus, the Arnold-Chiari II malformation, the tethered spinal cord, and prevention of infection significantly improve the prognosis of patients with myelomeningocele. McLone closely followed 100 patients aggressively treated over a 17-year period. He found that only 9% of the patients had IQs below 70 and that 75% had IQs above 80. Sixty-six percent of patients were in regular schools. Although 75% of the preadolescent patients were able to ambulate, the incidence of ambulation decreased to 50% with increasing age because of increased difficulty with mobility after weight gain. Intermittent catheterization of the bladder was necessary in 90% of the patients. Current studies show similar results.

Many neurosurgeons now recommend early aggressive treatment for all patients regardless of the level of the lesion unless there is a severe CNS anomaly, advanced hydrocephalus at birth, severe anoxic brain injury, active CNS infection, or congenital malformations or genetic syndromes incompatible with long-term survival. For neonates born with myelomeningocele, initial management has a profound effect on their survival and the handicaps with which they may have to cope.

Closure of the defect is usually done soon after birth to reduce the risk of infection and to limit postnatal neurologic deterioration. Prophylactic antibiotics are administered and repair is performed as soon as practical, but preferably before 48 to 72 hours of life. The arachnoid and skin are freed from the neural placode, which is usually sutured to form a neural tube. The dura is then freed and closed over the tube. The closure must be watertight, and a dural graft may be necessary. The skin is then closed either directly or by rotational flaps. Bony prominences, such as kyphus or gibbus deformities, which may inhibit skin closure or cause skin erosion, are removed.

Fetal Management

Intrauterine repair of myelomeningocele has been advocated as a means of improving neurologic outcome in fetuses with myelomeningocele; however, this method of treatment remains experimental. A recent single-institution, nonrandomized observational study by Bruner and colleagues, conducted between 1990 and 1999, compared outcomes, including the requirement for ventriculoperitoneal shunt placement, obstetrical complications, gestational age at the time of delivery, and birth weight, in patients who underwent intrauterine repair of myelomeningocele with those repaired postnatally. Although this study showed that intrauterine repair decreased the incidence of hindbrain herniation and shunt-dependent hydrocephalus, the study also demonstrated an increased risk of oligohydramnios and a need for hospital admission for preterm uterine contractions, an earlier gestational age at delivery (32 vs. 36 weeks), and a lower birth weight (2171 vs. 3075 g) in patients repaired in utero. Evaluation of outcomes was hampered by the small sample size and the short-term follow-up period. Lethal pulmonary hypoplasia has been observed after premature delivery at 32 weeks after in-utero repair of myelomeningocele during the 24th week gestation. Early repair has had little effect on postnatal distal sensorimotor function in survivors after fetal repair that showed decreased bladder capacity, increased detrusor storage pressures, and a significant post-void residual in four. Four infants had hydronephrosis, and three of the six had vesicoureteral reflux. These bladder and upper urinary tract findings are similar to those observed in patients with myelomeningocele repaired in the postnatal period. Until the long-term outcomes after this procedure are clarified by a randomized trial, prenatal repair must still be considered investigational.

HYDROCEPHALUS

Almost all children with myelomeningoceles will have some degree of hydrocephalus. A few (5% to 10%) will have clinically overt hydrocephalus at birth, but most will initially have only slightly enlarged ventricles. However, once the CSF-filled cystic mass in the back is eliminated by closure of the defect, the buffering action of this "cyst" is lost and the ventricles and the head progressively enlarge.

Pathophysiology

Cerebrospinal fluid is produced principally in the ventricular system by the choroid plexus. CSF flows from the lateral ventricles through the foramen of Monro into the third ventricle (Fig. 86-2). From the third ventricle, the CSF flows through the aqueduct of Sylvius into the fourth ventricle and then out through the lateral foramina of Luschka and median foramen of Magendie into the cisterna magna, where it flows into the spinal and cortical subarachnoid space for eventual reabsorption at the arachnoid villi granulations that extend into the dural venous sinuses.

Hydrocephalus develops if there is an overproduction of CSF, or if there is a failure of CSF reabsorption from a reduction in the ability of the arachnoid granulations to reabsorb CSF, or from failure of CSF to reach the site of reabsorption due to an obstruction in the CSF pathway. Overproduction of CSF is rare and usually due to a papilloma of the choroid plexus. Reduced absorption of CSF can occur as a result of scarring of arachnoid villi granulations from hemorrhage or infection. Obstruction is a common cause of hydrocephalus in infants and children and is the principal cause in patients with myelomeningocele. These obstructions result from malformations,

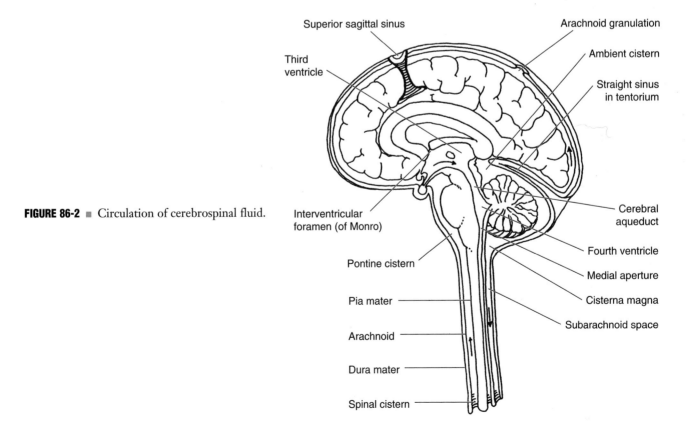

FIGURE 86-2 ■ Circulation of cerebrospinal fluid.

scarring, tumors, and infections. Essentially all children born with myelomeningoceles have Arnold-Chiari II malformations. The anatomic abnormalities associated with this malformations are responsible for the hydrocephalus. With the Arnold-Chiari II malformation there is obstruction of the outlet of the fourth ventricle, obstruction of flow of CSF into the cortical subarachnoid space, and compression leading to aqueductal stenosis.

Management

If progressive hydrocephalus is observed prenatally by ultrasound, the child is usually delivered by cesarean section as soon as lung maturity is ascertained. If there is significant enlargement of the ventricles, a ventriculoperitoneal shunt is placed. If the ventricles are less distended and hydrocephalus does not seem to be progressive, the criteria considered before operation include the thickness of the brain at the coronal suture visualized by ultrasonography, progressive developmental delay, symptomatic Arnold-Chiari II malformation, and the development of cystic dilation of the central spinal canal (syringomyelia).

The ventriculoperitoneal shunt is the current shunt of choice. It is relatively easy to place and is associated with a lower revision rate and fewer serious and late complications than other types of shunts (i.e., ventriculoatrial shunts). If a shunt is not placed shortly after birth, ongoing assessment of the infant's neurologic status and development and serial evaluation of the head circumference as well as serial determinations of ventricular size by ultrasonography are necessary. This approach results in 75% to 90% of infants with myelomeningoceles undergoing a shunt procedure within the first 2 to 3 weeks of life.

The major complications observed after ventriculoperitoneal shunt are malfunctions of the shunt (resulting in obstruction), infection, and overdrainage. Shunt malfunction has decreased with improved shunt hardware. The most common cause of shunt malfunction is now related to choroid plexus occlusion of the ventricular catheter. Placement of the catheter in the frontal horn or placement of an occipital catheter past the foramen of Monro avoids this complication. Seventy percent of shunt infections occur within the first month after insertion as a complication of the shunt procedure itself. Meticulous skin preparation, aseptic technique, and administration of perioperative antibiotics have reduced the infection rate to less than 1% in some centers, but in most reported series it ranges from 2% to 5%. The usual treatment of infection is complete removal of the shunt, temporary external ventricular drainage, administration of intravenous and/or intrathecal antibiotics, and later reinsertion of a new shunt catheter. Clinical signs of shunt infection are fever, irritability, changes in sensorium, and cutaneous erythema of the skin over the tubing and shunt. The diagnosis of infection is made by shunt tap. The majority of infections are caused by *Staphylococcus epidermidis* and *Staphylococcus aureus*. Gram-negative organisms include *Klebsiella* species, *Escherichia coli*, and *Proteus*. Finally, overdrainage of the ventricles can cause slit ventricle syndrome, subdural hematoma, trapped fourth ventricle, intracranial hypotension, and craniosynostosis. New flow-regulated valves have been designed to prevent overdrainage but still have not been proven. Intra-abdominal complications can also occur, including the development of a shunt cyst, catheter kinking or knot formation, and perforation of the shunt catheter into the bowel or bladder. If multiple revisions of the shunt are required and peritonitis ensues, a ventriculo-gallbladder shunt may be a reasonable alternative. The patient should receive cholecystokinin to ensure adequate gallbladder emptying in the early postoperative period and to prevent the buildup of back-pressure and avoid obstruction to flow of CSF. Ventriculoatrial shunts function well but are associated with more serious complications, such as shunt nephritis (an immune complex disease), pulmonary embolus, and pulmonary hypertension. Shunt-related pulmonary hypertension is associated with a high mortality rate.

A difficult group of patients to manage are very low-birth-weight infants who develop posthemorrhagic hydrocephalus after an intracranial hemorrhage. The efficacy of early surgical treatment is controversial. Ventriculostomy and use of shunts with valves have a high rate of complications, owing to shunt obstruction and infection. In those cases with rapidly progressive hydrocephalus that requires early drainage, the use of a temporary valveless shunt has been a valuable alternative.

Arnold-Chiari II Malformation

Almost all children born with myelomeningocele have an Arnold-Chiari II hindbrain malformation. With modern treatment controlling many of the complications of myelomeningocele, the Arnold-Chiari II malformation is now the leading cause of mortality and serious morbidity in children with myelomeningoceles. The major features of this malformation are caudal displacement of the cerebellar vermis, cervicomedullary junctions, pons, medulla, and fourth ventricle, with the cerebellar tonsils located at or below the foramen magnum, kinking of the medulla, obliteration of the cisterna magna, and a low-lying tentorium with a small posterior fossa.

Young infants with hydrocephalus can develop rapid neurologic deterioration with profound brainstem dysfunction within the first 2 months of life and die of brainstem involvement in 9 to 12 weeks. Life-threatening symptoms such as stridor, sleep apnea, apnea and bradycardia, and aspiration pneumonia often occur as a result of dysfunction of cranial nerves IX and X and medullary center involvement. Older infants and children present with potentially lethal breath-holding episodes, respiratory arrest, and cervical spinal cord involvement, leading to spasticity and weakness of the lower extremities. Although all infants and children with myelomenigoceles have the Arnold-Chiari II malformation, only 20% to 40% become symptomatic. Unfortunately however, one third of the symptomatic patients die.

Indications for surgery include stridor at rest, recurrent aspiration pneumonia, severe apnea and bradycardia, and cyanotic breath-holding spells. Treatment consists first of placing a shunt if this has not already been done. If the patient has been shunted, and the shunt is functioning adequately, then a craniocervical junction decompression is performed. The results of this operation

FIGURE 86-3 ■ Infants with a meningocele have a sac that contains only cerebrospinal fluid. The spinal cord is normal but may be tethered.

are highly variable, and a significant number of patients with serious respiratory symptoms fail to improve despite craniocervical decompression.

The Tethered Cord Syndrome

A tethered spinal cord results from the attachment of the spinal cord to congenitally abnormal structures in the lumbosacral area. Signs and symptoms of the tethered spinal cord develop in a significant number of patients with myelomeningocele because of adherence of the spinal cord to the area of the lumbar repair. Symptomatic tethered spinal cord usually develops by the fifth year, and signs and symptoms include back pain, changes in bladder tone, and sensory and/or motor loss in the lower extremities, spasticity, and scoliosis. Development of these signs and symptoms in patients with myelomeningocele necessitates an operation for untethering of the spinal cord in which the neural placode and spinal cord are freed from adherence to the overlying skin and dura. Tethered cord syndrome is also seen in up to 25% of patients with imperforate anus. In these patients, varying degrees of tethering are noted, and not all require surgical release. The diagnosis can be confirmed by ultrasound in the newborn and by MRI in other patients.

OTHER FORMS OF SPINAL DYSRAPHISM

Meningocele

Patients born with simple meningoceles are relatively rare. In patients with a meningocele, the spinal cord forms normally but the dura fails to fuse dorsally. This results in the formation of a cystic, skin-covered lesion that does not directly involve neural tissue (Fig. 86-3). In addition, meningoceles are a type of occult spinal dysraphism that may be associated with spinal cord tethering, but, unlike myelomeningoceles, are not typically associated with hydrocephalus or the Arnold-Chiari II malformation.

Lipomyelomeningocele

Patients with lipomyelomeningocele typically are born without neurologic deficits. They present with a skin-covered fatty mass in the lumbosacral area that passes through a midline defect in the lumbodorsal fascia, vertebral neural arch, and dura and merges with an

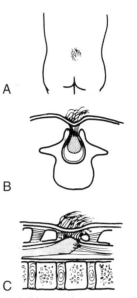

FIGURE 86-4 ■ Spina bifida occulta. **A,** Lumbrosacral depression with a cutaneous tuft of hair. **B,** The hair connects through the bifid spine with the dural sac. **C,** Lateral view.

abnormally low-lying tethered spinal cord. Without treatment, progressive neurologic deficits develop and eventually lead to paraplegia. Treatment involves releasing the tethered spinal cord, reducing the bulk of the lipoma, and repairing the dural defect, which often results in normal neurologic function. Magnetic resonance imaging is an excellent diagnostic modality that clearly demonstrates the extent of the lesion.

Spina Bifida with Cutaneous Manifestations

Cutaneous stigmata associated with occult spinal dysraphism include dimples, skin appendages, dermal sinuses, and a hairy patch or hemangioma over the lumbosacral area (Fig. 86-4). A tethered cord is common; however, other anatomic lesions may also be present. If neurologic signs develop, they can be relieved by untethering the spinal cord.

Congenital Dermal Sinus

Patients with congenital dermal sinus have a dimple in the midline, usually in the lumbosacral region. However, the dimple or sinus can occur anywhere along the spine from the craniocervical junction to the sacrum. The dimple or pit travels in a cephalad direction and may terminate in the extraspinal tissue but usually traverses through a bifid spine, into the dural sac, and then into the subarachnoid space. Frequently, it terminates in a dermoid tumor or an epidermoid cyst. Patients with congenital dermal sinuses may deteriorate from an infection traveling down the sinus intradurally, causing meningitis and/or intrathecal abscess, or from progressive growth of an epidermoid cyst or dermoid tumor, causing neural tissue compression. All patients with a visible dermal dimple in the midline should be investigated with an MRI, and if a dermal sinus is diagnosed it should be removed.

TABLE 86-2 ▪ Types of Craniosynostosis and Associated Issues

Disorder	Suture(s) Affected	Description of Head Shape	Congenital Brain Malformation	Intracranial Pressure	Frequency of Mental Retardation	Surgical Treatment	Comments
Scaphocephaly (also called dolichocephaly)	Sagittal	Long and narrow. "Boat-shaped." Anterior fontanelle is usually closed; narrow biparietal diameter of the skull with frontal bossing, occipital prominence, and ridging along the sagittal suture.	None. Cranial volume is normal.	Rarely elevated	Slight	Simple linear craniectomy of the closed sagittal suture should be carried out within first 3 months of life. A more involved operative procedure is required in children who are 6 months or older in which a portion of the calvarium is removed and the head is reshaped.	Scaphocephaly is a serious cosmetic defect. Strong male predominance 80%. Ridging along the fused sagittal suture is common. Most common type of craniosynostosis, accounting for approximately 50% of cases.
Brachycephaly	Bilateral coronal	Short, broad, and tall. The head is limited in the occipital frontal diameter, resulting in excessive lateral growth.	Usually none. Rarely there is agenesis of the corpus callosum.	Infrequently elevated	Slight to moderate	Treated early in infancy with opening of the sutures and advancement of the supraorbital margin. Frequently there is normal growth of the forehead and face. Children treated after 6 months usually require a formal craniofacial repair at 3 to 4 years of age to correct their proptosis and midface hypoplasia, which result from failure of full development of the anterior cranial fossa.	Coronal synostosis occurs in association with the autosomal dominant disorders of Apert's syndrome and Crouzon's syndrome. There is a slight female predominance.
Trigonocephaly	Metopic	"Bullet-shaped" forehead. Pointed and angular, narrowed forehead with a prominent midline bony ridge. The orbits are angled in, causing hypotelorism and posterior displacement of the lateral aspects of the orbits.	Occasionally has arrhenoencephaly, holoprosencephaly	Rarely elevated	Slight to moderate	Frontal bone is removed, metopic suture is opened, and the supraorbital margins are realigned.	Occasionally associated with other congenital abnormalities as well as intracranial abnormalities. If the metopic suture closes early, but after the age of 4 to 5 months, no surgical treatment is needed; this is usually familial.

Deformity	Suture(s)	Cranial appearance	Brain	ICP	Risk	Surgical treatment	Comments
Frontal plagiocephaly	Unilateral coronal	Involved side has a flattened frontal region with outward bulging of contralateral side. The nose is deviated toward the opposite side. The ipsilateral ear is moved forward and more inferior. The affected orbit is small.	No specific brain malformation but microencephaly is not rare.	Infrequently elevated	Slight to moderate	Frontal craniotomy with correction of the orbital deformity and unilateral fronto-orbital advancement	"Harlequin eye" is evident on plain radiographs, owing to elevation of the sphenoid ridge. Frontal plagiocephaly can also be caused by intrauterine constraint or torticollis, which can initially be treated with positioning and physical therapy but may require surgery.
Occipital plagiocephaly	Lambdoid	Flattening of the involved occipital region with prominence in the ipsilateral frontal region.	No specific brain malformation, but microencephaly is not rare.	Infrequently elevated	Slight to moderate	Multiple surgical procedures have been described from bilateral occipital craniectomies with reversal of the bone flaps to strip craniectomies	Closure of one or both lambdoid sutures causing a "flat occiput" is rare. Postural deformation, cranio-occipital malformation, cervical spine anomalies, and torticollis can have a similar appearance to lambdoid synostosis and can be treated with positioning, physical therapy, and/or helmet therapy.
Oxycephaly	Sagittal and coronal	"Tower head." The skull expands toward the vertex, giving it a long, narrow appearance with the top pointed or conical.	Sometimes agenesis of the corpus callosum.	Usually elevated	High	Surgical intervention required to allow for normal brain growth and to prevent the development of increased ICP.	Fusion of multiple sutures other than sagittal and coronal produces a conical head shape that varies, depending on the involved sutures. Surgical treatment is also dependent on the sutures involved.

Adapted from Carson BS: Craniosynostosis and neurocranial asymmetry. In Dufresne CR, Carson BS, Zinreich SJ (eds): Complex Craniofacial Problems. New York, Churchill Livingstone, 1992.

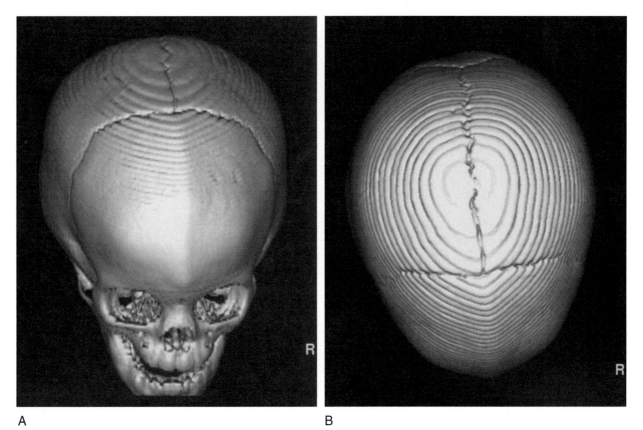

A   B

FIGURE 86-5 ■ Frontal (**A**) and cranial (**B**) views of a three-dimensional reconstruction of CT scans of a child who has craniosynostosis of the metopic suture.

CRANIOSYNOSTOSIS

Craniosynostosis was first identified and named in 1851 by Virchow. This term refers to a group of disorders characterized by premature closure of one or more cranial sutures. The name is derived from the suture or sutures involved. It is important to differentiate between primary and secondary craniosynostosis. Primary craniosynostosis is present at birth and results from premature fusion of one or more sutures; it sometimes restricts brain growth. In secondary craniosynostosis, the sutures close and the skull fails to grow, leading to brain agenesis or atrophy. The incidence is 1 in 1,900 live births, with a male predominance of 63%. Craniosynostosis can be detected by suture and fontanelle palpation as part of the newborn examination. It is important that the posterior fontanelle closes first, at approximately 3 months of life, and the anterior fontanelle closes at approximately 12 months. Prompt diagnosis and appropriate management of craniosynostosis can prevent disturbances in brain growth, increased intracranial pressure, and severe cosmetic defects. Table 86-2 delineates the characteristics of the more common abnormalities, and Figure 86-5 demonstrates the anatomy of the cranial sutures relative to the bones of the calvarium. Craniosynostosis may result from fetal exposure to maternal intake of sodium valproate. Fetal valproate syndrome affects 10% of infants born to mothers who take sodium valproate during pregnancy. This exposure results in trigonocephaly due to premature fusion of the metopic suture. Such patients' mean intelligence quotient is 75 (range 45-100). IQs are significantly higher if surgical correction of the craniosynostosis is performed before 6 months of age.

SUGGESTED READINGS

Bruner JP, Tulipan NB, Paschall RL, et al: Fetal surgery for myelomeningocele and the incidence of shunt-dependent hydrocephalus. JAMA 282:1819-1825, 1999.

This report details the largest series of intrauterine repairs for myelomeningocele to date with follow-up of various parameters.

Cohen AR, Robinson S: Early management of myelomeningocele. In McLone DG (ed): Pediatric Neurosurgery: Surgery of the Developing Nervous System, 4th ed. Philadelphia, WB Saunders, 2001, pp 241-259.

This is an excellent review of the management of myelomeningocele. The text also provides concise but thorough discussion of hydrocephalus, Arnold-Chiari II malformation, and tethered spinal cord.

Greenberg MS: Handbook of Neurosurgery, 5th ed. New York, Thieme, 2001.

This is an excellent current, comprehensive, user-friendly guide to neurosurgery. It contains thousands of literature citations and a thorough index for prompt access to answers on a multitude of neurosurgical topics.

Holmes NM, Nguyen HT, Harrison MR, et al: Fetal intervention for myelomeningocele: Effect of postnatal bladder function. J Urol 166:2383-2386, 2001.

Bladder function was not improved after fetal repair of myelomeningocele.

Lu GC, Steinhauer J, Ramsey PS, Faye-Peterson O: Lethal pulmonary hypoplasia after in-utero myelomeningocele repair. Obstet Gynecol 98:698-701, 2001.

This case demonstrates the potential risks of fetal repair of myelomeningocele.

Northrup H, Volcik KA: Spina bifida and other neural tube defects. Curr Probl Pediatr 30:313-332, 2000.

Excellent overview of the subject.

Park TS, Robinson S: Nonsyndromic craniosynostosis. In McLone DG (ed): Pediatric Neurosurgery: Surgery of the Developing Nervous System, 4th ed. Philadelphia, WB Saunders, 2001, pp 345-361.

Excellent review of the common types of craniosynostosis, including the surgical management of each type.

Walsh DS, Adzick NS, Sutton LN, Johnson MP: The rationale for in utero repair of myelomeningocele. Fetal Diagn Ther 16:312-322, 2001.

This report represents the current rationale for considering fetal surgical repair of myelomeningoceles.

Warf BC: Pathophysiology of the tethered cord syndrome. In McLone DG (ed): Pediatric Neurosurgery: Surgery of the Developing Nervous System, 4th ed. Philadelphia, WB Saunders, 2001, pp 282-288.

Concise concurrent review of tethered cord syndrome, including pathophysiology and treatment.

87

Cardiovascular Disorders

Congenital cardiovascular disorders in infants and children can be divided into four categories: (1) those that have a left-to-right shunt, which leads to congestive heart failure and failure to thrive (atrial septal defect, patent ductus arteriosus, ventricular septal defect, atrioventricular canal); (2) those with a right-to-left shunt from one of the "T's" (tetralogy of Fallot, tricuspid atresia, transposition of the great vessels, total anomalous pulmonary venous return, truncus arteriosus); (3) those with obstructive lesions, which are associated with ventricular hypertrophy and failure (aortic stenosis, coarctation, pulmonary stenosis, interrupted aortic arch); and (4) those with total mixing lesions (double-outlet right ventricle, hypoplastic left heart syndrome). The majority of the operations for cardiac anomalies can be distilled down to closing holes, relieving obstructions, and increasing or decreasing flow.

NONCYANOTIC CONGENITAL HEART DISEASE (LEFT-TO-RIGHT SHUNT)

This group of lesions represents congenital heart defects that cause congestive heart failure on the basis of left-to-right shunting in the heart.

Patent Ductus Arteriosus

Most infants born with patent ductus arteriosus (PDA) remain asymptomatic except those who are premature (Fig. 87-1). Their anomaly is usually discovered in later childhood on physical examination. In this situation, surgery can be carried out electively to prevent occurrence of later complications. In contrast, some patients show symptoms early in infancy, with severe congestive heart failure, but not usually until after 6 to 8 weeks of life when pulmonary vascular resistance falls. Many infants with PDA also have a coarctation of the aorta, an intracardiac defect such as ventricular septal defect (VSD), atrial septal defect (ASD), aortic or mitral valve anomaly, hypoplastic left heart syndrome (HLHS), or a combination of these conditions. In some of these cases the ductus may need to be kept open with prostaglandin E_1 to provide adequate pulmonary or systemic blood flow.

The incidence of PDA increases with smaller birth weight and earlier gestational age. Premature infants have persistent PDA in 7% to 38% of cases. Because pulmonary vascular resistance falls earlier than in full-term newborns, symptoms in premature newborns may be observed in the first week of life. At least 60% of these patients also have respiratory distress syndrome. The causative relationship between patent ductus and respiratory distress syndrome is not clear, but it is certain that infants with a large left-to-right shunt may have their respiratory problems worsened, and surgery in such patients may be beneficial if the ductus does not close spontaneously. The problem is to separate patients with congestive heart failure caused by large left-to-right shunts from those patients with predominant bronchopulmonary dysplasia, who are unlikely to benefit from operation. Some infants clearly have large left-to-right shunts with cardiomegaly and pulmonary plethora on chest film. Others have a radiographic pattern more typical of bronchopulmonary dysplasia with a normal heart size. Unfortunately, in many cases the radiographic pattern falls between these extremes.

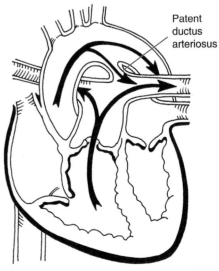

FIGURE 87-1 ■ Anatomy of a persistent PDA.

Diagnosis

The diagnosis of PDA is suspected in neonates with systolic murmur, wide arterial pulse pressure, hyperactive precordium, and increased pulmonary vascularity on chest film. The characteristic continuous murmur may not be present in neonates because their elevated pulmonary vascular resistance inhibits diastolic flow.

Although echocardiography is the mainstay of diagnostic imaging, because of the high incidence of associated anomalies, complete cardiac catheterization may be necessary in term infants and older children. Blood gas analysis will reveal the characteristic oxygen step-up in the pulmonary artery. Angiography will show dye escaping from the aorta into the pulmonary artery. In premature infants cardiac catheterization is technically difficult, limiting its usefulness. Fortunately, echocardiography is excellent in quantitating the size of the ductus and the amount of left-to-right shunting. The ratio between left atrial diameter and aortic diameter is determined. If this exceeds 1.15, the patent ductus is probably pathologic.

Treatment

In premature newborns indomethacin induces closure of the PDA in approximately 70% of patients. Oliguria is the biggest side effect of this therapy, and it should not be applied in those with underlying renal insufficiency. Other relative contraindications include active bleeding and necrotizing enterocolitis.

Operative Technique

The operation is frequently performed in the intensive care unit in premature newborns, especially those on high ventilator settings and/or high-frequency oscillatory ventilation. Although the patent ductus was often divided or ligated in the past, this is not necessary. Instead, the ductus is simply clipped, which has proven to be a safe and effective approach (Fig. 87-2).

A left-sided thoracotomy is performed, although in many cases this procedure is being performed thoracoscopically using 3-mm incisions, ports, and instruments. An incision in the fourth interspace provides adequate exposure. In premature infants an extrapleural approach is used because of the slight protection it may afford the lung.

If not, the mediastinal pleura is incised over the aorta. This incision should be carried right down to the adventitia of the aorta. Then the mediastinal soft tissues and recurrent laryngeal nerve will be readily retracted medially while the ductus is sharply and bluntly cleared of areolar tissue on all but the back side of the vessel. The ductus must not be lifted or handled roughly; it is especially vulnerable to being torn on its undersurface.

It is wise at this point to occlude the ductus temporarily to be sure that closure is tolerated, especially when no cardiac catheterization has been done and unrecognized cardiac anomalies may be present. A clip is then placed across the ductus while avoiding the recurrent laryngeal nerve. The wound is closed in layers. A chest tube is not typically inserted.

In older children the entire duct may be dissected and surrounded by ligatures. All the ligatures are tied down, again taking care not to lift the ductus and not to allow the ligatures to overlap. A 4- to 5-mm segment of ductus must be compressed within the ligatures to ensure that recanalization cannot occur. Small and medium-sized PDAs may be closed successfully in 80% to 90% of cases in older children through transcatheter coil embolization. Umbrella devices may also be used to close larger PDAs.

Although closure of a patent ductus in an older infant or child carries little risk, mortality is relatively high in neonates because of the associated anomalies.

Atrial Septal Defect

Atrial septal defects of the secundum and sinus venosus variety rarely produce symptoms in the newborn period or in early childhood (Fig. 87-3). In most cases the defect is identified on a routine examination when a murmur is heard. Because of the lower compliance of the left ventricle relative to the right, large ASDs can result in left-to-right shunting with pulmonary blood flow that may be four times systemic blood flow. Right ventricle overload may result. Operation is indicated when the ratio of pulmonary blood flow to systemic blood flow is more than 1.5. These defects are usually closed electively at 3 to 4 years of age.

An ostium primum atrial septal defect is located low in the atrial septum just above the atrioventricular valve.

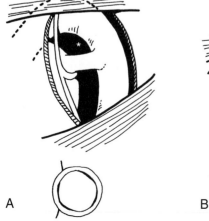
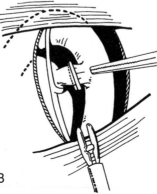

A   B

FIGURE 87-2 ■ **A,** Ligation of PDA in infancy. **B,** Note the clip placed across the ductus. Dissection is performed only over the anterior aspect and on either side, but not behind the ductus. (From Sherman NJ: Patent ductus arteriosus. In Rob and Smith's Operative Surgery: Pediatric Surgery, 5th ed. London, Chapman and Hall, 1992.)

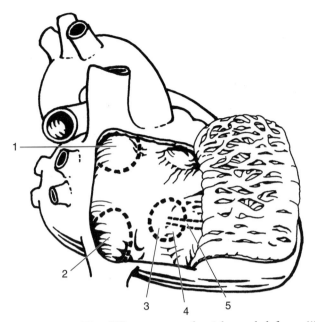

FIGURE 87-3 ■ The different types of atrial septal defects: (1) sinus venosus defect, (2) ostium secundum defect, (3) ostium primum defect, (4) ventricular septal defect of a complete atrioventricular canal, and (5) cleft septal leaflet of mitral valve. Together, 3, 4, and 5 complete the atrioventricular canal. (From Bahnson HT: Patent ductus arteriosus, coarctation of the aorta, and anomalies of the aortic arch. In Textbook of Surgery: The Biological Basis of Modern Surgical Practice. Philadelphia, WB Saunders, 1981.)

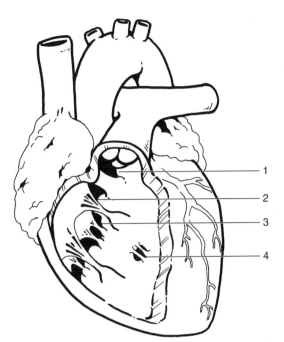

FIGURE 87-4 ■ Ventricular septal defects occur in four basic locations: (1) supracristal, (2) membranous (most common), (3) beneath the atrioventricular valves (the common endocardial cushion defect abnormality), and (4) within the muscular septum. (From Holder TM, Ashcraft KW: Cardiac Disease. In Pediatric Surgery, 4th ed. Chicago, Year Book Medical Publishers, 1986.)

Unlike the secundum defect, this anomaly often presents with symptoms in early childhood and requires repair. Mitral regurgitation may be present. The repair of this defect usually requires a patch and must be performed with care to avoid injury to the conduction system.

If an ASD is untreated, it will produce cardiac failure and severe arrhythmias in adult life with associated fixed pulmonary hypertension that will make correction at this stage in life impossible. Many of the small ASDs identified in the newborn period will close spontaneously. Studies have shown that a variety of devices can be used effectively to achieve transcatheter closure of an ASD in up to 98% of patients. These devices are of a variety of configurations, but, in general, consist of a central polyurethane or polyester occluder that is held in place by disks or arms that are deployed first on the left atrial and then on the right atrial side of the defect. Such devices are continuing to undergo clinical evaluation.

Ventricular Septal Defect

Most VSDs are located adjacent to the membranous portion of the ventricular septum (Fig. 87-4). Although a majority of membranous VSDs and small conoventricular and muscular VSDs close spontaneously within the first decade of life, a number persist, resulting in significant left-to-right shunting. If multiple muscular VSDs are present, they often will not close spontaneously and will require surgical closure. A large VSD can result in severe congestive heart failure during infancy. At birth there is usually no congestive failure; however, as pulmonary vascular resistance drops during the first several weeks of life, the left-to-right shunting increases and congestive heart failure develops. Growth retardation may be seen. Severe irreversible pulmonary vascular disease may develop as a result of increased pulmonary blood flow and pressure, although this usually occurs after 2 years of age. Often the congestive failure can be treated with vigorous medical therapy such as digitalization and diuresis. If medical therapy is unsuccessful, correction of the VSD should be carried out in infancy. Among symptomatic patients, two thirds currently undergo repair of the defect during the first year of life. The defect can be closed through a ventriculotomy or preferably by a transatrial approach. The mortality for this operation should be less than 1%. The only major complications of this procedure are recurrent VSDs because of a leak in the patch and heart block. As with ASDs, transcatheter closure of VSDs is being evaluated in clinical trials (Fig. 87-5).

Atrioventricular Canal Defect

In an atrioventricular canal defect the anatomic abnormalities are absence of the lower portion of the atrial septum (ASD) and upper portion of the ventricular septum (VSD), clefts in the septal leaflets of the mitral and tricuspid valves, and fusion of the anterior and posterior portions of these valves across the septal defects. These abnormalities result from inappropriate development of the endocardial cushions and the atrioventricular septum and are more frequently observed in the setting of Down syndrome. The valvular abnormalities may

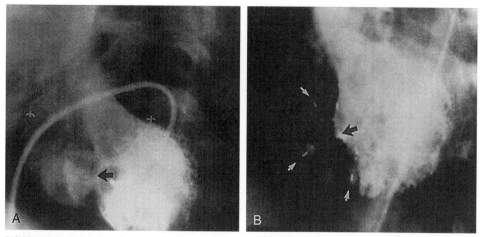

FIGURE 87-5 ■ Device closure of muscular VSD. **A,** Long axial oblique view of the left ventriculogram, which shows a midmuscular VSD (arrow). **B,** Post device placement, the VSD is closed. White arrows point to three of the four right ventricular arms, the left ventricular arms being obscured by contrast. The black arrow marks the site of the previously present VSD. (From Mandell V: Interventional procedures for congenital heart disease. Radiol Clin North Am 37:439-461, 1999.)

result in incompetence of both valves. These infants are usually symptomatic with severe congestive heart failure in early infancy owing to the large left-to-right shunt through the VSD. Echocardiography alone can be used to make the definitive diagnosis, although cardiac catheterization is often helpful to define the anatomy and to evaluate for valvular regurgitation. Corrective surgery is required within the first 3 to 6 months of life and consists of closure of the ASD and VSD with creation of competent atrioventricular valves. If untreated, 65% of these children succumb by 1 year and 96% by 5 years of age. If repair is delayed until 2 years of age, severe fixed pulmonary hypertension will be present and will preclude successful repair. Results are excellent unless left atrioventricular valve regurgitation occurs postoperatively, in which case the prognosis is less optimistic.

CYANOTIC CONGENITAL HEART DISEASE (RIGHT-TO-LEFT SHUNTING)

Right-to-left shunting of blood through intracardiac defects and lesions with abnormal intracardiac mixing will result in varying degrees of cyanosis. The most common congenital lesions that produce cyanosis are transposition of the great vessels, tetralogy of Fallot, tricuspid atresia, truncus arteriosus, and total anomalous pulmonary venous drainage, which will also produce cyanosis but to a much lesser degree. In addition, pulmonary atresia or stenosis may result in a right-to-left shunt with resulting cyanosis.

Transposition of the Great Arteries

In transposition of the great arteries the aorta arises from the right ventricle and the pulmonary artery arises from the left ventricle (Fig. 87-6). Thus the pulmonary and systemic vascular systems are in parallel rather than in series. Severe cyanosis results and postnatal survival requires the presence of an intracardiac or extracardiac

shunt such as an ASD, VSD, or PDA. Often an enlarged foramen ovale provides adequate mixing of pulmonary and systemic blood to allow the infant to survive. Diagnosis is initially made by echocardiography, which may also allow determination of the anatomy of the coronary arteries. Prostaglandin infusion is usually begun to maintain ductal patency and improve mixing. Unfortunately, mixing from a PDA may be inadequate, requiring cardiac catheterization and performance of a balloon atrial septostomy, which will provide immediate palliation for the infant.

Treatment

Total correction of transposition of the great arteries is performed in newborns using the arterial switch

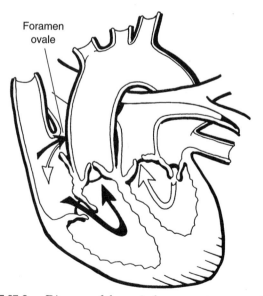

FIGURE 87-6 ■ Diagram of the typical anatomy in transposition of the great arteries. The atria and ventricles are normally situated. However, the great arteries are transposed.

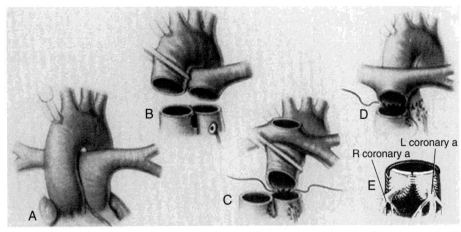

FIGURE 87-7 ■ **a,** Switch repair of transposition of the great arteries. **b,** The aorta and pulmonary artery are transected, and the orifices of the coronary arteries are excised with a rim of adjacent aortic wall. The aorta is brought under the bifurcation of the pulmonary artery, and the proximal pulmonary artery and the aorta are anastomosed without necessitating graft interposition. **c,** The coronary arteries are transferred to the pulmonary artery. **d,** The mobilized pulmonary artery is directly anastomosed to the proximal aortic stump. **e,** A closeup view of the coronary arteries anastomosed to the pulmonary artery is demonstrated. (Adapted from Castaneda AR, Jonas RA, Mayer Jr JE, Hanley FL: In D-transposition of the great arteries. Cardiac Surgery of the Neonate and Infant. Philadelphia, WB Saunders, 1994.)

operation (Fig. 87-7). With this technique the aorta and pulmonary artery are divided and switched such that the aorta arises from the pulmonary artery and vice versa. The coronary arteries are transferred to the new aorta. It is preferable to perform the procedure in the newborn period before exposure of the left ventricle to the low resistance pulmonary circulation alters its "systemic" characteristics. In a number of centers this has been highly successful with less than 3% operative mortality and good long-term results.

Tetralogy of Fallot

Although there are four characteristics to tetralogy of Fallot (TOF: right ventricular outflow stenosis, VSD, dextroposition of the aorta, and right ventricular hypertrophy), indeed all of these are caused by the single abnormality of right ventricular outflow obstruction caused by anterior (toward the right ventricle) displacement of the infundibular septum (Fig. 87-8). Conceptually, blood flows from the right ventricle across the VSD into the aorta rather than through the pulmonary outflow tract. Right ventricular hypertrophy develops in response to exposure of the right ventricle to systemic resistance. Stenosis of the pulmonary valve may also be present. Cyanosis is usually present in the newborn period. The degree of cyanosis is related to the amount of right-to-left shunting through the VSD. The greater the right ventricular outflow tract obstruction, the greater the right-to-left shunting. If severe right ventricular outflow tract obstruction is present, cyanosis may increase as the ductus closes. Severe spasm of the right ventricular outflow tract in otherwise pink patients results in deep cyanosis referred to as "tet spells."

Twenty-five percent of patients with TOF have a right-sided aortic arch, which is of major significance if there is associated esophageal atresia. This will often require that the esophageal atresia repair be carried out through the left side of the chest rather than the standard approach through a right-sided thoracotomy.

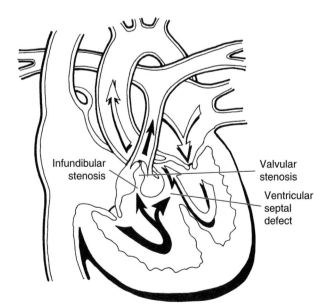

FIGURE 87-8 ■ Anatomy of tetralogy of Fallot. The infundibular pulmonic stenosis and preferential blood flow through the large VSD and overriding aorta are demonstrated.

Diagnosis

Patients with TOF are typically cyanotic with a prominent systolic ejection murmur. Chest radiography may reveal decreased pulmonary vascular markings. Echocardiography defines the anomaly, although catheterization is reserved for definition of unusual anatomy or anomalous coronary arteries. Children with TOF may squat to increase systemic vascular resistance, thus increasing pulmonary blood flow. If TOF is untreated, long-term survival is less than 10%.

Treatment

Correction of TOF is typically performed in the newborn period, which avoids prolonged cyanosis and development of right ventricular hypertrophy. An incision is made across the pulmonary valve and infundibulum (Fig. 87-9). The right ventricular outflow tract obstruction is managed with a transannular patch in most patients. A right ventricle-to-pulmonary artery conduit may be used in cases where pulmonary atresia is present. A temporary systemic-to-pulmonary artery shunt may be performed during the neonatal period in patients in whom a primary repair would be of high risk, such as those with other anomalies or more complex cardiac lesions (e.g., branch pulmonary artery obstruction), or in the presence of an anomalous left anterior descending coronary artery, which precludes a transannular pulmonary artery incision and widening with placement of a patch. Typically, a Blalock-Taussig end-to-side anastomosis between the proximal subclavian artery and the pulmonary artery or placement of a 5- to 6-mm Gore-Tex graft between the subclavian artery and the pulmonary artery is used for the systemic-to-pulmonary artery shunt. Elective correction of the anomaly can then be performed at 12 to 18 months of age.

Results

Elective total correction of TOF carries a less than 5% mortality with excellent relief of symptoms. Reoperation will be required in 5% to 10% of patients for residual VSD, right ventricular outflow tract obstruction, or pulmonary valvular insufficiency.

Tricuspid Atresia

Infants with tricuspid atresia are usually severely cyanotic at birth. Echocardiography provides an accurate diagnosis, and cardiac catheterization is usually only necessary to perform an atrial balloon septostomy for temporary palliation (Fig. 87-10). The patency of the ductus arteriosus is usually maintained in the newborn period by the administration of prostaglandin E_1. The right ventricle is often severely hypoplastic and of little functional use. Total correction of this defect involves application of the Fontan operation, in which the right ventricle is bypassed by directing blood from the cavae to the pulmonary artery (Fig. 87-11). Although the original Fontan operation used conduits for diversion of blood from the cavae to the pulmonary artery, current approaches involve direct cavopulmonary anastomoses often in a staged fashion with a bidirectional Glenn anastomosis performed first (see later and Figure 87-11).

Truncus Arteriosus

In truncus arteriosus both the right and left ventricle enter into a single vessel from which the aorta and pulmonary artery derive. There are four types of truncus arteriosus.

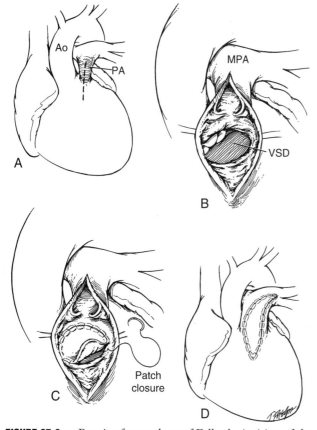

FIGURE 87-9 ■ Repair of a tetralogy of Fallot by incision of the pulmonary outflow tract (**A**), identification of the VSD (**B**), closure of the VSD (**C**), and patch reconstruction of the pulmonary outflow tract (**D**). (From Mee RB, Drummond-Webb JJ: Congenital heart disease. In Townsend C [ed]: Sabiston Textbook of Surgery, 16th ed. Philadelphia, WB Saunders, pp 1243-1265.)

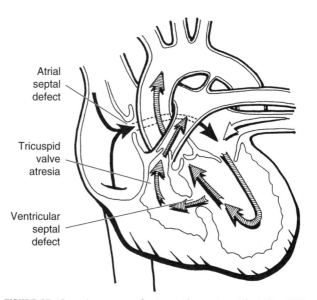

FIGURE 87-10 ■ Anatomy of tricuspid atresia with ASD, VSD, and a hypoplastic right ventricle.

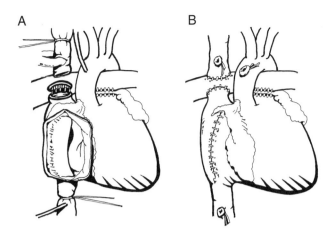

FIGURE 87-11 ■ Repair of tricuspid atresia via a modification of the Fontan operation. **A,** A conduit is placed in the right atrium, creating a uniform tunnel between the superior and the inferior vena cava. The main pulmonary artery is transected. The SVC is divided, and a bidirectional Glenn anastomosis is then performed between the cranial portion of the divided SVC and the right pulmonary artery. The atrial side of the divided SVC is then approximated to the underside of the right pulmonary artery. **B,** Completed total cavopulmonary connection. (From Stein DG, Laks H, Drinkwater DC, et al: Results of total cavopulmonary connection in the treatment of patients with a functionally single ventricle. J Thorac Cardiovasc Surg 102:280, 1991.)

In type 1 there is a single main pulmonary artery arising from the truncal vessel. In type 2 the vessels come off the back of the truncal vessel. In type 3 the right and left pulmonary arteries come off separately from the truncal vessel or the descending aorta. In type 4 the pulmonary arteries arise from the descending aorta. In all instances there is moderate cyanosis because saturated and desaturated blood mixes in the truncal vessel before being distributed to the systemic circulation. Because of the high flow to the pulmonary arteries, pulmonary hypertension is present and often becomes fixed by 1 year of age.

Treatment

Correction of this lesion should be carried out early, preferably in the first month of life. The correction involves closure of the VSD and insertion of a valved conduit from the right ventricle to the pulmonary artery. Results of surgery depend on the degree of pulmonary vascular resistance present at the time of the operation.

Total Anomalous Pulmonary Venous Drainage

There are three types of total anomalous pulmonary venous drainage (Fig. 87-12). The right and left pulmonary veins join together behind the heart and drain into the heart by way of either an ascending vein on the side opposite the vena cava (supracardiac type), the coronary sinus to the right atrium (cardiac type), or a descending vein that usually enters into the portal venous system (infracardiac type). The interposed hepatic venous system in the infracardiac type causes pulmonary venous hypertension, leading to pulmonary edema, severe hypoxia, and high mortality. Because the coronary sinus is small, pulmonary venous hypertension may also be seen in the cardiac type of this

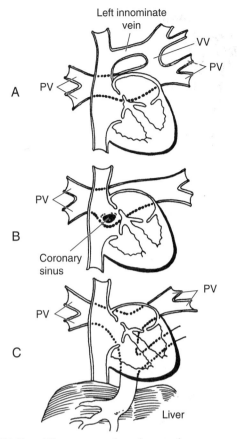

FIGURE 87-12 ■ Three types of total anomalous venous return. **A,** The supracardiac configuration in which pulmonary venous blood drains into the innominate vein through a vertical vein (VV), sometimes called a left vena cava. **B,** The cardiac type of drainage in which the pulmonary veins drain into the right atrium via the coronary sinus. **C,** The infracardiac type in which the pulmonary veins (PV) drain into the inferior vena cava via a connection to the portal vein. Severe pulmonary hypertension and edema frequently results with configuration C because of the resistance imposed by the liver vascular bed.

anomaly. Pulmonary venous hypertension is least commonly seen in the supracardiac type. All oxygenated venous blood mixes with systemic venous blood in the right atrium. An ASD must be present for survival of the infant, so an atrial balloon septostomy can be carried out at the time of catheterization. The diagnosis of this defect may be elusive in the newborn period because the chest film shows a normal heart size; no murmurs are audible; and identification may be difficult on echocardiography. If these patients are symptomatic in the newborn period, total correction must be carried out at that time, usually under deep hypothermia and circulatory arrest.

Critical Pulmonic Stenosis

Severe pulmonic stenosis associated with systemic or suprasystemic pressures in the right ventricle may produce cyanosis in newborns. These patients can be immediately managed by maintenance of patency of the ductus arteriosus with a prostaglandin E_1 infusion. A pulmonary valvulotomy or balloon dilatation is then carried out shortly after stabilization of the patient.

A systemic-to-pulmonary shunt as described earlier remains as an alternative for the immediate management of these newborns if right ventricular hypoplasia is present.

Pulmonary Atresia

Pulmonary atresia may occur with an intact ventricular septum and is almost always associated with significant right ventricular hypoplasia. The ductus is uniformly patent and maintained open with prostaglandin E_1 infusion. Most of these patients are managed in the immediate newborn period with a transventricular valvotomy and a systemic-to-pulmonary artery shunt.

If pulmonary atresia is associated with VSD, pulmonary artery hypoplasia is common. This entity is a variant of TOF and can be treated in the newborn period with a systemic-to-pulmonary artery shunt, followed at a later date by a conduit from the right ventricle to the pulmonary artery and VSD closure.

OBSTRUCTIVE LESIONS

Coarctation of the Aorta

Many infants born with uncomplicated coarctation of the aorta remain asymptomatic until their upper-extremity hypertension or diminished femoral pulses are discovered in later childhood. A substantial number, perhaps half of the total, however, develop heart failure in infancy. This group is distinguished by the high incidence of associated anomalies (89% in one series; usually a PDA but sometimes a VSD or aortic or mitral valve anomaly).

Coarctations may be classified according to their relationship to the patent ductus (or ligamentum arteriosum). In the uncomplicated postductal (postligamental) variety, the only physiologic abnormality is increased afterload to the left ventricle. Conversely, the physiologic relationships of the preductal form are much more complex because the descending aorta is perfused by the right ventricle through the ductus (Fig. 87-13). This form occurs most commonly in neonates.

When congestive heart failure does not promptly respond to vigorous medical therapy, operation should be undertaken.

Diagnosis

The classic diagnostic signs of coarctation are weak, delayed femoral pulses and upper-extremity hypertension. A discrepancy between upper and lower extremity blood pressure may be present. In the preductal form, however, the femoral pulses may be present, obscuring the diagnosis. An important diagnostic clue is that femoral pulses may vary in strength as the pulmonary artery pressure varies, appearing when the infant cries and disappearing with relaxation. Another clue is that arterial blood from the lower half of the body is more desaturated than that in the upper half (unless VSD is also present). Symptoms may increase after ductal closure. Those with severe coarctation may develop renal and intestinal ischemia and associated oliguria. A systolic murmur may be appreciated. In older children, heart failure and cardiomegaly may be present along with hypertension and rib notching on the chest radiograph owing to the enlarged collateral intercostal vessels on the underside of the ribs.

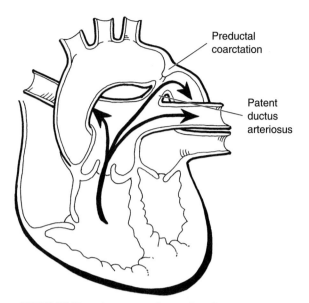

FIGURE 87-13 ■ Anatomy of a preductal coarctation.

Because the diagnosis of coarctation can sometimes be made with certainty on clinical grounds and because the most commonly associated anomaly (patent ductus) can be diagnosed and corrected by the same operative approach, operation is routinely performed after echocardiography confirms the diagnosis. In neonates, however, it may be preferable to have an accurate preoperative assessment of the anatomy and of associated anomalies as defined by an aortogram. The importance of a complete study in neonates with coarctation is exemplified by the frequently encountered combination of coarctation, PDA, and VSD in this group. When the VSD is large, a primary total correction of all three defects is most likely to be successful.

Operative Technique

Repair of a coarctation should be performed by age 1 to 2 years to avoid persistent hypertension. In those newborns with critical preductal coarctation, infusion of prostaglandin may maintain ductal patency, thus avoiding the need for emergent repair.

A number of techniques of repair have been developed: local resection and end-to-end anastomosis, prosthetic patch aortoplasty, subclavian patch angioplasty, or extended resection and anastomosis. A left posterolateral thoracotomy is performed entering the pleural cavity through the fourth interspace. The mediastinal pleura is incised and reflected medially with traction sutures to expose the aortic arch, subclavian artery, and ductus arteriosus. The anatomy of the arch must be clearly visualized, particularly in infants for whom the data may be incomplete.

In performing resection and anastomosis the surgeon must mobilize enough aorta proximally and distally to allow primary anastomosis. Synthetic grafts are not used in neonatal coarctation. Often one or two pairs of intercostal arteries must be divided with extreme care. Often the aorta between the origin of the left subclavian artery and the ductus (the so-called isthmus of the aorta) is hypoplastic even if uninvolved in the actual coarctation. If this is the case, it should be excised and the poststenotic segment should be brought up to the base of the subclavian artery. An extended aortic anastomosis may be necessary in children with a hypoplastic transverse arch.

When a resection of a coarctation with anastomosis is performed, parallel straight vascular clamps are placed above and below the coarctation. The ductus is ligated and the specimen excised (Fig. 87-14). The anastomosis is begun on the back row with a simple running 5-0 suture. The suture line of the anterior surface is interrupted two or three times to allow later growth. The use of absorbable 6-0 or 7-0 suture is preferred in neonates and infants.

Sometimes it is difficult to achieve adequate reconstruction after coarctation resection in small infants. The technique of subclavian patch angioplasty or prosthetic patch obviates many of the technical problems of resection and anastomosis in neonates (Fig. 87-15). The patent ductus is first ligated in situ. The aorta is clamped. Then the subclavian artery is divided at the apex of the chest after ligation of its branches, just as in a Blalock-Taussig shunt. The subclavian artery is split longitudinally, and this incision is carried down onto the aorta itself, well into the area of the poststenotic dilatation. If there is a diaphragm in the coarctation, it is excised. Finally, the subclavian flap is folded down and sutured in place with a 6-0 continuous suture. With prosthetic patch angioplasty, a prosthetic patch is used to augment the aorta at the site of coarctation. Reports of pseudoaneurysm formation have made the prosthetic patch angioplasty less favored.

Results

Recently, operative mortality after repair of coarctation by resection and anastomosis in neonates has been less than 5%. Almost all these deaths occur in patients with associated anomalies, but a few are related to the technical difficulty of achieving a good anastomosis. Persistent hypertension is one of the most common problems after repair. The incidence appears to be related to age at repair. Associated defects have included patent ductus (most often), VSD, transposition, and atresia of the aortic valve. In the group with coarctation and refractory failure, however, persistent medical therapy alone rarely succeeds, so surgery should be attempted despite the risk in the patient with multiple defects.

Recurrence of coarctation is common (as many as 34% in one series). Percutaneous balloon angioplasty may be successful in up to 70% of patients with recurrent coarctation. During aortic cross-clamping one generally relies on the collateral vessels around the coarctation to prevent ischemic damage to the spinal cord. Although neonates usually have poorly developed collaterals, paraplegia is rare. However, it may occur in 0.2% of older children and is a higher risk in those with repeat operations.

Aortic Arch Interruption

Fortunately rare, complete interruption of the aortic arch is a rapidly lethal congenital abnormality. Of affected children, 80% die within the first month of life. In 43% of patients the interruption occurs just distal to the left subclavian artery (type A); in 53% between the left carotid and left subclavian arteries (type B); and in 4% between the innominate and left carotid arteries (type C) (Fig. 87-16). Virtually all these patients also have a VSD and PDA, providing blood flow from the right ventricle to the aortic segment distal to the interruption. This anomaly may be part of the so-called hypoplastic left heart syndrome, which includes aortic and mitral valve hypoplasia and underdevelopment of the left ventricle (see later).

Choice of Operation

Complete repair with primary anastomosis is preferred with simultaneous correction of all associated lesions.

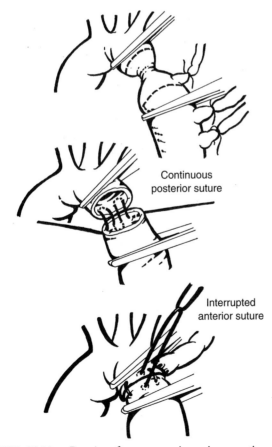

FIGURE 87-14 ■ Repair of a coarctation via resection and anastomosis.

Continuous posterior suture

Interrupted anterior suture

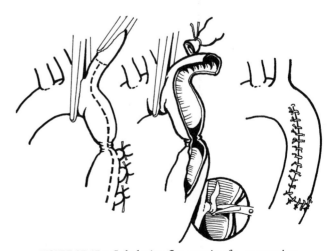

FIGURE 87-15 ■ Subclavian flap repair of a coarctation.

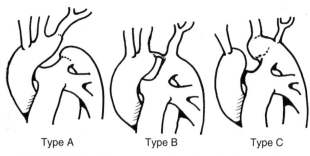

FIGURE 87-16 ■ Three types of aortic arch interruptions.

Type A lesions are best treated as one would treat a preductal coarctation, as discussed earlier. Some surgeons have used the subclavian artery plus or minus the left carotid artery to restore aortic continuity. The successful primary definitive repair of a type B defect with associated VSD can be carried out with a mortality of 5% to 8%.

MIXING LESIONS

Aortic Stenosis and Hypoplastic Left Heart Syndrome (HLHS)

Infants with aortic stenosis can develop severe congestive failure in the newborn period, which is not amenable to intensive medical therapy. Cardiac catheterization or echocardiography is frequently necessary to make a definitive diagnosis, which often demonstrates ventricular

pressures twice as high as systemic pressure. Correction of critical aortic stenosis in infancy is often an urgent or emergent procedure with a relatively high morbidity and mortality. If the obstruction is at the valve level, an aortic valvulotomy can be dramatic in relieving the congestive failure; however, if the annulus is small, the results of surgery are usually poor. In older patients, aortic valvuloplasty can be performed. Alternatives include aortic valve replacement with a mechanical or bioprosthetic valve or the Ross procedure in which the pulmonary valve is transferred to the aortic position, with implantation of the coronary arteries and the pulmonary artery reconstructed using homograft. Balloon valvotomy can also be performed in children with an 87% immediate and a 50% 8-year success rate. The most common complication of balloon valvotomy is femoral artery compromise in up to 60% of children younger than 2 years of age.

HLHS is a syndrome associated with severe aortic valve stenosis or atresia, hypoplasia of the ascending aorta, stenosis or atresia of the mitral valve, and a severely underdeveloped left ventricle (Fig. 87-17). The descending aorta is essentially a continuation of the ductus arteriosus, and the ascending aorta and aortic arch form a diminutive branch from this vessel. Pulmonary venous blood flows from the left into the right atrium via an ASD or incompetent foramen ovale and mixes in the right atrium with the venous blood. Pulmonary venous hypertension may occur if the communication between the left and right atria is not adequately patent. The large right ventricle is responsible for systemic blood flow,

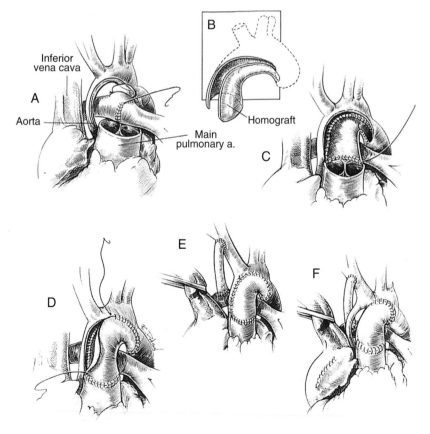

FIGURE 87-17 ■ The Norwood procedure for hypoplastic left heart syndrome. **A,** The distal divided main pulmonary artery may be closed by direct suture or with a patch. Note the diminutive aorta. **B,** The root of the aorta is opened in preparation for applying a homograft patch. **C,** The arterial wall allograft is used to supplement the anastomosis between the proximal divided main pulmonary artery and the ascending aorta, aortic arch, and proximal descending aorta. **D** and **E,** The procedure is completed by an atrial septectomy and a 3.5-mm modified right Blalock shunt. **F,** When the ascending aorta is particularly small, an alternative procedure involves placement of a complete tube of arterial allograft. The tiny ascending aorta may be left in situ, as indicated, or implanted into the side of the neoaorta.

typically through a PDA because a VSD is not usually present. The diminutive aortic arch and vessels, including the coronary arteries, are often perfused via the PDA unless a small aortic valve orifice is present to allow left ventricular flow. Newborns are typically cyanotic and may develop cardiogenic shock with hypoperfusion with partial closure of the PDA. The anomaly is typically identified on echocardiography where the diminutive left ventricle and aortic root along with an enlarged right atrium and right ventricle are noted. Associated noncardiac, especially neurologic, anomalies may occur in up to 30% of patients.

Treatment

Management includes maintenance of patency of the ductus with prostaglandin E_1 and dilation of the interatrial communication if necessary. Operative options include the Norwood procedure or transplantation. The former is performed in three stages in which the diminutive aortic arch is augmented with a patch; the pulmonary artery is transversely divided at its root; the aorta is transposed onto the root of the pulmonary artery; an atrial septectomy is performed; and a fixed-size conduit is interposed between the ligated pulmonary artery and the reconstructed aorta. In the second stage the superior vena cava (SVC) is connected to the pulmonary artery as a bidirectional Glenn anastomosis (Fig. 87-18), which allows SVC blood to flow directly into the pulmonary artery while the inferior vena cava (IVC) blood continues to flow into the right atrium as it did after the stage I repair. Finally, in the third stage a modified Fontan procedure is performed in which all SVC and IVC blood is isolated from the right atrium and routed directly into the pulmonary artery, thus converting the pulmonary and systemic circulations from parallel into serial configurations (see Fig. 87-11). At that procedure, the conduit between the aorta and the pulmonary artery is ligated. Data suggest that survival of the Norwood procedure in those patients with standard HLHS anatomy and no other anomalies through all stages may be as high as 70%.

Another option of operative management of HLHS is transplantation. The results of transplantation are approximately the same as with the Norwood procedure. Because of the shortage of infant organs and the risks of immunosuppression in this age group, the recent increase in survival with the Norwood procedure has made it the preferred approach in most centers. Transplantation is reserved, therefore, for those lesions that are a high risk for, or that have no options for, reconstruction (see later).

Double-Outlet Right Ventricle

In this anomaly both great arteries (all of one and at least 50% of the second great artery) arise from the right ventricle (Fig. 87-19). The outflow from the left ventricle is through a VSD, which can lie under the aorta (subaortic), the pulmonary artery (subpulmonic), both vessels (doubly committed), or remote from the vessels (noncommitted). The degree of cyanosis depends on the location of the VSD. If pulmonary stenosis is present, the physiology may be similar to that of TOF. The natural history of patients with double-outlet right ventricle is the development of pulmonary hypertension. Repair of this anomaly depends on the location of the VSD and can encompass placement of a baffle, which directs flow from the left ventricle to the aorta, an arterial switch operation, or complex reconstructions with conduits and modified Fontan procedures.

CARDIAC TRANSPLANTATION FOR CONGENITAL HEART DISEASE

Because of the great strides made in reconstructive surgery for congenital heart defects, cardiac transplantation is primarily reserved for those patients with severe cardiomyopathy or anatomic disorders that are not amenable to reconstructive surgery. Transplantation for congenital heart defects is carried out using the same techniques that are now standard for transplantation in older children and adults. At times the procedure must be modified to accommodate any underdeveloped cardiac chambers or to relieve any obstruction to pulmonary venous drainage. Results of transplantation in neonates have been excellent in centers with extensive experience in this area, and a 2-year survival over 80% has been reported. Furthermore, long-term survival of these patients is excellent at 60% to 75%.

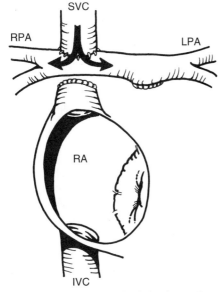

FIGURE 87-18 ■ The bidirectional Glenn shunt. An end-to-side anastomosis of the superior vena cava (SVC) to the right pulmonary artery (RPA) is perfomed. The proximal end of the SVC is divided at the cavoatrial junction. (From Bridges ND, Jonas RA, Mayer JE, et al: Bi-directional cavopulmonary anastomosis as interim palliation for high-risk Fontan candidates: Early results. Circulation 82 [Suppl IV]:IV-170, 1990. Copyright 1990, American Heart Association.)

EXTRACARDIAC ANOMALIES OF THE GREAT VESSELS

Vascular Rings

Anomalies of the aortic arch and its major branches can result in the formation of vascular rings about the esophagus and trachea, causing stridor and dysphagia.

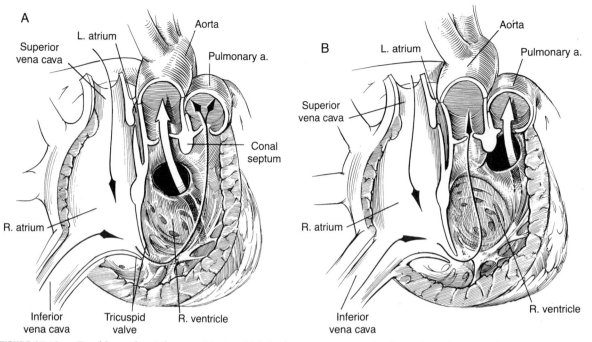

FIGURE 87-19 ■ Double-outlet right ventricle in which both great arteries arise from the right ventricle. **A,** A subaortic VSD favors flow of left ventricular blood to the aorta. **B,** The subpulmonary location of the VSD favors flow to the pulmonary artery. (From Castaneda A, Jonas RA, Mayer JE Jr, et al: Cardiac Surgery of the Neonate and Infant. Philadelphia, WB Saunders, 1994, p 446.)

Most common is the aberrant right subclavian artery from a left descending aorta that passes behind the esophagus, but this rarely causes serious symptoms in infancy (Fig. 87-20). Double aortic arch is the most important of these anomalies, often causing serious respiratory distress in young infants as it surrounds the trachea (Fig. 87-21). A right aortic arch with a left ligamentum arteriosum is the third most common form of vascular ring, usually presenting clinically much later in childhood than a double aortic arch.

Diagnosis

The diagnosis of vascular ring is suspected when feeding difficulty, coughing during feeding, or stridor is present. The infant tends to hold the neck extended to relieve compression. Plain chest radiographs are rarely helpful, but a barium swallow will reveal the characteristic filling defect

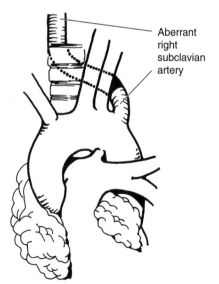

FIGURE 87-20 ■ Typical anatomy in the setting of an aberrant right subclavian artery.

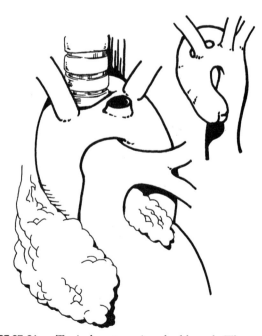

FIGURE 87-21 ■ Typical anatomy in a double arch. The anterior arch is larger in this example. However, in some instances the posterior arch is dominant.

in the mid esophagus. Cardiac catheterization and angiography may be done, primarily to establish the presence of associated abnormalities, but rarely do these procedures provide any additional useful information about the vascular ring itself. Magnetic resonance imaging in combination with echocardiography usually defines the anatomy clearly.

Operative Technique

No matter what the anatomy of the ring may be, it is best approached through an anterior left-sided thoracotomy unless tracheal stenosis is present, in which case a median sternotomy approach may be advantageous. The left lobe of the thymus gland is excised to expose the aortic arch. The entire aortic arch and its branches must first be dissected free so that the anatomy of the ring can be clearly understood. In the usual case of double arch, the right arch is typically posterior to, higher, and larger than the left arch, which forms the anterior portion of the ring. The smaller of the two arches (usually left) is generally divided to interrupt the constricting ring. The vessel should be occluded temporarily at the site of intended division to ascertain that flow to the carotids and descending aorta is not compromised by an unrecognized stricture in the other arch. In addition, it is essential to divide the ligamentum arteriosum or patent ductus and to dissect the esophagus and trachea free to the apex of the chest, dividing any constricting bands.

When the posterior arch is divided, further decompression of the trachea can sometimes be achieved by anchoring the major anterior arch to the back of the sternum with sutures, a so-called aortopexy. A right aortic arch and left ligamentum arteriosum are simply treated by dividing the ligament and dissecting the trachea and esophagus free.

Aberrant subclavian arteries may be simply divided, and other forms of rings may be treated by interruption of the ring at an appropriate site, taking care to free the trachea and esophagus completely.

In many cases stridor will not be immediately relieved because tracheomalacia may occur at the site of compression.

Pulmonary Artery Sling

A pulmonary artery sling is formed as a result of the left pulmonary artery originating from the right pulmonary artery and passing back to the left between the trachea and the esophagus. As it does so, the artery crosses the right main stem bronchus or the trachea just above the carina, leading to a stenosis of the trachea or bronchus. The ductus or ligamentum arteriosum may complete the ring of vessels surrounding the trachea. Patients demonstrate respiratory insufficiency due to airway compression or a tracheal stenosis with complete cartilage rings. The respiratory distress usually requires intubation, ventilation, and, in some instances, extracorporeal life support or extracorporeal membrane oxygenation. Operation to excise and reconstruct the portion of the trachea that is stenotic and to relocate the left pulmonary artery anterior to the trachea may be successful unless the length of the tracheal stenosis precludes primary tracheal resection and anastomosis (Fig. 87-22). In that case, augmenting

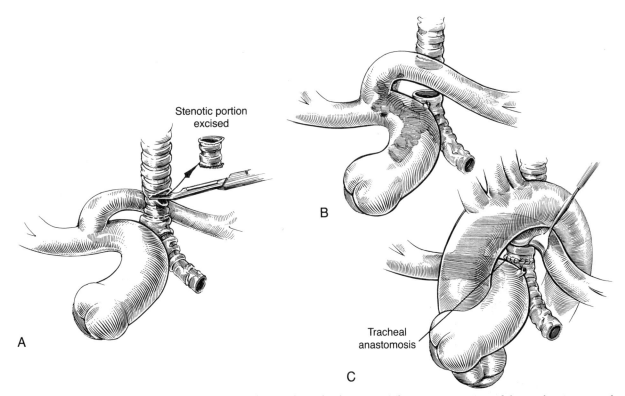

FIGURE 87-22 ■ Operation for a pulmonary artery sling with tracheal stenosis. The stenotic portion of the trachea is resected (**A**) and the left pulmonary artery transposed anteriorly (**B**). The ends of the trachea are then reapproximated (**C**). (From Castaneda AR, Jonas RA, Mayer JE, Hanley FL: Vascular rings, slings, and tracheal anomalies. In Cardiac Surgery of the Neonate and Infant. Philadelphia, WB Saunders, 1994.)

the trachea at the stenotic site with a rib cartilage graft may be the optimal strategy.

SUGGESTED READINGS

Gaynor JW, Spray TL: Congenital heart disease and anomalies of the great vessels. In O'Neill JA, Rowe MI, Grosfeld JL, et al (eds): Pediatric Surgery, 5th ed. Philadelphia, WB Saunders, 1998, pp 1835-1848.

Gross RE: Vascular anomalies in the thorax producing compression of the trachea or esophagus. In: The Surgery of Infancy and Childhood. Philadelphia, WB Saunders, 1953.

This is, even today, the best review of vascular rings.

Spray TL: Transplantation of the heart and lungs in children. Annu Rev Med 45:139, 1994.

This report summarizes the current status of cardiopulmonary transplantation and its place in the treatment of children with congenital heart disease.

Stark J, de Leval M: Surgery for Congenital Heart Defects, 2nd ed. Philadelphia, WB Saunders, 1994.

This is an excellent source of in-depth information on congenital cardiac disorders, diagnosis, and treatment.

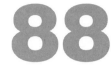

Musculoskeletal Disorders

Musculoskeletal disorders are common occurrences in infants and children. Some of the more frequent conditions encountered by pediatric physicians are discussed in this chapter.

CONGENITAL DISLOCATION OF THE HIP IN INFANCY

The term *developmental dysplasia of the hip* refers to the complete spectrum of abnormalities involved in the growing hip, with varied expression from dysplasia to subluxation to dislocation of the hip joint. Within this spectrum of congenital and developmental problems of the hip, the most common subset is congenital dysplasia or dislocation of the hip. The incidence of congenital dislocation of the hip is 1.5 per 1000 live births. This condition is more common in white female infants (4:1), is often unilateral, and occurs more frequently on the left side. High-risk factors include breech presentation, positive family history (20%), birth order (firstborn girls), and prenatal maternal oligohydramnios with fetal compression and deformation. It is believed that maternal hormones during pregnancy may contribute to joint capsule laxity, especially in the female fetus. The presence of any of these factors mandates an examination to exclude congenital dislocation of the hip at birth.

The diagnosis is suspected by the presence of an extra gluteal skin fold on the side of the dislocated hip (Fig. 88-1). The diagnosis can be made in the neonatal period by the Barlow test, which determines if the femoral head can be dislocated posteriorly, and the Ortolani maneuver, which reduces a dislocated hip. When performing the Ortolani maneuver, the examiner faces the infant, who is lying in a relaxed supine position with the hips flexed at 90 degrees (Fig. 88-2). As one hand stabilizes the pelvis, the other adducts the hip past the midline, while gentle outward pressure is applied with the thumb. As the hip is abducted and gently lifted toward the socket, a dislocated hip may be felt to relocate. In a dislocated hip, the femoral head is out of the acetabulum. In a hip able to be dislocated by the Barlow maneuver, the femoral head is reduced but also can be displaced. With a subluxated hip, the femoral head can be reduced and partially displaced. The affected infant usually manifests limited abduction. If the diagnosis is not made early, an adduction contracture may develop by 6 to 10 weeks of age,

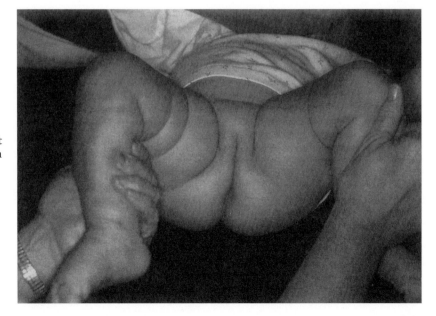

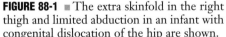

FIGURE 88-1 ■ The extra skinfold in the right thigh and limited abduction in an infant with congenital dislocation of the hip are shown.

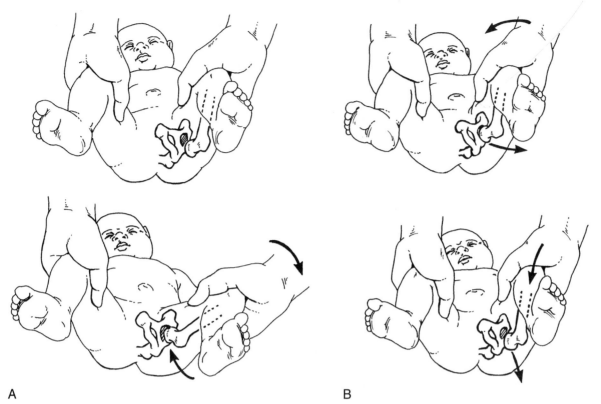

FIGURE 88-2 ■ Tests to evaluate hip stability. **A,** Ortolani maneuver. **B,** Barlow maneuver. (Copyright 2000 American Academy of Orthopaedic Surgeons. Reprinted from the Journal of American Academy of Orthopaedic Surgeons, Volume 8 (4), pp 232-242.)

and the examiner may not be able to reduce the hip. Radiographs of the hip in neonates are of little benefit. As a contracture develops, displacement of the femoral head may be seen, and an increased acetabular index is observed. The treatment of choice for congenital dislocation of the hip is early reduction in the neonatal period and dynamic splinting in the reduced position in a harness or spica. The success rate is greater than 80%. If reduction is unsuccessful, open reduction usually is required. Older children present with wide buttocks, an awkward gait, an unstable joint, and a lordotic stance. If the diagnosis is made after 18 months of age, little chance exists for a successful closed reduction. Congenital dislocation of the hip presenting in older patients almost always requires open reduction.

CLUBFOOT (TALIPES EQUINOCAVOVARUS)

The incidence of clubfoot is 1 to 2 per 1000 live births. In utero, pressure deformation, amniotic bands, oligohydramnios, and genetic predisposition all may play a role in the occurrence of clubfoot. Extrinsic clubfoot is readily correctable with nonoperative treatment. The more common intrinsic clubfoot with structural deformities of bones, tendon, ligaments, and muscles requires surgical

correction in most patients. The navicular is wedge-shaped and displaced medially. The talus and calcaneus are in equinus, and the posterior tibialis tendon, toe flexors, and Achilles tendon are shortened (Fig. 88-3). Although manipulation and casting may be tried early, operative release at 9 to 12 months of age constitutes normal treatment. Postoperatively the patient requires casting in the corrected position. A satisfactory result is achieved in 85% to 90% of patients.

ACUTE OSTEOMYELITIS

Acute hematogenous osteomyelitis occurs more frequently in young infants. Boys are affected more than girls (3:1), and the most common site of infection is the metaphysis of long bones. Sluggish flow in the sinusoidal veins near the physeal plate may be the underlying cause of bacterial proliferation at this site. The femur, tibia, humerus, fibula, and radius are the most frequently affected bones. *Staphylococcus aureus* is the most common infectious organism. Streptococci are the second most frequent organisms, with other organisms, including *Haemophilus influenzae*, being less prevalent. Presenting symptoms include the abrupt onset of fever, anorexia, and malaise or irritability. The affected bone is highly painful, and children often refuse to move the involved limb. Local swelling

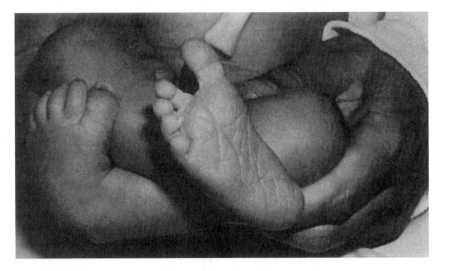

FIGURE 88-3 ■ Typical appearance of an infant with clubfeet.

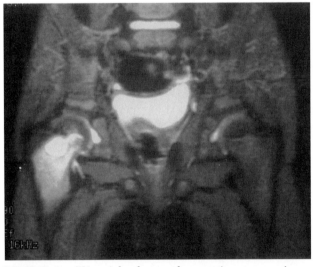

FIGURE 88-4 ■ T2-weighted coronal magnetic resonance image shows high signal edema with focal fluid collection in the right femoral metaphysis, which is consistent with osteomyelitis.

over the infected metaphysis may be noted early in the illness. In infants, swelling caused by infection, but in the absence of erythema, may affect the entire limb. Localized tenderness and limitation of motion are common findings.

Laboratory data show leukocytosis with a shift to the left on the differential count. The radiograph of the affected bone may be normal for 10 to 12 days after the onset of infection. After that time, increased radiolucency consistent with sequestrum may appear. The most sensitive and specific imaging technique available for differentiating osteomyelitis, cellulitis, and septic arthritis is magnetic resonance imaging (Fig. 88-4). Bone scintigraphy also can be useful early in the process before recognizable radiographic findings. Blood cultures are positive in 50% of patients. Aspiration at the point of maximum tenderness under the periosteum may recover purulent material. If purulent material is not recovered beneath the periosteum, the needle should be advanced into the bony metaphysis if possible. If purulent material is

recovered then, operative incision and drainage should be performed. Adequate treatment requires intravenous antibiotics, chosen according to the culture results, for at least 2 weeks without bone destruction and 2 to 6 weeks with smoldering infection and evidence of bone destruction. Oral antibiotics are given for 1 month after stopping parenteral administration. Chronic osteomyelitis is uncommon after the occurrence of osteomyelitis in infancy.

SEPTIC ARTHRITIS

Acute septic arthritis occurs primarily in infants, with a peak incidence between 1 and 2 years of age, and is almost always monarticular. The hip is the most frequently infected joint. The most common offending pathogen is *S. aureus*, which predominates in neonates and older children. *H. influenzae*, commonly seen in the past, has been eliminated by vaccine. Streptococci, gonococci, and pneumococci also may be responsible for some infections. Septic arthritis is the result of hematogenous infection affecting the joint synovium. Occasionally, septic arthritis may result from spontaneous decompression of metaphyseal osteomyelitis into the joint. The hip joint is particularly susceptible to this latter type of infection. Trauma with external entry into the joint is another mechanism of potential joint contamination.

The infection of the synovium results in an inflammatory response followed by a purulent exudate. The onset of illness is rapid and is associated with fever, tachycardia, and septicemia. Infants may be listless and lethargic and become irritable when handled, particularly if the affected joint is moved or touched. The major point of tenderness is directly over the infected joint.

The diagnosis of septic arthritis is confirmed by needle aspiration of the joint. The aspirate is cloudy and watery, containing numerous polymorphonuclear leukocytes (90%). Cultures for aerobes and anaerobes are obtained, and a Gram stain is performed. Radiographs frequently show joint effusion and a subluxated joint. Bone scintigraphy may show a "cold" femoral epiphysis as evidence of sepsis that has compromised the blood supply to the epiphysis. If the joint aspirate is watery, a trial of antibiotics without formal operative intervention may be adequate. If purulent material is recovered, however, the infected joint should be drained widely in the operating room and the patient given appropriate antibiotics based on Gram stain findings until culture report data are available. Postoperatively the patient is given antibiotics for 2 to 4 weeks and maintained on bed rest for a short time. The drainage catheter is removed on the second or third day. Prompt diagnosis and therapy result in a successful outcome. Delay of more than 5 days may result in avascular necrosis of the hip.

SUGGESTED READINGS

Dunre KB, Clarren SK: The origin of prenatal and postnatal deformities. Pediatr Clin North Am 33:1277, 1986.

This article describes the mechanism of intrauterine deformation as the cause of many congenital musculoskeletal anomalies.

Green NE, Mencio GA: Major congenital orthopedic deformities. In O'Neill JA, Rowe MI, Grosfeld JL, et al (eds): Pediatric Surgery, 5th ed. St. Louis, Mosby–Year Book, 1998, p 1859.

This chapter thoroughly reviews the major orthopedic problems seen in infants and children, including developmental dysplasia of the hip, congenital abnormalities of the feet, and congenital spinal anomalies.

Guille JT, et al: Development dysplasia of the hip from birth to six months. J Am Acad Orthop Surg 8:232, 2000.

This article describes the spectrum of disorders included in the new term developmental dysplasia of the hip.

Morrissey RT, Shore SL: Bone and joint sepsis. Pediatr Clin North Am 33:1551, 1986.

This article documents the virtual elimination of mortality related to bone and joint sepsis and emphasizes the importance of early diagnosis and treatment to avoid morbidity.

Craniofacial Disorders, Tonsils, and Adenoids

Craniofacial reconstruction emphasizes operative intervention during infancy and early childhood to maximize growth potential and minimize secondary distortion for most end-stage congenital facial anomalies. Advances in diagnosis and treatment planning were made possible by computed tomography (CT) with three-dimensional reconstruction of the craniofacial skeleton (Fig. 89-1). New challenges include understanding the biology of bone graft healing, mechanisms of distraction osteogenesis, the details of facial and skull growth, and the genetics of craniofacial anomalies. Operative techniques for correction of the morphogenetic defects were pioneered by Tessier. The primary concern in the timing of surgical intervention is the preservation and restoration of function.

Most craniofacial malformations may be categorized into the following major types:

1. Craniosynostosis (skull deformity alone)—plagiocephaly, skull deformity and midface hypoplasia (Crouzon's syndrome), or skull deformity with midface hypoplasia and extremity anomalies (Apert's syndrome)

2. Abnormalities of interorbital distance—hypertelorism or hypotelorism
3. Mandibulofacial dysostosis—Treacher Collins syndrome
4. First and second branchial arch deformity—hemifacial microsomia, Goldenhar's syndrome, or lateral facial dysplasia
5. Midface hypoplasia secondary to cleft lip or palate
6. Rare facial clefts
7. Miscellaneous craniofacial deformities

Additional patients with acquired defects secondary to tumor extirpation or trauma may require craniofacial reconstruction.

MAJOR CRANIOFACIAL MALFORMATIONS

Craniosynostosis

Craniosynostosis occurs in approximately 1 per 1000 births, with the facial skeleton affected in only 10%. Premature fusion of the sagittal suture prevents lateral

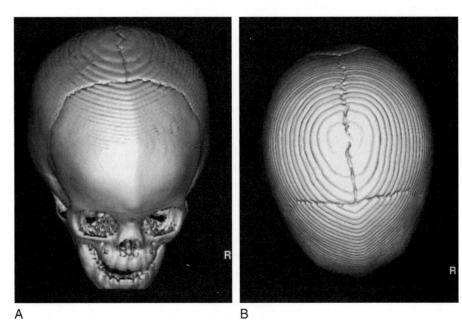

FIGURE 89-1 ■ Three-dimensional CT scans such as this one are crucial to planning surgical repair of craniofacial malformations because they not only define the pathology, but also possible repairs can be simulated. These two views show a typical case of craniosynostosis of the anterior or metopic suture, which results in trigonocephaly malformations. **A,** Frontal view. **B,** View from above.

A   B

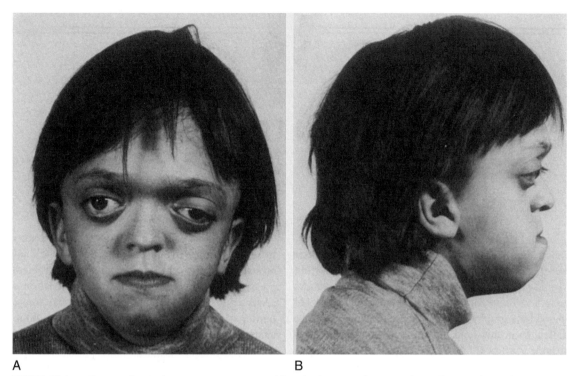

FIGURE 89-2 ■ Crouzon's syndrome in an 11-year-old girl, showing the typical exorbitism, hypoplasia of the maxilla and zygomatic regions, and relative prognathism.

expansion of the calvaria but permits expansion anteriorly at the coronal suture, resulting in a long narrow skull. Cranial sutures are passive sites of growth, allowing cranial expansion, and are not primary regulators of cranial growth. During the first year, the brain more than doubles in size and attains 60% of its adult weight.

In Crouzon's syndrome, craniosynostosis is accompanied by severe midface hypoplasia (Fig. 89-2). The shallow bony orbits produce exorbitism and divergent strabismus. Progressive visual loss may result from constriction of the osseous optic canals. Prolapse of the frontal sinus, inferior portion of the cribriform plates, and widening of the ethmoid sinuses may produce orbital hypertelorism. The maxilla is deficient, producing relative prognathism with a characteristic drooping lower lid and "parrot's beak" nose.

Apert's syndrome is a combination of craniosynostosis, midface hypoplasia, and extremity deformity. The facial anomalies are slightly different from those seen with Crouzon's syndrome, including an increased incidence of cleft palate and severe nasomaxillary hypoplasia. There is a complex mirror-image syndactyly of the hands and feet with interphalangeal synostosis. Crouzon's and Apert's syndromes are inherited as autosomal dominant traits with low penetrance.

Hypertelorism

Orbital hypertelorism denotes increased distance between the bony orbits and often is associated with other facial anomalies. Hypotelorism occurs less frequently than hypertelorism and often is associated with major intracranial anomalies, including microcephaly, Down syndrome, and others. The average adult interorbital distance is 25 mm for women, achieved by age 13 years, and 28 mm for men, achieved by 21 years. The principal pathologic change in hypertelorism is widening of the anterior ethmoid sinus and sometimes the inferior displacement of the cribriform plate.

Mandibulofacial Dysostosis (Treacher Collins Syndrome)

Mandibulofacial dysostosis occurs in 1 in 10,000 births and is inherited as an autosomal dominant trait with incomplete penetrance. The condition is symmetric with a downward cant of the palpebral fissure, frequently with a coloboma of the lower eyelids and absence of the eyelashes. The external ears are low set and hypoplastic, and there is a conductive hearing loss. Skin tags are often present along a line from the ear to the commissure of the mouth. The zygomatic bones and arches are hypoplastic. The mandibular rami are short with hypoplastic muscles of mastication. The teeth also are hypoplastic. The palate may be high and arched, with an overt cleft present in one third of patients.

Hemifacial Microsomia

Hemifacial microsomia, also called *lateral facial dysplasia,* *Goldenhar's syndrome, intrauterine facial necrosis, otomandibulovertebral anomaly,* or the *first and second branchial arch syndrome,* is similar to Treacher Collins syndrome but is predominantly a unilateral deformity. There is a progressive asymmetric growth of the normal side of the face, with an underdevelopment of the zygoma, maxilla, mandible, muscles of mastication, trigeminal nerve, external ear, and parotid gland of the involved side. Associated fifth or seventh cranial nerve deficits are common.

Correction of Congenital Craniofacial Anomalies

Surgical correction of craniofacial deformities requires a coordinated multidisciplinary team effort with each specialist contributing toward improving body image and function and leading the patient into the mainstream of society. A geneticist also should counsel the family regarding the inherited disorders and syndromes. Preoperative evaluation includes photographs, cephalometric radiographs, and CT scans for three-dimensional analysis of the craniofacial skeleton. The anatomic deformity; age; psychosocial situation; and other medical problems, such as increased intracranial pressure, ear infections, and velopharyngeal insufficiency, all are considered.

Early surgical correction facilitates subsequent facial growth and reduces secondary distortion of adjacent skeleton and soft tissues. Autologous bone for reconstruction is available from the iliac crest, ribs, tibia, and calvaria, the last-mentioned being preferred most often. Demineralized allogeneic bone implants also have been used widely in reconstruction procedures. Patients with craniosynostosis undergo reconstruction between 3 and 8 months of age. The Le Fort III osteotomy is the basic operation for correction of midface hypoplasia associated with Crouzon's and Apert's syndromes and is performed in early adolescence. Surgical correction of hypertelorism usually is performed before the child enters school. Treacher Collins syndrome usually is repaired before age 7 years, using autologous bone grafts.

The hypoplastic mandible in hemifacial microsomia, one of the most complex deformities for craniofacial repair, now commonly is treated by distraction osteogenesis in childhood. Internal (intraoral) or external devices are placed along the short mandible, an osteotomy is made, and the bone edges are distracted at 1 mm/day until an appropriate length is gained. The regenerating bone consolidates over the next 6 to 8 weeks with the distraction device left in place. Later in early adolescence at the time of skeletal maturity, conventional bone grafting or orthognathic surgery may be necessary to achieve improved symmetry and occlusion if necessary.

At operation, the airway is maintained by oral or nasal endotracheal tubes wired or sutured in place. Only rarely is tracheostomy necessary. Most patients remain intubated for 24 to 48 hours, after which the patient may be placed on a gradually increasing high-calorie, high-protein liquid diet. Prophylactic antibiotics are used. In a collected series of more than 1000 operative reconstructions, the mortality was less than 1.5% and the morbidity approximately 16%. Long-term follow-up shows marked improvement over the initial anomaly.

CONGENITAL ANOMALIES OF THE NOSE

The most common nasal anomaly is that associated with cleft lip. The unilateral cleft lip produces a short columella, flattening and lateral displacement of the alar cartilage, and deviation of the nasal septum. Bilateral cleft lip produces a short columella, a widened nasal tip, and lateral splaying of both alar cartilages. Nasal bridge hypoplasia often occurs with Down's syndrome and other craniofacial anomalies. In maxillonasal hypoplasia (Binder's syndrome), there is hypoplasia of the entire nose. Many nasal deformities cannot be corrected until the underlying orbital bony abnormalities are corrected.

Coloboma, or notching of the one alar rim, is the simplest form of cleft and usually has an associated displacement of the alar cartilage. Choanal atresia usually occurs posterior in the nasopharynx with a completely obstructing bilateral membranous or more commonly a solid bony obstruction. Surgical resection of the obstruction at an early age is usually curative.

Nasal anomalies and some nasal tumors may obstruct or deform the nasolacrimal drainage system. Excessive lacrimation can be evaluated by inserting isotope or radiographic contrast material into the conjunctival sac and noting the course of drainage.

NASAL TUMORS

Nasal tumors, either developmental or acquired, are fairly common and can be classified by embryonic derivation (Table 89-1). Congenital dermoid cysts of the nose are common and are located along the midline from the glabella to the columella. Often there is an associated dimple, usually with protruding hair. The stalk may enter the skull, producing a dumbbell cyst. Dermoid cysts and sinuses are lined by squamous epithelium with various dermal appendages, glands, and hair follicles. Repeated infections are common, and multiple sinus tracts may form, making total excision difficult.

During development, there is a projection of brain and meninges into the prenasal space, which usually becomes surrounded by bone and is called the *foramen cecum*. If the dural process does not become walled off, a meningocele results. If brain remains within the dural sac, it is termed an *encephalocele* (Fig. 89-3). The brain and dural contents may become walled off from the foramen cecum, in which case a nasal glioma remains. These tumors, either midline or asymmetric, are present at birth and often produce orbital hypertelorism, telecanthus, and nasal deformity. Meningoceles and encephaloceles are soft, compressible, and pulsatile, enlarging with crying. Nasal gliomas are firm. Treatment of nasal glioma is complete

---

TABLE 89-1 ■ Tumors of the Nose

Ectodermal
 Dermoid
 Dermoid sinus
Mesodermal
 Hemangioma
 Vascular malformation
Neural
 Meningocele
 Encephalocele
 Glioma
 Neurofibroma
 Chordoma
Mixed
 Teratoma ■

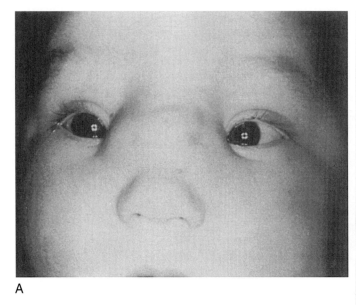

A

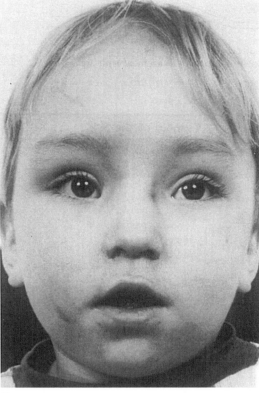

B

FIGURE 89-3 ■ Nasal encephalocele in a 2-month-old boy. **A,** Frontal view shows pseudo-orbital hypertelorism. **B,** Two years after removal of encephalocele and repositioning of the nasal bones.

excision after splitting the nasal bones. Meningoceles and encephaloceles require more complex reconstruction.

Hemangiomas of the nose have a proliferative and involutional phase similar to those in other areas of the body. Some of these lesions may become large and deforming, requiring wide resection and reconstruction using skin flaps. Resection of hemangiomas should be deferred until the involutional phase has been completed or a full course of steroids has been administered.

Teratomas of the nose are rare and may be benign or malignant. Giant teratomas present at birth are often massive lesions arising from the base of the skull and may pass through the nose into the mouth, resulting in a cleft palate and immediate postnasal respiratory obstruction.

CLEFT LIP

Cleft lip is one of the most common facial malformations, occurring in 1 in every 1000 births in the United States; it is more common in boys. Multiple genetic and, to a lesser extent, environmental factors seem to be involved. Many reconstructive procedures are available for the multiple variations of cleft lip deformity, with one of the most comprehensive reviews presented by Millard. Parents require extensive counseling when an infant is born with a cleft lip deformity. They should be reassured that operative reconstruction in most instances provides a near-normal appearance. Genetic counseling is helpful when there is concern about subsequent risk for further children being born with the same anomaly.

A cleft lip may be repaired immediately after birth or when the infant shows steady weight gain, usually between 6 and 12 weeks of age. The results of unilateral cleft lip repair are often excellent and are related closely to the severity of the original deformity (Fig. 89-4). Wide clefts, clefts with hypoplasia of the marginal tissues, clefts with a straight or an inverted alar rim, or clefts with gross deviation of the columellar base produce less desirable results. Often a cleft lip scar takes 6 to 12 months to resolve completely.

For bilateral cleft lip repair, more operative techniques are available with the reconstruction performed in one or two stages (Fig. 89-5). The results with the primary bilateral cleft lip repair are related closely to the severity and asymmetry present preoperatively. Patients with a small prolabium, a severely projecting premaxilla, wide alveolar gaps, and a short columella have less desirable results, and a few years may be necessary to achieve maximum benefit. Almost all patients require special orthodontic procedures to improve dentoalveolar and maxillary deformities. Prosthetic replacement of one and occasionally two missing permanent teeth in the line of the cleft is usually necessary in late adolescence. Later revision operations may be necessary for the lip and almost always for the nose.

CLEFT PALATE

Anomalies of the palate are often present in association with cleft lip. An embryologic system of classification of the various deformities has gained acceptance (Table 89-2).

Repair is concerned primarily with the anatomic deformity of the hard and soft palates, whereas improvement of speech and total rehabilitation of the patient also concerns the anatomy of the prepalate, tongue,

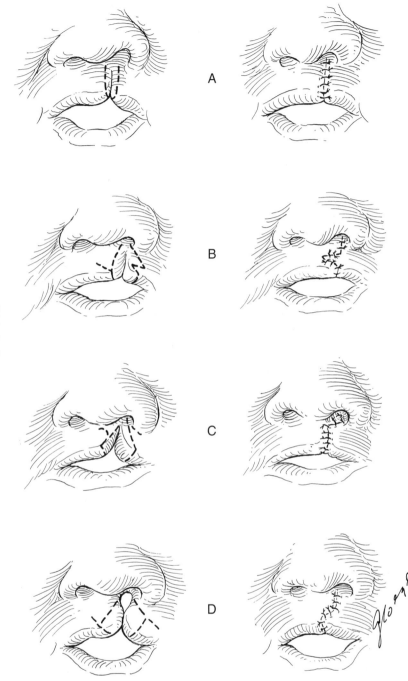

FIGURE 89-4 ■ Basic operations for repair of cleft lip. **A,** Straight-line operation. **B,** Lower one third triangular flap operation. **C,** Upper one third triangular flap operaton. **D,** Lower one third rectangular flap operation.

nasopharynx, and oropharynx. Variation in the transverse arching of the palate is common. The high arched palate often is a normal variation, but it frequently is associated with submucous cleft palate, craniosynostosis, and choanal atresia. Prepalatal clefts always involve the uvula and soft palate and usually involve the hard palate. Palatal clefts always involve the hard palate in addition to uvular and soft palate involvement. Palatal clefts also may develop dentoalveolar collapse of the posterior maxillary segments with crowding of the teeth.

The incidence of cleft palate and lip deformities is approximately 1 in every 750 live births. Females are more likely to develop isolated cleft palate deformities, whereas males develop cleft lip deformities. Associated anomalies are common and may be divided into two groups: (1) anomalies occurring in the immediate vicinity (e.g., Pierre Robin syndrome, Klippel-Feil syndrome, Psaume's syndrome) and (2) anomalies occurring elsewhere in the body (e.g., congenital heart disease and extremity anomalies [Ellis–van Creveld syndrome]). Less than 25% of patients with isolated cleft palate have a history of a similar lesion in the family.

Most infants with cleft palate deformities do not have respiratory problems. Most infants feed well using a long soft nipple with a large hole. Assisted feeding with a Brecht feeder may be helpful but has an increased risk of aspiration. Some food comes out through the nose until the palate is repaired. A few patients with difficulty in

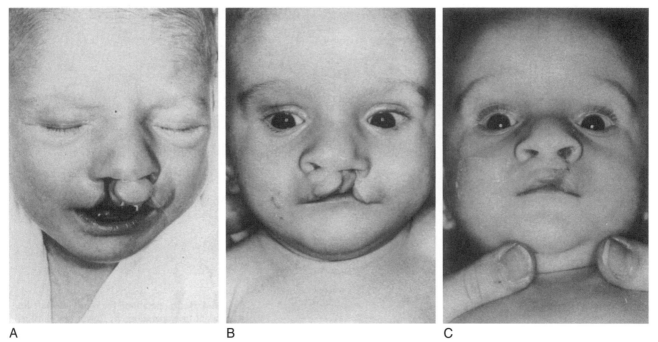

A　　　　　　　　　　　　B　　　　　　　　　　　　C

FIGURE 89-5 ■ **A,** Bilateral complete cleft lip in a 3-month-old boy. **B,** Six weeks after repair of the right side of the lip. **C,** Age 5 months, 2 weeks after repair of the left side of the cleft with lower one third triangular flap operation.

sucking or swallowing may require gavage or indwelling tube feedings.

The palate should be repaired by age 2 years, before the child has developed many speech abilities and habits. The two main approaches to reconstruction are approaches that produce adequate lateral mobilization to permit midline closure without tension and approaches that produce complete anterior detachment of the hard and soft palate to allow push-back of the whole palate (Figs. 89-6 and 89-7). Speech abilities with the two

TABLE 89-2 ■ Classification of Cleft Lip and Palate Deformities

Clefts of prepalate
　Cleft lip
　　Unilateral
　　Bilateral
　　Median
　　Congenital scars
　Cleft alveolar process
　　Unilateral
　　Bilateral
　　Median
　　Submucous
　Cleft lip and alveolar process
　Any combination of the foregoing types
　Premaxilla protrusion
　Premaxilla rotation
　Developmental arrestive prepalate
Clefts of palate
　Cleft soft palate
　Cleft hard palate
　Cleft soft and hard palate
Cleft of prepalate and palate
　Any combination of clefts and prepalate and palate
Facial clefts other than prepalatal or palatal
　Mandibular process clefts
　Nasal
　Oral

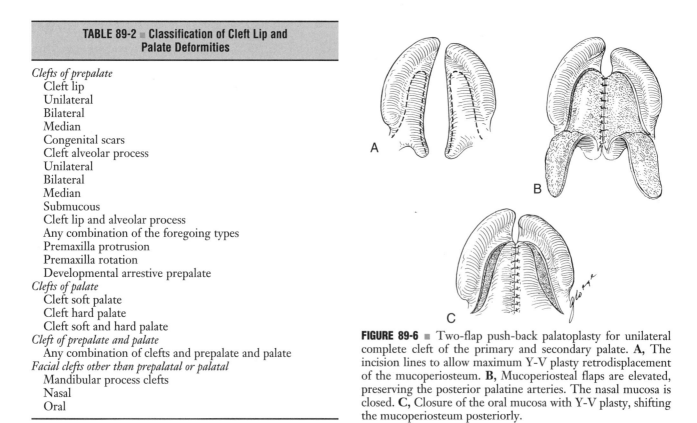

FIGURE 89-6 ■ Two-flap push-back palatoplasty for unilateral complete cleft of the primary and secondary palate. **A,** The incision lines to allow maximum Y-V plasty retrodisplacement of the mucoperiosteum. **B,** Mucoperiosteal flaps are elevated, preserving the posterior palatine arteries. The nasal mucosa is closed. **C,** Closure of the oral mucosa with Y-V plasty, shifting the mucoperiosteum posteriorly.

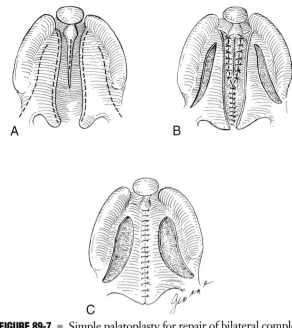

FIGURE 89-7 ■ Simple palatoplasty for repair of bilateral complete cleft of lip and palate. **A,** Incision lines to elevate the mucous membranes and inferior vomer. **B,** Mucoperiosteal flaps are elevated without anterior detachment. The cleft is usually wide. The nasal mucosa is closed. **C,** Closure of the oral mucosa with persistent cleft anteriorly.

procedures are approximately the same. Residual oronasal fistulas may be closed secondarily if they are a cause of foul odors, food impaction, or persistent escape of liquids into the nose. If the soft palate is short and immobile, and the pharynx is either of normal size or larger than normal, a palatopharyngoplasty may be indicated. Pharyngoplasty with insertion of free grafted material beneath the posterior pharyngeal wall may be useful in certain situations. Prosthetic speech appliances may be beneficial when surgery is contraindicated because of poor anesthetic risk.

Children with cleft palate have a higher than usual incidence of otitis media and hearing loss. Bilateral tube myringotomy and early treatment of ear infections are important. Tonsillectomy and adenoidectomy must be weighed carefully because removal of the tissue may enlarge the velopharyngeal space and affect speech. Children with cleft palate characteristically have a nasal quality of speech. Some cannot make the necessary closure between the soft palate and pharynx to prevent nasal escape of sound during phonation of many consonants and vowels. Speech therapy, when indicated, is valuable for children between 4 and 8 years old.

After cleft palate repair, approximately 70% of patients have acceptable speech. The remaining 30% require further speech therapy or palatopharyngeal reconstruction.

SURGERY OF THE TONSILS AND ADENOIDS

Controversy prevails regarding the indications for tonsillectomy and adenoidectomy. The most common childhood diseases of the tonsils and adenoids are (1) acute and chronic infections or secondary extension of microorganisms or toxins into the lymphatics or bloodstream; (2) direct spread of infection into the nose, paranasal sinuses, eustachian tubes, middle ear, or lower respiratory tract; and (3) enlargement of the tonsils and adenoids with obstruction of the airway.

Adenoidectomy alone is indicated when symptomatic adenoid disease is present without tonsillar infection. Acute adenoiditis may cause fever, sinusitis, and recurrent otitis media. Adenoid enlargement causes signs of obstruction, including oral breathing, snoring, nasal voice, accumulation of nasal secretions, and frequent head colds. Blockage of the eustachian tubes may produce conductive hearing impairment or chronic otitis media or both. Examination often reveals a large mass of adenoid tissue covered by mucopurulent discharge. In children younger than 4 years old, chronic adenoiditis may occur without chronic infection of the tonsils, and adenoidectomy is the operation of choice. Removal of tonsils and adenoids in young children occasionally stimulates hyperplasia of other lymphoid elements in the oropharynx. Recurrent inflammation of this tissue is difficult to treat and may cause persistent sore throat. In children older than 4 years of age, chronic adenoiditis generally is accompanied by chronic tonsillitis, and tonsillectomy with adenoidectomy is necessary.

Chronic adenoiditis must be distinguished from Tornwaldt's disease (infected nasopharyngeal bursa), retropharyngeal abscess, and vascular anomalies of the retropharynx. CT scans assist in determining the nature of nasopharyngeal and retropharyngeal masses. Although chronic adenoid infection may occur alone, chronic tonsillitis in children almost always is associated with chronic adenoiditis. With chronic tonsillitis, the cervical lymph nodes are usually enlarged, especially near the angle of the mandible. In the course of acute tonsillitis, bacteria may break through the tonsil capsule to form a peritonsillar abscess, causing trismus. Tonsillitis also commonly produces difficulty in swallowing.

Approximately 400,000 tonsillectomies are performed in the United States annually. Indications for combined tonsillectomy and adenoidectomy include the following:

1. Chronic recurrent tonsillitis
2. Peritonsillar abscess with history of recurrent pharyngitis
3. Nasal airway obstruction from hypertrophic adenoids, in association with chronic tonsillitis
4. Oropharyngeal obstruction
5. Conductive hearing impairment or recurrent otitis
6. Nephritis, rheumatic fever, iritis, and certain other systemic diseases
7. Congenital cardiovascular anomalies that may predispose to bacterial endocarditis
8. Recurrent sinusitis, bronchiectasis

Contraindications to tonsillectomy and adenoidectomy include the following:

1. Hemophilia and other blood dyscrasias, unless corrected

2. Disturbances of the bleeding and clotting mechanisms that resist correction
3. Active pulmonary tuberculosis, uncontrolled diabetes, acute nephritis, and active rheumatic fever
4. General debility
5. Acute bacterial illness and acute exanthemata
6. Peritonsillar hemangioma
7. Tumors of the tonsil and nasopharynx, which should be treated either by more extensive operation or by irradiation
8. Cleft palate
9. Congenitally short palate or submucous cleft

Tonsillectomy and adenoidectomy should be performed with the patient under general anesthesia with endotracheal intubation for control of the airway. After removal of the diseased tissue, thorough hemostasis should be achieved because postoperative hemorrhage is the major complication.

Tonsillectomy for appropriate indications returns to health children who previously have been repeatedly or chronically ill. Indiscriminate tonsillectomy subjects children to unnecessary risks and discomfort.

SUGGESTED READINGS

Imola MJ, Hamlar DD, Thatcher G, Chowdhury K: The versatility of distraction osteogenesis in craniofacial surgery. Arch Surg 4:8-19, 2002.

A good description is provided of modern approaches to the technical aspects of repair of craniofacial anomalies.

Kawamoto HK Jr: Craniofacial abnormalities. In O'Neill JA Jr, Rowe MI, Grosfeld JL, et al (eds): Pediatric Surgery, 5th ed. St. Louis, Mosby-Year Book, 1998, pp 853-861.

This is an extensive current review by a leading authority in the field of various craniofacial anomalies amenable to surgical reconstruction.

Lehman JA Jr: Cleft palate surgery for the 1990s: An overview of specific problems and treatment rationale. Probl Plast Reconstr Surg 2:1, 1992.

This review article discusses various up-to-date surgical approaches to the many different forms of cleft lip and palate.

McCarthy JG, Stelnicki EJ, Mehrara BJ, Longaker MT: Distraction osteogenesis of the craniofacial skeleton. Plast Reconstr Surg 107:1812–1827, 2001.

This is a comprehensive review of current distraction osteogenesis methods for treatment of the craniofacial skeleton.

Mullikan JB: Principles and techniques of bilateral complete cleft lip repair. Plast Reconstr Surg 75:477, 1985.

This article discusses approaches to the most complicated forms of cleft lip and palate and stresses indications for staged procedures in many instances.

Tessier P: The definitive plastic surgical treatment of the severe facial deformities of craniofacial dysostosis. Plast Reconstr Surg 48:419, 1971.

This is one of the most extensive reviews of craniofacial reconstruction by the leading authority in the field.

Index

Note: Page numbers followed by f indicate figures; those followed by t indicate tables.